General Thoracic Surgery

General Thoracic Surgery

Edited by

Thomas W. Shields, M.D., D.Sc. (Hon.)

Professor Emeritus of Surgery
Northwestern University Medical School
Formerly Chief of Thoracic Surgery
Veterans Administration Lakeside Medical Center
Attending Emeritus Surgeon
Northwestern Memorial Hospital
Chicago, Illinois

Volume 1
Fourth Edition

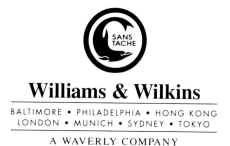

SANS
TACHE

Williams & Wilkins

BALTIMORE • PHILADELPHIA • HONG KONG
LONDON • MUNICH • SYDNEY • TOKYO

A WAVERLY COMPANY

Executive Editor: Carroll Cann
Production Coordinator: Mary Clare Beaulieu
Project Editor: Holly Lukens
Development Editor: Susan Hunsberger

Copyright © 1994
Williams & Wilkins
200 Chester Field Parkway
Malvern, PA 19355 USA

Accurate indications, adverse reactions, and dosage schedules for drugs are provided in this book, but it is possible they may change. The reader is urged to review the package information data of the manufacturers of the medications mentioned.

Printed in the United States of America

First Edition 1972

94 95 96 97 98
1 2 3 4 5 6 7 8 9 10

Dedication
To my wife, Ann; my children, Thomas William, John Leland, and Carol Ann; and my childrens' children: Jennifer, Alison, Steven, Nicole, Alexander, and Elizabeth

Preface

The fourth edition of General Thoracic Surgery is a continuum of the initial concept of the first edition published in 1972, which was updated in the second edition in 1983 and in the third edition in 1989. The present edition has been thoroughly revised, and the scope of coverage has been expanded to include not only the newer concepts in the knowledge and the practice of general thoracic surgery, but also in-depth descriptions of the technical aspects of the commonly, as well as the less frequently, performed pulmonary, chest wall, mediastinal, and esophageal surgical procedures by master surgeons in the specialty.

To accomplish the principal aim of extensive and comprehensive presentation of the field of general thoracic surgery, the fourth edition is composed of 136 chapters as well as an introduction that reviews the early history of the proud heritage of the specialty. One third of the 36 new chapters are primarily technical in scope, whereas the others provide comprehensive coverage of the newer aspects of the specialty and record and document more completely the present-day information in the many areas that are of concern to the general thoracic surgeon. Many of the previous chapters have been completely revised by either the original contributors or their successors to aid in attaining the goal of the text. Those few chapters that have not been extensively revised have been updated to be as current as possible. As with any text that becomes more inclusive, repetition and differences in opinion have become more common. These, within bounds, are fundamentally healthy. The reader is advised to make his or her own decision when opinions are divergent.

The overall organization of the text remains essentially unchanged, although there are now 24 sections in place of the previous 19. This has been done to enable a more precise and orderly presentation of the material presented. Cross-references are in abundance. A great effort has been made to expand the index appropriately so it will be a ready reference to all the important subjects in the text.

Once again, as in the first three editions, I have been fortunate to have the cooperation and aid of outstanding, knowledgeable thoracic surgeons, radiologists, anesthesiologists, oncologists, and physicians both here and abroad in Europe, Asia, and South America in the preparation of the text. I wish to thank all of them for their contributions, which are of inestimable value to the validity and importance of the text.

Chicago, Illinois   Thomas W. Shields

Contributors

Homeros Aletras, M.D.
Professor and Chairman of Surgery
Salonika University
Salonika, Greece

John C. Alexander, Jr., M.D.
Associate Professor of Surgery
Northwestern University Medical School
Chicago, Illinois

Robert W. Anderson, M.D.
Professor of Surgery and Biomedical Engineering
Northwestern University Medical School
Chicago, Illinois

Carl L. Backer, M.D.
Assistant Professor of Surgery
Northwestern University Medical School
Chicago, Illinois

Manjit S. Bains, M.D.
Associate Professor Surgery
Cornell University Medical College
New York, New York

Walter L. Barker, M.D.
Professor of Surgery
University of Illinois College of Medicine
Chicago, Illinois

Felix Battistella, M.D.
Assistant Professor of Surgery
School of Medicine
University of California, Davis
Sacramento, California

Arthur E. Baue, M.D.
Professor of Surgery, Cardiothoracic Division
St. Louis University School of Medicine
St. Louis, Missouri

Ronald H. R. Belsey, M.D.
Former Visiting Professor
University of Chicago Pritzken School of Medicine
Chicago, Illinois

John R. Benfield, M.D.
Professor and Chief of Cardiothoracic Surgery
Vice Chairman of Surgery
School of Medicine
University of California, Davis
Sacramento, California

Charles E. Blevins, Ph.D.
Professor of Anatomy
Indiana University School of Medicine
Indianapolis, Indiana

Simon C. Body, M.B.
Instructor in Anesthesia
Harvard Medical School
Boston, Massachusetts

Joan D. Boomsma, M.D.
Assistant Professor of Clinical Medicine
Northwestern University Medical School
Chicago, Illinois

Ralph Braunschweig, M.D.
Clinical Assistant Professor of Anesthesiology
Columbia School of Medicine
University of Missouri
Columbia, Missouri

Edward A. Brunner, M.D., Ph.D.
James E. Echenhoff Professor
Chairman of Anesthesia
Northwestern University Medical School
Chicago, Illinois

Peter H. Burri, M.D.
Professor of Anatomy
Institute of Anatomy
University of Berne
Berne, Switzerland

David P. Campbell, M.D.
Professor of Surgery and Pediatrics
Albany Medical College
Albany, New York

C. James Carrico, M.D.
Professor and Chairman of Surgery
University of Texas Health Science Center at Southwestern
    Medical Center
Dallas, Texas

Martin H. Cohen, M.D.
Director of Albert Einstein Cancer Center
Chairman of Medical Oncology
Professor of Medicine
Temple University School of Medicine
Philadelphia, Pennsylvania

Joel D. Cooper, M.D.
Professor of Surgery
Washington University School of Medicine
St. Louis, Missouri

Yvon Cormier, M.D.
Associate Professor of Medicine
Laval University Faculty of Medicine
Sainte-Foy, Québec, Canada

James D. Cox, M.D.
Vice President for Patient Care
M.D. Anderson Cancer Center
University of Texas Medical School at Houston
Houston, Texas

Robert M. Craig, M.D.
Associate Professor of Medicine
Northwestern University Medical School
Chicago, Illinois

Richard S. D'Agostino, M.D.
Attending Thoracic Surgeon
Lahey Clinic Medical Center
Burlington, Massachusetts

Thomas R. DeMeester, M.D.
Professor and Chairman of Surgery
University of Southern California School of Medicine
Los Angeles, California

Jean Deslauriers, M.D.
Professor of Surgery
Laval University Faculty of Medicine
Sainte-Foy Québec, Canada

Ronald B. Dietrick, M.D.
Formerly Director of Medical Services
Kwangju Christian Hospital
Kwangju, South Korea

André Duranceau, M.D.
Professor of Surgery
University of Montreal Faculty of Medicine
Montréal, Québec, Canada

Forrest C. Eggleston, M.D.
Formerly Professor and Head of Surgery
Christian Medical College
Ludhiana, Punjab, India

John A. Elefteriades, M.D.
Associate Professor of Surgery
Yale University School of Medicine
New Haven, Connecticut

F. Henry Ellis, Jr., M.D.
Clinical Professor of Surgery, Emeritus
Harvard Medical School
Boston, Massachusetts

Nabile M. El-Baz, M.D.
Associate Professor of Anesthesiology
Rush Medical College of Rush University
Chicago, Illinois

Bahman Emani, M.D.
Professor and Associate Director
Radiation Oncology Center
Washington University School of Medicine
St. Louis, Missouri

Gary R. Epler, M.D.
Associate Clinical Professor of Pulmonary Medicine
Boston University School of Medicine
Boston, Massachusetts

David H. Epstein, M.D.
Chief of Chest Radiology and Body Computed Tomography
Western Pennsylvania Hospital
Pittsburgh, Pennsylvania

L. Penfield Faber, M.D.
Professor of Surgery
Rush Medical College of Rush University
Chicago, Illinois

Ronald Feld, M.D.
Deputy Chief and Professor of Medicine
University of Toronto Faculty of Medicine
Toronto, Ontario, Canada

Stanley C. Fell, M.D.
Professor of Cardiothoracic Surgery
Albert Einstein College of Medicine
Bronx, New York

Peter F. Ferson, M.D.
Associate Professor of Surgery
University of Pittsburgh Medical Center
Pittsburgh, Pennsylvania

Jack Fisher, M.D.
Assistant Clinical Professor of Surgery
Vanderbilt University School of Medicine
Associate Clinical Professor of Surgery
Meharry Medical College School of Medicine
Nashville, Tennessee

Willard A. Fry, M.D.
Professor of Clinical Surgery
Northwestern University Medical School
Chicago, Illinois

Henning A. Gaissert, M.D.
Research Fellow
Harvard Medical School
Boston, Massachusetts

Gordon Gamsu, M.D.
Professor of Radiology and Medicine
University of California School of Medicine
San Francisco, California

Warren B. Gefter, M.D.
Professor of Radiology
University of Pennsylvania School of Medicine
Philadelphia, Pennsylvania

Gary G. Ghahremani, M.D.
Professor and Chairman of Diagnostic Radiology
Northwestern University Medical School
Chicago, Illinois

Joan Gil, M.D.
Professor of Pathology
Mt. Sinai School of Medicine of the City University of New York
New York, New York

Robert J. Ginsberg, M.D.
Professor of Surgery
Cornell University Medical College
New York, New York

Jeffrey Glassroth, M.D.
Marquardt Professor of Medicine
Northwestern University Medical School
Chicago, Illinois

Peter Goldstraw, F.R.C.S.
Honorary Senior Clinical Lecturer
University of London
London, United Kingdom

F. Anthony Greco, M.D.
Professor of Medicine
Vanderbilt University School of Medicine
Nashville, Tennessee

Hermes C. Grillo, M.D.
Professor of Surgery
Harvard Medical School
Boston, Massachusetts

Robert A. Gustafson, M.D.
Associate Professor of Surgery
West Virginia University School of Medicine
Morgantown, West Virginia

John D. Hainsworth, M.D.
Associate Director of Sarah Cannon Cancer Center
Centennial Medical Center
Nashville, Tennessee

Renee S. Hartz, M.D.
Professor of Surgery
University of Illinois College of Medicine
Chicago, Illinois

Stephen R. Hazelrigg, M.D.
Chairman and Associate Professor of Thoracic and Cardiovascular
    Surgery
Southern Illinois University School of Medicine
Springfield, Illinois

James R. Hemp
Instructor in Surgery
Rush Medical College of Rush University
Chicago, Illinois

Lauren D. Holinger, M.D.
Professor and Head of Pediatric Otolaryngology
Rush Medical College of Rush University
Chicago, Illinois

R. Maurice Hood, M.D.
Professor of Clinical Surgery
New York University School of Medicine
New York, New York

Babette J. Horn, M.D.
Assistant Professor of Clinical Anesthesiology
Northwestern University Medical School
Chicago, Illinois

Guo Jun Huang, M.D.
Professor of Thoracic Surgery
Chinese Academy of Medical Sciences
Beijing, People's Republic of China

Lynne Jahnke, M.D.
Fellow in Hematology/Oncology
Northwestern University Medical School
Chicago, Illinois

Robert W. Jamplis, M.D.
Clinical Professor of Surgery
Stanford University School of Medicine
Stanford, California

Kumar Jeyasingham, M.D.
Honorary Clinical Lecturer in Surgery
University of Bristol
Bristol, United Kingdom

Scott Johnson, M.D.
Clinical Instructor in Surgery
University of Southern California School of Medicine
Los Angeles, California

Axel W. Joob, M.D.
Assistant Professor of Surgery
Northwestern University Medical School
Chicago, Illinois

Thomas J. Keane, M.D.
Professor of Radiation Oncology,
University of Toronto Faculty of Medicine
Toronto, Ontario, Canada

Robert J. Keenan, M.D.
Assistant Professor of Thoracic Surgery
University of Pittsburgh Medical Center
Pittsburgh, Pennsylvania

Merrill S. Kies, M.D.
Associate Professor of Clinical Medicine
Northwestern University Medical School
Chicago, Illinois

Thomas J. Kirby, M.D.
Staff Surgeon and Director of Lung Transplantation
Cleveland Clinic Foundation
Cleveland, Ohio

Ritsuko Komaki, M.D.
Associate Professor of Radiotherapy
M.D. Anderson Cancer Center
University of Texas Medical School at Houston
Houston, Texas

Rodney J. Landreneau, M.D.
Head of Thoracic Surgery
University of Pittsburgh Medical Center
Pittsburgh, Pennsylvania

Pierre Leblanc, M.D.
Professor of Chest Medicine
Laval University Faculty of Medicine
Sainte-Foy, Québec, Canada

Richard W. Light, M.D.
Professor of Medicine
University of California, Irvine
Long Beach, California

Joseph LoCicero, III, M.D.
Associate Professor
Harvard Medical School
Boston, Massachusetts

Susan R. Luck, M.D.
Associate Professor of Clinical Surgery
Northwestern University Medical School
Chicago, Illinois

Michael J. Mack, M.D.
Clinical Assistant Professor
University of Texas Health Science Center at Southwestern
  Medical School at Dallas
Dallas, Texas

James W. Mackenzie, M.D.
Professor and Chairman of Surgery
University of Medicine and Dentistry of New Jersey-
  Robert Wood Johnson Medical School
New Brunswick, New Jersey

Kamal A. Mansour, M.D.
Professor of Cardiothoracic Surgery
Emory University School of Medicine
Atlanta, Georgia

Douglas J. Mathisen, M.D.
Associate Professor of Surgery
Harvard Medical School
Boston, Massachusetts

P. Michael McFadden, M.D.
Clinical Professor of Surgery
Tulane University School of Medicine
New Orleans, Louisiana

Joseph I. Miller, Jr., M.D.
Professor of Cardiothoracic Surgery
Emory University School of Medicine
Atlanta, Georgia

Wallace T. Miller, M.D.
Professor and Vice-Chairman of Radiology
University of Pennsylvania School of Medicine
Philadelphia, Pennsylvania

Wallace T. Miller, Jr., M.D.
Assistant Professor of Radiology
University of Pennsylvania School of Medicine
Philadelphia, Pennsylvania

Darroch W. O. Moores, M.D.
Clinical Associate Professor of Surgery
Albany Medical College of Union University
Albany, New York

Gordon F. Murray, M.D.
Professor and Chairman of Surgery
West Virginia University School of Medicine
Morgantown, West Virginia

Andrew P. Naef, M.D.
Honorary Professor
University of Lausanne Faculty of Medicine
Lausanne, Switzerland

Tsuguo Naruke, M.D.
Director of Surgery
Chief of Thoracic Surgery
National Cancer Center Hospital
Tokyo, Japan

Keith S. Naunheim, M.D.
Associate Professor of Surgery
St. Louis University School of Medicine
St. Louis, Missouri

John L. Nosher, M.D.
Clinical Professor and Chairman of Radiology
University of Medicine and Dentistry of New Jersey-Robert
  Wood Johnson Medical School
New Brunswick, New Jersey

Gerald N. Olsen, M.D.
Professor of Medicine
University of South Carolina School of Medicine
Columbia, South Carolina

Mark B. Orringer, M.D.
Professor and Head of Thoracic Surgery
University of Michigan School of Medicine
Ann Arbor, Michigan

Andranik Ovassapian, M.D.
Professor of Clinical Anesthesia
Northwestern University Medical School
Chicago, Illinois

Peter C. Pairolero, M.D.
Professor of Surgery
Mayo Medical School
Rochester, Minnesota

Kerry Paape, M.D.
Instructor of Clinical Surgery
Northwestern University Medical School
Chicago, Illinois

G. Alexander Patterson, M.D.
Professor of Surgery
Washington University School of Medicine
St. Louis, Missouri

David Payne, M.D.
Assistant Professor of Radiation Oncology
University of Toronto Faculty of Medicine
Toronto, Ontario, Canada

W. Spencer Payne, M.D.
Professor of Surgery (Retired)
Mayo Medical School
Rochester, Minnesota

Michail I. Perelman, M.D.
Professor of Surgery
Russian Academy of Medical Science and Sechenov's Moscow
    Medical Academy
Moscow, Russia

Carlos A. Perez, M.D.
Professor of Radiology (Radiation Oncology)
Mallinckrodt Institute of Radiology
Washington University School of Medicine
St. Louis, Missouri

Ronald B. Ponn, M.D.
Thoracic Surgeon
Hospital of St. Raphael
New Haven, Connecticut

Joe B. Putnam, Jr., M.D.
Assistant Professor of Thoracic Surgery
University of Texas Medical School at Houston
Houston, Texas

James A. Radosevich, Ph.D.
Associate Professor of Medicine
Northwestern University Medical School
Chicago, Illinois

Marleta Reynolds, M.D.
Associate Professor of Clinical Surgery
Northwestern University Medical School
Chicago, Illinois

Philip G. Robinson, M.D.
Assistant Professor of Clinical Pathology
University of Miami School of Medicine
Miami, Florida

R. Bernard Rochon, M.D.
Clinical Assistant Professor of Surgery
University of Texas Southwestern Medical Center
Dallas, Texas

Charles L. Rice, M.D.
Professor of Surgery
University of Illinois
Chicago, Illinois

Steven T. Rosen, M.D.
Associate Professor of Medicine
Northwestern University Medical School
Chicago, Illinois

Jack A. Roth, M.D.
Professor and Chairman of Thoracic Surgery
Bud S. Johnson Chair Professor of Tumor Biology
University of Texas Medical School at Houston
Houston, Texas

Martin Rothberg, M.D.
Staff Thoracic Surgeon
Trinity Medical Center
Minob, North Dakota

Valerie W. Rusch, M.D.
Associate Professor of Surgery
Cornell University Medical College
New York, New York

Steven A. Sahn, M.D.
Professor of Medicine
Director of Pulmonary and Critical Care Medicine
Medical University of South Carolina
Charleston, South Carolina

Dr. med. Joachim Schirren
Assistant Chief of Thoracic Surgery
Thoraxklinik Heidelberg-Rohrbach
Heidelberg, Germany

Stewart M. Scott, M.D.
Consulting Professor of Surgery
Duke University Medical Center
Durham, North Carolina

Robert C. Shamberger, M.D.
Associate Professor of Surgery
Harvard Medical School
Boston, Massachusetts

Frances A. Shepherd, M.D.
Associate Professor of Medicine
University of Toronto Faculty of Medicine
Toronto, Ontario, Canada

Thomas W. Shields, M.D.
M.D., D.Sc. (Hon)
Professor Emeritus of Surgery
Northwestern University Medical School
Chicago, Illinois

David B. Skinner, M.D.
Professor of Surgery
Cornell University Medical College
New York, New York

Herbert M. Sommers, M.D.
Professor of Pathology
Northwestern University Medical School
Chicago, Illinois

K. Eric Sommers, M.D.
Fellow in Cardiothoracic Surgery
University of Pittsburgh Medical Center
Pittsburgh, Pennsylvania

William G. Spies, M.D.
Associate Professor of Radiology
Northwestern University Medical School
Chicago, Illinois

Amit K. Srivastava, M.D.
Assistant Professor of Medicine
Northwestern University Medical School
Chicago, Illinois

Harold Stern, M.D.
Associate Clinical Professor of Surgery
Yale University Medical School
New Haven, Connecticut

John M. Streitz, Jr., M.D.
Clinical Assistant Professor
University of Minnesota Medical School—Duluth
Duluth, Minnesota

David J. Sugarbaker, M.D.
Associate Professor of Surgery
Harvard Medical School
Boston, Massachusetts

Panagiotis N. Symbas, M.D.
Professor of Surgery
Emory University School of Medicine
Atlanta, Georgia

Timothy Takaro, M.D.
Clinical Professor of Surgery
Duke University School of Medicine
Durham, North Carolina

Thomas R. J. Todd, M.D.
Professor of Surgery
University of Toronto Faculty of Medicine
Toronto, Ontario, Canada

Allan L. Toole, M.D.
Associate Clinical Professor of Cardiothoracic Surgery
Yale University School of Medicine
New Haven, Connecticut

Stephen Trainer, M.D.
Fellow in Thoracic Surgery
Thoraxklinik Heidelberg-Rohrbach
Heidelberg, Germany

Victor F. Trastek, M.D.
Associate Professor of Surgery
Mayo Medical School
Rochester, Minnesota

Harold C. Urschel, Jr., M.D.
Professor Cardiovascular and Thoracic Surgery
University of Texas Health Science Center at Southwestern Medical School
Dallas, Texas

Robert M. Vanecko, M.D.
Professor of Clinical Surgery
Associate Dean of Graduate Medical Education
Northwestern University Medical School
Chicago, Illinois

Alexander Vasilakis, M.D.
Instructor of Surgery
West Virginia University School of Medicine
Morgantown, West Virginia

Mohan Verghese, M.D.
Professor and Head of General and Cardiothoracic Surgery
Christian Medical College
Punjab, India

Prof. Dr. I. Vogt-Moykopf
Professor of Thoracic Surgery
Heidelberg University
Director of Thoraxklinik Heidelberg-Rohrbach
Heidelberg, Germany

Yoh Watanabe, M.D.
Professor and Chairman of Surgery
Kanazawa University School of Medicine
Kanazawa, Japan

William H. Warren
Associate Professor of Surgery and Pathology
Rush Medical College of Rush University
Chicago, Illinois

Paul F. Waters, M.D.
Professor of Surgery
University of California, Los Angeles, School of Medicine
Los Angeles, California

Ewald R. Weibel, M.D.
Professor of Anatomy
University of Berne
Berne, Switzerland

Earle W. Wilkins, Jr., M.D.
Clinical Professor of Surgery (Retired)
Harvard Medical School
Boston, Massachusetts

Hak Yui Wong, M.D.
Associate in Clinical Anesthesiology
Northwestern University Medical School
Chicago, Illinois

Cameron Wright, M.D.
Assistant Professor of Surgery
Harvard Medical School
Boston, Massachusetts

Manoel Ximenes, III, M.D.
Professor and Head of Thoracic Surgery Unit
Hospital de Base and Armed Forces Hospital
Brasilia, Brazil

Contents

Section V   Assessment of the Thoracic Surgical Patient

Section VI   Anesthetic Management of the General Thoracic Surgical Patient

Section VII   Postoperative Management of the General Thoracic Surgical Patient

Section VIII   Pulmonary and Tracheal Resections

Section IX   The Chest Wall

Section X   The Diaphragm

Section XI   The Pleura

Section XII   Thoracic Trauma

Section XIII   The Trachea

Section XIV   Congenital, Structural, and Inflammatory Diseases of the Lung

Section XV Carcinoma of the Lung

Section XVI Other Tumors of the Lung

THE ESOPHAGUS

Section XVII Anatomy

Section XVIII   Physiology

Section XIX   Diagnostic Studies

Section XX   Operative Procedures in the Management of Esophageal Disease

Section XXI   Trauma to the Esophagus

Section XXII   Benign Esophageal Disease

Section XXIII   Malignant Lesions of the Esophagus

THE MEDIASTINUM

Section XXIV   Infections, Tumors, and Cysts of the Mediastinum

Introduction

EARLY HISTORY OF THORACIC SURGERY

Andrew P. Naef

At the time of this writing, the St. Louis Lung-Transplant Registry records 1000 lung transplants, the number growing regularly in a typical exponential curve. To the outgoing generation of thoracic surgeons who remember their struggle with the complications of pulmonary and esophageal resections, and "blind" or "closed" heart surgery, and who were still aware of the even more primitive early twentieth century techniques of their teachers, today's transplantation success is miraculous. This miracle did not happen overnight, however; it took almost half a century, from early experimentation and Hardy's operation 30 years ago to Derom's lung transplantation in Belgium, surviving 10 months in 1968, until the finally successful struggle of the Toronto Group in the 1990s.

What is accomplished today under the leadership of general thoracic surgeons all over the world provides two important historical lessons: 1) Lung transplantation is the result of the combined know-how of general thoracic as well as cardiovascular surgeons; and 2) Even more importantly, lung transplantation owes its success to the tremendous advances in biomedical science and medical technique coupled to a unique team effort of many specialists.

The success story of pulmonary transplantation — or for that matter of cardiac surgery, an outgrowth of thoracic surgery — this amazing success is the result of the fascinating surgical adventure through the better part of this century. History can be told in a chronologic fashion according to events somehow bound to happen at a certain time, or in a more personalized manner, remembering the actors whose vision, courage, and skill made them happen under conditions hard to conceive of today. Because this history has been well told, I intend to highlight, somewhat anecdotally, only a few important events particularly relevant to general thoracic surgery, and honor some of the leading pioneers, Europeans as well as North Americans, the former having too often been overshadowed by the latter.

Medical history is intimately linked to the prevailing pathology at any given time, battle wounds at the time of Ambroise Paré, the "father of surgery," or Dominique Larey, Napoleon's army surgeon, or epidemics such as of anthrax, tuberculosis—TB, or syphilis fought by Pasteur, Koch, and Ehrlich. In analogy, thoracic surgery has gone through three pathology-related periods.

The first "thoracic" surgeons were the leading general surgeons around 1900 confronted with *pleuropulmonary suppuration* — empyema, lung abcess, and bronchiectasis — a pathologic process of epidemic proportions during and after World War I, and with the 1918 influenza epidemic. Lacking antibiotics, transfusion, and intensive care, they had to fight enormous odds to obtain the smallest success. As the roots of thoracic surgery actually go back to this time, almost a century ago, our historical introduction will essentially recall this all too often neglected first period.

The second period is marked by the explosive development of pulmonary *resection for TB* followed by the surgical treatment of lung cancer. This period resulted in the refinement of surgical technique and the growing number of specialized thoracic surgeons just before, during, and immediately after World War II, establishing thoracic surgery as an autonomous specialty.

The third period centers on the advance of pulmonary — essentially TB — surgeons toward *cardiac surgery*, culminating in the surgical treatment of *coronary artery disease*. This development eventually resulted in the divorce from general thoracic surgery of an independent, entirely new specialty: cardiovascular surgery.

Having thus established the pathology-related background, the soil on which thoracic surgery grew, we can turn to the key events and a few of the pioneers who had the vision, stamina, and dexterity to open up the road to thoracic surgery. Space does not permit discussion to do justice to all of them. Their story has been repeatedly and well told and my choice of a few is an entirely personal one. If I start by presenting a pioneer of fairly recent times, Clarence Crafoord, it is to illustrate the very foundation of our specialty, namely its interdisciplinary character, as exemplified by the close relationship of anesthesia, intensive care, and general thoracic and cardiovascular surgery.

Although Clarence Crafoord (1899–1984), perhaps the greatest European pioneer in thoracic surgery, has been claimed by cardiac surgeons* as one of their own, he started out as a truly general thoracic surgeon. His 1937 inaugural dissertation, *The Technique of Pneumonectomy in Man*, is a 147-page, carefully documented experimental and clinical study reporting 16 personal cases of pneumonectomy from 1934 on, placing him only 1 year behind the accounts of the 1933 pneumonectomy of Evarts Graham. In 1927, at 28 years of age, Crafoord created a medical sensation by reporting two successful Trendelenburg embolectomies. At about that time, in the early 1930s, his preoccupation with general surgical problems led to his pioneering in prophylactic anticoagulation with heparin — purified by his colleague Jorpes — and the development of positive pressure ventilation for anesthesia and "intensive care" — the Frenckner-Crafoord spiropulsator, later the Crafoord-Bjork-Engström respirator. It was this general thoracic surgical background that led to the first operation for coarctation in October 1944, as well as to the worldwide second open heart procedure in 1954 under extracorporeal circulation and hypothermia for the removal of a large intra-atrial myxoma, actually the first operation for a cardiac tumor. This patient not only survived the daring operation, but also today enjoys an active life at over 80 years of age! Clarence Crafoord was indeed one of the first and last, as well as one of the most brilliant, complete thoracic surgeons.

Paul Samson, who in his 1967 American Association for Thoracic Surgery — AATS — Presidential Address, *The Compleat Thoracic Surgeon*, used the old spelling, did not believe it necessary to add the adjective of "general" because he still definitely included cardiac surgery in his definition. He reported the result of a poll among 557 members of the AATS, the majority of 546 agreeing with his own definition. At the time, 25 years ago, *only a minority of 11 thought that cardiovascular surgery should become a separate specialty and that "general" thoracic surgery should be reabsorbed into general surgery!* As so many predictions, this one did not stand the test of time, and I would not venture to predict the situation 25 years from today!

In Europe, the historical beginning is usually identified with Ferdinand Sauerbruch (1875–1951), who published the first textbook on thoracic surgery around 1920. It is difficult to do justice to the historical importance of this typically German "Geheimrat." On the positive side is his stimulating influence on his pupils — who like Nissen became leaders in their own

right — as well as on the many young surgeons from abroad, especially North America, who visited his Charité Clinic in Berlin. Furthermore, Sauerbruch undoubtedly was the driving force behind the surgical treatment of pulmonary TB — at the time the essence of thoracic surgery. In Davos, Switzerland, the leading TB center in the world, Sauerbruch and his assistant, the Swiss surgeon Alfred Brunner, for many years developed the surgical treatment of TB as visiting surgeons. In fact, Sauerbruch's role as a TB surgeon was the foundation of his reputation as a "thoracic surgeon," although his venture toward intrathoracic surgery was hampered by his unhappy approach to anesthesia. Stimulated by his teacher, Joachim von Mikulicz, he published his research, *The Elimination of the Harmful Effects of Pneumothorax during Intrathoracic Operations*, in 1904. Having the choice between positive and negative pressure, admittedly the more physiologic approach, he chose the famous "negative pressure operative chamber," a practical disaster. Communication with the anesthetist at the head of the patient outside the chamber was difficult, and the inside heat for the surgeon and his team became almost unbearable as the operation proceeded. When finally Sauerbruch had to admit defeat and switch to "positive" pressure breathing, he used a tightly fitting face mask, presenting many other disadvantages such as gastric distention and retention of tracheobronchial secretions. It is amazing that Sauerbruch never took the logical step to the already well-known technique of intratracheal intubation.

Sauerbruch's most brilliant pupil Rudolf Nissen (1896–1981) — his 1931 pneumonectomy for non-neoplastic disease is an historical milestone and his fundoplication is still the best operation for gastroesophageal reflux — explains the retrograde state of anesthesia at the Sauerbruch Clinic: "Sauerbruch opposed subspecialization within the main specialty of surgery. He regarded such a development as a step towards the destruction of surgery and refused to acknowledge that anesthesia might develop into a subspecialty in its own right." This attitude was still prevalent in Europe's University Clinics after World War II. Nissen continued: "His [Sauerbruch's] influence delayed the development of thoracic surgical techniques that were coming into use in other countries."

Other surgeons, Brauer in Germany, Meyer, Green, and Janeway in New York, and Samuel Robinson at Massachusetts General Hospital, also wasted time trying to solve the "open pneumothorax problem" with complicated differential pressure machines.

In France, meanwhile, the leading surgeons, Péan, Duval, and Tuffier, sporadically approached the problems of intrathoracic surgery. In my opinion, one of the most innovative leaders at the turn of the century, especially during the early decades of the 1900s, was Theodore Tuffier (1857–1929). As early as 1896, he opted for intratracheal positive pressure anesthesia, instead of wasting time with the impossible negative pressure chamber. With Hallion, he published his

---

*Clifwood R: Crafoord and the first successful resection of a cardiac myoma. Ann Thorac Surg *154*:997, 1992.

experimental work in 1896, *Regulation de la pression intrabronchique et de la narcose,* and had one of the first intratracheal balloon catheters made. This research was probably stimulated by the worldwide first successful partial lung resection Tuffier had performed in 1891. To explain Tuffier's success and fame, he had, contrarily to others, the temerity to try a lung resection in an easy, that is, early case instead of struggling with a hopeless situation. To circumvent the danger of an open pneumothorax and a flapping mediastinum, he used an ingenious technique inspired by his experience with extrapleural plombage for cavitary tuberculosis. He freed the upper lobe extrapleurally and was eventually able to palpate the apical tuberculous lesions through a tear in the parietal pleura. He then clamped the apical parenchyma below the lesion and pulled it through the intercostal space outside the chest. The lung tissue was ligated under the clamp by a "chain ligature," which was then sutured to the inner chest wall. According to Tuffier, a collar of the torn parietal pleura around the apex to be resected prevented massive air entry into the pleura. The patient made an uneventful recovery and Tuffier concluded that for pulmonary resection to be successful, it should be done in early rather than late desperate cases! Although the indication was and remains controversial, and the operation by today's standards is not difficult, 100 years ago, it took courage and imagination to attempt it.

The daring and imaginative mind as well as the technical skill of Tuffier are also demonstrated by his foray into cardiac surgery. On July 13, 1912, he operated on a patient from Belgium with aortic stenosis. Before invaginating the aortic wall and pushing his finger far into the "hard stenotic ring," Tuffier felt the typical thrill that was considerably diminished after this miraculous attempt at dilatation of the valve ring. The patient recovered and Tuffier reported the case at an international congress in London the next year. Tuffier was aware, however, that animal experimentation was the key to any surgical progress. Therefore, in 1913, he spent a few weeks in Alexis Carrel's highly sophisticated facilities at the Rockefeller Center. This collaboration with Carrel resulted in their 1914 report on experimental cardiac surgery in the Presse Medicale.

Alexis Carrel (1873–1945), Nobel Prize laureate in 1912 and an exceptional pioneer, was a visionary, particularly disciplined experimental surgeon whose amazing results owe everything to his extraordinary dexterity, strict asepsis, and meticulous surgical technique. It is true that most of his spectacular contributions concern cardiovascular surgery and transplantation; however, the general thoracic surgeon should be aware of Carrel's decisive influence on the advent of a practical method for anesthesia during operations in the chest. In 1909, when Meltzer from the laboratory next to his at the Rockefeller Institute developed the method of intratracheal positive pressure ventilation and anesthesia, Carrel immediately adopted the method to anesthetize his laboratory animals during surgical experimentation. He then not only brought the method

to the attention of New York's clinical surgeons, such as Lilienthal and Elsberg, but also, at the 1910 meeting of the American Surgical Association, convinced the elite of North American surgeons of the superiority of Meltzer's positive pressure anesthesia over the cumbersome negative pressure operating chamber of Sauerbruch. I am convinced that he helped to open the road to "routine" operations in the chest!

The young Alexis Carrel was 21 years old when, in 1894, French President Sadi Carnot died in Carrel's hometown of Lyon from uncontrolled hemorrhage resulting from a vascular laceration inflicted by an assassin. This tragedy gave Carrel the idea to develop his method for suturing vessels, first in Lyon after Carnot's assassination and after his emigration to North America at the Hull Physiology Laboratory in Chicago (1904–1906). Carrel's technique is still basic to current vascular surgical practice.

Placed in the context of his time, Carrel's imagination and vision were boundless. In his memorable paper, *On the Experimental Surgery of the Thoracic Aorta and Heart,* presented to the American Surgical Association in 1910, he reported results of experiments involving almost all the operations that would make headlines in cardiac surgery 40 years later: digital exploration of cardiac chambers and mitral valve dilatation, brief open operations for mitral and aortic stenosis under temporary inflow occlusion, as well as an aortocoronary bypass for hypothetic coronary sclerosis in a dog. Carrel was able to accomplish the distal anastomosis in 5 minutes, but the dog's heart fibrillated after 3½ minutes, Carrel concluding that a technique had to be developed for doing the anastomosis in such a short time.

Carrel's main interest, however, concerned the field of transplantation, tissue culture, and organ preservation — thyroid gland — outside the body, the principal problem being the extracorporeal perfusion of the organ. This focus led to collaboration with the aviator Charles Lindbergh, who was also a mechanical genius and who became interested in extracorporeal circulation when his sister died of mitral stenosis. To Lindbergh, this was a simple mechanical, and thus solvable, problem. The result of their 5-year collaboration, an amazingly perfect perfusion machine, somewhere between extracorporeal circulation and an artificial heart, made the cover of Time Magazine in 1935.

Carrel presented experimental solutions at least 40 years before cardiac surgeons started treating patients. Somewhat condescendingly, he said: "I invent techniques, let others use them." This delay has never been explained. As clinical surgeons considered Carrel's visions unrealistic, it has been said that they "not only missed to carry the ball any further, but [also] simply dropped the ball"!

One last word about Carrel's controversial book entitled, "Man, the Unknown" published in 1935 and his subsequent "involvement" with the Vichy Government through his "Foundation for the Study of Human Relations." Carrel was accused of engendering a racist philosophy, but it should be remembered that at the time, the scientific world discovered the importance of genetics and that several countries and North American states enacted "eugenic" marriage laws.

Carrel, convinced by the importance of an elite for human progress, wrote in fact, "For the perpetuation of an elite, eugenics is indispensable." But his attitude should be appreciated in the context of his time, not according to 1990 standards. From our surgical standpoint, the man was a towering genius.

Although Carrel was of French ancestry, his sphere of influence was the North American continent, especially New York City. Before going on to review the explosive development of our specialty in North America, the remarkable level of thoracic surgery in Great Britain deserves discussion.

The story of the famous "Brompton Hospital" and Arthur Tudor Edwards (1890–1946), certainly the most important British chest surgeon between 1918 and 1939, is well known and has been told repeatedly—Abbey-Smith (1982); Bishop (1979). Tudor Edwards might soon be forgotten because of the brevity of his career — he died of heart disease at age 56 — and the scarcity of his publications. He was not a "writing" but a "cutting" surgeon, and according to his teacher, Gordon Taylor, "learned his chest surgery from no other pioneer . . . it was carved out of the hard rock of personal experience." He was appointed Chief Surgeon of the Brompton Hospital in 1922. From that day on, previously rare thoracic operations became more and more frequent: 33 cases in 1922, 62 in 1923, 128 in 1928. Early dissection lobectomies and pneumonectomies were performed by Tudor Edwards around that time, as early as anywhere else in the world. According to Price Thomas, the greatest contribution of Tudor Edwards to British chest surgery, however, was the part he played in the foundation of the Thoracic Society of Great Britain and Ireland. In essence, he may not have accomplished any revolutionary breakthrough like some of the North Americans, but he certainly inspired an entire British school of brilliant thoracic surgeons.

Following Tudor Edwards were three great surgeons: Russel Claude Brock (1903–1980), Holmes T. Sellors (1902–1989), and Clement Price Thomas (1893–1973). If Price Thomas remained a typical general thoracic surgeon — incidentally, a superb technician who performed the first bronchial sleeve lobectomy in 1947, about 20 years before everybody else — Sellors and especially Brock mark the passage of general thoracic toward cardiac surgery. Sellors was the first to recommend the face-down position, better known as the Overholt position, for TB resections to prevent contralateral spread in the preantibiotic era. He also performed the first pulmonic valvotomy in 1947, 2 months before Brock. Brock, also initially a lung surgeon, whose tenacity and energy were proverbial, published one of the earliest fundamental books on the anatomy of the bronchial tree with special reference to the surgery of lung abcess before going on to becoming the father of British heart surgery.

I would like to review, in somewhat more detail, the work of two remarkable surgeons whose careers were cut short or at least hampered by fate: Laurence O'Shaughnessy and Hugh Morriston Davis.

Laurence O'Shaughnessy (1900–1940) could have become the first British heart surgeon had his promising career not been cut short during the evacuation of the British Army at Dunkirk in 1940. A self-made man, he entered the Colonial Medical Corps in the Sudan at age 23 years, probably for economic reasons, where he became involved in the surgical treatment of pulmonary TB. At the time, Sauerbruch in Berlin was the world authority in that field and O'Shaughnessy, when on leave as well as at the end of his 7 years in the Sudan, spent much time at the Charité Hospital in Berlin. He considered Sauerbruch his "spiritual father." At least, he was his teacher, and in 1937, O'Shaughnessy published an excellent English edition of Sauerbruch's textbook with additional material from his own experience. A typical general thoracic, essentially TB, surgeon, O'Shaughnessy, however, already reported in 1936 his experimental and clinical experience of myocardial revascularization by cardio-omentopexy. It was his idea to bring the omentum up into the chest, initially to protect an esophageal anastomosis. Today, O'Shaughnessy's idea has been taken over by lung-transplant surgeons to provide collateral circulation to the tracheal anastomosis. Just as direct coronary revascularization replaced cardio-omentopexy, however, the revival of tracheal omentopexy was short-lived, soon to be followed by the logical solution of direct arterio-arterial revascularization of the trachea.

It should also be noted that in 1939, while already in Flanders, he wrote a paper concerning his animal experimentation with pulmonic valvotomy on the beating heart. Had he survived the Dunkirk debacle, he might have performed the operation in a patient before either Brock or Sellors.

Hugh Morriston Davies (1879–1965), according to the eulogy by Price Thomas, was the Doyen of British thoracic surgery, but to me, he is also a symbolic figure for the interdisciplinary integration of thoracic medicine as a whole. He introduced chest radiology against the resistance of radiologists who at the time declared chest radiographs useless and relegated him with his x-ray machine to a small basement room of the hospital. In 1912, his thesis was vindicated when a chest radiograph of one of his patients showed a large shadow in the right lower lobe. The presumptive diagnosis of lung cancer led to the first anatomic dissection lobectomy in the world.

Anesthesia was no problem for this all-round chest specialist. Having not opted for Sauerbruch's cumbersome negative pressure chamber in favor of the just published positive pressure approach of Meltzer, Davies constructed his own positive pressure anesthesia apparatus as early as 1910 or 1911, known jokingly as his "fire engine." Thus, his 1912 lobectomy was performed under positive pressure ether anesthesia. Although the patient died on the eighth postoperative day, this operation is of great historical interest, because at a time when lobectomies were still performed by the crude hilar mass ligation technique, he dissected vessels and bronchus separately, decades before such operations were reported by the North American pioneers Churchill, Kent, and others. In his publication, *Surgery of the Lung and Pleura*, Morriston Davies concluded in 1913: "Cancer of the lung is now accessible to surgical treatment and complete removal. But until all pulmonary cases are subjected to routine radiography the growths will not be recognized until they have extended beyond the possibilities of all treatment. In all doubtful cases at least an exploratory thoracotomy should be undertaken." A statement made 80 years ago and still true!

A few years later, at age 36 years, his surgical career was tragically interrupted. He contracted a septic infection during an empyema operation. Although an amputation was barely avoided, the infection resulted in crippling finger contractions. Forced by destiny, he resigned his hospital position, bought a TB sanitarium in Wales, and soon became the British authority for the medical treatment of the disease. Nevertheless, Davies remained a surgeon at heart. After visiting the 1910 congress of the German Surgical Society and listening to Sauerbruch and Willms describe their techniques, he performed the first thoracoplasty in Great Britain in 1912. Realizing that many of his sanitarium patients in fact needed surgical therapy, he trained again, using his left hand, and re-educated his crippled right hand. By 1922, he was again performing major surgery.

Having become, by destiny, an all-round chest specialist, he was the foremost promoter of interdisciplinary cooperation. In his 1948 *Provocative Talk on Tuberculosis*, he relates the following story reminding the reader that "in the 15th century medical faculties granted licenses to practice surgery to the 'less clever' pupils, so long as he did not exercise the art of medicine or call himself a physician." Morriston Davies continues: "In the 20th century, in 1915 to be exact, during a discussion of the treatment of tuberculosis at the London Medical Society, I attempted to talk on the surgical treatment but was ordered by the President to stand down on the ground that my remarks had nothing to do with the subject under discussion . . ." For Morriston Davies, then almost 70 years old, the very existence of the Thoracic Society of Great Britain and Ireland grouping many different specialists represented a tremendous change of spirit. In other words, at a time when most surgeons still behaved like demi-gods, Morriston Davies was an early promoter of team work, which proved to be the foundation of progress during our time.

It is not clear why the remarkable accomplishments of the British have remained in the shadow of the North American scene. The British trend to the "understatement" may have played a role, whereas the North American pioneers possibly had the drive of immigrants, or at least still their genetic make-up, to succeed and also to make their achievements known.

Finally, the destruction and deterioration of material conditions in Europe, resulting from the two great European wars and the loss of millions of young, potentially creative men, brought medical progress to a virtual standstill. Be that as it may, from that time on, the center of thoracic surgery moved across the Atlantic Ocean. Interestingly, however, the early pages of that story were still written by Europeans. Carrel, dissatisfied with conditions in France, had come to New York, as had Tuffier for a time. Many pupils of the great German medical and surgical tradition, such as Willy Meyer and Samuel Meltzer, had landed in New York during the 1880s for political as well as economic reasons. During the first decades of the twentieth century, this influx of European, especially German, medical culture made New York, main gateway to the New World, temporarily the center of medical and surgical progress. Logically, the first attempts at operations in the chest were performed in New York, by the coming leaders in thoracic surgery: Meyer, Torek, and Lilienthal.

Although thoracic surgery soon spread out to the traditional medical centers of Boston, Philadelphia, Baltimore, and beyond, it was certainly not by coincidence that the drive for the foundation of a New York, and soon thereafter, American Association for Thoracic Surgery originated in New York City. The New York association was founded on February 20, 1917 and the American association—AATS—on June 7, 1917. The New York surgeons who took this initiative were remarkable men whose memory should by no means fade behind the better known accomplishments of the no less brilliant surgeons one generation later, when thoracic surgery had developed from a sporadic branch of general surgery into a well-defined specialty of its own.

Three men are representative of this historical turning point: Willy Meyer, Samuel Meltzer, and Howard Lilienthal. Meyer and Meltzer were both German-trained immigrants; Lilienthal was a product of Harvard and the New York Mount Sinai Hospital. Meyer was unquestionably the enthusiastic driving force behind the foundation, leaving, however, the first presidency to the older, highly respected scholar Samuel Meltzer. Lilienthal, the brilliant all-round surgeon and daring explorer of a "new frontier," meanwhile contributed enormously to the life of the AATS.

Willy Meyer (1858–1932) represents, more than any other surgeon, the continuity between European — German — and North American surgery, and is a symbolic figure for the beginning of thoracic surgery in the United States of America. In a short history of the German — Lenox Hill — Hospital, one can read the somewhat grandiloquent overstatement that immigrants brought "the first fruits of the golden days of German medical education to their adopted land . . . a direct pipeline to the best European thought and practice of the day"!

Born and educated in Germany, Meyer came to the United States in 1884 and joined the staff of the German Hospital, built just 16 years before in 1868. For these early days, his outstanding accomplishments were the result of his enthusiasm and typically German energy. According to a contemporary portrayal, he arrived at the hospital promptly at 7.30 a.m., running up the steps, greeting the interns with his battle cry "Vorwärts

Kinder," which earned him the nickname "Marshal Vorwärts"! He died of a heart attack at age 74 while attending a meeting of the New York Surgical Society, having taken part in a discussion on cancer of the breast. This topic was of special interest to him because in 1894, he described the technique of radical mastectomy.

In 1884, while still in Germany, he assisted his teacher Friedrich Trendelenburg to work out and publish the method of elevating the patient's pelvis during certain lower abdominal operations — ultimately known as the Trendelenburg position.

Although active in every phase of surgery, thoracic surgery became his main interest. He performed some of the earliest esophageal and pulmonary operations in the United States. Unfortunately, he wasted precious time struggling with the "open pneumothorax problem" using Sauerbruch's "hypobaric operating chamber."

In 1908, Sauerbruch visited the United States to show his negative pressure chamber at the AMA Meeting. At the end of his visit, he did not take the bulky construction home to Germany, but left it with Willy Meyer, one of his unconditional admirers. The chamber was first installed at the Rockefeller Institute for experimental operations. During 1909 and 1910, Meyer and his brother Julius, an engineer, continued research and designed a "universal differential pressure chamber" combining Sauerbruch's negative chamber and Brauer's positive pressure compartment for the head of the patient only. The "universal chamber" allowed either negative pressure on the open chest with the surgeon inside the chamber, or positive pressure by means of a small box à la Brauer for the head of the patient with the surgical team working on the open chest outside at atmospheric pressure. In 1911, this highly complex machine was installed in the newly built thoracic surgical department of the German — Lenox Hill — Hospital and was used for a series of operations on patients. Meyer, however, was too intelligent a man to not understand eventually that Meltzer and Auer's intratracheal intubation for positive pressure ventilation was the method of choice.

Meltzer was an extraordinary scholar, and in gracious recognition of the older man's contribution to anesthesia in thoracic surgery, Meyer suggested Meltzer as the first President of the newly founded AATS. As for the "universal chamber," which had taken too much of his time and energy — actually worthy to be kept as a Smithsonian Museum piece — it had to be dismantled and sold as scrap metal in 1928 because the growing Lenox Hill Hospital had no space for it.

Another such cumbersome operating chamber was the "positive pressure cabin for thoracic surgery" of Samuel Robinson (1877–1947), also called "Sam Robinson's Box." Robinson, the fourth President of the AATS, initially a Massachusetts General Hospital surgeon, spent a year at the Sauerbruch clinic. After his return, he became the thoracic surgeon of Massachusetts General Hospital before moving to the Mayo Clinic, where he became the Chief of Thoracic Surgery in 1915.

The AATS, in a way a monument to the memory of Willy Meyer, has stood the test of time. According to a legend, Meyer's idea to provide a forum for surgeons interested in thoracic surgery to discuss their problems was triggered by the total lack of response when he presented the sensational case of Torek's total esophagectomy before the surgical section of the 1913 AMA convention. This forum, the AATS, was brought into life on June 7, 1917 at the Waldorf Astoria Hotel during another AMA Meeting in New York City, but it was far from easy to keep the Association alive through the difficult early war and post-war years. Most leading surgeons still were of the opinion that aside from the hopeless topics of bronchiectasis, tuberculosis, cancer, and syphilitic aortic aneurysm, the only true surgical problem deserving any discussion was empyema. By 1924, because of this lack of interest, only half of the founding members still belonged to the organization. Nevertheless, the enthusiasm of the remaining few was great, the scientific program being carried year after year by these early pioneers. One of them, Rudolf Matas (1860–1957), the New Orleans surgeon of Spanish origin, was indeed an active participant of the spectacular development of thoracic surgery since its beginning. Besides his many contributions to general as well as thoracic and vascular surgery, he was, as early as 1901, an early adept of positive pressure ventilation and anesthesia. Tracheal intubation was not yet easily performed and Matas resorted to the intralaryngeal tube of O'Dwyer, constructing his own Matas-O'Dwyer apparatus for artificial respiration and anesthesia. The third President of the Association, he contributed enormously to its early development. Appreciating the contribution of these pioneers, Evarts Graham later called Willy Meyer, Lilienthal, and Matas "the triumvirate that kept the Association alive."

Samuel Meltzer (1851–1921) was not a surgeon, but the stated goal of the AATS was to bring together physicians of different orientation — TB specialists, anesthetists, and broncoscopists interested in thoracic pathology. Thirty of the 50 charter members of the AATS were surgeons and 20 were not. Among them was Chevalier Jackson, whose name is synonymous with the development of diagnostic esophagobronchoscopy in North America.

Meltzer was born near Kovno, a little Lithuanian — at the time Russian — town. Destined to become a rabbi, he must have been an absolutely brilliant scholar. At 16 years of age, he was already an authority on Hebrew literature and was admired for his commentaries of biblical texts and the Talmud. He wanted more, however, and left for Königsberg and Berlin to study philosophy, chemistry, and finally medicine, graduating in 1882. His acquaintance in Berlin with one of the leaders in modern physiology, Hugo Kronecker, was crucial for Meltzer's future career.

He was 32 years old when he came to New York in 1883 and rapidly developed a busy practice. Physiology was his primary interest, however, and he continued his research in make-shift facilities on the side. In 1904, he was offered a part-time position at the Rockefeller Institute, and 3 years later, giving up his practice, he became a full-time physiologist at the Institute. Among his many contributions to the physiology of deglutition, tetanus, anaphylactic shock, bile secretion, and drainage stimulated by magnesium sulfate, we as thoracic surgeons are interested in his research on the toxic inhibition of the respiratory center by magnesium, leading Meltzer and his son-in-law John Auer to the technique of continuous intratracheal insufflation for ventilation and anesthesia (1909). The method was quickly adopted by Carrel in experimental surgery and then by Elsberg in clinical surgery. This revival of a method actually known for centuries since Vesalius (1555), certainly since Tuffier and Hallion (1896), placed in an environment such as Carrel's experimentation and the clinical surgeons' struggle with open pneumothorax, was indeed a breakthrough, condemning the Sauerbruch chamber to obsolescence. This practical method of anesthesia has certainly played an important role in the from thereon rapid development of thoracic surgery. Meyer and Meltzer knew each other well, and when Meyer at the German Hospital had no room for Sauerbruch's chamber after the 1908 Sauerbruch visit, Meltzer arranged space and the possibility for experimental surgery at the Rockefeller Institute. Their friendship and Meyer's admiration for Meltzer's scientific superiority was certainly the reason why Meltzer the scholar, and not Meyer the organizer, was elected as the first President of the AATS.

Howard Lilienthal (1861–1946), who founded what was probably the first North American Thoracic Surgical Service at the Mount Sinai Hospital in 1914, represents a pioneer who combined that rare mixture of technical skill, sound reasoning, and tenacity in the face of discouraging defeats. Trained as a typical all-round general surgeon, he belonged to the first generation of thoracic surgeons. As a general surgeon, he performed suprapubic prostatectomy before 1905 and described a "single and improved method of total nephro-ureterectomy in case of tuberculosis." He never avoided a difficult operation in favor of an easy one, and he was an early advocate of gastrectomy and cholecystectomy "en lieu" of gastroenterostomy, or the old-fashioned cholecystostomy, for retrieval of gallstones.

His most original contributions, however, were made in thoracic surgery. In 1921, he advocated extrapleural esophageal resection from the back to circumvent the disaster of intrapleural dehiscence, and was among the first to use Carrel's vascular suture in clinical surgical procedures. On February 20, 1910, he performed the first thoracotomy using intratracheal anesthesia at the Mount Sinai Hospital, the first step toward pulmonary resection, his most important historical contribution.

Charles Elsberg (1871–1948), 10 years Lilienthal's junior, constructed certainly one of the first positive pressure anesthesia machines (1909), giving the anesthesia himself for this first thoracotomy at the Mount Sinai Hospital. Interestingly, Elsberg abandoned anesthesia as well as thoracic surgery to become a pioneer

in neurosurgery and the Chief Surgeon of the New York Neurological Institute at its foundation in 1909.

Lilienthal, called "the father of lobectomy," performed a "one-stage lobectomy" as early as 1914, an enormous advance compared to the ghastly two-stage technique leaving the necrotic lobe to slough out after hilar strangulation. From 1914 to 1922, long before penicillin or even the sulfa drugs, he performed 31 cases of one-stage lobectomy for bronchopulmonary suppuration, accepting a mortality rate of approximately 50%. Even at a time when a certain risk was accepted for any type of surgery, Lilienthal's colleagues were critical of this high mortality rate. Retrospectively, one might wonder if surgical progress might not have been considerably delayed were it not for men like him. Lilienthal himself, quite aware of the dilemma, explained those disappointing results by the desperate cases he felt morally compelled to take on: "Patients have threatened suicide if refused the chance of operation. . . . To refuse to operate on a wretched patient, otherwise incurable, merely because the statistics may be unfavorable seems hardly fair. . . ." Still relying on hilar mass-suture ligation, he thought that individual dissection-ligation would take too long. Under the precarious conditions of anesthesia and instrumentation in the 1920s, every operation was still a race with death, and Lilienthal said that "a lobectomy taking more than 45 minutes would almost certainly result in the loss of the patient."

As most pioneers, he was also an enthusiastic and gifted teacher. His two-volume text entitled, *Thoracic Surgery*, published in 1925, was still considered "a classic" by Graham 20 years later, and according to Ravitch, he was the first person to present a motion picture to the American Surgical Association in 1917! The title of that movie was "The Technique of Thoracotomy and Lung Mobilisation in Empyema."

These men and their contemporaries dominated the scene well into the 1930s, when the next extremely dynamic generation took over and established routine pulmonary and esophageal surgery as we know it today.

Until 1931, no surgeon had dared perform a total pneumonectomy, interestingly for fear of producing a severe pulmonary embolus-like syndrome by ligating the main pulmonary artery. In 1931 and 1932, Nissen in Berlin and Cameron Haight in Ann Arbor performed a two-stage left pneumonectomy by the crude, today incredible technique of separately strangulating the lobar pedicles, gauze-packing the pleural cavity, and letting the grossly bronchiectatic lobes slough out after about 2 weeks. Miraculously, both patients, 12- and 13-year-old girls, survived and were cured. By today's standard, they were good operative risks.

Evarts A. Graham (1883–1957) was the daring surgeon who, on April 5, 1933, performed the first one-stage pneumonectomy for cancer on a 48-year-old gynecologist — also a good risk. Although he resected the lung in one stage, he also used the hilar mass ligation-suture technique, the same technique Lilienthal used for his lobectomies 20 years before.

It was Brunn (1929), Rienhof (1933), and Archibald (1934) who introduced routine anatomic dissection for lobectomy and pneumonectomy. Rienhof, along with Crafoord, are remembered for describing an experimentally and clinically tested technique for bronchial closure, a decisive step toward the prevention of the ever-present danger of bronchial fistula.

Churchill, Chamberlain, and Overholt, almost simultaneously, developed the technique of anatomic segmentomy, replaced today by the certainly less anatomic stapling technique. Lingulectomy was actually suggested in 1939 by Churchill and Belsey, but segmental resection for all pulmonary segments had to wait until after the war when Chamberlain and Overholt developed this technique on a large scale in the treatment of bronchiectasis and especially tuberculosis. "TB resection" was really the take-off for routine pulmonary resection. Overholt and Chamberlain, soon followed by many others, operated on thousands of TB patients until, a few years later, streptomycin "definitely" took care of an outgoing epidemic. The lung cancer epidemic soon took the place of TB, however, and led not only to further refinements of surgical technique, but also to the commitment of leading chest surgeons, such as Alton Ochsner and R.H. Overholt, to the antitobacco crusade.

Meanwhile, the esophagus, always a borderline territory between otolaryngologists, abdominal surgeons, and thoracic surgeons, presented a formidable challenge. Lilienthal (1921) resected an esophageal cancer through a posterior mediastinal extrapleural approach to prevent the dreaded complication of intrapleural dehiscence and fistulization. Although recommended later by Cameron Haight for repair of an esophageal atresia with tracheoesophageal fistula, the posterior extrapleural approach was certainly inadequate for any extensive esophageal resection and repair.

The first milestone on the road to surgery of esophageal carcinoma was the successful total esophagectomy by Franz Torek (1861–1938) on March 4, 1913. At age 11 years, he had arrived with his parents from Wroclaw — at the time Breslau — a Prussian University town. After his graduation from the College of Physicians and Surgeons, he joined the staff of the German Hospital as Willy Meyer's colleague. He had the reputation of being a brilliant, totally silent, and unemotional surgeon. He had to be, to undertake this difficult operation under the operating conditions of 1913. "The tumor was fairly fixed just below the transverse portion of the aortic arch. . . . The dissection of that part of the esophagus, which passes behind the aortic arch offered great difficulties. They were finally overcome by *dislodging the aorta and lifting it forward after having ligated and divided a number of its intercoastal branches.* . . . The tumor was also attached to the left bronchus which sustained a longitudinal cut . . . repaired with a silk suture." This difficult operation took Torek only 1 hour and 45 minutes, and it was apparently a radical one, the patient surviving 13 years! The time was not ripe, however,

and 16 years later, when Torek reported the Lenox Hill experience at the American Surgical Association in 1929, there were only two more survivors, operated upon by Carl Eggers among 23 attempts. Meade recounts that when Garlock presented two cases of esophagectomy for cancer at the New York Surgical Society in 1937, Torek, who had never had the chance to do another successful esophagectomy, at 76 years of age sat in the front row of the audience. He had shown the way to younger men, fulfilling his work.

It also has been said that this operation triggered the idea of founding the AATS. Meyer, who reported Torek's case 3 months later before the Surgical Section of the AMA, was deeply frustrated by a total lack of interest for his presentation and decided that surgeons interested in thoracic disease needed a forum before which they could discuss their problems.

Thirty-one years after Torek's historical operation, on September 20, 1944, R.H. Sweet successfully performed his first supra-aortic esophagogastrostomy after freeing the esophagus behind the arch à la Torek and placing the proximal esophagus in front of the arch, an operation later known as the Sweet operation.

Richard H. Sweet (1901–1960), an exceptional pioneer, deserves to be remembered in more detail. Although born and trained in New Jersey and New York, he became a typical Bostonian, his reserved distinction earning him the nickname of "Sir Richard." To my generation, he was the quintessence of a master surgeon. The speed of his operations was impressive and watching his elegant, meticulous technique, never showing any hasty movements, one was surprised that it took him less than 2 hours to complete an esophagectomy "from skin to skin." This dogmatic left thoracotomy esophagectomy, an easy operation for the master, was the source of many complications for the patients and difficulties for the average surgeon. It was therefore with great relief that almost everyone switched from the Sweet approach to the right thoracotomy-abdominal technique of Lewis (1946), still later replaced by the "pull-through"-no thoracotomy technique of Denk (1913), Gray Turner (1931), and Orringer (1978).

Sweet also was a great teacher. As a trained general surgeon, he considered operating simply a technical problem, and in the introduction to his remarkable textbook, *Thoracic Surgery* (1950), he wrote: "The present volume is based upon the concept that any properly qualified surgeon can acquire with relative ease a satisfactory proficiency in thoracic surgery employing the techniques herein described."

As we reached midcentury, other general thoracic surgeons, Blalock, Gross, Bailey, and Harken to name only a few, opened the road to cardiovascular surgery, a chapter beyond the domain of this history of general thoracic surgery. All of these more recent developments belong to a well-documented, not very distant past repeatedly described in textbooks and individual memoirs. Avoiding telling this well-known story again in detail, the purpose of this historical introduction is to retrace the scattered roots of general thoracic surgery grown out of the still somewhat crude field of general surgery at the turn of the century. The men who moved things along, first in Europe and then after crossing the Atlantic Ocean, were trained in general abdominal, urologic, and orthopedic surgery. They had to improvise their techniques for anesthesia themselves to overcome the "open pneumothorax problem." With scanty, newly developed asepsis, and the lack of antibiotics, routine blood transfusion, and intensive care, they opened the road to thoracic surgery that represented their new frontier. Today, the fascinating territory of scientific organ transplantation and the amazing potential of video-assisted endoscopic thoracic surgery — and its limits — represent the challenge for a new generation of dynamic thoracic surgeons worthy of their forefathers.

The Lung, Pleura, Diaphragm, and Chest Wall

Anatomy

CHAPTER 1

ANATOMY OF THE THORAX

Charles E. Blevins

The thorax is a flexible, airtight cage whose framework comprises the most continuously active combination of skeletal, muscular, and articulating tissues in the body. Its primary function is to produce movements responsible for ventilation of the lungs. It also affords protection for thoracic viscera and support for the upper extremities, but such responsibilities are secondary to the vital function of producing the alternating changes in pressure required for inflation and deflation of the lungs. Such pressure changes must be orderly, well-coordinated, and accompanied by close compliance of the lungs with changes in thoracic dimensions. The volume and rate of air movement must be compatible with vital needs for oxygen under a variety of conditions. To meet such requirements, a uniquely functional anatomic apparatus is required.

RESPIRATORY MOVEMENTS

Movements of the thorax are the result of both active and passive events. During inspiration, the thorax is actively enlarged by coordinated muscle contractions. As a direct result of increased thoracic dimensions, intrathoracic, intrapleural, and intrapulmonic pressures are sequentially reduced so that atmospheric air is forced into the lungs. Expiration is a passive event, largely owing to the relaxation of forces generated during inspiration. It is marked by the return of thoracic dimensions to resting levels, and by increased pressure within the chest, pleural cavities, and lungs. Muscle activity may facilitate the expiratory phase of breathing, but it is not essential.

Inspiratory movements enlarge the thorax in all dimensions. They are a blend of efforts directed in the anteroposterior, bilateral, and superoinferior axes. Increase in anteroposterior dimensions is marked by forward and upward movement of the lower part of the sternum, which is called the "pump-handle" movement. The sternum is more firmly anchored at its upper extent by relatively short ribs and costal cartilages than at its lower limits where both ribs and cartilages are longer.

Because the points of pivot of the ribs are located at their vertebral articulations, elevation of the ribs lifts the body of the sternum outward and forward. The greatest excursion occurs at the level of the longest ribs, that is, ribs five to seven. The axis for such movement is on a line drawn through the head, neck, and tubercle of each rib (Fig. 1–1).

During normal quiet respiration, the ribs are elevated by contraction of the intercostal muscles. Taylor (1960) and Campbell (1955) reported that the scalene muscles also aid in elevation in some individuals. Jones and associates (1953) reported that the effect of muscles

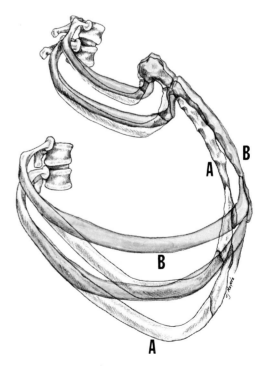

Fig. 1–1. The "pump-handle" movement in breathing. Compare position of sternum and ribs at the beginning (A) and the end (B) of inspiration. Note the increase in anteroposterior dimensions.

within individual intercostal spaces is apparently small, but synchronous contraction of all intercostal muscles is sufficient to elevate the rib cage as a unit. The resultant increase in anteroposterior dimension is greatest at the level of ribs five to seven (see Fig. 1–1).

Increase in bilateral dimensions is marked by upward and lateral excursion in the vicinity of the midaxillary line. The greatest degree of movement is noted in ribs seven to ten, whose costal cartilages descend and then ascend before articulation with the sternum. Because the middle of each rib-cartilage unit is lower than either costovertebral or costosternal articulations, elevation swings each unit upward and laterally, much like the action of lifting a bucket handle upward toward the middle of its arc of swing (Fig. 1–2). This action is accomplished by contraction of intercostal muscles also, but Cherniack and Cherniack (1961) suggested that it is facilitated by muscle fibers of the diaphragm that are perpendicular to the costal margin.

The greatest increase in thoracic dimensions during inspiration is in the superoinferior dimensions. It is accomplished by contraction of the diaphragm, which is generally described as "dome-shaped." The dome, however, is uneven; its anterolateral attachments are at higher levels than its posterolateral attachments. Furthermore, it is indented by the heart and may present

two domes, one related to the liver and one related to the stomach and spleen. Contraction of the majority of its muscle fibers flattens the diaphragm against the abdominal viscera, thereby increasing vertical intrathoracic dimensions. Contraction of its peripheral or costal muscle fibers may also produce an outward flaring of the lowest costal margin. During quiet respiration, the diaphragm undergoes an excursion of about 1 to 2 cm, but it may move as much as 6 to 7 cm during deep breathing. The lower ribs are believed to be helpful in resisting upward and medial pull of the diaphragm as a result of stabilization by the serratus posterior inferior muscles. The quadratus lumborum may stabilize the twelfth rib, but its effect on respiration is probably insignificant.

The diaphragm and intercostal muscles are therefore the primary muscles of inspiration. Movements of the diaphragm account for 75 to 80% of pulmonary ventilation during quiet respiration compared to 20 to 25% contributed by the intercostal muscles — mainly the external intercostals and the anterior portions of the internal intercostals. During severe or labored breathing, however, other skeletal muscles may be used. The sternocleidomastoid, serratus posterior superior, and levatores costarum may be active in elevation of the ribs. Muscles of the extremities may also be helpful in moments of severe need. With the torso in fixed position, movement of the arms and shoulders away from the thorax may be sufficient to enlarge thoracic dimensions to a small but sometimes necessary degree. Deltoid, trapezius, pectoral, and latissimus dorsi muscles are involved in such activity.

Expiration can occur only when intrapulmonic pressure exceeds that of the atmosphere. At the end of inspiration, the lungs are inflated and stretched. Inspiratory muscles have reached optimal efficiency in expanding the rib cage against atmospheric pressure. At this point, elastic resistance of lung tissue is at first equal to and then greater than muscular forces that would retain the expanded state of the thorax. The lungs recoil elastically and the consequent rise in intrapulmonic pressure is sufficient to force air out of the lungs. Both soft and hard tissues of the thoracic wall comply passively with the reduction of lung volume, aided by atmospheric pressure directed against them. Expiration stops when intrapulmonic pressure is once again equal to atmospheric pressure. In quiet breathing, expiration is accomplished almost exclusively by elastic recoil of the lungs and the rib cage. During vigorous or carefully controlled expiration, however, such as while singing, shouting, abdominal straining, or playing a wind instrument, muscles of the abdominal wall may aid in the reduction of thoracic dimensions by compression of abdominal viscera against the diaphragm.

Although the change from inspiratory to expiratory efforts thus represents a shift from active to passive events, the change in airflow is not a chaotic event. Rather, it is well regulated by the diaphragm, which continues to contract with decreasing efficiency, but does not reach the zero point until the middle of

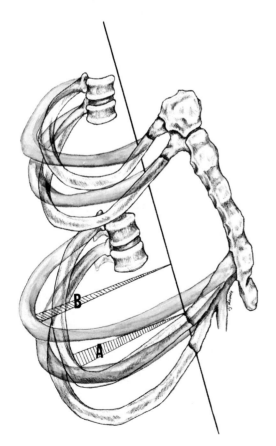

Fig. 1–2. The "bucket-handle" movement in breathing. Compare distance of the ribs from central axis of the thorax at the beginning (A) and the end (B) of inspiration. Note increase in lateral dimensions.

expiration. In this respect, it is similar to the action of limb musculature, in which gradual relaxation of flexor muscles prevents uncoordinated movement of an extremity in the opposite direction by antagonistic extensors. As described by Agostini and Torri (1962), during maximal breathing efforts, the diaphragm also contracts toward the end of vigorous expiration, limiting the extent to which the lungs can collapse.

SURFACE LANDMARKS AND STRUCTURES SUPERFICIAL TO THE THORAX

The thoracic surgeon is primarily concerned with the thoracic wall and the thoracic contents; however, a few overall considerations of structures related to surface features are helpful in orientation to deeper structures of the thorax itself (Fig. 1–3). In all but the most obese subjects, the outline of the sternum can be visualized in the thoracic midline. Extending laterally and slightly upward from the jugular notch of the sternum, the clavicles curve forward and then backward toward the shoulders. From the lowermost margin of the body of the sternum, the lower margin of the rib cage diverges bilaterally to reach its lowest level at the midaxillary line.

The outline of the sternocleidomastoid muscles may be seen extending diagonally upward from the upper part of the anterior surface of the manubrium of the sternum and the medial one third of the clavicle toward the base of the skull. Immediately below the clavicle, the outline of the pectoralis major muscle is evident. These muscles extend bilaterally from broad clavicular, sternal, and costal origins, converge toward the axilla, and form a bilaminar, U-shaped tendon that attaches to the lateral lip of the intertubercular sulcus of the humerus. The lower margin of each pectoralis major muscle forms the anterior fold of the axilla. The pectoralis major muscles are supplied by medial and lateral pectoral nerves from the brachial plexus and are versatile in function. They adduct and rotate the arm medially and in addition may elevate it — clavicular portion — or depress it — sternocostal portion. If the shoulder girdle is held in fixed position, these muscles may also elevate the upper ribs in forced inspiration. During artificial respiration, pulling the flexed upper extremity toward the head may also force the pectoralis major muscles to elevate the upper ribs.

Deep to the pectoralis major muscles lie the pectoralis minor muscles. They originate by slips from the second to fifth ribs and converge upward to a tendon that inserts on the coracoid process of the scapula. Supplied also by the medial and lateral pectoral nerves, these muscles are active in depressing and rotating the shoulders downward.

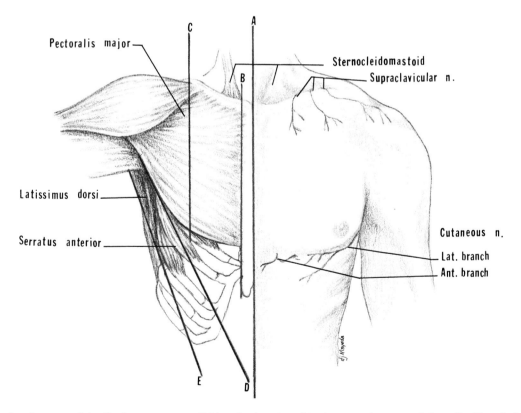

Fig. 1–3. Surface features and details of structures superficial to the thoracic wall in the pectoral region and the axilla. Musculoskeletal features are shown on the left. Surface features and cutaneous innervation are shown on the right. Cutaneous branches of the fifth intercostal space are illustrated as typical of other intercostal spaces not shown. Common lines of reference are shown. A = midsternal line; B = lateral sternal line; C = midclavicular line; D = anterior axillary fold; E = posterior axillary fold.

In thin, muscular subjects, the serratus anterior muscles can be visualized along the anterolateral aspects of the thoracic wall. They originate by slips from the upper eight ribs. They are closely applied to the thoracic wall as they pass upward and laterally to attach to the anterior surface and medial border of the scapula on either side. They hold the scapulae toward the thoracic wall and are important in adduction and elevation of the arms above the horizontal position during scapulohumeral movement. On each side, the serratus anterior is supplied by the long thoracic nerve, which passes downward in the midaxillary line on the external surface of the muscle.

In men, the nipple lies near the lower border of the pectoralis major muscles, just lateral to the midclavicular line, over the fourth intercostal space or fourth or fifth ribs. Nipple position is inconsistent in women owing to the variable size of the mammary gland, which lies generally over the second to sixth ribs. The "axillary tail" extends upward into the axilla along the lower border of the pectoralis major muscle.

Cutaneous innervation of the anterolateral thoracic wall is supplied by supraclavicular nerves and terminal filaments of thoracic spinal nerves. Skin above, overlying, and slightly below the clavicle is supplied by supraclavicular nerves, which arise as terminal filaments of spinal nerves C3 and C4. The remainder of the thoracic wall is supplied by anterior cutaneous and lateral cutaneous branches of thoracic spinal nerves.

The posterior aspect of the thorax is almost completely covered by superficial muscles of the back, but a few bony landmarks are either visible or palpable (Fig. 1–4). In the midline, the spinous process of the seventh cervical vertebra — vertebra prominens — stands out clearly. Below this process, the spine of the first thoracic vertebra may be equally visible. Spines of the remaining 11 thoracic vertebrae extend downward so that the tip of each overlies the body of the vertebra below. In the midthoracic levels, the vertebral spines may be sufficiently long to overlie the intervertebral disc below the subjacent vertebra. The medial border of each scapula lies lateral to the midline at the level of the second to seventh ribs. The spine of the scapula extends diagonally upward from the medial border at about the third thoracic vertebra to end in the acromion at the shoulder.

Surface contours of the back of the thorax are formed by muscles of the shoulder and scapular region; these muscles support and help move the upper extremity. Posterolateral margins of the neck and uppermost limits of the shoulder are marked by the trapezius muscles. Each of these arises from broad origins, including the superior nuchal line of the occipital bone, the ligamentum nuchae of the neck, the spine of the seventh cervical vertebra, and spines and supraspinous ligaments of all thoracic vertebrae. Fibers sweep downward, laterally, and upward toward the shoulder, where they insert on the spine and acromion of the scapula and on the lateral one third of the clavicle. In lower cervical

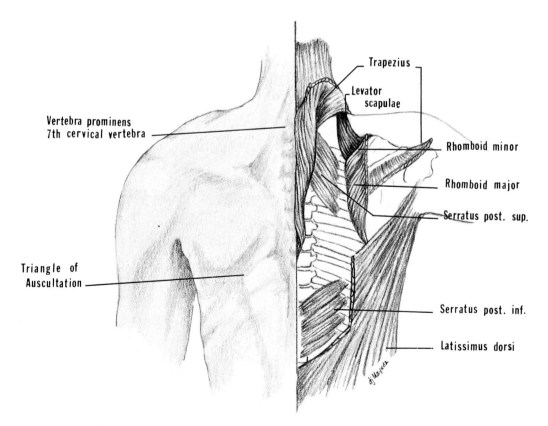

Fig. 1–4. Surface features and details of structures superficial to the posterior aspect of the thorax. The scapula has been displaced upward and laterally on the right side to permit a better view of muscles superficial to the thorax.

and upper thoracic levels, their aponeurotic origin is sufficiently devoid of muscle fibers to allow spines of thoracic vertebrae to be easily palpable. The trapezius muscles are supplied by spinal accessory nerves and by filaments from cervical spinal levels C3 and C4. They are powerful stabilizers of the scapulae and shoulders and can elevate, depress, or adduct the scapulae, thereby aiding in the entire spectrum of scapulohumeral movements.

Lower and lateral parts of the back of the thorax are covered by the latissimus dorsi muscles. These muscles arise by broad aponeurotic origins, from spines of lower thoracic vertebrae, the lumbodorsal fascia, and the iliac crests. Additional slips of muscle also arise from outer surfaces of the lower three or four ribs and blend with overlying components. Muscle fibers converge upward to insert by tendons into the intertubercular groove of the humerus on each side. In their upper thirds, these muscles converge with the teres major muscles to form the posterior folds of the axillae. The latissimus dorsi muscles are adductors, extensors, and medial rotators of the arm. Each is supplied by a thoracodorsal nerve from the posterior cord of the brachial plexus. Because of attachment to the ribs, the latissimus dorsi muscles can also be considered accessory muscles of respiration.

The lower border of the trapezius muscle overlies the upper border of the latissimus dorsi. Near the point of overlap, a triangle is formed by the lateral border of the trapezius, the upper border of the latissimus dorsi, and the medial border of the scapula. Save for lower fibers of the rhomboid muscles, this area is free of an intervening mass of muscle tissue. Because a stethoscope placed over this triangle can detect respiratory sounds relatively free of distortion, it is called the *triangle of auscultation.*

Deep to the trapezius and latissimus dorsi muscles lies a layer of muscles involved in scapular movements and, to a lesser degree, movements of the ribs. Those related to the scapula are the levator scapulae, rhomboid major, and rhomboid minor muscles. The thin levator scapulae extends from the transverse processes of the first three or four cervical vertebrae diagonally downward to attach at the superior angle of the scapula on each side. The rhomboid minor may be fused with the rhomboid major. It extends from spines of the seventh cervical vertebra and first thoracic vertebra to the medial border of the scapula near the base of its spine. The rhomboid major arises from the spines of the second to the fifth thoracic vertebrae and the supraspinous ligament between these vertebrae and is attached to the medial border of the scapula, usually below the spine of the scapula. The levator scapulae, rhomboid major, and rhomboid minor elevate, adduct, and retract the scapula. All are supplied by the dorsal scapular nerve, but the levator scapulae is supplied also by branches from C4 and C5.

The serratus posterior muscles are said to be inspiratory muscles and thus merit brief attention. The serratus posterior superior muscles arise by aponeuroses from the ligamentum nuchae and spinous processes of the seventh cervical vertebra and the first to third thoracic vertebrae, and are attached to the upper borders of the first three to the first five ribs. They are supplied by ventral rami of segmental spinal nerves — intercostal nerves — and are said to be active in elevation of the upper ribs. The serratus posterior inferior muscles take aponeurotic origins from spinous processes of the lower two thoracic and upper two lumbar vertebrae; they insert by muscular slips on the lower three or four ribs. They are also supplied by ventral rami of segmental spinal nerves and are presumably able to prevent upward displacement of their ribs during inspiration.

Innervation of skin over the back is provided by medial cutaneous branches of dorsal rami of C4, C5, C8, T1, and T2 and by medial and lateral cutaneous branches of T3 to T10. Considerable overlap and asymmetry of these nerves have been described by Johnston (1908).

ANATOMIC FEATURES

Firm structural support for the thorax is provided by the sternum, 10 pairs of costae — ribs and costal cartilages, 2 pairs of ribs without cartilage, and 12 thoracic vertebrae and their intervertebral discs. Collectively, these components surround a cavity that is reniform in cross section, related to the neck above by a narrow thoracic inlet and to the abdominal cavity below by a larger thoracic outlet. The inlet is surrounded by the manubrium of the sternum, the first ribs, and the first thoracic vertebra. Its anterior boundaries lie about 1 inch below the posterior limits. The inlet is roofed by bilateral thickened endothoracic fascia — Sibson's fascia or suprapleural membrane — and subjacent parietal pleura, which project upward into the base of the neck. Additional details of soft tissue relations of the thoracic inlet are considered at the end of this chapter in the section on *Surface Anatomy.* The outlet is formed by the xiphoid process, fused costal cartilages of ribs seven to ten, the anterior portions of the eleventh ribs, the shafts of the twelfth ribs, and the body of the twelfth thoracic vertebra. The anterior margin of the outlet is at the level of the tenth thoracic, the lateral limits at the second lumbar, and the posterior margin at the twelfth thoracic vertebra. The outlet is therefore higher at its anterior margin than at its posterior limit and reaches its lowest level in the lateral aspect near the midaxillary line. It is sealed off from the abdominal cavity by the diaphragm.

The Sternum and Its Joints

The sternum is an elongated, flat bone that lies in the anterior midline. It is 15 to 20 cm long and is formed from cartilaginous precursors that ossify separately to form three components: the manubrium, the body, and the xiphoid process (Fig. 1–5).

The manubrium is about 5 cm wide in its upper half and 2.5 to 3 cm wide in its lower half. Its upper border

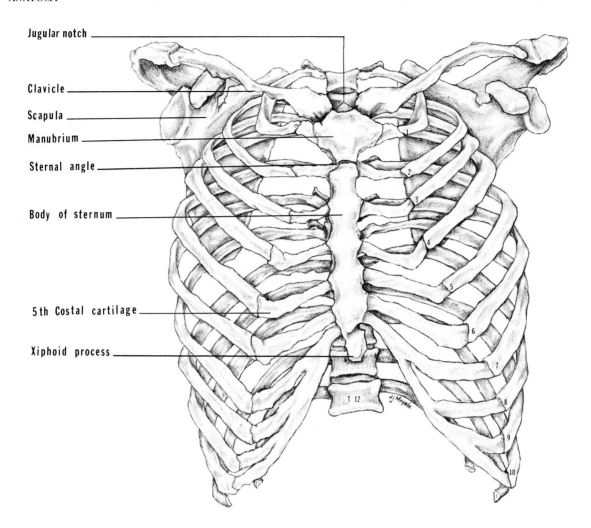

Jugular notch

Clavicle

Scapula

Manubrium

Sternal angle

Body of sternum

5th Costal cartilage

Xiphoid process

Fig. 1–5. Anterior view of the skeleton of the thorax and bones of the pectoral girdle. Bilateral asymmetry is evident in the body and xiphoid process of the sternum. The left subcostal arch is slightly higher than the right one.

is thickened and marked on either side by a notch for articulation with the clavicle. Centrally, an indentation is present, which together with the sternal ends of each clavicle forms the jugular — suprasternal — notch. The widest portion of the manubrium is marked by bilateral indentations — costal incisura — to accommodate articulation of the first costal cartilage. At the lower limits, each lateral margin of the bone is indented by a demifacet for articulation of the upper half of the second costal cartilage. The lower margin of the manubrium articulates with the body of the sternum.

The body or longest portion of the sternum is slightly more than twice the length of the manubrium. It is slanted at a steeper angle than the manubrium; hence its articulation with that bone forms an angle, called the sternal angle. The outer border of this angle is readily palpable and lies at the level of the fourth to fifth thoracic vertebrae or their intervening intervertebral disc. The joint is a synchondrosis: articular surfaces of each bone are covered with hyaline cartilage and are united by fibrocartilage. It is sufficiently flexible to allow movement of the body on the more stable manubrium during respiratory movements. Ossification of the joint may form a synostosis during adult years, thus limiting

flexibility, but, as noted by Trotter (1934), correlation is not observed between age and its incidence.

Lateral margins of the body exhibit segmental incisurae for articulation of costal cartilages two to seven. The incisura for the second costal cartilage is incomplete, for it represents only the lower half of the articulation surface that is completed by the demifacet on the lower margin of the manubrium. The body ends at about the level of the tenth to eleventh thoracic vertebrae, where it forms a cartilaginous joint with the xiphoid process.

The xiphoid is a cartilaginous process that is usually ossified by middle age. It is the shortest and thinnest part of the sternum and may occasionally be bifid or perforated. It extends downward for a variable distance to end in the sheath of the rectus abdominis muscle. Its posterior surface is even with that of the sternal body; its anterior surface is somewhat recessed. The xiphoid is flexible at the xiphisternal joint, but it moves with the sternum during respiratory movements. Supportive costoxiphoid ligaments, extending from its anterior surface to the front of the seventh costal cartilage, prevent its backward displacement by contractions of the diaphragm.

The midline of the sternum is almost completely subcutaneous and is therefore easily accessible for sternal puncture, sternal transfusion, or incision during thoracic surgery. Its lateral margins are covered by origins of the sternal components of the pectoralis major muscles.

Ribs and Their Joints

The size and shape of the thorax are largely determined by the ribs and costal cartilages. A rib and its associated cartilage are properly termed a costa. The costae form continuous arches that extend backward for a short distance in relation to the vertebrae, turn forward at the angle, and extend toward the sternum, with which all but two pairs of them articulate directly or indirectly. Developmentally, the costae arise as arched, cartilaginous struts extending serially and horizontally from their respective vertebral bodies to the sternum. As development proceeds, the vertebral ends of each costal pair migrate cephalad. This shift in position is more pronounced in costal pairs two to nine and, as a result, the head of each of these ribs becomes pressed against the body of the vertebra immediately above. At the end of the growth period, ribs two to nine articulate with both their own and the immediately suprajacent vertebrae. The tenth rib may migrate sufficiently to articulate with the ninth and tenth thoracic vertebrae or it may remain low enough to articulate only with the body of the tenth thoracic vertebra. The eleventh and twelfth ribs migrate only slightly and thus form joints only with their own vertebrae. The angle of costal elements of the thoracic wall relative to the vertebrae and the sternum is therefore the result of cephalic migration of vertebral extremities and relative retention of sternal extremities at their original levels.

Ossification is initiated at the bend or angle of the costae. It spreads posteriorly toward the vertebrae and anteriorly toward the sternum. By the time bone deposition stops, the short vertebral portion is completely ossified. Because that part of the costa from the angle forward is longer, its ossification is not complete by the time bone formation ceases. The ossified portion of each costa becomes the rib proper and the unossified part remains as costal cartilage.

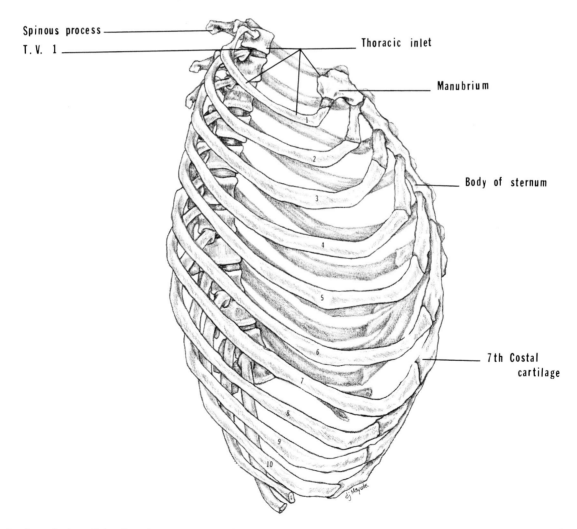

Fig. 1–6. Lateral view of the thoracic cage.

Relations of ribs and their costal cartilages to the sternum and to each other vary at different levels (Figs. 1–5, 1–6). The upper seven pairs of ribs articulate directly with the sternum by way of costal cartilages and are therefore called "true" or vertebrosternal ribs. In contrast, the lower five pairs are called "false" ribs, because they do not articulate with the sternum at all. Of the false ribs, three pairs — the eighth, ninth, and tenth — are called vertebrocostal because their associated cartilages articulate with immediately suprajacent cartilages. The remaining pairs — eleven and twelve — terminate in cartilaginous tips, ending in muscles of the abdominal wall. Because their only articulation is with the vertebrae, they are called vertebral ribs.

The costal cartilages change sequentially in length and direction. The first and second costal cartilages are short and follow a slightly downward course. The third and fourth gradually increase in length and are horizontal, or nearly so. The fifth to seventh cartilages extend downward from the tip of their ribs and then turn upward to meet the sternum. Because both ribs and cartilages of these costae are the longest and most flexible, they are maximally involved in the "bucket-handle" rib movement. The fused cartilages of ribs seven to ten course diagonally upward to the lower end of the sternum to form the infrasternal angle.

Ribs exhibit many similar features, but their form is variable at different levels. They increase in length from the first to the seventh and then gradually shorten to the twelfth. The most common features are characteristic of ribs three to nine, which are frequently called "typical ribs." From their vertebral to sternal ends, each of these ribs is formed by a head, a neck, and a shaft (Fig. 1–7). The head is enlarged and marked by two facets, separated by an interarticular crest. The upper facet articulates with a facet on the body of the suprajacent vertebra. A slightly larger inferior facet articulates with a facet on the body of the adjacent

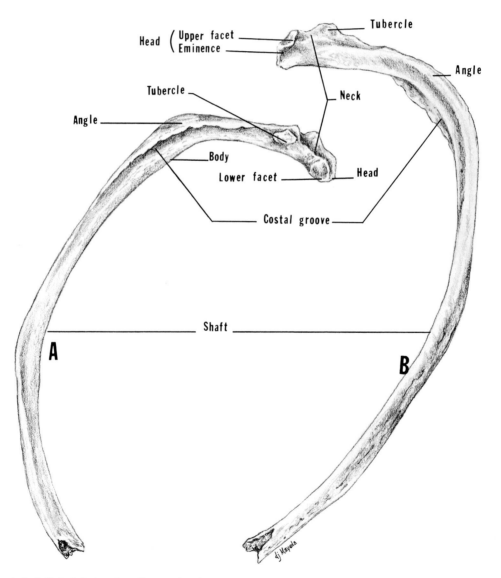

Fig. 1–7. A "typical rib." *A*, Inferior view; *B*, superior view.

vertebra whose number corresponds with that of the rib. The joint formed between costal facets, suprajacent, and adjacent vertebral bodies is termed a costovertebral joint.

The neck of each rib extends dorsolaterally for about 2.5 cm, and is marked by a crest on its upper border. The end of the neck and beginning of the shaft are marked by a tubercle. The tubercle bears a roughened elevation and a smooth articular surface. The elevation serves as an attachment for costotransverse ligaments. The articular surface meets a facet on the transverse process of the corresponding vertebra to form the costotransverse joint.

The shaft of the rib extends dorsolaterally for an additional 5 to 7.5 cm and then turns gradually forward and downward. The accentuated portion of this forward curvature is called the angle of the rib. The angle marks the lateral extent of the erector spinae muscles of the back. Throughout its course, the shaft is twisted slightly so that its superolateral border is rounded and convex. The lower margin of the inferomedial surface is scored by a costal groove for the intercostal vessels and nerves. This groove is most clearly defined on the inner aspect of the posterior half of each rib. The shaft terminates in a small indentation, which forms a hyaline-cartilaginous joint with its costal cartilage.

The less typical ribs differ in the following respects. The first rib is shorter than the rest and, beyond its neck, is wider and more curved. The head is small and bears only one facet for articulation with the body of the first thoracic vertebra. The upper and lower surfaces of the shaft are flat and its edges are sharp. Near the middle of the shaft, a rounded tubercle is present that serves as an attachment for the anterior scalene muscle. Behind the tubercle is a depression where the first rib is crossed by the subclavian artery. A smaller depression for the subclavian vein may sometimes be noted in front of the tubercle.

The second rib is nearly twice the length of the first and articulates with the bodies of the first and second thoracic vertebrae. Its shaft is curved but not twisted and is marked by a roughened tubercle for upper digitations of the serratus anterior muscle.

The eleventh and twelfth ribs are sequentially shorter than suprajacent ones and bear only one articular surface for their corresponding vertebrae. They exhibit poorly defined or completely absent necks, angles, and costal grooves. The length of the twelfth rib is of consequence in renal surgery. Although it is often shorter in a woman than in a man, Hughes (1949) has shown that longer ones, 11 to 14 cm, are more common than shorter ones, 1.5 to 6 cm. The posterior margin of parietal pleura normally crosses the twelfth rib at the lateral margin of the erector spinae muscles. If the twelfth rib is short, the surgeon may inadvertently palpate the lower border of the eleventh rib to determine the level for the initial incision. Such an incision risks entering the thoracic cavity instead of extraperitoneal tissue or renal fascia behind the kidneys.

Variations in rib structure may be of clinical significance. The first rib may be fused with the second at the scalene tubercle. This union is usually associated with other variations in the second rib, sternum, or associated thoracic vertebrae. The seventh cervical vertebra may bear a cartilaginous or ossified rib called a cervical rib. Such a rib may be short or it may be attached to the first costal cartilage or to the manubrium. Variations in the thoracic inlet or the presence of a cervical rib can produce compression of the subclavian artery and the brachial plexus resulting in compromise of neurovascular supply to the upper extremity. Occasionally, the sternal extremity of the third or fourth rib may be bifid, and the eighth rib may reach the sternum on one or both sides. A lumbar rib may be associated with the first lumbar vertebra.

The structure of the heads of ribs two through nine and the associated vertebrae shows that the costovertebral joints consist of two joint cavities, each composed of costal and vertebral facets. The cavities are separated by a ligament extending from the interarticular crest of the rib to the intervertebral disc. Articular surfaces are covered with fibrous cartilage; joint cavities are surrounded by a synovial articular capsule. The capsule is thickened by radiate ligaments that fan out from the head of the rib to adjacent vertebral bodies.

Costotransverse joints, between the articular tubercle and the transverse process of the rib, are also synovial. Articular surfaces are covered with hyaline cartilage and the joint is enclosed by a fibrous capsule. The capsule is reinforced by costotransverse ligaments, which connect the neck and tubercle of the rib to the transverse process of its own vertebra and to that immediately above. Motions involved in both the "bucket-handle" and "pump-handle" movements of breathing are permitted by the flexibility of both the costovertebral and costotransverse joints. Fixation of these joints adversely affects pulmonary function.

Intercostal Spaces

The frequency with which the spaces between ribs are used in surgical approaches to the thorax prescribes an understanding of their muscular, fascial, and neurovascular features (Figs. 1–8 to 1–11). Lying deep to the skin, superficial fascia — tela subcutanea — and muscles related to the thoracic girdle and upper extremity, each intercostal space is traversed by three layers of muscle and their related deep fascia. Both muscles and fascia are attached to periosteum at the upper and lower borders of the ribs. During thoracoplasty, an incision over the body of the rib and subsequent retraction of its periosteum during removal of the rib will not violate the contents of the intercostal spaces.

From the surgical approach, the first layer of tissue to be encountered within the intercostal space is composed of the external intercostal muscles. Their fibers extend diagonally downward and forward from the lower margin of each rib to the upper margin of the subjacent rib. Musculature of this layer is continuous

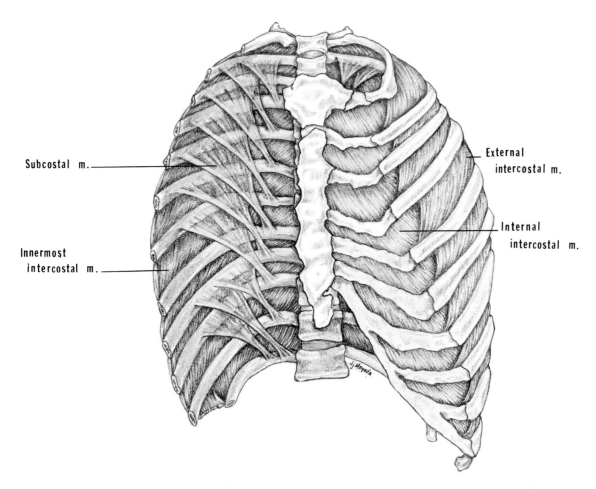

Subcostal m.

Innermost
intercostal m.

External
intercostal m.

Internal
intercostal m.

Fig. 1–8. Anterior view of the thoracic wall and muscles of the intercostal spaces. The left side of the thorax is intact. The anterior half of the right side has been removed to demonstrate the inner aspect of the posterolateral thoracic wall.

from a posterior position at the tubercle of the rib and posterior fibers of the costotransverse ligament (Figs. 1–9, 1–11, 1–12) to an anterior position at or near the costal cartilages. At this point, the investing fascia of the muscle continues further anteriorly to the sternum as the external — anterior — intercostal membrane (Figs. 1–12, 1–13). Intercostal muscles of the lower seven intercostal spaces interdigitate with the external oblique muscle of the abdominal wall. The next layer encountered consists of the internal intercostal muscles and their fascia. Muscle fibers extend downward and backward between costal cartilages in the anterior-medial part of the intercostal space and between the ribs proper further laterally and posteriorly in the intercostal space. The reverse direction of these muscle fibers from those of the external intercostal muscle lends a cross-diagonal supportive force. Musculature of this layer extends from the sternum (Figs. 1–12, 1–13) as far posteriad as the angle of the ribs (Figs. 1–11, 1–12). At this point, their investing fasciae form the internal-posterior-intercostal membrane, which attaches to the tubercle of each rib and the adjacent vertebra (Fig. 1–11). Neurovascular components of the intercostal spaces are encountered immediately deep to these two

layers. From above downward, the intercostal vein, artery, and nerve enter the posterior part of the intercostal space (see Figs. 1–11, 1–12). In this region, they lie within the endothoracic fascia deep to the internal intercostal membrane and just superficial to parietal pleura (see Fig. 1–12). They remain in this position for a distance of 4 to 6 cm whereupon they gain the space between the internal and innermost intercostal muscles along the costal groove near the angle of the ribs (see Figs. 1–7, 1–10 to 1–12). The neurovascular component, therefore, lies in the upper limits of the intercostal space, in contrast to the collateral branches, which lie in the lower limits. The origin and distribution of these neurovascular elements are considered in detail later. Their position with respect to the ribs is important during incision of the intercostal space. Because major intercostal vessels and nerves lie in close relation to the lower border of each rib, incisions near this level are to be avoided. A preferable site is along the upper margin of each rib. Although accessory nerves and vessels may be sectioned at this level, loss of function or sensitivity is negligible. It is equally important, however, to understand that the overlap of adjacent nerves is so great that paralysis and complete

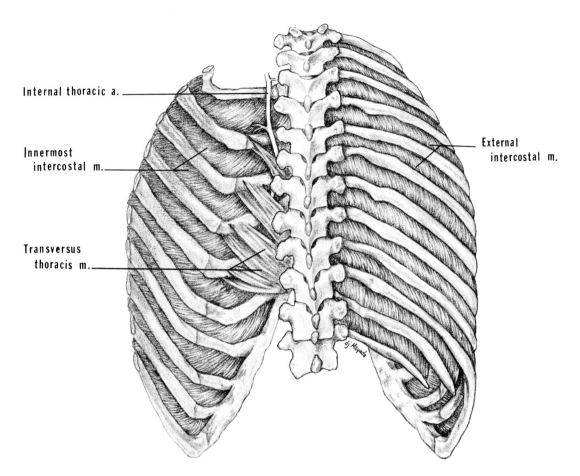

Internal thoracic a.

Innermost intercostal m.

Transversus thoracis m.

External intercostal m.

Fig. 1–9. Posterior view of the thoracic wall and muscles of the intercostal spaces. The right side of the thorax is intact. The posterior half of the left side has been removed to show the inner aspect of the anterior thoracic wall.

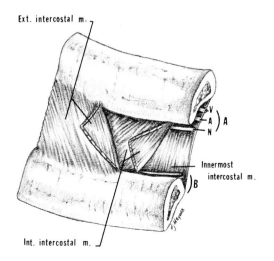

Ext. intercostal m.

V
A
N

A

Innermost intercostal m.

B

Int. intercostal m.

Figure 1–10. Relations of structures within an intercostal space. Intercostal vessels and nerves are shown at A. Collateral vessels are shown at B. V = vein, A = artery, N = nerve.

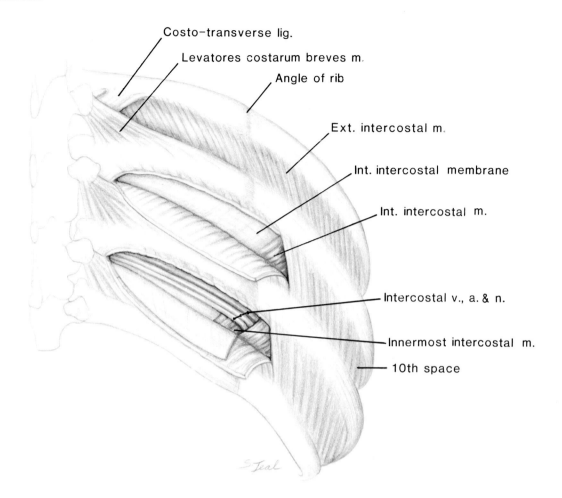

Costo-transverse lig.

Levatores costarum breves m.

Angle of rib

Ext. intercostal m.

Int. intercostal membrane

Int. intercostal m.

Intercostal v., a. & n.

Innermost intercostal m.

10th space

Fig. 1–11. Exposure of the posterior part of intercostal spaces 8, 9, and 10. Note that the intercostal vein, artery and nerve lie between the internal intercostal muscle and the innermost intercostal muscle layers. From the intervertebral foramen to the angle of the rib, the intercostal vessels and nerves are covered by the internal intercostal membrane.

anesthesia are seldom produced within one intercostal space unless its nerve, the one above, and the one below are all severed.

The next layer of tissue encountered is less well defined. It consists of the innermost intercostal, subcostal, and transversus thoracis muscles and their fasciae. The innermost intercostals are best developed in the middle portion of the intercostal space (see Figs. 1–9 to 1–12) and may be absent completely in the upper regions of the thoracic wall. They extend between adjacent ribs in the same direction as the internal intercostal muscles. Davies and associates (1932) considered them inner laminae of the internal intercostal muscles. The subcostal muscles extend as a variable number of slips from the lower margin of the angle of the ribs, diagonally across more than one intercostal space to the upper margin of the second or third rib below. The transversus thoracis is a thin layer of muscle on the inner aspect of the anterior thoracic wall. Aponeurotic slips of this muscle extend diagonally upward from the body and xiphoid process of the sternum to costal cartilages. The lowermost fibers of the transversus thoracis are almost horizontal and are con-

tinuous with the transversus abdominis muscle of the abdominal wall.

Deep to the third layer of muscles is the endothoracic fascia. It consists of variable amounts of areolar connective tissue, affording a natural cleavage plane for separation of the subjacent pleura from the thoracic wall.

The arterial supply of the intercostal spaces consists of posterior and anterior intercostal arteries. The posterior intercostal arteries of the first and second intercostal spaces arise from the highest intercostal arteries, which are branches of the subclavian artery; those of the remaining nine intercostal spaces are branches of the thoracic aorta. These arteries supply most of their respective intercostal spaces except the anteriormost limits. Each gives rise to a posterior branch supplying the spinal cord and deep muscles and skin of the back, an anterior branch running between the vein and nerve in the costal groove, and a collateral branch arising near the angle of the rib and descending to the upper border of the rib below. In the midaxillary line, each anterior branch gives rise to a lateral cutaneous branch, which perforates the intercostal space to supply overlying skin. The posterior intercostal artery coursing below the

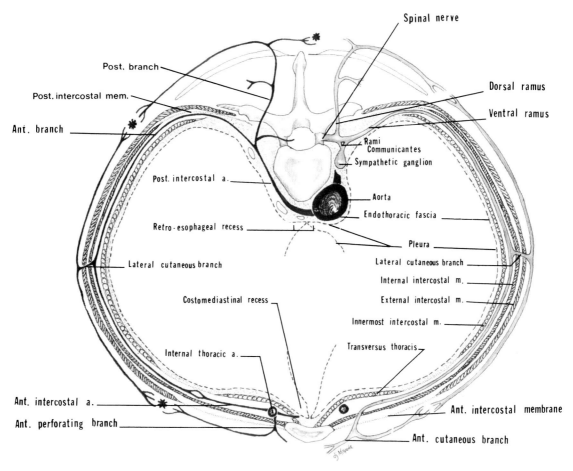

Fig. 1–12. Summary scheme of structures within an intercostal space. Arteries are shown on the left, nerves on the right.

twelfth rib is called the subcostal artery. It follows a course similar to those above but has no collateral branches.

The anterior intercostal arteries arise as segmental branches of the internal thoracic arteries in the first five or six intercostal spaces and as branches of the musculophrenic arteries in the lower intercostal spaces. Two such arteries are given off in each intercostal space, one passing toward the upper rib and one toward the lower. They continue laterally to anastomose with terminal branches of anterior and collateral branches of the posterior intercostal arteries.

The intercostal spaces are drained by eleven pairs of posterior intercostal veins and one pair of subcostal veins. These vessels follow the course of the posterior intercostal arteries and for the most part are tributary to the azygos or hemiazygos venous system. They lie above the nerve and artery throughout their course. Major blood flow is directed posteriorly by valves, but terminal vessels may also be tributary to the internal thoracic veins by way of small anterior intercostal veins. Posterior intercostal veins of the first intercostal space may be tributary to the brachiocephalic, vertebral, or superior intercostal veins. The second, third, and fourth posterior intercostal veins drain into the superior in-

tercostal vein on each side; these in turn drain into the brachiocephalic vein on the left and into the azygos vein on the right. Right and left subcostal veins join the ascending lumbar veins on their respective sides of the thorax and ascend as the azygos and hemiazygos veins, respectively.

Lymphatic drainage of the anterior limits of the upper four or five intercostal spaces enters the sternal — internal thoracic — nodes, which lie along the internal thoracic arteries. Their efferent vessels are tributary to a single vessel that joins the bronchomediastinal trunk. These nodes may commonly be invaded by metastases from breast carcinoma. Posterolateral portions of the intercostal spaces are drained by lymphatics that are tributary to one or two nodes near the vertebral ends of each intercostal space. Such nodes also receive lymphatic tributaries from the pleura. Nodes of upper intercostal spaces drain into the thoracic duct; those of the lower spaces are tributary to the cisterna chyli.

The thoracic wall is innervated segmentally by twelve pairs of thoracic spinal nerves. Upper thoracic spinal nerves also supply innervation to the axilla and upper extremity. Lower thoracic spinal nerves also supply portions of the abdominal wall and are called thoracoabdominal nerves. The midthoracic spinal nerves —

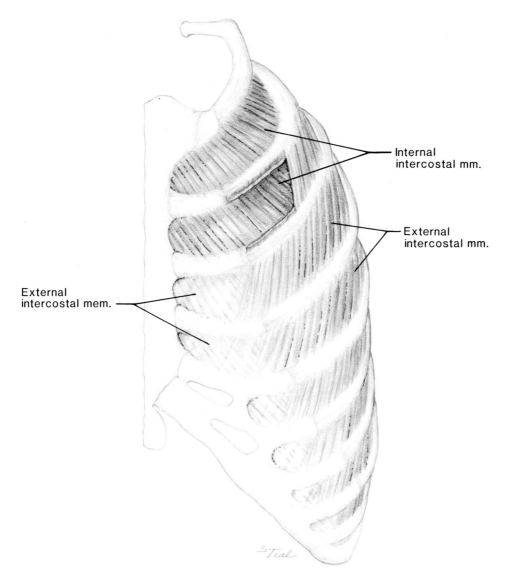

Internal
intercostal mm.

External
intercostal mm.

External
intercostal mem.

Fig. 1–13. Anterior view of the left half of the thorax. Note the opposing diagonal course of the external intercostal muscle fibers vs. those of the internal intercostal muscle fibers. The external — anterior — intercostal membrane extends from the costochondral junction to the sternum in the intercostal spaces.

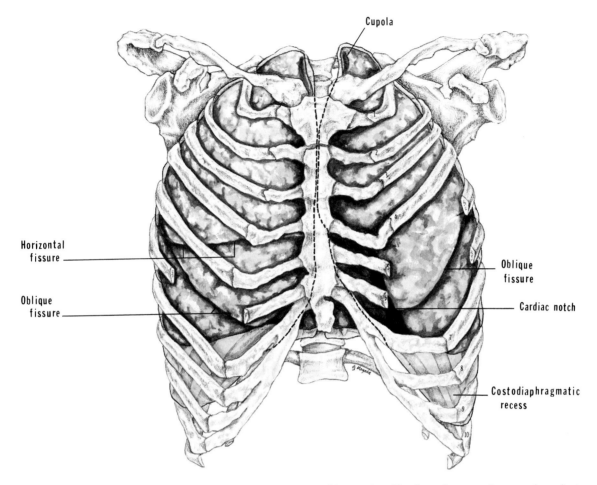

Cupola

Horizontal fissure

Oblique fissure

Oblique fissure

Cardiac notch

Costodiaphragmatic recess

Fig. 1–14. Anterior view of the thorax showing surface relations of pleura and lungs. Pleural borders subjacent to bone are shown by interrupted lines.

T4 to T6 — exhibit the most common pattern and are considered as typical nerves to the thoracic wall. Each spinal nerve is formed from a dorsal and a ventral root. The dorsal root contains sensory neurons that are distributed to posterior gray columns of the spinal cord. The ventral root contains somatic motor neurons originating in anterior gray columns of the spinal cord. Near the intervertebral foramen, the dorsal and ventral roots unite to form a mixed spinal nerve. Each spinal nerve gives rise to a small meningeal nerve and then passes out of the intervertebral foramen, to branch into a dorsal and ventral ramus (see Fig. 1–12).

The dorsal ramus of the thoracic spinal nerve passes backward to supply paravertebral back muscles and skin of the back. It forms medial and lateral cutaneous branches. Medial branches supply periosteum, ligaments, and joints of the vertebra, as well as deep muscles of the back before terminating in cutaneous filaments. Lateral branches supply the small levator costae muscles and deep back muscles, and follow a long descending course before becoming cutaneous. Extensive terminal overlap and anastomoses occur among medial and lateral cutaneous branches of dorsal rami from different spinal levels. Consequently, cutaneous pain is difficult to localize in this region.

Just lateral to the intervertebral foramen, the ventral ramus of the thoracic nerve establishes communications with the sympathetic chain by two branches or rami communicantes (see Fig. 1–12). The white ramus contains preganglionic sympathetic fibers, and the gray ramus contains postganglionic sympathetic fibers. Beyond this point, the ramus continues as the intercostal nerve and is responsible for segmental distribution to skin, muscle, and serous membranes of the thoracic wall. Each intercostal nerve passes backward below the rib in the vicinity of costotransverse ligaments and then gains the costal groove. It continues its course in the plane between the innermost intercostal and internal intercostal muscles. Near the angle of the rib, a collateral branch is given off. This branch passes laterally and then forward in the lower part of the intercostal space, terminating as a lower anterior cutaneous nerve.

Near the midaxillary line, a lateral cutaneous branch is given off. It pierces the intercostal muscles, passes through the serratus anterior muscles, and then forms anterior and posterior cutaneous branches.

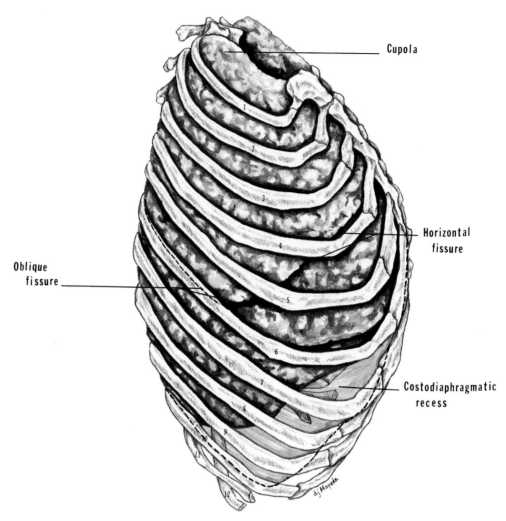

Fig. 1–15. Lateral view of the thorax showing surface relations of pleura and lungs.

Just lateral to the sternal margin, the intercostal nerve lies between transversus thoracis and internal intercostal muscles. At this point, it pierces overlying internal and external intercostal muscles, becomes subcutaneous, and forms anterior and median cutaneous branches.

Each segment of the thoracic wall is thus supplied circumferentially from behind forward by branches of the dorsal ramus and collateral, lateral, and anterior branches of the ventral ramus. The ventral rami — intercostal nerves — supply the intercostal, subcostal, serratus posterior superior, and tranversus thoracis muscles and the skin overlying the intercostal spaces. Although the pattern of innervation for each intercostal space is basically similar, considerable intersegmental overlap is characteristic. For that reason, complete paralysis or anesthesia in only one intercostal space does not occur unless the nerve of that space, as well as those of the intercostal spaces above and below, is sectioned.

SURFACE ANATOMY

Knowledge of the surface relations of lobes and fissures of the lungs is important in percussion, auscultation, and radiographic evaluation of the pulmonary field. Although the lungs are in constant motion during respiration, the surface relations observed by Brock (1954) are essentially as described in Chapter 6. Knowledge of the topography of the various fissures of the lung is helpful in localizing abnormal pulmonary sounds as well as in localizing abnormal densities in radiographs of the chest (Figs. 1–14, 1–15).

For surgical purposes, the lungs and pleura may be considered coextensive, with their respective costal, mediastinal, and diaphragmatic surfaces separated only by a film of serous fluid. In quiet respiration, those parts of the lung within the costomediastinal and costodiaphragmatic recesses are insufficiently inflated to be identified by percussion. Percussible limits of the lower border of the lung normally lie at slightly higher levels than the lower limits of the pleura. The frequency with which indwelling lines or catheters are surgically inserted into the subclavian veins and the consequence of damaging nearby pleura or neurovascular structures require special knowledge of soft tissue relations at the thoracic inlet (Figs. 1–16, 1–17). On both sides of the thorax, the subclavian vein lies deep to the clavicle and crosses the first rib anterior to the attachment of the

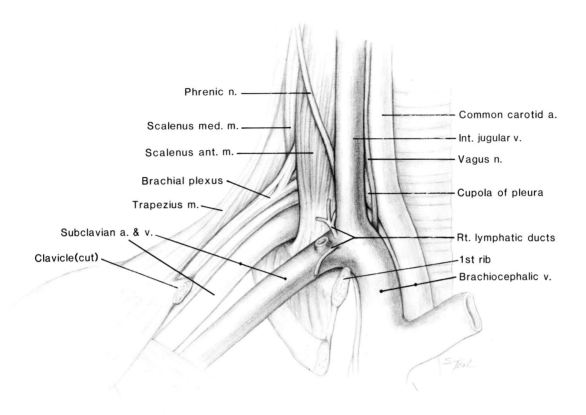

Phrenic n.
Scalenus med. m.
Scalenus ant. m.
Brachial plexus
Trapezius m.
Subclavian a. & v.
Clavicle(cut)

Common carotid a.
Int. jugular v.
Vagus n.
Cupola of pleura
Rt. lymphatic ducts
1st rib
Brachiocephalic v.

Fig. 1–16. Relations of the pleural cupola on the right side. Note the position of the cupola near the inferior and medial border of the scalenus anterior muscle, where it is crossed by the phrenic and vagus nerves. The subclavian artery passes anterior to the insertion of the scalenus anterior muscle on the first rib. The subclavian artery and the brachial plexus lie posterior and lateral to the muscle.

Fig. 1–17. Relations of the pleural cupola on the left side. Note the position of the cupola near the inferior and medial border of the scalenus anterior muscle. The cupola is crossed by the phrenic and vagus nerves. The vagus nerve lies between the internal jugular vein and the common carotid artery, but it is not visible in this dissection.

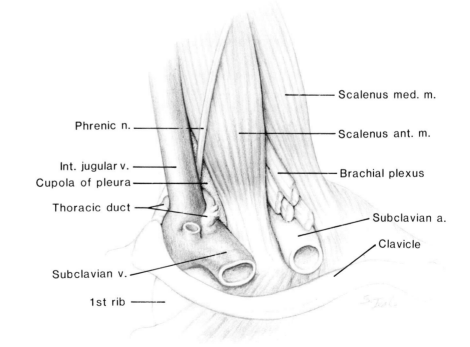

Phrenic n.
Int. jugular v.
Cupola of pleura
Thoracic duct
Subclavian v.
1st rib

Scalenus med. m.
Scalenus ant. m.
Brachial plexus
Subclavian a.
Clavicle

serratus anterior muscle on the scalene tubercle of the first rib. The second part of the subclavian artery passes posterior to the scalenus anterior muscle and its third part lies lateral to the attachment of muscle on the first rib. Likewise, components of the brachial plexus pass behind and then lateral to the scalenus anterior muscle. More importantly, in relation to pulmonary function, the cupola of the pleura is consistently related to the inferior and medial border of the scalenus anterior muscle. In this position, the cupola reaches its most superficial position and therefore is susceptible to damage during invasive surgical procedures. This portion of the cupola is also crossed superficially by the phrenic nerve and the vagus nerve. On the right side, the vagus nerve descends within the carotid fascia between the internal jugular vein and the common carotid artery and subsequently crosses the first part of the subclavian artery to enter the thorax between the common carotid and subclavian arteries. On the left side, the vagus nerve lies on the cupola of the pleura between the internal jugular vein and the common carotid artery to enter the thorax between the common carotid and subclavian arteries.

REFERENCES

Agostini E, Torri G: Diaphragm contraction as a limiting factor to maximum expiration. J Appl Physiol 17:427, 1962.

Brock RC: The Anatomy of the Bronchial Tree: With Special Reference to the Surgery of Lung Abscess. 2nd Ed. London: Oxford University Press, 1954.

Campbell ETM: The role of the scalene and sternomastoid muscles in breathing in normal subjects. An electromyographic study. J Anat 89:378, 1955.

Cherniack RM, Cherniack L: Respiration in Health and Disease. Philadelphia: WB Saunders, 1961.

Davies F, Gladstone RJ, Stibbe EP: Anatomy of intercostal nerves. J Anat 66:323, 1932.

Hughes FA: Resection of twelfth rib in surgical approach to renal fossa. J Urol 61:159, 1949.

Johnston HM: The cutaneous branches of the posterior primary divisions of the spinal nerves and their distribution in the skin. J Anat Physiol 43:80, 1908.

Jones DS, Beargie RT, Pauly TE: Electromyographic study of some muscles of costal respiration in man. Anat Rec 117:17, 1953.

Taylor A: The contribution of the intercostal muscles to the effort of respiration in man. J Physiol (Lond:) 151:390, 1960.

Trotter M: Synostosis between manubrium and body of sternum in Whites and Negroes. Am J Phys Anthropol 18:439, 1934.

READING REFERENCES

Gardner E et al: Anatomy. 3rd Ed. Philadelphia: WB Saunders, 1969.

Basmajian JV: Grant's Method of Anatomy. 10th Ed. Baltimore: Williams & Wilkins, 1980.

Healy JE, Seybold WD: A Synopsis of Clinical Anatomy. Philadelphia: WB Saunders, 1969.

Hollinshead WH, Rosse C: Textbook of Anatomy. 4th Ed. Philadelphia: JB Lippincott, 1985.

Lachman E: Comparison of posterior boundaries of lungs and pleura as demonstrated on cadaver and on roentgenogram of the living. Anat Rec 83:521, 1942.

Mainland D, Gordon ET: Position of organs determined from thoracic radiographs of young adult males, with study of cardiac apex beat. Am J Anat 68:457, 1941.

Woodbourne RT: Essentials of Human Anatomy. 7th Ed. New York: Oxford University Press, 1983.

CHAPTER 2

ANATOMY OF THE PLEURA

Thomas W. Shields

EMBRYOLOGY

The paired pleural cavities are derivatives of the intraembryonic portion of the primitive coelom. The primitive coelom arises by splitting of the lateral mesoderm on either side of the embryo into splanchnic and somatic layers. These paired cavities are subsequently separated by three partitions into three subdivisions: the pericardial cavity, the pleural cavities, and the peritoneal cavity. The partitions are the unpaired septum transversum, the paired pleuropericardial folds, and the paired pleuroperitoneal folds. The right and left coelomic chambers dorsal to the septum transversum for a period remain relatively unexpanded as the so-called pleural canals; these lie on either side of the mediastinal region. The development of the pleuroperitoneal folds complete the separation of the pleural canals from the other two body cavities: the pericardial cavity and the peritoneal cavity. At the fourth week of development, the laryngotracheal outgrowth from the floor of the pharynx is noted, and in the fifth week, the two lung buds begin to enlarge into the respective pleural canals. According to Patten (1968), the pleural spaces open up in advance of lung growth and the lungs move — bulge — into the space prepared to receive them. With growth, the lungs and the pleuropericardial membranes come to lie on either side of the heart and the pleuroperitoneal folds become part of the diaphragm. In this process of expansion of the lungs into the pleural canals, the splanchnic mesoderm is pushed out as a covering over the mesenchyma-packed bronchial trees (Fig. 2–1). The splanchnic mesoderm becomes thinned to form the mesothelial layer of the pleura, and the mesenchymal tissue immediately beneath this layer becomes the connective tissue of the pleura. The splanchnic mesoderm is thus the origin of the visceral pleura and the somatic mesoderm is the origin of most of the parietal pleura.

HISTOLOGY

The two pleural layers have similar histologic structures. The surface is composed of a single mesothelial layer resting on an elastic basal membrane. The mesothelial cells, according to Wang (1982, 1985), vary in thickness from less than 1 to over 4 μm and from 16.4 ± 6.8 to 41.9 ± to 9.5 μm in diameter. Their shape may vary according to their location in the pleural membrane.

Ultrastructurally, the mesothelial cells demonstrate microvilli. Tight apical junctions are present, but gap junctions, desmosomes, or half desmosomes occur infrequently on the basal part of the cell membrane.

Immunohistochemically, the mesothelial cells, as reported by Dervan (1986) and Bolen (1986) and their associates, express both low- and high-molecular weight cytokeratin. The normal mesothelial cells are negative for reaction to vimentin, epithelial membrane antigen — EMA, carcino embryonic antigen — CEA, and Factor VIII-related antigen.

Beneath the basal membrane of the mesothelial layer is a collection of loose connective tissue. This submesothelial layer contains collagen tissue, elastic fibers, small blood vessels, lymphatic networks, and nerve fibers. The mesenchymal cells in this layer, according to Keating (1978), Said (1984), and England (1989) and their co-workers, have the characteristics of fibroblasts. The cells are negative for cytokeratin, CEA, and Factor VIII-related antigen.

The thickness of the visceral and parietal pleural layers are approximately the same, on the average of 30 to 40 μm according to Staub and colleagues (1985). Large dehiscences, or stomata, have been documented in the parietal pleura. Chretien and Huchon (1990) state that these stomata, ranging from 2 to more than 6 μm in diameter, connect the pleural cavity with the subpleural lymphatic network and permit egress of material into the lymphatics from the pleural space. Wang (1985)

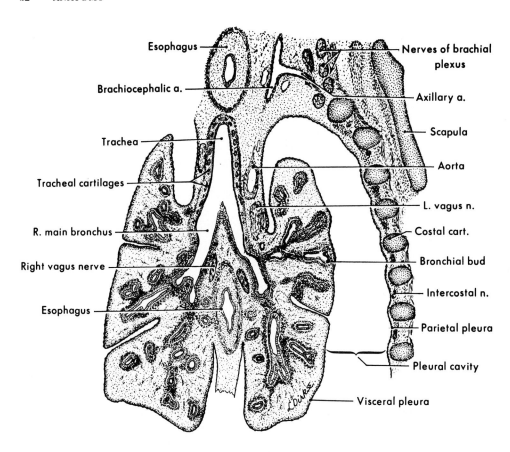

Esophagus

Brachiocephalic a.

Trachea

Tracheal cartilages

R. main bronchus

Right vagus nerve

Esophagus

Nerves of brachial plexus

Axillary a.

Scapula

Aorta

L. vagus n.

Costal cart.

Bronchial bud

Intercostal n.

Parietal pleura

Pleural cavity

Visceral pleura

Fig. 2–1. Frontal section through the developing lungs in an 8-week-old embryo. Projection drawing (×25) from University of Michigan Collection, EH 352, CR 25 mm. *From* Patten BM: Human Embryology. 3rd Ed. New York: McGraw-Hill Book, 1968.

has described focal accumulations of macrophages, along with pluripotential mesenchymal, lymphoid, and plasma cells — called Kampmeier's foci — in the caudal portions of the mediastinal pleura that may be functionally related to the aforementioned stomata.

GROSS ANATOMIC FEATURES

The visceral pleura is closely applied to the lung surfaces from the hila outward. It lines the major and minor fissures to the extent that each is developed; the minor fissure on the right may be incomplete to absent in 50% of humans. It also may delineate the various accessory fissures (see Chapter 6) when present. The pulmonary ligament, which extends caudad from each hilus to near the diaphragm, consists of two apposed layers of visceral — splanchnic — pleura and becomes continuous with the parietal pleura.

The visceral pleura is adherent to the lung parenchyma. A naturally occurring cleavage plane is absent. When the visceral pleura is stripped from the lung parenchyma, a raw surface with innumerable air leaks, and at times small bleeding vessels, is left behind.

The parietal pleura lines the chest wall — the costal pleura — the mediastinum, and the diaphragm and forms the cupula or plural dome at the thoracic inlet bilaterally. The mediastinal pleura extends from the sternum ventrally to the thoracic spine dorsally and

covers the mediastinal structures and the pericardium. The diaphragmatic pleura adheres tightly to the diaphragmatic tissues, and a cleavage plane between the two is basically nonexistent. Similarly, the mediastinal pleura is densely adherent to the pericardium. In contrast, the remainder of the mediastinal pleura, the pleura of the cupula, and the costal pleura can be readily dissected from the underlying tissues. The plane of cleavage from the chest wall is between the loose connective tissue layer and the endothoracic fascia attached to the underlying osseous, muscular, and vascular structures of the chest wall.

Topographically, the borders of the pleura are formed by continuity of the outer surface of costal, mediastinal, and diaphragmatic pleurae. A sharp anterior border of the pleura is defined along the line at which costal and mediastinal pleurae meet, subjacent to the sternum. The inferior border of the pleura is formed by the line of union between costal and diaphragmatic pleurae. The posterior border is outlined by the meeting of costal pleura with the posterior margin of mediastinal pleura near the thoracic vertebrae. The anterior reflection of mediastinal and costal pleurae forms a thin, sharp costomediastinal recess within the pleural sac. A similar recess, the costodiaphragmatic recess, form at the base of the pleural sac by reflections of costal and diaphragmatic pleurae, may be related to overlying structures of the thoracic cage. The topographic localization of the anterior, inferior, and posterior borders of the pleura vary somewhat. The anterior pleural borders of the pulmonary cupulae are separated by visceral structures at the base of the neck. As they descend medially behind the sternum, they appose one another at the sternal angle and form the anterior mediastinal line seen on the chest radiograph in Figure 2–2. The right anterior border continues downward close to the mid-

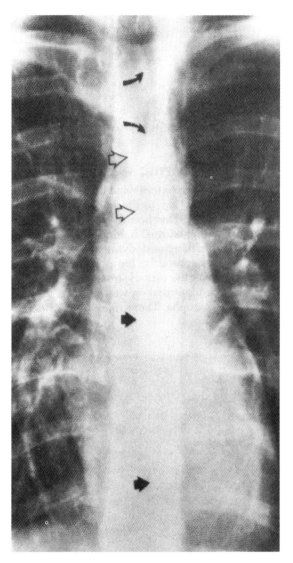

Fig. 2–2. Chest radiograph (PA) reveals the azygoesophageal recess, superior esophageal recess, and anterior mediastinal line. A slightly curved shadow convex to the right (solid arrows) projected in front of the thoracic spine from below the right main bronchus and extending down to just above the diaphragm is the azygoesophageal recess. Superiorly, a second curved linear shadow convex to the left (curved arrows) projected over the tracheal air column represents the superior esophagopleural recess. Between the two is a third linear shadow projected over the lower half of the tracheal air column (open arrows) representing the anterior mediastinal line. *From* Fraser RG, Pare JAP: Diagnosis of Diseases of the Chest. 2nd Ed. Philadelphia: WB Saunders, 1983.

line. At the lower limits of the body of the sternum, it diverges laterally along the sixth or seventh costal cartilage to become the inferior pleural border. The left anterior pleural border may follow a similar course, but more commonly, it diverges laterally at the fourth costal cartilage, lies at the lateral sternal margin at the fifth, courses still further laterally at the sixth cartilage, and then diverges laterally with increasing severity at the seventh costal cartilage. The lateral displacement of the left anterior pleural border between the fourth and sixth costal cartilages forms the cardiac notch — the cardiac incisura. Radiographically, a lateral view demonstrates this area as a soft tissue shadow bounded by an interface between lung and the heart and adjacent fat. The interface has been termed the retrosternal line by Whalen and associates (1973).

The inferior borders of both pleural sacs diverge laterally along the seventh costal cartilage and then cross ribs eight, nine, and ten. They reach their lowest level at about the middle of the eleventh rib in the midaxillary line. From this point, they follow an almost horizontal course, cutting across the twelfth rib to meet the posterior pleural border at the twelfth thoracic vertebra. If the twelfth rib is short, the posterior pleural border may lie below it. In some individuals, as noted by Melnikoff (1923), the inferior border may be sufficiently high so that it does not cross the twelfth rib at all, instead, meeting the posterior borders of the pleura at the eleventh thoracic vertebra.

The posterior pleural borders ascend alongside or in front of the bodies of thoracic vertebrae until they diverge superiorly near the pulmonary cupulae. They are rounded, in contrast to either anterior or inferior borders. Right and left posterior borders may be in close apposition in front of the vertebral bodies. Where this situation occurs, thin retroesophageal recesses are formed behind the esophagus and in front of the aorta and the hemiazygos and azygos veins.

As a result of these recesses, lines, usually two, are visible within the mediastinal contour on a well-exposed frontal chest radiograph. These lines have been termed the azygoesophageal recess and the superior esophageal recess (see Fig. 2–2). The left paraspinal line, which also is frequently seen, is related to the reflection of the parietal pleura from the vertebral bodies over the descending aorta (Fig. 2–3). Fraser and colleagues (1989) discuss in detail the explanations for these lines as seen on radiographs of the chest.

BLOOD SUPPLY

The visceral pleura was believed to be supplied by both the bronchial and pulmonary arterial systems. The investigations of Albertine and associates (1982) in sheep, however, revealed that the visceral pleural blood supply was entirely from the bronchial arterial system. There is no reason to believe it is otherwise in the human. Venous drainage is by way of the pulmonary veins. The blood supply to the parietal pleura is from

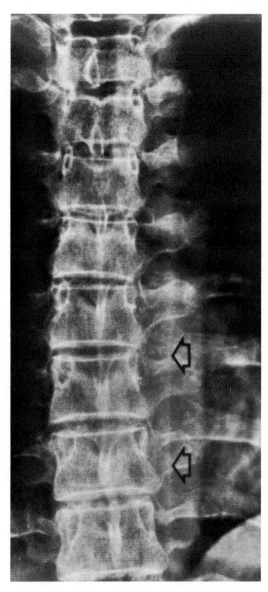

Fig. 2–3. Radiograph of the mediastinum (AP, with patient supine) reveals the longitudinal shadow (arrows) extending from the arch of the aorta to the diaphragm representing the paraspinal line. *From* Fraser RG, Pare JAP: Diagnosis of Diseases of the Chest. 2nd Ed. Philadelphia: WB Saunders, 1983.

the various systemic arterial vessels supplying the chest wall, diaphragm, and mediastinum, as well as from vessels to the cupula from the subclavian arteries in the neck. Venous drainage is to the corresponding veins and, at times, directly into the superior vena cava.

Lymphatic Drainage

The subpleural space of the visceral pleura has a large network of lymphatic channels, but only rarely is a subpleural lymph node identified. Trapnell (1964) reported the incidence of intrapulmonary lymph nodes to be 18%, but no nodes were found in a subpleural location. Greenberg (1961), however, described a lymph node in this location that was removed surgically because it had been identified radiographically as a coin lesion.

The lymphatic drainage of the visceral pleura is primarily to the deep pulmonary plexus located in the interlobar and peribronchial spaces. Riquet and associates (1989) however, described direct subpleural lymphatic connections to the mediastinal nodes in approximately 22 to 25% of lung segments studied. These subpleural connections were present more often in the upper lobes than in the lower lobes.

The lymphatic drainage of the parietal pleura is into the parietal pleural lymphatic channels. The aforementioned stomata and Kampmeier's foci play important roles in this process. The lymphatic networks of the chest wall drain into the internal mammary chain anteriorly and the intercostal chain posteriorly. The drainage of the diaphragmatic pleura is to the retrosternal and mediastinal lymph nodes as well as to the celiac lymph nodes in the abdomen.

NERVE SUPPLY

The parietal pleura is innervated by both somatic and sympathetic and parasympathetic fibers via the intercostal nerves. The diaphragmatic pleura is supplied by the phrenic nerves. The visceral pleura is devoid of somatic innervation.

REFERENCES

Albertine KH, et al: Structure, blood supply and lymphatic vessels of the sheep's visceral pleura. Am J Anat 165:277, 1982.

Bolen JW, Hammer SP, McNutt MA: Reactive and neoplastic serosal tissue. A light microscopic, ultrastructural, and immunocytochemical study. Am J Surg Pathol 10:34, 1986.

Chretien J, Huchon GJ: New contributions to the understanding of pleural space structure and junction. *In* Deslauriers J, Lacquet LK (eds): Thoracic Surgery: Surgical Management of Pleural Diseases. International Trends in General Thoracic Surgery. Vol. 6. St. Louis: C.V. Mosby, 1990.

Dervan PA, Tobin B, O'Connor M: Solitary (localized) fibrous mesothelioma: Evidence against mesothelial cell origin. Histopathology 10:867, 1986.

England DM, Hochholzer L, McCarthy MJ: Localized benign and malignant fibrous tumors of the pleura. A clinicopathologic review of 223 cases. Am J Surg Pathol 13:640, 1989.

Fraser RG, et al: Diagnosis of Diseases of the Chest. 3rd Ed. Philadelphia: WB Saunders, 1989.

Greenberg HB: Benign subpleural lymph node appearing as a pulmonary "coin" lesion. Radiology 77:97, 1961.

Keating S, et al: Solitary fibrous tumor of the pleura: An ultrastructural and immunohistochemical study. Thorax 42:976, 1978.

Melnikoff A: Die chirurgische Anatomie des Sinus costodiaphragmaticus. Arch Klin Chir Berl 123:133, 1923.

Patten BM: Human Embryology. New York: McGraw-Hill Book, 1968, pp. 87, 406.

Riquet M, Hidden G, Debesse B: Direct lymphatic drainage of lung segments to the mediastinal nodes. An anatomic study on 260 adults. J Thorac Cardiovasc Surg 97:623, 1989.

Said JW, et al: Localized fibrous mesothelioma: An immunohistochemical and electron microscopic study. Hum Pathol 15:440, 1984.

Staub NC, Wiener-Kronish JP, Albertine KM: Transport through the pleura: Physiology of normal liquid and solute exchange in the pleural space. *In* Chretien J, Bignon J, Hirsch A (eds): The Pleura in Health and Disease. New York: Marcel Dekker, 1985, pp. 169-193.

Trapnell, D.H.: Recognition and incidence of intrapulmonary lymph nodes. Thorax *19*:44, 1964.

Wang, N.S.: Morphological data of the pleura: Normal conditions.

In Chretien J, Hirsch A (eds): Diseases of the Pleura. Paris: Masson, 1982, pp. 10-24.

Wang NS: Mesothelial cells in situ. *In* Chretien J, Bignon J, Hirsch J (eds): The Pleura in Health and Disease. New York: Marcel Dekker, 1985, pp. 23-24.

Whalen JP, et al: The retrosternal line: A new sign of an anterior mediastinal mass. AJR Am J Roentgenol *117*:861, 1973.

CHAPTER 3

EMBRYOLOGY AND ANATOMY OF THE DIAPHRAGM

Thomas W. Shields

The diaphragm serves as the anatomic division between the thoracic and the abdominal cavities and, as such, is a muscular structure that is dealt with by both abdominal and thoracic surgeons. The surgical correction of acquired and congenital abnormalities of the diaphragm may be made from either abdominal or thoracic approaches, depending on the nature of the lesion, the location of the lesion, other abnormalities of the chest or abdomen, and the particular training and experience of the involved surgeon. The diaphragm exists as an anatomic barrier but is not a surgical barrier; the competent surgeon should be able to handle any surgical problem involving the diaphragm and, therefore, should be versatile enough to approach diaphragmatic lesions from either above or below.

EMBRYOLOGY

The diaphragm originates from an unpaired ventral portion — the septum transversum; from paired dorsal lateral portions — the pleuroperitoneal folds; and from an irregular medial dorsal portion — the dorsal mesentery (Fig. 3–1). The septum transversum, formed during the third week of gestation, separates the pericardial region from the rest of the body cavity. This part of the diaphragm grows dorsad from the ventral body wall and moves caudad with the other contributors to the diaphragm to reach the normal position of the diaphragm at about 8 weeks. The pleuroperitoneal folds arise on the lateral body walls, at the level where the cardinal veins swing around to enter the sinus venosus of the heart. These folds extend medially and somewhat caudally to join with the septum transversum and the dorsal mesentery to complete the development of the diaphragm at about the seventh week; the right pleuroperitoneal canal closes somewhat earlier than the left. Muscle fibers migrate from the third, fourth, and fifth cervical myotomes, carrying along their innervation, and grow between the two membranes to complete the structures of the diaphragm. During the tenth week, the intestines return from the yolk sac to the abdominal

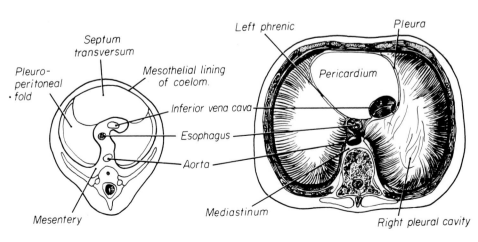

Fig. 3–1. Embryologic components of the diaphragm. *Redrawn from* Shields TW: The diaphragm. *In* Nora P (ed.): Operative Surgery: Principles and Techniques. Philadelphia: Lea & Febiger, 1972.

Septum transversum

Left phrenic

Pleura

Pleuro-peritoneal fold

Mesothelial lining of coelom.

Pericardium

Inferior vena cava

Esophagus

Aorta

Mesentery

Mediastinum

Right pleural cavity

cavity and, at about 12 weeks, rotation and fixation of the intestines occur.

A delay or variation in the described timetable may result in a variety of congenital hernias with or without a hernial sac, or may even result in a congenital "eventration" of a hemidiaphragm. Early return of the intestines to the abdomen prior to closure of the pleuroperitoneal membrane results in a hernia through this opening — a so-called foramen of Bochdalek hernia. A sac usually is not present, but if it is, the return of the intestines may have occurred after the closure of the pleuroperitoneal membrane but prior to the migration of the cervical myotomes between the membranes. Foramen of Morgagni hernias occur anteriorly, almost always have a sac, and therefore probably result from lack of ingrowth of the cervical myotomes. A congenital short esophagus is related to late closure of the diaphragm and early return of the intestine to the abdomen. Congenital "eventration" may be a total error of ingrowth of cervical myotomes in one or both hemidiaphragms, and therefore, is really a large congenital diaphragmatic hernia and not an eventration. An absent diaphragm probably represents an error of growth of the septum transversum and other embryologic elements. Duplication of a hemidiaphragm can occur. The fusion and formation timetable variations also may involve defects in the diaphragm in association with certain vascular anomalies of the lungs and heart.

ANATOMY

Gross Features

The diaphragm is a dome-shaped structure of muscular fibers radiating out from either side of an irregularly shaped central tendon; it consists of the right and the left hemidiaphragms. In structure and function, the diaphragm differs from any other muscle in the body. It is a muscular septum between the abdominal and thoracic cavities, serving as the major muscle of respiration. Its domelike shape allows important abdominal structures, such as the liver and the spleen, to have the protection of the lower ribs and the chest wall. Voluntary muscular fibers originate from the xiphisternum, from the lateral lower six ribs on each side, and from the external and internal arcuate ligaments that arise from the upper three lumbar vertebrae. Bilaterally, the muscle fibers insert into the central tendon of the diaphragm. The muscle mass of the diaphragm is considered by DeTroyer and associates (1982) and Rochester (1985) as comprising two distinct parts — a thin costal muscle mass and a thicker crural portion. Although both muscle masses are innervated by the phrenic nerves, their activity on stimulation are different. The differences that result in diaphragmatic and lower chest wall movement are discussed in Chapter 45. Suffice to mention that the movement of the crural portion has the lesser effect on ventilatory exchange.

The central tendon is a thin aponeurosis of closely interwoven fascial fibers in the form of a three-leaf clover. The two lateral leaves form the dome of the diaphragm and the third — anterior — leaf is fused with the diaphragmatic surface of the pericardium.

Major interest in the muscular portion of the diaphragm centers about the two crura, which play varying roles in the formation of the esophageal hiatus. The right crus arises from the bodies of the first and second lumbar vertebrae, and the fibers divide as they pass to the left, normally overlapping in front and behind to form the entire esophageal hiatus. Collis and associates (1954), however, found this arrangement in only a little more than half of their subjects. In the others, the left crus contributed to a varying degree to the makeup of the hiatus, and in approximately 2%, the left crus made up the major portion of the esophageal hiatus.

The hiatal opening is situated at the level of the tenth thoracic vertebra just to the left of the midline and just ventral to where the aorta passes into the abdomen. The inferior vena cava passes through the tendinous portion of the right side of the diaphragm between the anterior leaf and the right lateral leaf at the level of the eighth thoracic vertebra. The other normal openings are the parasternal foramina — the foramina of Morgagni — through which the internal mammary arteries pass into the abdomen to become the superior epigastric arteries (Fig. 3–2).

The thoracic side of the diaphragm is covered with the parietal pleura, and the abdominal surface with peritoneum, except at the naturally occurring openings.

Blood Supply

The principal blood supply of the diaphragm is derived directly from the aorta or from its most superior abdominal branches (Fig. 3–3), and its venous drainage empties into the inferior vena cava. Both the arterial supply and the venous drainage — the right and left inferior phrenic veins — are found on the undersurface of the diaphragm (Fig. 3–4). The inferior phrenic artery usually bifurcates posteriorly near the dome of the diaphragm and the branches course along the margins of the central tendon. The smaller posterior division courses laterally above the dorsal and lumbocostal origin of the diaphragm, where it has collateral anastomes with the lower five intercostal arteries. The larger anterior division runs anterosuperiorly to the edge of the central tendon, where it anastomoses freely with the pericardiacophrenic artery. The venous pattern is similar except that the veins generally course along the posterior aspect of the central tendon to join the inferior vena cava. Veins on the inferior surface of the diaphragm communicate with the hepatic veins through the left triangular and coronary ligaments of the liver.

Nerve Distribution

The right and left phrenic nerves arise from their respective third, fourth, and fifth cervical nerve roots and constitute the total nerve supply for the ipsilateral hemidiaphragm. The distribution of each nerve is

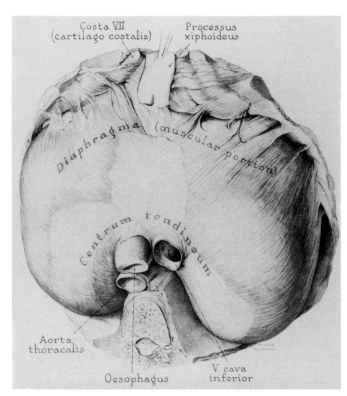

Fig. 3–2. The diaphragm as seen from above. Normal apertures and topographic landmarks are shown. *Reproduced with permission from* Anson BJ: Atlas of Human Anatomy. Philadelphia: WB Saunders, 1950, p. 210.

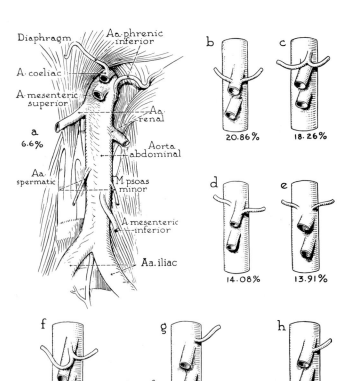

Fig. 3–3. The arterial supply of the diaphragm from the abdominal aorta with variations in the origin of the inferior phrenic arteries. *Redrawn with permission from* Anson BJ, McVay C: Surgical Anatomy. 5th Ed. Philadelphia, WB Saunders, 1971.

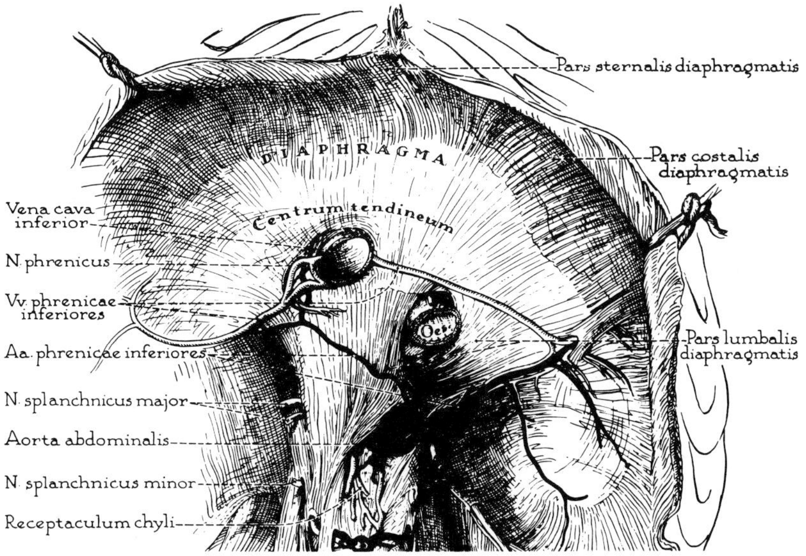

Pars sternalis diaphragmatis

DIAPHRAGMA

Centrum tendineum

Pars costalis diaphragmatis

Vena cava inferior

N phrenicus

Vv. phrenicae inferiores

Aa. phrenicae inferiores

Pars lumbalis diaphragmatis

N. splanchnicus major

Aorta abdominalis

N. splanchnicus minor

Receptaculum chyli

Fig. 3–4. The arterial and venous distribution on the undersurface of the diaphragm. *Redrawn with permission from* Anson BJ, McVay C: Surgical Anatomy. 5th Ed. Philadelphia: WB Saunders, 1971.

important in reference to incisions into the diaphragm. The course of each has been described by Merendino and co-workers (1956). The right phrenic nerve reaches the diaphragm just lateral to the inferior vena cava, and the left just lateral to the left border of the heart. Generally, the nerves divide, either just above or at the level of the diaphragm, into several terminal branches. Some are distributed to the pleural and peritoneal surfaces, but the great bulk of each nerve passes into, or through, the diaphragm and most often divides into four major rami to supply the various muscular portions. Usually, two of the rami share a common trunk for a varying distance so that three muscular branches arise from each phrenic nerve: one anteromedially, one laterally, and the remaining one posteriorly (Fig. 3–5). Injury to any of these branches

causes paralysis of the supplied portion of the hemidiaphragm.

Surgical Incisions

Incisions into the diaphragm must be made so as to avoid injury to the major branches of the phrenic nerves. Incision through the central tendon rarely causes diaphragmatic paralysis (Fig. 3–6a and b), but this approach provides only minimal exposure of the adjacent compartment. A more satisfactory access is provided by a circumferential incision at the periphery of the diaphragm, which permits excellent exposure of the upper abdominal contents from the thorax and vice versa with little or no possibility of injury to any major branch of the ipsilateral phrenic nerve (Fig. 3–6c). On the left, the incision may be started at the esophageal hiatus and

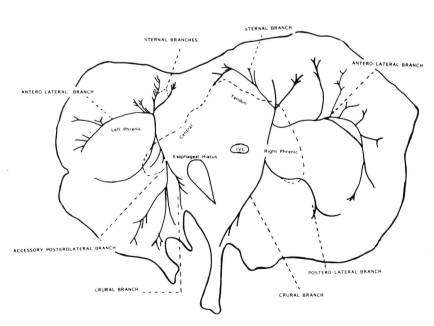

STERNAL BRANCH

STERNAL BRANCHES

ANTERO-LATERAL BRANCH

ANTERO LATERAL BRANCH

Left Phrenic

Tendon

Central

Esophageal Hiatus

IVC

Right Phrenic

ACCESSORY POSTEROLATERAL BRANCH

CRURAL BRANCH

POSTERO LATERAL BRANCH

CRURAL BRANCH

Fig. 3–5. Distribution of the phrenic nerves as seen from above. *Redrawn with permission from* Merendino KA, et al: The intradiaphragmatic distribution of the phrenic nerve with particular reference to the placement of diaphragmatic incisions and controlled segmental paralysis. Surgery 39: 189, 1956.

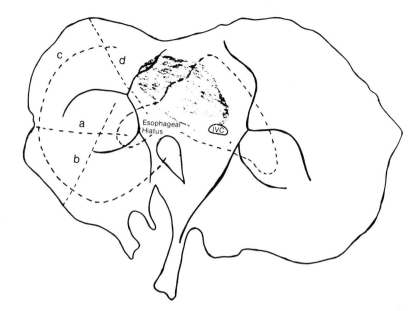

Fig. 3–6. Safe areas for incision into the diaphragm. *Redrawn with permission from* Merendino KA, et al: The intradiaphragmatic distribution of the phrenic nerve with particular reference to the placement of diaphragmatic incisions and controlled segmental paralysis. Surgery 39:189, 1956.

carried from behind forward circumferentially 2.5 to 3 cm away from the attachment of the diaphragm to the chest wall. The crural or posterior branch of the phrenic nerve is divided but this division is of little consequence. The main branch of the left inferior phrenic artery is usually encountered with this incision and requires division and ligation. Alternatively, the incision may be started anteriorly just lateral to the pericardium and extended circumferentially as far posteriorly as necessary. The ipsilateral hemidiaphragm may then be raised as a trapdoor and retracted medially for exposure. Closure of the incision is accomplished readily by approximating the cut edges of the hemidiaphragm with multiple interrupted simple or mattress sutures of 0 or 2-0 nonabsorbable material of the surgeon's choice. A similar incision may also be carried out on the right.

When a combined abdominothoracic approach is used, the incision in the diaphragm may be extended medially between the pericardial attachment to the diaphragm and the entrance of the phrenic nerve into the diaphragm, with severence of only the small sternal division of the nerve (Fig. 3–6d). The incision is then carried to the apex of the esophageal hiatus. To ensure adequate exposure, the phrenic nerve and pericardiacophrenic vessels must be freed from the pericardium proximally and retracted laterally. Care must be exercised to prevent injury to these structures during this retraction. This incision is closed the same as a circumferential incision. Sicular (1992) reported the use of this latter incision with the use of the 90 GIA stapling instrument in more than 50 patients with no compromise

of exposure. Moreover, he reported no clinical evidence of phrenic nerve injury postoperatively. Incisions in the diaphragm other than a circumferential or a very medial one must be avoided because the anterolateral and posterolateral branches of the nerve are likely to be divided.

REFERENCES

Collis JL, Kelly TD, Wiley AM: Anatomy of the crura of the diaphragm and the surgery of hiatus hernia. Thorax 9:175, 1954.

De Troyer A, et al: Action of costal and crural parts of the diaphragm on the rib cage in dogs. J App Physiol 53:30, 1982.

Meredino KA, et al: The intradiaphragmatic distribution of the phrenic nerve with particular reference to the placement of diaphragmatic incisions and controlled segmental paralysis. Surgery 39:189, 1956.

Rochester DF: The diaphragm: Contractile properties and fatigue. J Clin Invest 75:1397, 1985.

Sicular A: Direct septum transversum incision to replace circumferential diaphragmatic in operations on the cardia. Am J Surg 164:167, 1992.

READING REFERENCES

Anson BJ: Atlas of Human Anatomy. Philadelphia: WB Saunders, 1950.

Anson BJ, McVay C: Surgical Anatomy. 5th Ed. Philadelphia: WB Saunders, 1971.

Patten B: Human Embryology. 3rd Ed. New York: McGraw-Hill Book, 1968, p. 406.

Shields TW: The diaphragm. *In* Nora P: Operative Surgery: Principles and Techniques. Philadelphia: Lea & Febiger, 1972.

CHAPTER 4

EMBRYOLOGY OF THE LUNGS

Charles E. Blevins

EVOLUTIONARY NOTES

The development of an efficient mechanism for exchange of respiratory gases between air and circulating blood gives testimony to a community of descent among vertebrates. Although lungs are characteristic of all vertebrates and found only in tetrapods, some species of Dipnoi or lungfish have a pharyngeal region of the gut that is modified to form a primitive lung or air bladder. Indeed, Pattle and Hopkinson (1963) provided evidence for the presence of surfactant in the lungfish Protopterus. Although a diversity of lung forms exist in amphibians and birds, perhaps the most extensive information concerning the mechanism of oxygen uptake and carbon dioxide has come from experiments on amphibians. The importance of amphibians in the evolution of lungs from primitive gills lies in the role of the skin in the exchanges of respiratory gases. Krogh (1904) demonstrated the importance of cutaneous respiration in frogs by showing that most of the carbon dioxide leaves through the skin while the lung is primarily responsible for oxygen uptake. This work was later confirmed by Hughes (1967) while working in the laboratory of Rahn in Buffalo, New York. Further support for this view involves cardiovascular dynamics. Poczopko (1957) demonstrated an increase in cutaneous circulation during immersion of frogs, and Whitford and Hutchison (1963) and Vinegar and Hutchison (1965) showed that rising temperature resulted in an 80 to 90% increase in carbon dioxide loss through the skin.

According to Hughes (1967), cutaneous respiration played an important role in the origin of terrestrial vertebrates. His reasoning is that fish ancestors, who supplemented gill respiration by visits to the surface to take in air, evolved to the extent of developing diverticula of the pharynx to supplement gill respiration. These diverticula became the main source of oxygen for the animal, but carbon dioxide release took place through the gills. As the adult animal increasingly came to land for food, the gills were lost and the skin became the main surface for the release of carbon dioxide. Because the skin was permeable to carbon dioxide and also to water, moist swampy conditions were conducive to survival. Furthermore, the loss of scales was accompanied by the ability to secrete mucus and thus prevent water loss. Once on land, the organism lost its permeable skin to reduce water loss permitting further evolution of the lungs. Presumably, morphologic adaptations allowed a graded evolution of physiologic factors associated with increased Pco_2 in the lung, that is, reduction of the effect of carbon dioxide on the oxygen-hemoglobin dissociation curve, an improved blood-buffering mechanism, and reduced sensitivity of the respiratory center to carbon dioxide. Assuming a moist environment, by these means, Hughes believed it was possible for the organism to adjust for oxygen uptake first, and subsequently evolve to manage increased carbon dioxide in the lung.

EARLY DEVELOPMENT

O'Rahilly and Boyden (1973) documented the first appearance of the lung bud 26 days after fertilization, during the fourth week of human development. Its appearance is presaged by the formation of bilateral grooves that run longitudinally in the floor of the pharynx, just caudal to the pharyngeal pouches. As noted by Moore (1988), proliferation of the endodermal cells lining the interior of these grooves forms tracheoesophageal folds, which fuse across the midline to pinch off a ventral laryngeotracheal diverticulum, or ridge, from the more dorsally placed esophagus. With further differentiation, the proximal end of the diverticulum develops into the larynx. The caudal end enlarges into the lung bud, which bifurcates to form two smaller knoblike bronchial buds (Fig. 4–1A and B). The bronchial buds subsequently elongate and migrate dorsally on either side of the esophagus, where they differentiate further and grow laterally into the pericardioperitoneal canals.

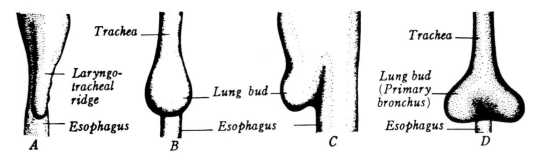

Fig. 4–1. Early stages of the human respiratory primordium (after Grosser and Heiss), ×75. *A*, at 2.5 mm, in ventral view; *B* and *C*, at 3 mm, in ventral and lateral views; *D*, at 4 mm, in ventral view. *Reproduced with permission from* Arey LB: Developmental Anatomy. 7th Ed. Philadelphia: WB Saunders, 1965, p. 265.

By the first part of the fifth week, enlargement of the bronchial buds forms the primordia of primary bronchi. A larger right primary bronchus extends caudally in contrast to a more obliquely divergent left bronchus (Fig. 4–2*A*) This asymmetric pattern between the right and left primary bronchi persists after birth, which accounts for the greater liability if a foreign object enters the right rather than the left bronchus. Although it is tempting to think that the more obliquely placed left bronchus arrives in this position to leave more space for the developing heart, the asymmetry occurs too early to account for the predatory position of the heart on the left side.

Subsequent to this event, during the fifth week of development, another type of asymmetry establishes the basic pattern of pulmonary lobes in the right and left lungs. The right primary bronchus gives rise to two lateral secondary buds; the left bronchus forms only one (Fig. 4–2*B* and *C*). These lateral secondary buds have different spatial destinies. On the right side, the upper lateral secondary bud differentiates into the upper —apical— lobe, and the lower secondary bud forms the middle lobe of the right lung. On the left side, the lateral secondary bronchial bud forms the upper lobe of the left lung. The lower lobes of both the right and left lungs are formed from the terminal

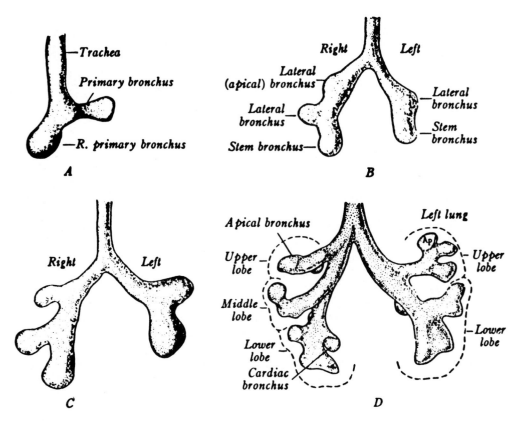

Fig. 4–2. Development of primary and secondary bronchi of the human lung in ventral views (after Heiss and Merkel). ×50. *A*, at 5 mm; *B*, at 7 mm; *C*, at 8.5 mm; *D*, at 10 mm. (Ap-apical bronchus-homologue of left lung.) *Reproduced with permission from* Arey LB: Developmental Anatomy 7th Ed. Philadelphia: WB Saunders, 1965, p. 265.)

blind ends — stem bronchi — of the right and left primary bronchi.

A third order of branching of these simple epithelial tubes forms the tertiary or segmental bronchi, 10 on the right side and 8 on the left. With subsequent condensation and differentiation of the mesenchyme that surrounds these tertiary branches, the precursor tissues for cartilage, bronchial smooth muscle, connective tissue, and blood vessels, the basic ingredients for bronchopulmonary segmentation are in place. According to the agreements reached at the International Congress of Anatomists in Leningrad, 1970 (Nomina Anatomica, 1970), the events concluded at the end of the fifth week mark the termination of the embryonic period of lung development.

LATER DEVELOPMENT

Pseudoglandular Period

From the end of the fifth week until the end of the sixteenth week, the lung is said to be in the *pseudoglandular period* of development. During this period, intrasegmental bronchial division continues at a remarkable rate. Indeed, in an extensive study, Bucher and Reid (1961a) found that 70% of the generations of bronchi present at birth are formed between the tenth and fourteenth week. In the shorter apical segments of the upper lobes, some 14 to 18 generations of branches are formed, compared to 17 to 28 generations of buds reached in the longer segments — such as the lingula and middle lobe and anterior and posterior basal segments — which continue to grow until the end of the sixteenth week. This period of growth is designated the pseudoglandular period because the characteristic cuboidal epithelium of the bronchial tube gives the developing lung the histologic appearance of an exocrine gland.

Canalicular Period

The next formal period of development recognized by the Commission on Embryological Terminology (1970) is the *canalicular period*, during which the future respiratory part of the bronchopulmonary segments are both more clearly defined and, most importantly, vascularized. Before definitive establishment of this period, however, Boyden (1974) described a precanalicular phase of growth during the sixteenth week. Studying peripheral branches of the medial segment of the right lung, he found prospective terminal bronchioles, each followed by three generations of presumptive respiratory bronchioles, each of which ended in three to five closely packed generations of buds that he identified as future alveolar sac elements. He concluded that the ends of the bronchiolar tree were in a hurry to complete the respiratory unit pattern just before canalization occurred.

Short (1950) presented evidence that the canalicular period begins between weeks 16 and 17. During this time, the respiratory unit of the lungs is formed.

Pulmonary acini are outlined by thinned out connective tissue that forms the septa interacinosa (Fig. 4–3). Campiche and associates (1963), Boyden (1974), and Looslie and Baker (1962) documented the invasion of acini by developing capillaries (Figs. 4–3, 4–4). The essential components of the acini are clearly evident, in addition to the surrounding capillaries. These components include (1) a terminal bronchiole, (2) two to four prospective respiratory bronchioles, and (3) a cluster of six to seven generations of closely packed buds that become the saccules of the terminal sac period.

The invasion of pulmonary acini by capillaries apparently is not rapid. Boyden (1976) observed in the macaque fetus that canalization by capillaries takes place in a centripetal pattern, first involving small distal generations of acini, then prospective respiratory bronchioles that are still growing in length. Campiche and associates (1963) demonstrated with light microscopy that during canalization, capillary processes are inserted between adjoining cuboidal endothelial cells and, in some instances, may bulge out into the acinar lumen (Fig. 4–4). Their electron microscopic observations indicate, however, that the capillaries are always covered by extended cytoplasm of thinned out endothelial cells (Fig. 4–5).

While canalization establishes essential surface relations between endothelial cells and capillaries, an equally important event occurs — the differentiation of endothelial cells or future pneumocytes. Two types of

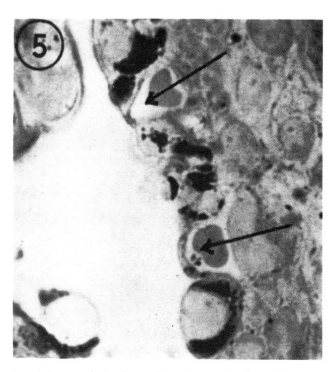

Fig. 4–3. Developing human lung tissue at 4 to 5 months. Note the invasion of capillaries (arrows) penetrating into the epithelium in wedge-like fashion to separate flattened epithelial cells. Os/Ag; ×1300. *Reproduced with permission from* Campiche MA, et al: An electron microscopic study of the fetal development of human lung. Pediatrics 32:978, 1963.

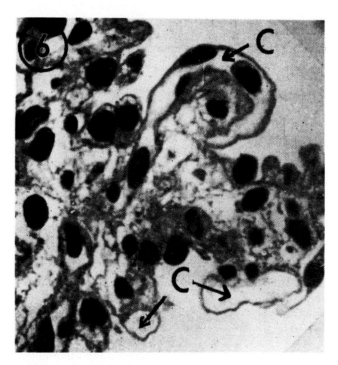

Fig. 4–4. Developing human lung tissue at 5–6 months. Note the bulging of capillaries (c) into the lumen of the alveolus. (Hemalume-erthrosine, ×100. *Reproduced with permission from* Campiche MA, et al: An electron microscopic study of the fetal development of human lung. Pediatrics 32:978, 1963.

pneumocytes are formed, as described by Campiche and colleagues (1963) and Meyrick and Reid (1977). In earlier phases of development, the endothelial cells appear to contain an abundance of glycogen. During the canalization process, as capillaries approach the surface, those endothelial cells in which thin cytoplasm extends to cover the capillaries and that exhibit reduced glycogen and pinocytotic vesicles are designated as type I pneumocytes (Fig. 4–5). The other distinctly identifiable cell type is the type II pneumocyte. This cell continues to exhibit considerable glycogen content, but more importantly, contains so-called lamellar inclusions, which have been demonstrated to be the source of pulmonary surfactant.

Terminal Sac Period

The last antenatal period of lung development recognized by the 1970 Commission on Embryological Terminology is the *terminal sac period*. This name replaces the term "alveolar" period suggested by Loosli and Potter (1959). The terminal sac period extends from week 26 of gestation to term. Our understanding of this phase is once again the meticulous work of Boyden (1959), who studied the lung of a premature infant of 30 to 32 weeks gestation. His observations at the light microscopic level revealed that respiratory bronchioles are lined on one side by capillarized epithelium, and the other side is covered by ciliated cuboidal epithelium. Respiratory bronchioles that were previously rapidly growing tubes of buds lined by cuboidal epithelium form clusters of thin-walled saccules that arise from the third respiratory bronchioles via transitional ducts. The clusters are five or six generations of capillary-coated endothelium. Connective tissue septa between saccules appears much the same as in the canalicular period, but they become thinner as the potential air spaces enlarge.

PERINATAL EVENTS

At birth, the transition of lungs from a secretory tissue to a functional respiratory organ capable of exchange of respiratory gases between ambient air and circulating blood is one of the most remarkable phenomena of living organisms. Despite extensive experimental work, physiologic factors controlling these events are still not well defined. It is known, however, that fetal lungs are both physically and metabolically active, because breathing movements are prominent and surfactant and fluids are secreted into future air spaces.

Respiratory Movements

Dawes and co-workers (1970) demonstrated that fetal sheep exhibit regular breathing movements. Later, Boddy and Dawes (1975) and Patrick (1980) recorded that such movements also occur in the human fetus during periods of low voltage electrocortical activity. As stated by Rigatto (1992), these observations mean that what had traditionally been called the initiation of breathing at birth should be called the establishment of continuous breathing at birth.

Experiments with fetal breathing by Moss and Scarpelli, (1979), Jansen (1982), and Rigatto (1988) establish that the fetal breathing apparatus responds well to chemical agents that are known to alter breathing postnatally. For instance, increased $Paco_2$ results in an increase in breathing. Administration of hypoxic mixtures abolishes fetal breathing, but this response is associated with decrease in the amplitude of electrocortical activity and a decrease in body movements. In reverse relation, Baier and associates (1988) found that arterial Po_2 at levels above 200 mgHg — via tracheal intubator — induced continuous breathing in fetal sheep. Rigatto (1992) believes these findings suggest that low partial pressure of O_2 could be a normal mechanism in inhibiting breathing in utero.

Despite these responses to concentrations of the respiratory gases, some evidence suggests that the actions of CO_2 and hypoxia are central. Jansen and colleagues (1981) and Rigatto (1987) showed that resection of the carotid bodies does not alter fetal breathing, nor does it affect the initiation of continuous breathing at birth. It seems, therefore, that the precise role of peripheral chemoreceptors in both intrauterine and neonatal breathing remains unknown. Rigatto (1992) speculates that continuous breathing at birth may depend on a hormone or chemical mediation more than low oxygen, or that sensory stimuli or increased arterial oxygen tension may trigger mediators in the lung or brain to induce continuous breathing.

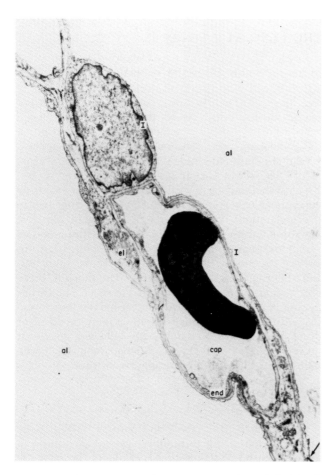

Fig. 4–5. Electron micrograph of a type I alveolar endothelial cell (pneumocyte) and a capillary from part of the human alveolar wall. Note how the delicate, thinned cytoplasmic extension of the type I cell (I) completely covers the capillary (cap) that contains a red blood cell. ×4800. al = alveoli; end = endothelium of capillary. *Reproduced with permission from* Meyrick B, Reid, L: Development of the lung. *In* Hodson WA (ed): Lung Biology in Health and Disease. Vol 6. New York: Marcel Dekker, 1977.)

Removal of Fetal Lung Liquid Near Birth

Normal intrauterine lung growth depends on balance between production and controlled drainage of luminal liquid. Alcorn and colleagues (1977) demonstrated that obstruction of tracheal outflow increases lung size, distends terminal respiratory units, and decreases the number of type II epithelial cells, and unimpeded leakage of tracheal fluid results in the opposite effects. In a review of formation and removal of fetal liquids, Bland (1992) indicated that the following events contribute significantly to the clearance of fluids from the late fetal and neonatal lung. First, a high protein concentration compared to little or no protein in future pulmonary air spaces creates a transepithelial osmotic difference greater than 10 cm H_2O. Second, epithelial sodium pumps that actively transport sodium in the direction of the lung lumen during gestation suddenly stop, thus aiding osmotic forces conducive to removal of fluid to interstitial tissue. Thus, epithelial sodium pumps and transpulmonary pressure associated with lung inflation drive liquid from the lung lumen into the interstitium. Air entry into the lungs displaces liquid and decreases hydrostatic pressure in the pulmonary circulation, which improves pulmonary blood flow and in turn increases lung blood volume and vascular surface for fluid uptake. Apparently about 10% of luminal liquids exit the lung through pulmonary lymphatics. The process may be aided by reduction of intrathoracic pressure occasioned by spontaneous breathing. Most of the pulmonary fluid, however, enters lung microcirculation. Increased microvascular pressure, attributable to hypoxemia or left ventricular failure, or conditions contributing to low plasma protein concentration may slow this process of fluid reabsorption, potentially contributing to the development of neonatal respiratory distress.

THE LUNG AT BIRTH

Boyden and Tompsett (1965) and Boyden (1967) have provided the most detailed description of postnatal changes in the lungs at various ages — to 7 years. Hislop and Reid (1974) summarized this work in diagrammatic form (Fig. 4–6). In this figure, the acinus is defined as all structures distal to the terminal bronchiolus. At birth, three generations of respiratory bronchioli, one generation of a transitional duct, and three generations of saccules, each ending in a terminal sac, are present. In other acini, more or fewer generations are present. The respiratory bronchioli are increasing in length. The saccules have increased the pulmonary surface area through the presence of shallow depressions in their walls. These depressions are considered only primitive alveoli at this stage, because the true cup shape of the adult alveoli has not been reached. The primitive alveoli demonstrate variation in size and depth when seen in wax reconstructions (Fig. 4–7). The entire acinus at this stage exhibits an axial length of about 1.1 mm.

Rapid development of true alveoli occurs between the sixth and eighth postnatal week. Elongation of the respiratory bronchioli also occurs. Saccules and transitional ducts become alveolar ducts by increasing in length and deepening of the primitive alveoli in their walls.

THE LUNG AT 2 MONTHS

By this stage of growth, Boyden and Tompsett (1965) observed three generations of respiratory bronchioli and four generations of alveolar ducts that represented remodeled saccules. The axial length of the acinus is about 1.75 mm, and the terminal saccules are all lined by alveoli (Fig 4–6e). Hislop and Reid (1974) believe that the increase in number of alveoli is attributable to development of new alveoli along alveolar ducts. After birth, little terminal branching occurs, but each terminal saccule produces one to four alveolar sacs within the same generation, each containing many alveoli. Furthermore, the proximal part of the terminal saccule

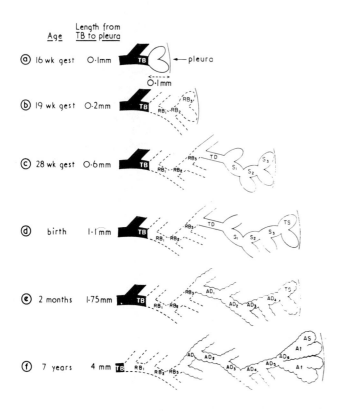

Age | Length from TB to pleura

(a) 16 wk gest   0·1mm

(b) 19 wk gest   0·2mm

(c) 28 wk gest   0·6mm

(d) birth   1·1mm

(e) 2 months   1·75mm

(f) 7 years   4 mm

Fig. 4–6. Schematic representation of the growth of the acinus (subpleural). a, At 16 weeks gestation, the airways terminate as a tubule close to the pleura. TB = terminal bronchiole. b, By 19 weeks gestation, the last generation of airway shows thinned epithelium and forms the first respiratory bronchiolus (RB) and a second generation of respiratory bronchioli has formed by branching. c, By 28 weeks gestation, three generations of respiratory bronchioli and one generation of transitional duct (TD) have arisen by further branching. The transitional duct gives rise to two primitive saccules (S). d, By birth, three generations of saccules are found, all ending in terminal saccules. No true alveoli are present, although indentations representing future alveoli are found. e, By 2 months, alveoli have developed in the walls of respiratory bronchioli, transitional ducts, and saccules. f, By 7 years, remodeling of respiratory bronchioli and alveolar ducts has occurred. Also, the terminal sac has formed the adult atrium (At), which has given rise to alveolar sacs (AS) that formed by budding. This pattern is similar to that found in the adult. Any further development is probably attributable to an increase in size. *Reproduced with permission from* Hislop A, Reid L: Development of the acinus in the human lung. Thorax 29:90, 1974.

becomes an alveolar duct, and the distal part the atrium. The atrium is that part of the airway beyond the last muscles in its walls.

It is believed that considerable remodeling of the airways occurs. Boyden and Tompsett (1965) describe "centripetal alveolization" in which terminal bronchioli may be transformed into an extra generation of respiratory bronchioli. It is also possible that distal respiratory bronchioli may be transformed into alveolar ducts by increasing alveolarization in their walls. Other possibilities include further branching of alveolar ducts, giving rise to another one or two generations, or that an increase in length of all generations can occur without an increase in their numbers.

THE LUNG AT 7 YEARS

Boyden (1971) added a new technique of observation to his previously successful method of graphic reconstruction and wax models made from serial sections of the lungs. By tracing serial sections on transparent plastic sheets, which were then viewed as stacked translucent objects, he gained further knowledge of the pulmonary acini. His material was the lung of a 6-year, 8-month-old child, scaled at the age of 7 years in the diagram of Hislop and Reid (1974) (Fig. 4–6f). By both methods of reconstruction, he observed three generations of respiratory bronchioles and from two to five generations of alveolar ducts, ending in saccules. He also found the acinus to be "replete with numerous variations, such as dilated atria and saccules, supernumerary structures, recurrent ducts, irregular branches, and differing lengths of airways." He thought these observations bore out the "fight for space" in earlier periods of lung growth. Boyden recorded the impression that no two acini are alike in either their proximal or distal parts. Such variation, he believed, made it questionable to be able to quantitate mathematically the diffusion of gases in the peripheral airways.

HISTOGENESIS

According to Arey (1989) and Sorokin (1965), tissue differentiation in the respiratory system takes place in a proximodistal direction, thus speaking of "histogenetic gradients" in the development of both endoderm and mesenchyme.

Endodermal Differentiation

During the glandular phase of development, epithelium of the primitive trachea is stratified in identical fashion to that of the esophagus. The cells are vertically oriented and their thinner portion is squeezed next to adjacent cells near their basal borders. With subsequent growth of the bronchial tree, a gradient of epithelium is evident by 10 weeks of gestation, from pseudostratified to columnar to cuboidal cells. Bucher and Reid (1961 b) documented the presence of ciliated cells throughout the bronchial tree by 13 weeks. Sorokin (1965) reported that cilia first appear in the trachea and then progressively at more distal levels. These changes, as well as those occurring in subjacent mesenchyme, are summarized diagrammatically by Burri and Weibel (1973), in Figure 4–8.

During the seventeenth to twenty-sixth week of gestation, as stated previously, two types of alveolar epithelial cells differentiate, type I and type II cells. Their cytologic features are best appreciated by electron microscopy. Type I cells cover most — 80 to 90% — of the alveolar surface by long cytoplasmic extensions containing pinocytotic vesicles. These cells are poor in mitochondria and endoplasmic reticulum, and exhibit only a small Golgi complex (Fig. 4–9). Type II cells, on the other hand, exhibit microvilli and cover less of

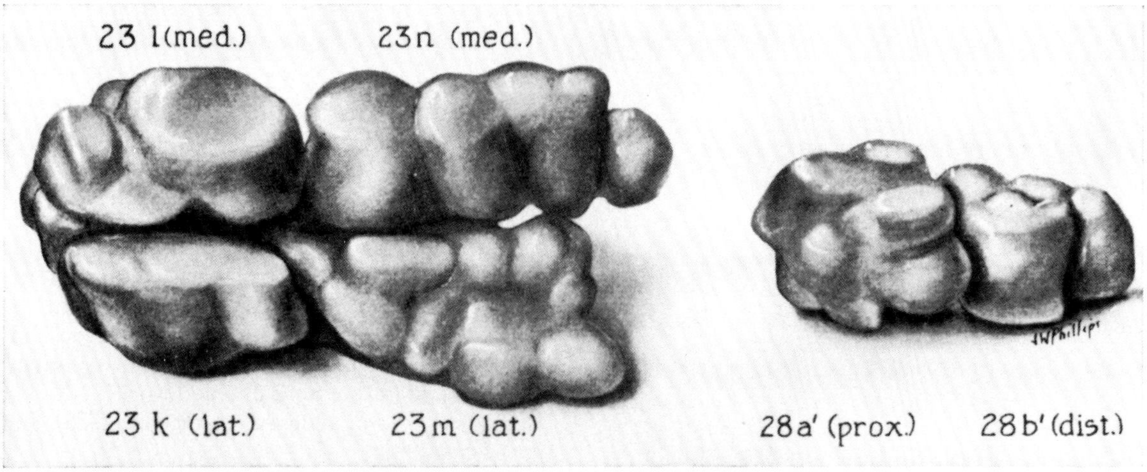

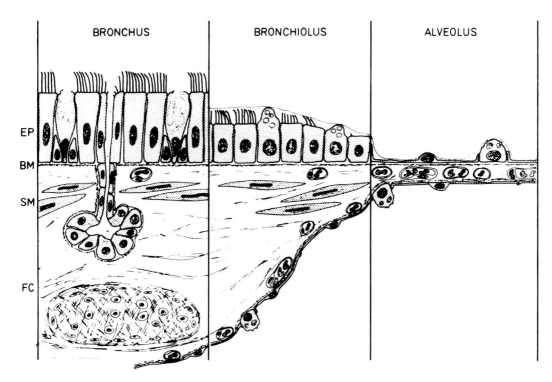

Fig. 4–7. Wax reconstructions of terminal air sacs in a 2-day-old infant (×85). Note the shallowness and variations in size of the pulmonary alveoli that appear as smaller elevations on the surface of the terminal air sacs during the perinatal period. *Reproduced with permission from* Boyden EA, Tompsett DH: The changing patterns in the developing lungs of infants. Acta Anat *61:*182, 187, 1965.

the alveolar surface. Their organelle population is extensive, including rough endoplasmic reticulum, ribosomes, multivesicular bodies, and numerous large mitochondria. The most strikingly consistent feature of type II cells is their lamellated bodies. These are membrane-bound stacks of phospholipid material, the

osmophilic nature of which makes them easily recognizable at the ultrastructural level (Figs. 4–5, 4–10).

The differing cytoplasmic features of type I and type II cells have inevitably led to studies concerning their respective function. The early ultrastructural work of Low (1953) demonstrated that the stretched-out cyto-

Fig. 4–8. The change of airway wall structure at the three principal levels. The epithelial layer (EP) gradually becomes reduced from pseudostratified to cuboidal and then to squamous, but retains its organization as a mosaic of lining and secretory cells. The smooth muscle layer (SM) disappears in the alveoli. The fibrous coat (FC) contains cartilage only in bronchi and gradually becomes thinner as the alveolus is approached. BM = basement membrane. *Reproduced with permission from* Weibel ER: The Pathway for Oxygen. Cambridge: Harvard University Press, 1984.

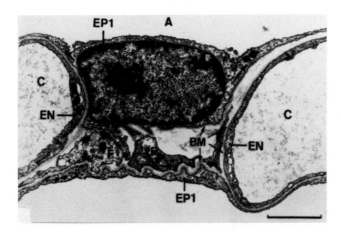

Fig. 4–9. Electron micrograph of a type I alveolar epithelial cell (EP1) from human lung. (Scale marker = 2 μm). The nucleus (N) is surrounded by little cytoplasm, which extends as thin leaflets (arrows) to cover the capillaries (C). Note the basement membranes (BM) of the epithelium and endothelium (En) that fuse in a minimal barrier. The interstitial space contains fibroblast processes (F). *Reproduced with permission from* Weibel ER: The Pathway for Oxygen. Cambridge: Harvard University Press, 1984.

plasm of type I cells covers lung interstitium that in turn covers capillary epithelium, confirming that alveolar capillaries are not exposed directly to capillary air.

Resolution of type II cell function was to come later, however. It was known from the observations of Pattle (1958) that bubbles expressed from lungs of mature animals were more stable than those from fetal lungs. Clements (1957) emphasized the importance of a bubble stabilizing factor — surfactant — in the prevention of atelectasis. Buckingham and Avery (1962) then found that surfactant does not appear until late in gestation, coincidental with the appearance of lamellar bodies in type II cells. Further observations by Clements (1962) showed that surface tension at the alveolae-air interface is extremely low at low lung volumes. In 1954, Macklin had correctly proposed that type II cells are the source of surfactant and that this material functioned to maintain a favorable surface tension during all phases of alveolar activity, to remove particulate matter, and to prevent alveolar surfaces from desiccation. Further details of the lamellar bodies as sources of surfactant as well as the synthesis and biochemistry of surfactant are available in the more detailed works of Meyrick and Reid (1977), Van Golde and associates (1988), and Polin and Fox (1992).

Additional endodermal derivatives include goblet cells in the surface epithelium and tubuloacinar glands, which lie deep to the smooth muscle layer of bronchioles and open onto the surface by an excretory duct. Bucher and Reid (1961b) observed *goblet cells* in the trachea and larger bronchi as early as 13 weeks of gestation. Between 12 and 24 weeks, surface goblet cells are found only in the most proximal intrasegmental bronchi, never reaching as far distally as the glands or a bronchiolus. Goblet cells are numerous, however, in the crypts of excretory ducts of the glands. Developing glands are evident by the fourteenth week as invaginating derivatives of the epithelium. They continue to develop through week 28. Gland density is highest in proximal bronchi and decreases toward the periphery, being more concentrated at bifurcations.

With the aid of the electron microscope, Jeffrey and Reid (1977) described still other cell types in the

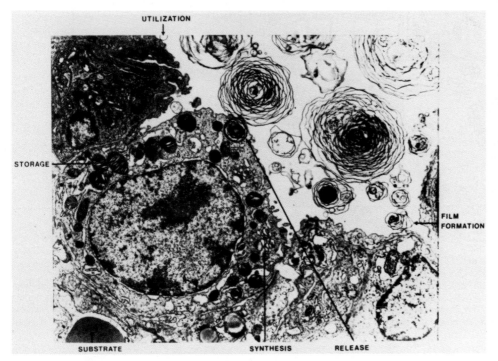

Fig. 4–10. Electron micrograph of a type II alveolar epithelial cell showing stages of synthesis, storage, release, and surface films formation of surface active material (surfactant). Note the densely stained osmophilic nature of the lamellated membrane-bound organelles, the phospholipid contents of which are in various stages of compactness. (Original magnification = ×100.) *Reproduced with permission from* Taeusch HW, Avery ME: Development of the lung. *In* Hodson WA (ed): Lung Biology and Health and Disease, Vol 6. New York; Marcel Dekker, 1977.

epithelium. The Clara cell is nonciliated with cytoplasm containing secretory granules, smooth endoplasmic reticulum, and mitochondria. The serous cell resembles a serous cell of the submucosal gland and presents numerous electron-dense, membrane-bound granules of uniform diameter, as well as much rough endoplasmic reticulum. So-called Kultschitsky cells are found at 16 weeks of gestation and in prematurely born infants. These cells have electron-dense cytoplasm and abundant glycogen in fetal life, but electron-lucent cytoplasm and no glycogen are found in the adult. Well-defined dense core vesicles are also present in the basal portion of this type of cell.

Mesodermal Differentiation

Coincident with differentiation of the endoderm, developmental changes occur in the mesenchyme surrounding the developing airways. The early suggestions of Rudnick (1933) and confirming experiments of Sampaolo and Sampaolo (1961) and Dameron (1961) demonstrated that mesenchyme is absolutely essential to elongation and budding of the bronchial tree. Mesenchyme investing the developing endodermal tubes of the lung, and first visible at 7 weeks of gestation, is the precursor tissue for cartilage, blood vessels, smooth muscle, and the lymphatics.

Cartilage

Bucher and Reid (1961a) have shown that cartilage appears in the trachea and main bronchi at 10 weeks of gestation, but does not reach the segmental bronchi until the twelfth week, some 6 weeks after the segmental bronchi are formed. The rate of cartilage growth does not parallel bronchial branching because it does not demonstrate the same burst of activity. Most bronchial branching occurs between the tenth and fourteenth weeks. Cartilage first appears as precartilaginous plates, the cell borders of which gradually become PAS positive. Gradually, extracellular ground substance appears and an irregular net of intercellular reticulum becomes evident in the perichondrial region. Cellular formation of cartilage occurs within 2 weeks on average, but development of final characteristics of the extracellular matrix takes from 15 to 20 weeks. Even at term, distal plates of cartilage do not exhibit a mature extracellular matrix.

Smooth Muscle

Looslie and Hung (1977) recorded that smooth muscle first appears at 6 to 8 weeks gestation, first in the tracheal, bronchi, and lobar bronchi and subsequently in developing segmental bronchi, terminal and respiratory bronchioles, and alveolar ducts. Smooth muscle of the pulmonary arteries appears in immature form at 12 weeks and gradually matures over the next 10 weeks. At birth, arterial smooth muscle extends as far as the terminal bronchioles. Towers (1968) and Hislop and Reid (1974) observed that arterial smooth muscle cells grow peripherally as the arteries become larger and longer, but cease to extend into the alveolar walls.

DEVELOPMENTAL DETERMINANTS

The dramatic transition of epithelium of the primitive gastrointestinal tract into a bulging diverticulum representing the precursor of a functional pulmonary system suggests unique morphogenetic activities that could be associated with inductive or histochemical events. Sorokin (1965) observed that both in vitro and in vivo experiments with developing lung explants demonstrate that all characteristics of pulmonary form are implicit in the epithelium and mesenchyme associated with the tracheal bud. Rudnick (1933) found that once started, lung development from explants seems to go on as a matter of course in a self-determined manner. The older the culture, however, the better the chances for obtaining adult-like harvests.

In vitro cultures do not permit the development of blood vessels to the same degree as occurs in vivo. Initially, cultures grown on optimal media keep up with in vivo controls, but within several days, even the best cultures fall behind. Such regression results from a progressively slowing mitotic rate in the epithelium rather than in the surrounding mesenchyme. As a consequence, epithelial branching slows. It is important to recognize, however, that it is growth rather than differentiation that becomes limited in cultured specimens. Chemical and structural differentiation of pulmonary cells are so well matched in vivo and vitro that the relative independence of differentiation from growth is readily evident.

Inductive Activity

Although it is widely held that formation of the tracheal buds is a response to inductive forces, solid experimental evidence confirming this belief is still to be found. Sorokin (1965) reports, however, that inductive activity is demonstrated in lung tissue mature beyond the early tracheal bud stage of development. When mesenchyme is removed from lung explants, budding of the bronchial tree ceases. Once the mesenchyme is regenerated, however, bronchial budding resumes. When isolated from mesenchyme, epithelium forms spherical masses that spread over the culture surface.

If mesenchyme is removed from the developing bronchial tree and placed on plasma clots some distance from the denuded bronchial tree, it migrates backward to envelop the epithelium. If a section of mesenchyme from the tracheal bud is removed from a bronchial bud and the grafted lung is cultivated in vitro, a supernumerary bud grows from the epithelium beneath the graft. When mesenchyme from the normally budding lateral side of a primary bronchus is grafted onto the normally inactive medial side, a supernumerary branch is induced. In such induction, the mesenchyme found nearest the normally budding regions is most able to stimulate the epithelium. This response appears to be through cell division, because epithelial mitotic figures are most abundant in terminal buds of the bronchial tree.

The aforementioned inductive influences are specific to pulmonary mesenchyme, however; mesenchyme introduced to developing epithelium from other regions of the body checks or permits only an inferior degree of bronchial development.

An additional factor to consider is that in short-term cultures of dissociated cells from embryonic chick lung, the cells tend to reaggregate into one mass, with epithelial cells in the center. These cells resume function within 48 hours, optimally when the dissociated cells are obtained from 11- to 12-day-old chicks. The effectiveness of this reassociation decreases, however, with the age of tissue from which the dissociated samples are taken. During tissue dissociation, epithelium is combined with varying amounts of mesenchyme. Under these conditions, optimal histogenesis seems to depend more on proper balance between epithelium and mesenchyme than on the time at or in which they are cultured.

As summarized by Arey (1989), the foregoing review of a variety of experimental efforts concerning the developing lung bud clearly indicates: (1) the operation of a true inductive force at the appropriate time in development; (2) the ability of dissociated cells of epithelium and mesenchyme to recognize others of the same kind and to reassociate separately into homogeneous tissue masses; (3) the existence of a chemotactic influence, separate from induction, that attracts separated mesenchyme to migrate toward epithelium; and (4) an ability of such recombined tissues to resume the branching type of tubular bronchial development.

Histochemical Activity

Sorokin and associates (1959) and Sorokin (1961) confirmed that glycogen is deposited in two definite patterns, one in epithelium and another in mesenchyme. The epithelial pattern is thought to be more significant because glycogen is deposited as new cells form. Mesenchymal deposits of glycogen appear to be more important in the carbohydrate metabolism of the fetus. Histochemical studies reveal changes in enzyme activities. For example, alkaline phosphatase, found initially in relation to tracheal bud epithelium, continues to be active during the early development of terminal buds, developing glands, vascular epithelium, and other regions characterized by intense cell proliferation. Succinic dehydrogenase is weakly active in embryonic lung tissue, but its histologic reactivity increases in maturing epithelium from the trachea to bronchioles. Increased cytoplasmic ribonucleoprotein is also reported.

Despite such histochemical observations, experimental evidence confirming causative sequential histochemical events for pulmonary development is still lacking. It is known that the fetus develops at low oxygen tension. Villee (1954) showed, however, that the rate of oxidative metabolism increases with gestation between 7.5 weeks and term. In organ cultures of rat and guinea pig lung, Sorokin (1961) demonstrated that lung tissue is capable of developing to an advanced degree even in the presence of metabolic inhibitors.

On the basis of the preceding histochemical events, Sorokin (1965) put forth the following as yet unsubstantiated scenario, worthy of future investigation and interpretation. Glycogen storage and rapid cell division are promoted during early inductive development. Thus, glycogen is the main form of energy during early development when relatively undifferentiated cells of the bronchial tree are developing. Energy derived from glycolysis is devoted to the synthesis of the cytoplasm and cell division. With subsequent increase in the citric acid cycle, the cytochrome system, and the hexose-monophosphate shunt, cellular differentiation becomes evident in the epithelium, which is now diverted to operating newly emerging cell machinery. Consequently, the rate of cell division decreases. From histochemical localization of succinic dehydrogenase, indophenol oxidase, and glucose-6-phosphate dehydrogenase, one would expect that epithelium would be more affected than mesenchyme by a decrease in initial activity. Therefore, branching would no longer occur in more differentiated locations but would continue in undifferentiated terminal buds. In the more mature regions of the epithelium, glycogen storage decreases at about the time when activity of the three oxidative pathways increases.

ANOMALIES

According to Arey (1989), variations may occur in the size and number of the major pulmonary lobes, but pulmonary agenesis or a reduction in lung size rarely occurs. Variations in the bronchopulmonary segments and in their component bronchi have been observed. Rarely, there is a third true upper lobe with a corresponding epiarterial bronchus that may be found on the left side. As observed in other forms, that is, sheep, pig, and ox, the right epiarterial bronchus may arise directly from the trachea. Infrequently, a cardiac lobe of the lung may occur in man as well as in mammals, including some primates. A variety of more serious complications, pulmonary agenesis and aplasia, sequestration, and tracheoesophageal fistulas, are considered in detail in Chapters 72 and 102.

DEVELOPMENT OF THE PULMONARY VESSELS

Arey (1989) observed that pulmonary blood vessels arise as early as the fifth week of gestation. Pulmonary arteries and veins develop together. Before birth, their development is closely related to growth of the bronchial tree. Hislop and Reid (1972) found that after birth, vascular development occurs rapidly and synchronously with the multiplication of alveoli. Final and complete vascularity of the lungs is said to be complete with the intimate association of capillaries and the extensive and complex surface of the alveoli (Fig. 4–11).

Pulmonary Arteries

In their early development, the pulmonary arteries are associated with the primitive branchial arch system.

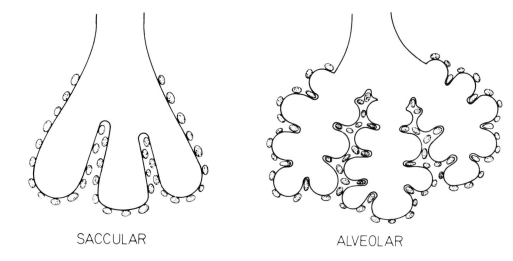

SACCULAR   ALVEOLAR

Fig. 4-11. The manner in which a saccular lung is transformed into an alveolar lung. *Reproduced with permission from* Weibel ER: The Pathway for Oxygen. Cambridge: Harvard University Press, 1984.

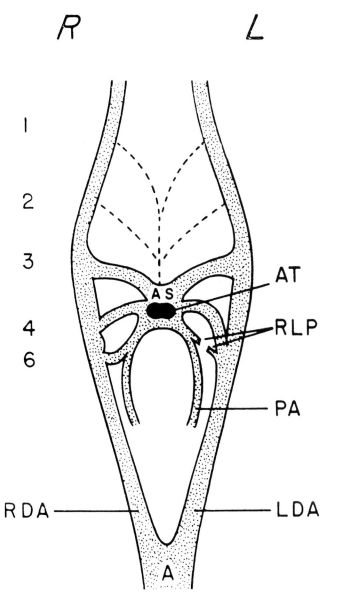

Fig. 4-12. Diagram of the branchial arch arteries connecting the ventral aortic sac (AS) with the right dorsal aorta (RDA) and the left (LDA) in a 5-mm embryo (redrawn after Congdon, 1922). The first and second arches have retrogressed, the third and fourth are complete. On the left, the dorsal and ventral sprouts of the sixth (pulmonary) arch have nearly met (RLP), and on the right side, the arch is complete. From the ventral sprouts, plexiform vessels (PA) pass to the lung bud. A = aorta; AT = aortic trunk opening. *Reproduced by permission from* Hislop A, Reid L: Growth of the Respiratory System — Anatomical Development. *In* Davis JA, Dobbing (eds): Scientific Foundations of Paediatrics. Philadelphia: WB Saunders, 1974, p. 217.

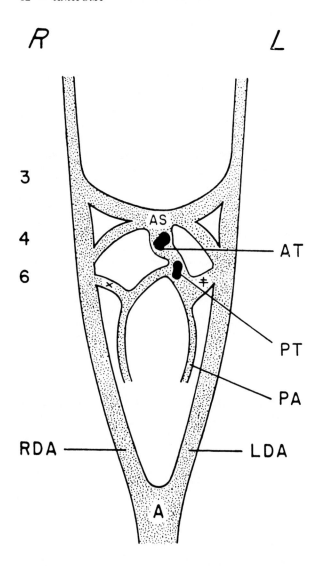

Fig. 4–13. Diagram of the branchial arch arteries in an 11-mm embryo (redrawn after Congdon, 1922). The opening from the aortic sac (AS) is double, the aortic trunk (AT) leads to the third and fourth arches and the pulmonary trunk (PT) leads to the sixth. The left fourth arch is increasing in size more than the right. The left sixth arch (‡) is increasing in size considerably while the dorsal part of the right sixth arch (X) is disappearing. The right dorsal aorta (RDA) between the fourth arch and its junction with the left dorsal aorta (LDA) disappears and blood can only flow to the main dorsal aorta (A) via the fourth and sixth arches on the left. PA = pulmonary artery; A = aorta. *Reproduced with permission from* Hislop A, Reid L: Growth of the Respiratory System — Anatomical Development. *In* Davis JA, Dobbing J (eds): Scientific Foundations of Paediatrics. Philadelphia: WB Saunders, 1974, p. 217.

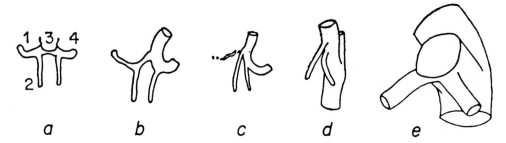

Fig. 4–14. Development of the pulmonary artery and ductus arteriosus (redrawn after Congdon, 1922). Degeneration of the distal or dorsal part of the right arch is apparent (b and c) while the proximal or ventral part is incorporated into the right pulmonary artery. The dorsal part of the left sixth arch (4) becomes larger and remains in connection with the dorsal aorta to form the ductus arteriosus (d and e). The right and left pulmonary approach each other (d) and together join the main pulmonary trunk, which is made up mainly of the ventral part of the left sixth arch. a, 7-mm embryo; b, 11 mm; c, 13 mm; d, 18 mm; e, 43 mm. 1 = right pulmonary arch; 2 = right pulmonary artery; 3 = communication with aortic sac. *Reproduced by permission from* Hislop A, Reid L: Growth of the Respiratory System — Anatomical Development. *In* Davis JA, Dobbing J (eds): Scientific Foundations of Paediatrics. Philadelphia: WB Saunders, 1974, p. 217.

In the 4-mm embryo — 4 weeks — the aortic sac, or truncus arteriosus region, lies just ventral to the third and fourth pharyngeal pouches. The aortic sac gives rise to primitive segmental paired aortic arches that arch between the pharyngeal pouches to join the dorsal aorta. Although six pair of arterial arches form, they form sequentially, and are not all present at any one time. The fifth arches are inconstant, incomplete, and transitory. They disappear shortly after the 11-mm stage without a trace. By the 5-mm stage — 32 days — the first and second arches have retrogressed and the third and fourth are intact. Outgrowths of the sixth arch pass caudally toward angiogenic tissue forming about the lung buds (Fig. 4–12). The sixth arches are rendered complete when sprouts from each dorsal aorta fuse with those originating from the aortic sac. Fusion of these arches occurs first on the right side and then on the left (Fig. 4–13). The right arch then becomes thinner and disappears; the left arch is destined to form the pulmonary artery. By the 11-mm stage, the aortic sac is divided into aortic and pulmonary streams by partitioning of the aortic sac and primitive bulbs so that the aortic trunk is continuous with the third and fourth arches on the left side and the pulmonary artery opens into the left sixth arch (see Fig. 4–13). The left sixth arch enlarges while the right sixth arch disappears. The right dorsal aorta then disappears between the fourth arch and its union with the left dorsal aorta, leaving the main flow of blood to the main dorsal aorta via the fourth and sixth arches on the left side.

In the development of the pulmonary artery and ductus arteriosus, the distal — dorsal — part of the right arch degenerates, while the proximal — ventral — part is incorporated into the right pulmonary artery. Meanwhile, the dorsal part of the left sixth arch enlarges to form the ductus arteriosus. Subsequently, the right and left pulmonary arteries approach each other and join the main pulmonary trunk, which is forming mainly from the ventral part of the left sixth arch (Fig. 4–14).

Bronchial Arteries

In embryos of 10 to 11 mm, the lung buds are supplied by paired segmental branches arising from the dorsal aorta superior to the celiac arteries. These communications disappear, however, so that bronchial arteries arise from the aorta between weeks 9 and 12 as noted by Boyden (1970).

Pulmonary Veins

As presented by Neil (1956), the development of pulmonary veins is heralded by the appearance of a rich collection of angioblasts and vascular channels around the developing lung buds and a small endothelial evagination growing toward the lung bud from the superior margin of the left atrium as the primordium of the pulmonary vein (Fig. 4–15). On days 28 to 30, the evagination becomes canalized and connects with the vascular plexus (Fig. 4–16). During days 30 to 32 — 7 to 8 mm, the common pulmonary vein drains

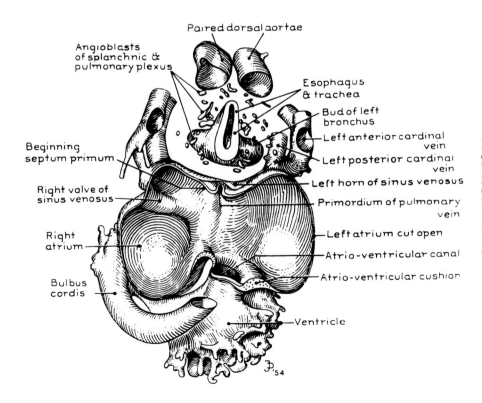

Fig. 4–15. Anterosuperior view of the heart, great vessels, and lung bud; human embryo of Horizon XIII (4 mm crown-rump length), Carnegie No. 836. ×50. In the heart, the endocardium only is represented. *Reproduced with permission from* Neil CA: Development of the pulmonary veins. Pediatrics *18*:882, 1956.

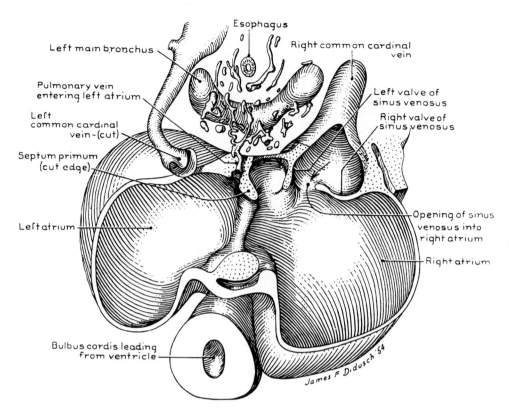

Esophagus

Left main bronchus

Right common cardinal vein

Pulmonary vein entering left atrium

Left valve of sinus venosus

Right valve of sinus venosus

Left common cardinal vein-(cut)

Septum primum (cut edge)

Left atrium

Opening of sinus venosus into right atrium

Right atrium

Bulbus cordis leading from ventricle

James F. Didusch '54

Fig. 4–16. Posteroinferior view of the heart; human embryo of Horizon XV (6 mm crown-rump length), Carnegie No. 7598. ×25. *Reproduced with permission from* Neil CA: Development of the pulmonary veins. Pediatrics *18*:882, 1956.

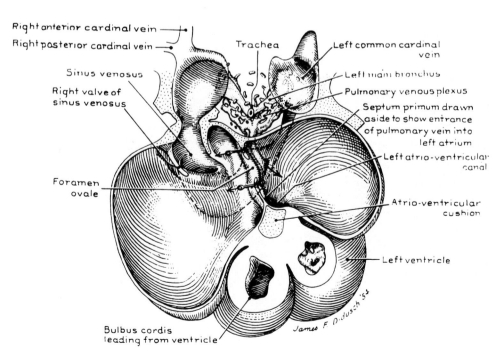

Right anterior cardinal vein

Right posterior cardinal vein

Trachea

Left common cardinal vein

Sinus venosus

Left main bronchus

Right valve of sinus venosus

Pulmonary venous plexus

Septum primum drawn aside to show entrance of pulmonary vein into left atrium

Left atrio-ventricular canal

Foramen ovale

Atrio-ventricular cushion

Left ventricle

Bulbus cordis leading from ventricle

James F. Didusch '54

Fig. 4–17. Posteroinferior view of the heart; human embryo of Horizon XV (7 mm crown-rump length), Carnegie No. 721. ×25. *Reproduced with permission from* Neil CA: Development of the pulmonary veins. Pediatrics *18*:882, 1956.

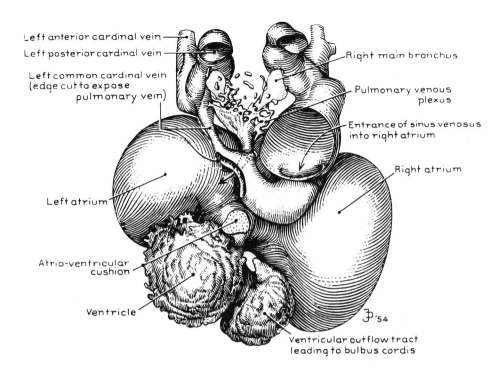

Left anterior cardinal vein

Left posterior cardinal vein

Left common cardinal vein
(edge cut to expose
pulmonary vein)

Left atrium

Atrio-ventricular
cushion

Ventricle

Right main bronchus

Pulmonary venous
plexus

Entrance of sinus venosus
into right atrium

Right atrium

Ventricular outflow tract
leading to bulbus cordis

Fig. 4–18. Anterosuperior view of the heart, same embryo as in Figure 4–17. ×25. *Reproduced with permission from* Neil CA: Development of the pulmonary veins. Pediatrics *18:* 882, 1956.

the pulmonary plexus into the left atrium, just caudal to the entry of the sinus venosus (Figs. 4–17, 4–18). Subsequently, the common pulmonary vein is absorbed into the left atrium along with its tributary veins.

NERVE SUPPLY TO THE LUNGS

As reported by Streeter (1912a, b), the essential features of the sympathetic and parasympathetic innervation of the lungs are established by 6 weeks gestation. Sympathetic ganglia destined for the lungs arise segmentally from neural crest cells on each side of the neural tube at upper thoracic levels. Neuroblast precursors of preganglionic neurons originate from the intermediolateral cell column of spinal segmental levels T1 to T4 and migrate peripherally toward segmental ganglia, where they connect with neuroblasts within the ganglia. With maturation, neuroblasts within the ganglia follow the developing bronchial system as postganglionic sympathetic neurons of the pulmonary plexus.

Neuroblasts in the vagal level of the brain stem migrate peripherally through greater distances to reach the developing lung bud. Still others migrate further with supporting sheath cells to form ganglia within the pulmonary plexus and along the bronchial tree. With maturation and formation of synapses within the ganglia, the pre- and postganglionic components of the parasympathetic supply to the lungs are completed.

REFERENCES

Alcorn D, et al: Morphological effects of chronic tracheal ligation and drainage in the fetal lamb lung. J Anat *123:*649, 1977.

Arey LB: Embryology of the lungs and esophagus. *In* Shields TW (ed): General Thoracic Surgery. 3rd Ed. Philadelphia: Lea & Febiger, 1989, p. 8.

Baier RO, et al: The effects of continuous distending airway pressure under various background concentrations of oxygen, high frequency oscillatory ventilation, and umbilical cord occlusion on fetal breathing and behavior in sheep. Proceedings of the Society for the Study of Fetal Physiology, Cairns, Australia, 1988, p. 26.

Bland RD: Formation of fetal lung liquid and its removal near birth. In Poplin RH, Fox WW (eds): Fetal and Neonatal Physiology. Vol. 1. Philadelphia: WB Saunders, 1992, pp. 782-789.

Boddy K, Dawes GS: Fetal breathing. Br Med Bull *31:*3, 1975.

Boyden EA, Tompsett DH: The changing patterns in the developing lung of infants. Acta Anat *61:*164, 1965.

Boyden EA: Notes on development of the lung in infancy and early childhood. Am J Anat *121:*749, 1967.

Boyden EA: The pattern of the terminal air spaces in a premature infant of 30-32 weeks that lived nineteen and a quarter hours. Am J Anat *126:*31, 1969.

Boyden EA: The developing bronchial arteries in a fetus of the twelfth week. Am J Anat *129:*357, 1970.

Boyden EA: The structure of the pulmonary acinus in a child of six years and eight months. Am J Anat *132:*275, 1971.

Boyden EA: The mode of origin of pulmonary acini and respiratory bronchioles in the fetal lung. Am J Anat *141:*317, 1974.

Boyden EA: The development of the lung in the pigtail monkey (*Macaca nomestrina L.*) Anat Rec *186:*15, 1976.

Bucher U, Reid L: Development of the intrasegmental bronchial tree. Thorax *16:*207, 1961a.

Bucher U, Reid L: Development of the mucous-secreting elements in the human lung. Thorax *16:*219, 1961b.

Buckingham S, Avery ME: Time of appearance of lung surfactant in the foetal mouse. Nature *193:*688, 1962.

Burri PH, Weibel ER: Funktionelle Aspekte der Lungenmorphologie. *In* Rontgendiagnostik der Lunge: Aktuelle Probleme der Rontgendiagnostik. 2nd Ed. (Fuchs WA, Voegli E, eds). Berne: Huber, 1973, pp. 1-17.

Campiche MA, et al: An electron microscope study of the fetal development of human lung. Pediatrics *32:*976, 1963.

Clements JA: Surface tension of lung extracts. Proc Soc Exp Biol Med *95:*170, 1957.

Clements JA: Surface phenomena in relation to pulmonary function. Physiologist 5:11, 1962.

Congdon ED: Transformations of the aortic arch system during the development of the human embryo. Contrib Carnegie Inst 14:47, 1922.

Commission on Embryological Terminology (1970)

Dameron FL: Etude experimental de l'organogenese de poumon: Nature et specificite des interactions epithelio-mesench-mateuses. J Embryol Exp Morphol 20:151, 1968.

Dawes GS, et al: Respiratory movements and paradoxical sleep in the fetal lamb. J Physiol 210:47P 1970.

Hislop A, Reid L: Intrapulmonary arterial development during fetal life-branching pattern and structure. J Anat 113:35, 1972.

Hislop A, Reid L: Development of the acinus in the human lung. Thorax 29:90, 1974.

Hughes GM: Evolution between air and water. In De Reuck Avs, Potter R (eds): Ciba Foundation Symposium: Development of The Lung. Boston: Little, Brown and Co., 1967, pp. 64-81.

Jansen AH, et al: Effects of carotid chemoreceptors denervation on breathing in utero and after birth. J Appl Physiol 51:630, 1981.

Jansen AH: Influence of sleep state on the response to hypercapnia in fetal lambs. Respir Physiol 48:125, 1982.

Jeffrey PK, Reid LM: Ultrastructure of airway epithelium and submucosal gland during development. In Hodson WA (ed): Development of the Lung. New York: Marcell Dekker, 1977, pp. 87-134.

Jones AW, Radnor CJP: The development of the chick tertiary bronchus. II. The origin of the surface lining system. J Anat 113:325, 1972.

Krogh A: On the cutaneous and pulmonary respiration of the frog: a contribution to the theory of gas exchange between the blood and the atmosphere. Skand Arch Physiol Leipz 15:328, 1904.

Loosli CG, Baker RF: The human lung: Microscopic structure and diffusion. In De Ruch AVS, O'Connor J (eds): Ciba Foundation Symposium: Pulmonary Structure and Function. London: Churchill, 1962, pp. 194-204.

Loosli CG, Hung SS: Development of pulmonary innervation. In Hodson WA (ed): Development of the Lung. New York: Marcel Dekker, 1977, pp. 269-306.

Loosli CG, Potter EL: Pre- and postnatal development of the human lungs. Am Rev Respir Dis 80 (Part 2): 5, 1959.

Low FN: The pulmonary alveolar epithelium of laboratory animals and man. Anat Rec 117:241, 1953.

Macklin CC: The pulmonary alveolar cells and the pneumocytes. Lancet 1:1099, 1954.

Meyrick B, Reid LM: Ultrastructure of airway epithelium and submucosal gland during development. In Hodson WA (ed): Development of the Lung. New York: Marcel Dekker, 1977, pp. 87-134.

Moss IR, Scarpelli EM: Generation and regulation of breathing in utero: Fetal response test. J Appl Physiol 47:527, 1979.

Moore LL: The Developing Human. 4th Ed. Philadelphia: WB Saunders, 1988, pp. 208-210.

Neil CA: Development of the pulmonary veins. Pediatrics 18:880, 1956.

Nomina Anatomica. 5th Ed. Baltimore: Williams & Wilkins, 1983, p. E38.

O'Rahilly R, Boyden EA: The timing and sequence of events in the development of the human respiratory system during the embryonic period proper. Z Anat Entwicklungsgesh 141:237, 1961.

Patrick J, et al: Patterns of human fetal breathing during the last ten weeks of pregnancy. Obstet Gynecol 56:24, 1980.

Pattle RE: Properties, function, and origin of the alveolar lining layer. Proc R Soc Lond [Biol] 148:217, 1958.

Pattle RE, Hopkinson DAW: Lung lining in bird, reptile, and amphibia. Nature 200:894, 1963.

Pattle RE: The development of the fetal lung. In Wohlstenholme EGW, O'Connor M (eds): Fetal Autonomy. Ciba Foundation Symposium. London: Churchill, 1969, pp. 132-144.

Poczopko P: Further investigations on the cutaneous vasomotor reflexes in the edible frog in connection with the problem of regulation of the cutaneous respiration in frogs. Zool Polaniaio 8:161, 1957 (1958).

Polin RA, Fox WW: Fetal and Neonatal Physiology. Vol. 2. Philadelphia: WB Saunders, 1992.

Rigatto H, et al: The effect of total peripheral chemodenervation on fetal breathing and on the establishment of breathing at birth. Proceedings of the International Symposium on Fetal and Neonatal Development, Oxford, 1987.

Rigatto H, et al: Effect of increased arterial CO_2 on fetal breathing and behavior in sheep. J Appl Physiol 65:2544, 1988.

Rigatto H: Control of breathing in fetal life and onset and control of breathing in the neonate. In Polin RH, Fox WW (eds): Fetal and Neonatal Physiology. Vol. 1. Philadelphia: WB Saunders, 1992.

Rudnick D: Developmental capacities of the chick lung in chorioallantoic grafts. J Exp Zool 66:125, 1933.

Sampaolo G, Sampaolo CL: Indagini spermantle sullo sviluppo del polomone embrionale (pollo e coniglio). Quad Anat Pratl 17:1, 1961.

Short RH: Alveolar epithelium in relation to the growth of the lungs. Philos Trans R Soc Lond [Biol] 235:35, 1950.

Sorokin SP, Padykula HA, Herman F: Comparative histochemical patterns in developing lungs. Dev Biol 1:125, 1959.

Sorokin SP: A study of organ cultures of mammalian lungs. Dev Biol 3:60, 1961.

Sorokin SP: Recent work on developing lungs. In DeHaan RL, Ursprung H (eds): Organogenesis. New York: Holt, Rinehardt, and Winston, 1965.

Streeter GL: Sympathetic nervous system. In Keibel F, Mall JB (eds): Manual of Human Embryology. Vol. 2. Philadelphia: Lippincott, 1912a, pp. 144-156.

Streeter GL: The histogenesis of nervous tissue. In Keibel F, Mall JB (eds): Manual of Human Embryology. Vol. 2. Philadelphia, Lippincott, 1912b, pp. 1-28.

Taeusch, HW, Avery ME: Development of the lung. In Hodson WA (ed): Lung Biology and Health and Disease. Vol. 6. New York: Marcel Dekker, 1977.

Towers B: The fetal and neonatal lung. In Assali NS: Biology of Gestation. Vol. 2. New York: Academic Press, 1968, pp. 189–223.

Tyler WS, Pangborn J: Laminated membrane surface and osmophilic inclusion in avian lung epithelium. J Cell Biol 20:157, 1964.

Van Golde LMG, Batenburg JJ, Robertson B: The pulmonary surfactant system: Biochemical aspects and functional significance. Physiol Rev 68:374, 1988.

Villee CH: The intermediary metabolism of human fetal tissue. Cold Spring Harbor Symp Quant Biol 19:186, 1954.

Vinegar A, Hutchison VH: Pulmonary and cutaneous gas exchange in the green frog Rana clamitans. Zoologica (New York) 50:47, 1965.

Weibel ER: The Pathway for Oxygen. Cambridge: Harvard University Press, 1984.

Whitford WG, Hutchison VH: Cutaneous and pulmonary gas exchange in the spotted salamander, Amblystoma maculatum. Biol Bull Woods Hole Marine Biol Station 124:344, 1963.

CHAPTER 5

ULTRASTRUCTURE AND MORPHOMETRY OF THE HUMAN LUNG

Peter H. Burri, Joan Gil, and Ewald R. Weibel

ORGANIZATION OF THE LUNG

The application of electron microscopy and of quantitative methods in morphology — morphometry — has widened the general understanding of lung structure and has set the course for a more functional approach to the study of pulmonary architecture.

It cannot be the aim of this chapter, however, to cover all aspects of lung microanatomy; in this respect, the reader is referred to the specialized literature. We would rather present the morphologic and quantitative background needed to understand the functioning of the gas exchange apparatus.

The lung is composed of three phases: air, tissue, and blood. The tissue forms a complete barrier between air and blood; it is a stable structural framework, whereas air and blood are continuously exchanged. In describing the ultrastructure of the lung, we emphasize the specializations of the tissue in forming boundary spaces for air and blood. Morphometry deals with the quantitative relations among these three phases.

From the functional point of view, the organization of the lung may be defined in relation to the hierarchy of airways and blood vessels, from the trachea down to alveoli, or from the main stem of the pulmonary artery through the capillary network to the pulmonary veins entering the left atrium.

All of this is jointly considered in the scheme of Figure 5–1. Besides showing the three phases, the diagram introduces the three major functional zones of the lung; first, the *conductive zone* consisting of air channels and blood vessels, the function of which is to guide and distribute air and blood into the peripheral lung units; second, the *respiratory zone* comprised of alveoli and capillaries; and third, the *intermediate* or *transitory zone* containing elements of both.

FINE STRUCTURE OF THE LUNG

Fine Structure of Conducting Airways

The conducting airways are a system of tubes, which multiply toward the periphery by division according to the principle of irregular dichotomy. From the trachea to bronchi to bronchioles, the structure of the airway gradually changes. What is common to all is the general scheme of a three-layered wall made of a *mucosa*, a *muscle layer*, and a *connective tissue sheath* (Fig. 5–2), and the presence of a typical ciliated epithelium, which is described first.

The Lining Epithelium of Conductive Airways

The inspired air must be humidified and warmed before it reaches the delicate gas-exchange area; furthermore, air pollutants and dust, as well as airborne microorganisms, must be removed. Although the upper

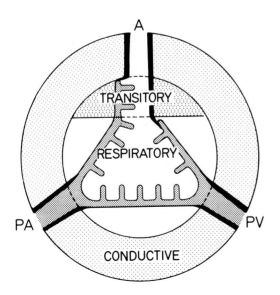

Fig. 5–1. Schematic representation of lung zones. A = airways, PA = pulmonary artery, PV = pulmonary vein.

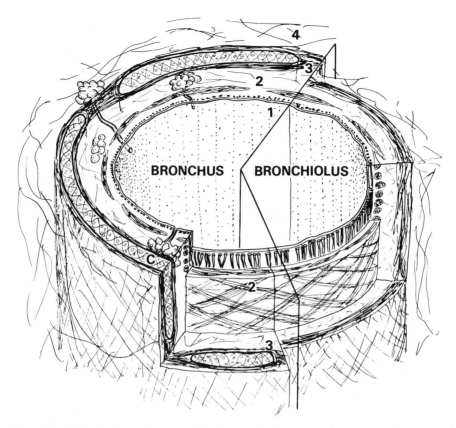

Fig. 5–2. Structure of bronchi and bronchioles. 1, Mucosa with epithelium and elastic fibers; 2, smooth muscle layer; 3, fibrous layer contains cartilage (C) in the bronchi; 4, peribronchial sheath of loose connective tissue.

respiratory tract — in particular the nasal portion — is especially designed for these functions, the respiratory epithelium (Fig. 5–3) of all conducting airways shows special features for the handling of airborne particles. It is a ciliated pseudostratified columnar epithelium with numerous scattered goblet cells. Ciliated cells occur from the trachea down to the last respiratory bronchiole, but their height decreases with the reduction of the airway diameter; ciliated cells of the trachea are columnar (Fig. 5–4), whereas those of the respiratory bronchioles are cuboidal (Fig. 5–5). The frequency of goblet cells also decreases toward the periphery; in bronchioles, they are replaced by Clara cells (Fig. 5–5), whose secretory role is not yet clear. They have, however, been shown to be the source of some pulmonary surfactant apoproteins, as reported by Plopper and co-workers (1991). Cytologic, kinetic, and histochemical studies by Breeze and Wheeldon (1977), Jeffery and Reid (1977), Jeffery (1983), and Spicer (1983) and St. George (1985) and their co-workers have provided insights into the cell types of the airway epithelium of various species, including man. Great emphasis is also being put on the investigation of the endocrine cells interspersed in the epithelium, often called Feyrter, Kulchitsky, APUD — *a*mine *p*recursor *u*ptake and *d*ecarboxylation — or small granule cells. These endocrine cells are present in the respiratory tract of all vertebrate species investigated so far. Lauweryns and Cokelaere (1973) found them thinly scattered along the airways, either isolated or clustered in neuroepithelial bodies. Suspected to be involved in the secretion of vasoactive substances in the lung, they most likely represent, according to Sorokin and co-workers (1983), a heterogeneous population of cells. The formation of neuroepithelial bodies in the developing hamster lung has been investigated by Hoyt and co-workers (1990). From labeling studies with ^{3}H-thymidine, the authors conclude that the pulmonary endocrine epithelial cells are derived from the endoderm and not from the neural crest.

The frequently found basal cells represent a proliferative pool of undifferentiated cells, which are thought to replace the overlying cells upon differentiation and maturation. Less common are the brush cells and migratory cells. Finally, one should mention the occurrence of naked nerve endings between individual cells, more frequently in the trachea and large bronchi. They are thought to be irritant receptors.

Figure 5–3 shows a schematic representation of a portion of the respiratory epithelium of a bronchus. The function of this epithelium is to capture airborne particles in a sticky mucous layer and to remove them efficiently from the lung. For this purpose, cilia show a synchronized rhythmic beat within a thin layer of fluid

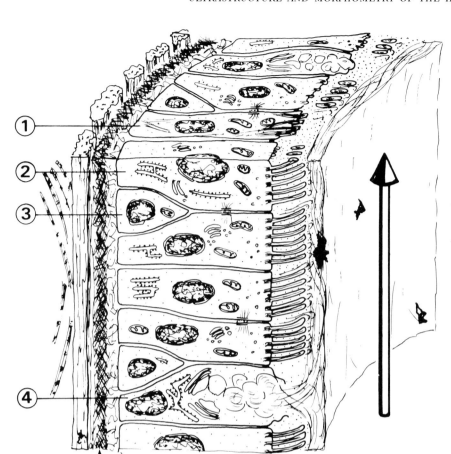

Fig. 5–3. Pseudostratified epithelium of bronchus with brush (1), ciliated (2), basal (3), and goblet cells (4). The cilia beat in a serous fluid that is topped by a mucous layer secreted partly by goblet cells. A strong basement membrane (BM) and a layer of longitudinal elastic fibers form the basis of the epithelium.

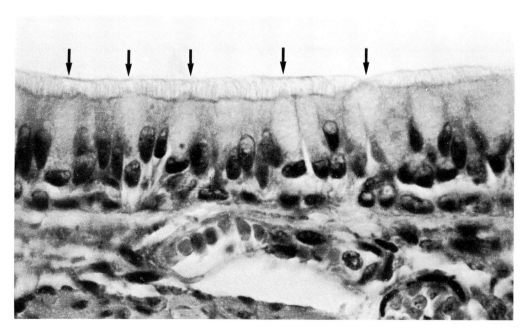

Fig. 5–4. Pseudostratified epithelium from bronchus. Note goblet cells (arrows). ×600.

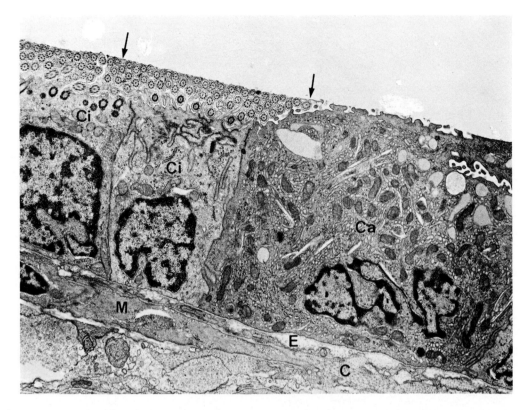

Fig. 5–5. Electron micrograph of bronchiolar wall with simple cuboidal epithelium made up of ciliated cells (Ci) and Clara cells (Ca). In place of the mucous layer is a fine osmiophilic film (arrows) at the air-liquid interface. A smooth muscle cell (M) and collagenous (C) and elastic (E) fibers are seen in the subepithelial tissue. Rat lung fixed by vascular perfusion. ×9200.

of low viscosity. On top, a blanket of mucus is moved in the direction of the pharynx, carrying along intercepted particles. This cleaning mechanism can be compared with a conveyor belt and is often called the mucociliary escalator. The mechanism of mucus propulsion has been described in detail by Sleigh (1991). The mucous layer is secreted onto the epithelial surface by goblet cells and by seromucous glands located in the walls of trachea and bronchi (Fig. 5–2). The small bronchioles are most likely devoid of mucus, as their wall contains neither goblet cells nor glands. Their surface is formed by a fluid layer of low viscosity that is sometimes topped by a thin osmiophilic film (Gil and Weibel, 1971). Finally, the presence in the bronchial secretion of several humoral agents, which would protect the airways against infections, has been reported.

Trachea and Bronchi

Trachea and bronchi are characterized by the presence of cartilage within the fibrous sheath of their walls (Fig. 5–2). In the trachea and stem bronchi, the cartilage is in the form of incomplete rings; in the trachea, these cover the ventral and lateral aspects, whereas the dorsal wall contains a strong layer of transverse smooth muscle. After about the second or third generation, these rings are gradually replaced by irregular cartilage plates and a layer of smooth muscle appears between mucosa and cartilage.

All conducting airways are surrounded by an external, loose connective tissue sheath (Fig. 5–2), which is continuous with the other connective elements of the lung. It is a structure of considerable physiologic significance, as it contains bronchial vessels, to supply the bronchial wall with blood from the systemic circulation, as well as nerves and lymphatic vessels. Only a small part of the arterial bronchial flow, in some species as little as 25%, is drained by the bronchial veins. Most of it goes into the peribronchial venous plexus and from there into the pulmonary veins forming a small right-to-left shunt. The bronchus is usually accompanied by a branch of the pulmonary artery, which is enveloped by connective tissue continuous with the peribronchial sheath.

Lymphatic vessels contained in these peribronchial and perivascular sheaths, as well as in the subpleural and septal connective tissue, constitute the main drainage path for the interstitial fluid.

Bronchioles

A bronchiole is an airway devoid of cartilage and seromucous glands; goblet cells are rare. Because airway structure does not change abruptly, either seromucous glands or goblet cells may still be present in transitional zones. Bronchioles are rather small conducting airways, measuring about 1 mm or less in diameter. Their added cross-sectional area is such, however, that they are not supposed to contribute substantially to the flow resistance of the airways in the normally breathing healthy individual. Their walls are generally thin and molded into the surrounding parenchyma. They are supplied with blood from the lesser circulation, rather than from bronchial arteries. The bronchiolar mucosa is lined by a simple cuboidal epithelium (Fig. 5–5) composed of ciliated cells and of Clara cells, which have the characteristic features of secreting cells: their cytoplasm contains many mitochondria, rough and smooth endoplasmic reticulum, and typical membrane-bounded granules of low electron density that are considered storage vacuoles for a secretory product of still unknown composition. These cells seem to take the place of goblet cells of larger airways.

In bronchioles, the *smooth muscle cells* form a well-developed, relatively thick layer arranged in a geodesic network, capable of narrowing the airway.

Resistance to Airflow in Conducting Airways

The partition of airflow resistance between large and small airways both in health and disease had been controversial. It is universally accepted that, in the healthy lung, the major site of resistance is the large, central airways, whereas the bronchioles contribute less than 20%, but it is important to know that pathologic increases of resistance always occur in the bronchiolar region. Airflow in the trachea is turbulent, in the bronchioles laminar. In between, it is often referred to as transitional, implying an admixture of both, although experimental studies are difficult to perform. One of the major contributions to the understanding of the pathophysiology of emphysema was the clarification of the mechanisms of early airway closure. A priori, examination of the bronchiolar anatomy immediately reveals the factors that account for their active and passive narrowing: smooth muscle, compression by neighboring parenchyma during inflation, and internal surface tension. The elements that counteract the above and act to cause bronchiolar dilatation are less evident, however, made possible only by the radial insertion of alveolar walls in their periphery and by the principle of mechanical interdependence. The integrity of alveolar walls is therefore essential in keeping bronchioles open during deflation. In conditions like emphysema, in which alveolar walls are lost, the loss of bronchiolar support causes a calamitous early collapse of small bronchioles at the onset of expiration, with trapping of air in all areas of the parenchyma located behind the obstruction.

Fine Structure of Transitory Airways

Respiratory Bronchioles

The last generation of exclusively conducting bronchioles is the terminal bronchioles. These branch to form about three generations of respiratory bronchioles (see Fig. 5–22), which have essentially the same structure as other bronchioles except that, here and there and increasingly toward the periphery, the continuity of their wall is interrupted by areas of typical gas-exchanging tissue. Contrary to common textbook descriptions, the cuboidal epithelial cells of respiratory bronchioles are in most cases ciliated; short cilia can even be demonstrated in close proximity to alveoli.

Alveolar Ducts and Sacs

The mammalian airways form a blind-ending system. Dichotomy as a branching pattern can be demonstrated up to the last ranks of the airway system, the alveolar ducts and alveolar sacs (see Fig. 5–22). These structures differ from the bronchioles described previously in that they lack a proper wall; instead, their wall is formed by the openings of alveoli (Fig. 5–6); their epithelial lining is nothing more than extensions of squamous alveolar epithelial cells. It is generally admitted that three generations of alveolar ducts immediately follow the last respiratory bronchioles. Finally, the last ducts give rise to two alveolar sacs. An alveolar sac represents the blind end of the airway branching system (see Fig. 5–22).

Fine Structure of the Gas-Exchange Region

In the respiratory zone of the lung, the blood is spread in capillaries in the walls of the alveoli. The air-blood contact becomes intimate and gas exchange can take place.

The Alveoli

Alveoli are small pouches placed in groups around respiratory bronchioles, alveolar ducts, and alveolar sacs. They are polyhedral structures lacking one side — the mouth, which opens into the airways — and they have been compared with the cells of a honeycomb (Fig. 5–6) or with the air bubbles in a foam. A polygonal shape in general is economical, for it allows a close packing of the alveoli. Haefeli-Bleur's and one of our (E.R.W.) (1987) studies on human pulmonary acini revealed that the shape of alveoli is not simple and that often an "alveolus" appears like a cluster of several connected pouches, as in Figure 5–6B. Furthermore, alveolar shape also depends on the degree of lung inflation, according to one of us (J.G.) and co-workers (1979). Only in fully inflated lungs has the alveolar configuration some similarity with the cells of a honeycomb. At lower inflation degrees, alveoli are often cup-like.

The alveolar wall is always common to two adjacent alveoli and is called the alveolar or interalveolar septum (Fig. 5–6B). The most conspicuous feature of the septum is a single but dense network of capillaries, which is shown in Figure 5–7 in face view. Sometimes, the septa are interrupted by pores of Kohn, which provide a path of communication between adjoining alveoli. The septa also contain a skeleton of connective tissue fibers that is specially well developed around the mouth of alveoli, where it forms a polygonal ring (see Fig. 5–6) and may contain smooth muscle fibers. The collagenous and elastic fibrous elements form a three-dimensional continuum that extends from the pleura to the hilus. This continuum assures transmission of chest

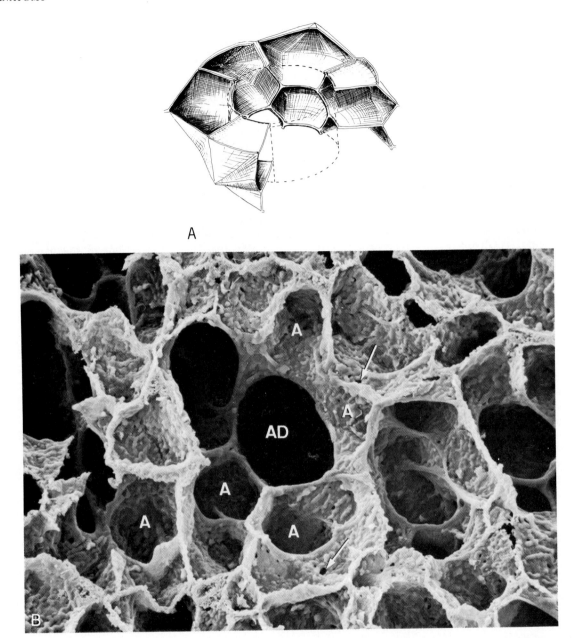

A

B

Fig. 5–6. *A*, Schematic representation of arrangement of alveoli around the alveolar duct. *Reproduced with permission from* Weibel, E.R.: Morphometry of the Human Lung. Heidelberg: Springer, 1963, p. 57. *B*, Scanning electron micrograph of human lung. ×150. AD = alveolar duct; A = alveoli; arrows point to pores of Kohn.

and diaphragmatic movements into the deeper regions of the lung, but it contributes only a smaller part to the retractive force of the lung, the major part being due to surface forces. We (E.R.W. and J.G.) (1977) and one of us (E.R.W.) (1984) discussed the arrangement of the connective tissue in detail.

The Alveolocapillary Tissue Barrier

Figure 5–8 shows a section of a small portion of an interalveolar septum with a capillary. The septum is lined on both sides by alveolar epithelial cells, which, in this instance, are thin. The capillary is also lined by a single squamous cell layer, the endothelium. Together

with the intercalated connective tissue, these two cell layers constitute the alveolocapillary tissue barrier, which is the structure separating air and blood in the pulmonary gas-exchange region. It is supplemented by an extremely thin extracellular lining layer that contains macrophages (Figs. 5–9, 5–10). The morphometric characteristics of the cell population that constitutes this tissue barrier in the human lung are shown in Table 5–1.

Epithelium. The epithelium of the alveoli is continuous, although its thickness in places only reaches 0.1 to 0.3 µm, which is at the limit of resolution of the light microscope. The study by Low

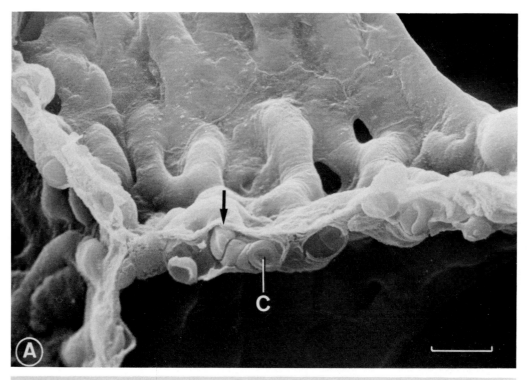

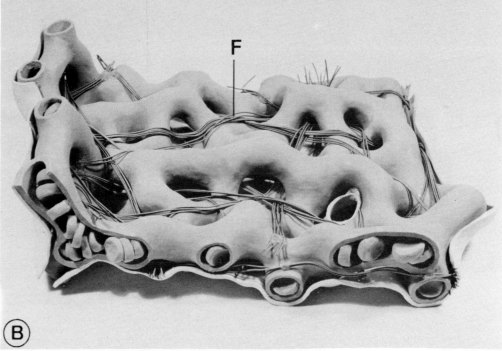

Fig. 5–7. Capillaries in the alveolar wall of human lung are shown in a scanning electron micrograph *(A)* and in a model *(B)*. Note thin tissue barrier separating air and blood (arrow) and fibers (F) interwoven with capillary network (C). Scale marker = 10 μm. *Reproduced with permission from* Weibel ER: The Pathway for Oxygen. Cambridge Harvard University Press, 1984.

(1952) brought the first conclusive evidence for an uninterrupted epithelial lining of alveoli. It consists of the following cell types (see Table 5–1).

Alveolar epithelial cells type I (Fig. 5–11), also called squamous cells, send out broad, thin cytoplas-

mic extensions. Although they are some 30 to 40% less numerous than the type II cells, they cover between 92 and 95% of the total alveolar surface. The nuclei lie in depressions between two capillaries. These cells are poor in organelles — such as mitochondria or endo-

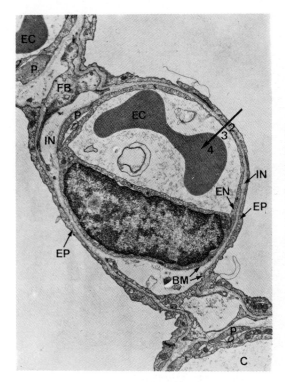

Fig. 5–8. Electron micrograph of alveolar capillary (C) from monkey lung with erythrocyte (EC). Note endothelial cell lining of capillary (EN), processes of pericytes (P) and the thin extensions of squamous alveolar epithelial cells (EP) covering the alveolar surface. The interstitial space (IN) is bounded by two basement membranes (BM) and contains some fibroblast processes (FB) as well as a few connective tissue fibrils. This lung was fixed by instillation of fixative into airways resulting in a loss of the surface lining layer; hence only parts 2 (tissue barrier), 3 (blood plasma), and 4 (erythrocyte) of the gas exchange pathway are preserved. ×8600. *Reproduced with permission from* Weibel ER: Morphometric estimation of pulmonary diffusion capacity. I. Model and method. Respir Physiol *11*:54, 1970/71.

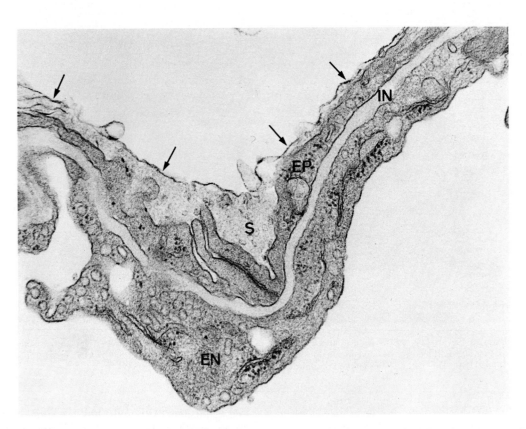

Fig. 5–9. Air-blood barrier of rat lung fixed by vascular perfusion to preserve surface lining layer (S) made up of base layer and osmiophilic surface film (arrows). IN = interstitial space; EP = squamous alveolar epithelial cells; EN = endothelial cell lining of capillary. ×38,700: *Reproduced with permission from* Weibel ER: Morphometric estimation of pulmonary diffusion capacity. I. Model and method. Respir Physiol *11*:54, 1970/71.

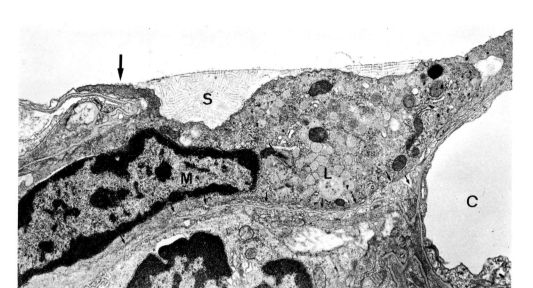

Fig. 5–10. Alveolar macrophage (M) with pseudopods and groups of lysosomal vesicles (L) in cytoplasm submerged beneath surface lining layer (S) and closely stuck to the alveolar epithelium (arrows). The base-layer of the surface lining layer contains so-called tubular myelin figures. The capillary (C) is empty because of fixation by vascular perfusion. ×10,500. *Reproduced with permission from* Gil J: Ultrastructure of lung fixed under physiologically defined conditions. Arch Intern Med *127*:896, 1971.

plasmic reticulum — which are confined to the peri-nuclear cytoplasm, whereas the cytoplasmic extensions essentially contain only pinocytotic vesicles. Crapo and associates (1982) found that in man, a single type I cell covers some 5000 μm² of the alveolar surface, on the average.

Alveolar cells type II are cuboidal (Fig. 5–12). These cells have also been called granular pneumocytes, septal cells, alveolar cells, and great alveolar cells, although they are smaller than type I cells. They have no cytoplasmic extensions and typically are in niches between capillaries of the alveolar septum. Their free surface is covered by somewhat irregular microvilli. The cells occupy from 5 to 8% of the alveolar surface and form junctional complexes with neighboring alveolar cells type I. Compared with alveolar cells type I, the granular pneumocyte is rich in mitochondria, endoplasmic reticulum, Golgi apparatus, and multivesicular bodies. Their most distinctive morphologic feature, however, is the presence of lamellar osmiophilic inclu-

sions — "lamellated bodies" — which are now known to be the sites of storage of the surface-active phospholipids. At the light microscopic level, alveolar cells type II may be easily confounded with macrophages.

A third pneumocyte, the brush cell, was described by Meyrick and Reid (1968). In the rat, this cell can be found in terminal bronchioles; it is, however, rare in the gas-exchange zone. The brush cell is characterized by a spray of rather thick and regular cylindric microvilli at the surface and by thick bundles of microfibrils in the cytoplasm. Brush cells are large, but only a small part of their membrane reaches the epithelial surface. Similar cells occur in larger airway epithelia and in other organs also; their significance is still obscure.

Alveolar macrophages — dust cells — are the cells of the alveolar lining layer (see Fig. 5–11). They are large cells exhibiting many vacuolar inclusions and lysosomes. Most of their phagosomes are filled with dark, lipid-rich inclusions. In their functional location, they are closely apposed to the alveolar epithelial surface

Table 5–1. Morphometric Characteristics of Cell Population in the Human Alveolar Septal Tissue

| | Cell Number | | Average Cell | |
	Absolute n × 10⁹	Relative %	Volume μm³	Apical Surface μm²
Pneumocytes I	19	8.3	1,763	5,098
Pneumocytes II	37	15.9	889	183
Endothelial cells	68	30.2	632	1,353
Interstitial cells	84	36.1	637	—
Macrophages	23	9.4	2,491	—

After Crapo JD, et al: Cell numbers and cell characteristics of the normal human lung. Am Rev Respir Dis *126*:332, 1982.

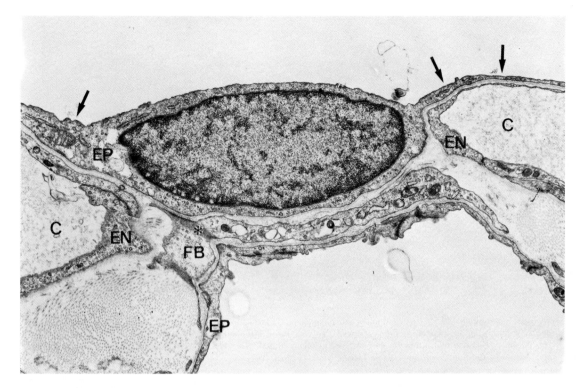

Fig. 5–11. Type I alveolar cell with thin cytoplasmic extensions (arrows). C=alveolar capillary; EP=squamous alveolar epithelial cells; EN=endothelial cell lining of capillary; FB=fibroblast process with an intracytoplasmic bundle of contractile filaments (*). ×8600.

and are submersed under the surfactant film of the lining layer (see Fig. 5–10); their bodies are in depressions of the alveolar wall and they send out large extensions. In conventional histologic preparations, they have been removed from their original position on the alveolar wall; they appear to float in the alveolar space and their surface is generally rounded-off so that they acquire the appearance of large, spherical cells. Contrary to previous views that alveolar macrophages are derivatives of the epithelium, it has been shown convincingly that they derive from blood monocytes.

Interstitium. The interstitium is the space between the basal laminae of alveolar epithelium and capillary endothelium (see Fig. 5–8). It contains connective tissue and interstitial fluid. The connective tissue comprises cells, fibers, and amorphous substance containing proteoglycans allegedly in a gel matrix. Its distribution can vary considerably. In places where the air-blood barrier is thin, connective tissue may be reduced to a few isolated, fine fibrils or may even be absent, in which instance the adjoining basement membranes fuse. These latter regions are particularly important for gas exchange. In lung edema, they usually are not widened by interstitial fluid and can therefore be called "restricted" as opposed to those "unrestricted" thicker portions of interstitium between capillaries, where interstitial fluid can accumulate under pathologic conditions. The interstitial fibroblasts have been demonstrated to contain contractile filaments (see Fig. 5–11), so Kapanci and co-workers (1974, 1976) suggested that they could regulate blood flow through the alveolar septum. In view of the interstitial

structure described, one of us (E.R.W.) and Bachofen (1979) proposed an alternative function for these cells: they could control the compliance of the unrestricted interstitial regions by regulating the width of the septum. In the postnatal rat lung, the interstitial cells form two distinct populations of cells: a lipid-containing — LIC, and a non-lipid-containing type — NLIC. The lipid droplets of LIC disappear, however, before weaning; the fate of the LIC remains unclear, according to Maksvytis and co-workers (1984). Lymphatic vessels are never found in alveolar septa; nevertheless, a continuous path of the interstitial fluid toward the lymphatics of the subpleural space and of the peribronchial and perivascular connective sheaths has been postulated; the fluid probably follows connective fibers.

Endothelium. The endothelial cells form a capillary wall that is similar in structure to the endothelium in some other organs (Figs. 5–8, 5–9, 5–13). The cells form thin cytoplasmic extensions and hence resemble the alveolar epithelial cells of type I. A single cell covers between 1000 and 1500 μm^2 of the capillary lumen. Lung capillaries have no fenestrations. Further details are discussed subsequently.

Extracellular Lining Layer and Pulmonary Surfactant

On the basis of theoretic considerations, as early as 1929, von Neergaard predicted that the alveolar surface must be lined by a layer of surface-active fluid, now commonly called pulmonary surfactant. It is an essential element, assuring the stability of the air-filled lung. Its basic characteristics are twofold: first, it lowers the

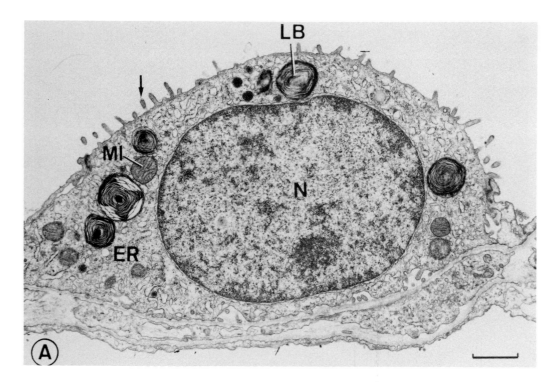

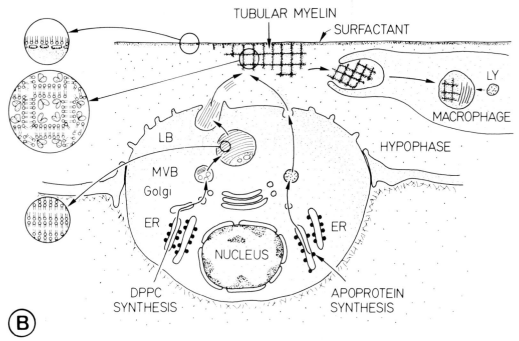

Fig. 5–12. *A*, In a type II epithelial cell, the abundant cytoplasm surrounding the nucleus (N) contains the characteristic osmiophilic lamellar bodies (LB), which store surfactant, and a rich complement of organelles such as endoplasmic reticulum (ER) and mitochondria (MI). The surface membrane carries microvilli (arrow), and junctions (J) with neighboring type I cells. *Reproduced with permission from* Weibel ER: Design and structure of the human lung. *In* Fishman AP (ed): Pulmonary Diseases and Disorders. New York: McGraw-Hill, 1971. *B*, Diagram of pathways for synthesis and secretion of surfactant DPPC and apoproteins by a type II cell, and for their removal by macrophages and by recycling. Note the arrangement of phospholipids in the lamellar bodies, in tubular myelin, and in the surface film. Dashed line depicts possible alternative route of apoprotein secretion. *Modified with permission from* Weibel ER: The Pathway for Oxygen. Cambridge: Harvard University Press, 1984.

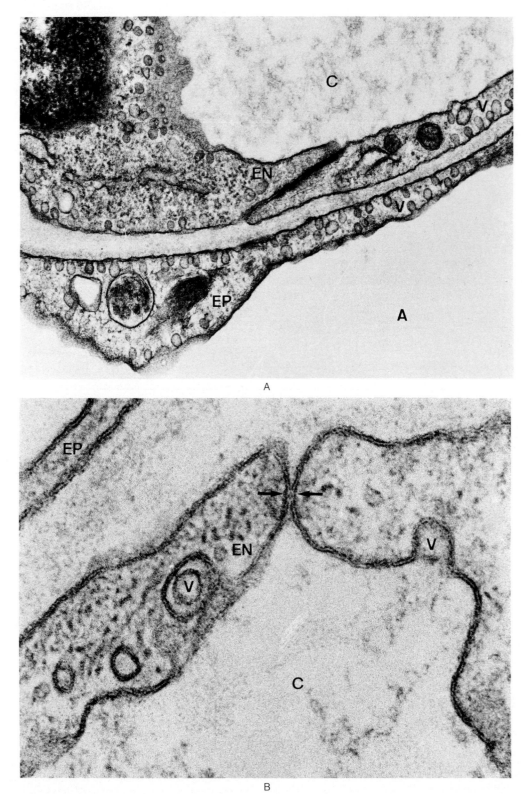

A

B

Fig. 5–13. *A*, Air-blood barrier showing thin cytoplasmic extensions of alveolar epithelium type I (EP) and of endothelial cells (EN) with intercellular junction. Note abundance of pinocytotic vesicles (V). ×37,000. *B*, High-power view of junction between two capillary endothelial cells. The triple-layered structure of the cell membranes is apparent. In the junction the membranes are closely apposed over a very short stretch (arrows). Note pinocytotic vesicles (V). A=alveolus; C=capillary, ×184,800.

surface tension at the air-liquid interface of the alveoli; and second, its surface tension is variable with the degree of inflation of alveoli.

Morphologic demonstration of pulmonary surfactant is only possible with the electron microscope. In routine preparations, usually no traces of this material are found (see Fig. 5–8). In lungs fixed by vascular perfusion, an extracellular duplex lining layer on the alveolar surface can be preserved (see Fig. 5–9), which two of us (J.G. and E.R.W.) (1969/70) supposed to contain the alveolar surfactant system fixed in situ. Much of this material forms pools in pits and irregularities of the alveolar wall, which it smooths out. These pools are polymorphous: sometimes they are of moderate electron density with dark specks, or they may contain lipid micelles or tubular myelin, a liquid crystal made up of surface active lipoproteins.

The synthesis and secretion of pulmonary surfactant is the function of the type II pneumocytes. Figure 5–12B shows how the organelles of this cell are involved in synthesizing, storing and secreting the surfactant phospholipids and the specific apoproteins. The single most abundant component of surfactant is the phospholipid dipalmitoyl phosphatidylcholine — DPPC — whereas the surfactant apoprotein A — SP A — quantitatively prevails over the others — SP B, SP C, and SP D. It appears that tubular myelin figures (see Fig. 5–10) are an extracellular reserve form of surfurcant, which can spread on the surface when alveoli enlarge. For further details and references, see Weibel (1985), Mason and Williams (1991), and Hawgood (1991).

Fine Structure of Pulmonary Blood Vessels

Alveolar Capillaries

The dense capillary network (see Fig. 5–7) that is intercalated between adjoining alveoli and forms part of the interalveolar septa is lined by an uninterrupted endothelial cell layer (see Fig. 5–8). Characteristically, these endothelial cells are formed of two parts: 1) a region of cytoplasm surrounding the nucleus and containing the majority of cellular organelles, such as mitochondria, endoplasmic reticulum, Golgi complex, and various granules; and 2) thin cytoplasmic extensions, which are 0.1-μm thick and virtually free of organelles. In the thinnest regions — <0.1 μm — they are composed of two cell membranes and some intercalated cytoplasm (see Fig. 5–8); the portions of average thickness contain numerous pinocytotic vesicles that are, in part, attached to either of the cell membranes (Figs. 5–8, 5–13). These vesicles are involved in the transport of materials, mainly of proteins, across the endothelial cell. In connection with passage of macromolecules, the main problem, however, is the different permeability between endothelium and epithelium. There is general agreement that the epithelium represents the chief permeability barrier of the lung. Endothelium can be permeated under a variety of circumstances. The explanation for this difference was provided by compar-

ative freeze-fracture studies of endothelial versus epithelial junctions. The epithelial tight junctions consist of a continuous network of three to five interconnected ridges and grooves; the endothelial junctions have only one to three rows of particles with few interconnections and even some discontinuities, as discussed by Schneeberger (1991). Because it is believed that an inverse correlation exists between the number of strands constituting a tight junction and its permeability, it follows that epithelial junctions are "tight" while endothelial junctions are relatively "leaky."

Alveolar capillaries are associated with pericytes. Pericytes seem to be less frequent in the alveolar capillaries than in the systemic capillaries and less densely branched. Their function is still debated: they are supposed to be contractile cells or phagocytic elements, or both.

Ultrastructure of Larger Pulmonary Vessels

The endothelial lining of pulmonary arteries and veins differs from that of alveolar capillaries in that the cytoplasmic extensions are thicker (Fig. 5–14).They are likewise rich in pinocytotic vesicles and may contain numerous cellular organelles. These endothelial cells also contain a characteristic rod-shaped granule (see Fig. 5–16) known to occur in all vascular endothelia of all vertebrate species thus far investigated by one of us (E.R.W.) and Palade (1964). In the mammalian vascular system, these organelles are particularly numerous in medium-sized and larger branches of pulmonary arteries and veins, whereas they occur less frequently in systemic vessels of the same size. Based on indirect evidence, two of us (P.H.B. and E.R.W.) (1968) proposed that these organelles contain a procoagulative substance. This assumption proved to be correct. Wagner and associates (1982) and Warhol and Sweet (1984), using immunocytochemical techniques, demonstrated that the endothelial specific organelles contained Factor VIII–related antigen, also called von Willebrand factor. More recently, Bonfanti and co-workers (1989) and McEver and associates (1989) showed that the granule membrane carries the leukocyte-binding protein P-selectin, also found in the α-granules of platelets.

The electron microscopic study of intima and media of pulmonary vessels does not reveal many features that are not manifest by light microscopy. The circular smooth muscle cells of peripheral vessels of the muscular type are long, slender, and rather densely arranged (Fig. 5–14). In elastic vessels — larger pulmonary arteries — the connective tissue elements prevail (Fig. 5–15); the space between the prominent elastic laminae contains much collagenous tissue and relatively short smooth muscle cells, which extend from one elastic lamina to the next in an oblique course and appear to insert on the elastic laminae with ramified ends (Fig. 5–15). In Figure 5–16; a portion of a longitudinal section of a medium-sized pulmonary vein is shown; its thin wall is made up of an endothelium, a few irregularly arranged smooth muscle fibers, and collagenous as well as elastic fibers.

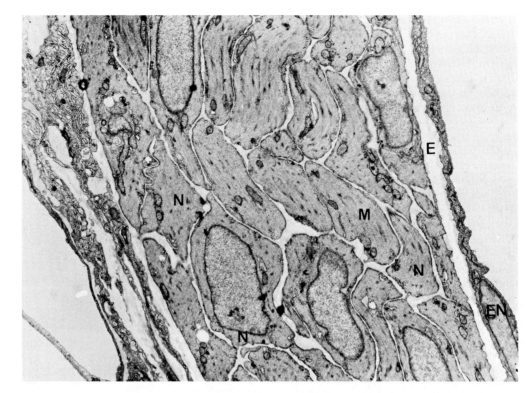

Fig. 5–14. Electron micrograph of longitudinal section of medium-sized pulmonary artery of muscle type. The endothelium (EN) lies over a strong elastic membrane (E). The smooth muscle fibers (M) are obliquely sectioned; their cytoplasm shows a very fine filamentous structure. Some muscle cells (labeled N) show intercellular contacts (nexus), serving spread of excitation among the cells. ×5850.

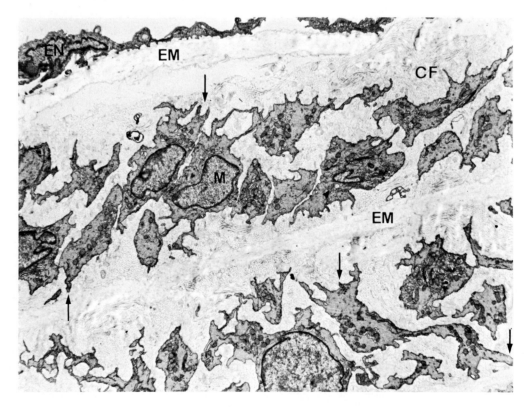

Fig. 5–15. Electron micrograph of pulmonary artery of elastic type. Note three strong elastic membranes (EM) paralleling the endothelium (EN), and ramified smooth muscle cells (M), which take an oblique course reaching from one elastic membrane to the next (arrows). Direction of muscle fibers alternates from one layer to the next. Collagen fibrils (CF) are abundant and mixed with elastic fibers. ×4850.

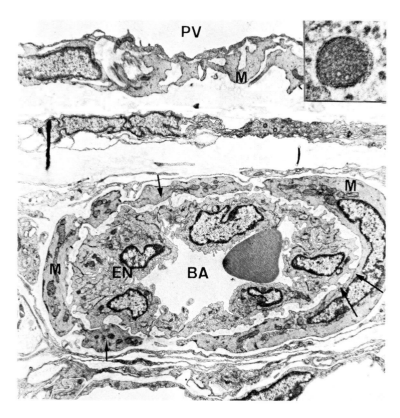

Fig. 5–16. Bronchial arteriole (BA) in a semicontracted state with thick endothelium (EN), and a simple layer of smooth muscle cells (M). Note numerous contacts between endothelial and muscle cells (arrows). At top, section of wall of small pulmonary vein (PV) with loose smooth muscle layer (M) and endothelium. ×4850. Inset shows sample of specific endothelial organelles (also called Weibel-Palade bodies) at higher power. Note membrane and internal tubules. ×83,200.

One interesting feature is that smooth muscle cells of these vessel walls not only form close intercellular contacts in form of patches or nexus (see Figs. 5–14, 5–15), but also have close cell-to-cell contact with endothelial cells by means of short extensions across the internal elastic membrane (see Fig. 5–16). It is assumed that cell-to-cell contacts between endothelial or epithelial cells and smooth muscle or interstitial cells are important in inducing and regulating various cell functions.

Bronchial Vessels. The arteries of the bronchial wall are of the "muscle type." Figure 5–16 shows a small bronchial arteriole with one layer of circular smooth muscle and typically thick endothelial layer. Note the many contacts between muscle and endothelial cells. Bronchial arteries are often characterized by intimal longitudinal smooth muscle bundles that one of us (E.R.W.) (1959) found to be related to the stretch strain to which these vessels are frequently exposed rather than to a special regulatory function.

MORPHOMETRY OF THE LUNG

The application of morphometric methods in analyzing lung tissue has yielded new insights into lung structure and its dimensions, and has opened the possibility of a morphologic approach to the study of lung function.

Compartmental Distribution of Lung Volume

Any morphologic analysis of the functional capacity of the gas-exchange apparatus involves exact knowledge of the total lung volume and of its compartmental distribution.

To illustrate the distribution of the lung volume among the various zones and constituents, we consider the lung of a medium-sized adult inflated to about three-fourths total lung capacity; the total lung volume would then amount to about 5.7 L. Table 5–2 gives the approximate distribution of this volume among the lung compartments as derived from morphometric analysis of fixed lungs. The greatest compartment is the air space, of which about two thirds is in alveoli, and only a small fraction in conductive airways — representing the anatomic dead space.

Number and Size of Alveoli and Capillaries

Alveoli

In spite of its ability to supply the organism with enough oxygen, the lung of the newborn is still immature structurally. Besides primitive air sacs, which have often been misinterpreted as alveoli, only a fraction of the final number of alveoli is present at birth. Two of us (P.H.B., E.R.W.) with a co-worker (1974), and Kauffman and associates (1974), studied the postnatal development of alveoli previously, using the rat lung as a model. It showed that alveoli were formed by outgrowth of new, so-called secondary septa from the sides of the primary ones present at birth. This occurrence transformed the smooth-walled channels and saccules of the newborn lung into alveolar ducts and alveolar sacs. This process was followed by an important

Table 5–2. Approximate Distribution of Total Lung Volume in Milliliters for Adult Human Lung at Three-Fourths Total Lung Capacity*

Zones	Air Channels	Tissue	Blood	
Conducting	Bronchi 170	Walls Septa Fibers	Arteries 150	Veins 150
Transition	Respiratory bronchioles Alv. ducts 1500	Lymph 200	Arterioles 60	Venules 60
Respiratory	Alveoli 3150	Barrier 150	Capillaries 140	

*Total lung volume = 5.7 liters

Reproduced with permission from Weibel ER: Normal Values for Respiratory Function in Man (Arcangeli P, et al, eds). Milano, Panminerva Medica, 1970, p. 242.

remodeling of the septal structure. Indeed, in contrast to the mature septum containing a single capillary network interlaced with a fibrous skeleton, the primary and secondary septa presented a three-layered structure: a capillary network was found on both sides of a thick central sheet of connective tissue. The restructuring now consisted in a massive reduction of the interstitial tissue, probably accompanied by fusions of capillary segments. Zeltner and co-workers and Zeltner and one of us (P.H.B.) (1987) obtained similar findings in studies on human lung growth. At about 1 month of age, a human lung compared well structurally with the lung of a 1-week-old rat. Although alveolar formation in man starts during late fetal life, according to Langston and co-workers (1984), more than 80% of all alveoli are formed postnatally. Following alveolization, the septal structure is altered much in the same way as in the rat lung: a remodeling of the parenchymal microvas-

culature reduced the double capillary network to a single one. Figure 5–17 summarizes the findings of these studies and proposes a new staging and timing of lung development and growth. It appears that alveolization proceeds at a faster pace than assumed so far: bulk alveolar formation seems to be terminated at about 1½ years of age. It is further accompanied and followed, respectively, by a stage of microvascular maturation lasting from a few months after birth to the age of 2 or 3 years. One of us (E.R.W.) (1963) found that, in the adult, the number of alveoli averages 300 million. According to Angus and Thurlbeck (1972), the number is related to body length and may vary largely between 200 and 600 million.

For a lung of an adult inflated to three fourths of its maximal volume, one of us (E.R.W.) (1963) found that the average alveolar diameter lies between 250 and 290 µm. Glazier and associates (1967), however, demon-

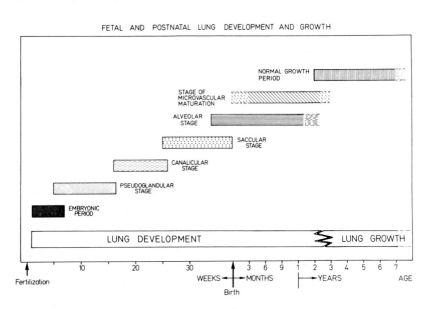

Fig. 5–17. Stages and timing of human lung development. Open-ended bars indicate that exact start and end of the stages are still unknown. *Reproduced with permission from* Zeltner TB, Burri PH: The postnatal development and growth of the human lung. II. Morphology. Respir Physiol 67:269, 1987.

strated, on dog lungs, that alveolar size is not identical in all parts of the lung, but that in an erect lung, the upper parts contain larger alveoli than the dependent parts, owing to the weight of the lung tissue.

Capillaries

As shown previously, capillaries form a dense network spreading over the surface of alveoli (see Fig. 5–7). On average, this network is made up of hexagonal meshes, which means that usually three capillary segments are connected to each other at a junction point. The capillary network seems to be continuous over many interalveolar facets, perhaps even over a whole lobule or more. The number of small capillary segments in the adult human lung is of the order of 300×10^9. One of us (E.R.W.) (1963) noted that this figure implies that each alveolus is surrounded by a network composed of 1800 to 2000 capillary segments. In an electron microscopic morphometric analysis of eight normal human lungs by Gehr and co-workers (1978a), the total capillary volume varied between 125 and 387 ml — mean 213 ml — and the capillary surface area from 74 to 189 m^2 — mean 126 m^2. During lung growth, capillary volume showed the steepest increase among all the parameters relevant for gas exchange. During the first 6 months, capillaries held only 22% of the volume of the interalveolar septa; this value reached 42% in adult lungs, according to Zeltner, one of us (P.H.B.), and co-workers (1987).

Between 1 month of age and adulthood, capillary volume increases about 35 times and capillary surface area about 20 times in the human lung. With the capillary density being about equal, new capillaries have to be continuously added to the existing network. Caduff, Fischer, and one of us (P.H.B.) (1986) and one of us (P.H.B.) and Tarek (1990) demonstrated by scanning electron microscopy and by ultrastructural analysis of serial sections that the pulmonary capillary network grows by formation of new intercapillary meshes rather than by sprouting of new capillaries. The process has been termed intussusceptive growth — growth within itself — in analogy to the growth of cartilage. It consists in the formation of transcapillary tissue pillars that divide existing capillary segments. The newly formed and originally small individual tissue pillars — diameter <1.5 µm — subsequently increase in diameter and thus give rise to new intercapillary meshes. Recently, Patan, one of us (P.H.B.), and co-workers (1992) proposed that intussuceptive growth may be a mode of capillary network expansion common to many organ systems and not only to lung.

The Gas Exchange Surface and the Air-Blood Barrier

The alveolocapillary air-blood barrier is composed of a surface-lining layer, epithelium, interstitium, and endothelium that have to be crossed by the oxygen molecules on their way from air to blood. As it will be developed, the following dimensions of this barrier are of greatest importance for gas exchange: first, the surface area of air-tissue interface; second, the surface area of tissue-blood interface; and third, the thickness of the barrier and of its components.

The alveolar surface area of the adult human lung has been found to vary between 97 and 194 m^2 — mean 143 m^2.

This range is in contrast to previously published results, where, by light microscopic morphometry, values between 70 and 80 m^2 had been obtained. This discrepancy is due to the higher resolution of the electron microscope, which allows one to measure the complex free surface of the epithelial cells. With the light microscope, one could analyze only a smoothed surface of the alveolar wall.

In most species investigated, the total capillary surface area did not differ from the alveolar surface area by more than 10 to 12%. In the rat lung, the capillary-to-alveolar surface ratio is 1.05 to 1.1, which means that the capillary surface area of the rat lung is 5 to 10% higher than the alveolar surface. In the human and in the dog lung, where the capillaries are less dense, the quotient is about 0.88.

Thickness and Composition of the Alveolocapillary Barrier

From Figure 5–8, it is evident that the width of the alveolocapillary barrier can vary from about 0.3 to several microns. The thickness of this tissue barrier is important because it determines, together with other parameters, the diffusion resistance of the barrier that oxygen molecules moving from the alveolus to the capillary must overcome. This resistance is low in thin and higher in thick parts, so that the flux of gas at each point is inversely proportional to local barrier thickness. Hence, the thin parts of the barrier contribute most to gas exchange. In estimating an overall average thickness, this factor is best taken into account by determining the harmonic mean thickness of the air-blood barrier, that is, the average of the reciprocal value of thickness, rather than the arithmetic mean, which estimates the tissue mass building the barrier. The arithmetic and harmonic mean thickness vary relatively little in various mammalian species. It appears that, on the average, the harmonic mean thickness is about one third of the arithmetic mean thickness. Estimates on human lungs give values of about 0.6 µm for the harmonic mean barrier thickness, whereas the arithmetic mean thickness lies around 2 µm.

Morphometric Estimation of Diffusing Capacity

The term "diffusing capacity of the lung" — D$_L$ — has been introduced by physiologists, as noted by Forster (1964), to estimate the conductance of the pulmonary gas exchange apparatus for gaseous diffusions between alveolar air and capillary blood. The physiologic definition uses Ohm's law and states that, for oxygen,

$$D_{L_{O_2}} = \dot{V}_{O_2}/\Delta P_{O_2}$$

in which $\dot{V}_{O_2}$ is the O$_2$ uptake and ΔP_{O_2} the mean gradient of O$_2$ partial pressure between alveoli and capillaries.

It is implicit in the definition that a major part of D$_L$ is determined by structural properties of the lung, mainly by the available gas-exchange surfaces, by the thickness of the air-blood barrier, and by the capillary blood volume. One of us (E.R.W.)(1970/71) noted that refinements in morphometric methods have made it possible to estimate D_L from measurements of lung structure performed on electron micrographs. To this end, the air-hemoglobin barrier must be subdivided into three partial restances — or conductances, that is, the reciprocal of the resistances — which are arranged in series, as shown in Figures 5–8 and 5–18. We then find D_L from the sum of the partial resistances

$$\frac{1}{D_L} = \frac{1}{D_t} + \frac{1}{D_p} + \frac{1}{D_e}$$

whereby D_t, D_p, and D_e are the diffusion conductances in tissue, plasma, and erythrocytes, respectively. D_L can be calculated if we measure the alveolar and capillary surface areas, S_a and S_e, the capillary volume V_c, and the harmonic mean thicknesses τ_h of tissue — t — and plasma — p. In addition, we need to know appropriate values for the physical coefficients of permeability — αD — and of the rate of O_2 binding by the blood — θ.

Table 5–3 presents the results obtained by Gehr and associates (1978a) in a morphometric study of adult human lungs. Using "most reasonable" estimates of the physical coefficients, one of us (E.R.W.) (1984) found $D_{L_{O_2}}$ to amount to about 205 ml O_2/min/mm Hg. In more recent studies, one of us (E.R.W.) (1993) attempted to reduce a number of uncertainties in the model, for example, by taking tissue and plasma to form a single diffusion barrier. This effort resulted in a somewhat lower $D_{L_{O_2}}$ estimate of about 160 ml O_2/min/mm Hg.

For comparison, the currently available or accepted physiologic values of D_L at rest amount to about 30 ml O_2/min/mm Hg. This value is hence far below the morphometric estimates. It should be noted that two different things are measured: morphometry estimates the size of the gas-exchange apparatus that is maximally available for gas exchange. Its values refer to a fully expanded lung. This can lead to an overestimation of D_L by as much as 25 to 50%, because one of us (J.G.)

Table 5–3. **Basic Morphometric Parameters and Diffusing Capacity in Human Lung**

Weight	74	kg
Alveolar surface	143	m^2
Capillary surface	126	m^2
Capillary volume	213	ml
Tissue barrier	0.62	μm
Plasma barrier	0.15	μm
$D_{L_{O_2}}$	205	ml O_2
		min/mm Hg

and associates (1979) showed that in lungs inflated with air and fixed by vascular perfusion, parts of the diffusion barrier are folded away from the surface even at highest inflation and thus do not contribute to gas exchange. Furthermore, we suppose that a gradient from air to blood exists at every point along the alveolar capillary. Under resting conditions, this is most certainly not the case; in fact, it is probable that the capillary blood is saturated before it leaves the capillary, as Karas and associates (1987) showed for the lungs of animals performing heavy exercise. We would therefore expect that the physiologic estimates of D_L at rest should amount to only 20 to 40% of the maximal or "true" diffusing capacity. That this reasoning is probably correct is shown by the findings of Bitterli and co-workers (1971) in man that, in exercise, physiologic estimates may yield values of D_L between 70 and 100 ml O_2/min/mm Hg. The morphometric estimate of pulmonary diffusing capacity in man is therefore about two times larger than the physiologic estimate. One of us (E.R.W.) and colleagues (1983) confirmed this difference by direct measurement of the physiologic and morphometric values of D_L in animals. We concluded from this that the lung provides a gas-exchange apparatus that is large enough to allow O_2 to diffuse to the blood in sufficient quantity when O_2 consumption is elevated owing to work. Destruction of lung tissue, as occurs in emphysema, would tend to reduce the "true" diffusing capacity by reduction of the gas-exchange surfaces and, possibly, by thickening of the barrier.

Figure 5–19 shows the results of a comparative study of D_L in mammalian species ranging from the smallest mammal, the Etruscan shrew, weighing only 2 g, to the horse. It is apparent that D_L is directly related to body mass; in contrast, maximal O_2 consumption — $\dot{V}_{O_2}$ mass — varies with the 0.8 power of body mass. Consequently, the lung's capacity for O_2 uptake is not matched to the body's need for O_2 when one compares animals of different body size.

On the other hand, the lung can respond to increased O_2 demands, or to reduced environmental O_2 at high altitude, by enlarging the pulmonary diffusing capacity, as we (P.H.B. and E.R.W.) (1971) and Hugonnaud (1977) and Gehr (1978b) and their associates showed. One of us (E.R.W.) and colleagues (1987) found that athletic animals, such as dogs or horses, have a larger diffusing capacity than animals of the same size but lower O_2 needs. The question of how the lung's morphometric

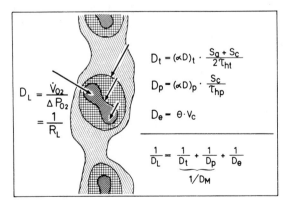

Fig. 5–18. Model for estimating pulmonary diffusing capacity from physiologic (left) and morphometric information (right).

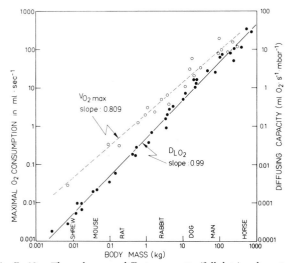

Fig. 5–19. The pulmonary diffusing capacity (full dots) and maximal O_2 consumption (open circles) scale with body mass at a different slope on a double-logarithmic plot. *Reproduced with permission from Weibel ER: The Pathway for Oxygen. Cambridge: Harvard University Press, 1984.*

properties are related to the body's O_2 needs is still a matter of scientific debate, as one of us (E.R.W.) (1984) and Taylor and co-workers (1987) noted.

Morphometry of Conducting and Transitory Airways and Blood Vessels

Figure 5–20 shows a plastic cast of a human lung; in the right lung, only the airways have been modeled, whereas in the left lung, pulmonary arteries and veins have also been demonstrated. It is apparent that the airways branch toward the periphery by systematically dividing in two, that is, by dichotomy. This dichotomy, however, is not regular; the two branches arising from a parent branch may differ considerably in both length and diameter. This is called irregular dichotomy. Figure 5–21 shows a similar cast of an acinus from a human lung in which the casting material, silicon rubber, has filled the airways out to the most peripheral alveoli. On such preparations, Haefeli-Bleuer and one of us (E.R.W.) (1987) showed that the most peripheral airways, the respiratory bronchioles and alveolar ducts, also branch by irregular dichotomy.

The pattern of dichotomous branching provides a scheme with respect to which the systematic progression of the increase in the number of branches and of the reduction in dimensions can be described. If we first disregard the irregularities, we can estimate the average

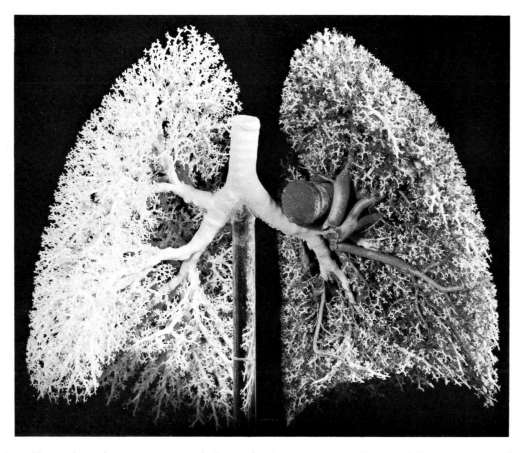

Fig. 5–20. Cast of human lung, showing airways in right lung and pulmonary arteries and veins in left lung. Note irregular dichotomy of all branches.

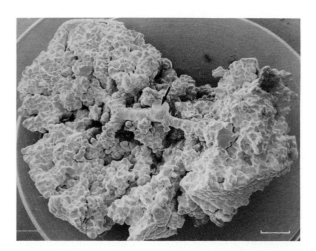

Fig. 5–21. Scanning electron micrograph of a silicon rubber cast of a human pulmonary acinus. Part of the alveolar ducts have been trimmed off to show the transitional bronchiole (arrow) and the first few orders of respiratory bronchioles. Note that alveolar ducts and sacs are densely covered by alveoli. Scale marker = 1 mm.

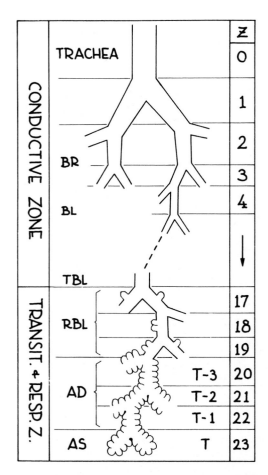

Fig. 5–22. Schematic representation of the sequence of airway branches as a function of generation z. Bronchi (BR), bronchioles (BL), terminal (TBL), and respiratory (RBL) bronchioles are followed by alveolar ducts (AD) and sacs (AS) in the terminal generation. T = 23. *Reproduced with permission from* Weibel ER: Morphometry of the Human Lung. Heidelberg: Springer, 1963, p. 111.

number of generations necessary to provide a sufficient number of terminal airway channels to carry alveoli for gas exchange, namely, alveolar ducts and sacs. One of us (E.R.W.) (1963) alone and with Haefeli-Bleuer (1987) estimated this average number of generations at 23. Figure 5–22 shows that the first 16 generations are purely conducting airways, leading from the trachea to the terminal bronchioles. From generation 17 on, alveoli are progressively incorporated into the airway wall until, in the twentieth generation, the entire wall is occupied by them. On the basis of more recent information, the transition from terminal to alveolated bronchioles may occur at generation 14, so that a total of nine generations carry alveoli. It must be stressed that these are average values and that, because of the irregularity, airways will terminate in alveolar sacs anywhere from about generations 15 to 30.

This irregularity becomes apparent if length and diameter of the bronchial branches are measured on casts. Nevertheless, average dimensions can be calculated from these size distributions. If the average diameters — d — are plotted semilogarithmically against generations — z (Fig. 5–23), we find them to follow an exponential function, namely,

$$d(z) = d_o \cdot 2^{-z/3}$$

Therefore, with each generation, the average airway diameter is reduced by $\sqrt[3]{1/2}$ — which, as pointed out by Thompson (1942), is known in hydrodynamics to be a function of optimal size relationship between parent and daughter branches. But Figure 5–23 also reveals that the diameters of peripheral or transitory airways that are provided with alveoli do not fit on this function; they are considerably larger than one would expect from their position in the bronchial tree. This difference can be explained by their different roles in conveying oxygen from ambient air to alveoli. In conducting airways, air

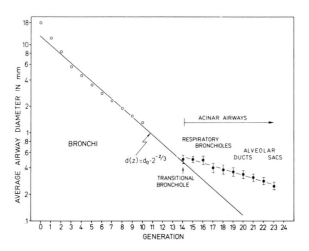

Fig. 5–23. Progressive reduction by cube root of ½ of average diameter of conducting airways in regularized dichotomy model contrasts with the slow decrease of diameter of acinar airways with progressive generations of branching. Compare text. *Reproduced with permission from* Haefeli-Bleuer B, Weibel ER: Morphometry of the human pulmonary acinus. Anat Rec *220*:401, 1988.

Table 5–4. Dimensions of Human Airway Model (Average Adult Lung with Volume 4800 ml at about Three-fourths Maximal Inflation)

Generation z	Number per Generation $n(z)$	Diameter $d(z)$ cm	Length $l(z)$ cm	Total Cross Section $A(z)$ cm^2	Total Volume $V(z)$ cm^3	Accumul. Volume $\sum_{i=0}^{z} V(i)$ cm^3
0	1	1.8	12.0	2.54	30.50	30.5
1	2	1.22	4.76	2.33	11.25	41.8
2	4	0.83	1.90	2.13	3.97	45.8
3	8	0.56	0.76	2.00	1.52	47.2
4	16	0.45	1.27	2.48	3.46	50.7
5	32	0.35	1.07	3.11	3.30	54.0
6	64	0.28	0.90	3.96	3.53	57.5
7	128	0.23	0.76	5.10	3.85	61.4
8	256	0.186	0.64	6.95	4.45	65.8
9	512	0.154	0.54	9.56	5.17	71.0
10	1024	0.130	0.46	13.4	6.21	77.2
11	2048	0.109	0.39	19.6	7.56	84.8
12	4096	0.095	0.33	28.8	9.82	94.6
13	8192	0.082	0.27	44.5	12.45	106.0
14	16384	0.074	0.23	69.4	16.40	123.4
15	32768	0.066	0.20	113.0	21.70	145.1
16	65536	0.060	0.165	180.0	29.70	174.8
17	131072	0.054	0.141	300.0	41.80	216.6
18	262144	0.050	0.117	534.0	61.10	277.7
19	524288	0.047	0.099	944.0	93.20	370.9
20	1048576	0.045	0.083	1600.0	139.50	510.4
21	2097152	0.043	0.070	3220.0	224.30	734.7
22	4194304	0.041	0.059	5880.0	350.00	1084.7
23*	8388608	0.041	0.050*	11800.0	591.00	1675.0

*Adjusted for complete generation.

is transported en masse; that is, a solution of O_2 in nitrogen is flowing through the tubes, and hydrodynamic principles prevail. Toward the periphery, however, O_2 molecules have to advance toward the alveolar surface by diffusion in the gas phase — and this, as emphasized by Gomez (1965), requires a greater cross-sectional area of the peripheral airways.

From this detailed information, we can construct a first model of the lung that may be useful for some general considerations on structure-function relationship in the airway system. The model assumes regular dichotomy over 23 generations. Its most pertinent dimensional properties are given in Table 5–4. It may be noted that the anatomic dead space of 150 ml, as estimated by physiologic methods, is reached at about generation 16, which corresponds to terminal bronchioles.

Irregular dichotomous models can also be constructed. Figure 5–24 reveals the numbers of generations necessary to arrive at airways of 2-mm diameter, as well as the distribution of distances from these branches to the trachea; these branches were located between generations 4 and 13 and at 18 to 31 cm from the root of the trachea. Each of these about 400 branches of 2-mm diameter leads through an average of 14 subsequent branchings until alveolar sacs are reached. The units of lung tissue that they supply have a volume of some 12 ml and contain approximately 740,000 alveoli each. This consideration of irregularity can be carried

further, but one should refer to the original publications by one of us (E.R.W.) (1963) and Haefeli-Bleuer and (E.R.W.) (1987) for additional information.

Different models of the airway tree have been proposed. Horsfield (1991) considers the airway tree as a system of confluent tubes originating in parenchymal airways and ending in the trachea; this minimizes the effects of branching irregularities but otherwise leads to the same type of conclusions on the physiologic effects of airway design. West and co-workers (1986) used the principles of fractal geometry to arrive at a different description of the airway branching pattern.

The blood vessels undergo, in principle, the same sequence of branching as the airways, with some differences in detail. Pulmonary arteries are topographically closely associated with the airways (Fig. 5–20); down to the respiratory bronchioles their branching would therefore seem to parallel that of the airways, but this is only partially true. It is well known that relatively large pulmonary arteries may send smaller branches to the capillary network of adjacent groups of alveoli. These "accessory" branches are called supernumerary arteries and cause, on the one hand, a more rapid progression of arterial branching and, on the other, greater irregularity in the arterial dimensions per generation.

At present, no extensive data on the morphometry of the pulmonary vascular tree are available. A preliminary model can be derived by comparing pulmonary

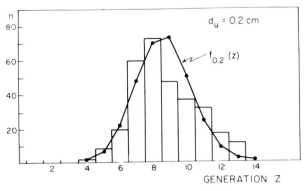

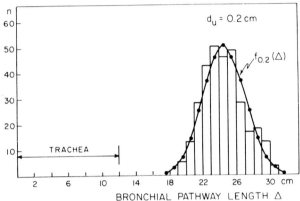

Fig. 5-24. Distribution of airways of 2-mm diameter with respect to generation z and distance from larynx Δ. *Modified with permission from* Weibel ER: Morphometry of the Human Lung. Heidelberg: Springer, 1963, p. 126.

arteries with airways and by determining the average generation number of dichotomous branching. The larger branches of the pulmonary artery, perhaps down to 2-mm diameter and reaching to the eighth generation on the average, have dimensions closely approximating those of the accompanying bronchi. In a first approximation, we may therefore use the measurements obtained on the bronchial tree to describe the major pulmonary arterial tree. We would therefore claim that these branches reduce their dimension with each generation to obey the hydrodynamic law of optimal size reduction described previously (Fig. 5–23). Next, we may determine the total number of precapillaries, that is, of the terminal arterial branches that lead into the capillary network, and calculate from that the average generation number of dichotomous branching needed to reach this number; one of us (E.R.W.) and Gomez (1962) found this to be of the order of 28 generations, hence about five generations more than the airways. The diameter of these precapillaries is between 20 and 30 μm; if this range is plotted on Figure 5–23, it falls on the function for dimensional reduction by $\sqrt[3]{1/2}$ fitted to the major branches, which suggests that the pulmonary arterial tree reduces the dimension of its branches progressively following a hydrodynamic law for optimal reduction of diameters in a dichotomous branching system all the way out to the terminal branches.

This seems logical, as mass flow of blood occurs throughout, the diffusion of gases in the blood phase playing a negligible role for transport along the vessel axis. All this is highly conjectural, however, as long as it is not substantiated by more extensive actual measurement.

REFERENCES

Angus GE, Thurlbeck WM: Number of alveoli in the human lung. J Appl Physiol 32:483, 1972.

Bitterli J, et al: Repeated measurements of pulmonary O_2 diffusing capacity in man during graded exercise. *In* Scherrer M: Pulmonary Diffusing Capacity on Exercise. Stuttgart: H. Huber, 1971, p. 139.

Bonfanti R, Furie BC, Furie B, Wagner, DD: PADGM (GMP140) is a component of Weibel-Palade bodies of human endothelial cells. Blood. 73:1109-1112, 1989.

Breeze RG, Wheeldon EG: The cells of the pulmonary airways. Am Rev Respir Dis 116:705, 1977.

Burri PH: The postnatal growth of the rat lung. III. Morphology. Anat Rec 180:77, 1974.

Burri, P.H., and M.R. Tarek. A novel mechanism of capillary growth in the rat pulmonary microcirculation. Anat. Rec. 228:35-45, 1990.

Burri PH, Weibel ER: Beeinflussung einer spezifischen cytoplasmischen Organelle von Endothelzellen durch Adrenalin. Z Zellforsch 88:426, 1968.

Burri PH, Weibel ER: Morphometric estimation of pulmonary diffusion capacity. II. Effect of P_{O_2} on the growing lung. Respir Physiol 11:247, 1971.

Burri PH, Dbaly J, Weibel ER: The postnatal growth of the rat lung. I. Morphometry. Anat Rec 178:711, 1974.

Caduff, JH, Fischer LC, Burri PH: Scanning electron microscope study of the developing microvasculature in the postnatal rat lung. Anat. Rec. 216:154-164, 1986.

Crapo JD, et al: Cell numbers and cell characteristics of the normal human lung. Am Rev Respir Dis 125:332, 1982.

Forster RE: Diffusion of gases. *In* Fenn WD, Rahn H: Handbook of Physiology, Section 3, Respiration, Vol. I. Washington, DC: American Physiological Society, 1964, p. 839.

Gehr P, Bachofen H, Weibel ER: The normal human lung: Ultrastructure and morphometric estimation of diffusion capacity. Respir Physiol 32:121, 1978a.

Gehr P, et al: Adaptation of the growing lung to increase $\dot{V}_{O_2}$: III. The effect of exposure to cold environment in rats. Respir Physiol 32:345, 1978b.

Gil J: Ultrastructure of lung fixed under physiologically defined conditions. Arch Intern Med 127:896, 1971.

Gil J, Reiss OK: Isolation and characterization of lamellar bodies and tubular myelin from rat lung homogenates. J Cell Biol 58:152, 1973.

Gil J, Weibel ER: Improvements in demonstration of lining layer of lung alveoli by electron microscopy. Respir Physiol 8:13, 1969/70.

Gil J, Weibel ER: Extracellular lining of bronchioles after perfusion-fixation of rat lungs for electron microscopy. Anat Rec 169:185, 1971.

Gil J et al: The alveolar volume to surface area relationship in air and saline-filled lungs fixed by vascular perfusion. J Appl Physiol 47:990, 1979.

Glazier JB, et al: Vertical gradient of alveolar size in lungs of dogs frozen intact. J Appl Physiol 23:694, 1967.

Gomez DM: A physico-mathematical study of lung function in normal subjects and in patients with obstructive pulmonary diseases. Med Thorac 22:275, 1965.

Haefeli-Bleuer B, Weibel ER: Morphometry of the human pulmonary acinus. Anat Rec 220:401, 1988.

Hawgood, S. Composition, structure, and metabolism. In: The Lung Scientific Foundation, Vol. 1. Edited by R.G. Crystal and J.B. West, Raven Press, New York, 1991. p. 247.

Horsfield, K. Pulmonary airways and blood vessels considered as confluent trees. In: The Lung Scientific Foundation, Vol. 1.

Edited by R.G. Crystal and J.B. West, Raven Press, New York, 1991. p. 721.

Hoyt, RF Jr, McNelly N, Sorokin SP: Dynamics of neuroepithelial bodies (NEB) formation in developing hamster lung: Light microscopic autoradiography after 3H-thymidine labeling in vivo. Anat. Rec. *227*:340-350, 1990.

Hugonnaud C, et al: Adaptation of the growing lung to increased oxygen consumption. II. Morphometric analysis. Respir Physiol *29*:1, 1977.

Jeffery PK: Morphologic features of airway surface epithelial cells and glands. Am Rev Respir Dis *128*:14S, 1983.

Jeffery PK, Reid LM: The respiratory mucous membrane. *In* Brain JD, Proctor DF, Reid LM: Respiratory Defense Mechanisms, Part I. New York: Marcel Dekker, 1977.

Kapanci Y: Location and function of contractile interstitial cells of the lungs. *In* Bonhuys A: Lung Cells in Disease. New York: Elsevier North-Holland, 1976, p. 69.

Kapanci Y, et al: "Contractile interstitial cells" in pulmonary alveolar septa. J Cell Biol *60*:375, 1974.

Karas RH, et al: Adaptive variation in the mammalian respiratory system in relation to energetic demand. VII. Flow of oxygen across the pulmonary gas exchanger. Respir Physiol *69*:101, 1987.

Kauffman SL, Burri PH, Weibel ER: The postnatal growth of the rat lung. II. Autoradiography. Anat Rec *180*:63, 1974.

Langston C, et al: Human lung growth in late gestation and in the neonate. Am Rev Respir Dis *129*:607, 1984.

Lauweryns JM, Cokelaere M: Hypoxia sensitive neuroepithelial bodies. Intrapulmonary secretory neuroreceptors modulated by the CNS. Z Zellforsch *145*:521, 1973.

Low FN: Electron microscopy of the rat lung. Anat Rec *113*:437, 1952.

Maksvytis HJ, et al: In vitro characteristics of the lipid-filled interstitial cell associated with postnatal lung growth: Evidence for fibroblast heterogeneity. J Cell Physiol *118*:113, 1984.

Mason, R.J., and M.C. Williams. Alveolar type II cells. In: The Lung Scientific Foundation, Vol. 1. Edited by R.G. Crystal and J.B. West, Raven Press, New York, 1991. p. 235.

McEver, R.P., H.J. Beckstead, K.L. More, L. Marshall-Carlson, and D.F. Bainton. GMP-140, a platelet α-granule membrane protein, is also synthetized by vascular endothelial cells and is localized in Weibel-Palade bodies. J. Clin. Invest. *84*:92-99, 1989.

Meyrick B, Reid L: The alveolar brush cell in rat lung: A third pneumocyte. J Ultrastruct Res *23*:71, 1968.

Patan, S, Alvarez MJ, Schittny JC, Burri PH: Intussusceptive microvascular growth: A common alternative to capillary sprouting. Arch. Histol. Cytol. Vol. 55, Suppl., 1992, p. 65-75.

Plopper, C.G., D.M. Hyde, and A.R. Buckpitt. Clara cells. In: The Lung Scientific Foundation, Vol. 1. Edited by R.G. Crystal and J.B. West, Raven Press, New York, 1991. p. 215.

Schneeberger, E.E. Airway and alveolar epithelial cell junctions. In: The Lung Scientific Foundation, Vol. 1. Edited by R.G. Crystal and J.B. West, Raven Press, New York, 1991. p. 205.

Sleigh, M.A. Mucus propulsion. In: The Lung Scientific Foundation, Vol. 1. Edited by R.G. Crystal and J.B. West, Raven Press, New York, 1991. p. 189.

St. George JA, et al: An immunohistochemical characterization of Rhesus monkey respiratory secretions using monoclonal antibodies. Am Rev Respir Dis *132*:556, 1985.

Sorokin SP, et al: Comparative biology of small granule cells and neuroepithelial bodies in the respiratory system: Short review. Am Rev Respir Dis *128*:26S, 1983.

Spicer SS, et al: Histochemical properties of the respiratory tract epithelium in different species. Am Rev Respir Dis *128*:20S, 1983.

Taylor CR, et al: Adaptive variation in the mammalian respiratory system in relation to energetic demand. VIII. Structural and functional limits to oxidative metabolism. Respir Physiol *69*:117, 1987.

Thompson D'Arcy W: Growth and Form. New York: Cambridge University Press, 1942, p. 448.

Von Neergaard K: Neue Auffassungen über einen Grundbegriff der Atemmechanik. Die Retraktionskraft der Lunge, abhängig von der Oberflächenspannung in den Alveolen. Z Gesamte Exp Med *66*:373, 1929.

Wagner DD, Olmsted JB, Marder VJ: Immunolocalization of von Willebrand protein in Weibel-Palade bodies of human endothelial cells. J Cell Biol *95*:355, 1982.

Warhol MJ, Sweet JM: The ultrastructural localization of von Willebrand factor in endothelial cells. Am J Pathol *117*:310, 1984.

Weibel ER: Die Blutgefässanastomosen in der menschlichen Lunge. Z Zellforsch *50*:653, 1959.

Weibel ER: Morphometry of the Human Lung. Heidelberg: Springer, 1963.

Weibel ER: Morphometric estimation of pulmonary diffusion capacity. I. Model and method. Respir Physiol *11*:54, 1970/71.

Weibel ER: The Pathway for Oxygen: Structure and Function in the Mammalian Respiratory System. Cambridge MA: Harvard University Press, 1984, pp. 1-425.

Weibel ER: Lung cell biology. *In* Fishman AP, Fisher AB: Handbook of Physiology. Section 3, The Respiratory System, Vol. I. Bethesda: American Physiological Society, 1985, p. 47.

Weibel ER, Bachofen H: Structural design of the alveolar septum and fluid exchange. *In* Fishman AP, Renkin EM: Pulmonary Edema. Bethesda: American Physiological Society, 1979.

Weibel ER, Gil J: Structure function relationship at the alveolar level. *In* West JG: Bioengineering Aspects of the Lung. New York: Marcel Dekker, 1977.

Weibel ER, Gomez DM: Architecture of the human lung. Science *137*:577, 1962.

Weibel ER, Palade GE: New cytoplasmic components in arterial endothelia. J Cell Biol *23*:101, 1964.

Weibel ER, et al: Maximal oxygen consumption and pulmonary diffusing capacity: A direct comparison of physiologic morphometric measurements in canids. Respir Physiol *54*:173, 1983.

Weibel ER, et al: Adapative variation in the mammalian respiratory system in relation to energetic demand. VI. The pulmonary gas exchanger. Respir Physiol *69*:81, 1987.

Weibel ER, et al: Morphometric model for pulmonary diffusing capacity. I. Membrane diffusing capacity. Submitted for publication.

West BJ, V Bhargava V, Goldberg AL: Beyond the principle of similitude; Renormalization in the bronchial tree. J Appl Physiol *60*:1089, 1986.

Zeltner TB, Burri PH: The postnatal development and growth of the human lung. II. Morphology. Respir Physiol *67*:269, 1987.

Zeltner TB, et al: The postnatal development and growth of the human lung. I. Morphometry. Respir Physiol *67*:247, 1987.

READING REFERENCES

Ballard PL: Hormones and Lung Maturation. Berlin: Springer, 1986.

Burri PH: Development and growth of the human lung. *In* Fishman AP, Fischer AB: Handbook of Physiology, Section 3, The Respiratory System, Vol. I. Bethesda: American Physiological Society, 1985, p. 1.

Burri PH: Development and regeneration of the lung. *In* Fishman AP: Pulmonary Diseases and Disorders. Vol. 1. New York: McGraw-Hill Book, 1988, p. 61-78.

Burri PH: Postnatal development and growth of the pulmonary microvasculature. *In* Motta PM, Murakami T, Fujita H: Scanning Electron Microscopy of Vascular Casts: Methods and Applications. Boston: Kluwer Academic Publishers, 1992, p. 139-156.

Gil J: Models of Lung Disease. Vol. 47. New York: Marcel Dekker, 1990.

Murray JF: The Normal Lung. 2nd Ed. Philadelphia: WB Saunders, 1986.

Scarpelli EM, Mantone AJ: The pulmonary surfactant system. *In* Robertson B, van Golde LMG, Batenburg JJ: Pulmonary Surfactant. Amsterdam: Elsevier Science Publishers, 1984; p. 119.

Thurlbeck WM: Pathology of the lung. New York: Thieme, 1988.

Von Hayek H: Die menschliche Lunge. 2. Auflage. Heidelberg: Springer, 1970.

Weibel ER: Functional morphology of lung parenchyma. *In* Macklem PT, Mead J: Handbook of Physiology, Section 3, The Respiratory System, Vol. III. Part 1. Bethesda: American Physiological Society, Bethesda, 1986, p. 89.

CHAPTER 6

SURGICAL ANATOMY OF THE LUNGS

Thomas W. Shields

Until recent decades, the anatomy of the lungs was a little understood and seemingly unimportant subject. With the development of radiographic and endoscopic techniques and the advancement of pulmonary surgery, detailed anatomic knowledge of the lungs became a necessity.

The essential anatomic unit of the lung, the bronchopulmonary segment, was established as that portion of the lung substance that represents the total branching of a major — segmental — subdivision of a lobar bronchus. These units are named for their topographic position in the lung.

THE LOBES AND FISSURES

The right lung is composed of three lobes — the upper, middle, and lower — and is the larger of the two lungs. The left is made up of only two lobes — the upper and lower. Two fissures are usually present on the right. The oblique — major — fissure separates the lower lobe from the upper and middle lobes, and the horizontal — minor — fissure separates the other two (Fig. 6–1). In life, the oblique fissure on the right begins posteriorly at the level of the fifth rib or intercostal space, runs downward and forward approximating the course of the sixth rib, and ends at the diaphragm in the vicinity of the sixth costochondral junction. The horizontal fissure begins in the oblique fissure in the region of the midaxillary line at the level of the sixth rib and runs anteriorly to the costochondral junction of the fourth rib. On the left, the oblique — major — fissure is found (Fig. 6–2). This begins at a somewhat higher level posteriorly, between the third and fifth ribs, and runs downward and forward to end in the region of the sixth or seventh costochondral junction.

Variations in the fissures do occur, and often part or all of a fissure fails to develop. This is commonly seen as a more or less complete fusion of the middle lobe and the anterior portion of the upper lobe in over 50% of lungs examined. Accessory fissures occur also, and

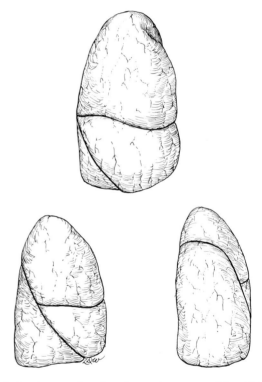

Fig. 6–1. Anterior, lateral, and posterior aspects of the right lung. *Redrawn and modified by permission from* Anson BJ: Atlas of Human Anatomy. Philadelphia: WB Saunders, 1950, p. 199.

certain portions of the lung may be demarcated into so-called accessory lobes. On occasion, such fissures are visible as linear shadows on the radiograph of the chest, and the accessory lobe may appear less radiolucent than the surrounding portions of the lung. The usual accessory lobes are the posterior accessory, the inferior accessory, the middle lobe of the left lung, and the azygos lobe (Fig. 6–3). In contrast to the first three named, which are true accessory lobes made up of specific bronchopulmonary segments, the azygos lobe is not a true accessory lobe because it is formed of

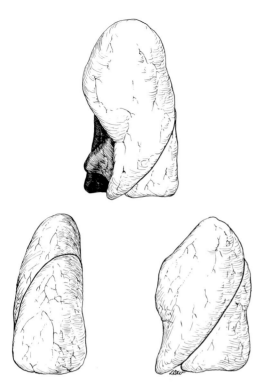

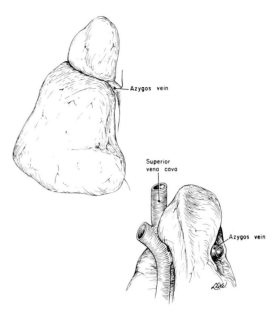

Fig. 6–4. Anterior and posterior views of the azygos lobe formed by an aberrant loop of the azygos vein. *Redrawn and modified by permission from* Anson BJ: Atlas of Human Anatomy. Philadelphia: WB Saunders, 1950, pp. 203-204.

Fig. 6–2. Anterior, lateral, and posterior aspects of the left lung. *Redrawn by permission from* Anson BJ: Atlas of Human Anatomy. Philadelphia: WB Saunders, 1950, p. 199.

varying portions of one or two segments — apical and posterior — of the right upper lobe. The fissure is formed by an aberrant loop of the azygos vein and its mesentery of two layers of the parietal pleura and two of the visceral pleura (Fig. 6–4). On the radiograph, this fissure may appear as an inverted comma to the right of the mediastinum (Fig. 6–5). This anomaly is seen in 0.5 to 1.0% of the anatomic dissections and routine radiographs of the chest.

BRONCHOPULMONARY SEGMENTS

Each lobe of the right and left lungs is subdivided into several individual anatomic units, the broncho-

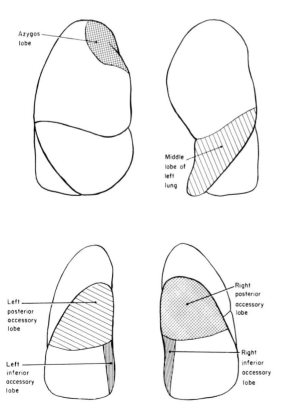

Fig. 6–3. Accessory lobes of the lungs.

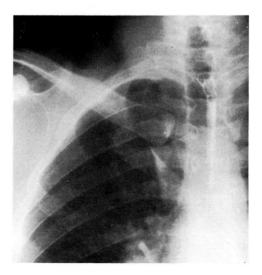

Fig. 6–5. Radiograph of the chest showing an azygos lobe.

Table 6–1. Bronchopulmonary Segments

	Right Lung		Left Lung	
		Upper Lobe		
Apical	1	Superior Division		
Anterior	2	Apical Posterior	1 + 3	
Posterior	3	Anterior	2	
		Inferior Division — Lingula		
		Superior Lingular	4	
		Inferior Lingular	5	
		Middle Lobe		
Lateral	4			
Medial	5			
		Lower Lobe		
Superior	6	Superior	6	
Medial Basal	7	Anteromedial Basal	7 + 8	
Anterior Basal	8	Lateral Basal	9	
Lateral Basal	9	Posterior Basal	10	
Posterior Basal	10			

pulmonary segments. The general pattern is that of 18 segments, 10 in the right lung and 8 in the left. The terminology proposed by Jackson and Huber (1943) is accepted by most and is listed in Table 6–1. The topographic positions of the segments are shown in Figure 6–6. Knowledge of the detailed anatomic features of the bronchial distribution and the vascular supply of each segment is essential for the surgeon. Although there is a general pattern to the anatomic features in each segment, variation is the rule. The usual pattern and the most common deviations from it are best portrayed by separate descriptions of the bronchial, arterial, and venous systems.

BRONCHIAL TREE*

The trachea bifurcates at about the level of the seventh thoracic vertebra into the right and left main stem bronchi. Compared with the left bronchus, which arises at a sharper angle, the right bronchus arises in a more direct line with the trachea — an important factor in the localization of aspirated material.

The Right Bronchial Tree

The length of the right main bronchus from the trachea to the point where the right upper lobe bronchus branches from its lateral wall is about 1.2 cm. The upper lobe bronchus, approximately 1 cm in length, in turn gives off three segmental bronchi, one to the apical, one to the posterior, and one to the anterior segment. The branching may be a simple trifurcation or with varying combinations of the three major branches. The segmental bronchi further subdivide to supply the various portions of the segments.

---

*The described anatomic patterns and variations of the bronchi and pulmonary arteries and veins have been selected by the author primarily from the studies of Birnbaum (1954), Bloomer, Liebow, and Hales (1960), and Boyden (1955).

Proceeding distally from the takeoff of the upper lobe bronchus, the primary bronchus is known as the bronchus intermedius, over which the main stem pulmonary artery crosses, thus giving rise to the term "eparterial bronchus" to designate the right upper lobe bronchus. After a distance of approximately 1.7 to 2 cm, the middle lobe bronchus arises from the anterior surface of the bronchus intermedius. It varies in length between 1.2 and 2.2 cm before it bifurcates into lateral and medial branches. The superior segmental bronchus of the lower lobe arises from the posterior wall of the bronchus intermedius, slightly distal to the middle lobe bronchus. The superior segment is called the posterior accessory lobe when a fissure is present. This bronchus most often arises as a single branch and divides into three rami, usually by bifurcation or rarely by trifurcation. Distal to the superior bronchus, the basal stem bronchus sends off segmental bronchi to the medial — the inferior accessory lobe when a fissure is present — anterior, lateral, and posterior basal segments. The medial basal bronchus arises anteromedially and is distributed to the anterior and paravertebral surfaces of the lower lobe. The anterior basal branch arises on the anterolateral aspect of the basal trunk approximately 2 cm distal to the superior segmental bronchus and divides into two major rami. The lateral basal bronchus and the posterior basal bronchus most often arise as a common stem. Each of these bronchi, in turn, divides typically into two major subdivisions (Fig. 6–7).

Numerous variations occur, but the basic pattern encountered is as described. Infrequently, the upper lobe bronchus on the right undergoes two separate bifurcations to form the three bronchopulmonary segments. Of more interest is the rare occurrence of a tracheal bronchus that arises above, or at the level of, the main stem carina and supplies the apical bronchopulmonary segment of the right upper lobe (Fig. 6–8). The variations in the middle lobe bronchus and its branchings, other than an occasional superoinferior spatial relationship of the segments rather than lateral and medial arrangements, are of little interest. In the division of the lower lobe bronchus, the presence of a subsuperior or an accessory subsuperior bronchus is a frequent finding. One to three such bronchi may be identified.

The Left Bronchial Tree

The left main bronchus is longer than the right and its first branch arises anterolaterally as the left upper lobe bronchus approximately 4 to 6 cm distal to the main stem carina. This bronchus is approximately 1 to 1.5 cm long and divides into superior and inferior — lingular — branches. The superior division ascends and the inferior descends. The superior branch most often bifurcates into an apical posterior segmental bronchus and an anterior segmental bronchus. Occasionally, the anterior segment migrates inferiorly to create a trifurcate pattern. The inferior or lingular bronchus — the analog of the middle lobe — is variable in length — 1 to 2 cm — and subsequently divides into superior and

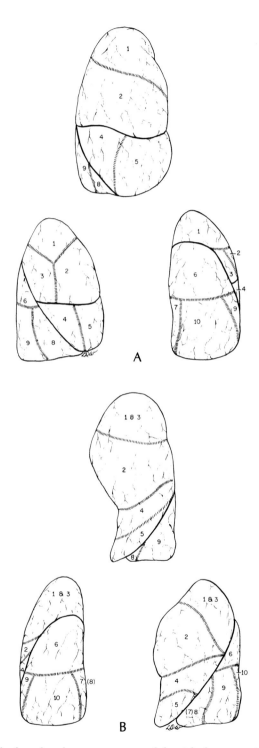

Fig. 6–6. *A*, Topographic positions of the bronchopulmonary segments of the right lung seen in anterior, lateral, and posterior views. *B*, Topographic positions of the bronchopulmonary segments of the left lung seen in anterior, lateral, and posterior views.

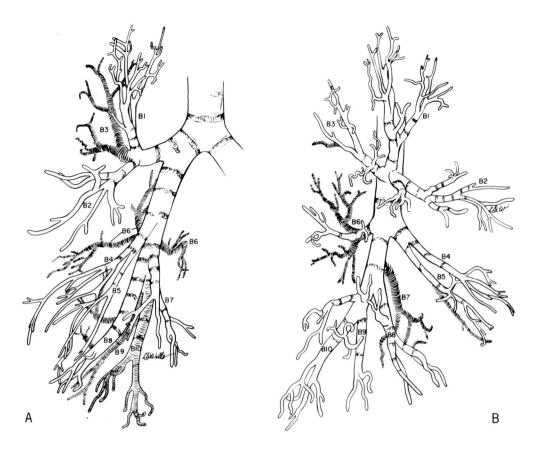

Fig. 6–7. *A* and *B*, Right bronchial tree, anterior and lateral views. Boyden's modification of numerical nomenclature used. (Redrawn and modified from Brock, R.C.: The Anatomy of the Bronchial Tree, 2nd ed. London, Oxford University Press, 1954, pp. 190-191.)

inferior divisions, the former of which in turn subdivides into posterior and inferior rami.

Approximately 0.5 cm distal to the left upper lobe orifice, the lower lobe stem bronchus gives off its first branch, the superior segmental bronchus. This bronchus arises posteriorly and bifurcates in most instances, but trifurcation does occur. After giving off the superior branch, the basal trunk continues for an average distance of 1.5 cm as a single trunk. The bronchus then usually bifurcates into an anteromedial basal segmental bronchus and a common stem bronchus for the lateral basal and posterior basal bronchi. These branches further subdivide into numerous rami for their respective segments (Fig. 6–9).

On the left side, the common variations are in the distribution of the segmental bronchi from the superior and inferior divisions of the left upper lobe bronchus and the presence of a subsuperior or accessory subsuperior bronchus arising from the lower lobe bronchus. Many of these deviations from normal have little clinical importance, but are significant at the time of surgical resection of the various portions of the lungs.

THE PULMONARY ARTERIAL SYSTEM

The main pulmonary artery arises to the left of the aorta and passes superiorly and to the left. It occupies a position anterior to the left main bronchus and divides into the right and left main pulmonary arteries. These two vessels lie in an oblique line that is parallel, and slightly superior, to the pulmonary veins. The right main pulmonary artery is longer than the left, but its extrapericardial length up to its first branch is less than that of the left. The branching pattern of the pulmonary arteries is more variable than that of the bronchi, although the arteries tend to lie closely adjacent to the segmental bronchi and to follow their branching. No one pattern for either the right or the left pulmonary artery may be described as standard. A relatively typical distribution of the segmental arteries is often encountered, however, and from this, the multitude of variations may be readily understood (Figs. 6–10, 6–11).

The Right Pulmonary Artery

As it leaves the pericardial sac, the right pulmonary artery is anterior and inferior to the right main bronchus and posterior and superior to the superior pulmonary vein. The first branch is the truncus anterior — the major vessel carrying blood to the right upper lobe. It arises superolaterally and divides into two branches. The more superior branch of the truncus anterior again divides to form an apical branch that loops posteriorly over the upper lobe bronchus to supply a variable

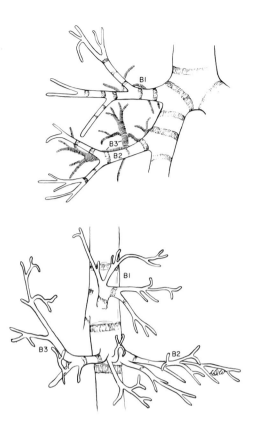

Fig. 6–8. Tracheal bronchus supplying the apical segment of the right upper lobe. (Redrawn and modified with permission from Bloomer, W.E., Liebow, A.A., and Hales, M.R.: Surgical Anatomy of the Bronchovascular Segments. Springfield, IL, Charles C Thomas, 1960, p. 25.)

lobar portion of the artery, the vessel is considered the common basal trunk. The medial basal segmental artery may arise independently or may arise in common with the anterior basal branch. The remainder of the basal trunk then terminates with its division into the lateral and posterior segmental branches, the mode of actual branching being variable.

The major variations in the right arterial system occur with almost each of the aforementioned branchings. In as many as 20% of the population, two arteries arise from the anterior trunk. These vessels are designated as the truncus anterior superior and the truncus anterior inferior. When they are present, the recurrent posterior branch is almost always a branch of the truncus anterior superior. Infrequently, more than one ascending branch to the upper lobe arises from the interlobar portion of the artery; the more proximal branch supplies a portion of the anterior segment. On occasion, the posterior ascending artery arises from the superior segmental artery or, even more rarely, from the middle lobe artery. The middle lobe artery, as well as the superior segmental artery, although usually a single vessel, may be represented by two or, at times, even three vessels. Last, in addition to the variable branchings of the common basal trunk, a subsuperior or accessory subsuperior artery may arise from either the common stem or the posterior basal branch.

The Left Pulmonary Artery

The left pulmonary artery ascends to a higher level, passes more posteriorly, and has a greater length before giving off its first segmental branch to the lung than does the right pulmonary artery. The branches to the left upper lobe arise from the anterior, the posterosuperior, and the interlobar portions of the vessel. The number of branches may vary from two to seven, but four branches to the lobe form the most common pattern. Generally, the first branch arises from the anterior portion of the artery to supply the anterior segment, a part of the apical segment, and occasionally, the lingular division of the lobe. The first branch of this anterior segmental artery supplies the anterior segment and also may give off a lingular branch. Usually, it also branches to provide a vessel carrying blood to the apical segment. The second and, infrequently, a third branch from this first anterior trunk give rise to a vessel, or vessels, going to the anterior segment, to the apical segment, and uncommonly, to the posterior segment. This anterior trunk is generally short, and often the branches may appear as separate vessels arising from a common opening from the main artery. A second branch from the main artery as it passes distally and posterosuperiorly over the left upper lobe bronchus and into the interlobar fissure is present in almost 80% of instances. This second arterial branch, and occasionally a third, is given off anterosuperiorly to the apical posterior segment. Posteriorly, as the artery passes into the interlobar fissure, it branches to form a vessel going to the superior segment of the lower lobe. This vessel usually is a single one that bifurcates or, infrequently,

portion of the posterior segment. The latter vessel is known as the posterior recurrent artery. The more inferior branch of the truncus anterior goes to the anterior segment, but also may give off a branch to the apical segment. The truncus anterior carries the entire blood supply to the right upper lobe in one out of ten individuals. In most persons, one or more ascending vessels from the interlobar portion of the pulmonary artery are also present. The interlobar portion crosses over the bronchus intermedius. Generally, only one ascending vessel to the upper lobe is present. This branch, frequently small in caliber, supplies almost exclusively the posterior segment and is referred to as the posterior ascending artery. At the same level, or even either slightly proximal or distal to the posterior ascending artery, the middle lobe artery arises anteromedially from the interlobar portion of the pulmonary artery. The site of origin is usually at the level of the junction of the horizontal and oblique fissures. The artery is usually single and bifurcation of the vessel is the rule, but the subdivisions are variable. The arterial branch to the superior segment of the lower lobe arises posteriorly and opposite to the middle lobe artery at the same level or slightly distal to it. The superior segmental artery is usually a single trunk that bifurcates. Distal to the aforementioned branchings of the inter-

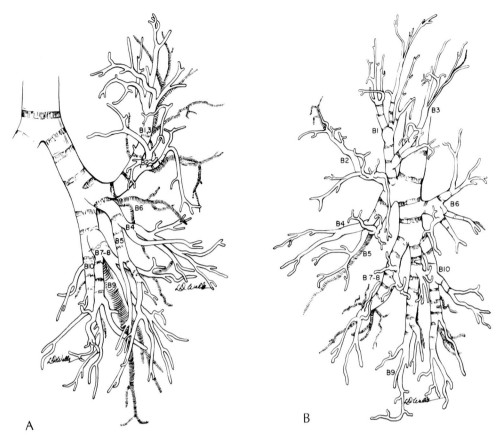

Fig. 6–9. *A* and *B*, Left bronchial tree, anterior and lateral views. Boyden's modification of numerical nomenclature used. (Redrawn and modified from Brock, R.C.: The Anatomy of the Bronchial Tree, 2nd ed. London, Oxford University Press, 1954, pp. 191-192.)

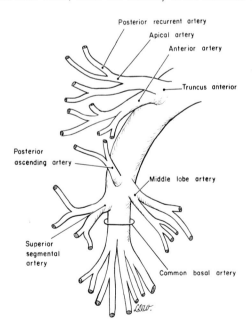

Fig. 6–10. Common pattern of branching of the right pulmonary artery.

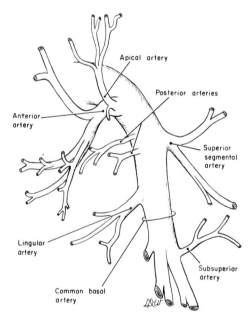

Fig. 6–11. Common pattern of branching of the left pulmonary artery.

trifurcates at a variable distance from its takeoff from the main stem arterial trunk. Most often, the lingular artery originates from the interlobar portion of the pulmonary artery distal to the superior segmental artery

and constitutes the lingular arterial supply in toto in 80% of persons. At a variable distance from the origin of the lingular vessel, the pulmonary stem artery, now the common basal trunk, most commonly divides into two major branches. The more anterior branch supplies the anteromedial basal segment, and the posterior one supplies the lateral basal and posterior basal segments. The patterns of branching of the common basal trunk and its major divisions are variable.

Likewise, major variations may occur in all the segmental branches of the left pulmonary artery. As mentioned, the first anterior branch may supply the lingular division as well as other portions of the upper lobe, and, although in less than one in ten individuals, this branch may carry all the blood supplying the lingular division. Another variation is that the first anterior branch may carry only the blood supplying the apical segment; the anterior segment in this situation receives its arterial supply from the interlobar portion of the artery. As noted, the superior segmental artery usually arises proximal to the branch, or branches, going to the lingula, but in as many as one in three persons, the superior segmental branch may be distal to the lingular artery takeoff. Both these vessels may be multiple. Again, in one of three persons, a branch of one of the lingular vessels or even a direct branch from the interlobar portion of the artery may supply some blood to the anterior segment of the left upper lobe. Rarely, this vascular branch carries the entire arterial supply to this segment. As on the right, branches to the subsuperior segmental region are often found arising as single or multiple vessels from the common basal stem or, more frequently, from the posterior basal branch. Last, a vessel may arise from the common basal stem or one of its branches to contribute to the lingular blood supply.

PULMONARY VENOUS SYSTEM

The venous drainage pattern of the lung reveals a greater number of variations than does the arterial pattern. The usual two major venous trunks from both lungs are the superior and inferior pulmonary veins. The tributaries of these veins are intersegmental and form various combinations to create the major trunks (Figs. 6–12, 6–13).

Right Pulmonary Veins

The superior pulmonary vein lies anterior and somewhat inferior to the pulmonary artery. It usually is made up of four major branches, which drain the upper and middle lobes. The first three branches from above downward drain the upper lobe and are identified as the apical anterior, anterior-inferior, and posterior branches. The posterior branch is composed of central and interlobar divisions. The fourth and most inferior trunk drains the middle lobe and generally is made up of two branches. Although the middle lobe vein most often joins the superior pulmonary vein, on occasion, it may enter the pericardium and drain into the atrium as a separate vessel. Rarely, it becomes a tributary of the inferior pulmonary vein.

The inferior pulmonary vein is inferior and posterior to the superior vein. It drains the lower lobe and as a rule is made up of two major trunks. The first is the

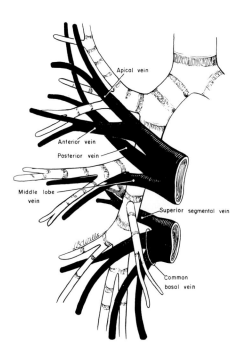

Fig. 6–12. Schematic representation of the tributaries of the right superior and inferior pulmonary veins. *Adapted with permission from Kubick S: Klinische Anatomie, Ein Farbfoto-Atlas der Topographie 2. Aufl (Band III-Thorax). Stuttgart: Georg Thieme, 1971, p. 97.*

superior segmental vein, which drains the superior segment. The other branch, known as the common basal vein, is made up of superior basal and inferior basal tributaries, and these vessels drain the various basal segments of the lower lobe.

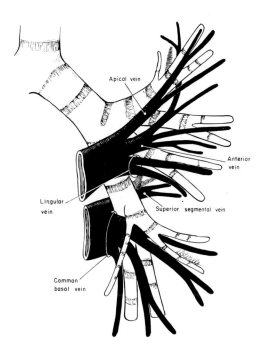

Fig. 6–13. Schematic representation of the tributaries of the left superior and inferior pulmonary veins *Adapted with permission from Kubick S: Klinische Anatomie, Ein Farbfoto-Atlas der Topographie 2. Aufl (Band III-Thorax). Stuttgart: Georg Thieme, 1971, p. 97.*

Left Pulmonary Veins

On the left, the superior pulmonary vein is closely applied to the anteroinferior aspect of the pulmonary artery, and, as a result, obscures the anterior branches of the artery. This vein is made up of three to four tributaries that drain the entire upper lobe. The first division, the apical posterior vein, is made up of an apical ramus and a posterior ramus. The second division represents the anterior vein, which may have three rami: a superior, inferior, and posterior rami. The third and fourth divisions represent the superior and inferior lingular veins. A single trunk may represent these veins in about 50% of persons. This trunk, as seen with the middle lobe vein on the right, may drain into the inferior pulmonary vein; this variant occurs more commonly on the left than on the right.

The inferior pulmonary vein, as on the right, is located inferior and posterior to the superior vein and has two similar tributaries: the superior segmental and the common basal veins. The latter is made up of superior and inferior basal divisions, which drain the basal segments of the lobe.

INTRAPERICARDIAL ANATOMY

The right pulmonary artery passes from the left to the right behind the ascending aorta and constitutes the superior border of the transverse sinus. It then lies behind the superior vena cava and forms the superior border of the postcaval recess of Allison (Fig. 6–14); the medial and inferior borders of this recess are the superior vena cava and right superior pulmonary vein. Although the right pulmonary artery is longer than the left pulmonary artery, it is not as accessible as the left. The left pulmonary artery passes inferior to the aortic arch and forms the superior border of the left pulmonary

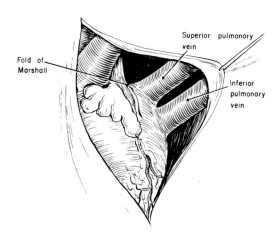

Fig. 6–15. Intrapericardial anatomy on the left. (Redrawn with permission from Healey, J.E., Jr., and Gibbon, J.H., Jr.: Intrapericardial anatomy in relation to pneumonectomy for pulmonary carcinoma. J. Thorac. Surg. *19*:864, 1950.)

recess. The medial border of this recess is formed by the fold of Marshall (Fig. 6–15).

The superior and inferior pulmonary veins bulge into the pericardium and are invested to a greater, or lesser, extent by the pericardium's serous layer. On the right, these two vessels most often enter into the left atrium separately, although rarely they form one vessel. In contrast, on the left, the two veins form a common trunk in one out of four persons.

The serous — parietal — pericardial investments of the vessels are important because these fibrous tissue layers must be divided to obtain free access to the entire circumference of the individual vessel. On the right, the serous layer leaves the lateral and posterior surfaces of the superior vena cava and comes to lie upon the artery in the postcaval recess. At this point, only about one fifth of the circumference of the vessel is free. In contrast, three fourths of the circumference is free in the transverse sinus medial to the superior vena cava. From the artery, the serous layer passes inferiorly and reflects upon the superior, anterior, and inferior surfaces of the superior vein; approximately one third of this vessel is not free posteriorly. The layer then descends to cover most of the inferior pulmonary vein and then passes down to envelop the inferior vena cava. On the left, the reflection of the serous pericardium passes over the anterior and inferior surfaces of the left pulmonary artery, and approximately one half of the vessel is free in the pericardial sac. The layer then descends inferiorly to the superior vein, so that only the posterior surface is not free in the sac. It then passes downward to envelop the inferior vein, which is subsequently almost totally free within the sac, except for a small surface located posteriorly.

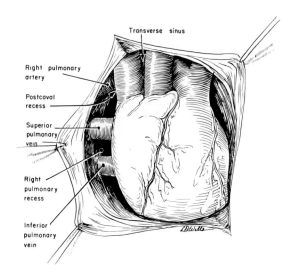

Fig. 6–14. Intrapericardial anatomy on the right. (Redrawn with permission from Healey, J.E., Jr., and Gibbon, J.H., Jr.: Intrapericardial anatomy in relation to pneumonectomy for pulmonary carcinoma. J. Thorac. Surg. *19*:864, 1950.)

BRONCHIAL ARTERIES AND VEINS

The bronchial arterial system arises from the systemic circulation and accounts for approximately 1% of the cardiac output. It empties mainly into the pulmonary veins and a lesser bronchial vein system that enters the azygos venous system on the right and the hemiazygos on the left. The origins of the arteries are variable from the aorta, intercostal arteries, and, occasionally, from the subclavian or innominate arteries. Rare origin from other systemic vessels of the chest — internal mammary artery — or even from a coronary artery has been recorded.

The most extensive anatomic study was reported by Caudwell and associates (1948). These investigators recorded nine patterns of origin. In 90% of the 150 autopsy specimens studied, the pattern was one of four types (Fig. 6–16), and the remaining 10% were distributed in five other less common variations (Table 6–2).

The level of origin of the bronchial arteries was from the third to eighth vertebral bodies, most commonly between the levels of the fifth and sixth thoracic vertebrae, and arose from the descending thoracic aorta and rarely from the arch. Most of the bronchial vessels arose separately — 74% of specimens — and only in

Table 6–2. Origins and Number of Bronchial Arteries in 150 Dissected Autopsy Specimens

Anatomic Variation	Number of Right Bronchial Arteries	Number of Left Bronchial Arteries	% Incidence
I	1	2	40.8
II	1	1	21.3
III	2	2	20.8
IV	2	1	9.7
V	1	3	4.0
VI	2	3	2.0
VII	3	2	0.6
VIII	1	4	0.6
IX	4*	1	0.6

*A branch from the left bronchial artery anterior to the esophagus passing to the right bronchus plus two right bronchial arteries from the aorta and one right bronchial artery from the subclavian artery. *From* Caudwell EW, et al: The bronchial arteries. An anatomic study of 150 human cadavers. Surg Gynecol Obstet 86:395,1948.

26% did two vessels have a common origin. The right bronchial arteries arose from the anterolateral or lateral surface of the aorta and rarely from its posterior aspect. In 88.7% of specimens, the right bronchial artery arose in common with an aortic intercostal vessel: 78% from the first, 7.3% from the second, and 1.3% from the third. Nathan and colleagues (1970) described the anatomy of this major right bronchial artery. They found that it arose anywhere from 0.5 to 5 cm from the origin of the intercostal artery from its origin from the aorta and courses upward and forward toward the right main stem bronchus. In its courses on the right anterolateral aspect of the vertebral column, it passes to the right of the thoracic duct and crosses the esophagus to terminate at the lower level of the trachea near the origin of the right main stem bronchus. At the level of the trachea, it crosses lateral to the vagus nerve. In its mediastinal course, the right bronchial artery generally runs parallel to the arch of the azygos vein by which it is overlapped.

On the left, the bronchial arteries are more variable in their courses to the bronchus and, according to Caudwell and associates (1948), 94% arise directly from the aorta. Only 4% are associated with an intercostal vessel, which invariably is a right intercostal artery. In most instances, the bronchial vessels that arise from the aorta pass in back of the trachea, and in only a few cases does one pass in front of the trachea. Rarely, such a branch to the right may be in close proximity to the tracheal carina. It is possible a branch of such an anatomically situated vessel could be injured during a mediastinoscopy as suggested by Miller and Nelems (1989).

These anatomic studies by the aforementioned investigators have been confirmed by the angiographic observations of Olson and Athanasoulis (1982) and other interventional radiologists. Deffebach and associates (1987) reviewed the distribution of the bronchial arteries once they entered the hilus of the lung and course within the bronchial tree. Essentially, the arteries to either side form a communicating arc around the main bronchus.

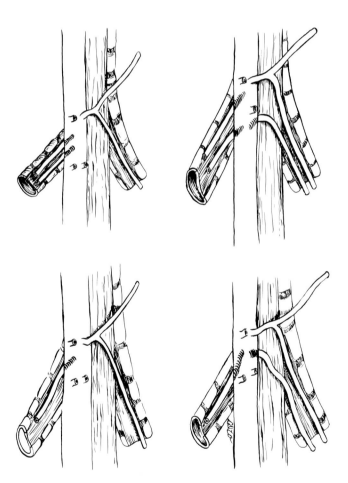

Fig. 6–16. The four most common sites of origin and numbers of bronchial arteries to the right and left lung (see Table 6–2 for percentage of occurrence of each). *From* Caudwell, EW, et al: The bronchial arteries. An anatomic study of 150 human cadavers. Surg Gynecol Obstet 86:395, 1948.

From here, the main arterial divisions radiate along the major bronchi. These vessels are closely applied to the bronchial wall, with generally two divisions, an anterior and posterior branch, along each bronchus. The vessels follow the course of the bronchus and divide as do the bronchi. Networks of intercommunicating vessels are often present on the bronchial walls. It has been assumed that two thirds of this blood supply empties into the pulmonary veins, and that the rest empties into the bronchial veins. The bronchial veins are present in the mucosa and also external to the bronchial cartilage. The direction of flow is to the venous plexus of the perihilar regions and then subsequently into either the azygos or hemiazygos systems.

REFERENCES

Anson BJ: Atlas of Human Anatomy. Philadelphia: WB Saunders, 1950.

Birnbaum, GL: Anatomy of the Bronchovascular System. Its Application to Surgery. Chicago, Year Book Medical Publishers, 1954.

Bloomer WE, Liebow AA, Hales MR: Surgical Anatomy of the Bronchovascular Segments. Springfield, IL: Charles C Thomas, 1960.

Boyden EA: Segmental Anatomy of the Lungs. New York: McGraw-Hill Book, 1955.

Caudwell EW, et al: The bronchial arteries. An anatomic study of 150 human cadavers. Surg Gynecol Obstet 86:395, 1948.

Deffebach ME, et al: The bronchial circulation, small but a vital attribute of the lung. Am Rev Respir Dis 135:463, 1987.

Jackson CL, Huber JF: Correlated applied anatomy of bronchial tree and lungs with system nomenclature. Dis Chest 9:319, 1943.

Kubick S: Klinische Anatomie, Ein Farbfoto — Atlas der Topographie 2. Aufl (Band III — Thorax). Stuttgart: Georg Thieme, 1971.

Miller RR, Nelems B: Mediastinal lymph node necrosis: A newly recognized complication of mediastinoscopy. Ann Thorac Surg 48:247, 1989.

Nathan H, Barkay M, Orda R: Anatomic observations on the origin and course of the aortic intercostal arteries. J Thorac Surg 59:372, 1970.

Nathan H, Orda R, Barkay M: The right bronchial artery, anatomical considerations and surgical approach. Thorax 25:328, 1970.

Olson PR, Athanasoulis CA: Hemoptysis: Treatment with transcatheter embolizations of the bronchial arteries. In Athanasoulis CA, et al: Interventional Radiology. Philadelphia: WB Saunders, 1982, p. 196.

READING REFERENCES

Allison PR: Intrapericardial approach to the lung root in the treatment of bronchial carcinoma by dissection pneumonectomy. J Thorac Surg 15:99, 1946.

Barrett RJ, Day JC, Tuttle WM: The arterial distribution to the left upper pulmonary lobe. J Thorac Surg 32:190, 1956.

Barrett RJ, O'Rourke PV, Tuttle WM: The arterial distribution to the right upper pulmonary lobe. J Thorac Surg 36:117, 1958.

Brock RC: The Anatomy of the Bronchial Tree. 2nd Ed. London: Oxford University Press, 1954.

Cory RAS, Valentine EJ: Varying patterns of the lobar branches of the pulmonary artery. Thorax 14:267, 1959.

Cudkowicz L: The Human Bronchial Circulation in Health and Disease. Baltimore: Williams & Wilkins, 1968.

Healey JE Jr, Gibbon JH Jr: Intrapericardial anatomy in relation to pneumonectomy for pulmonary carcinoma. J Thorac Surg 19:864, 1950.

Kent EM, Blades B: The surgical anatomy of the pulmonary lobes. J Thorac Surg 12:18, 1942.

Kubik S, Healey JE: Surgical Anatomy of the Thorax. Philadelphia: WB Saunders, 1970.

Milloy FJ, Wragg LE, Anson BJ: The pulmonary arterial supply to the right upper lobe of the lung based upon a study of 300 laboratory and surgical specimens. Surg Gynecol Obstet 116:35, 1963.

Milloy FJ, Wragg LE, Anson BJ: The pulmonary arterial supply to the upper lobe of the left lung. Surg Gynecol Obstet 126:811, 1968.

CHAPTER 7

LYMPHATICS OF THE LUNGS

Thomas W. Shields

The lung has an extensive network of lymphatic vessels that are situated in the loose connective tissue beneath the visceral pleura, in the connective tissue in the interlobular septa, and in the peribronchial-vascular sheaths.

In the pulmonary parenchyma, the lymphatic capillaries form extensive plexuses within the connective tissue sheaths that surround the airways and the blood vessels. The origin of these channels is believed to be at the level of the terminal and respiratory bronchioles and they do not extend into the interalveolar septa according to Leak and Jamuar (1983). The channels begin as blind-end tubes and saccules. As these channels extend proximally toward the hilar area associated with the enlarging airways and blood vessels, they have been designated as juxta-alveolar lymphatics by Lauwreyns (1971) and Leak (1980). These networks drain into larger collecting vessels with thicker walls and contain monocuspid, conical valves that direct the flow of lymph toward the hilar area in a centripetal direction. The physiologic mechanisms controlling this lymphatic flow are little understood.

Lymphatic channels that also drain the periphery of the lung lobules run in the lobular septa along with the pulmonary veins. With the occurrence of extra-alveolar interstitial edema, some of these may be recognized as Kerley's B lines radiographically as noted by Steiner (1973) (Fig. 7–1).

The extensive subpleural network drains primarily by the channels in the interlobular septa to the hilar area, but direct connections to the mediastinum have been recorded by Rouvière (1932), Borrie (1952, 1965), and more recently by Riquet and associates (1989). The channels in the lobular septa have multiple connections with the channels in the bronchovascular sheaths. These connecting channels are frequently up to 4 cm in length and lie midway between the hilus and the periphery of the lung. When distended, they are recognized as Kerley's A lines (see Fig. 7–1).

Collections of lymphatic cells may be seen along the course of the lymphatic channels and within the bron-

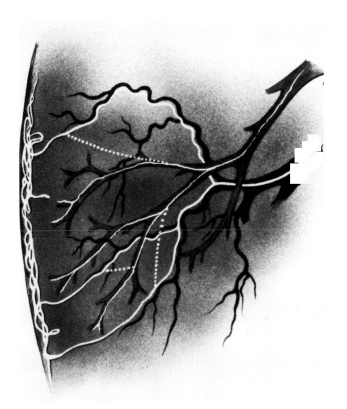

Fig. 7–1. Lymphatic drainage of the lung and pleura is shown in a drawing of a coronal section through the middle of the lung. Lymphatic channels from the pleural plexus enter the lungs at the interlobular septa and extend medially to the hilus along the venous radicals (dark vessels). Lymphatic channels originating in the peripheral parenchyma extending medially in the bronchovascular bundles (lighter shaded vessels). Communicating lymphatics (dotted lines) extend between the peribronchial and perivenous lymphatics. *From* Fraser RC, Paré JAP: Diagnosis of Diseases of the Chest. 2nd Ed. Philadelphia: WB Saunders, 1977.

chial structures, but recognizable intrapulmonary lymph nodes are recognized only infrequently in contrast to the common presence of bronchopulmonary lymph nodes.

PULMONARY LYMPH NODES

The pulmonary lymph nodes are divided into the intrapulmonary and the bronchopulmonary nodes. The latter are subdivided into the lobar and hilar lymph nodes.

Intrapulmonary Lymph Nodes

The intrapulmonary lymph nodes are located infrequently just beneath the visceral pleura. Rarely, a peripheral lymph node may present as a solitary peripheral nodule as reported by Greenberg (1961). Trapnell (1964) was able to identify radiologically peripheral lymph nodes in only 1 of 92 inflated lungs obtained at autopsy, an incidence of just over 1%. With high-resolution computed tomography — CT, some of the small lesions identified in patients with multiple metastases to the lung are subsequently proved to be small peripheral lymph nodes.

In addition to these rare, radiographically identified intrapulmonary lymph nodes, Trapnell (1963) reported the identification of other intrapulmonary lymph nodes in the substance of the lung by a combined technique of injection of the subpleural lymphatics and subsequent radiologic evaluation of autopsy lung specimens. Intrapulmonary nodes were observed in 5 of 28 injected specimens; an incidence of 18%. The actual location of these nodes was undocumented, but Nagaishi (1972) noted that such lymph nodes are related to the bifurcation of the segmental bronchi or may lie in the bifurcation of the branches of the associated pulmonary arteries and may extend out to the fifth or sixth order segmental bronchi.

Bronchopulmonary Lymph Nodes

The lobar bronchopulmonary lymph nodes are found at the angles formed by the origins of the various lobar bronchi and lie in close association with the bronchus or the adjacent pulmonary vessels. The hilar lymph nodes are situated alongside the lower portions of the main bronchi or the respective pulmonary artery and the pulmonary veins lying within the visceral pleural reflections.

The number of bronchopulmonary lymph nodes is variable. These lymph nodes more frequently are present in greater numbers in children than in adults. Borrie (1965) suggests that the maximal development of these nodes is reached by the end of the first decade of life and then atrophy and disappearance of these lymph nodes occur gradually during adulthood. The presence of pulmonary infection or malignancy greatly affects the number of bronchopulmonary lymph nodes that may be identified.

In a study of 200 operative specimens of lungs containing lung cancer, Borrie (1965) identified lymph nodes in 13 locations in the right lung and in 15 locations in the left lung that are now considered bronchopulmonary lymph nodes. These sites are listed in Table 7–1, and shown schematically in Figures 7–2 and 7–3. The incidence of bronchopulmonary lymph nodes present in each location is listed in Table 7–2.

Hilar Lymph Nodes

The hilar lymph nodes are contiguous with the lobar lymph nodes distally as well as with the mediastinal lymph nodes proximally. The hilar lymph nodes lying superior to the right main stem bronchus classically have been considered to extend up to the inferior border of the azygos vein, but this concept was questioned by Tisi and associates (1983) in their recommendations as to the location of the various mediastinal lymph node stations. The lymph nodes medial to the right main stem bronchus may be considered as hilar nodes when located away from the tracheal carina, but as they become subadjacent to this structure, they are best termed

Table 7–1. Distribution of Bronchopulmonary Lymph Nodes*

Right Lung	Left Lung
1. Between upper and middle lobe bronchi	1. Angle between left upper and lower lobe bronchi
2. Below middle lobe bronchus	2. Above upper lobe bronchus
3. Medial to upper lobe bronchus	3. Medial to left main bronchus
4. Above upper lobe bronchus	4. Medial to superior segmental bronchus
5. Junction of oblique and transverse fissure lying on right pulmonary artery	5. Medial to upper lobe bronchus
6. Medial to superior segmental bronchus	6. Above superior segmental bronchus
7. Behind upper lobe bronchus	7. Anterior to left main bronchus
8. Medial to middle lobe bronchus	8. Behind left main bronchus
9. Between superior segmental bronchus and lower lobe bronchus	9. Medial to lower lobe bronchus
10. Medial to lower lobe bronchi	10. Behind upper lobe bronchus
11. Above superior segmental bronchus	11. Lateral to left main bronchus
12. Between anterior and medial basal bronchi	12. Lateral to lower lobe bronchus
13. Lateral to lower lobe bronchus	13. Lateral to upper lobe bronchus
	14. Between segmental bronchi of left upper lobe
	15. Between superior segmental bronchus and basal bronchi

*Listed in order of decreasing frequency of the number of times lymph nodes identified in each location. *From* Borrie J: Lung Cancer. Surgery and Survival. New York: Appleton-Century-Crofts, 1965.

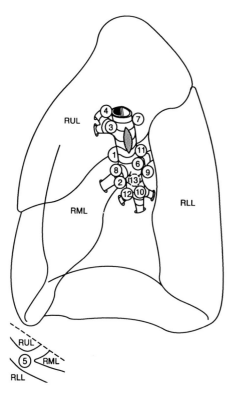

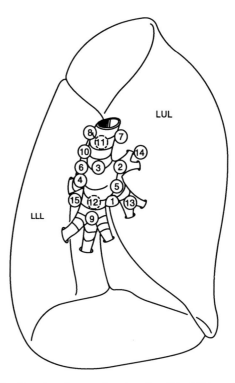

Fig. 7–2. Bronchopulmonary lymph nodes of the right lung. Drawing of the medial aspect of the right lung shows the 13 most common locations of lymph nodes identified in 93 specimens by Borrie. The sites are numbered in the order of decreasing frequency in which lymph nodes were identified in each respective site (see Tables 7–1 and 7–2). Inset at bottom shows the lateral view of the junction of the oblique and transverse fissures. At this site, lymph nodes are lateral to the origins of the middle and lower lobe branches of the right pulmonary artery. *Redrawn from* Borrie J: Lung Cancer: Surgery and Survival. New York: Appleton-Century-Crofts, 1965.

Fig. 7–3. Bronchopulmonary lymph nodes of the left lung. Drawing of the medial aspect of the left lung shows the 15 most common locations of bronchopulmonary lymph nodes identified in 101 specimens by Borrie. The sites are numbered in the order of decreasing frequency in which lymph nodes were identified in each respective site (see Tables 7–1 and 7–2). *Redrawn from* Borrie J: Lung Cancer Surgery and Survival. New York: Appleton-Century-Crofts, 1965.

subcarinal lymph nodes and thus belong to the lymph nodes of the mediastinal compartment.

On the left side, the anatomic separation between the hilar and the mediastinal lymph nodes proximally is at an imaginary plane connecting the lateral surfaces of the ascending and descending portions of the thoracic aorta. The left hilar nodes are located medial, anterior, posterior, and lateral to the left main stem bronchus in the order of decreasing frequency in number. The hilar nodes located anteriorly are found in relationship to the left main stem pulmonary artery. Proximally, these latter nodes are contiguous with the subaortic lymph nodes of the mediastinum, including the lymph node located at the site of the ligament arteriosum — the so-called Bartello's node. The nodes on the medial surface of the main stem bronchus as their position advances upward become subcarinal in location.

Lobar Lymph Nodes

The two most common locations in which lobar lymph nodes are found in the right lung are between the upper lobe bronchus and middle lobe bronchus: the area that

Borrie (1952) termed the right bronchial sump — the superior interlobar lymph node of Rouvière (1932) — and the region just below the middle lobe bronchus adjacent to the lower lobe bronchus — the inferior interlobar lymph node of Rouvière (1932). In the left lung, the most common location is at the angle of the left upper lobe bronchus and the lower lobe bronchus. Borrie (1952) designated this area as the left lymphatic sump and the nodes found here correspond to the left interlobar node of Rouvière (1932).

Right Lymphatic Sump

The lymph nodes in the lymphatic sump of the right lung lie in relationship to the bronchus intermedius (Fig. 7–4). According to Nohl-Oser (1989), a constant lymph node is found at the upper posterior end of the major fissure in the angle between the right upper lobe bronchus and the bronchus intermedius. A branch of the bronchial artery coursing over the posterior aspect of the right main bronchus leads to it (Fig. 7–5). Another lymph node is found on the interlobar portion of the pulmonary artery where this vessel gives off the posterior ascending segmental branch to the posterior segment of the upper lobe and the superior segmental artery to the superior segment of the lower lobe. Inferiorly, this lymph node is contigu-

Table 7–2. Bronchopulmonary Nodes

Right Lung		Left Lung	
Area	% Nodes Present*	Area	% Nodes Present†
1	100	1	97
2	65.5	2	49
3	42	3	33
4	40	4	32
5	29	5	29
6	25	6	22
7	22.5	7	21
8	22.5	8	17
9	21.5	9	16
10	10	10	14
11	7.5	11	13
12	3	12	8
13	2	13	6
		14	6
		15	4

*Percent of 93 right lung specimens containing bronchopulmonary lymph nodes in each area.

†Percent of 101 left lung specimens containing bronchopulmonary lymph nodes in each area.

Adapted from Borrie J: Lung Cancer. Surgery and Survival. New York: Appleton-Century-Crofts, 1965.

ous with a constant node lying above the superior segmental bronchus of the lower lobe. Other lymph nodes of the sump are found at the base of the major fissure lying closely alongside the interlobar portion of the pulmonary artery or in the bifurcations of its branches. Frequently, lymph nodes are identified more

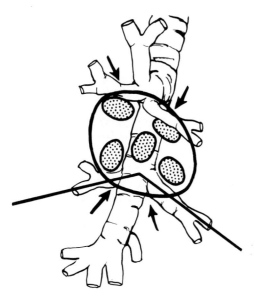

Fig. 7–4. The collection of lymph nodes lying within the right lymphatic sump. The line drawn through the axis of the superior segmental bronchus of the lower lobe and the middle lobe bronchus represents the level below which nodes are not involved by malignant disease in the upper lobe. Arrows indicate the tendency of lymphatic drainage. *From* Nohl-Oser HC: Lymphatics of the Lung. *In* Shields TW (ed): General Thoracic Surgery. 3rd Ed. Philadelphia: Lea & Febiger, 1989.

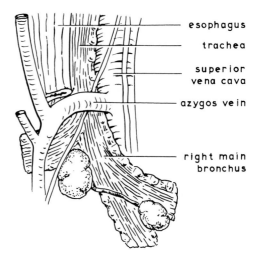

Fig. 7–5. The posterior aspect of the right main bronchus, as seen when the lung is pulled forward during dissection. The subcarinal lymph nodes and the node below the right upper lobe bronchus are seen. A constant bronchial artery leading to the latter node is shown. *From* Nohl-Oser HC: Lymphatics of the Lung. *In* Shields TW (ed): General Thoracic Surgery. 3rd Ed. Philadelphia: Lea & Febiger, 1989.

anteriorly, lying among the upper lobe branches of the superior pulmonary vein.

Other Interlobar Lymph Nodes of the Right Lung

In addition to the sump nodes, the other interlobar lymph nodes can be grouped according to Borrie (1965) into those of the upper, middle, and lower lobes. The lymph nodes of the right upper lobe are located above the upper lobe bronchus, medial to it and just behind it. Those lying above the bronchus merge with the hilar nodes of the distal portion of the right main stem bronchus. The lymph nodes of the middle lobe, in addition to the subadjacent node below the middle lobe bronchus — the inferior interlobar node of Rouvière (1932) — are located lateral to the middle lobe bronchus near its confluence with the lower lobe bronchus, as well as medial to it. The right lower lobe lymph nodes, in addition to the aforementioned superior and inferior sump nodes, are found medial to the superior segmental bronchus or between it and the basal bronchi. Lymph nodes are also present in relationship to the basal stem of the lower lobe bronchus and lay on its medial aspect, lateral to it and between the anterior and medial basal bronchi.

Left Lymphatic Sump

The collection of lymph nodes described by Nohl (1956, 1962) — Nohl-Oser (1972) — as comprising the left lymphatic sump lies between the upper and lower lobes in the main fissure (Fig. 7–6). A constant node is present in the bifurcation between the upper and lower lobe bronchi in close relationship to the origin of the lingular — inferior division — branch of the upper lobe (Fig. 7–7). A small bronchial arterial branch passing across the membranous portion of the left main

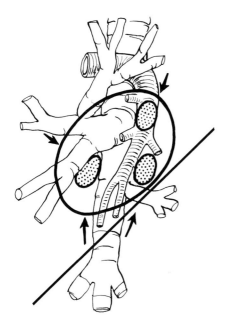

Fig. 7–6 The left lymphatic sump (see text), found by opening the main fissure. The straight line, drawn through the superior — apical — segmental bronchus of the left lower lobe, represents the level below which lymphatic drainage from the upper lobe does not occur. Arrows indicate tendency of lymphatic drainage. *From* Nohl-Oser HC: Lymphatics of the Lung. *In* Shields TW (ed): General Thoracic Surgery. 3rd Ed. Philadelphia: Lea & Febiger, 1989.

bronchus leads to it. Other lymph nodes are found lying on the interlobar portion of the left pulmonary artery in the fissure and in the angles formed by its branches. Another constant node is described, which is found above and posterior to the left main stem bronchus. This node is contiguous with a node lying in the angle formed by the main stem bronchus and the takeoff of the bronchus to the superior segment of the lower lobe.

Other Interlobar Lymph Nodes of the Left Lung

In addition to the left lymphatic sump nodes, Borrie (1965) noted that lymph nodes of the left upper lobe are present medial, posterior, and lateral to the upper lobe bronchus. Lymph nodes are also present between the segmental divisions of this bronchus.

The lymph nodes of the left lower lobe are located more commonly in the vicinity of the superior segmental bronchus of the lobe. They are found medial, above, and inferior to it, between it and the basal bronchi. The other lobar nodes of the lower lobe are found medial or lateral to the basilar stem of the lower lobe bronchus.

LYMPHATIC DRAINAGE OF THE LOBES OF THE LUNG TO THE BRONCHOPULMONARY LYMPH NODES

The lymphatic drainage of the lobes of the lungs is primarily to the bronchopulmonary nodes, although direct lymphatic drainage to the mediastinal lymph nodes was described by Rouvière (1932), Borrie (1952),

and Cordier (1958) and Riquet (1989) and their colleagues. This direct drainage is discussed subsequently.

The right upper lobe lymphatic drainage, as deduced from the study of Borrie (1956), is commonly to one of the superior interlobar lymph nodes — the sump nodes — on the lateral aspect of the bronchus intermedius, to the nodes above the right upper lobe bronchus and to those medial to it. Subsequent drainage is proximal to the azygos or subcarinal lymph nodes. Drainage has not been described as occurring to any lymph nodes below the level of the right lymphatic sump.

The middle lobe lymphatics drain to lymph nodes of the superior sump region, although drainage to the inferior sump node also occurs. Drainage from the right lower lobe is to the inferior interlobar node and to the superior sump nodes, primarily those lying on the medial surface of the bronchus intermedius.

Drainage of the left upper lobe from all segments may occur to the left sump nodes. Nodes about the upper lobe bronchus and the left main stem bronchus also receive drainage from this lobe. Lymphatic drainage of the lower lobe is to the subadjacent peribronchial nodes and to the interlobar sump nodes. From here, drainage is proximal to the hilar or mediastinal lymph node groups, or both.

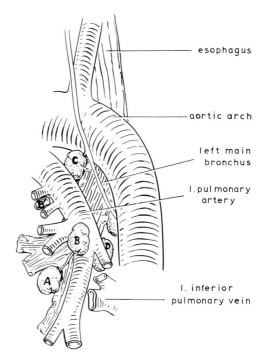

Fig. 7–7. The lymph nodes most frequently seen on opening the main fissure of the left lung. A constant node (A) lies in the angle between the upper and lower lobe bronchi, with a bronchial artery leading to it. Other lymph nodes (B and B′) are found on the main pulmonary artery and in the angles of the branches. The constant node (C) behind and above the pulmonary artery, before it enters the fissure, is shown. Another node (D) above the inferior pulmonary vein is seen with its connections to the inferior tracheobronchial nodes higher up. *From* Nohl-Oser HC: Lymphatics of the Lung. *In* Shields TW (ed): General Thoracic Surgery. 3rd Ed. Philadelphia: Lea & Febiger, 1989.

Lymphatic drainage from the middle and right lower lobes and the left lower lobe also occurs to the nodes in the respective pulmonary ligament. These lymph nodes are considered mediastinal. The incidence of nodes identified in Borrie's work (1965) was 12% in the right pulmonary ligament and 47% in the left.

MEDIASTINAL LYMPH NODES

The mediastinal lymph nodes that are important in the lymphatic drainage of the lungs can be divided into four distinct but interconnected groups: the anterior — prevascular — lymph nodes in the anterior mediastinal compartment and the tracheobronchial lymph nodes, the paratracheal lymph nodes, and the posterior lymph nodes in the visceral compartment of the mediastinum.

Anterior Mediastinal Lymph Nodes

These lymph nodes are in the prevascular compartment of the mediastinum and override the upper portions of the pericardium and great vessels as these extend upward. On the right side, the nodes lie parallel and anterior to the right phrenic nerve. They extend upward to and along the superior vena cava to the area beneath the right innominate vein. On the left, they are in close proximity to the origin of the pulmonary artery and the ligamentum arteriosum. They extend upward near the left phrenic nerve to lymph nodes lying along the inferior border of the left innominate vein in the region where it is joined by the left superior intercostal vein.

Tracheobronchial Lymph Nodes

These nodes lie in three groups about the bifurcation of the trachea. The right and left superior tracheobronchial nodes are located in the obtuse angles between the trachea and the corresponding main stem bronchus. These nodes lie outside of the pretracheal fascia. The lymph nodes of the right superior tracheobronchial group are medial — beneath — the arch of the azygos vein and above the right pulmonary artery. These nodes are contiguous with the right superior hilar nodes distally and the right paratracheal nodes proximally. On the left side, the superior tracheobronchial nodes lie deep within the concavity of the aortic arch. Some are closely related to the left recurrent laryngeal nerve; others are situated slightly more anteriorly and are contiguous with the node at ligamentum arteriosum and the root of the left pulmonary artery. Their association with these nodes constitutes the link between the nodes in the visceral compartment and those in the anterior mediastinal lymph node group.

The inferior tracheobronchial nodes — more commonly referred to as the subcarinal nodes — lie in the angle of the bifurcation of the trachea (Fig. 7–8).

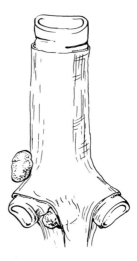

Fig. 7–8. The location of the inferior tracheobronchial nodes within the pretracheal fascial envelope and the superior tracheobronchial nodes outside this fascial layer. *Redrawn from* Sarrazin R, Voog R: La Mediastinoscopie. Paris: Masson 1968.

Although these nodes, in contrast to the superior tracheobronchial groups, lie within the pretracheal fascial envelope, they lie outside the relatively dense bronchopericardial membrane. These nodes are contiguous with the hilar nodes on the medial aspect of both the right and left main stem bronchi. Some of the subcarinal lymph nodes lie more posteriorly in relationship to the tracheal bifurcation and are on the anterior surface of the esophagus and are thus connected with the posterior group of lymph nodes. In addition, Brock and Whytehead (1955) described a low anterior tracheal group lying in front of the lower end of the trachea, which constitutes a bridge between the right superior tracheobronchial lymph nodes and the subcarinal — inferior tracheobronchial — lymph nodes.

Paratracheal Lymph Nodes

These lymph nodes are situated on the right and left sides of the trachea above the respective superior tracheobronchial nodes and extend upward along the trachea. The right paratracheal lymph nodes lie anterolaterally to the trachea and to the right of the innominate artery. Inferiorly, these nodes are overlapped by the superior vena cava. More superiorly, these nodes lie behind and above the innominate artery to the right of the midline of the trachea and extend to the inlet of the chest. Inferiorly, the left paratracheal nodes lie above the tracheobronchial angle to the left of the midline of the trachea behind the aortic arch. More superiorly, they are situated above the arch but behind the great vessels and extend to the inlet of the chest. The left paratracheal lymph nodes are generally smaller in size and number as compared to the right paratracheal lymph nodes.

Table 7–3. AJC Classification of Regional Lymph Nodes

Mediastinal (N₂) Nodes	Bronchopulmonary (N₁) Nodes
Superior mediastinal nodes	10. Hilar
1. Highest mediastinal	11. Interlobar
2. Upper paratracheal	12. Lobar
3. Pre- and retrotracheal	13. Segmental
4. Lower paratracheal	
(including azygos nodes)	
Aortic nodes	
5. Subaortic (aortic window)	
6. Para-aortic (ascending	
aorta or phrenic)	
Inferior mediastinal nodes	
7. Subcarinal	
8. Paraesophageal (below	
carina)	
9. Pulmonary ligament	

Posterior Mediastinal Lymph Nodes

These nodes may be separated into two groups: the paraesophageal nodes and those located in either pulmonary ligament. These posterior nodes are identified less commonly in the superior portion than in the inferior portion of the mediastinum. A paraesophageal node is occasionally found retrotracheally at the level of the arch of the azygos vein. The paraesophageal nodes as a group are more numerous in the inferior portion of the mediastinum and are found more frequently on the left than on the right side. The inferiorly located nodes have connections with the para-aortic nodes beneath the diaphragm. In the pulmonary ligament on either side, usually two or more small lymph nodes may be present. A relatively constant node, and usually the largest, lies in close proximity to the inferior border of the inferior pulmonary vein and is often termed the sentinel node.

Mediastinal Lymph Node Maps

Naruke and associates (1978) suggested the use of an anatomic map with the aforementioned conventional lymph node stations numbered so that the various lymph node stations involved by tumor could be uniformly recorded in lung cancer patients (Fig. 7–9). This mapping scheme is used by most Japanese surgeons and has been used with minor modifications by the Sloan-Kettering Memorial group and others in North America. The American Joint Committee for Cancer Staging and End Results Reporting — AJC — published a similar map in its 1983 fascicle. The lymph node stations are defined in Table 7–3. The American Thoracic Society — ATS — in a report by Tisi and colleagues (1983), however, noted what they believed to be

Table 7–4. Proposed Definitions of Regional Nodal Stations for Prethoracotomy Staging

X	Supraclavicular nodes.
2R	Right upper paratracheal (suprainnominate) nodes: nodes to the right of the midline of the trachea between the intersection of the caudal margin of the innominate artery with the trachea, and the apex of the lung. (Includes highest R mediastinal node.) (Radiologists may use the same caudal margin as in 2L.)
2L	Left upper paratracheal (supra-aortic) nodes: nodes to the left of the midline of the trachea between the top of the aortic arch and the apex of the lung. (Includes highest L1 mediastinal node.)
4R	Right lower paratracheal nodes: nodes to the right of the midline of the trachea between the cephalic border of the azygos vein and the intersection of the caudal margin of the brachiocephalic artery with the right side of the trachea. (Includes some pretracheal and paracaval nodes.) (Radiologists may use the same cephalic margin as in 4L.)
4L	Left lower paratracheal nodes: nodes to the left of the midline of the trachea between the top of the aortic arch and the level of the carina, medial to the ligamentum arteriosum. (Includes some pretracheal nodes.)
5	Aortopulmonary nodes: subaortic and para-aortic nodes, lateral to the ligamentum arteriosum or the aorta or left pulmonary artery, proximal to the first branch of the LPA.
6	Anterior mediastinal nodes: nodes anterior to the ascending aorta or the innominate artery. (Includes some pretracheal and preaortic nodes.)
7	Subcarinal nodes: nodes arising caudal to the carina of the trachea but not associated with the lower lobe bronchi or arteries within the lung.
8	Paraesophageal nodes: nodes dorsal to the posterior wall of the trachea and to the right or left of the midline of the esophagus. (Includes retrotracheal, but not subcarinal nodes.)
9	Right or left pulmonary ligament nodes: nodes within the right or left pulmonary ligament.
10R	Right tracheobronchial nodes: nodes to the right of the midline of the trachea from the level of the cephalic border of the azygos vein to the origin of the right upper lobe bronchus.
10L	Left peribronchial nodes: nodes to the left of the midline of the trachea between the carina and the left upper lobe bronchus, medial to the ligamentum arteriosum.
11	Intrapulmonary nodes: nodes removed in the right or left lung specimen plus those distal to the main stem bronchi or secondary carina. (Includes interlobar, lobar, and segmental nodes.)

From Tisi GM, et al: Clinical staging of primary lung cancer. Am Rev Respir Dis *127*:659, 1983.

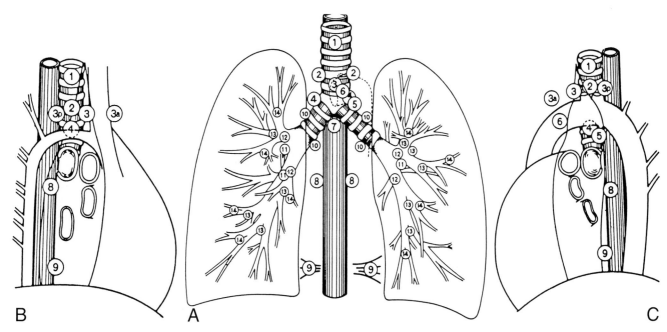

Fig. 7–9. Modified lymph node map of Naruke and the American Joint Committee (see Table 7–3 for definitions). *A,* Frontal view. *B,* Right lateral view. *C,* Left lateral view. *From* Naruke T, et al: Lymph node mapping and curability at various levels of metastasis in resected lung cancer. J Thorac Cardiovasc Surg 76:832, 1978.

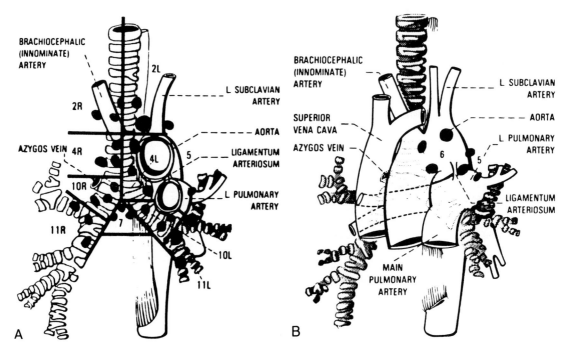

Fig. 7–10. *A,* ATS map of regional pulmonary nodes (see Table 7–4 for definitions). *B,* ATS map of regional nodes in stations 5 and 6. *From* Tisi GM, et al: Clinical staging of primary lung cancer. Am Rev Respir Dis 127:659, 1983.

deficiencies in the commonly accepted specific anatomic definition of each nodal station when determined by mediastinoscopy, mediastinotomy, and CT examinations of the chest. Although some of the points were minor, a major area of conflict was the recommendation that the hilar stations — the right and left stations 10 of the Naruke and AJC maps — be deleted because of the ambiguity of the radiologic definition of these areas. It was suggested that these areas be redesignated as peribronchial on the left and tracheobronchial on the right, and be assigned to the mediastinal compartments, both stations being outside of the pleural reflection. The ATS suggested the anatomic stations as listed in Table 7–4 and located as represented in Figure 7–10. The ATS map has been adopted by many investigators in North America. The validity of one schema over the other is moot. In reviewing data presented in the literature, however, cognizance of the differences in the method of recording the data must be borne in mind for their proper interpretation.

Number and Size of Lymph Nodes in the Various Mediastinal Locations

The first major report of the number of lymph nodes in the mediastinum was published by Beck and Beattie (1958). In cleared specimens of the mediastinum from 5 autopsies, they reported an average of 3 nodes in the anterior mediastinum and an average of 50 in the tracheobronchial area of the mediastinum. Of the latter, an average of 16 nodes were located in the peribronchial region, 11 in the subcarinal, and 23 in the paratracheal regions. These data were essentially nonspecific anatomically as were the data recorded by Genereux and Howie (1984). These authors, however, were among the first investigators, which include Baron (1982), Osborne (1982), Ekholm (1977) and Moak (1982) and their colleagues, to record the size of normal mediastinal lymph nodes as identified by CT scanning. From 89 to 95% of normal lymph nodes identified in these studies were less than 11 mm in size. Genereux and Howie's data were essentially similar to that of the other early investigators.

Glazer and associates (1985) not only reported the size of normal nodes but also correlated the number of lymph nodes usually identified by CT and their size in each of the superior mediastinal stations and the subcarinal region as described by the ATS map (Fig. 7–10, A and B). The data were generated by a retrospective review of 56 CT scans of patients without primary inflammatory pulmonary disease or primary lung neoplasm. The largest normal mediastinal nodes were found in the subcarinal and right tracheobronchial regions and, as a rule, the nodes were larger on the right side than on the left side. The maximum number of nodes and the size above which a node was considered enlarged are listed in Table 7–5 for each of the mediastinal stations. From these data, it was suggested that 10 mm be considered the upper limit for the short axis of normal mediastinal lymph nodes. An anatomic study by Kiyono and associates (1988) in which the dissection of the

Table 7–5. Normal Lymph Nodes in the Mediastinum as Identified on CT Examination in 56 Patients

	% Patients with Nodes Present	Mean Number of Nodes Present*	Short Axis Measurement Above Which Node Is Considered Enlarged
2R	95%	2	7 mm
2L	75	2	7
4R	100	3	10
4L	81	3	10
5	59	1	9
6	86	5	8
7	95	2	11
8R	57	1	10
10L	45	1	7
10R	100	3	10
11L	70	1	7

*Approximate mean without standard deviation. *Adapted from* Glazer GM et al: Normal mediastinal lymph nodes: number and size according to American Thoracic Society mapping. AJR Am J Roentgenol *144*: 261, 1985.

mediastinal lymph nodes in 40 cadavers was carried out produced similar results (Table 7–6). These authors suggested the normal size for the diameter of the short axis of the lymph nodes in stations 2, 5, 6, 8, 9, and 10L to be 8 mm; for station 4 and 10R to be 10 mm; and for station 7 to be 12 mm.

Relative to the number of lymph nodes, it may be noted that CT examination may fail to identify all the nodes present, particularly in the subaortic and subcarinal regions, and does not demonstrate nodes present in either of the pulmonary ligaments or those in the inferior paraesophageal area. The use of endoscopic ultrasound examination, which is particularly sensitive

Table 7–6. Number of Mediastinal Lymph Nodes Dissection of the Mediastinum of 40 Cadavers

Node Station*	% with Nodes Present	Number of Nodes Max	Number of Nodes Mean	Short Transverse Diameter (in mm) Max Standard†
2R	80	11	2.5	7.8
2L	68	7	2.1	5.6
4R	98	11	4.8	9.2
4L	98	16	4.5	9.2
5	58	6	1.1	8.5
6	85	15	4.7	7.2
7	100	6	2.9	12.3
8R	58	6	1.2	8.2
8L	50	5	1.1	6.1
9R	10	2	0.1	3.9
9L	35	3	0.5	6.5
10R	95	10	3.5	10.8
10L	90	7	2.4	6.8

*Stations as defined by the ATS map.
†Maximum standard was set at +2 SD from mean. *From* Kiyono K, et al: The number and size of normal mediastinal lymph nodes: A postmortem study. AJR Am J Roentgenol *150*: 771, 1988.

Table 7–7. Number of Nodes Identified in the Inferior Compartment of the Mediastinum* by Transesophageal Ultrasound — TEUS — versus CT

	Stations 7, 8, and 10	R9	L9
TEUS	274	8	22
CT	96	1	2

*Naruke map. *Adapted from* Kondo D, et al: Endoscopic ultrasound examination for mediastinal lymph node metastases of lung cancer. Chest 98:587, 1990.

for the detection of mediastinal nodes in these latter areas, was reported by Kondo and colleagues (1990). These investigators, although the patients studied had carcinoma of the lung, were able to identify lymph nodes in these latter areas, but the data are incomplete as to the actual number of normal nodes identified in the various regions (Table 7–7). Again, however, most lymph nodes considered normal were less than 10 mm in size — 97%.

LYMPHATIC DRAINAGE OF THE LUNGS TO THE MEDIASTINAL LYMPH NODES

The lymphatic drainage of the lungs to the mediastinal lymph nodes has been studied extensively. Various techniques of injection of dyes into the lymphatic channels of lungs from autopsy specimens of stillborn infants and adults without pulmonary disease have been used in the studies of Rouvière (1932), Cordier and associates (1958), and, more recently, by Riquet and colleagues (1989). Borrie (1952, 1965) and Nohl (1962) studied the drainage patterns by dissection of the operative specimens from lungs of cancer patients, as have many investigators subsequently, including Naruke (1978), Martini (1983), Libshitz (1986), Watanabe (1990, 1991), and Ishida (1990) and their associates. In addition to these studies, Nohl-Oser (1972) and Greschuchna and Maassen (1973) published their findings from the evaluation of the superior mediastinum by mediastinoscopy in patients with lung cancer. Also in living patients, but without known pulmonary disease, the lymphatic drainage of the lungs was studied by the technique of lymphoscintigraphy using antimony sulfide colloid or rhenium colloid labeled with ^{99m}Tc injected into the various bronchopulmonary segments via the fiberoptic bronchoscope by Hata and associates (1981).

Although the terminology for the lung segments and the mediastinal lymph nodes, as well as their locations, per se varied considerably in these multiple studies, relatively consistent drainage patterns for each lung and its respective lobes and segments can be identified reasonably.

The patterns of "normal" lymphatic drainage from the lungs to the mediastinum are relatively consistent despite minor variations suggested by different workers, which may be the result of the methods of investigation used and the selection of the subjects studied. The dynamic study by the use of lymphoscintigraphy in normal healthy subjects as reported by Hata and associates (1981) and summarized in 1990 appears to be a highly satisfactory schemata to recommend. The patterns of drainage from the right and left lung segments are seen in Figure 7–11. A summary of the findings is directly quoted in essence.*

Right Lung

The lymphatic drainage from the apical and posterior segments of the right upper lobe flows via the hilar nodes into the right superior tracheobronchial nodes and further into the paratracheal nodes and up into the neck in the right scalene nodes through ipsilateral upper paratracheal nodes. About one half of the lymph from the anterior segment of the upper lobe flows via the same route. The other half flows into the subcarinal nodes or into the right anterior mediastinal nodes. Lymph that passes through the subcarinal nodes may flow further into the right scalene nodes through the pretracheal and ipsilateral paratracheal nodes, and a small amount of lymph is observed to flow into the left paratracheal nodes. Lymph that goes to the right anterior mediastinal nodes flows along the left brachiocephalic vein into the left anterior mediastinal nodes and into the left scalene nodes.

The routes of lymphatic drainage from the bronchi of the middle lobe and the superior segment of the right lower lobe are similar. Most of the lymph from these segmental bronchi flows into the subcarinal or right superior tracheobronchial nodes and then to the right upper paratracheal nodes. Some of the lymph from the bronchi of the middle lobe also flows into the subcarinal and left paratracheal nodes, or into the right anterior mediastinal nodes, as mentioned for lymphatic drainage from the anterior segment of the right upper lobe.

A dominant flow of the lymphatic drainage occurs from the basal segments of the right lower lobe into the subcarinal nodes through the bronchopulmonary nodes. The lymph then flows into the ipsilateral lower and upper paratracheal nodes and further into the right scalene nodes.

Left Lung

Four major routes are described by Hata and associates (1990) for the lymphatic drainage from the segmental bronchi of the left lung. The first passes through the subaortic nodes. This route divides into two pathways: one runs along the left vagus nerve to the left scalene nodes, the other runs along the left recurrent laryngeal nerve to the highest left mediastinal nodes. The second route runs through the para-aortic nodes upward along the left phrenic nerve via the anterior mediastinal nodes to the left scalene nodes. The third route runs along the left main bronchus to the left superior tracheobronchial nodes and the paratracheal

---

*From Hata E, et al: Rationale for extended lymphadenectomy for lung cancer. Theor Surg 5:19, 1990.

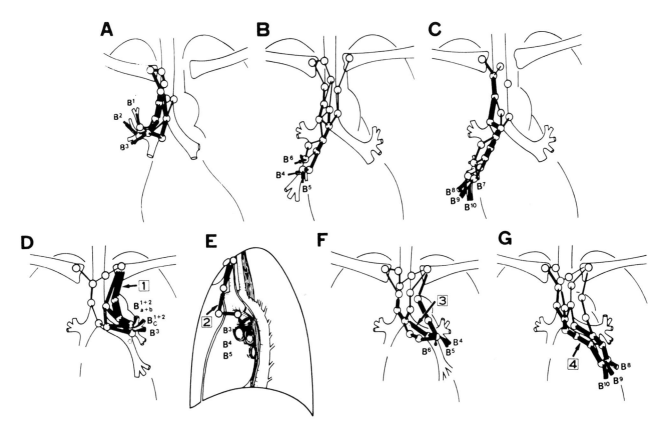

Fig. 7–11. Standard patterns of lymphatic drainage of the lungs. *A*, From segments of the right upper lobe; *B*, From segments of the middle lobe and superior segment of the right lower lobe; *C*, From basal segments of the right lower lobe; *D*, Route 1 from the left lung; *E*, Route 2 from the left lung; *F*, Route 3 from the left lung; *G*, Route 4 from the left lung. See text for explanation. *From* Hata E, et al: Rationale for extended lymphadenectomy for lung cancer. Theor Surg 5:19, 1990.

nodes. From the left tracheobronchial nodes, this route divides into two branches. One extends to the right side of the mediastinum through the right upper pretracheal node, the other runs upward along the left side of the trachea to the highest left mediastinal nodes. The fourth route runs under the left main bronchus to the subcarinal nodes. After passing the subcarinal nodes, this route extends to the right superior tracheobronchial nodes or through the lower pretracheal node to the right upper paratracheal nodes. Some branches extend upward along the left side of the trachea to the highest left mediastinal nodes.

As a consequence, the lymphatic drainage from the left lung is variable; however, the major routes of lymphatic drainage from each segment are as follows. The most important route of lymphatic drainage from the apicoposterior segmental bronchus of the upper lobe is the first route. Although the second route is the most common for lymphatic drainage from the anterior and lingular bronchi of the upper lobe, the other routes are used as well for lymphatic drainage from these bronchi. Lymph from the superior segmental bronchus of the lower lobe drains commonly along the first, third, and fourth routes. The most important route of drainage from the basal segmental bronchi of the lower lobe is the fourth route.

Significance of the Lymphatic Drainage Patterns

These routes, as described by Hata (1990), agree in most details with the patterns described by Rouvière (1932) and Nohl (1956). In addition, other significant features of the lymphatic drainage from the various lobes of the lungs to the mediastinal lymph nodes, as well as re-emphasis of some of the aforementioned observations, must be pointed out. 1) The drainage from the right lung is essentially unilateral and crossover to lymph nodes in the contralateral mediastinum is infrequent. Hata and colleagues (1981) noted drainage from the right upper lobe into the left paratracheal nodes and sequentially from the right prevascular nodes into the left prevascular — anterior — nodes. Similar pathways were observed infrequently from the middle lobe and superior segment of the lower lobe. Drainage from the basilar segments of the right lower lobe rarely progressed to the left side of the mediastinum, although Riquet and colleagues (1989) recorded the presence of one direct drainage channel from the right basal segments to the left pulmonary ligament. In patients with known carcinoma of the lung studied by prethoracotomy mediastinoscopy, contralateral drainage from the right lung to the mediastinum was likewise observed with minimal frequency. Nohl-Oser (1972) and Greschuchna and Maassen (1973) reported the incidence of contralateral metastases from tumors of the right upper lobe with metastatic mediastinal node disease were 5 and 9%, respectively. From tumors of the right lower lobe with associated metastatic mediastinal node disease, the incidences of contralateral disease were 7 and 5%, respectively. When the total number of tumors of the right lung — less than one half with metastatic mediastinal node involvement — are used as the denominator in the series reported by Nohl-Oser (1972), the incidences of crossover from the right upper and right lower lobes are reduced to 2 and 3%, respectively. 2) In contrast, contralateral mediastinal drainage from the left lung is relatively common, occurring most frequently via the subcarinal nodes, as initially pointed out by Rouvière (1932) and reconfirmed by all of the subsequent studies. Occasionally, crossover occurs by means of the lower pretracheal node in drainage from the left lower lobe. Again, Riquet and associates (1989) identified a direct channel from the left to a right paratracheal node. These workers also described direct channels from the left lower lobe to the opposite side of the lower portion of the inferior mediastinum. In the mediastinoscopy data of Nohl-Oser (1972) and Greschuchna and Maassen (1973), contralateral involvement from tumors of the left upper lobe to the right side of the mediastinum in patients with mediastinal node involvement was 22 and 21%, respectively. From the left lower lobe, the figures were 40 and 33%, respectively. Again, to put these data into perspective, 28% of the patients in Nohl-Oser's (1972) study had metastatic mediastinal nodal involvement from tumors of the left lung so that the 22 and 40% incidences represent an actual 6 and 11% incidence of crossover from the left upper and lower lobes to the right side of the mediastinum. These percentages are in agreement with the findings of Hata et al (1990), who found 7 and 11% incidences, respectively, in patients who had undergone bilateral mediastinal node dissection for left lung tumors. 3) Drainage from the lower lobes on either side to the ipsilateral superior mediastinal lymph nodes is common. 4) Drainage to the inferior mediastinum — to the subcarinal lymph nodes — from the right upper lobe does occur. This finding was first observed by Rouvière (1932) and, although discounted by Nohl (1962) — Nohl-Oser (1972) — it has been amply reconfirmed by the studies of Borrie (1965) and Hata (1981, 1990), Riquet (1989), Watanabe (1990), and their associates. Watanabe and colleagues (1990) reported a 13% incidence of subcarinal lymph node involvement in 45 patients with right upper lobe tumors. Libshitz and co-investigators reported a similar 14% incidence of such involvement. 5) Drainage of the superior division of the left upper lobe to the subcarinal area is unusual but, as noted by Hata and colleagues (1981), commonly occurs from the inferior — lingular — division of that lobe. 6) Direct lymphatic channels from either lung drain to the mediastinal lymph nodes, bypassing the bronchopulmonary nodes in a significant number of lungs. This phenomenon was observed previously and

has been described as "skip" metastases in lung cancer patients by Martini (1987), Libshitz (1986), Ishida (1990), and their associates, among others. Skip metastases from the right upper lobe were seen in the superior tracheocarinal nodes most frequently; a few occurred in the paratracheal node group and infrequently to the subcarinal lymph nodes. Right lower lobe tumors exhibited skip metastases to the subcarinal nodes and to the inferior pulmonary nodes. On the left side, upper lobe lesions tended to show skip metastasis to the subcarinal and aortic window areas; the lower lobe lesion showed a similar pattern as seen on the right; that is, the subcarinal and inferior pulmonary ligament nodes. Riquet and colleagues (1989) used injection studies of the subpleural lymphatics of adult lungs obtained at autopsy to identify direct lymphatic channels running from the subpleural plexus of the lobar segments to the various mediastinal lymph nodes without passing through the bronchopulmonary nodes. Most of these channels were superficial, but a few penetrated the lung substance. On occasion, these direct but separate channels coexisted with other channels draining into the bronchopulmonary lymph nodes. These direct channels were observed in 22% of the segments injected in the right lung and 25% of the segments in the left lung. In all other specimens, the dye followed the classic patterns and filled the respective bronchopulmonary lymph nodes. A summary of the study by Riquet and colleagues (1989) is found in Table 7–8. 7) Drainage to the ipsilateral pulmonary ligament nodes from the right and left lower lobes and subsequently to the inferior paraesophageal lymph nodes was pointed out by Borrie (1952) and others of the aforementioned investigators. 8) Drainage from the superior mediastinum continues to progress cephalad to the scalene lymph nodes in the neck, more often involving the right than the left scalene area. 9) Lastly, lymphatic drainage from the lower regions of the mediastinum may progress caudad to the para-aortic lymph nodes below the diaphragm. Riquet and associates (1988, 1990) described a direct channel from the basal segments of both lungs to juxtaceliac nodes. This drainage pathway had been noted by Meyer (1958).

All of the aforementioned points must be remembered in the overall consideration of the lymphatic drainage from the lungs. The clinical relevance of the lymphatic

Table 7–8. Direct Pathways to Mediastinal Lymph Nodes from the Lungs

Site	Percent	Total % for Each Lung
Right upper lobe	36.3	
Middle lobe	18.6	22.2
Right lower lobe	22.3	
Left upper lobe	38.6	25.0
Left lower lobe	21.1	

Adapted from Riquet M, Hidden G, Debesse B: Direct lymphatic drainage of lung segments to the mediastinal nodes. An anatomic study of 260 adults. J Thorac Cardiovasc Surg 97:623, 1989.

drainage and the various lymph node groups are discussed in the respective chapters relating to infections and tumors of the lungs.

REFERENCES

Baron RL, et al: Computed tomography in the preoperative evaluation of bronchogenic carcinoma. Radiology *145*:727, 1982.

Beck E, Beattie EJ: The lymph nodes in the mediastinum. J Int Coll Surg 29:247, 1958.

Borrie J: Primary carcinoma of the bronchus: Prognosis following surgical resection (Hunterian Lecture). Ann R Coll Surg Engl *10*:165, 1952.

Borrie J: Lung Cancer: Surgery and Survival. New York: Appleton-Century-Crofts, 1965.

Brock R, Whytehead LL: Radical pneumonectomy for bronchial carcinoma. Br J Surg *43*:8, 1955.

Cordier G, et al: Les lymphatiques des bronches et des segments pulmonaires. Bronches 8:8, 1958.

Ekholm S, et al: Computed tomography in preoperative staging of bronchogenic carcinoma. J Comput Assist Tomogr *4*:763, 1977.

Genereux GP, Howie JL: Normal mediastinal lymph node size and number: CT and anatomic study. AJR Am J Roentgenol *142*:1095, 1984.

Glazer GM, et al: Normal mediastinal lymph nodes: Number and size according to American Thoracic Society mapping. AJR Am J Roentgenol *144*:261, 1985.

Greenberg HB: Benign subpleural lymph node appearing as a pulmonary "coin" lesion. Radiology *77*:97, 1961.

Greschuchna D, Maassen W: Die lymphogenen Absiedlungswege des Bronchialkarzinoms. Stuttgart: Georg Thieme, 1973.

Hata E, et al: Rationale for extended lymphadenectomy for lung cancer. Theor Surg 5:19, 1990.

Hata E, Troidl H, Hasegawa T: In vivo Untersuchungen der Lymphdrainage des Bronchialsystems beim Menchen mit des Lympho-Szintigraphie: Eine neue diagnostische Technik. *In* Hamelmann H, Troidl H (eds):Behandlung des Bronchialkarzinoms. Stuttgart: Georg Thieme, 1981.

Ishida T, et al: Strategy for lymphadenectomy in lung cancer three centimeters or less in diameter. Ann Thorac Surg *50*:708, 1990.

Kiyono K, et al: The number and size of the mediastinal lymph nodes: A postmortem study. AJR Am J Roentgenol *150*:771, 1988.

Kondo D, et al: Endoscopic ultrasound examination for mediastinal lymph node metastases of lung cancer. Chest 98:587, 1990.

Lauweryns JM: The blood and lymphatic microcirculation of the lung. *In* Sommers SC (ed): Pathology Annual. New York: Appleton-Century-Crofts, 1971, p 365.

Leak LV: Lymphatic removal of fluids and particles in mammalian lung. Environ Health Perspect 35:55, 1980.

Leak LV, Jamuar MP: Ultrastructure of pulmonary lymphatic vessels. Am Rev Respir Dis *128*:559, 1983.

Libshitz HI, McKenna RJ, Mountain CF: Patterns of mediastinal metastases in bronchogenic carcinoma. Chest 90:229, 1986.

Martini N, Flehinger BJ: The role of surgery in N$_2$ lung cancer. Surg Clin North Am 67:1037, 1987.

Martini N, et al: Results of resection in non-oat cell carcinoma of the lung with mediastinal lymph node metastases. Ann Surg *198*:386, 1983.

Manual for Staging Cancer: American Joint Committee for Cancer Staging and End-results Reporting. Chicago, 1983.

Meyer KK: Direct lymphatic connections from the lower lobes of the lung to the abdomen. J Thorac Surg 35:726, 1958.

Moak GD, et al: Computed tomography versus standard radiology in the evaluation of mediastinal adenopathy. Chest 82:69, 1982.

Nagaishi C: Functional Anatomy and Histology of the Lung. Baltimore: University Park Press, 1972.

Naruke T, Suemasu K, Ishikawa S: Lymph node mapping and curability at various levels of metastasis in resected lung cancer. J Thorac Cardiovasc Surg 76:832, 1978.

Nohl HC: An investigation into the lymphatic and vascular spread of carcinoma of the bronchus. Thorax *11*:172, 1956.

Nohl HC: The Spread of Carcinoma of the Bronchus. London: Lloyd-Luke Ltd, 1962.

Nohl-Oser HC: An investigation of the anatomy of the lymphatic drainage of the lungs. Ann R Coll Surg Engl *51*:157, 1972.

Osborne DR, et al: Comparison of plain radiography, conventional tomography and computed tomography in detecting intrathoracic lymph node metastases from lung carcinoma. Radiology *142*:157, 1982.

Riquet M, Hidden G, Debesse B: Abdominal nodal connections of the lymphatics of the lung. Surg Radiol Anat *10*:251, 1988.

Riquet M, Hidden G, Debesse B: Direct lymphatic drainage of lung segments to the mediastinal nodes. An anatomic study of 260 adults. J Thorac Cardiovasc Surg 97:623, 1989.

Riquet M, et al: Direct metastases to abdominal lymph nodes in bronchogenic carcinoma (letter to the editor). J Thorac Cardiovasc Surg *100*:153, 1990.

Rouvière H: Anatomie des Lymphatics de le homme. Paris: Masson et Cie, 1932.

Steiner RE: The radiology of the pulmonary circulation. *In* Shanks CS, Kerley P (eds): A Textbook of X-Ray Diagnosis. London: HK Lewis, 1973, p. 121.

Tisi GM, et al: Clinical staging of primary lung cancer. Am Rev Respir Dis *127*:659, 1983.

Trapnell DH: The peripheral lymphatics of the lung. Br J Radiol 36:660, 1963.

Trapnell DH: Recognition and incidence of intrapulmonary lymph nodes. Thorax 19:44, 1964.

Watanabe Y, et al: Mediastinal spread of metastatic lymph nodes in bronchogenic carcinoma. Mediastinal nodal metastases in lung cancer. Chest 97:1059, 1990.

CHAPTER 8

ANATOMY OF THE THORACIC DUCT

Joseph I. Miller, Jr.

Embryologically, the thoracic duct is a bilateral structure and has the potential of having many varied anatomic patterns. The pattern and anatomy of the thoracic duct is considered standard, as reported by Davis (1915), in only 65% of humans. Many anatomic variations occur in lymphatic and lymphaticovenous anastomosis (Fig. 8–1).

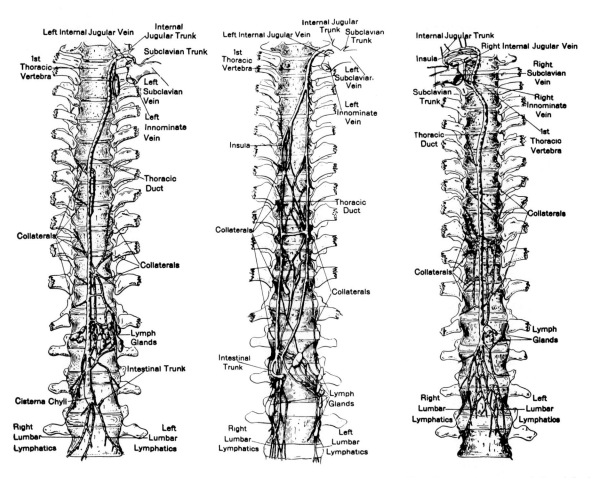

Fig. 8–1. Variations of the thoracic duct. *Left*, A duct conforming to the usual description. *Middle*, Absence of a cisterna chyli and duplication of much of the course of the duct. *Right*, Absence of a cisterna, and right-sided termination. *From* Edwards EA, Malone PD, Collins JJ Jr: Operative Anatomy of the Thorax. Philadelphia: Lea & Febiger, 1972.

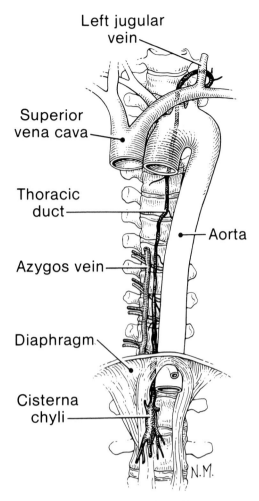

Left jugular vein

Superior vena cava

Thoracic duct

Azygos vein

Diaphragm

Cisterna chyli

Aorta

N.M.

Fig. 8–2. Usual anatomic pattern of the thoracic duct.

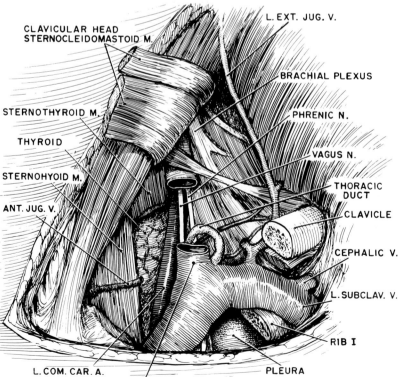

CLAVICULAR HEAD STERNOCLEIDOMASTOID M.

L. EXT. JUG. V.

BRACHIAL PLEXUS

PHRENIC N.

STERNOTHYROID M.

THYROID

VAGUS N.

STERNOHYOID M.

THORACIC DUCT

ANT. JUG. V.

CLAVICLE

CEPHALIC V.

L. SUBCLAV. V.

RIB I

L. COM. CAR. A.

PLEURA

L. INT. JUG. V.

Fig. 8–3. Termination of the thoracic duct. *From* Edwards EA, Malone PD, Collins JJ Jr: Operative Anatomy of the Thorax. Philadelphia: Lea & Febiger, 1972.

TYPICAL PATTERN OF THE THORACIC DUCT

The usual anatomic pattern of the thoracic duct is shown in Figure 8–2. The thoracic duct is the main collecting vessel of the lymphatic system and is far larger than the right terminal lymphatic duct. Most commonly, the thoracic duct originates from the cisterna chyli in the midline at the level of the second lumbar vertebra. The cisterna chyli is 3 to 4 cm long and 2 to 3 cm in diameter. It is generally found along the vertebral column at the level of L2, but may be found anywhere between T10 and L3, generally to the right side of the aorta.

From the cisterna chyli, the thoracic duct ascends to enter the chest through the aortic hiatus at the level of T10 to T12, just to the right of the aorta. Above the diaphragm, the duct lies on the anterior surface of the vertebral column behind the esophagus and between the aorta and the azygos vein. The duct usually lies in front of the right intercostal arteries with the nerves close by. The duct continues upward on the right side of the vertebral column to approximately the level of the fifth or sixth thoracic vertebra, where it crosses behind the aorta and aortic arch into the left posterior portion of the visceral compartment of the mediastinum. From there, it passes superiorly in close approximation to the left side of the esophagus and the pleural reflection into the neck. Before exiting the mediastinum, the duct receives tributaries from the bronchomediastinal trunk of the right lymphatic duct. Once the duct enters the neck, it arches 2 to 3 cm above the clavicle and swings laterally anterior to the subclavian artery and thyrocervical arteries. It continues deeper into the neck in front of the phrenic nerve and the scalenus anticus muscle. At this point, it passes behind the left carotid sheath and jugular vein before anastomosing with the left subclavian-jugular junction (Fig. 8–3). The anatomic manner in which the thoracic duct ends varies. It may enter the jugular vein as a single trunk or as multiple trunks. It most commonly enters at the junction of the left internal jugular and subclavian veins.

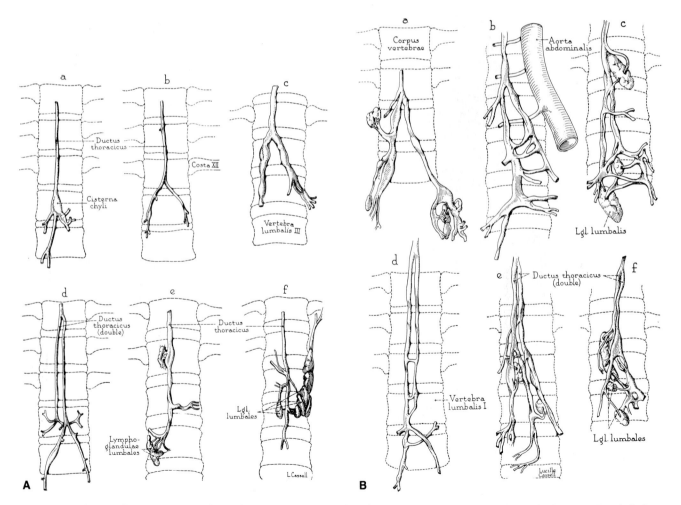

Fig. 8–4. Thoracic duct. Variations and vertebral relations. *A, a* and *c,* ducts possessing sacculations of considerable size; *b* and *d,* ducts of slender form; *e* and *f,* ducts of elongated form. *B, a,* duct of common, Y-shaped form; *b* through *d,* ducts possessing numerous anastomoses between the bilateral tributaries; *e* and *f,* trifid ducts. *From* Anson BJ: An Atlas of Human Anatomy. Philadelphia: WB Saunders, 1963.

MAJOR VARIATIONS OF THE THORACIC DUCT

The only thing constant about the anatomy of the thoracic duct is the numerous anatomic variations. Davis (1915) reported nine major variations, and Anson (1950) listed 12 different anatomic variations of the lower portion of the thoracic duct (Fig. 8–4).

Major variations of the thoracic duct itself include doubling, left-sidedness, and right or bilateral termination, as well as the rare azygos vein termination. The embryologic basis for these variations is the plexiform nature of the trunks from which the duct arises. Doubling was reported in 4.7% by Adachi (1953), and in 39% in a larger series by Van Pernis (1949); the lower figure is probably correct for extensive duplication. In a few instances, the abdominal components of the trunk may pass upward to both sides or only to the left of the aorta. Rarely, as noted by Adachi (1953) as well as Davis (1915), the duct may be left-sided throughout its course. Adachi also reported that only the upper part of the duct may be double so that it terminates in both the right and left sides of the neck — 1.8% — or the right side alone — 1.6%. At its termination, the duct may enter into a short plexus with its tributary trunks so that in about 20% it enters the vein by two or more branches. Termination of the duct in the azygos system is rare. Edwards (1972) reported, in an autopsy subject, that he had observed the duct to enter the hemiazygos vein. In its cervical course, Adachi (1953) noted that the duct may run posterior rather than anterior to the vertebral or the subclavian artery.

In 1922, Lee reported a detailed study of the collateral circulation of the lymphatic system in the mediastinum. He identified various connections between the thoracic duct and the azygos vein, as well as other connections between intercostal veins and the thoracic duct within the chest. The thoracic duct contains valves in various locations throughout its entire course.

Lymph from the right side of the head, neck, and chest wall, as well as from the right lung and the lower half of the left lung, through the bronchomediastinal trunk, drain into the right lymphatic duct. This duct also carries lymph from the heart and the dome of the liver, and from the right diaphragm. Bessone and colleagues (1971) pointed out that the right lymphatic duct is small and is rarely visualized.

REFERENCES

Adachi B: Der Ductus Thoracicus des Japaner. Tokyo: Kenkyursha, 1953.

Anson BJ: An Atlas of Anatomy. Philadelphia: WB Saunders, 1950, pp 336-337.

Bessone LN, Ferguson TB, Burford TH: Chylothorax: A collective review. Ann Thorac Surg 12:527, 1971.

Davis MK: A statistical study of the thoracic duct in man. Am J Anat 171:212, 1915.

Edwards AE: The Thoracic Duct In Edwards EA, Malone PD, Collins JJ Jr: Operative Anatomy of Thorax. Philadelphia: Lea & Febiger, 1972, p 227.

Lee FC: The establishment of collateral circulation following ligation of the thoracic duct. Johns Hopkins Hosp Bull 33:21, 1922.

Van Pernis PA: Variations of the thoracic duct. Surgery 26:806, 1949.

Physiology of the Lungs

CHAPTER 9

PULMONARY GAS EXCHANGE

Joan D. Boomsma and Jeffrey Glassroth

LOCUS OF BLOOD-GAS INTERFACE

The alveolocapillary membrane is where inspired air and pulmonary blood meet and gas transfer occurs. This membrane is made up of the attenuated cytoplasm of an alveolar lining cell — alveolar type I cell — and its basement membrane plus the attenuated cytoplasm of the capillary endothelial cell and its basement membrane. Divertie and Brown (1964) described a space of variable width between the two basement membranes, the interstitial space. The majority of disease processes that alter the alveolocapillary membrane interfere with gas transport across this membrane and probably produce their deleterious effects by interfering with pulmonary ventilation, pulmonary blood flow, or the homogeneous distribution of blood and air, or by some combination of these distribution defects.

PHYSICS AND PHYSIOLOGY OF GASES

Pressure and temperature changes alter the volume of all gases in a predictable manner. Because of marked variation in solubility and chemical reaction rates in body fluids, the behavior of different gases in a liquid phase in vivo varies widely.

Laws Pertaining to Gases in the Gas Phase

At constant pressure, the volume of a gas is directly proportional to the temperature — Charles' law. At constant temperature, the volume is inversely proportional to the pressure — Boyle's law.

The combination of Charles' and Boyle's laws gives the relationship: $PV = nRT$, in which n is the number of moles of gas, R is a constant having the same value for all perfect gases, and T is the absolute temperature in degrees Kelvin — K. $T = t° C + 273$. At 0°C and 760 mm Hg pressure, 1 mole of any perfect gas will have a volume of 22.41 liters.

The partial pressure of one gas in a mixture of gases of volume V is equal to the pressure that the gas would exert if it occupied the same volume V in the absence of other gases — Dalton's law. The partial pressure of each gas in a mixture is proportional to the fraction of the mixture made up by that gas; for example, the fraction of oxygen in room air is 0.21, and the sum of the partial pressures of all the gases in a mixture equals the total pressure of the gas mixture.

The partial pressure of any gas in a mixture is the product of the total or barometric pressure — P_B — times the fraction of the gas in the mixture — F: $P = P_B \times F$. If there is water vapor in the mixture, the partial pressure of water vapor must be subtracted from the barometric pressure. Water vapor pressure is assumed to equal 47 mm Hg when a gas is fully saturated at 37°C: $P = (P_B - 47) \times F$. For example:

Barometric pressure = 760 mm Hg
Oxygen concentration = 20.93%
$P_{O_2} = (760 - 47) \times 0.2093 = 149$ mm Hg

Environmental Conditions and Measurement of Gases

Body Temperature and Pressure, Saturated With Water Vapor — BTPS

Under this condition, the temperature of the gas is 37°C and the partial pressure of water vapor is 47 mm Hg.

Ambient Temperature and Pressure, Saturated — ATPS

Under most circumstances, the ambient temperature is lower than body temperature. A gas at ambient conditions usually contains less water vapor than under BTPS conditions, depending on ambient temperature and relative humidity.

Standard Temperature and Pressure, Dry — STPD

Oxygen, carbon dioxide, and carbon monoxide volumes are expressed at Standard Temperature and Pressure, Dry — STPD conditions. This manner of expression is customary for any gas undergoing metabolic exchange. Lung volumes and ventilation are expressed at BTPS conditions. A minute ventilation of 10 L/min STPD is equivalent to 12 or 13 L/min BTPS.

Conversion from ATPS Volumes to BTPS Volumes

As air temperature increases from ambient — ATPS — to BTPS conditions, gas volumes increase because of thermal expansion. If a fluid reservoir such as that within the lung is present, the water vapor pressure will increase to 47 mm Hg. The expansion due to heat and the increase in volume due to the addition of water vapor are expressed in the formula:

$$V_{BTPS} = V_{ATPS} \times \frac{273 + 37}{273 + t_A} \times \frac{P_B - P_{H_2O}}{P_B - 47}$$

273 = melting point of ice in °K
37 = body temperature in °C (degrees centigrade)
t_A = ambient temperature °C
P_B = barometric pressure, in mm Hg
P_{H_2O} = water vapor pressure at t_A
47 = water vapor pressure at 37°C (saturated)

Laws Pertaining to Gases in Liquids

Partial Pressure

A gas in contact with a liquid will exchange molecules with the liquid. When equilibrium is reached, the number of gas molecules entering the liquid phase equals the number leaving to enter the gas phase, and the partial pressures of the gas in both the liquid and the gas phase are equal.

Volume

The volume of a gas contained in a liquid is expressed in volumes percent — ml per 100 ml of liquid. These volumes are usually expressed under STPD conditions. The gas may be merely physically dissolved, in chemical combination, or both. For example, the oxygen content of the arterial blood of a healthy subject with a hemoglobin concentration of 14 g percent while breathing room air will be about 19 volumes percent — 19 ml oxygen STPD per 100 ml of whole blood. All but 0.3 volumes percent of the oxygen is in chemical combination with hemoglobin.

UNIQUE PROPERTIES OF SPECIFIC GASES

Different gases have special biologic properties. Some gases — oxygen and carbon dioxide — undergo metabolic exchange, other gases are insoluble in the pulmonary membrane and remain in the gas phase, and other gases have specific effects on the body that make them valuable as anesthetic agents.

Gases That Undergo Metabolic Exchange

Oxygen

This essential component of cellular respiration is carried in the blood in two forms: in physical solution in the plasma and in chemical combination with hemoglobin. The quantity of oxygen that can be carried in physical solution is minimal — about 1.5% of the total — compared with the large amount of oxygen that exists in chemical combination with hemoglobin. The quantity of oxygen combined with hemoglobin depends on the partial pressure of oxygen in the blood. This relationship (Fig. 9–1), the oxyhemoglobin dissociation curve, has a sigmoid shape with a steep slope between 10 and 60 mm Hg Po₂. The curve is comparatively flat between 70 and 100 mm Hg (Fig. 9–1). The characteristics of this curve must be considered when treating hypoxemia.

Changes in Po₂ at the upper portion of the curve have little effect on the arterial oxygen saturation. At the lower end of the curve where the oxygen pressures are equivalent to the Po₂ in the capillaries, large quantities of oxygen are available for tissue metabolism. Both acidosis and temperature elevation shift the oxyhemoglobin saturation curve to the right (Fig. 9–1). This rightward shift makes oxygen more readily available in the more acid environment of the tissues. The quantity of dissolved oxygen is directly proportional to the partial pressure of oxygen in blood and equals 0.003 ml of oxygen per 100 ml of blood per mm Hg Po₂. With an arterial Po₂ of 90 mm Hg, the amount of dissolved oxygen in the blood is equal to 0.27 ml per 100 ml; but if the subject breathes 100% oxygen and achieves an arterial Po₂ of 600 mm Hg, the amount of dissolved oxygen would be 1.8 ml per 100 ml of blood.

Even during 100% oxygen breathing, the dissolved oxygen contributes little to the total blood oxygen content if hemoglobin values are near normal. One gram of hemoglobin combines chemically with 1.34 ml of oxygen. If the blood hemoglobin is 15 g/100 ml, then 20.1 ml of oxygen/100 ml of blood can be carried in association with hemoglobin at saturation. The actual

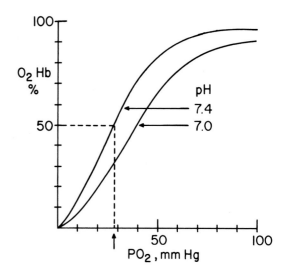

Fig. 9–1. Oxyhemoglobin (O₂ Hb) dissociation curve. The sigmoid relationship between Po₂ and percent saturation of hemoglobin with oxygen is shown together with the rightward shift of the curve that occurs with acidosis. The arrow denotes the p50 (see text).

quantity of oxygen in combination with hemoglobin depends on the partial pressure of oxygen and the amount of available hemoglobin (Fig. 9–2). The blood hemoglobin that is combined with oxygen — oxyhemoglobin — divided by the oxygen capacity of the blood sample — hemoglobin concentration × 1.34 — gives the percent saturation of the hemoglobin with oxygen. Oxygen partial pressures in excess of 60 mm Hg add comparatively little to the oxygen content of the blood (see Fig. 9–1).

The oxygen combining characteristics of hemoglobin may be expressed in terms of the p50 (see Fig. 9–1). The p50 is the partial pressure of oxygen at which hemoglobin is 50% saturated. When measured under the following conditions: temperature 37°C, pH 7.40, and P_{CO_2} 40 mm Hg, the p50 is normally 27 mm Hg. Certain diseases or conditions may change the p50. For example, as noted previously, an increase in either hydrogen ion concentration, temperature, or both, will shift the oxygen-hemoglobin dissociation curve to the right and increase the p50. An increase in carbon dioxide tension or in the enzyme 2,3 diphosphoglycerate — 2, 3 DPG — will also shift the curve to the right. The opposite change in temperature, hydrogen ion concentration, carbon dioxide tension or 2,3 DPG shifts the curve to the left and lowers the p50 below 27 mm Hg. An increase in 2,3 DPG occurs in the presence of chronic hypoxemia, for example, at high altitudes and in chronic severe anemia, and shifts

the curve to the right. This action facilitates the release of oxygen in the tissues since rightward movement of the oxygen-hemoglobin dissociation curve results in a lower saturation of hemoglobin at higher partial pressures of oxygen. In addition to an increase in 2,3 DPG, other compensations for chronic hypoxemia improve the delivery of oxygen to the tissues, such as an increase in cardiac output and secondary polycythemia. Substantial carboxyhemoglobinemia, as in acute carbon monoxide poisoning, has a physiochemical effect on the oxygen-hemoglobin curve and shifts it to the left and up. This action lowers the p50, increases the affinity of hemoglobin for oxygen, and compounds the problem of tissue hypoxemia initially caused by the combination of a significant amount of hemoglobin with carbon monoxide. The shift in the oxygen-hemoglobin dissociation curve contributes to the acute lactic acidosis that often follows tissue hypoxia irrespective of the cause.

Carbon Dioxide

Contrary to its limited capacity for oxygen, blood can accommodate enormous quantities of carbon dioxide (Fig. 9–3). Carbon dioxide is carried in the blood as a dissolved gas, as bicarbonate ions, carbonic acid, carbaminohemoglobin, and as other carbamino compounds. Reduced — unoxygenated — hemoglobin has a greater affinity for carbon dioxide than does oxyhe-

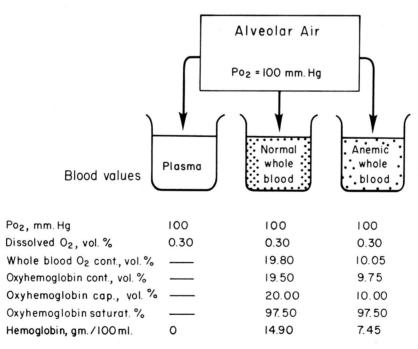

Blood values	Plasma	Normal whole blood	Anemic whole blood
P_{O_2}, mm. Hg	100	100	100
Dissolved O_2, vol. %	0.30	0.30	0.30
Whole blood O_2 cont., vol.%	——	19.80	10.05
Oxyhemoglobin cont., vol.%	——	19.50	9.75
Oxyhemoglobin cap., vol. %	——	20.00	10.00
Oxyhemoglobin saturat. %	——	97.50	97.50
Hemoglobin, gm./100 ml.	0	14.90	7.45

Fig. 9–2. Oxygen solubility and hemoglobin binding. Plasma in contact with oxygen contains only that amount of gas that can dissolve (0.00003 ml oxygen/ml plasma/mm Hg P_{O_2}). Each gram/100 ml blood of hemoglobin combines with 1.34 ml oxygen. With 14.90 g percent hemoglobin, the oxygen capacity is 20.00 volumes percent. At a P_{O_2} of 100 mm Hg and with this hemoglobin, blood will contain 19.50 volumes percent oxygen. When the oxygen dissolved in the plasma is added to the oxygen bound to hemoglobin, the total oxygen content becomes 19.80 volumes percent. Were this patient anemic with only 7.45 g percent of hemoglobin, the saturation at the same P_{O_2} would be identical. The whole blood oxygen content exceeds the oxyhemoglobin capacity in the anemic patient because of the relatively greater contribution of dissolved oxygen to the whole blood oxygen content. *From* Preston FW, Beal JM (eds): Basic Surgical Physiology. Chicago: Year Book, 1969.

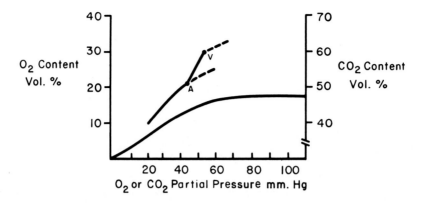

Fig. 9–3. Oxygen and carbon dioxide dissociation curves for whole blood. Oxyhemoglobin saturation of this blood at any P_{O_2} can be determined by dividing the corresponding oxygen content into the oxygen capacity (18.0 volumes percent in this case). The carbon dioxide dissociation curve is relatively linear over the range of partial pressures usually encountered in clinical practice. The difference in the carbon dioxide curve for the arterial (A) and venous (V) blood is due to a greater carbon dioxide carrying capacity of unoxygenated hemoglobin — Haldane effect. *From* Preston FW, Beal JM (eds): Basic Surgical Physiology. Chicago: Year Book, 1969.

moglobin. This upward shift in the carbon dioxide dissociation curve at low P_{O_2} is called the Haldane effect and facilitates transfer of carbon dioxide from tissue to capillary blood, where the P_{O_2} is low, and transfer of carbon dioxide from the capillary into the pulmonary alveolus where the P_{O_2} is higher (Fig. 9–3).

Gases That Are Soluble but Metabolically Inactive

Carbon Monoxide

Coburn (1970) noted that carbon monoxide is produced by the body in small quantities and is therefore involved in metabolic exchange, but we will consider it a foreign and inactive gas. Carbon monoxide is moderately soluble in the pulmonary membrane and has an affinity for hemoglobin 210 times greater than does oxygen. Because of these properties, carbon monoxide in low concentrations and for brief exposure periods is highly useful in the measurement of the diffusion capacity. Even brief exposure to high concentrations or prolonged exposure to relatively low levels of carbon monoxide can be highly toxic, because large amounts of carboxyhemoglobin, which is a stable compound, are produced and prevent hemoglobin from participating in oxygen transport.

Nitrogen

Nitrogen diffuses across the pulmonary membrane and is present in body tissues at the same partial pressure as in alveolar air. Inhalation of 100% oxygen rapidly eliminates nitrogen from the alveolar air, but a small amount of nitrogen continues to diffuse into the alveolar air from the large body tissue stores. Prolonged breathing of 100% oxygen eventually eliminates nitrogen stores from the body.

Gases That Are Insoluble in the Pulmonary Membrane

Helium and Neon

At low concentrations, helium and neon are essentially insoluble in tissue and within brief time intervals do not diffuse across the pulmonary membrane. Because they can be confined to the pulmonary gas compartment, concentration changes of these gases can be used to calculate the size of lung volume compartments.

Anesthetic Gases

All gases used for inhalation anesthesia are highly soluble in both blood and tissue and therefore diffuse rapidly through the pulmonary membrane. Nitrous oxide is a common example, and is the most widely used inorganic gas in anesthesia. The blood concentration required to produce surgical anesthesia in man varies but is approximately 23 volumes percent. To achieve this concentration, the inspired nitrous oxide percentage must be high, so an increased inspired oxygen concentration must be given along with it to avoid hypoxemia. Nitrous oxide is carried in solution in the blood, not in combination with hemoglobin, and is almost completely eliminated from blood and tissue promptly on termination of nitrous oxide inhalation. A minute quantity diffuses through the skin of anesthetized subjects.

Multiple Inert Gases

A variety of other inert gases of varying solubilities, for example, ethane, sulfur hexafluoride, have been used in the study of ventilation and perfusion relationships within the lung. Tests using this so-called multiple inert gas technique popularized by Wagner (1974) are generally available only in research laboratories, but in that setting, they have proved to be useful in increasing our understanding of gas exchange in the lung.

MEASUREMENTS OF GAS EXCHANGE

Total pulmonary gas exchange may be measured by collecting expired air and calculating the amount of oxygen consumed and carbon dioxide produced per unit of time. The normal resting adult male consumes approximately 275 ml of oxygen and produces 230 ml of carbon dioxide per minute. Such measurements give little information about the actual efficiency of gas exchange.

Pulmonary Diffusing Capacity

Whether in the gas phase, dissolved in the plasma, or in chemical association, gases move from regions of higher to lower pressures. The diffusing capacity is a measure of the capacity of the pulmonary membrane to transfer gas between alveolar air and pulmonary capillary blood. Carbon dioxide diffuses from the pulmonary capillary blood into the alveolar air because the capillary P_{CO_2} is higher than the alveolar P_{CO_2}. Carbon dioxide is highly soluble in the pulmonary membrane, and its diffusion is rarely impaired despite extensive lung disease. Retention of carbon dioxide occurs whenever alveolar ventilation is ineffective, resulting in an alveolar P_{CO_2} increase and a reduction of the gradient for carbon dioxide across the pulmonary membrane. Limitations of oxygen diffusion do result in clinically significant disease. Although oxygen diffusion can be determined, carbon monoxide is a more convenient agent for diffusion measurements.

Carbon monoxide diffusion can be measured by three basic methods: single breath, rebreathing, and steady state or continuous breathing. The term "diffusion capacity" may well be a misnomer. Many processes are involved in the transfer of carbon monoxide from inspired air to pulmonary capillary blood. Diffusion is only one part of this system, and diffusion may not be measurable apart from other factors that influence gas transfer.

Results of measurements of the carbon monoxide diffusing capacity are influenced by the method used, the volume of blood in the pulmonary capillary bed, the blood hemoglobin level, and the breathing pattern. Finley and colleagues (1962) noted that abnormal carbon monoxide diffusion values may result from ventilation/perfusion imbalance. As an example of this concept — exaggerated to absurdity — consider a patient with completely normal lungs, one of which is perfused but not ventilated and the other ventilated with air containing trace amounts of carbon monoxide but not perfused. No carbon monoxide uptake will occur even though the pulmonary membrane is normal. A reduction in the blood gas interface secondary to a loss of capillary surface area, as occurs when pulmonary capillary volume is reduced, is one basis for the impaired diffusion in some lung diseases. Because the diffusing capacity measures more than just gas diffusion, the term "transfer factor" has been adopted to describe the overall process. Irrespective of the gas used, the diffusion capacity or transfer factor calculation requires a determination of gas uptake per unit of time and a measurement of the pressure difference between the alveolus and the pulmonary capillary. The result is expressed in ml/min/mm Hg.

The diffusion defects noted in diffuse lung diseases are the result of a combination of factors including a reduction in the pulmonary capillary bed volume, a decrease in the surface area of the blood gas interface,

and imbalances in the ventilation and perfusion of the pulmonary parenchyma secondary to nonuniform distribution of the pathologic changes within the lung parenchyma. The classic concept of the "alveolar capillary block" — a uniform increase in the thickness of the pulmonary membrane that retards the movement of gas — is probably inaccurate, particularly in the resting state.

Arterial Blood Gases

An indirect but useful method of estimating the adequacy of pulmonary gas exchange is the measurement of arterial blood gas tensions and pH. In the normal resting state, with the subject breathing room air, blood gas and pH values are maintained within narrow limits. The arterial P_{O_2} is greater than 75 to 80 mm Hg, depending on the subject's age, the arterial P_{CO_2} is between 38 and 42 mm Hg, the pH is 7.38 to 7.42, and the plasma bicarbonate ion is 20 to 28 mEq/L. The position of the normal subject at the time the blood sample is taken has little effect on the results, but in persons with considerable abdominal obesity or diaphragmatic paralysis, significant changes in arterial blood gas composition may occur when the individuals move from the erect to the supine position. Hyperventilation reduces alveolar P_{CO_2}, increases alveolar P_{O_2}, and has similar effects on arterial blood gas composition. In the normal subject, mild exercise has no significant effect on the arterial P_{O_2}; a mild rise in the P_{O_2} occurs if the exercise is vigorous. In diseases associated with ventilation/perfusion imbalance, however, an acute fall in the arterial P_{O_2} may occur with exercise. The arterial blood gas and pH in various states are illustrated in Table 9–1.

When interpreting arterial P_{O_2} — Pa_{O_2} — measurements, the alveolar oxygen tension — PA_{O_2} — should be estimated. This can be accomplished as follows:

$$PA_{O_2} = FI_{O_2} \times (P_B - 47) - \frac{(PA_{CO_2})}{R}$$

in which FI_{O_2} is the inspired fraction or percentage of oxygen, P_B is barometric pressure — assume 760 mm Hg at sea level, 47 is water vapor pressure at 37°C, PA_{CO_2} is the alveolar CO_2, which is assumed to equal the measured arterial CO_2 — Pa_{CO_2}, and R is the respiratory quotient, assumed to be 0.8.

The equation may be simplified to:

$$PA_{O_2} = FI_{O_2} - (Pa_{CO_2} \times 1.25)$$

The alveolar-arterial oxygen difference — PA_{O_2}–Pa_{O_2} — of a person breathing room air averages about 8 mm Hg in young persons and increases with age to values over 20 mm Hg in the eighth decade. Calculation of this difference will correct for changes in level of ventilation — that is, Pa_{CO_2}. A PA_{O_2}–Pa_{O_2} value should never be negative or near zero. Such a calculation suggests a laboratory error.

Table 9–1.   Blood Gases and Acid-Base Status in Various Conditions

Condition (Clinical Example)	Breathing Pattern	Status	Po₂ (mm Hg)	Pco₂ (mm Hg)	pH	HCO₃⁻ (mEq/L)
Normal	—	—	75–90	38–42	7.38–7.42	20–28
Resp. alkalosis (anxiety)	Hypervent.	Acute	High	Low	High	Normal
Resp. acidosis (narcotic overdose)	Hypovent.	Acute	Low	High	Low	Normal
Resp. alkalosis (pulm. fibrosis)	Hypervent.	Chronic	Low or normal	Low	High norm	Low
Resp. acidosis (obstructive dis.)	Hypovent.*	Chronic	Low	High	Low norm	High
Metab. acidosis (diabetic acid.)	Hypervent.	Acute	High	Low	Low	Low
Metab. alkalosis (prolonged vomiting)	Hypovent.*	Chronic	Low	High	High	High

*May not be clinically apparent. Po_2 = partial pressure of oxygen; Pco_2 = partial pressure of carbon dioxide; HCO_3^- = bicarbonate.

Acid-Base Balance

An acute change in arterial Pco_2 is accompanied by an acute change in arterial pH in the opposite direction. The pH shift approximates 0.01 units per mm Hg change in Pco_2. Under acute conditions, the serum bicarbonate concentration exerts little influence on the relationship of pH and Pco_2. It takes from hours to days for the renal compensatory mechanisms to alter the bicarbonate level and thus correct the pH following an abrupt and persistent change in Pco_2. Such compensation does not occur with brief changes in ventilation, but is present whenever hyperventilation or alveolar hypoventilation is chronic. Renal buffering mechanisms respond to chronic increases in arterial Pco_2 and concomitant decreases in pH by retaining bicarbonate. Chronic hyperventilation leading to sustained hypocapnia and an elevated pH stimulates compensatory renal bicarbonate excretion. Some examples of acid-base derangements are shown in Table 9–1. Acid-base balance and its relationship to pulmonary gas exchange will be described further. It may be misleading to attempt an interpretation of arterial blood gas and pH changes without some knowledge of the status of the patient and prior treatment. Combined respiratory and metabolic acid-base problems may become complex and the acid-base status can be unraveled only with full knowledge of the clinical condition of the patient.

FACTORS AFFECTING PULMONARY GAS EXCHANGE

Partition of Ventilation

Each inspiration has a useful component that bathes the alveoli with fresh air and a component that "goes along for the ride" and ventilates only the conducting tubes — alveolar and dead-space fractions of the tidal volume. That portion of the ventilation distributed to alveoli where gas exchange occurs is the alveolar ventilation. Ventilation of lung regions with anatomically intact but nonfunctioning alveoli is equivalent to ventilation of the conducting airways — dead-space ventilation. The normal subject, breathing quietly at rest, has approximately 1 ml of dead-space volume per pound of body weight. The total minute ventilation measured at the mouth reveals little regarding effective alveolar ventilation. But, if one also knows the respiratory rate, it is possible to estimate alveolar ventilation, assuming that most alveoli are functioning. For example, two patients breathe a total of 5 L/min. One patient, however, breathes 25 times per minute with a tidal volume of 200 ml, whereas the other patient breathes 10 times a minute with a tidal volume of 500 ml. The patient with a 200-ml tidal volume mainly ventilates his dead space. The actual dead-space volume — V_D — and the ratio between dead space and tidal volumes — V_D/V_T — can be measured if the alveolar and expired concentrations of a gas undergoing metabolic exchange and the tidal volume are known. Carbon dioxide is customarily used, and it is assumed that the arterial and alveolar Pco_2 are equivalent. The formula for these measurements, as shown, merely states that the ratio of dead-space volume to tidal volume is the same as the ratio of alveolar — arterial — CO_2 to expired CO_2.

$$V_D/V_T = \frac{Pco_2 \text{ (arterial)} - Pco_2 \text{ (expired)}}{Pco_2 \text{ (arterial)}}$$

Distribution of Ventilation

Several methods are available to evaluate the uniformity or nonuniformity of the distribution of inspired air. One method requires that the patient inhale 100% oxygen for 7 minutes, thereby washing out the nitrogen in the lungs. With a nitrogen meter and continuous sampling of the expired air stream, a continuous plot of the breath-by-breath exhaled nitrogen concentration is obtained. In the normal subject, a rapid decrease of nitrogen occurs within the first minute or two of oxygen breathing. Patients with gross alveolar hypoventilation or marked maldistribution of ventilation will have a slow washout curve. When ventilation abnormalities are marked, the washout curve has an erratic pattern with much variation in the breath-to-breath concentration of exhaled nitrogen. In the presence of localized areas of marked hypoventilation, as in bullous disease, the nitrogen concentration in the forced expiratory air sample delivered at the end of the 7-minute washout period will be elevated. Another method for evaluating ventilation uniformity uses a single-breath nitrogen washout. The patient inspires 100% oxygen to total lung capacity and exhales completely while the nitrogen concentration and volume of the single expirate are monitored. The alveolar portion of the expiration should have a nearly constant nitrogen concentration if inspired oxygen is uniformly distributed within the lung.

A single-breath nitrogen washout curve is shown in Figure 9–4. The initial portion of the expirate contains no nitrogen as it consists solely of the terminal portion of the previous inhaled oxygen — phase 1. As expiration continues, the nitrogen concentration rises rapidly as the dead space is rinsed with alveolar gas — phase 2. A nitrogen plateau then appears, which rises slowly, at a rate of 1.0 to 1.5% nitrogen per liter expired, in normal subjects — phase 3. A steep — concentration increase of greater than 1.5% N_2/L — or irregular phase 3 occurs whenever ventilation is nonuniform. In obstructive lung disease, values of 10% N_2/L or greater are not unusual. Most adults have a fourth phase. The onset of phase 4 is apparent from an abrupt increase in nitrogen concentration. This sudden rise occurs when the lung volumes are small and airways to the dependent portions of the lung close. The lung volume corresponding with the onset of phase 4 is known as the closing volume. Because of a gradation of intrapleural pressure from apex to base in the upright subject, small airways in the dependent lung zones are subjected to higher transpulmonary pressures than those at the apex. The basal airways close at small lung volumes, producing the characteristic phase 3–4 junction that defines the closing volume. The rise in nitrogen concentration during phase 4 is attributable to the lesser dilution of upper zone nitrogen during the previous oxygen inhalation. Also, basal lung zones, with a lower N_2 concentration, cease contributing to expiration after the onset of phase 4. The closing volume enlarges and the phase 4 onset moves up in the vital capacity, toward total lung capacity with age and in the presence of small airway pathology. As the closing volume point rises

progressively in the patient's lung volume, it eventually exceeds the resting end-expiratory lung volume, which is the functional residual capacity — FRC. Thus, some dependent airways close at the end of every breath. During normal resting tidal ventilation, ventilation of dependent lung zones is reduced, creating a ventilation/perfusion imbalance. This imbalance increases with age and is one of the factors responsible for a decline in the arterial oxygen tension of the elderly.

Distribution of Blood Flow

Pulmonary blood flow can be considered uniform in anatomic terms if every alveolus receives equivalent blood flow. In functional terms, physiologic uniformity exists when blood flow is distributed to each alveolus in proportion to its ventilation. Blood flow nonuniformity occurs to some degree in normal individuals. In an upright subject breathing normally at rest, the lung bases are perfused, whereas the apices are minimally perfused owing to gravity and the low hydrostatic pressures in the pulmonary circuit. The apical areas of the lung receive considerable ventilation but are poorly perfused. This mismatch is not sufficiently great to be physiologically significant in the normal individual.

The distribution of blood flow to various portions of the lung can be evaluated by several methods. The chest radiograph may demonstrate relative hyperlucency of one parenchymal region, suggesting a local reduction in pulmonary blood flow as may occur with a pulmonary embolus. Perfusion scans using radioactive tagged macroaggregated albumin that lodges in the pulmonary capillaries provide good evidence of the gross distribution of blood flow within the pulmonary vascular bed (see Chapter 14). More precise visualization of pulmonary blood flow requires catheterization and contrast visualization of the vascular bed. Arterial blood gas determinations are not particularly useful for estimating abnormalities in the distribution of pulmonary blood flow. In most instances in which nonuniformity of blood flow is the sole functional abnormality, arterial blood gas values are within normal limits.

Relationship of Ventilation and Perfusion

Effective gas exchange within the lung requires a close approximation of the distribution of ventilation and pulmonary capillary blood flow. Major nonuniformity or mismatching between ventilation — V — and perfusion — Q — will be reflected in arterial blood gas abnormalities. In normal individuals, the distribution of blood flow and ventilation to various areas of the lung is neither completely homogeneous nor equally matched. Some regions of lung, for example, tend to receive relatively more ventilation than blood flow. Normally, no adverse consequences follow from this relationship. Major physiologic disturbances occur primarily when blood flow to regions that are relatively underventilated, i.e., low V/Q, is substantial. In such situations, of which atelectasis and pneumonitis are examples, severe hypoxemia may occur. Elimination of carbon dioxide tends to be unaffected because other,

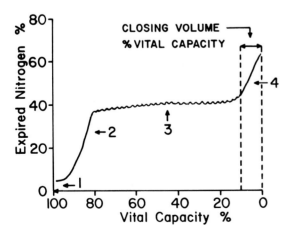

Fig. 9–4. Tracing of expired nitrogen concentration and expired volume from total lung capacity to residual volume. The four phases of the curve (see text) are shown. Oscillations of the nitrogen tracing during phase 3 are synchronous with the heart beat and are caused by cardiac churning of gases in the airways.

more normal, lung regions are usually overventilated in compensation. This allows maintenance of a normal or low arterial carbon dioxide tension. Compensation for a fall in oxygen tension, on the other hand, is limited by the shape of the oxyhemoglobin dissociation curve (see Fig. 9–1).

Shunts and Venous Admixture

A "right-to-left shunt" exists whenever blood passing through the pulmonary capillaries is not exposed to ventilated alveoli and is not oxygenated. Thus, as noted by Robin and associates (1977), a shunt can be considered an area of lung in which V/Q is zero. Shunts occur in such conditions as lobar pneumonia and with acute atelectasis of a lobe or entire lung. The fraction of total pulmonary blood flow that is shunted can be approximated by measurement of arterial Po_2. With minor degrees of shunting, the Po_2 with the subject at rest and breathing room air may be normal. Up to 6% right-to-left shunt occurs in healthy subjects, and this "physiologic" shunt results from venous blood normally entering the pulmonary veins, left atrium, or left ventricle. Whenever there is a greater than normal degree of shunting, hypoxemia will be present and inhalation of 100% oxygen for 10 to 20 minutes will fail to increase the Po_2 above 550 mm Hg, which would be expected in normal individuals. The ratio of shunted to total pulmonary blood flow can be estimated as follows if the arterial Po_2 is greater than 150 mm Hg during oxygen breathing:

$$\frac{\text{Shunt Flow}}{\text{Total Flow}} = \frac{[Po_2 \text{ (alv.)} - Po_2 \text{ (art. blood)}] \times 0.003}{\begin{array}{c}(\text{art.} - \text{mixed ven. } O_2 \text{ cont.}) + \\ [Po_2 \text{ (alv.)} - Po \text{ (art.)}] \times .003\end{array}}$$

Po_2 (alv.) = the alveolar Po_2 while breathing 100% oxygen. Alveolar Po_2 is estimated from the barometric pressure minus water vapor pressure (47 mm Hg) and alveolar Pco_2 (approximately 40 mm Hg).
Thus, Po_2 (alv.) = (760 − 47) − 40 = 673 mm Hg.
0.003 = the solubility factor for converting Po_2 into oxygen content in volume percent (see Fig. 9–2).
Art.-mixed ven. O_2 cont. = the difference in oxygen content between mixed venous and arterial blood. It is usually from 4 to 6 volumes percent and can be assumed for the purpose of estimating shunt flow.

The assumed value for the difference between mixed venous and arterial oxygen content has a definite effect on the calculated shunt. The larger the difference between alveolar and arterial Po_2, the greater the effect of the assumed value of arterial-mixed venous difference on the calculated shunt flow.

Venous admixture is a variant of right-to-left shunt that involves a relative but not total lack of ventilation to the involved area, i.e., V/Q is low but greater than zero. Ventilation of a lung region may be normal, but, if blood flow is increased, ventilation may be relatively inadequate; or ventilation may be decreased in the presence of normal blood flow. Venous admixture results from relative ventilation/perfusion imbalances. Unlike a

true shunt, the arterial Po_2 deficit of venous admixture can be corrected by 100% oxygen breathing. Studies with the multiple inert gas technique of Wagner and co-workers (1974) have shown that, contrary to past assumptions, extremely low ventilation/perfusion ratios can produce hypoxemia that is not corrected with 100% oxygen breathing. Furthermore, the use of high oxygen concentrations to measure shunt may cause absorptive atelectasis in those regions with a low V/Q and, thereby, increase the shunt. Nevertheless, measurement of the "shunt fraction" has practical application; for example, for monitoring the progress of acutely ill patients with the adult respiratory distress syndrome. This practical utility is especially true when samples of mixed venous blood are available from a central — Swan-Ganz — catheter line allowing accurate determination of the mixed venous and arterial oxygen content difference.

MANAGEMENT OF PATIENTS WITH IMPAIRED GAS EXCHANGE

The diagnosis and proper management of impaired gas exchange requires accurate measurement of arterial blood gases and pH. Minimal or subclinical defects in gas transport or distribution may require measurements of diffusion, and alveolar and arterial Po_2 at rest and with exercise. It has been estimated that a 50% reduction in the exercise carbon monoxide diffusing capacity is needed before a significant reduction in the exercise arterial Po_2 will be noted. Nevertheless, the majority of clinically significant problems can be evaluated by obtaining data from a careful history and physical examination supplemented by arterial blood measurements.

Proper interpretation of arterial blood gas and pH values requires a thorough knowledge of the patient's previous history of lung disease, or other medical and surgical problems that might alter pulmonary gas transport. Diuretics, steroids, and sedative drugs are frequent causes of abnormal arterial blood gas composition. Knowledge of prior use of sedatives and analgesics is most important in evaluating blood gas data, particularly in patients with pulmonary disease, because they may be unduly sensitive to respiratory depression from small doses that are usually well tolerated. Calculation of the $PA_{O_2}-Pa_{O_2}$ difference assists the clinician in identifying aberrations in arterial blood gas values that are attributable to primary disturbances of ventilation without accompanying changes in the lung parenchyma. Patients with abnormal breathing patterns who are thought to have abnormal gas transport may have acid-base disturbances instead. For example, hypoventilation with an attendant rise in arterial Pco_2 and fall in Po_2 may occur because of severe metabolic alkalosis.

Many therapeutic options are available for the management of patients with alterations in pulmonary gas exchange. Selection of the appropriate program should be based on a careful evaluation of the patients and their metabolic status, particularly their arterial blood gases. Important goals include optimization of tissue oxygenation and maintenance of relatively normal acid-base balance. To achieve adequate oxygenation, oxygen-carrying capacity — hemoglobin concentration, cardiac output, and regional blood flow — must be maintained. Arterial P_{O_2} should, ideally, be at least 65 to 75 mm Hg to completely saturate hemoglobin. This value may be achievable with relatively low concentrations of $F_{I_{O_2}}$. When gas exchange is seriously deranged, concentrations exceeding an $F_{I_{O_2}}$ of 0.50 may be needed, raising the possibility of pulmonary oxygen toxicity. As pointed out by Weisman and co-workers (1982), positive airway pressure, either as continuous positive airway pressure — CPAP — or positive end-expiratory pressure — PEEP, may allow significant reductions in the amount of supplemental oxygen needed to maintain acceptable arterial P_{O_2} levels. Excessive levels of positive pressure, however, particularly in patients with volume depletion, may cause a reduction in cardiac output. Thus, careful monitoring of these patients is essential. In patients who appear unlikely to maintain adequate levels of ventilation, as indicated by a rising arterial P_{CO_2} or unusual degree of ventilatory effort, mechanical ventilation is advisable. Methods such as assist-control, intermittent mandatory ventilation —

IMV, synchronized IMV, and pressure support are available to facilitate optimal mechanical support.

REFERENCES

Coburn RF: Current concepts: Endogenous carbon monoxide production. N Engl J Med *282*:207, 1970.

Divertie MB, Brown AL Jr: The fine structure of the normal human alveolar-capillary membrane. JAMA *187*:938, 1964.

Finley TN, Swenson EW, Comroe JH Jr: The cause of arterial hypoxemia at rest in patients with "alveolar-capillary block syndrome." J Clin Invest *41*:618, 1962.

Robin ED, et al: A shunt is (not) a shunt is (not) a shunt. Am Rev Respir Dis *115*:553, 1977.

Wagner PD, Saltzman HA, West TB: Measurement of continuous distributions of ventilation-perfusion ratios: Theory. J Appl Physiol *36*:588, 1974.

Weisman IM, Rinaldo JE, Rogers RM: Current concepts: Positive end-expiratory pressure in adult respiratory failure. N Engl J Med *307*:1381, 1982.

READING REFERENCES

Bates DV: Respiratory Function in Disease. 3rd Ed. Philadelphia: WB Saunders, 1989.

West JB: Respiratory Physiology: The Essentials. 3rd Ed. Baltimore: Williams & Wilkins, 1985.

CHAPTER 10

MECHANICS OF BREATHING

Joan D. Boomsma and Jeffrey Glassroth

The term "mechanics of breathing" refers to the elastic properties of the lung and chest wall and to airflow resistance. These properties are described and related to lung volume and airflow measurements — the standard tests of ventilatory function (Table 10–1). The subdivisions of the lung volume referred to are shown in Figure 10–1.

Table 10–1. Subdivisions of the Lung Volume

Gas Volumes Commonly Reported

Vital capacity (VC) is the maximum volume that can be expired following a maximal inspiration.

Total lung capacity (TLC) is the volume in the lungs after a maximal inspiration.

Residual volume (RV) is the volume remaining in the lungs after a maximal expiration. In normal individuals, RV is approximately 25 to 30% of TLC.

Functional residual capacity (FRC) is the volume in the lungs at the end of a normal expiration.

Tidal volume (TV) is the volume of a spontaneous breath.

Other Volumes

Inspiratory capacity (IC) is the maximal volume that can be inspired from the resting end-expiratory position to TLC.

Expiratory reserve volume (ERV) is the volume that can be expired from a spontaneous end-expiratory position — that is, from FRC to RV.

Inspiratory reserve volume (IRV) is the volume that can still be inspired from a spontaneous end-inspiratory position.

ELASTIC PROPERTIES OF THE LUNG

The inflated lung is an elastic structure that tends to deflate itself. The deflation force exerted by an expanded lung is the elastic recoil pressure. This recoil pressure increases with increasing lung volume, and the pressure required to maintain inflation equals the elastic recoil pressure. Irrespective of the manner in which it is measured, the recoil pressure of the lung is always considered positive because it is always directed toward deflation. The elastic recoil pressure is expressed as the pressure difference between the alveolar lumen and the pleural space. Alveolar pressure is equivalent to atmospheric pressure when the glottis and mouth are open and there is no airflow. Therefore, under these conditions, the intrapleural pressure is equal but opposite in sign to the elastic recoil pressure.

Pleural pressure changes can be conveniently and reliably measured in the upright subject by placing a small tube with an attached balloon in the esophagus. Under static conditions, that is, in the absence of airflow, a given degree of lung inflation is maintained either by inspiratory muscle contraction, by the elasticity of the chest wall resisting inward collapse, or both. The "resting" lung volume or FRC is the result of the balance between equal but opposite forces generated by the inward elastic recoil of the lungs and the outward recoil of the chest cage.

A pressure-volume plot made under static conditions (Fig. 10–2) defines the elastic properties of the lung. Multiple measurements of the elastic recoil pressure or the intrapleural pressure and corresponding intrathoracic gas volume over the entire range of lung volumes are necessary to describe the entire pressure-volume curve of the lung. The pressure-volume relationship of the lung is often described in terms of lung compliance. If measured over the tidal volume portion of the curve, it is almost linear, and is expressed as the change in volume per unit change in pressure — ml/cm H_2O.

The pressure-volume relationship is basic to an understanding of the fundamental relation between the work of breathing and lung mechanics. The "stiffer" lung displays a more horizontal curve (Fig. 10–2C), meaning that it takes a greater pressure to achieve the same inflation volume compared with a normal lung (Fig. 10–2A). These lungs are called less compliant. At lung volumes approaching total lung capacity, considerably more pressure per liter of inspired volume is required than at smaller lung volumes. In both health and disease, the tidal volume occurs on the steepest part

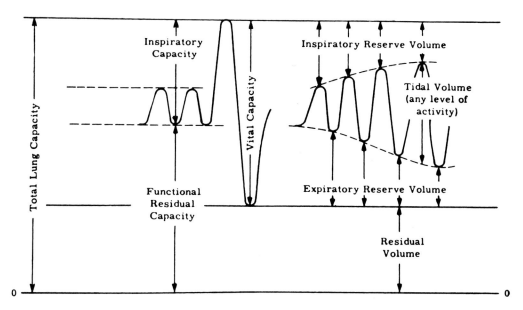

Fig. 10–1. Lung volumes. *From* Standardization of definitions and symbols in respiratory physiology. Fed Proc 9:602, 1950.

of the pressure-volume curve where the largest volume change is accomplished with a minimal pressure change. For any given ventilatory requirement, every person has an optimal pattern of tidal volume and breathing frequency at which the work of breathing is minimal. When the lungs are stiff, a pattern of rapid, shallow breathing is adopted and this pattern minimizes the work of breathing. Even so, more effort than normal is required to ventilate stiff lungs (Fig. 10–2C). Although it would appear that the patient with emphysema is at an advantage because less effort is required to deform the lungs (Fig. 10–2B), work of breathing is increased because of obstruction to airflow and because hyperinflation requires that tidal breathing be shifted to a less advantageous position on the pressure-volume curve.

The elastic properties of the lung reside mainly in the alveolar walls and their liquid lining. The walls contain a network of collagen, elastic, and reticular fibers in addition to their capillary network and epithelial lining. The thin liquid film on the luminal surface of the alveolar epithelium creates a surface tension that accounts in part for lung elasticity. Surface tension forces tend to reduce the surface to the smallest possible area. In the bubble-like alveolus, surface tension increases as the size of the bubble decreases, and, if unopposed, would lead to alveolar collapse. A lipid substance in the alveolar lining fluid reduces surface tension at the gas-liquid interface, thereby protecting the lungs against alveolar collapse. This substance, surfactant, can be extracted from normal lung tissue and is absent or reduced in persons with pulmonary atelectasis, hyaline membrane disease, or infarction. Surfactant maintains surface-tension forces relatively constant despite varying degrees of lung inflation and alveolar size.

Although pressure changes in the lung are similar everywhere during inflation, ventilation is not evenly distributed throughout the normal organ. At successive horizontal levels of the lung, from apex to base, the volume change produced by a given pressure change becomes progressively greater. The most dependent portions of the lung receive more ventilation per unit of lung tissue than the uppermost levels. The reason for this discrepancy is the effect of gravity. Although pressure changes producing inflation are essentially the same over the normal lung surface, the absolute pres-

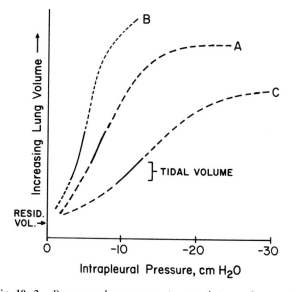

Fig. 10–2. Pressure-volume curves: A, normal; B, emphysema; C, pulmonary fibrosis. The solid line represents the tidal volume in these three conditions.

sure is not. In the upright position, the weight of the lung makes the intrapleural pressure at the lung base less negative than it is at the apex. With a less negative intrapleural pressure at the bases, the elastic recoil pressure and the volume of each alveolus at the base are less than in higher regions at the onset of inspiration (Fig. 10–3). With inflation, the pressure change transmitted to all lung tissue is the same, but different regions inflate to different volumes depending on where, on the pressure-volume curve, inflation commences. A dependent portion has a lesser recoil pressure to begin with; therefore, a normal breath will inflate a basal region more than other areas because its behavior is confined to a steeper portion of the pressure-volume curve. Fortunately, perfusion of the normal lung is similarly affected by gravity so that a fairly good match between ventilation and perfusion is maintained throughout the lung.

In diseases of the lungs in which the elastic properties are not uniformly the same, regional ventilation becomes nonuniform. Adjacent lung regions, even neighboring alveoli, have different pressure-volume characteristics. Thus, the same pressure change, even when beginning at the same absolute level of intrapleural pressure, produces different volume changes in neighboring areas. The pressure-volume characteristics as measured with an esophageal balloon are those of the whole lung and are averages that may obscure regional differences. Diffuse infiltrative disease, such as diffuse pulmonary fibrosis, produces inequalities not only in inspired gas distribution, but also in the distribution of blood flow, resulting in abnormal gas exchange. The overall adverse effects of these diseases can best be assessed by measurements of gas exchange and arterial blood gas content (see Chapter 9).

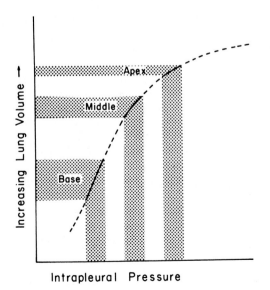

Fig. 10–3. Effect of gravity in the upright position. As one approaches the base of the lung, there is a greater volume change per unit of lung tissue for the same pressure change.

ELASTIC AND MECHANICAL PROPERTIES OF THE CHEST WALL

Lung inflation and deflation are accomplished by changes in the dimensions of the chest wall. These dimensional changes are determined by the elastic properties of the bony and soft tissue structures of the thorax and by the muscle forces that impart motion to the respiratory system. Like the lung, the chest wall exerts a recoil pressure proportional to its volume of expansion. This recoil pressure is measured as the difference between pleural pressure and body surface pressure under static conditions when the muscles of respiration are completely relaxed. By plotting this pressure against the thoracic gas volume, one obtains the pressure-volume relationship of the chest wall. The compliance of the chest wall, as described by the slope of this relationship, is normally high enough so that the rib cage and soft tissue structures do not restrict respiratory movement.

Certain factors, however, may restrict movement of the chest wall and reduce its compliance. An increase in the longitudinal dimension of the thorax is primarily determined by movement of the diaphragm. Diaphragmatic movement may be restricted by conditions that increase intra-abdominal pressure, such as pregnancy, obesity, ascites, and intra-abdominal tumors. Changing from the erect to the supine position may also restrict the diaphragm by shifting the weight of the abdominal contents toward the diaphragm. These conditions generally reduce vital capacity, total lung capacity, and functional residual capacity.

Changes in the anteroposterior and transverse dimensions of the chest wall are primarily effected by the intercostal muscles and accessory muscles of respiration, and depend on the mobility of the rib cage. Thus, conditions that result in deformation or fixation of the thorax, such as kyphoscoliosis or ankylosing spondylitis, may also restrict expansion. Obesity may also reduce chest wall compliance by increasing the soft tissue mass of the thorax. Moreover, because respiratory movement ultimately depends on the action of the respiratory muscles, conditions that result in paralysis or weakness of the respiratory muscles severely limit ventilation and often cause respiratory failure. Because of the difficulties of measuring chest wall compliance, muscle strength, and leverage, as well as intra-abdominal pressure and gravitational forces, it is customary to rely on measurements of their consequences, such as changes in lung volumes, gas exchange, ventilation, and perfusion. The results of these tests plus knowledge of the clinical status of the patient are usually adequate to determine whether the chest wall or underlying lung disease is at fault.

LUNG VOLUME MEASUREMENTS

An isolated decrease in a lung volume does not affect health as long as adequate volume remains to permit normal ventilation of the alveoli. Although the tidal volume normally increases with exercise, the ventilation necessary for a given level of exercise can be achieved by increasing either tidal volume or breathing frequency. Thus, compensation for a limited lung volume can be attained by increasing the breathing frequency. In the presence of lung diseases characterized by airway obstruction, however, ventilation is maintained by a relatively greater increase in tidal volume than in frequency. This interrelation between tidal volume and frequency is further considered subsequently in the section *Work of Breathing.*

The reduction of lung volumes occurring with diseases of the chest wall, lungs, or pleura provides a crude guide to the severity of the disease. Thus, volume measurements may be useful for deciding when therapeutic intervention is appropriate or in judging the response or lack of response to therapy. Lung volume measurements are made easily, and their reproducibility renders them useful for longitudinal studies in a given patient. For example, a loss of 500 ml on serial testing of a patient with an initial vital capacity of 4 or 5 L would be significant. Unfortunately, a single measurement is not a sensitive indicator of early disease because of an approximately 20% variation in lung volumes among persons of the same age, height, and sex.

Although no specific diagnosis is suggested by a lung volume decrease, simple volume measurements, particularly the vital capacity, are just as sensitive an index of disease as the direct measurement of mechanical factors that determine static lung volumes, such as the lung compliance.

Vital Capacity

The vital capacity can be determined either by adding separate measurements of the maximal expired volume and maximal inspired volume starting from the resting lung volume, or by using a single expiratory effort starting from total lung capacity (see Fig. 10–1). The maneuver may be performed in a leisurely or slow manner as distinct from the "forced" vital capacity. In the forced maneuver, the patient empties the lungs as rapidly as possible starting from total lung capacity. In patients with obstructive lung disease, this forced maneuver may increase expiratory obstruction and produce a spuriously low measurement of vital capacity (see *Airway Resistance During Expiration*).

Functional Residual Capacity

The FRC is the volume of gas remaining in the lungs at the end of normal expiration. Two methods are used for measurements of functional residual capacity: inert gas dilution or washout and body plethysmography. Nitrogen, argon, and helium are the inert gases customarily used. For an accurate determination, the gas must be evenly distributed or washed out from all air-containing units of the lung. This may not occur, or may occur only slowly, in the presence of bullous disease, airway obstruction, or other conditions in which portions of the lung are poorly ventilated.

For the plethysmographic method of measuring functional residual capacity, the subject sits in an airtight cabinet, the body plethysmograph. Measurements of changes in alveolar pressure and lung volume are made simultaneously while the patient is panting against an obstruction to airflow that is interposed briefly at the mouth. Alveolar pressure is equivalent to the pressure at the mouth under these circumstances. With this method, all of the gas within the chest, even in the presence of airway obstruction or bullous disease, is measured. The test is simple to perform but relatively elaborate, and costly equipment is required. The same apparatus can be used, however, for the direct measurement of airway resistance. Discrepancies between plethysmographic and inert gas volume determinations may reflect the volume of poorly ventilated lung that is present.

Residual Volume

The RV, air remaining in the lungs after complete expiration, is calculated by subtracting the expiratory reserve volume (see Fig. 10–1) from the functional residual capacity determined by any of the preceding methods, and is therefore no more accurate than the functional residual capacity.

Total Lung Capacity

The TLC is usually computed by merely adding the separately determined vital capacity and residual volume. It is less reproducible than the vital capacity because the variability in the separately measured volume components may be additive. The TLC can also be calculated from chest radiographs and includes all the gas within the lungs, similar to the plethysmographic measurements.

AIRFLOW RESISTANCES

To generate airflow, the bellows action of the chest wall must overcome the elastic properties of the lungs and chest wall plus frictional resistances to motion. These frictional resistances consist of pressure losses from air flowing through the airways and to friction within the tissues of the lung and chest wall during breathing movements. Unlike measurements of elastic recoil pressures made under static conditions, resistances are a dynamic property and must be measured while there is airflow. The components of total airflow resistance within the lungs and thorax are: airway resistance, lung tissue resistance, and chest wall resistance. The sum of the last two resistances is about equal to the airway resistance. The resistances of lung tissue and chest wall tend to be minimally affected by disease and are overshadowed by the magnitude of the changes in airway resistance. The majority of airway resistance occurs in large airways — those 2 mm or larger in diameter.

Increases in airflow resistance are attributable primarily to increases in airway resistance; thus, indirect

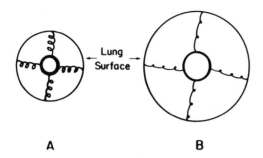

A   **B**

Fig. 10–4. Effect of inspiration on an intrapulmonary airway: *A*, End-expiration; *B*, End-inspiration. The inner circle could also represent an alveolus.

measurements of airflow resistance, such as the maximum midexpiratory flow rate, volume expelled in the first second of the forced vital capacity maneuver, and maximum voluntary ventilation, may be used as an index of airway resistance.

Measurements of airflow resistance provide an "average" value for the entire system of airways. In any generalized obstructive lung disease, some airways have a higher resistance to airflow than others, and flow is greater into alveoli whose conducting airways have the lowest resistance. The result is a nonuniform distribution of inspired air creating a mismatch between ventilation and perfusion and impairment of gas exchange.

Airway Resistance During Inspiration

Airway diameter varies depending on the gradient between intra- and extralumenal airway pressures. These gradients function in an opposite manner for intrathoracic and extrathoracic airways. The extrathoracic airway diameter increases during *e*xpiration, whereas the intrathoracic airway increases in diameter on *in*spiration. An exception is a fixed orifice type of obstruction such as occurs in association with a tumor completely encircling an airway. Airway dilatation on inspiration is produced by radial traction provided by elastic forces of the lung tissue surrounding the airway (Fig. 10–4). A loss of elastic recoil, such as that occurring in emphysema, results in a decrease of airway caliber. Conversely, an increase in elastic forces increases traction on the airway, enlarging airway dimensions.

Inspiratory airflow increases in direct proportion to the force or effort applied. Patients with chronic obstructive pulmonary disease, in whom impaired expiratory airflow is invariably present, may have decreased inspiratory flow as well. Inspiratory flow is reduced in patients with chronic bronchitis and in those with asthma because the bronchial lumen is narrowed by secretions and edema, bronchospasm, or both. Inspiratory flow is also reduced when airways become stiff and less expansile because of inflamed bronchial walls or become narrow owing to decreased radial traction (Fig. 10–4). Inspiratory flow measurements, usually made

from an inspiratory flow-volume loop (see Fig. 10–7), are primarily useful in unusual, but often remedial, localized obstructions of major airways, because limitation of inspiratory flow may equal or exceed expiratory flow limitation. In patients with the usual types of obstructive lung diseases, inspiratory flow limitation is not clinically important, whereas expiratory flow limitation is invariably severe.

Airway Resistance During Expiration

Unlike inspiratory flow, which depends to a major extent on the muscular effort generated, expiratory flow depends primarily on the mechanical properties of the lungs and is related to effort only up to a certain point. Beyond this point, further increases in effort do not increase expiratory flow and in some instances may decrease it. This concept is illustrated in the isovolume pressure-flow curves in Figure 10–5. These curves are obtained by performing a series of active expirations with increasing effort at a particular lung volume and by plotting flow rates against corresponding pleural pressure. In this instance, pleural pressure represents the driving pressure or force related to muscular effort. In Figure 10–5 curves obtained at three different lung volumes are represented. Between total lung capacity — TLC — and 75% of TLC, flow increases with effort and depends not only on effort but also on the patency of airways and high elastic recoil of the lung at high volumes. At volumes below approximately 75% of TLC, expiratory flow increases with effort up to a point, at which further increases in effort do not lead to a higher flow rate. Flow reaches a maximal level at this point because further increases in pleural pressure resulting from effort tend to compress airways and limit flow to the same extent that they tend to drive flow. This dynamic compression occurs because intrathoracic airways are exposed to pleural pressures. This concept is illustrated by the model in Figure 10–6. In this model, the "lung" or "alveolus" and airway are suspended in a box representing the thorax. The lung is

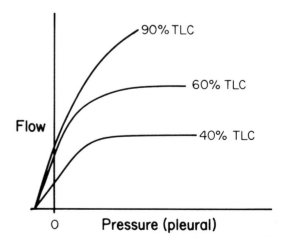

Fig. 10–5. Isovolume pressure flow plot at three different lung volumes.

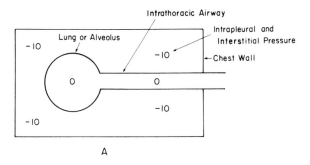

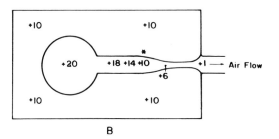

Fig. 10–6. See text for discussion. Static recoil pressure is +10 cm H$_2$O. *A*, Static conditions; *B*, Dynamic conditions. Airway is compressed downstream from point marked by asterisk.

separated from the chest wall for descriptive purposes only, and the space between the lung and chest wall should be considered the airless pleural space. The numbers represent pressure in centimeters of water. In Figure 10–6A, the pleural pressure is equal to the pressure surrounding the airways. At this level of lung inflation, the pleural pressure is equal and opposite in sign to the elastic recoil pressure of the lung — +10; no pressure gradient is present to produce airflow, and net alveolar pressure is atmospheric, or zero. During active expiration (Fig. 10–6B), pleural pressure becomes less negative. Because alveolar pressure is equal to the sum of pleural pressure and lung recoil pressure, it will increase by an amount equal to the increase in pleural pressure. At this point, the difference between alveolar pressure — +20 — and airway opening pressure — 0 — represents the total pressure producing expiratory flow. It follows that at some point between the alveolus and the airway opening, airway intraluminal pressure is equal to pleural pressure, and intraluminal pressures downstream from this point will be less than pleural pressure. This downstream segment will tend to collapse and limit flow. With any further increase in effort, the downstream segment tends to collapse even further. In this case, any additional increase in driving pressure resulting from greater effort is merely dissipated in keeping the collapsed segment open.

Maximal flow over most of the vital capacity is thus effort independent, but it is dependent on the lung recoil pressure and the resistance of peripheral airways upstream from the collapsible segment. Therefore, diseases such as emphysema that reduce the elasticity

of airways and lung tissue tend to produce flow limitation by reducing the driving pressure and by making airways more collapsible. Diseases such as chronic bronchitis and asthma produce flow limitation by increasing the resistance of upstream or peripheral airways. Because maximal expiratory flow over the effort-independent range of the vital capacity — below 75% of TLC — depends on the resistance of peripheral airways, tests of forced expiration have become a useful means of detecting airway disease in its early stages.

Because of the pressure, volume, and flow relationships of the lung, the presence of airway obstruction can be determined by measuring maximal expiratory flow. Because maximal flow is relatively independent of effort and primarily dependent on the recoil pressure of the lung, and because the recoil pressure of the lung is dependent on lung volume, one need only relate the measured flow to the lung volume at which it is measured; this relationship is called a flow-volume curve (Fig. 10–7).

The initial acceleration phase of the expiratory half of the loop represents the inertia of the system. Thereafter, maximal flow decreases as lung volume decreases. The initial portion of the curve between TLC and approximately 75% of TLC is the effort-dependent portion. Beyond this point, maximal flow is relatively independent of effort and dependent on lung recoil and the resistance of airways upstream from the collapsible segment. By measuring flow at a particular volume, such as 50% or 25% of the vital capacity, and comparing it to established normal standards, one can detect the presence of airflow limitation. Measurements made from the maximal expiratory flow-volume curve can identify patients with early expiratory airflow limitation before abnormalities occur in their timed vital capacity measurements. Although such measurements are more sensitive, they are neither as reproducible nor as specific as spirometric tests of forced expiration that relate expired volume to the time of expiration, such as the timed vital capacity.

Timed Vital Capacity

This measurement is obtained from the conventional spirogram, a graph of expired volume and time. The patient makes a forced expiration from TLC (Fig. 10–8). Because the effort must be maximal, the patient must be cooperative and the technician capable must be able to coax the patient to do his or her best. The slope of a tangent to the volume-time curve at any point represents airflow at that point. Because airflow is maximal as long as a certain minimal effort is exceeded, portions of the forced vital capacity curve are reproducible, provided the patient exerts his or her best effort. Both reproducibility and appearance of the tracing can be used to judge the dependability of the results obtained.

Other analyses from the timed vital capacity include the volume expired in the first second of the forced vital capacity maneuver, the FEV$_1$. It includes the earliest part of expiration, which is effort dependent, and a later

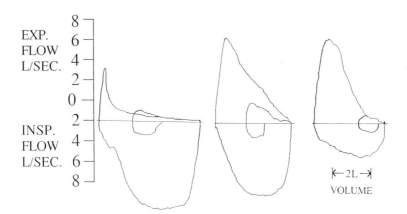

EXP.
FLOW
L/SEC.

INSP.
FLOW
L/SEC.

←2L→

VOLUME

Fig. 10-7. Flow-volume loops from three subjects. The small, inner loop represents flow and volume changes during a normal, resting tidal breath. For each tracing, the residual volume is to the right, and total lung capacity to the left. On the left, the patient has a large vital capacity and severe expiratory airflow limitation throughout the entire vital capacity, but no problem with inspiratory airflow. Note that dynamic airway compression occurs during a forced expiratory maneuver — airflow in the mid vital capacity is greater during a relaxed, tidal breath than it is during the forced vital capacity. A normal, healthy subject is shown in the middle panel. On the right, the patient has inspiratory airflow limitation, but very good expiratory airflow. This pattern reflects an extrathoracic airway defect, which can occur with tracheal tumors, vocal chord lesions, or tracheomalacia.

portion, which is less so. If airflow is diminished because of disease, flow tends to decrease throughout expiration. Measurement of airflow in the first 2 and first 3 seconds of the expiratory effort helps verify the 1-second value. If the 1-second volume is low but the 2- and 3-second volumes are normal, one suspects poor performance. Some laboratories report the volume expired at 0.75 or even 0.5 second. These volumes have the same significance as the 1-second volume. Reduced 1-second volumes are particularly meaningful when the patient's total vital capacity is normal, because airflow obstruction is then likely. If the total vital capacity is reduced, then the forced 1-second volume may also be reduced, whether or not airflow obstruction is present. Therefore,

it is useful to report the 1-second volume, or other timed fractional volumes, as a percentage of the total forced vital capacity, the so-called FEV_1/FVC ratio.

Another derived index of airflow is the forced expiratory flow between 25 and 75% of vital capacity, $FEF_{25-75\%}$, also called the maximum mid-expiratory flow rate — MMF. This rate is calculated by measuring the time required to expire the middle 50% of the vital capacity. Because it is an estimate of the average rate of airflow over the middle half of the vital capacity, it is expressed in units of flow. Hence, the middle 50% of the vital capacity in liters is divided by the time taken to expire it (see Fig. 10-8). Because this measurement is derived from the effort-independent portion of the forced vital capacity, it primarily reflects the flow characteristics in peripheral airways upstream from or proximal to the collapsible segment. For this reason, the $FEF_{25-75\%}$ is considered a useful test of small airway function.

Peak Flow

Peak flow can be measured either from the flow-volume loop (see Fig. 10-7) or with a simple hand-held anemometer type of device such as the Wright Peak Flow Meter. These two methods do not give comparable results and both depend on patient effort. Despite these limitations, determination of peak flow is one test that young children are often able to perform well and may be the only way of measuring their airflow.

Maximum Voluntary Ventilation

Maximum voluntary ventilation — MVV — is determined by having the patient breathe as fast and as deep as possible for a fraction of a minute. The expired volume is measured and the ventilation is expressed in liters per minute. The determination depends on both adequate inspiratory and expiratory airflow plus con-

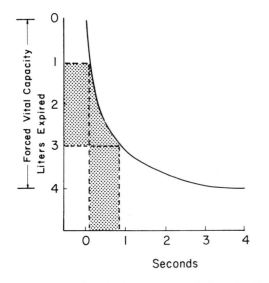

Forced Vital Capacity
Liters Expired

Seconds

Fig. 10-8. The forced vital capacity curve. Both the mid-half of the forced vital capacity and the time required to deliver this mid-half volume are shaded.

siderable endurance and patient cooperation. When properly performed, it provides an excellent index of overall ventilatory ability. It also serves as an alternate test of airflow and as a check on the results of other expiratory flow measurements. Because the maximum midexpiratory flow rate and timed fractions of the forced vital capacity are calculated from the same volume-time curve (see Fig. 10–8), both will be spuriously low if the performance is poor.

Relation of the Functional Residual Capacity and Residual Volume to Airflow Obstruction

Functional residual capacity and residual volume may increase in obstructive lung disease by two mechanisms. First, there may be a loss of lung tissue and therefore lung elasticity. The chest wall forces that counterbalance lung elastic recoil are less opposed and expand the thorax to a larger volume. Second, if airway resistance is increased to such a degree that the patient cannot exhale the inspired volume before inspiring the next breath, the patient will increase the intrathoracic gas volume until expiratory resistance has decreased sufficiently to allow satisfactory exhalation (Fig. 10–9).

Measurements of Airway Resistance and Airflow

The pressure drop from the alveoli to the mouth and the airflow at the mouth can be measured and provide a direct measure of airway resistance — resistance = pressure/flow. Airway resistance — R_{aw} — depends on the lung volume at which it is measured, as would be expected because airways narrow at decreasing lung volumes (see Fig. 10–4) independent of the dynamic narrowing previously described. Proper interpretation of an airway resistance value requires knowledge of the lung volume at which it was measured, particularly in the presence of airflow obstruction, because lung volumes are often increased. Lung volumes range so widely among normal subjects that both airway resistance and the corresponding lung volume must be measured. With the body plethysmograph method, both volume and resistance are determined simultaneously. The relationship between airway resistance and lung volume (see Fig. 10–9A) is curvilinear, whereas the relationship between the reciprocal of airway resistance, airway conductance, and lung volume is nearly linear (see Fig. 10–9B). The slope of this conductance-lung volume plot is the specific conductance. The specific conductance is relatively insensitive to changes of resistance in the peripheral airways until it has increased severalfold, because changes in small airway resistance are masked by the relatively higher resistance of the upper airways. Direct resistance or conductance measurements are seldom more sensitive for defining airway obstruction than is a well-performed forced vital capacity determination.

WORK OF BREATHING

Breathing requires that the respiratory muscles or a mechanical ventilator generate a pressure — force — sufficient to move the volumes of air required for ventilation. Force is required to stretch tissue, to counteract gravity, and to overcome frictional resistances of tissues and airways. There is an optimal combination of breathing frequency and tidal volume at which the work of breathing is minimal. This combination varies between subjects and for specific metabolic requirements. If tidal volume is increased, the pressures required become disproportionately large (see pressure-volume curve in Fig. 10–2). If breathing frequency increases, the airway resistance increases owing to additional flow turbulence and to increased expiratory airway narrowing because of dynamic airway compression. Attempts to drive the respiratory system faster than it will respond, using pressures greater than those required for maximum expiratory airflow, represent wasted effort. In both health and disease, each person spontaneously selects whatever combination of

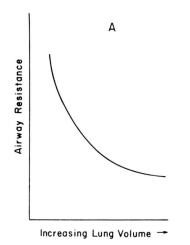
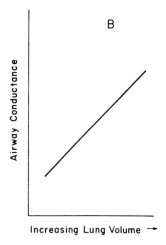

Fig. 10–9. *A*, The airway resistance is dependent on the lung volume at which it is measured and is non-linear. *B*, The reciprocal of airway resistance, airway conductance, is linearly related to lung volume. The slope of this line is the specific conductance.

tidal volume and breathing frequency achieves the required ventilation at a minimal work of breathing. In normal man, the work of breathing requires little energy, approximately 1 ml of oxygen per liter of ventilation. In disease, the oxygen cost of breathing increases greatly and may represent a large portion of the metabolic needs of the patient, thereby limiting the proportion of total oxygen uptake available for muscles not involved in ventilation. Thus, exercise capacity is limited when lung disease causes a substantial increase in the work of breathing.

PRACTICAL APPLICATION OF PULMONARY MECHANICS

An understanding of pulmonary mechanics is extremely useful when applied to the management and monitoring of ventilated patients. Ventilation depends on volume changes driven by pressure gradients, and it does not matter whether the force is generated by respiratory muscles or by a mechanical ventilator.

In ventilated patients, for example, it is useful to evaluate and monitor maximal dynamic, or peak pressure — PD, and static, or plateau pressure — PS. Peale pressure is that required to distend the entire respiratory system at a given inspiratory flow and tidal volume. In ventilated patients, this system includes the machine circuitry and tubing in addition to the lung and chest wall. Therefore, increases in PD may be related to a variety of conditions that either decrease respiratory system compliance or increase resistance to gas flow, including parenchymal lung disease, fluid or air in the pleural space, or increased airway resistance — for example airway secretions, kinked tubing, and so forth. Plateau pressure is that required to distend the respiratory system at peak inspiration in the absence of gas flow. Any additional pressure that has been added to the system — PEEP — is subtracted; PS is measured by imposing a transient airway occlusion, or inspiratory pause, of approximately 1 second. Under these "no-flow" conditions, PS reflects alveolar pressure rather than the entire respiratory system and thus is not influenced by conditions such as bronchospasm or airway secretions.

Respiratory system or static compliance characterizes the pressure-volume relationship of the lung and can be determined in a mechanically ventilated patient once plateau pressure is measured.

$$\text{Compliance} = \frac{\text{Tidal volume}}{\text{PS-PEEP}}$$

$$\text{Normal} = 60\text{--}100 \text{ ml/cm } H_2O$$

Measuring respiratory system compliance is worthwhile in diseases such as adult respiratory distress syndrome — ARDS — which is characterized by severely reduced compliance. Compliance can be used to monitor progress or modify PEEP therapy in ARDS. For example, compliance should improve with increases in PEEP as alveoli are recruited, but it may be reduced when PEEP is increased to the point of overdistention. Additionally, the difference between the peak and static — no-flow — pressures provides an estimate of the pressure required to overcome airflow resistance. Increases in peak-static pressure difference suggest increasing resistance to airflow. A firm understanding of the mechanics of breathing can be valuable in optimizing the management of critically ill patients.

READING REFERENCES

General

Bates DV: Respiratory Function in Disease. Philadelphia: WB Saunders, 1989.
Chusid EL: The Selective and Comprehensive Testing of Adult Pulmonary Function. Mt. Kisco, NY: Futura Publishing, 1983.
Murray JF: The Normal Lung. 2nd Ed. Philadelphia: WB Saunders, 1986.
West JB: Respiratory Physiology: The Essentials, 3rd Ed. Baltimore: Williams & Wilkins, 1985.
Wilson AF: Pulmonary Function Testing — Indications and Interpretations. Orlando: Grune & Stratton, 1985.

Chest Wall and Lung Elasticity

Gibson GJ, Pride NB: Lung distensibility. Br J Dis Chest 70:143, 1976.
Rahn H, et al: The pressure-volume diagram of the thorax and lung. Am J Physiol 146:161, 1946.
Turner JM, Mead J, Wohl ME: Elasticity of human lungs in relation to age. J Appl Physiol 25:664, 1968.

Airflow Resistance

Fry DQ, Hyatt RE: Pulmonary mechanics: A unified analysis of the relationship between pressure, volume and gasflow in the lungs of normal and diseased human subjects. Am J Med 29:672, 1960.
Hogg JC, Macklem PT, Thurlbeck WM: Site and nature of airway obstruction in chronic obstructive lung disease. N Engl J Med 278:1355, 1968.
Hyatt RE, et al: Expiratory flow limitation. J Appl Physiol 55:169, 1983.
Mead J, et al: Significance of the relationship between lung recoil and maximum expiratory flow. J Appl Physiol 22:95, 1967.
Pride NB, et al: Determinants of maximum expiratory flow from the lungs. J Appl Physiol 23:646, 1967.

Practical Application of Pulmonary Mechanics

Marini JJ: Lung mechanics determinations at the bedside: Instrumentation and clinical application. Resp Care 35:669, 1990.
Suter PM, Fairley HB, Isenberg MO: Optimal end-expiratory airway pressure in patients with acute pulmonary failure. N Engl J Med 292:284, 1975.

Thoracic Imaging

CHAPTER 11

RADIOGRAPHIC EVALUATION OF THE LUNGS AND CHEST

Wallace T. Miller

For the physician interested in diseases of the chest, the chest radiograph is of paramount importance in identifying the presence of such disease and in providing clues about its nature.

THE ROUTINE EXAMINATION

Adequate radiographic examination of the chest necessitates at least two projections to provide a three-dimensional view of the thorax. The number of projections considered adequate varies with the individual physician. The views commonly used are straight posteroanterior — PA — and lateral projections.

The PA radiograph can be made at 60 to 80 kilovolts — kV — at a tube film distance of 72 inches without a grid. A high kilovoltage technique, however, is now generally accepted practice. This technique involves the use of x rays above the 125-kV range with a fine line grid, creating a radiograph that has more information by providing less contrast but more penetration. An added advantage of this high-kV technique is the decreased time required for exposure, reducing patient motion.

The lateral radiograph is of considerable importance in the routine examination of the chest, because some lesions in the chest are apparent only in the lateral view. Examples include small mediastinal lesions, some masses in the anterior portions of the lung adjacent to the mediastinum (Fig. 11–1), lesions in the vertebral column, lesions behind the heart and diaphragm on the PA view, and small pleural effusions (Fig. 11–2). Thus, adequate examination of the chest in other than routine screening procedures requires a lateral image.

SUPPLEMENTARY RADIOGRAPHS

The routine examination of the chest allows discovery of most chest lesions. Additional projections or different types of radiographs, however, may be necessary to make an accurate assessment of the character of a particular lesion.

Oblique views are helpful in localizing a suspected lesion and then projecting it free from overlying structures. The oblique radiograph is particularly helpful in determining whether a lesion is in the lung or in the chest wall. It is also helpful in investigating mediastinal lesions, particularly with barium in the esophagus (Fig. 11–3). The oblique radiograph is designated right or left anterior or right or left posterior on the basis of the patient's relationship to the film cassette. In a right anterior oblique position, the right side of the patient is closer to the film and the patient is facing the film cassette.

The oblique view can be confusing to interpret. It is helpful to remember that the heart is an anterior structure and thus moves to the left in a right anterior oblique or to the right in the left anterior oblique view. The aortic arch appears "closed" in the right anterior oblique and "open" in the left anterior oblique view.

It is helpful when examining oblique radiographs to remember that posteriorly placed lesions in the lung maintain a constant relationship with the spine and anteriorly placed lesions in the lung maintains a constant relationship with the heart.

Figures 11–4C and 11–4D demonstrate some of the normal anatomic structures seen on the oblique radiograph.

Lateral decubitus radiographs are extremely important in the investigation of suspected pleural effusion or in demonstration of air fluid levels in pulmonary cavities. The decubitus radiograph is made with the beam projected in a horizontal plane, with the patient lying on his or her side. In a right lateral decubitus radiograph, the patient lies on the right side and free pleural fluid will layer along the right lateral chest wall (see Fig. 11–2C). Amounts of fluid as small as 50 to

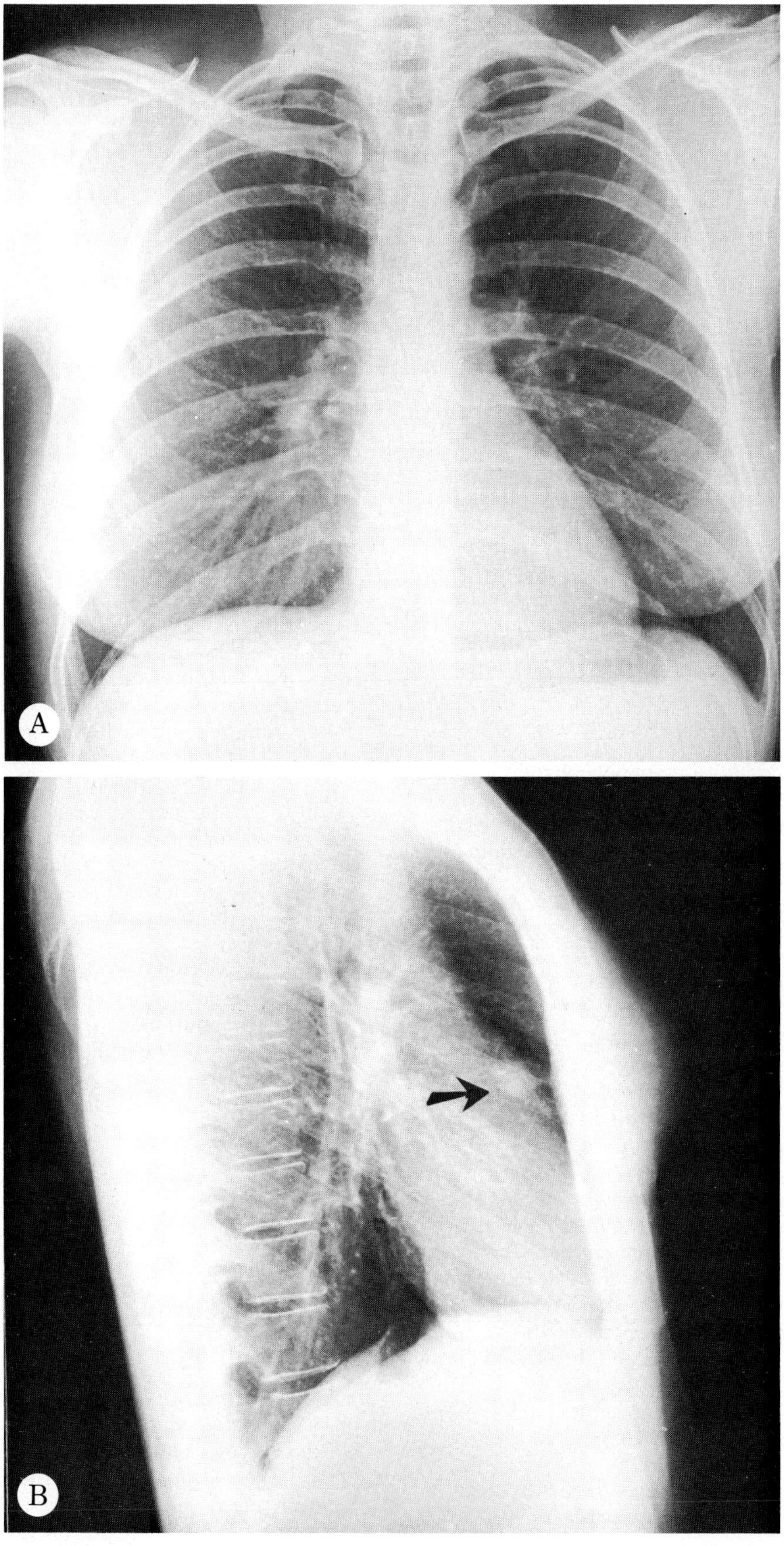

Fig. 11–1. Carcinoma of the lung. The posteroanterior (PA) radiograph *(A)* apparently shows no abnormality, but the lateral view *(B)* demonstrates an unsuspected mass adjacent to the anterior mediastinum (arrow). This mass was subsequently seen to lie in the right upper lobe and was a primary carcinoma of the lung. This finding demonstrates the value of the lateral radiograph in the survey examination.

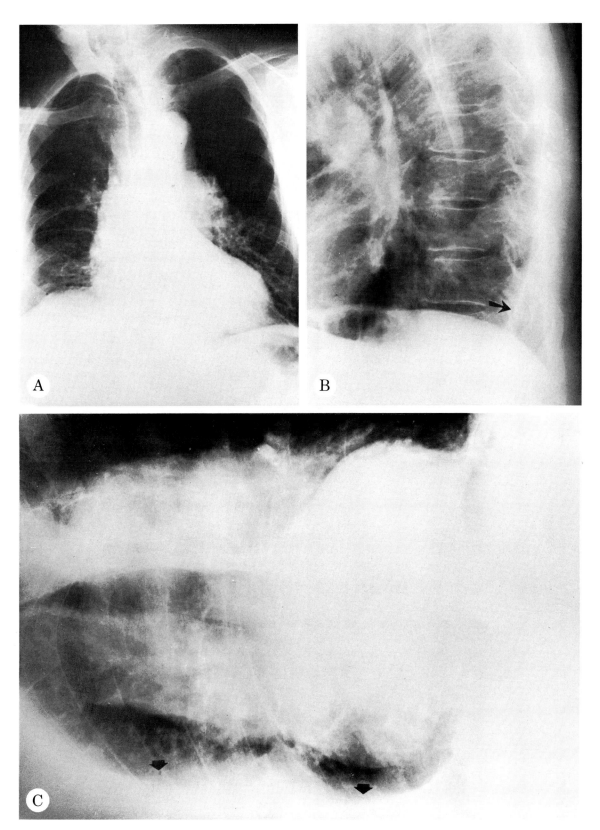

Fig. 11–2. Pleural effusion. No apparent abnormality is noted on the PA radiograph *(A)*. The lateral view *(B)* demonstrates blunting of the posterior costophrenic sulcus (arrow), suggesting a pleural effusion. The right lateral decubitus view *(C)* demonstrates a large effusion on the right (arrows).

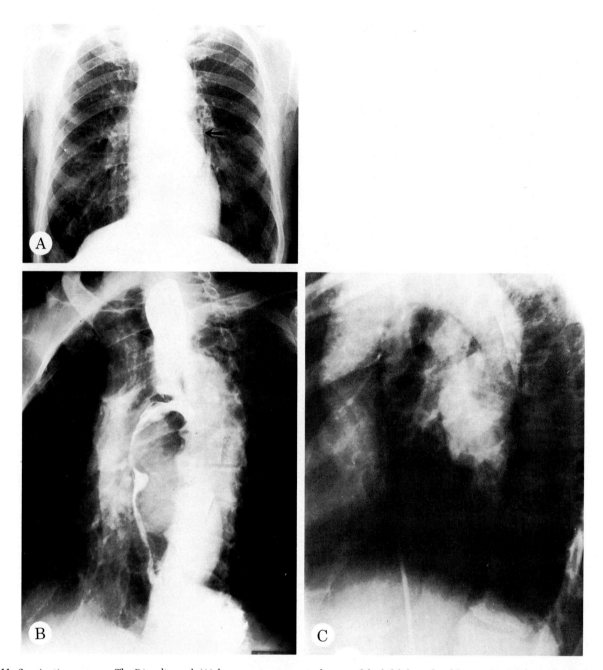

Fig. 11–3. Aortic aneurysm. The PA radiograph *(A)* demonstrates a mass in the area of the left hilus. The oblique view *(B)* shows the displacement of the esophagus by the mass and also shows the intimate relationship of the mass to the descending aorta. An aortogram *(C)* (lateral projection) confirms the diagnosis of an aortic aneurysm.

100 ml can be identified in the lateral decubitus position. If pneumothorax is present and the examination is being made to investigate the air-outlined pleura, the x-ray beam should be centered on the elevated rather than the recumbent side.

The lordotic view is a useful projection in investigating the apical portions of the lungs that may be obscured by overlying shadows of the anterior first rib and the clavicle in the routine PA projection. It is used for confirmation of a suspected lesion identified in the apex (Fig. 11–5). In this view, lesions located anteriorly

appear to move upward and those located posteriorly appear to move downward. A lordotic radiograph may also be useful in demonstrating disease in the right middle lobe, particularly if the right middle lobe is collapsed.

Stereoscopic views of the chest may be useful in studying lesions adjacent to the mediastinum or partially obscured by overlying bony structures. Stereoscopy can be particularly useful in investigating apical lesions and in recognizing cavities. The physician experienced in stereoscopy may prefer stereoscopic radiographs for

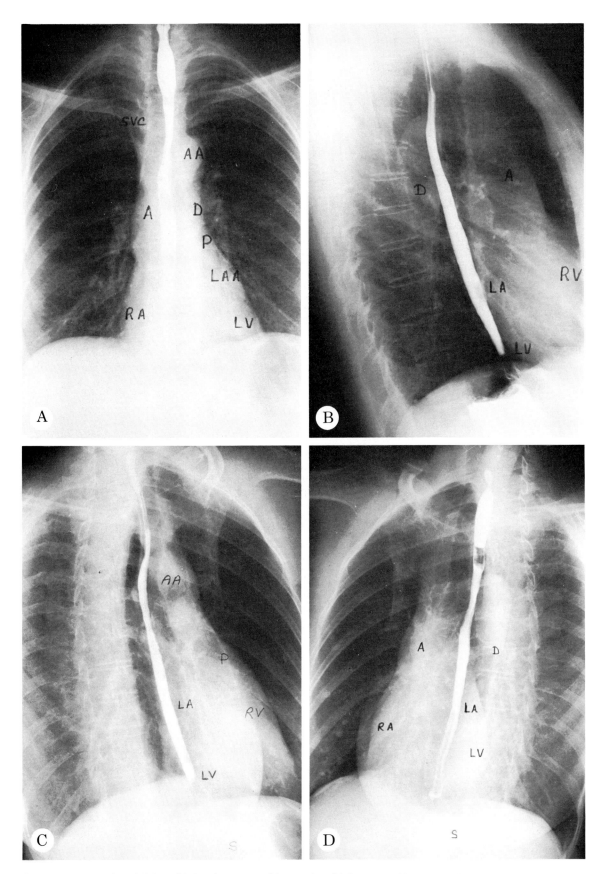

Fig. 11–4. Normal PA *(A)*, lateral *(B)*, right anterior oblique *(C)*, and left anterior oblique *(D)* radiographs. A = ascending aorta; D = descending aorta; AA = aortic arch; RA = right atrium; RV = right ventricle; LA = left atrium; LV = left ventricle; LAA = left atrial appendage; P = main pulmonary artery; SVC = superior vena cava; S = stomach.

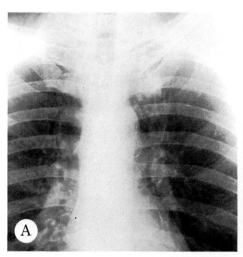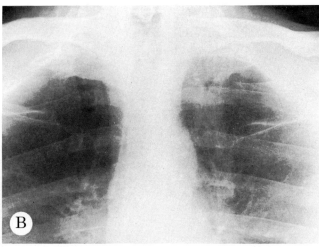

Fig. 11–5. Carcinoma of the lung. The presence of the mass in the left apex can only be suspected on viewing the PA radiograph *(A)*. Note the increased density under the first anterior rib on the left. An apical lordotic view *(B)* demonstrates a definite mass in the left apex, which subsequently proved to be a carcinoma of the lung.

localization of lesions of the chest rather than oblique or lordotic projections.

Expiratory radiographs may be helpful in assessing pulmonary air trapping, either local or diffuse. They can be helpful in the investigation of endobronchial neoplasms or particularly in the localization of endobronchial foreign bodies in children. A foreign body usually manifests as an emphysematous lobe or lung so that, on the expiratory radiograph, the mediastinum will shift to the side opposite the lesion. The expiratory radiograph is also useful in investigating a suspected pneumothorax that is poorly recorded with routine inspiration.

Penetrated grid radiographs are exposed at higher kV or ma, or both, and a fixed or moving — Bucky — grid is used between the patient and the film to remove scattered radiation. This practice allows better penetration and improved radiographic contrast, aiding in investigation of mediastinal or bony lesions. This radiograph is useful in identifying a suspected lesion behind the heart or diaphragm and poorly seen on the routine radiograph because of inadequate penetration (Fig. 11–6).

The supine radiograph is made when the patient is unable to sit or stand and is the routine projection in infants, owing to the difficulty of obtaining satisfactory erect images in the very young. Interpretation of this radiograph should take into consideration the magnification of mediastinal structures that occurs with the subject in the recumbent position and also the increase in pulmonary perfusion in the upper lobes, which may give the appearance of pulmonary vascular engorgement. The supine radiograph can be helpful in investigating pleural effusion, although decubitus views are more reliable.

Magnification radiographs can be made by using a very small focal spot — 0.3 mm — and increasing the patient-film distance, thus magnifying pulmonary structures without undue sacrifice of detail. Magnification techniques can occasionally be helpful in evaluating diffuse lung disease. High-resolution CT is now the standard procedure for evaluating diffuse lung disease.

LAMINOGRAPHY

Laminography — tomography, body section radiography, planigraphy — uses reciprocal movement of the x-ray tube and film about a fixed fulcrum to create a radiograph in which a plane of several millimeters' thickness is in focus and the remainder of the details of the anatomy of the patient are blurred. This study essentially allows radiographic investigations of a thin slice of the body of the patient and it is useful in the study of chest lesions, both pulmonary and mediastinal. Laminographs are useful: 1) to obtain better visualization of a poorly understood shadow seen on the chest radiograph; 2) to demonstrate the presence or absence of calcification within a pulmonary nodule; and 3) to demonstrate the presence or absence of cavitation within a pulmonary lesion. Laminography is helpful in the study of pulmonary tuberculosis (Fig. 11–7). Favis (1955) showed that laminography revealed cavitation in 10.7% of patients in whom no suggestion of a cavitation was seen on the conventional radiograph. The primary role of laminography is in better demonstration of a lesion poorly shown or poorly understood on the routine radiograph. It is of little value in a blind search for a clinically suspected lesion not shown on the routine radiographic study.

Laminograms are usually made in the AP or lateral position, but the oblique position can sometimes be useful, particularly when evaluating the hilar area. Oblique hilar tomography may clearly demonstrate or exclude adenopathy in a hilum that is suspiciously large on routine images.

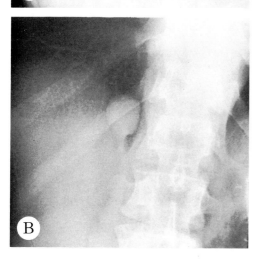

Fig. 11–6. Pulmonary granuloma. The routine PA radiograph (A) appears normal. An overpenetrated grid radiograph (B) demonstrates a pulmonary nodule seen through the left diaphragm.

Laminography was widely used in the study of pulmonary and mediastinal lesions. It has largely been supplanted by computed tomography — CT. It may still be used to demonstrate cavitation or calcification within a lesion. It may also be used to demonstrate additional nodules where a solitary pulmonary nodule is identified. CT is more useful in this regard.

COMPUTED TOMOGRAPHY

Computed tomography — CT — is a widely used radiologic technique for imaging cross-sectional anatomy of the body. In this technique, a pencil-thin beam of x-rays passes through the body, and the transmitted radiation is measured by a sodium iodide crystal. A series of measurements is made as the beam rotates around the body. These measurements are then fed into

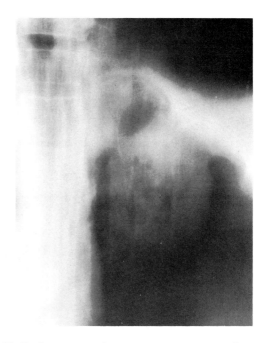

Fig. 11–7. Laminogram demonstrates cavitation in pulmonary tuberculosis. This cavity is thick walled and is more characteristic of carcinoma than tuberculosis. Resection proved this mass to be a large tuberculoma.

a computer, which reconstructs the x-ray absorption characteristics of each small area in the plane of the scan. The resultant image is an accurate measurement of the x-ray transmission of each part of the imaged body plane. Density differences of 0.5% can be recognized by this technique, whereas density differences of 4 to 5% are necessary for recognition on the usual radiograph.

In the chest, CT scanning is particularly useful in the mediastinum, where absorption characteristics of various masses may yield useful information. It is particularly useful in identifying mediastinal nodes when the routine chest radiograph is equivocal or normal.

CT scanning is sensitive in detecting pulmonary nodules. Using CT scanning, Schaner and associates (1978) identified 48% more nodules than with whole lung tomography, although 60% of the newly detected nodules were granulomata or subpleural lymph nodes, and the CT scan is unable to differentiate these from metastases.

CT scanning is helpful in assessing the degree of mediastinal and chest wall involvement of a peripheral carcinoma of the lung (Fig. 11–8). CT scanning is discussed in greater detail in Chapter 12.

MAGNETIC RESONANCE IMAGING

Magnetic resonance imaging uses radio waves modified by a magnetic field to produce images that contain somewhat different information than is obtained in the standard radiograph or CT scan. By varying the excitation time of the radio signal and the repetition time between the signals, information can be obtained about

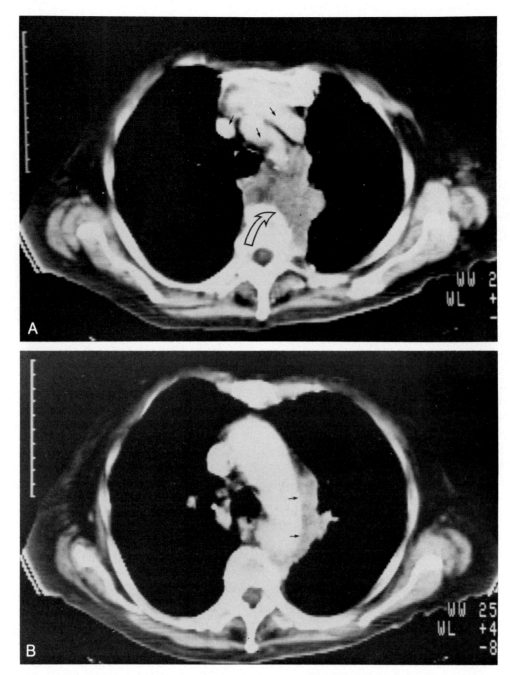

Fig. 11–8. CT scan demonstrating invasion of the aorta and vertebral body by carcinoma of the lung. *A,* A large mass is invading the T3 vertebral body (open arrow). This mass was not apparent on the routine chest radiograph. The great vessels are opacified by contrast material (small arrows). *B,* CT scan at a level inferior to that in *A* shows opacification of the aortic arch with tumor adherent to the aortic arch (arrows).

the material that is being imaged that may be useful in assessing the character of the tissue being evaluated — it may allow one to distinguish between tumor, cyst, blood, and various normal tissues. It also allows one to assess blood flow in various vessels, because the flowing blood contains no signal and usually shows as a void (Fig. 11–9*A* and *C*).

Magnetic resonance imaging in the chest is particularly useful in studying mediastinal structures, for which it competes with CT in degree of usefulness. It has major applications and potential in imaging the heart, the cardiac chambers, and great vessels.

Magnetic resonance imaging is discussed in greater detail in Chapter 13.

DIGITAL RADIOGRAPHY

Digital radiography is a technique in which a charged plate — rather than film — is used to record the radiographic image. The information on the plate is then

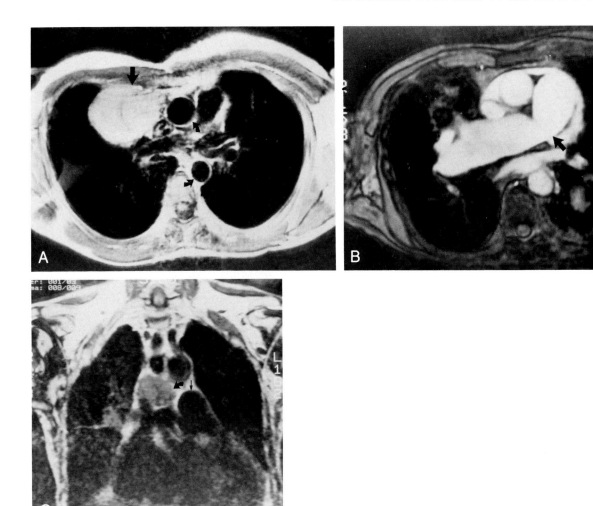

Fig. 11–9. MR scan in a patient with carcinoma of the lung and atrial septal defect. *A*, A large mass (large arrow) invades the mediastinum. The ascending and descending aorta (curved arrows) show no signal and are seen as a dark image or void. The pulmonary artery and its branches are also visible as dark structures between the ascending and descending aorta. These are surrounded by mediastinal fat, which appears white. *B*, A different technique allows the blood vessels to show as white structures rather than black. No contrast material is used. A massively dilated pulmonary artery (arrow) is noted, secondary to this patient's atrial septal defect. *C*, A coronal section shows metastatic adenopathy (curved arrow) adjacent to the dilated main pulmonary artery (small arrow) and above the right main pulmonary artery. The distinction between adenopathy and the normal vascular structures had been difficult to see on a CT scan but is easy to see on this MR image.

converted into digital form, which may then be displayed as a television image or converted to "hard copy" (film). Digital radiography is gaining acceptance as a chest imaging technique, but it is limited in resolution when compared to film. It is probably the imaging technique of the future for a number of reasons.

FLUOROSCOPY

Historically, fluoroscopy of the chest has been used as a screening procedure in the determination of disorders and diseases of the chest. It is no longer acceptable for screening. Small lesions are easily missed and no permanent record of the fluoroscopic procedure is usually made. The amount of visual information available on a radiograph is infinitely greater than that

available even with an image-intensified fluoroscope. In addition, the patient radiation exposure is many times greater with fluoroscopy.

Fluoroscopy is still useful in evaluating a lesion that has been identified by radiography; it is especially useful in studying pulmonary or cardiac dynamics. Fluoroscopic observation of the patient during breathing and rotation can localize a lesion to the lung or to the chest wall and can also identify the position of the lesion.

Fluoroscopy is also the ideal technique for needle aspiration biopsy of pulmonary lesions. Being able to visualize the lesion in "real time" is a significant advantage over CT-guided biopsy.

Air trapping is readily identified fluoroscopically, and limitation of diaphragmatic motion or paralysis of a hemidiaphragm can be appreciated. These observations are helpful in the investigation of an elevated hemidiaphragm seen on the routine chest radiograph or in investigating a suspected subphrenic abscess.

Evaluation of diaphragmatic motion fluoroscopically must be done with the subject in both the PA and lateral positions. Partial eventration of the diaphragm is a common finding and it is frequently misinterpreted as diaphragmatic paralysis if the patient is fluoroscoped only in the PA position. The dome of the diaphragm may move paradoxically with the patient in this position, but in the lateral position, a portion of the diaphragm — usually the posterior — will be seen to move normally. This finding indicates a localized diaphragmatic weakness — eventration — rather than true paralysis.

True paralysis of the diaphragm may be overlooked if fluoroscopy is done with the patient breathing quietly. Asking the patient to take a quick "sniff" may demonstrate a previously overlooked paralysis.

Fluoroscopy may also be useful in recognizing pulmonary emphysema and in evaluating the extent of this disease. Intracardiac calcification can be readily identified fluoroscopically, and a pericardial effusion occasionally can be seen fluoroscopically or in a cinefluorographic film strip.

The character of a mediastinal lesion may be better understood following fluoroscopy, particularly when the esophagus is outlined with barium sulfate. The esophagus is a mobile structure and is frequently displaced by mediastinal masses. The character and the location of the displacement can aid in the differential diagnosis of a mediastinal mass and in determining the surgical approach to such a mass.

It is useful to observe a mediastinal mass for pulsation because many middle mediastinal masses are vascular. Unfortunately, it frequently is impossible to differentiate between the true expansile pulsation of a vascular mass and the transmitted pulsation of a mass adjacent to the aorta. The Valsalva and Müller maneuvers can sometimes be useful in distinguishing between an avascular and a vascular mass. A nonvascular mass will not change with the Valsalva or Müller maneuver; the vascular mass may become smaller with the Valsalva and larger with the Müller maneuver.

THE LUNG

The anatomic positions of the lung and the normal fissures are described in Chapter 6. The interlobar septa are frequently visible on the chest radiograph (Fig. 11–10) and are of great help in assessing loss of volume in any of the lobes. Anomalous septa are not uncommon. Any pulmonary segment may have an anomalous fissure between that segment and the remainder of the lobe, resulting in an accessory lobe. The most common anomalous fissures are the superior and inferior accessory fissures. The superior accessory fissure occurs in 5% of anatomic specimens and separates the superior segment of the lower lobe from the basilar segments.

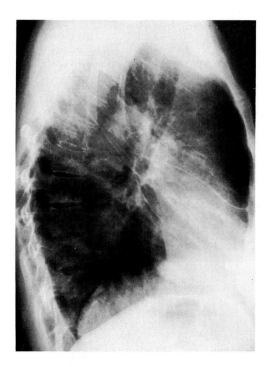

Fig. 11–10. Interlobar septa. The major fissures bilaterally and the minor fissure on the right are seen in this chest radiograph of the patient with interstitial edema and fluid in the fissures.

The inferior accessory fissure occurs in approximately 30% of anatomic specimens and separates the medial basal segment of the right lower lobe from the remainder of the right lower lobe. Another commonly seen anatomic fissure is the azygos fissure, which extends supralaterally from the azygos vein to the apex of the right lung. This fissure is seen in 1% of specimens and does not create a true accessory lobe, as do most other anomalous fissures.

Each lobe of the lung is divided into several pulmonary segments, each of which is supplied by a segmental bronchus. Various names have been applied to the pulmonary subsegments. The widely used classification of Jackson and Huber (1943) and the numeric classification of Boyden (1955) are presented in Table 6–1 and are illustrated in Figure 6–6. The pulmonary segments may undergo consolidation or atelectasis. The characteristic configuration of pulmonary consolidation of the various segments is schematically presented in Figures 11–11 through 11–15. Occasionally, consolidation of an anomalous pulmonary segment can be recognized on the routine radiograph. More commonly, segmental variations are demonstrated by bronchography.

The pulmonary arteries accompany the bronchial tree and exhibit a segmental distribution similar to that of the bronchial tree. The pulmonary veins are slightly larger than the arteries and lie lateral to them in the upper lobes and somewhat more horizontal in the lower lobes. It frequently is possible to distinguish between the arteries and veins on the routine radio-

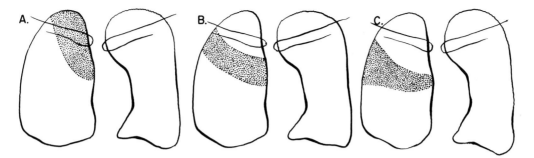

Fig. 11–11. Consolidation of the right upper lobe. *A*, Apical segment; *B*, Posterior segment; *C*, Anterior segment.

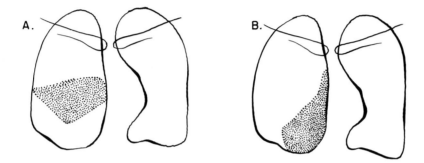

Fig. 11–12. Consolidation of the right middle lobe. *A*, Lateral segment; *B*, Medial segment.

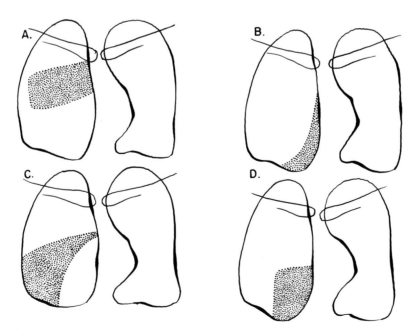

Fig. 11–13. Consolidation of the right lower lobe. *A*, Superior segment; *B*, Medial basal segment; *C*, Lateral basal segment; *D*, Posterior basal segment.

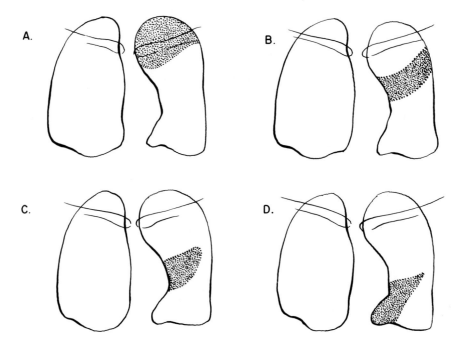

Fig. 11–14. Consolidation of the left upper lobe. *A*, Apical posterior segment; *B*, Anterior segment; *C*, Lingular segment, superior division; *D*, Lingular segment, inferior division.

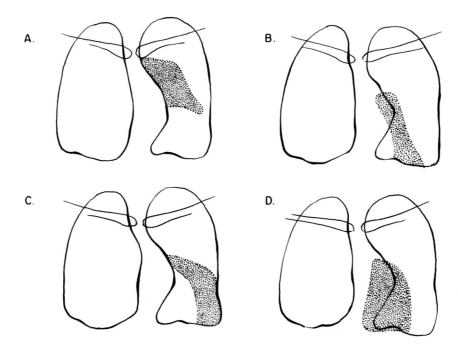

Fig. 11–15. Consolidation of the left lower lobe. *A*, Superior segment; *B*, Lateral basal segment; *C*, Anteromedial basal segment; *D*, Posterior basal segment.

graph of the chest. Laminography makes this identification simple.

THE MEDIASTINUM

The heart occupies the major part of the lower half of the mediastinum anterior to the spine. On the PA radiograph, the transverse diameter of the heart is normally one half of the transverse diameter of the chest or less. Detailed discussion of the anatomy and pathology of the heart is beyond the scope of this text. Figure 11–4 demonstrates the normal position of the cardiac chambers and the great vessels in the PA and lateral projections.

The mediastinum is divided by anatomists into the superior and inferior mediastinum and into the anterior, middle, and posterior compartments. For the surgeon, designation of superior and inferior compartments is of little importance. What is important, however, is the division of the mediastinum into three compartments: the anterior, middle — visceral — and paravertebral compartments, as seen on the lateral radiograph.

In the anatomic division of the mediastinum, the anterior compartment is bounded anteriorly by the sternum and posteriorly by the heart, aorta, and brachiocephalic vessels. The middle mediastinum contains the heart, ascending aorta, great vessels, trachea and main bronchi, and the esophagus. The "posterior mediastinum" in reality is nonexistent and should be considered to be the two paravertebral sulci.

The radiologic classification of mediastinal lesions becomes simple when one includes the descending aorta and the esophagus in the middle — visceral — compartment and those structures that lie posterior to the anterior spinal ligament in the paravertebral areas or posterior compartment. Thus, arbitrary divisions can be made on the lateral radiograph (Fig. 11–16) to divide the mediastinum into these three compartments.

Various lines or stripes occur about the mediastinum on the PA radiograph. Displacement of these stripes is often indicative of mediastinal pathology.

The paraspinal line, as Brailsford (1943) described, is a longitudinal density lying to the left of the thoracic spine (Fig. 11–17). It is related to the left-sided position of the descending aorta and will be seen on the right side if the descending aorta is present on the right. Ordinarily, no paraspinal line is seen on the right, but in patients with large hypertrophic spurs, the spurs may push the paraspinal line out, making it visible. Tumors or inflammatory processes involving the paravertebral bodies will characteristically displace the paraspinal line (Fig. 11–18). The line is ordinarily less than 1 cm from the left border of the vertebral column, but in some people, it may lie normally as far as 3 cm to the left of the vertebral column (Fig. 11–17).

The anterior mediastinal stripe is an oblique linear density presenting from right to left downward over the trachea for a distance of several centimeters (Fig. 11–19). The stripe is produced by the contiguous pleura

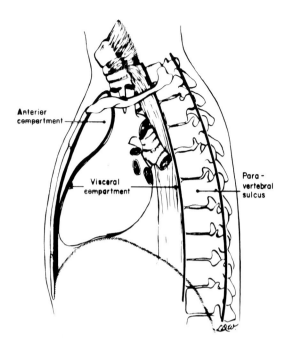

Fig. 11–16. The mediastinal compartments. Imaginary lines drawn along the anterior border of the trachea extended to the xiphoid and the anterior border of the spine divide the mediastinum into three compartments: anterior, visceral (middle), and paravertebral (posterior). (As described by Shields 1972.)

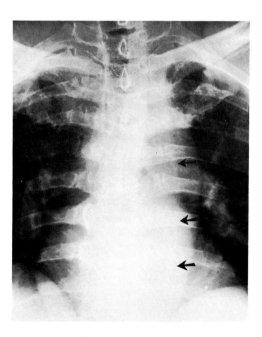

Fig. 11–17. Paraspinal line is seen only on the left in most patients. In this patient, it is unusually wide but normal.

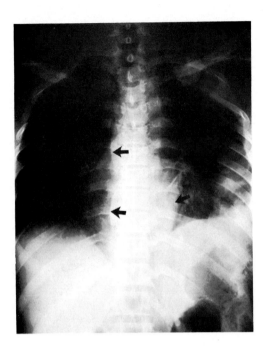

Fig. 11–18. Tuberculosis of the spine. Note displacement of the paraspinal line on the left and also on the right by tuberculous abscess.

of the right and left upper lobes as they touch anterior to the great vessels.

The inferior esophageal pleural stripe lies posterior to the heart and represents the right side of the distal esophagus (Fig. 11–19). The superior esophageal pleural stripe is slightly higher than the anterior mediastinal stripe and is slightly to the left. It represents the apposition of the two lungs against the esophagus in the retrotracheal area of the upper mediastinum. All of these mediastinal stripes can be displaced by lesions in the adjacent mediastinum.

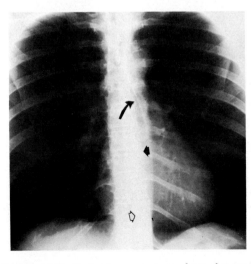

Fig. 11–19. Mediastinal stripes: anterior mediastinal stripe (curved arrow), paraspinal stripe (short closed arrow); inferior esophageal stripe (short open arrow).

THE DIAPHRAGM AND CHEST WALL

The diaphragm is a musculotendinous structure that separates the thorax from the abdomen. It is divided into right and left hemidiaphragms. The hemidiaphragm is usually lower on the side where the heart is anatomically placed in the absence of displacement due to some pathologic process. Thus, the right hemidiaphragm is usually higher than the left. Felson (1973) found, in a series of 500 normal chests, that the left hemidiaphragm was at a level even with or higher than the right in 9% of the subjects.

Variations of diaphragmatic contour are frequent. Most commonly, a segment of the diaphragm is elevated because of a lack of muscle in the segment — localized eventration. Fluoroscopically, paradoxic motion often is observed in such a localized segment and, in all instances, that portion of the diaphragm moves less well than the normal diaphragm.

The chest wall is composed of the bones and muscles of the thoracic cage. The bones are readily identifiable radiographically owing to the differences in density, but the muscular shadows are not readily identifiable unless a large mass of muscle is absent, either owing to a surgical procedure or to congenital anomaly. Thus, bony abnormalities can be easily identified on the chest radiograph, but soft-tissue abnormalities are seldom seen. The soft tissues of the chest wall can be studied by CT scanning or magnetic resonance imaging.

THE ABNORMAL CHEST

Abnormalities of the Lung

Radiographic images are made possible by the different coefficients of absorption of the various body tissues. Thus, air, fat, bone, and soft tissues can be distinguished one from another. The chest is admirably suited for detection of pathology for one major reason. The lung contains air in the bronchi and alveoli, making excellent contrast between the lung and the adjacent structures. In addition, the lung is a common site of pathology — manifest on the chest radiograph as areas of increased or decreased density — and frequently gives clues to the nature of systemic diseases as well as localized pulmonary conditions. Further, the air in the lung surrounds the mediastinum and the heart and allows fairly accurate evaluation of these structures. Of course, CT and magnetic resonance imaging allow even better visualization. It is important for the radiologist and the surgeon to recognize certain primary patterns occurring in the lungs as these patterns often indicate the nature of the patient's illness.

Atelectasis

Atelectasis is loss of volume of the lung, lobe, or segment from any cause. Fraser and Paré (1989) list five mechanisms of atelectasis. Resorption atelectasis occurs secondary to obstruction of a major bronchus or multiple small bronchi. For the surgeon, this type of atelectasis is the most important because it is often secondary to obstruction of a major bronchus by tumor, foreign body, or bronchial plug. Passive atelectasis occurs secondary to a space-occupying process in the thorax, particularly pneumothorax or hydrothorax. Compression atelectasis is a localized parenchymal collapse contiguous to a space-occupying pulmonary mass or bulla. Adhesive atelectasis or mitral atelectasis denotes collapse occurring in the presence of patent bronchi, presumably secondary to abnormalities of surfactant. This form of atelectasis occurs in association with pneumonia. Cicatrization atelectasis results from pulmonary fibrosis, either localized or general.

Several radiographic signs suggest atelectasis. The most reliable sign of collapse is displacement of interlobar fissures. Localized increase in density of the collapsed lobe is another reliable sign of atelectasis. Indirect signs of atelectasis include: elevation of the hemidiaphragm of the ipsilateral side; deviation of the trachea and other mediastinal structures toward the involved side; compensatory hyperaeration of the rest of the ipsilateral lung, and sometimes of the contralateral lung, with herniation of the contralateral upper lobe across the mediastinum; displacement of the hilum toward the collapsed lobe or segment; and decrease in size of the bony hemithorax of the involved side. These indirect signs are ordinarily seen only with atelectasis of major segments of the lung. They are less reliable than the direct signs and can occasionally be simulated by normal anatomic variations.

Certain fundamental observations can be made about lobar collapse. The proximal portion of the lobe is tethered to the hilus and consequently the radiographic shadow of the collapsed lobe will always point toward the hilus. Lobar collapse always occurs toward the mediastinum on the PA view. On the lateral radiograph, the upper lobe collapses anteriorly, the lower lobe collapses posteriorly, and the middle lobe symmetrically decreases in volume.

Robbins and Hale (1945), as well as Lubert and Krause (1951), described the radiographic patterns of lobar collapse. The patterns of lower lobe collapse are similar on the right and left sides, whereas the patterns of upper lobe collapse are slightly different. Figures 11–20 through 11–24 show schematic representations of lobar collapse, as described by Lubert and Krause (1951).

Recognition of the presence of a collapsed lobe is frequently difficult, particularly if the collapse is almost complete (Figs. 11–25 through 11–28). Of great help in identifying the presence of atelectasis is the silhouette sign, popularized by Felson (1973). The sign is based on the premise that consolidation of a segment or lobe of a lung contiguous with the border of the heart, aorta, diaphragm, or mediastinum will obliterate that portion of the border of the radiograph. Frequently, this obliteration of a heart border or a fuzziness of the diaphragm is the first clue to the presence of atelectasis.

Diffuse Pulmonary Disease

Pulmonary pathology can manifest as density occurring in the pulmonary alveoli or in the interstitial space or both. It is frequently helpful to distinguish alveolar from interstitial disease, although in some instances, this distinction cannot be made or can be made only with great difficulty. In pure alveolar or interstitial disease, certain radiographic appearances aid in the distinction.

The radiographic findings that can be helpful in recognizing alveolar disease are, first and frequently, a

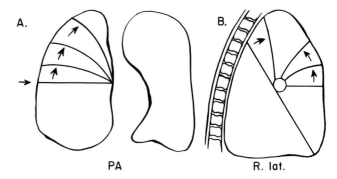

Fig. 11–20. Lobar collapse of the right upper lobe. *After* Lubert M, Krause GR: Patterns of lobar collapse as observed radiographically. Radiology 56:165, 1951.

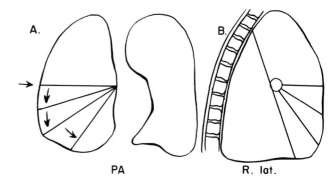

Fig. 11–21. Lobar collapse of the right middle lobe. *After* Lubert M, Krause GR: Patterns of lobar collapse as observed radiographically. Radiology 56:165, 1951.

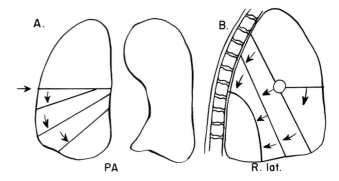

Fig. 11–22. Lobar collapse of the right lower lobe. *After* Lubert M, Krause GR: Patterns of lobar collapse as observed radiographically. Radiology 56:165, 1951.

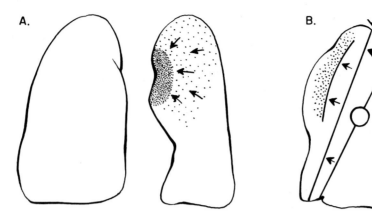

Fig. 11–23. Lobar collapse of the left upper lobe. *After* Lubert M, Krause GR: Patterns of lobar collapse as observed radiographically. Radiology 56:165, 1951.

confluence of alveolar shadows creating large homogeneous densities (Fig. 11–29). Second, an air bronchogram is frequently present (Fig. 11–30). The air bronchogram was described originally by Fleischner (1948) and has been popularized by Felson (1973). Parenchymal consolidation results in visualization of the bronchi when the air in the bronchi is not displaced by endobronchial fluid, such as in pneumonia. The air in the bronchi — usually not visible because of surrounding alveolar air — is now obvious because the alveoli are filled with fluid. Third, a small fluffy, rosette-shaped shadow may be seen diffusely through the lungs. This is the "acinar shadow" Aschoff (1924) described and is probably representative of consolidation of a single pulmonary acinus. Fourth, certain patterns of distribution may be seen in alveolar disease, for example, lobar or segmental consolidation and the "butterfly" pattern of perihilar increase in density (see Fig. 11–29). Fifth, rapidity of change of pulmonary

lesions favors alveolar disease over interstitial disease, which tends to change more slowly.

Common causes of a diffuse alveolar pattern are pneumonia, pulmonary edema, bleeding into the alveoli, or aspiration of blood or gastric contents into the alveoli. Less common causes of diffuse alveolar consolidation include parenchymal sarcoidosis, pulmonary alveolar proteinosis, metastatic carcinoma — from many causes, but especially breast carcinoma — and occasionally bronchioloalveolar cell carcinoma.

Interstitial disease has several radiographic characteristics. Kerley lines are frequently present, creating a series of fine linear densities throughout the lungs (Fig. 11–31). Shanks and Kerley (1951) described A, B, and C lines, which they attributed to lymphatic dilatation. The A lines are thin, straight lines several centimeters in length radiating from the hili. The B lines are transverse lines 1 to 2 cm long, seen at the lung bases and extending to the pleura. The C lines form a fine, interlacing network throughout the lungs, producing a reticular pattern. These lines may indicate dilatation of lymphatics, but may also represent interstitial fibrosis or edema.

Discrete nodules of varying sizes are also indicative of interstitial disease. These nodules may vary from minute to large and usually show a lack of confluence and have sharply defined margins (Fig. 11–32). A reticulonodular pattern may also be present in interstitial disease. A slow rate of change of a diffuse process favors interstitial over alveolar disease.

Common diseases causing a diffuse interstitial pattern include interstitial pulmonary edema, pneumoconiosis, sarcoidosis, metastatic tumor — both nodular and lymphangitic form, diffuse interstitial pneumonia, collagen disease — scleroderma and rheumatoid lung, eosinophilic granuloma of the lung, and idiopathic pulmonary fibrosis.

High-resolution or thin-slice CT scanning may yield additional information about diffuse lung disease, beyond that seen on the routine chest radiograph. This technique is discussed in detail in Chapter 12.

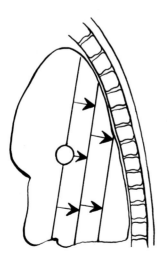

Fig. 11–24. Lobar collapse of the left lower lobe (PA) view. *After* Lubert M, Krause GR: Patterns of lobar collapse as observed radiographically. Radiology 56:165, 1951.

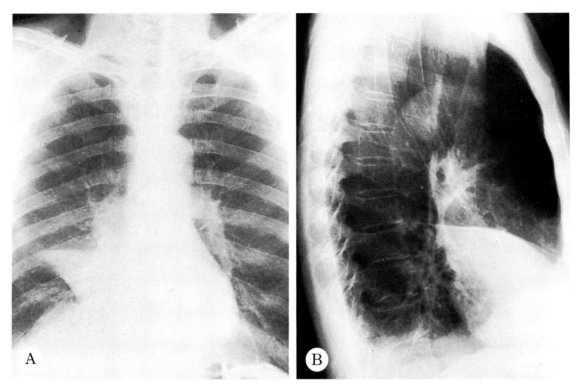

Fig. 11–25. Carcinoma with right middle lobe collapse. PA radiograph *(A)* shows obliteration of the right cardiac border by the collapsed right middle lobe (silhouette sign) with an associated mass in the right hilus. The approximation of major and minor fissures can be noted on the lateral view *(B)*.

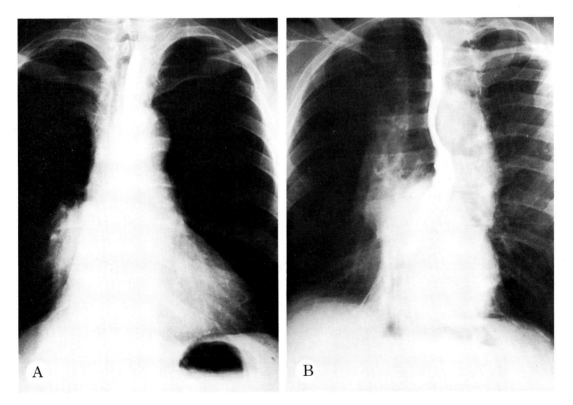

Fig. 11–26. Right lower lobe atelectasis. On the PA radiograph *(A)*, a mass is noted in the right hilus, as is increased density behind the right side of the heart indicating right lower lobe collapse. (Note preservation of the silhouette of the border of the right side of the heart.) Right lower lobe collapse is confirmed on the oblique view *(B)*.

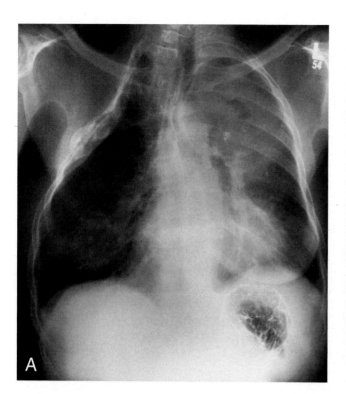

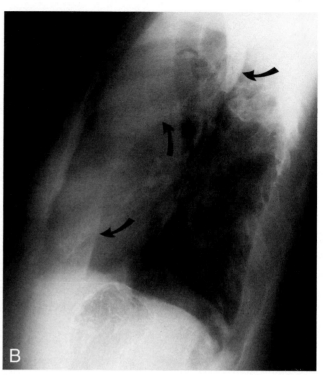

Fig. 11–27. *A,* Left upper lobe atelectasis related to tumor. PA radiograph shows an old thoracoplasty on the right side. On the left, note hazy density over the left upper lung field with loss of definition of the left cardiac border, characteristic of left upper lobe atelectasis. A small collection of air can be seen over the left second anterior rib, representing a cavity within necrotic tumor. *B,* Lateral view shows the fissure (arrows) to be pulled forward in its lower portion but bulging in its upper portion. This characteristic "s = sign" is seen when a lobe collapses around a tumor. The tumor is a large cavitary mass in the upper lobe but not involving the lingula, which collapses anteriorly.

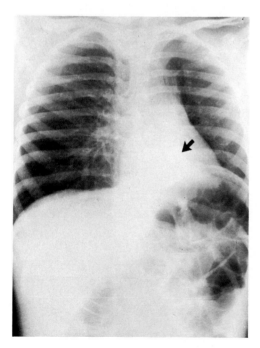

Fig. 11–28. Postoperative left lower lobe atelectasis. The wedge-shaped density of the collapsed left lower lobe is seen behind the heart (arrow). Note also a shift of the mediastinum and elevation of the left hemidiaphragm. The silhouette of the medial border of the left hemidiaphragm behind the heart is lost.

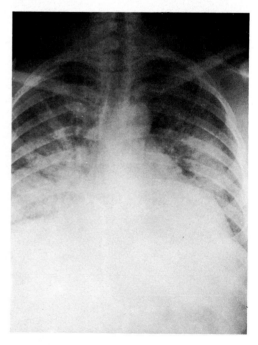

Fig. 11–29. Pulmonary edema. Note the patchy confluence of this diffuse alveolar pattern.

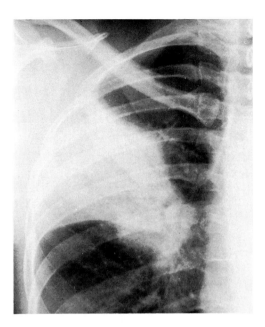

Fig. 11–30. Pneumonia. Notice the confluence of this alveolar pattern with the prominent air bronchogram. Lobar distribution is also in favor of an alveolar process.

Localized Pulmonary Densities

These densities may have poorly circumscribed or discrete margins. If the margins are poorly circumscribed, a solitary density most likely denotes pneumonia or pulmonary infarction. Primary lung tumor may

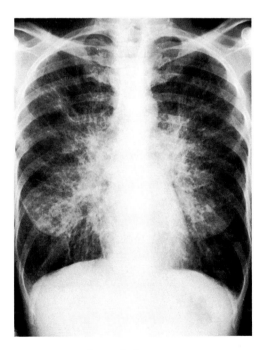

Fig. 11–31. Interstitial spread of metastatic pancreatic carcinoma. Note the reticular and linear pattern of this diffuse interstitial disease. Prominent Kerley lines are present.

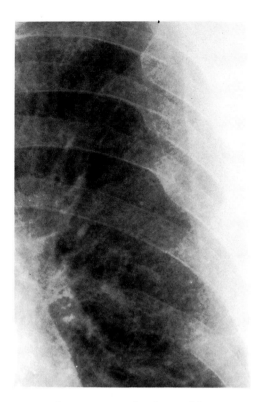

Fig. 11–32. Silicosis. Notice the fine nodular pattern of this interstitial process.

present in this fashion so that it is important to follow a poorly circumscribed density to complete clearing to be certain that it does not represent a tumor. Pulmonary tuberculosis and other chronic inflammatory diseases also manifest as poorly localized pulmonary density. A chronic infiltrate in the apical or posterior segment of the upper lobe or in the superior segment of the lower lobe should make one suspect tuberculosis. Cavitation is also suggestive of tuberculosis.

The sharply circumscribed pulmonary density most likely is a tumor or a granuloma. Primary or metastatic carcinoma commonly manifests in this fashion. Tuberculous granuloma, histoplasmosis and other fungal diseases, benign pulmonary tumors, and occasionally pneumoconiosis may present as a sharply circumscribed pulmonary density. Also to be considered are pulmonary infarct, pneumonia, arteriovenous malformation (Fig. 11–33), bronchial cyst, and bronchial adenoma. It is sometimes possible to ascertain the nature of a solitary pulmonary nodule by appropriate clinical tests, but a transthoracic lung biopsy or thoracotomy is usually necessary to make a definitive diagnosis (see Chapter 87).

Multiple sharply circumscribed densities almost invariably indicate metastatic malignant disease. Occasionally, however, rheumatoid nodules, fungal disease, Wegener's granulomatosis, or alveolar sarcoidosis may produce a similar pattern. Septic emboli may appear as multiple pulmonary nodules, but these are usually cavitary (Fig. 11–34).

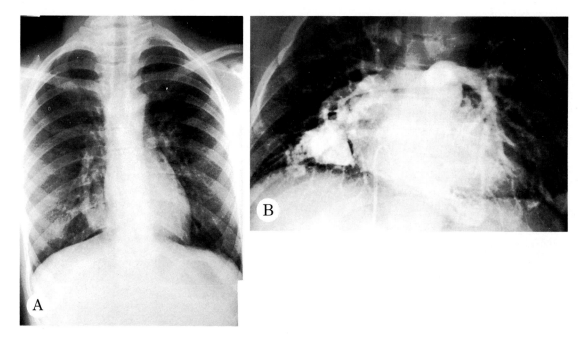

Fig. 11–33. Pulmonary arteriovenous (AV) malformation. Several nodular densities are seen in the lung fields, the largest of which is along the right cardiac border *(A)*. A pulmonary angiogram *(B)* demonstrates multiple malformations.

Cavitation of a solitary pulmonary density usually indicates a lung abscess, primary bronchial carcinoma, tuberculosis (Fig. 11–35), or fungal disease. Tumors and lung abscesses ordinarily have thick, shaggy walls, whereas often fungal disease and tuberculosis often have thin, smooth walls. If a lung abscess is chronic, the wall that initially was thick and shaggy generally becomes thin and smooth. Multiple cavitary lesions in the chest suggest septic emboli, metastatic tumor, tuberculosis, fungal disease, or Wegener's granulomatosis.

Calcification within a solitary pulmonary nodule can help to point to its etiologic basis. Certain types of calcification are strong evidence of benign disease. Central calcification or concentric ringlike calcification suggests granuloma. Multiple punctate calcifications throughout the lesion suggest granuloma or hamartoma. Eccentric calcification is most commonly seen in granuloma, but it can also be seen in primary lung car-

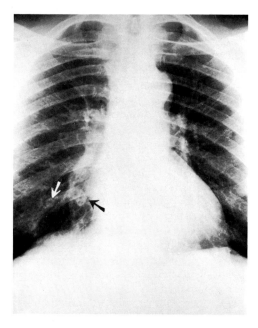

Fig. 11–34. Septic emboli. Several pulmonary nodules are present in both lungs with cavitation of two right lower lobe nodules (arrows).

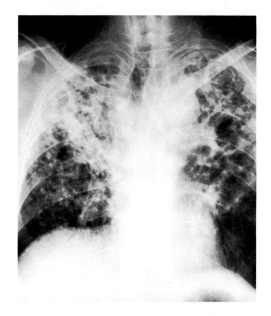

Fig. 11–35. Widespread cavitary pulmonary tuberculosis.

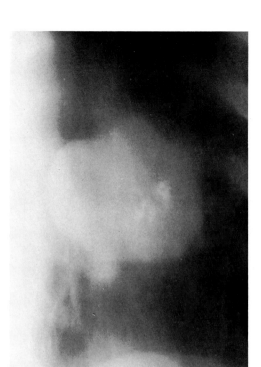

Fig. 11–36. Hamartoma. A laminogram shows "popcorn" calcification in this large hamartoma.

cinoma. Thus, an eccentric calcification cannot be taken as an indication of benign disease. Multiple pulmonary calcifications usually indicate healed pulmonary infections such as histoplasmosis, tuberculosis, and varicella pneumonia.

In the study of localized pulmonary densities, laminography is helpful in identifying suspected or unsuspected cavitation or calcification within the density (Fig. 11–36). High-resolution CT scanning is even more helpful. Comparison of CT numbers of a solitary nodule with those of a phantom of known CT density may definitively indicate a benign lesion and obviate surgical excision.

Determination of the rate of change of a pulmonary density is also important. If previous radiographs can be obtained for comparison, they may reveal that the lesion is changing rapidly or slowly or not at all. If prior radiographs cannot be obtained, follow-up examination in one or several weeks may reveal the growth rate of the pulmonary process.

Abnormalities of the Pleura

Pleural Effusion

A collection of fluid within the pleural space is the most common pleural abnormality. Fluid in the pleural cavity appears radiographically as a homogeneous opacity that is ordinarily in a dependent position in the pleural cavity. The fluid may be exudate, transudate, blood, pus, or chyle. Small amounts of free pleural fluid may be difficult to detect radiographically. Careful observation of the posterior costophrenic sulcus on the

lateral radiograph often shows minor blunting of the sulcus with as little as 50 to 100 ml of fluid. A lateral decubitus view may confirm the presence of free pleural fluid (see Fig. 11–2).

With larger pleural effusions, the lateral costophrenic sulcus is also blunted. On occasion, the fluid may remain infrapulmonary and displace the lung upward so that the lateral costophrenic angle remains sharp (Fig. 11–37). This infrapulmonary location of fluid can be suspected if the apparent hemidiaphragm is elevated, if the costophrenic sulcus is blunted posteriorly, or if the gas bubble in the gastric fundus lies some distance below the dome of the apparent hemidiaphragm. Decubitus views demonstrate that fluid is free and not loculated. CT scanning commonly identifies pleural effusion not seen on the routine radiograph.

As the amount of pleural effusion increases, passive atelectasis occurs in the underlying lung and eventually the mediastinum may be displaced to the contralateral side.

Fluid may become loculated in the pleural space, in which instance it may be difficult to differentiate from localized pleural thickening. Loculated pleural fluid generally has a convex border toward the hilus. Pleural thickening is more likely to have a concave border toward the hilus. Loculated pleural effusion may appear in the interlobar fissure, where it assumes a cigar-shaped configuration. Localized pleural tumor may masquerade as localized pleural thickening or pleural fluid. On occasion, loculated fluid may assume a lobar shape (Fig. 11–38) or simulate a mass (Fig. 11–39).

Common causes of pleural effusion are tuberculosis, pneumonia, viral pleural infection, metastatic tumor, primary lung or primary pleural tumor, lymphoma and leukemia, pulmonary infarction, chest trauma, collagen vascular disease, congestive heart failure, and intra-abdominal problems such as subphrenic abscess or pancreatitis.

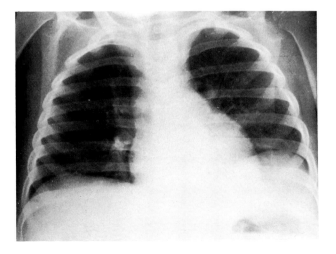

Fig. 11–37. Left pleural effusion. The separation of the stomach bubble from the lung is due to a large left pleural effusion in this child who has nephrosis. Note that the costophrenic sulcus is not blunted laterally by this free "infrapulmonary" effusion.

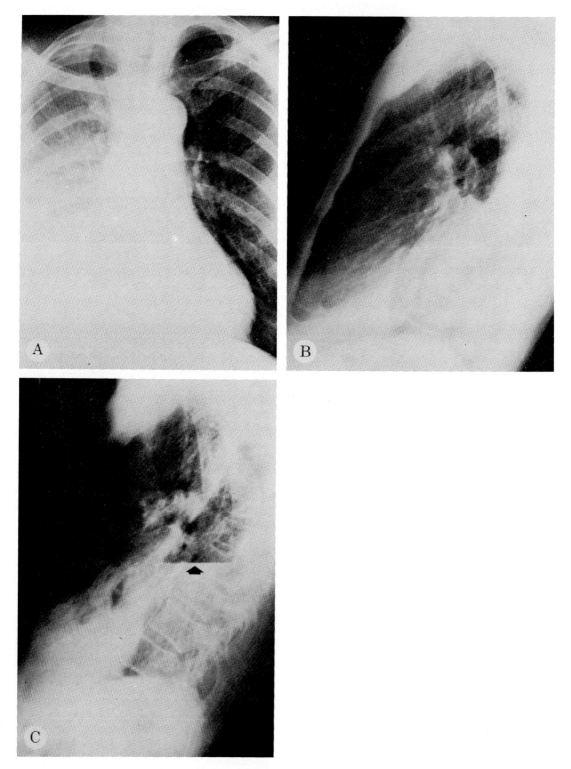

Fig. 11–38. Tuberculosis with loculated pleural effusion. The loculated effusion seen on the PA *(A)* and the lateral *(B)* radiographs simulated collapse of the right lower lobe. A right lateral decubitus radiograph showed no evidence of free effusion. After thoracentesis, however, a large collection of loculated fluid with an air fluid level (arrow) was apparent *(C)*.

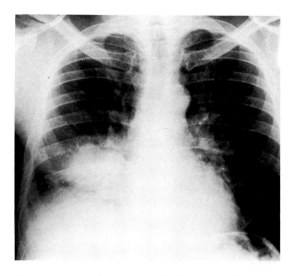

Fig. 11–39. Loculated empyema. This loculated collection of fluid near the border of the right side of the heart simulates a lung mass.

Pleural Thickening

Pleural thickening represents a localized fibrosis of the pleura that may be secondary to several causes. It is commonly seen at both apices, at the costophrenic angles, and occasionally along the lateral chest wall. It can be distinguished from free pleural fluid in a radiograph made with the subject in the decubitus position. Distinguishing pleural thickening from loculated pleural fluid may be more difficult, even by CT scan. The lack of change over a long period of time suggests pleural thickening rather than loculated fluid.

Causes of localized pleural thickening are usually old infection, particularly tuberculosis, or remote pulmonary infarction. Generalized pleural thickening occurs following the healing of hemothorax or pyothorax and is commonly associated with tuberculosis. Asbestosis or talc pneumoconiosis may also cause diffuse pleural thickening. Diffuse pleural mesothelioma may be difficult to distinguish from pleural thickening although pleural effusion and pleural nodulation are often present with mesothelioma. Diagnostic pneumothorax (Fig. 11–40) may help make the differentiation.

Apical pleural thickening may be difficult to distinguish from superior sulcus tumor. This distinction can be made radiographically only if rib destruction can be demonstrated or if the pleural density shows significant change over a short period of time. Magnetic resonance imaging is particularly useful in identifying or excluding a superior sulcus tumor.

Calcification of the pleura is usually secondary to old hemothorax, pyothorax, or tuberculosis. It is seen in asbestos exposure in the diaphragmatic pleura, pericardium, and chest walls. It may occur in one or multiple areas.

Pneumothorax

The presence of air within the pleural cavity is easily detected radiographically by identifying a thin line of visceral pleura surrounding the partially collapsed lung. This feature is best seen at the apex of the lung when the patient is upright, but sometimes is seen only laterally or at the lung base if the patient is supine. It may be necessary to obtain a radiograph following expiration to be absolutely certain that a small pneumothorax is present. The expiratory image accentuates the pneumothorax because the pleural cavity is decreased in volume in expiration. Fluid in the pleura in association with pneumothorax demonstrates the straight line of an air-fluid level rather than the curved line — meniscus — seen when no pneumothorax is present. A straight air-fluid level may on occasion be the finding that makes the radiologist aware that a pneumothorax is present.

Abnormalities of the Mediastinum

The radiographic features of mediastinal tumors are discussed in detail in Chapter 133 and are not dealt with here. Several aspects of mediastinal disease might be emphasized, however. In all mediastinal lesions, it is important to determine the location of the mass because the differential diagnosis varies considerably for each of the three mediastinal compartments. The one mass that commonly occurs in all three compartments is lymph node enlargement. It is often possible to determine the probable etiologic basis for the enlargement of lymph nodes by using certain helpful radiographic criteria.

Sarcoidosis has a characteristic pattern when it causes enlarged nodes. This pattern has been called the 1–2–3 sign because three prominent areas of enlarged nodes are identified—in both hili and in the right paratracheal area. In sarcoidosis, the hilar nodes also tend to be more peripherally situated or peribronchial with discrete nodes identifiable rather than one large amorphous mass tight against the mediastinum as is more commonly seen in association with metastatic tumor or lymphoma.

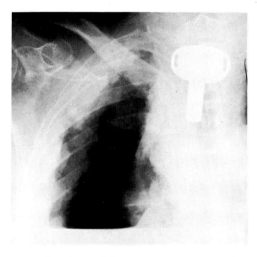

Fig. 11–40. Pleural mesothelioma. Diagnostic pneumothorax demonstrates diffuse pleural involvement by mesothelioma.

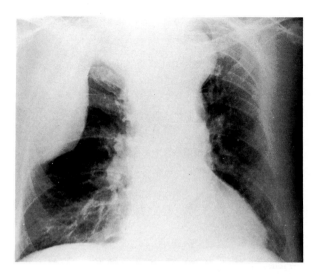

Fig. 11–41. Aortic dissection with extrapleural collection of blood. The widened contour of the aortic arch is strong presumptive evidence of a dissecting aneurysm in this patient with back pain. The mass in the right side of the chest has the characteristic configuration of an extrapleural lesion and in this instance represents a large extrapleural hematoma. A left-side hematoma would be more characteristic.

Lymphoma usually presents in only one node-bearing area rather than in several, and this area is commonly the anterior mediastinum. Lymph node enlargement in one nodal area alone or in one hilus and the mediastinum in a younger individual should make the clinician suspect lymphoma. In an older person, this same pattern should make one suspect a small cell carcinoma of the lung.

Middle mediastinal node enlargement may be identifiable only on films exposed during barium swallow or especially by CT scanning. Enlargement of nodes in the middle mediastinum is usually indicative of metastatic tumor, most commonly from the lung.

Primary tuberculosis commonly manifests as node enlargement in one hilus or in the mediastinum, but it usually occurs in children and commonly in association with a parenchymal pulmonary lesion. It occurs frequently in the immunocompromised adult, in which instance the pattern is similar to that seen with lymphoma.

Early lymph node enlargement may be difficult to detect. The importance of previous radiographs for comparison must be emphasized once again. A slightly widened mediastinum that has not changed for several years is not significant, whereas a minor alteration of mediastinal outline can be important if not present on radiographs made at an earlier date. CT is invaluable in demonstrating mediastinal adenopathy if there is any reason to expect it.

Masses occurring in the anterior cardiophrenic angle are almost invariably benign and so probably do not merit further investigation. These masses include pericardial cysts, foramen of Morgagni hernia, prominent pericardial fat pad, and pericardial fat necrosis.

Abnormalities of the Diaphragm and Chest Wall

The radiographic features of abnormalities of the diaphragm are covered in Chapters 45 to 51 in Section X and are not discussed here.

The most common chest wall abnormalities identifiable radiographically involve the ribs. Abnormalities of the chest wall that protrude into the thorax create a characteristic radiographic appearance that has been labeled the extrapleural sign by Felson (1973). These extrapleural lesions are smooth, seen well in only one projection—in which they are tangential to the x-ray beam—and usually have an acute angle at their borders, where the parietal pleura is being stripped from the thoracic cage (Fig. 11–41). Metastatic malignant disease of the rib is the most common cause of the extrapleural sign. Myeloma, primary rib tumor, fracture, or osteomyelitis may be responsible for this finding. Primary tumor of the chest wall or extrapleural hematoma may also present in this fashion.

Abnormalities of the soft tissues of the chest may also be discernible on the radiograph of the chest but are better visualized by CT scanning. The nipple of the breast frequently creates a shadow simulating a pulmonary nodule and must be considered when the nodule overlies the breast area.

CONTRAST EXAMINATIONS

Air in the bronchi and in the pulmonary alveoli provides an excellent contrast medium and makes the plain film examination of the chest fruitful. Nonetheless, in many instances, artificial contrast material introduced into a thoracic structure yields information that cannot be obtained from the routine chest radiograph. Positive contrast material can be readily introduced into the esophagus, trachea and bronchi, pulmonary vasculature, aorta and mediastinal arteries, superior vena cava, and mediastinal veins — and, with some degree of difficulty, into the mediastinal lymphatics. Negative contrast material — air or other gases — can be introduced into the pleural cavity, the peritoneal cavity, the mediastinum, or the heart. CT and magnetic resonance imaging, with their superior ability to demonstrate mediastinal structures, have to a considerable degree eliminated the need for many contrast-enhanced examinations.

Barium Swallow

Contrast examination of the esophagus is made by means of a simple technique that is best carried out under fluoroscopic guidance. A thick mixture of barium outlining the esophageal contour readily demonstrates any displacement of the esophagus by adjacent mediastinal structures on routine radiographs. Abnormalities of the esophagus itself, such as achalasia or esophageal tumor, can be readily demonstrated. Considerable information about the location and nature of a mediastinal mass, particularly one in the visceral compartment, can be obtained by studying the displacement of the esophagus by such a mass. Barium swallow is useful in evaluating patients with primary bronchial carcinoma in that it may identify previously unsuspected mediastinal lymph node metastases. Barium in the esophagus is also helpful in evaluating enlargement of the cardiac chambers. Whereas barium swallow was at one time an important diagnostic tool in mediastinal disease, it has been replaced in large part by CT.

Bronchography

Instillation of positive contrast material into the trachea for visualization of the bronchial tree may be accomplished by one of several methods. The contrast material can be dripped over the patient's extended tongue into the trachea; it can be introduced by a catheter inserted through the patient's nose or mouth into the trachea; or it can be introduced by an indwelling catheter inserted into the trachea through a puncture made in the cricothyroid membrane. The contrast medium generally used is aqueous or oily propyliodone — Dionosil.

Following the advent of fiberoptic bronchoscopy, bronchography was used almost exclusively to identify bronchiectasis or to assess the extent of known bronchiectasis. Bronchoscopy is ordinarily employed as investigative procedure for suspected bronchial abnormalities. Bronchoscopy is ordinarily used as an investigative procedure for suspected bronchial abnormalities. High-resolution CT scanning has now supplanted bronchography in the diagnosis of bronchiectasis. Consequently, there is little indication for bronchography today.

Angiography

Opacification of the vasculature of the chest is often helpful in the investigation of a pulmonary or mediastinal abnormality. It is currently used when CT or magnetic resonance imaging yields an equivocal diagnosis.

Pulmonary Angiography

Pulmonary angiography can be accomplished by introducing a catheter into the main pulmonary artery or one of its branches or by introducing a catheter into the great veins or heart proximal to the pulmonary artery. It can also be carried out by direct injection into the veins of one or both arms.

Pulmonary angiography is most commonly used to investigate thromboembolic disease of the lungs. Large thrombi are seen as negative filling defects within the opacified pulmonary arterial tree and poor perfusion of the vessels distal to these thrombi is usually evident (Fig. 11–42).

Congenital abnormalities of the pulmonary vascular tree, such as hypoplasia or agenesis of the pulmonary artery, arteriovenous malformation (see Fig. 11–33), pulmonary varix, or anomalous pulmonary venous return, also are identified by angiography. These abnormalities ordinarily can be suspected on the routine radiographic examination of the chest, but angiography

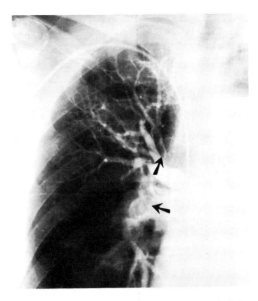

Fig. 11–42. Pulmonary embolus. Multiple large emboli (arrows) in the right pulmonary artery are demonstrated by pulmonary arteriography. Lack of perfusion of the right middle and lower lobes is apparent.

may be necessary for confirmation. Pulmonary angiography may be useful in determining resectability of primary carcinoma of the lung by demonstrating invasion of important mediastinal structures (Fig. 11–43).

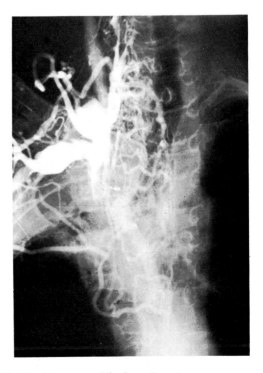

Fig. 11–43. Carcinoma of the lung. Superior vena cavagram demonstrates complete obstruction of the superior vena cava with extensive collateral circulation in this patient with a nonresectable bronchial carcinoma.

Magnetic resonance imaging has become a major rival for angiography and may well largely replace angiography for vascular and mediastinal imaging in the future.

Opacification of the chambers of the heart — angiocardiography — is used to study intracardiac malformations and pericardial effusions. Discussion of angiographic findings of intracardiac abnormalities is beyond the scope of this text.

Aortography

Positive contrast material can be used to opacify the aorta by either selective catheterization of the aorta itself or by injection of the venous system, either directly or by catheter, and study of opacification of the aorta after contrast material passes through the heart. Because the aorta is an important structure in the visceral mediastinal compartment, opacification of the aorta can be useful in evaluating masses in this area.

Aneurysms of the thoracic aorta are usually readily identifiable by routine chest radiography. Most aortic aneurysms are fusiform and conform to the shape of the aorta. Dissecting aneurysm of the aorta and saccular aneurysms of the aorta, however, may present difficult diagnostic problems. Dissecting aortic aneurysms can usually be suspected on clinical grounds. The routine radiograph is helpful if it shows a change in the aortic contour from earlier images or widening of the aortic shadow even without earlier radiographs. Aortography, CT, or magnetic resonance imaging is necessary to be certain that a dissection is present, however. The false channel of the dissection can ordinarily be shown as a negative defect that subsequently opacifies (Fig. 11–44).

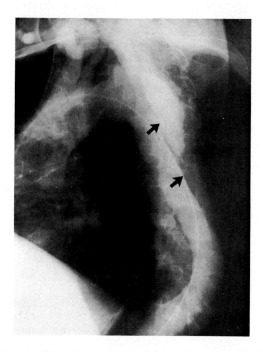

Fig. 11–44. Dissecting aneurysm of the aorta. Aortography clearly demonstrates the presence of the false channel of the aortic dissection (arrows).

Most aneurysms of the abdominal aorta are fusiform but thoracic aortic aneurysms frequently take a saccular form, in which case they can pose a diagnostic problem. An aortic aneurysm can be suspected by proximity of a mass to the aorta and by ringlike calcification in the wall of the mass. Aortography, CT, or magnetic resonance imaging is usually necessary to make certain that this mass is an aneurysm. It is important to recognize that an aneurysm may be filled with clot and may not opacify during aortic injection. Irregularities of the contour of the aortic wall in the area of the aneurysm usually indicate its presence.

Aortography may also be useful in identifying aneurysms of the great vessels or anomalies of the great vessels. Tortuous great vessels may simulate superior mediastinal masses (Fig. 11–45). Noninvasive CT scanning or, in particular, magnetic resonance imaging have largely supplanted aortography in vascular imaging.

Selective Catheterization of the Aortic Branches

Catheterization of the bronchial arteries was initially thought to be helpful in the diagnosis of primary carcinoma of the lung. Subsequent investigation, however, revealed changes in patients with inflammatory lesions of the lung that are difficult to distinguish from those due to tumor. Bronchial arteriography may be helpful in documenting bronchial collateral circulation in patients with pulmonary artery stenosis. Bronchial artery embolization has been performed to control massive bleeding in patients with tumor or pulmonary aspergilloma.

Venography

The superior vena cava can easily be opacified by injecting the veins of one or both upper extremities. This opacification may yield information about masses in the superior mediastinum. Invasion of the superior vena cava by bronchial carcinoma or displacement of vena cava by enlarged mediastinal lymph nodes ordinarily indicates inoperability. Superior vena cavagraphy may also be useful in investigation of the superior vena cava syndrome.

The azygos vein is another thoracic vein that can be opacified readily. This opacification is accomplished by injecting contrast material into a rib or a vertebral spinous process or by refluxing contrast material into the azygos vein following direct catheterization of this vein from the superior or inferior vena cava. Azygography has been used in the past in evaluating the operability of primary carcinoma of the lung. It may also be helpful in investigating mediastinal masses or in the investigation of liver disease.

Selective catheterization of the thymic vein was described by Kreel (1967) and has been used in the investigation of thymic masses. Selective sampling of thymic and other mediastinal veins is sometimes useful in identifying small, functioning mediastinal neoplasms that are secreting various endocrine products.

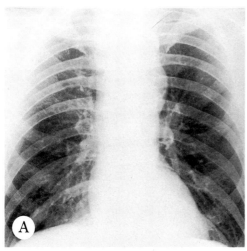

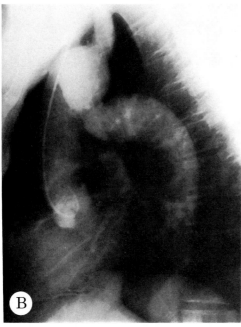

Fig. 11–45. Pseudocoarctation of the aorta. Aortography *(B)* demonstrates that a suspected mediastinal mass *(A)* is a tortuous and kinked aorta.

Air Contrast Studies

Air contrast studies can be made by injecting air or some other gas into various compartments of the chest. These procedures are not as popular as the angiographic techniques, but often can yield equally important information.

Diagnostic Pneumothorax

This procedure is useful in investigating pleural lesions (Fig. 11–40). It is simple to introduce some air into the pleural space following diagnostic thoracentesis. Radiographs made with the patient in various positions may yield helpful clues about the nature of the disease involving the pleura.

Diagnostic Pneumoperitoneum

This study may be used to investigate anomalies of the diaphragm. It is most useful in investigating diaphragmatic hernias or subphrenic abscess.

Diagnostic Pneumomediastinum

Although infrequently used, diagnostic pneumomediastinum has been used to investigate anterior mediastinal masses, particularly those in the thymus. In patients with myasthenia gravis, in whom a thymic tumor is strongly suspected, pneumomediastinography may reveal a tumor where none could be seen on the routine radiograph. CT scanning, however, is the procedure of choice in searching for occult thymomas or thymic carcinoids, and so diagnostic pneumomediastinum is rarely performed.

REFERENCES

Aschoff L: Lectures on Pathology. New York: Paul B. Hoeber, 1924.
Boyden EA: Segmental Anatomy of the Lungs. A Study of the Patterns of the Segmental Bronchi and Related Pulmonary Vessels. New York: McGraw-Hill Book, 1955.
Brailsford JF: The radiographic posteromedial border of the lung or the linear thoracic paraspinal shadow. Radiology 41:34, 1943.
Favis EA: Plainigraphy (body section radiography) in detecting tuberculosis pulmonary cavitation. Dis Chest 27:688, 1955.
Felson B: Chest Roentgenology. Philadelphia: WB Saunders, 1973.
Fleischner FG: The visible bronchial tree: A roentgen sign in pneumonic and other pulmonary consolidations. Radiology 5:184, 1948.
Fraser RG, Paré JAP: Diagnosis of Diseases of the Chest. Philadelphia: WB Saunders, 1989.
Jackson CL, Huber JF: Correlated applied anatomy of the bronchial tree and lungs with a system of nomenclature. Dis Chest 9:319, 1943.
Kreel L: Selective thymic venography: New method for visualization of the thymus. Br Med J 1:406, 1967.
Lubert M, Krause GR: Patterns of lobar collapse as observed radiographically. Radiology 56:165, 1951.
Robbins LL, Hale CH: The roentgen appearance of lobar and segmental collapse of the lung. Radiology 44:107; 45:120, 260, 347, 1945.
Schaner EG, et al: Comparison of computed and conventional whole lung tomography in detecting pulmonary nodules. AJR Am J Roentgenol 131:51, 1978.
Shanks SC, Kerley P: A Textbook of X-ray Diagnosis. Vol II. Philadelphia: WB Saunders, 1951.

READING REFERENCES

Brock RC: The Anatomy of the Bronchial Tree. London: Oxford University Press, 1954.
Cimmino CV: Further notes on the esophageal-pleural stripes. Radiology 77:74, 1961.
Felson B: The roentgen diagnosis of disseminated pulmonary alveolar disease. Semin Roentgenol 12:3, 1967.
Foster-Carter AF, Hoyle C: The segments of the lungs: A commentary on their investigation and morbid radiology. Dis Chest 11:511, 1945.
Gefter WB, et al: Semi-invasive aspergillosis: A new look at the spectrum of Aspergillus infection of the lung. Radiology 140:313, 1981.
Genereaux GP: Radiologic assessment of diffuse lung disease. In Tavaras JM, Ferrucci JT: Radiology: Diagnosis Imaging, Intervention. Philadelphia: JB Lippincott, 1986.
Genereaux GP: The posterior pleural reflections. AJR Am J Roentgenol 141:141, 1983.

Heitzman ER: The Lung: Radiologic-Pathologic Correlations. St. Louis: CV Mosby, 1984.

Heitzman ER: The Mediastinum: Radiologic Correlations with Anatomy and Pathology. St. Louis: CV Mosby, 1977.

Lee JKT, Segel SS, Stanley RT: Computed Body Tomography with MRI Correlation. New York: Raven Press, 1989.

Liebow AA, et al: The genesis and functional implications of collateral circulation of the lungs. Yale J Biol Med 22:637, 1950.

Lynch PA: A different approach to chest roentgenography: Triad technique (high kilovoltage, grid wedge filter). AJR Am J Roentgenol 93:965, 1965.

Ormond RS, Jaconette JR, Templeton AW: The pleural esophageal reflection: An aid in the evaluation of esophageal disease. Radiology 80:738, 1963.

Osborne DR, et al: Comparisons of plain radiography, conventional tomography, and computed tomography in detecting intrathoracic lymph node metastases from lung carcinoma. Radiology 142:157, 1982.

Parkes WR: Occupational Lung Disorders. London: Butterworths, 1982.

Ravin CE: Pulmonary vascularity: Radiographic considerations. J Thorac Imaging 3:1, 1988.

Reid L: The lung: Its growth and remodeling in health and disease. AJR Am J Roentgenol 129:777, 1977.

Rosai J, Levine GD: Tumors of the thymus. Fasicle 13, Atlas of Tumor Pathology. AFI (Armed Forces Institute of Pathology), 1975.

Schatz M, Patterson R, Fink J: Immunologic lung disease. N Engl J Med 300:1310, 1979.

Storch CB: Fundamentals of Clinical Fluoroscopy. New York: Grune & Stratton, 1951.

Viamonte M Jr: Angiography evaluation of lung neoplasm. Radiol Clin North Am 3:529, 1965.

Wittenborg MH, Aviad I: Organ influence on a normal posture of the diaphragm: A radiological study of inversions and heterotaxis. Br J Radiol 136:280, 1963.

CHAPTER 12

COMPUTED TOMOGRAPHY OF THE LUNGS AND CHEST

Wallace T. Miller, Warren B. Gefter, and David H. Epstein

Computed tomography — CT — is now firmly established as an indispensable radiologic technique for the evaluation of the chest. Computed tomography can provide cross-sectional images with exceptional anatomic detail and far greater tissue contrast than can be obtained by conventional radiography. Although the major contribution of CT in the thorax is in the evaluation of the mediastinum, CT has also found applications in the evaluation of the lung, pleura, and chest wall. Magnetic resonance — MR — imaging has become a competing method for cross-sectional imaging of the chest. Currently, however, MR imaging evaluates the pulmonary parenchyma poorly. Consequently, CT remains the standard cross-sectional evaluation of the chest, with MR imaging used primarily as a problem-solving tool with specifically tailored examinations.

TECHNIQUE

Computed tomography passes multiple, highly collimated x-ray beams at various angles through the anatomic plane of interest to expose an array of electronic detectors rather than a radiographic film. The density of the tissue that each beam traverses determines the beam's degree of attenuation and consequently the output from the detectors. These projections of tissue density obtained from the detectors are then mathematically reconstructed by a computer into an image that is essentially a map of tissue densities. Density differences of only 1 to 2% can be recognized by this technique, whereas differences of 4 to 5% are required for recognition on standard radiographs.

The standard thoracic CT examination is performed with 10-mm thick contiguous axial slices from lung apex to base. Examinations performed for staging of lung carcinoma should include imaging of the adrenal glands, because of the propensity for adrenal metastases. The judicious and appropriately timed administration of intravenous iodinated contrast agents is particularly important in evaluating the pulmonary hila and mediastinum. Intravenous contrast enhancement is also critical to proper evaluation of the aorta and great vessels, particularly in patients with suspected dissection of those vessels. In certain situations, the examination may be tailored to evaluate a specific problem. For example, if a small hilar mass is suspected, 5-mm thick slices through the hilum will provide improved spatial resolution and improve detection of such masses.

Conventional CT evaluates the pulmonary interstitium poorly because of diminished spatial resolution relative to conventional chest radiographs. High-resolution CT — HRCT — of the thorax was developed to circumvent this problem. In this examination, 1-mm slice thicknesses are used to increase spatial resolution. The mathematical reconstruction is altered to increase edge enhancement — "bone algorithm." Retrospective targeting with smaller fields of view also increases spatial resolution.

Two significant recent advances in CT technology include ultrafast — cine — CT and spiral — helical — CT. Both of these techniques make it possible to obtain multiple contiguous slices in a time brief enough to permit breath holding. Unlike conventional CT scanning, with ultrafast CT, the x-ray tube does not mechanically move around the patient. Rather, an electron beam is electromagnetically swept across stationary target rings, resulting in a rotating fan beam of x-rays. Scans can be obtained as rapidly as 50 msec per slice. In the dynamic mode, multiple rapid sequential images are acquired at the same anatomic level, allowing for the dynamic display of physiologic events. Examples of thoracic applications of such a technique include the differentiation of fixed versus dynamic narrowing of the trachea; that is, tracheal stenosis versus tracheomalacia, and in the assessment of blood flow within vascular lesions such as pulmonary arteriovenous malformations.

Alternatively, multiple contiguous anatomic slices can be acquired during a breath hold, resulting in a three-dimensional, volumetric data set from which tomographic images can be reformatted in any desired plane, or three-dimensional displays can be created.

Spiral CT, which represents a modification of a conventional CT scanner, enables the x-ray tube to rotate continuously around the patient as the table moves through the scanner. The x-ray beam therefore traces out a spiral path, so that a continuous volume of tissue can be scanned within a breath hold. Such a technique is ideal for imaging small lung nodules, because there are no gaps and no respiratory motion between slices. Again, using postprocessing software, the images can be reconstructed in any selected plane or three-dimensional displays can be rendered. As with ultrafast CT, these volumetric displays provide a vivid and useful means of evaluating abnormalities of both the airways and the pulmonary vasculature, which, because of their branching structure, are particularly difficult to evaluate when limited to the axial orientation of conventional scans. Examples of potential applications include the pre- and postoperative evaluation of the tracheobronchial tree in connection with bronchoplastic procedures, endobronchial stent placement, and, evaluating the bronchial anastomosis after lung transplantation (Fig. 12–1).

Differences in tissue density are expressed in terms of CT numbers. Typical CT numbers range from −1000 — air — to +1000 — dense cortical bone. Structures of the same density as water have a CT

number of approximately zero; in contrast, fat is approximately −100. Because many technical variables can affect a CT number, a relative comparison of CT numbers between structures is usually far more informative than any absolute value. The full scale of CT numbers generated by the CT reconstruction process cannot be displayed in a single image because current electronic display systems use only a limited number of shades of gray. The operator has to select, through manipulation of the electronic windows at the CT console, the portion of the CT number range to display. All CT images of the chest should be viewed with at least two, and optimally three, window settings: one for the lungs, one for the mediastinum and chest wall, and one for the bony structures.

CLINICAL APPLICATIONS

Mediastinum

Mediastinal Masses

The evaluation of mediastinal masses seen on conventional radiographs is enhanced by CT by more subtle density discrimination as well as clarification of relationships to other vital structures and visualization of tissue planes. Solid lesions can be separated from those that are cystic or fatty, and areas of necrosis or calcification are detected more easily with CT than with plain film radiography.

The thymus gland normally appears as a bilobed, arrowhead-shaped structure, often best visualized at the level of the aortic arch but frequently seen extending from the left brachiocephalic vein to the root of the aorta and pulmonary artery. Moore and colleagues (1983) reported that normal thymic measurements vary with age. Because of fatty infiltration, patients older than 30 years tend to have atrophic glands; however, the thymic contours are usually preserved. In patients older than 40 years, the presence of a spherical or ovoid mass in the expected location of the thymic gland or deformity of the adjacent pleura is suggestive of thymoma (Fig. 12–2). Diffuse enlargement of the thymic gland with preservation of its normal shape is more suggestive of hyperplasia. Well-circumscribed thymic tumors are typically benign, whereas tumors showing infiltration into adjacent fat are usually malignant. CT, however, cannot differentiate consistently benign from malignant thymoma unless evidence of metastatic disease to the mediastinum, pleura, or lungs is present (Fig. 12–3). Thymoma is seen in 10 to 15% of patients with myasthenia gravis. It is also associated with red cell aplasia.

Brown and associates (1982) reported CT to be helpful in localizing thymic carcinoid tumors in patients suspected of having ectopic production of ACTH. Imaging with CT may also help to identify mediastinal parathyroid adenomas in patients with unexplained hypercalcemia.

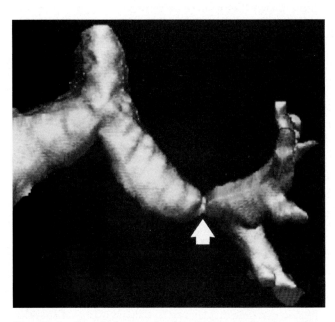

Fig. 12–1. Bronchial stenosis after lung transplantation. This shaded-surface three-dimensional display of the bronchial tree was created from multiple, contiguous slices obtained by ultrafast CT during breath holding. Note the area of stenosis (arrow) at the anastomosis between the native left main bronchus and the bronchus of the left lung transplant.

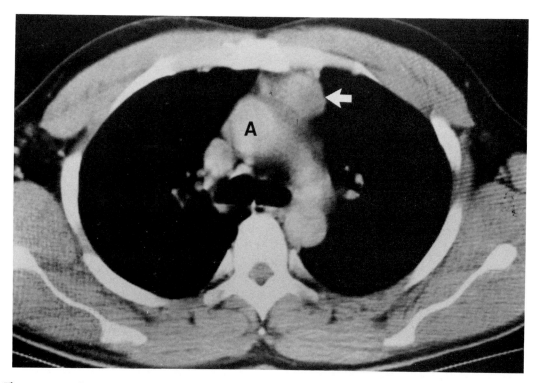

Fig. 12–2. Thymoma. A well-circumscribed ovoid soft tissue mass (arrow) anterior to the ascending aorta (A) in patient with myasthenia gravis is consistent with thymoma.

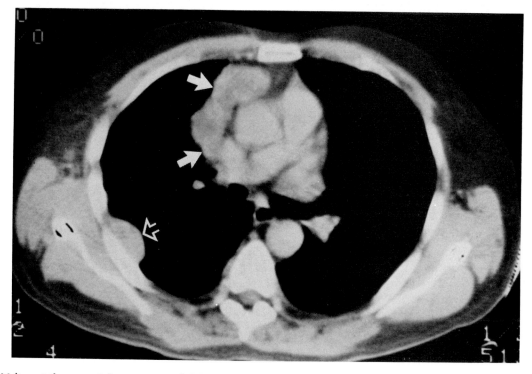

Fig. 12–3. Malignant thymoma. Inhomogeneous, slightly irregular anterior mediastinal mass (closed arrows) with a pleural metastasis on the right (open arrow) indicates a malignant thymoma.

Teratomas and other mediastinal germ cell tumors are difficult to distinguish from thymic lesions by CT criteria alone. Both are usually solid masses and may contain calcifications. Teratomas, however, more frequently than thymomas, show areas of low density within the mass because of either cystic or fatty components. A predominantly low-density mediastinal mass suggests a cystic teratoma or mediastinal germ cell tumor (Fig. 12–4).

The iodine content of a substernal thyroid on CT scans that are not contrast enhanced is diagnostically helpful because of its higher density than other solid mediastinal

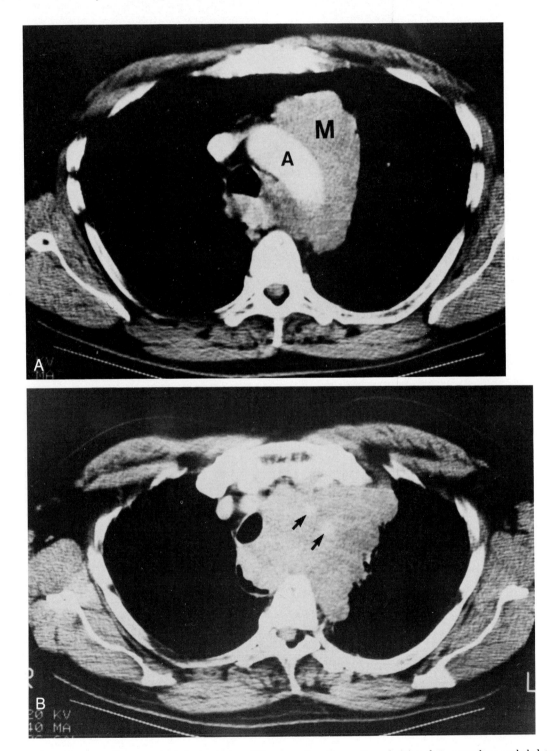

Fig. 12–4. Mediastinal germ cell tumor. *A*, Soft tissue mass (M) surrounding the aortic arch (A) and *B*, extending cephalad to encase the great vessels (arrows) and displace the trachea to the right. This mass cannot be distinguished from extensive lymphadenopathy due to lymphoma or metastatic tumor.

masses. Imaging with CT can also confirm the presence of a substernal thyroid by showing direct extension of the mass from the neck into the mediastinum on contiguous sections. Occasionally, a substernal thyroid may appear to have low density because of a relative lack of iodine in areas of cystic degeneration. Imaging with CT cannot exclude malignancy of the thyroid gland.

Perhaps the greatest utility of CT in evaluation of the mediastinum has been in the detection, extent, and distribution of lymphadenopathy. Lymph nodes appear as discrete or confluent regions of soft tissue density separable from other mediastinal structures, particularly after intravenous contrast administration. Lymphadenopathy may manifest as regions of lower density because of necrosis or high-density calcification from granulomatous disease, chemotherapy, or radiation therapy. The identification of lymph nodes does not indicate their histologic characteristics or even the presence of disease. Anatomic and pathologic studies reported by Genereux and Howie (1984) of patients with no known chest disease frequently identified lymphadenopathy in all regions of the mediastinum. Lymph node size tended to vary with location; however, 95% of normal lymph nodes were less than 11 mm in diameter. Enlarged lymph nodes may have a variety of causes, including metastatic tumor, lymphoma, sarcoidosis, and other granulomatous or inflammatory causes.

Most benign cystic lesions of the mediastinum are homogeneous and water equivalent in density. They are not enhanced after intravenous contrast media administration. Bronchogenic cysts are typically round or ovoid, low-density structures — water equivalent — in the subcarinal or right paratracheal regions (Fig. 12–5). Pericardial cysts occur in both the right and left cardiophrenic angle. Either mass may be higher in density owing to hemorrhage or proteinaceous contents; in these cases, MR imaging may be a useful supplementary technique to confirm the fluid content of the lesions.

Homer and associates (1978) reported that localized benign mediastinal fat collections can be diagnosed with absolute certainty using CT. Their low density permits easy distinction from lymphadenopathy. Epicardial fat pads, and paravertebral and retrocrural lipomatosis are easily identified by their low CT numbers in the fat range. Rare fatty mediastinal tumors such as lipomas and thymolipomas may also be identified by their fat content on CT examinations (Fig. 12–6).

Neurogenic tumors, the most common paravertebral masses, are very well evaluated by CT, allowing precise localization, detection of vertebral body destruction, and recognition of intraspinal tumor extension. The latter, however, may be shown to better advantage by MR imaging.

Mediastinal Widening

The evaluation of a widened mediastinal contour on the plain film radiograph is ideally suited for CT as reported by Baron and colleagues (1981a). Imaging with CT can distinguish normal variants — abundant fat or tortuous vessel — from aneurysms, aortic dissections,

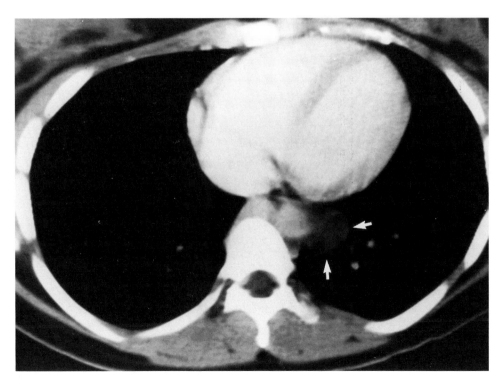

Fig. 12–5.   Foregut cyst of the mediastinum. CT scan shows a well-circumscribed, fluid-containing density (arrows) adjacent to the descending aorta. Its fluid density is typical of a benign mediastinal cyst.

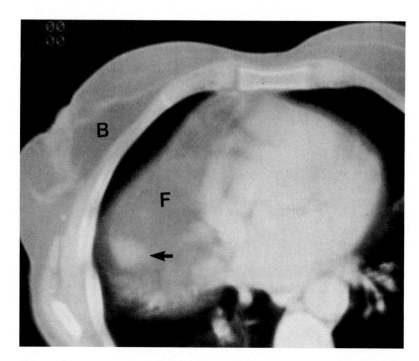

Fig. 12–6. Thymolipoma. CT scan demonstrates a partially fatty (F), partially soft tissue density mass (arrow) adjacent to the right side of the heart. This appearance is suggestive of the rare fatty tumor of the thymus, a thymolipoma. Note that the fat of the mass has similar attenuation to the fat of the breast tissue (B).

or soft tissue masses. Abundant fat in the mediastinum is readily diagnosed because of its characteristic low CT density. It is a common finding in patients taking corticosteroids or with Cushing's syndrome. With the administration of intravenous iodinated contrast material, Baron and associates (1981b) noted that tortuous great vessels and congenital vascular anomalies of the aortic arch were readily demonstrated (Fig. 12–7).

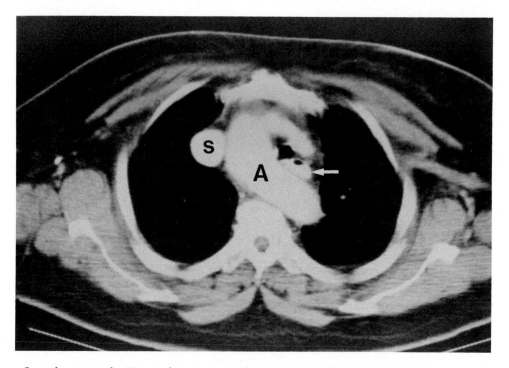

Fig. 12–7. Circumflex right aortic arch. CT scan shows a congenital anomaly of the aortic arch (A) with the aorta passing to the right and behind the trachea and esophagus (arrow). The superior vena cava (S) is identified laterally on the right.

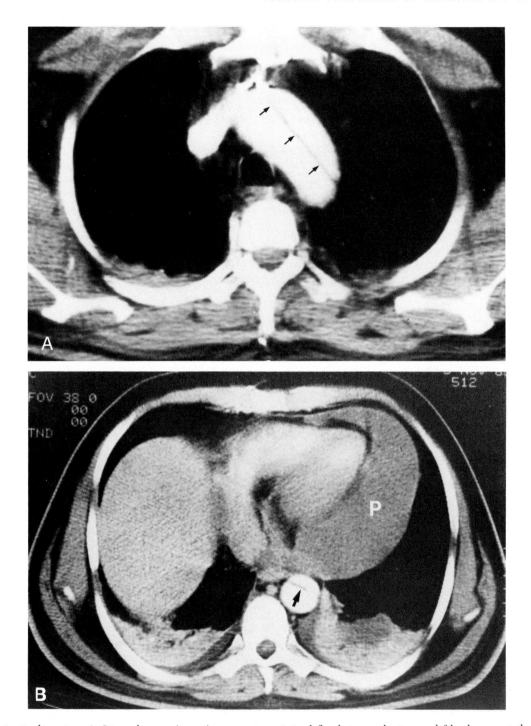

Fig. 12–8. Aortic dissection. *A*, Linear lucency (arrows) represents an intimal flap between the true and false lumens at the level of the aortic arch. *B*, The intimal flap (arrow) is again identified in the descending aorta. A large pericardial effusion (P) is also identified. Posteriorly, note the small bilateral pleural effusions and passive atelectasis in the lung bases.

Gross and co-workers (1980) found CT to be useful in detecting aortic dissection in individuals who are hemodynamically stable. Medial displacement of intimal calcification, high-density intramural hematoma, or both, may be identified on the precontrast CT scan. After intravenous contrast administration, one may identify a thickened aortic wall, a septum between two opacifying lumens, or a differential time density be-tween opacification of the two lumens suggesting an aortic dissection. The origin of the dissection, as well as any associated hemothorax or hemopericardium, can be visualized (Fig. 12–8). MR imaging provides information similar to that demonstrated by CT with similar accuracy. It has the additional advantages of not requiring intravenous contrast agents, the ability to image in the coronal, sagittal, or oblique planes, and the ability to assess the aortic valve for regurgitation. Choice of imaging technique largely depends on local availability of MR or CT scanning, as well as local surgical philosophy. In a comprehensive comparison of noninvasive imaging for thoracic aortic dissections, Nienaber and colleagues (1993), however, demonstrated MR imaging to be the method of choice in hemodynamically stable patients. If the patient is hemodynamically unstable, it is advisable to resort directly to aortography rather than CT or MR imaging.

Computed tomography is being used increasingly in the evaluation of blunt chest trauma to evaluate for potential traumatic aortic tears, with the following caveats. In patients who are unstable or in whom the clinical suspicion of traumatic aortic laceration is high, angiography or direct surgical intervention is recommended as the initial evaluation. In stable patients with low to moderate possibility of traumatic aortic laceration, however, CT examination is a reliable screening examination before angiography. Raptopoulos and colleagues (1992) noted that use of CT as a screening examination would have decreased the need for aortography by 56% in their series of 191 patients. A normal CT scan, however, does not exclude traumatic aortic tears. Morgan and associates (1992), in a review of five recent studies, demonstrated a 1% false-negative rate for CT in a population of 523 patients.

Unlike aortic dissections, the defect in the aorta produced by traumatic aortic lacerations is only rarely visualized directly on the CT examination. Instead, the usual finding is the presence of a mediastinal hematoma as a soft tissue density in the mediastinum or streaking of the mediastinal fat. Because mediastinal hematomas may be a result of other mediastinal vascular injuries, in particular lacerations of minor veins, an abnormal CT scan is not specific for aortic injury. In the study of Raptopoulos and colleagues (1992), an aortic laceration was detected at angiography in only 21% of positive CT examinations.

Diffuse mediastinal infection or fibrosing mediastinitis is difficult to distinguish from infiltrating metastatic tumor or lymphoma in the mediastinum. The confirmation of infiltrating soft tissue abnormality, however, should lead to biopsy and appropriate tissue diagnosis.

Mediastinal contours may be distorted by esophageal neoplasms. CT can be helpful in defining the extent of tumor and detecting metastasis to lymph nodes, liver, and lung (Fig. 12–9). Computed tomographic staging of esophageal carcinoma remains controversial, however, with reported accuracies from a low of 33% as reported by Quint and associates (1985) to a high of 95% reported by Thompson and co-workers (1983). Staging of adenocarcinoma of the gastroesophageal junction is particularly poor as noted by Freeney and Marks (1982). Computed tomographic staging of distal esophageal carcinomas should include images through the celiac axis — the normal lymphatic drainage region for the distal esophagus — because occasionally metastatic adenopathy to the celiac nodes will be detected. After

esophagectomy with gastric interposition, the mediastinal contour is widened in most patients, owing to the intrathoracic stomach; CT has been helpful in detecting postoperative complications including mediastinal abscess or hematoma in these patients and in distinguishing these lesions from the normal postoperative intrathoracic stomach. Becker and associates (1987) found CT was the most effective imaging technique for the detection of tumor recurrence in such patients (Fig. 12–10).

Determination of aortic and tracheobronchial invasion by tumor is also problematic. Contiguity of the tumor mass with the aorta or major airways raises the suspicion of tumorous involvement. The greater the length that tumor mass is contiguous with the major mediastinal structures, the greater the likelihood of tumorous invasion; however, proof requires surgical and histologic evaluation.

Lungs

Pulmonary Nodule

Advances in CT technology have concentrated on various disorders of the pulmonary parenchyma. Using conventional radiology, the distinction between a benign and malignant solitary pulmonary nodule depends on its growth pattern and the presence of calcification. A nodule that fails to grow over a 2-year interval, or a nodule that has diffuse, central, "popcorn," or concentric rings of calcification is presumed to be benign. Eccentric calcification may be seen in some carcinomas, and therefore the presence of calcification alone does not specifically indicate benignancy.

In those patients in whom calcification is not demonstrated, thoracotomy or biopsy is usually required to exclude malignancy. Patients with smooth, round, or oval solitary nodules measuring 3 cm or less in diameter, who have no previous radiographs, are potential candidates for a CT phantom study. This examination detects occult, microscopic calcification within the nodule by comparing CT attenuations between the patient and a reference phantom (Fig. 12–11). Zerhouni and associates (1986) and Huston and Muhm (1989) and others have shown this technique to be effective in establishing the benign character of the nodule. Imaging with CT rarely yielded a confident diagnosis of benign disease in larger nodules and in those with an irregular or spiculated border. Swensen and associates (1991) argued that the number of false-positive benign diagnoses is higher than previously reported; however, this has yet to be confirmed by other researchers.

Computed tomography is also useful in proving the solitary nature of a pulmonary nodule. Particularly in patients with a known extrathoracic malignancy, the detection of a solitary nodule on the chest radiograph should prompt the clinician to obtain a CT examination in order to determine whether other nodules are present.

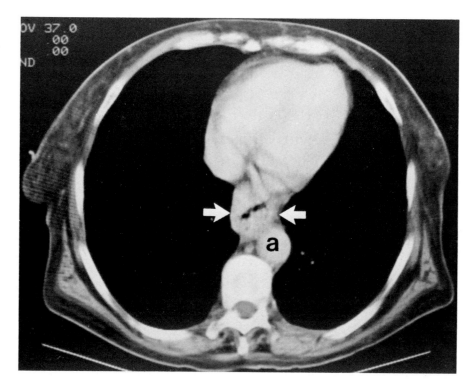

Fig. 12–9. Esophageal carcinoma. CT scan reveals esophageal wall thickening (arrows) and contiguity of the mass with the descending aorta (a).

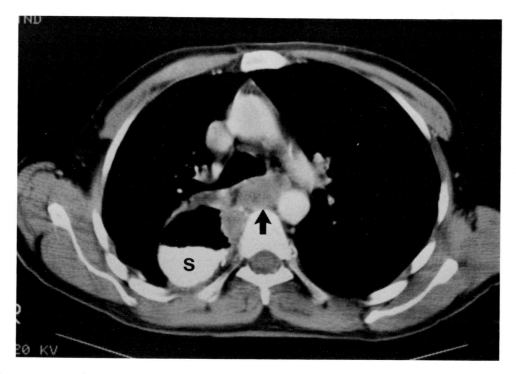

Fig. 12–10. Recurrent tumor after esophagectomy. CT scan shows soft tissue density (arrow) behind the carina and medial to the intrathoracic stomach (S). These findings are characteristic of recurrent tumor.

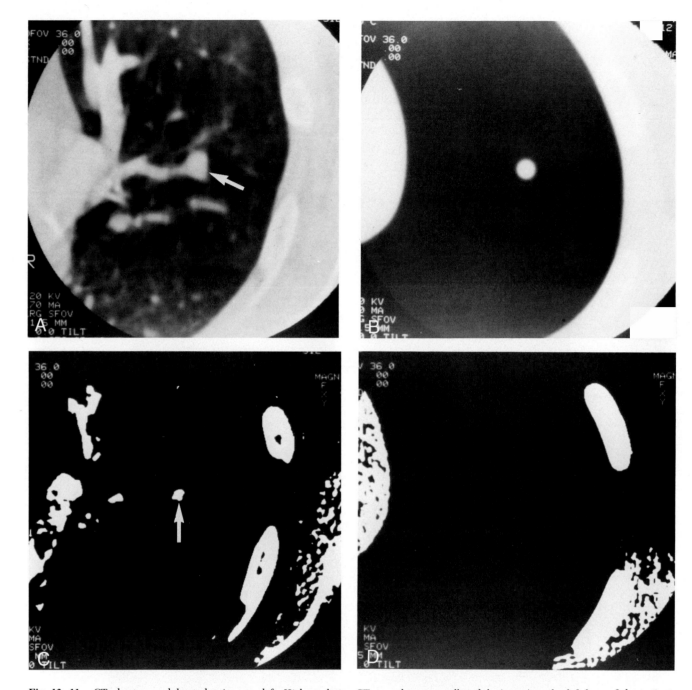

Fig. 12–11. CT phantom nodule study. *A upper left,* High-resolution CT scan shows a small nodule (arrow) in the left lung of the patient. *B upper right,* CT image of the phantom shows reference nodule corresponding to size and position of patient's nodule. *C lower left,* CT image of the patient's nodule is compared with *D lower right,* CT image of the phantom nodule at the window level setting at which the phantom nodule disappears. Note persistent density of the patient's nodule, which indicates the presence of calcification (not evident on conventional radiographs) and is consistent with a benign lesion. The nodule, likely a granuloma, has remained stable on follow-up studies.

Lung Carcinoma

Computed tomography has become a routine part of the preoperative staging of lung carcinoma. An understanding of the uses and limitations of chest CT allows the surgeon to manage patients with lung carcinoma appropriately. Imaging with CT provides information about size of the primary lesion; direct extension of tumor to the contiguous structures of the chest wall, mediastinum, and diaphragm; presence of hilar and mediastinal adenopathy; and hematogenous dissemination of tumor to the remaining lung, liver, and adrenals. Webb and associates (1991) of the Radiological Diagnostic Oncology Group — RDOG — showed that CT and MR imaging have similar overall accuracy in the staging of lung carcinoma.

Computed tomography is neither sensitive nor specific for direct invasion of the chest wall or mediastinum. In one study of chest wall invasion reported by Glazer and colleagues (1985) CT was shown to have an 87% sensitivity, 59% specificity, and a 68% accuracy. In this study, local chest wall pain was shown to be both more specific — 94% — and more accurate — 85%. Contiguity of tumor with the pleural surface does not imply parietal pleural invasion; however, demonstration of a mass within the soft tissue of the chest wall or adjacent rib destruction in a patient with lung carcinoma is specific for chest wall invasion (Fig. 12–12). Obliteration of the extrapleural fat plane has been shown by Ratto and co-workers (1991) to be 85% sensitive, 87% specific, and 86% accurate for the detection of chest wall invasion. They also demonstrated that a length of tumor-pleura contact to tumor diameter ratio of greater than 0.9 has a sensitivity of 83%, specificity of 80%, and accuracy of 81%.

In the case of superior sulcus — Pancoast — tumors, the axial plane of orientation of CT slices limits evaluation of chest wall extension at the lung apex. Magnetic resonance imaging is better suited for the local staging of such tumors, including potential involvement of the brachial plexus, subclavian vessels, and vertebral involvement.

Like chest wall invasion, contiguity of tumor with the mediastinum cannot be equated with mediastinal invasion. Displacement or compression of mediastinal vessels, trachea, or esophagus, or obliteration of normal fat planes, however, is indicative of mediastinal invasion (Fig. 12–13). Glazer and colleagues (1989) noted that

CT can reliably determine resectability of lung cancers adjacent to the mediastinum if three criteria are met: 1) less than 90° of contact with the aorta; 2) presence of mediastinal fat between the mass and the major mediastinal organs; and 3) less than 3 cm of contact with the mediastinum. In their series, 97% of tumors that met these criteria were technically resectable. Most patients had no mediastinal invasion; the minority had limited focal invasion that did not preclude surgical resection. Cross-sectional imaging, therefore, can play an important role in identifying gross involvement of major mediastinal structures that would render a patient unresectable — stage IIIB.

The CT assessment of mediastinal lymphadenopathy is important in the preoperative staging of bronchial carcinoma, particularly in comparison to surgical staging. One inherent difficulty posed for CT in this regard is that even though lymph nodes containing tumor are apt to be larger than normal, no absolute size criterion is known above which a lymph node must contain tumor, and, conversely, microscopic metastases occur in lymph nodes that are normal in size. The sensitivity and specificity of CT in detecting enlarged lymph nodes caused by metastatic disease have been variably reported in the literature, as noted by Libschitz and colleagues (1984), and is influenced by patient selection, prevalence of disease, lymph node size construed as abnormal, and method of surgical sampling.

Most surgeons recognize that enlarged lymph nodes need not harbor metastases, and that normal-sized lymph nodes may contain metastases, as confirmed by one of us (D.M.E.) and co-workers (1986). The ad-

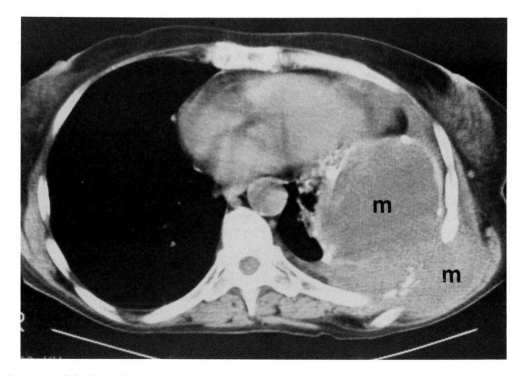

Fig. 12–12. Carcinoma of the lung. CT scan shows extension of a large mass (m) originating in the left lung through the chest wall with rib destruction. A soft tissue mass within the chest wall and rib destruction are the most specific CT findings for chest wall invasion.

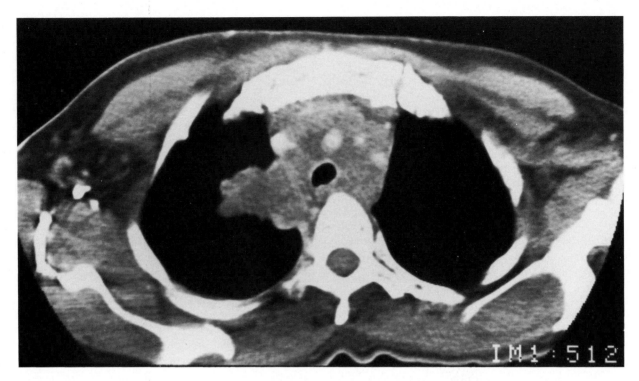

Fig. 12–13. Carcinoma of the lung. This CT scan of the chest demonstrates contiguous spread of tumor throughout the mediastinum from a medially positioned bronchogenic carcinoma of the right lung. Note that the tumor surrounds all of the great vessels, precluding surgical therapy.

vantage of CT over chest radiography is its ability to identify the precise mediastinal location of enlarged lymph nodes that should undergo biopsy for presence of metastasis prior to resection (Fig. 12–14). A normal mediastinum on CT examinations frequently eliminates the need for surgical staging — mediastinoscopy or mediastinotomy. In 10% of these patients, however, histologic evidence of metastatic tumor in nodes may be anticipated at thoracotomy. To summarize, enlarged lymph nodes identified by CT require histologic confirmation. Imaging with CT should serve as a guide for selecting the appropriate staging procedure to sample enlarged lymph nodes. No patient should be denied surgery on the basis of node size alone.

Staging CT of the chest may also detect the presence of hematogenous metastasis to adrenals, liver, and the contralateral lung. Because of the propensity of lung carcinoma to metastasize to the adrenal glands, imaging to the level of the adrenals should be performed in all staging chest CTs. Unfortunately, not all lesions of the liver, lung, and adrenals detected prove to be metastases. Hemangioma is a common benign mass that may mimic metastasis in some individuals. MR imaging of the liver distinguishes hemangiomas from other hepatic tumors and is indicated in individuals with one or a few hepatic lesions demonstrated on staging CT.

Like hemangiomas in the liver, benign cortical adenomas of the adrenal glands are a frequent normal finding seen in 3 to 5% of the general population and may be confused with adrenal metastasis. Adenomas

frequently contain a large amount of lipid material and therefore are of low attenuation on CT examinations, which may be a clue to the diagnosis. In large part, however, definitive diagnosis has required tissue confirmation. Mitchell and co-workers (1992) using chemical shift MR imaging, were able to identify 26 of 27 benign adrenal masses because of their lipid content. They had no false-positive results among the 45 masses imaged. This preliminary work suggests that chemical shift MR imaging may replace invasive testing in excluding adrenal metastasis.

Pulmonary Metastases

In patients known to have an extrapulmonary malignancy, CT provides a sensitive means of identifying small pulmonary metastases (Fig. 12–15). Schaner and colleagues (1978) noted that the major problem in using CT imaging for the detection of occult metastasis is its lack of specificity. Granulomas or subpleural lymph nodes may constitute up to 25% of lung nodules in geographic areas endemic for histoplasmosis. These nodules, unless calcified, are generally indistinguishable from pulmonary metastases.

Rounded Atelectasis

Rounded atelectasis consists of a masslike area of atelectatic lung occurring in the setting of adjacent pleural reaction, most often in the setting of pleural and parenchymal asbestos-related changes. The lesion can be difficult to differentiate from primary carcinoma of

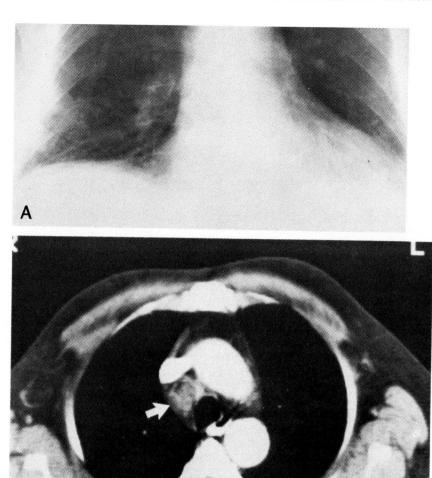

Fig. 12–14. Carcinoma of the lung. *A,* PA chest radiograph reveals no evidence of mediastinal adenopathy. *B,* CT scan reveals a 2-cm right paratracheal lymph node (arrow) behind the superior vena cava. At mediastinoscopy, this lymph node contained metastatic tumor.

the lung, frequently requiring biopsy for definitive diagnosis; however, CT scanning can be useful in suggesting the diagnosis when the following criteria of McHugh and Blaquiere (1989) are present: 1) rounded or oval mass, 3.5 to 7 cm, abutting the pleural surface; 2) curving bronchovascular structures — "comet tail" — entering the mass; and 3) associated pleural thickening. Other CT features that suggest the diagnosis include volume loss in the involved lobe as described by Lynch and associates (1988), and the presence of uniform, dense enhancement — at least 200% increase — during dynamic contrast-enhanced examinations, as reported by Westcott (1991).

Diffuse Lung Diseases

The chest radiograph is normal in 10 to 15% of patients with biopsy-proven diffuse interstitial lung disease and in 20 to 60% of patients with emphysema.

High-resolution CT, which can resolve the fine interstitial structures of the lung, has provided a new means of evaluating this group of diseases. It is now recognized that various diseases follow characteristic CT patterns. Some researchers, such as Mathieson and colleagues (1989), have shown improved accuracy of diagnosis using high-resolution CT compared with conventional chest radiography.

Interstitial lung diseases can be divided into several basic patterns. The *bronchovascular pattern* demonstrates thickening of the interstitial structures surrounding the small bronchioles. Lymphangitic carcinomatosis and sarcoidosis are the diseases that most commonly produce this pattern (Fig. 12–16). The *septal* or *perilobular pattern* demonstrates thickening of the fine septa that separate groups of acini into the secondary lobules. Characteristically, thickening of the interstitium is evident in a rim of tissue adjacent to the

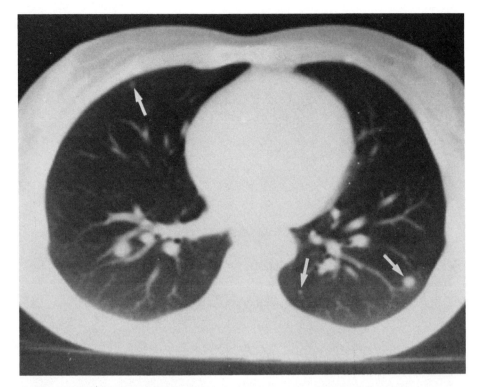

Fig. 12–15. Multiple pulmonary nodules. CT scan reveals multiple small pulmonary nodules (arrows) that were occult with conventional radiography. In a patient with a known extrathoracic malignancy, these nodules are suggestive of, although not definitive for, metastatic disease.

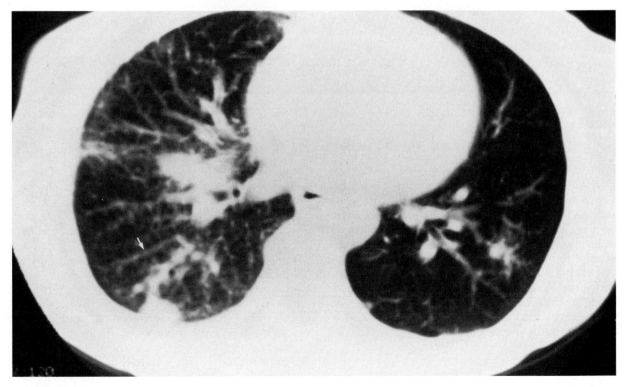

Fig. 12–16. Lymphangitic carcinomatosis. CT scan of the chest reveals nodular thickening along the course of the pulmonary arteries and bronchi, seen as increased numbers of lines in the right lung as compared to the left lung. This finding is characteristic of the bronchovascular pattern of interstitial disease and was attributed to lymphangitic carcinomatosis in this woman with breast cancer.

chest wall. Idiopathic pulmonary fibrosis, asbestosis, and collagen vascular diseases such as scleroderma and rheumatoid arthritis are the interstitial diseases that most commonly produce this pattern (Fig. 12–17). Some interstitial diseases manifest as numerous small, millimeter-sized nodules, including sarcoidosis, miliary tuberculosis, hypersensitivity pneumonitis, silicosis, and coal workers' pneumoconiosis (Fig. 12–18).

The pattern of interstitial disease on CT scans can also be used to determine the most efficacious means of obtaining tissue for diagnosis. Because diseases producing the bronchovascular pattern affect the tissues adjacent to the bronchi, transbronchial biopsy has a high diagnostic yield for these diseases. Diseases demonstrating a septal pattern usually require surgical biopsy for diagnosis because the area of most active disease is not adjacent to the bronchi. Although interstitial diseases may affect large regions of pulmonary parenchyma, the disease may be patchy in distribution. Imaging with CT can help to determine the most appropriate area for surgical biopsy. In addition, Müller and associates (1984) showed that regions of "ground glass" opacity correlate with regions of active disease. Biopsies may be targeted toward these areas to improve diagnostic yield.

Computed tomography is also useful in evaluating diseases with decreased attenuation, such as emphysema and bullous lung disease. High-resolution CT has been shown by some — Kinsella (1990) and Kuwano (1990) and their colleagues among them — to be more accurate than pulmonary function tests in the detection of early pulmonary emphysema. Emphysema characteristically demonstrates diffuse regions of low attenuation without definable walls. Computed tomography is also capable of exactly defining the size and location of bullae, which is helpful in the preoperative planning of surgical bullectomy.

Air-Space Disease

Naidich and associates (1985) described the CT appearance of air-space disease. The findings include: 1) air-space nodules that are poorly marginated opacities ranging up to 1 cm, caused by sublobular accumulations of fluid, hemorrhage, or cells; 2) coalescent densities that are usually the result of confluence of air-space nodules; 3) air bronchograms and air alveolargrams; and 4) ground-glass opacity defined as a zone of increased lung density. Several disease processes can produce air-space patterns identified with CT. Pneumonia or aspiration, hemorrhage, pulmonary edema, alveolar proteinosis, and alveolar cell carcinoma may have an identical CT appearance (Fig. 12–19). In general, CT adds little to the characterization of alveolar processes, although it may be better than plain-film radiography in defining the extent of disease, particularly important for demonstrating the spread of lobar alveolar cell

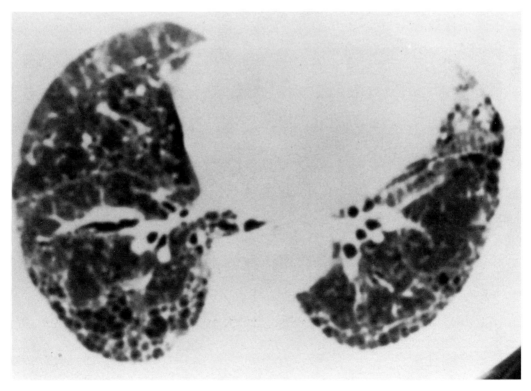

Fig. 12–17. Idiopathic pulmonary fibrosis. This high-resolution CT scan demonstrates interstitial thickening and honeycombing in a peripheral, septal pattern that is characteristic of idiopathic pulmonary fibrosis. Differential diagnosis would include asbestosis and the interstitial lung disease seen in collagen vascular diseases such as scleroderma and rheumatoid arthritis.

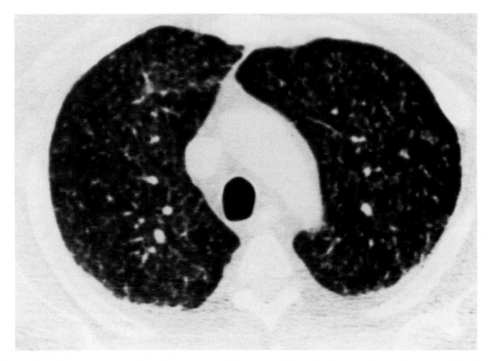

Fig. 12–18. Miliary tuberculosis. Numerous, less than 1-mm nodules are noted in this high-resolution CT scan of the chest. These nodules were due to miliary tuberculosis.

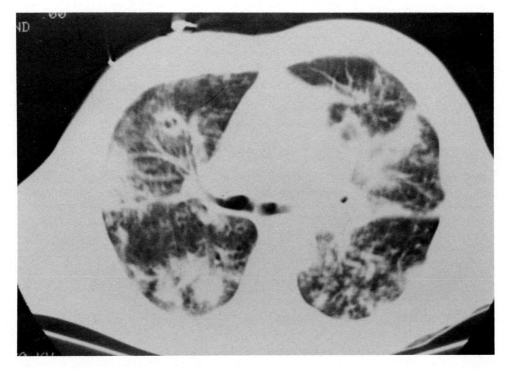

Fig. 12–19. Aspiration pneumonia. CT scan shows bilateral patchy air-space infiltrates consistent with pneumonia. Air-space infiltrates from a variety of etiologies are indistinguishable with CT.

carcinoma to the contralateral lung, as reported by one of us (DME) and associates (1982). Alveolar infiltrates resulting from amiodarone toxicity are characteristically hyperdense relative to muscle on unenhanced CT scans, as noted by Kuhlman and colleagues (1990). This finding appears to be specific for this disease process.

Tracheobronchial Tree Involvement

CT can provide valuable information in the assessment of a variety of disorders of the trachea, because the lumen, wall, and extraluminal structures are all visualized. In particular, the presence and extent of extraluminal involvement by primary neoplasms can be defined and plays an important role in the preoperative assessment of these tumors. The craniocaudal extent of lesions can also be determined, and this process will likely be facilitated with the continuous scanning capability of spiral CT. Direct invasion of the trachea by adjacent neoplasms, frequently from esophageal carcinoma, can be identified (Fig. 12–20). Whereas fluoroscopy is used for functional evaluation of the trachea — that is, tracheomalacia — ultrafast CT can evaluate fixed stenoses versus nonfixed tracheal obstructions, particularly in pediatric patients, as described by Ell (1986) and Brasch (1987) and their colleagues. Unfortunately, this method is not widely available.

Computed tomography using thin sections and high-resolution technique has virtually eliminated the use of bronchography in the evaluation of patients with suspected bronchiectasis (Fig. 12–21). Using 1.5-mm thick slices obtained at 10-mm intervals, Grenier and colleagues (1986) demonstrated a sensitivity of 97% and a specificity of 93% for CT. Naidich (1991) has emphasized that CT is particularly valuable in patients with definite evidence of bilateral bronchiectasis, since unnecessary surgery can be obviated in such cases. Bronchography now may be limited to a select group of surgical candidates in whom CT has demonstrated localized disease.

Computed tomography has proven to be highly accurate in the identification of endobronchial lesions, especially with the use of thin sections, as demonstrated by Naidich (1987) and Mayr (1989) and their associates. However, as pointed out by Naidich (1991), CT cannot precisely differentiate mucosal from submucosal or extrinsic involvement. The ability of CT to be of value in evaluating peribronchial disease is complementary to fiberoptic bronchoscopy. Imaging with CT has proven efficacious in guiding transbronchial needle aspiration and biopsy and in selecting patients for endobronchial laser therapy. In selected instances of endobronchial disease, Shepard and McLoud (1991) have reported that CT can suggest a specific diagnosis; that is, the calcification of broncholiths and the intravenous contrast enhancement of carcinoid tumors.

Computed tomography has also proven valuable in screening patients presenting with a history of hemoptysis. In a study by Naidich and associates (1990) comparing fiberoptic bronchoscopy and CT in such patients, all focal airway lesions seen on bronchoscopy were identified on CT, including all malignancies.

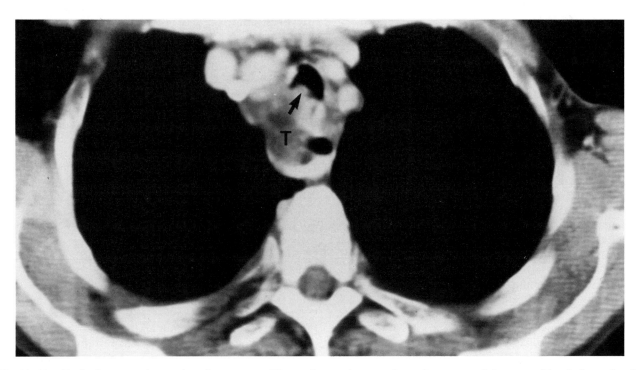

Fig. 12–20. Tracheal invasion by esophageal carcinoma. CT scan depicts direct mediastinal extension of the tumor (T), which invades the posterolateral wall of the trachea (arrow).

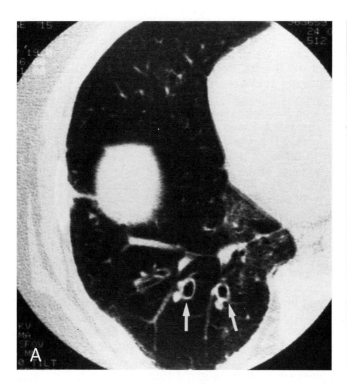

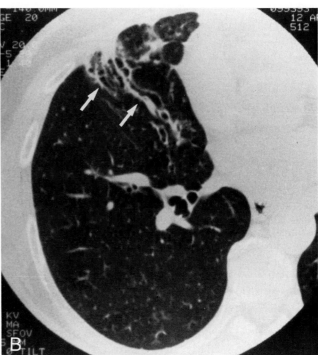

Fig. 12–21. Bronchiectasis. *A,* Dilated, thick-walled bronchi (arrows) in the right lower lobe are seen in cross-section on this high-resolution CT scan. Note that the bronchi are larger in diameter than their adjacent pulmonary vessels, indicative of bronchiectasis. This appearance has been referred to as the "signet ring" sign. *B,* Right middle lobe bronchiectasis in another patient. Here, the bronchiectatic airways are oriented parallel to the high-resolution CT slice. The thickened walls of these dilated bronchi (arrows) give the appearance of "tram lines."

Moreover, CT demonstrated bronchiectasis as a cause of hemoptysis in a significant percentage of these patients.

Pulmonary Vascular Lesions

Computed tomography can be extremely useful in the noninvasive diagnosis of vascular lesions of the lung, including pulmonary arteriovenous malformation — AVM, pulmonary varix, scimitar syndrome — partial anomalous venous return, and sequestration. Contrast-enhanced studies, particularly with the use of the new spiral and ultrafast technology, can demonstrate the vascular morphology of these lesions. The diagnosis of an AVM is established by identifying the feeding artery and draining vein, as well as contrast enhancement of the lesion — unless it is thrombosed (Fig. 12–22). In patients with a chronic, lower lobe paravertebral mass or focal consolidation suspected of representing sequestration, the diagnosis of this entity can be established using CT if the abnormal systemic artery supplying the lesion is identified — and in some cases the venous drainage as well. The need for more invasive conventional aortography may therefore be obviated in such cases. Magnetic resonance imaging has also proven useful in the evaluation of all of these pulmonary vascular lesions, offering the advantages of flow sensitivity without the need for intravenous contrast, media administration and the ability to image directly in multiple planes. The principal disadvantage of MR

imaging relative to CT is the poorer signal-to-noise ratio of MR in imaging parenchymal lung detail.

In general, CT has not played a significant role in the diagnosis of pulmonary embolism. In selected instances, conventional CT has been used to diagnose large central emboli (Fig. 12–23); however, the long scan times and motion artifacts have limited its use in the detection of more peripheral emboli. Preliminary studies using ultrafast CT and spiral CT technologies, as shown by Remy-Jardin (1992) and Geraghty (1992) and their associates, have demonstrated the potential to diagnose pulmonary emboli in second to fourth-division pulmonary vessels 0.7 mm in diameter. Napel and co-workers (1992) reported that three-dimensional angiographic displays of the pulmonary vasculature from breath-hold spiral CT data yielded resolution of peripheral vessels less than 2 mm in diameter. Although these techniques show exciting promise in providing noninvasive pulmonary angiograms, further clinical experience to document their utility is required.

Computed tomography may prove particularly valuable in patients being evaluated for chronic thromboembolic pulmonary hypertension. In this disorder, acute emboli fail to undergo normal lysis, become organized and fibrotic, and may ultimately become incorporated within the walls of the pulmonary arteries. Such chronic thromboemboli may lead to the development of pulmonary arterial hypertension. Patients with this disorder often show dramatic improve-

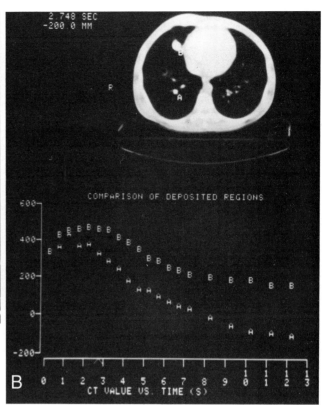

Fig. 12–22. Pulmonary arteriovenous malformation (AVM). *A,* The lesion appears as a lobulated nodule (arrow) in the right middle lobe on this ultrafast CT image. *B,* Using dynamic, ultrafast scans after administration of a bolus of intravenous contrast agent, CT attenuation measurements were obtained over time from the lesion ("B") as well as a right lower lobe artery ("A") for reference. The temporal enhancement pattern of the lesion (upper curve on graph), which parallels that of the pulmonary artery (lower curve), is consistent with an AVM.

ment after surgical thromboendarterectomy, only patients with clots in the proximal pulmonary arteries, however, are candidates for surgery. The presence and extent of such central mural clots may be underestimated on conventional pulmonary arteriograms. On the other hand, studies by one of us (W.B.G.) and Hatabu (1993) using MR and by Remy-Jardin (1992) using CT suggest that these techniques are advantageous in demonstrating proximal mural thromboemboli (Fig. 12–24), and thus can be a useful adjunct to conventional angiography.

Miscellaneous Conditions

Bronchial adenomas are low-grade malignancies that are often endobronchial and frequently extend beyond the bronchus into the surrounding lung or mediastinum. Characteristically, they are extremely vascular tumors and most endoscopists will not perform a biopsy of such a lesion because of the danger of extensive bleeding. Because most bronchial adenomas arise in the central airways, CT can identify these lesions and define extrabronchial extension. Moreover, because of their vascular nature, contrast enhancement has been reported by Aronchick and collaborators (1986) in three bronchial carcinoids. This enhancement pattern should alert the endoscopist to the possibility of a bronchial adenoma.

In patients with suspected noninvasive or semi-invasive aspergillosis, CT may demonstrate occult mycetomas, which are not detected on chest radiographs.

Pleura

Abscess versus Empyema

Computed tomography may provide valuable information in evaluating disease processes of the pleura and in distinguishing pleural from parenchymal lung disease. Familiarity with the CT appearance of the pleural fissures is helpful in localizing lung infiltrates and nodules and in distinguishing loculated pleural fluid from parenchymal consolidation. This application is particularly helpful in differentiating lung abscesses from empyema with bronchopleural fistula. Empyemas are enclosed within the pleural cavity and conform to the shape of the chest wall. Most empyemas have thin, smooth walls, especially along their inner margins. Abscesses, however, because they originate within the pulmonary parenchyma, remain spherical (Fig. 12–25). Most abscesses tend to have thickened, irregular walls and margins. Ancillary findings of empyema include compressed lung adjacent to the inner margin of an empyema, as well as displacement of vessels and bronchi by large pleural fluid collections. The accurate iden-

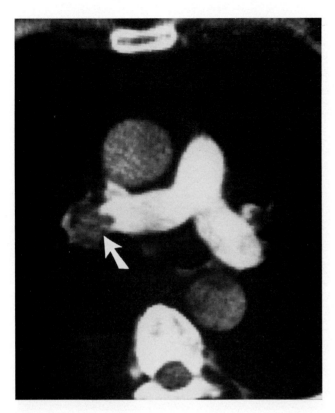

Fig. 12–23. Acute pulmonary embolus. Intense opacification of the pulmonary arteries obtained on this ultrafast CT scan clearly depicts the large intraluminal clot in the right pulmonary artery (arrow).

tification of loculated empyemas by CT also provides useful guidance for tube thoracostomy.

Effusion versus Ascites

The differentiation of pleural effusion from ascites is sometimes difficult. Halvorsen and colleagues (1986)

reported four CT signs that are useful. The following criteria suggest ascites: 1) fluid is inside — below — the diaphragm; 2) fluid does not elevate the crus of the diaphragm; 3) the interface between fluid and the liver is distinct; and 4) fluid is only posterior or lateral to the liver at the level of the bare area. Pleural effusion, on the other hand, is suggested by the following criteria: 1) fluid is outside — above — the diaphragm; 2) fluid elevates the crus of the diaphragm; 3) the interface between fluid and the liver is indistinct; and 4) fluid is posterior or medial to the liver at the level of the bare area. Used individually, each of these signs may be indeterminate or misleading. If all four criteria are fulfilled, accurate distinction of pleural fluid from ascites is possible (Fig. 12–26).

Mesothelioma

Malignant mesothelioma often appears on CT examinations as a thick, pleurally based rind of soft tissue encasing the lung (Fig. 12–27). A nodular contour to the pleural thickening, involvement of the medial pleural surface along the mediastinum, and spread into the interlobar fissures are helpful features in differentiating diffuse malignant mesothelioma from benign pleural thickening. A variable quantity of fluid, usually loculated, is generally present. The density of this fluid is usually less than that of the rind of soft tissue. At times, mesothelioma may appear as loculated pleural fluid with or without scattered soft tissue masses attached to the visceral or parietal pleural surfaces (Fig. 12–28). Pleural metastasis may appear identical to mesothelioma and is the major differential diagnosis when either of these findings are observed. Malignant mesothelioma may spread directly to involve the mediastinum, pericardium, contralateral lung, or chest wall. It may also spread through the diaphragm to

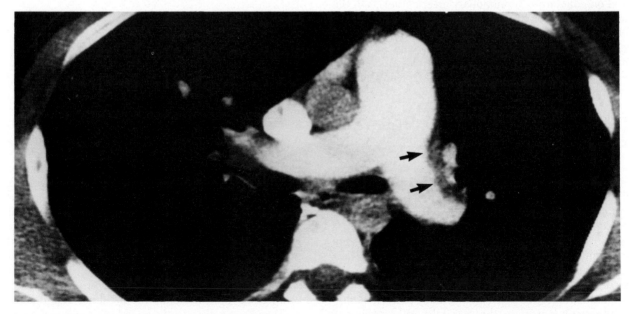

Fig. 12–24. Chronic pulmonary embolus. Mural thrombus along the wall of the proximal left pulmonary artery is evident on this ultrafast CT scan. Such CT scans may complement conventional angiography in the preoperative evaluation of patients with chronic thromboembolic pulmonary hypertension.

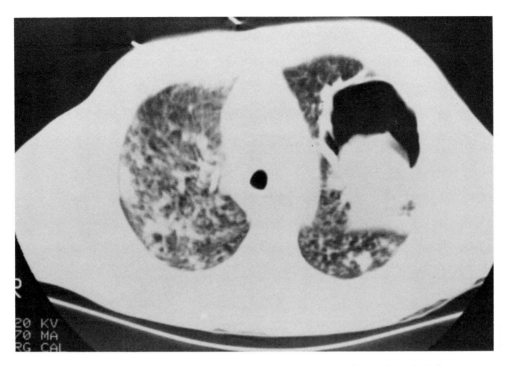

Fig. 12–25. Lung abscess. A large necrotic left lung abscess with debris has a thickened and irregular wall while retaining its spherical shape. An empyema would conform to the shape of the chest wall.

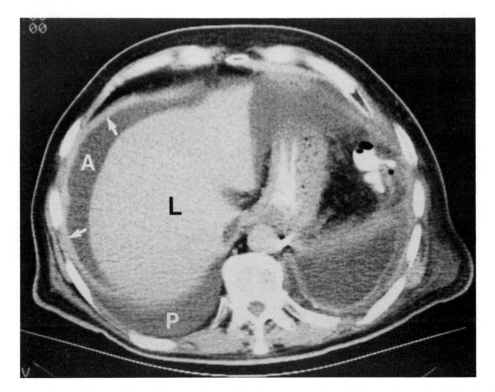

Fig. 12–26. Ascites and pleural effusion. CT scan shows evidence of both ascites and pleural effusion. The ascites (A) lies inside the diaphragm (arrows) and has a distinct interface with the liver (L). Pleural fluid (P) is identified posteriorly behind the diaphragm and has an indistinct interface with the liver.

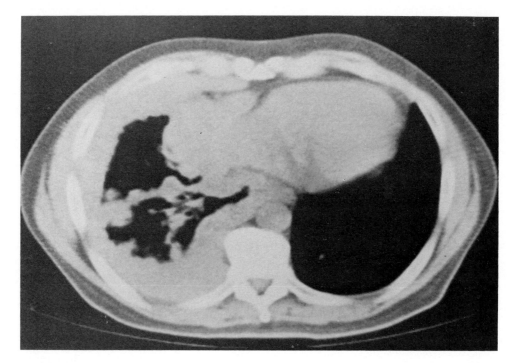

Fig. 12–27. Mesothelioma. A thick rind of pleurally based soft tissue encases the entire right hemithorax and is consistent with a malignant mesothelioma.

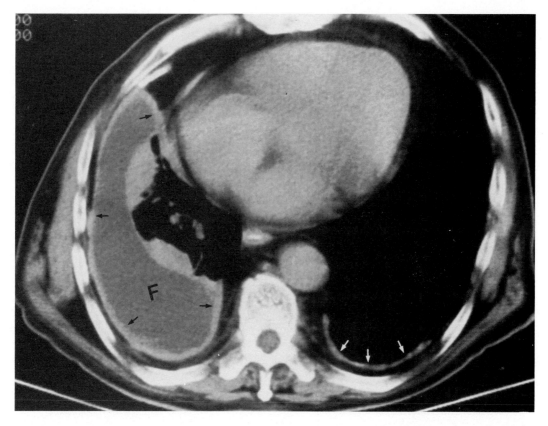

Fig. 12–28. Mesothelioma can demonstrate a moderate pleural effusion seen as fluid density (F) and a thin excess rind of tissue coating the surface of the visceral and parietal pleura (black arrows). Note the asbestos-related pleural plaque in the left hemithorax (white arrows).

involve the abdominal and retroperitoneal viscera. Computed tomography is the most effective form of imaging available to identify the extent of involvement with malignant mesothelioma.

Miscellaneous Conditions

Some benign processes involving the pleura are well evaluated with CT. This technique is useful in confirming subtle pleural plaques noted on the chest radiograph in patients who have a history of exposure to asbestos (Fig. 12–28). The pleural plaque caused by asbestos-related disease can also be confidently distinguished from pulmonary nodules. Computed tomography may be useful in distinguishing rounded atelectasis from carcinoma in patients with evidence of asbestos-related pleural disease, as described by Mintzer and associates (1981). Well-circumscribed, localized pleural tumors such as fibrous mesothelioma — solitary localized fibrous tumor — and pleural lipoma can be identified with CT. Only in the case of a lipoma, however, can a specific diagnosis be made (Fig. 12–29). Computed tomography is useful in identifying a lipoma because of its characteristic lower density.

Chest Wall

Because of its soft-tissue contrast and multiplanar capabilities, MR imaging has become the method of choice for evaluating processes that primarily involve the chest wall or diaphragm; CT, however, remains an excellent means of evaluating the chest wall, particularly in processes that involve both the chest wall and pulmonary parenchyma.

Metastatic Tumor

As with primary lung cancer, mesothelioma and metastatic tumor from extrathoracic primary tumors may cause rib destruction. The oblique orientation of the ribs on axial images, however, hampers the accurate evaluation of rib destruction, which is often better visualized on conventional rib radiographs.

Computed tomography does provide precise anatomic definition of many chest wall lesions. In patients with chest wall neoplasia, previously unsuspected areas of involvement may be visualized. It also may be difficult to distinguish between chest wall tumor and infection, because of their similar CT appearance. Biopsy is often required.

Postoperative Evaluation

Computed tomography has been used to evaluate complications of median sternotomy. Unfortunately, the sensitivity and specificity of CT for sternal osteomyelitis and mediastinitis after median sternotomy is limited. Browdie and associates (1991) noted 4 true-positive, 4 false-positive, 14 true-negative, and 2 false-negative CT examinations in 6 proven poststernotomy wound infections following 737 cardiac operations. They found that indium-111 leukocyte scanning and epicardial pacer cultures were a more accurate means of detecting poststernotomy wound infections. Despite the limitations of CT, however, it is a useful means of

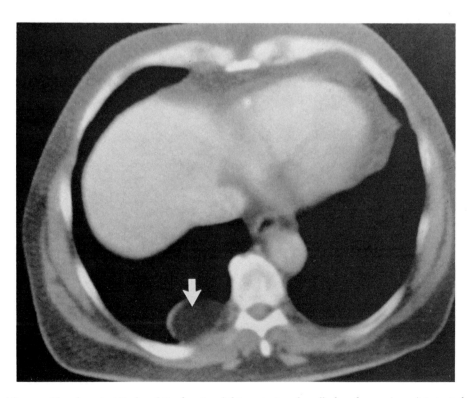

Fig. 12–29. Pleural lipoma. The characteristic low fatty density of this posterior pleurally based mass (arrow) is typical of a pleural lipoma.

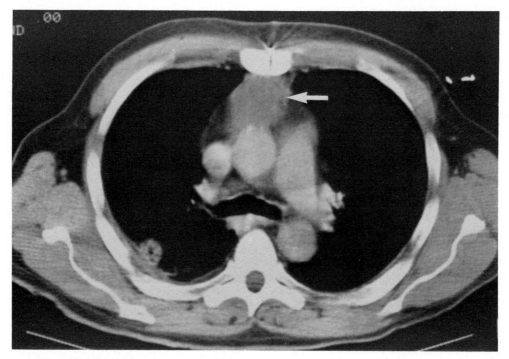

Fig. 12-30. Postoperative infection. Fluid density in the mediastinum (arrow) 2 weeks after median sternotomy proved to be a localized mediastinal abscess.

detecting substernal and mediastinal wound collections that would benefit from surgical drainage as opposed to mediastinitis, which does not require surgical intervention (Fig. 12-30). Computed tomography has also been useful in the detection of tumor recurrence after pneumonectomy for lung cancer, as reported by Glazer and colleagues (1984).

Miscellaneous Conditions

Evaluation of the posterior paraspinal region is facilitated by CT. Distinction is usually made between enlarged lymph nodes, vessels, and anatomic variants such as lipomatosis. Paraspinal hematomas and involvement of vertebral bodies by extension of paraspinal masses caused by infection or metastatic tumor can also be identified. In certain situations, MR imaging of paraspinal masses may be the preferred technique because it more accurately evaluates involvement of intraspinal contents, particularly the spinal cord. It is often difficult, however, to distinguish paraspinal infection from tumor, and CT-guided biopsy may provide a definitive diagnosis in this instance.

REFERENCES

Aronchick J, et al: Computed tomography of bronchial carcinoid. J Comput Assist Tomogr 10:71, 1986.

Baron RL, et al: Computed tomography in the evaluation of mediastinal widening. Radiology 138:107, 1981a.

Baron RL, et al: CT of anomalies of the mediastinal vessels. AJR Am J Roentgenol 137:571, 1981b.

Becker CD, et al: Patterns of recurrence of esophageal carcinoma after transhiatal esophagectomy and gastric interposition. AJR Am J Roentgenol 148:273, 1987.

Brasch RC, et al: Upper airway obstruction in infants and children evaluated with ultrafast CT. Radiology 165:459, 1987.

Browdie DA, et al: Diagnosis of poststernotomy infection: Comparison of three means of assessment. Ann Thorac Surg 51:290, 1991.

Brown LR, et al: Roentgenologic diagnosis of primary corticotropin-producing carcinoid tumors of the mediastinum. Radiology 142:143, 1982.

Ell SR, Jolles H, Galvin JR: Cine CT demonstration of nonfixed upper airway obstruction. AJR Am J Roentgenol 146:669, 1986.

Epstein DM, et al: Value of CT in the preoperative assessment of lung cancer: A survey of thoracic surgeons. Radiology 161:423, 1986.

Epstein DM, Gefter WB, Miller WT: Lobar bronchioloalveolar cell carcinoma. AJR Am J Roentgenol 139:463, 1982.

Freeny PC, Marks WM: Adenocarcinoma of the gastroesophageal junction: Barium and CT examination. AJR Am J Roentgenol 138:1077, 1982.

Gefter WB, Hatabu H: Evaluation of pulmonary vascular anatomy and blood flow by magnetic resonance. J Thorac Imag, In press.

Genereux GP, Howie JL: Normal mediastinal lymph node size and number: CT and anatomic study. AJR Am J Roentgenol 142:1095, 1984.

Geraghty JJ, et al: Ultrafast computed tomography in experimental pulmonary embolism. Invest Radiol 27:60, 1992.

Glazer HS, et al: Utility of CT in detecting postpneumonectomy carcinoma recurrence. AJR Am J Roentgenol 142:487, 1984.

Glazer HS, et al: Pleural and chest wall invasion in bronchogenic carcinoma: CT evaluation. Radiology 157:191, 1985.

Glazer HS, et al: Indeterminate mediastinal invasion in bronchogenic carcinoma: CT evaluation. Radiology 173:37, 1989.

Grenier P, et al: Bronchiectasis: Assessment by thin-section CT. Radiology 161:95, 1986.

Gross SC, et al: Computed tomography in dissection of the thoracic aorta. Radiology 136:135, 1980.

Halvorsen RA, et al: Ascites or pleural effusion? CT differentiation: Four useful criteria. RadioGraphics 6:135, 1986.

Homer MJ, Wechsler RJ, Carter BL: Mediastinal lipomatosis. Radiology 128:657, 1978.

Huston III J, Muhm JR: Solitary pulmonary nodules: Evaluation with a CT reference phantom. Radiology *170*:653, 1989.

Kinsella M, et al: Quantitation of emphysema by computed tomography using a "density mask" program and correlation with pulmonary function tests. Chest *97*:315, 1990.

Kuhlman JE, et al: Amiodarone pulmonary toxicity: CT findings in symptomatic patients. Radiology *177*:121, 1990.

Kuwano K, et al: The diagnosis of mild emphysema. Correlation of computed tomography and pathology scores. Am Rev Respir Dis *141*:169, 1990.

Libshitz HI, et al: Mediastinal evaluation in lung cancer. Radiology *151*:295, 1984.

Lynch DA, et al: Asbestos-related focal lung masses: Manifestations on conventional and high-resolution CT scans. Radiology *169*:603, 1988.

Mathieson JR, et al: Comparison of diagnostic accuracy of CT and chest radiography. Radiology *171*:111, 1989.

Mayr B, et al: Tumors of the bronchi: Role of evaluation with CT. Radiology *172*:647, 1989.

McHugh K, Blaquiere RM: CT features of rounded atelectasis. AJR Am J Roentgenol *153*:257, 1989.

Mintzer RA, et al: Rounded atelectasis and its association with asbestos-induced pleural disease. Radiology *139*:567, 1981.

Mitchell DG, et al: Benign adrenocortical masses: Diagnosis with chemical shift MR imaging. Radiology *185*:345, 1992.

Moore AV, et al: Age-related changes in the thymus gland: CT-pathologic correlation. AJR Am J Roentgenol *141*:241, 1983.

Morgan PW, et al: Evaluation of traumatic aortic injury: Does dynamic contrast-enhanced CT play a role? Radiology *182*:661, 1992.

Müller NL, et al: Role of computed tomography in the recognition of bronchiectasis. AJR Am J Roentgenol *143*:971, 1984.

Naidich DP, et al: Computed tomography of the pulmonary parenchyma. Part 1. Distal air-space disease. J Thorac Imaging *1*:39, 1985.

Naidich DP, et al: Comparison of CT and fiberoptic bronchoscopy in the evaluation of bronchial disease. AJR Am J Roentgenol *148*:1, 1987.

Naidich DP, et al: Hemoptysis: CT-bronchoscopic correlations in 58 cases. Radiology *177*:357, 1991.

Napel SA, et al: Maximum and minimum intensity projection of spiral CT data for simultaneous 3D imaging of the pulmonary vasculature and airways. Radiology *185*:126, 1992.

Nienaber CA, et al: The diagnosis of thoracic aortic dissection by noninvasive imaging procedures. N Engl J Med *328*:1, 1993.

Quint LE, et al: Esophageal carcinoma: CT findings. Radiology *155*:171, 1985.

Raptopoulos V, et al: Traumatic aortic tear: Screening with chest CT. Radiology *182*:667, 1992.

Ratto GB, et al: Chest wall involvement by lung cancer: Computed tomographic detection and results of operation. Ann Thorac Surg *51*:182, 1991.

Remy-Jardin M, et al: Central pulmonary thromboembolism: Diagnosis with spiral volumetric CT with the single-breath-hold technique — comparison with pulmonary angiography. Radiology *185*:381, 1992.

Schaner EG, et al: Comparison of computed and conventional whole lung tomography in detecting pulmonary nodules: A prospective radiologic-pathologic study. AJR Am J Roentgenol *131*:51, 1978.

Shepard JO, McLoud TC: Imaging the airways. Computed tomography and magnetic resonance imaging. Clin Chest Med *12*:151, 1991.

Swensen SJ, et al: CT evaluation of solitary pulmonary nodules: Value of 185-H reference phantom. AJR Am J Roentgenol *156*:925, 1991.

Thompson WM, et al: Computed tomography for staging esophageal and gastroesophageal cancer: Re-evaluation. AJR Am J Roentgenol *141*:951, 1983.

Webb WR, et al: CT and MR imaging in staging non-small cell bronchogenic carcinoma: Report of the Radiologic Diagnostic Oncology Group. Radiology *178*:705, 1991.

Westcott JL, Hallisey MJ, Volpe JP: Dynamic CT of round atelectasis. Radiology *181*:182, 1991.

Zerhouni EA, et al: CT of the pulmonary nodule: A cooperative study. Radiology *160*:319, 1986.

READING REFERENCES

Bergin CJ, Müller NL: CT in the diagnosis of interstitial lung disease. AJR Am J Roentgenol *145*:505, 1985.

Goodman LR, et al: Complications of median sternotomy: Computed tomographic evaluation. AJR Am J Roentgenol *141*:225, 1983.

Klein JS, Webb WR: The radiologic staging of lung cancer. J Thorac Imaging *7*:29, 1991.

Naidich DP, Zerhouni EA, Siegelman SS: Computed Tomography and Magnetic Resonance of the Thorax. New York: Raven Press, 1991.

Pennes DR, et al: Chest wall invasion by lung cancer: Limitations of CT evaluation. AJR Am J Roentgenol *144*:507, 1985.

Petasnick JP: Radiologic evaluation of aortic dissection. Radiology *180*:297, 1991.

Zerhouni EA, et al: Computed tomography of the pulmonary parenchyma. Part 2. Interstitial disease. J Thorac Imaging *1*:54, 1985.

CHAPTER 13

MAGNETIC RESONANCE IMAGING OF THE THORAX

Gordon Gamsu

Magnetic resonance — MR — imaging has, since the late 1970s, generated considerable interest as a safe technique for human imaging. As Pykett (1982) and Crooks and colleagues (1982a) showed, the sensitivity of MR imaging for demonstrating human disease is impressive. Magnetic resonance imaging uses physical properties of matter that are different from those that result in x-ray-based radiographic images, and thus can provide unique diagnostic information. Magnetic resonance imaging has outstanding tissue contrast resolution and excellent separation of blood vessels from soft tissues. At present, MR imaging of the heart and mediastinum are clinically practical alternatives to other imaging methods. Imaging of the lungs with MR still has limited application because of magnetic susceptibility-induced inhomogeneity, which causes signal loss in the lungs. Sufficient information is now available to detail the strengths and weaknesses of MR imaging relative to computed tomography — CT — and other modes of imaging.

TECHNIQUES

General Principles

Atomic nuclei with an odd number of nucleons — protons and neutrons — act as magnetic dipoles. They align within a strong magnetic field, producing a net magnetic vector parallel to the magnetic field. To date, most MR imaging uses hydrogen protons. Perturbation of the aligned protons by a radio frequency — RF — pulse of a specific frequency displaces the magnetic vector by a predictable amount, dependent on the strength and duration of the RF pulse. As the protons return to their original orientation, they emit a detectable RF signal. If the magnetic field contains a gradient, the emitted RF signal varies with the proton's position within the magnetic field. By suitable signal detection, the proton's precise position within the magnetic field can be plotted. In biologic tissues, various MR imaging techniques are used to define the position of protons in three dimensions within the imaged body part.

Several nuclei found in biologic systems can be imaged with MR, including hydrogen, phosphorus-31, sodium-23, carbon-13, and fluorine. Hydrogen is used most commonly because of its abundance and suitability for MR imaging. The MR image represents the intensity of the MR signal within the imaged volume and depends on a variable combination of four parameters. These parameters are hydrogen density, two relaxation times called T1 and T2, and motion of the hydrogen protons within the imaged volume.

As the hydrogen density increases, increasing numbers of hydrogen nuclei align within the magnetic field, producing a more intense MR signal. The T1 or "spin-lattice" relaxation time depends on the interaction of the hydrogen nucleus with its molecular environment. The T1 relaxation time characterizes a time within which the proton aligns itself in a given magnetic field. The T2 or "spin-spin" relaxation time reflects magnetic interactions between protons. During realignment of the perturbed proton, the MR signal decays as the resonance of the protons becomes unsynchronized. The time of decay of the MR signal is the T2 relaxation time.

The last parameter affecting the intensity of the image signal is bulk motion of the protons within the imaging volume. For instance, in thoracic imaging, rapidly flowing blood or the beating heart are not imaged with the usual imaging sequences. The time required for MR in the human is between 10 and 60 msec for the shortest component of an imaging sequence. Moving protons are subjected to different events than are stationary protons. Their emitted signal thus differs, depending on the MR sequence used to obtain the image. Motion of protons within the imaging volume increases or decreases the intensity of the MR signal.

Imaging Techniques

Radiographic images reveal little intrinsic contrast between normal and abnormal soft tissues. Changing radiographic imaging parameters produces only small changes in tissue contrast. On the other hand, MR imaging uses tissue properties that can be manipulated extensively. Crooks and colleagues (1982b) demonstrated that hydrogen density varies only by about 20% for most soft tissues. The T1 and T2 relaxation times of different tissues, however, can vary by over 1000%. Magnetic resonance imaging uses techniques that allow these differences in tissue properties to be translated into major differences in tissue contrast. Techniques such as free induction decay, spin-echo, inversion recovery, and partial saturation can change the extent to which the T1 and T2 relaxation properties of different tissues affect the relative contrast between these tissues. The most commonly used technique for MR imaging is spin-echo — SE — which is both T1- and T2-dependent over a wide range of tissue relaxation times. Spin-echo imaging is also sensitive to flow and hydrogen density.

Contrast between tissues is relative when an SE technique is used. The degree to which T1 and T2 affect tissue intensity can be altered by two excitation properties called the repetition time — TR — and the echo time — TE. The TR is the time between excitations. The specific time used for the TR allows expression of differences in T1 relaxation of the tissues. The TR can be set on MR units at times between 10 and 5000 msec. If two tissues have different T1 relaxation times, the appropriate TR setting allows images that demonstrate contrast differences between the two tissues. The tissue with the longer T1 does not have sufficient time to realign itself completely within the magnetic field before the next pulse sequence is initiated, and it will have less signal strength than a tissue with a shorter T1 relaxation time. For instance, as I and co-workers (1983) showed, most malignant neoplasms have a longer T1 — 800 to 1200 msec — than mediastinal fat — less than 400 msec — when imaged at field strengths of 0.3 to 1.5 Tesla. With a TR of 500 msec, mediastinal fat is more intense than a mediastinal neoplasm and the latter is readily identified. Images performed with a short TR are thus called T1 dependent. On spin-echo images performed with a long TR — more than 2000 msec — tissues with both short and long T1 relaxation times have equal signal intensity and may not be distinguishable.

The TE or echo time can also be controlled and is set in milliseconds. On most MR imaging units, it can be varied between 4 and 200 msec. Provided the TR is sufficiently long, the decay differences — T2 relaxation times — between tissues control their contrast. This is demonstrated by varying the TE, and the subsequent images are called T2 dependent or "T2-weighted." Thus, with a long TE — more than 60 msec — the signal from tissue with a short T2 time diminishes more than the signal from tissue with a long T2 relaxation time. The tissue with a long T2 shows greater signal intensity on the T2-weighted image.

With most MR imaging units, SE images are obtained at multiple levels during any single scanning sequence. The levels that can be obtained and the time taken for image acquisition depend on the TR and TE used. Typically, 5 to 15 slices or levels are obtained, each slice being 1.5- to 10-mm thick. The usual time for the multiple image acquisition is about 5 to 15 minutes. For most body imaging purposes, the MR scan is composed of a 256^2 matrix with each pixel element about 1.5 mm^2. During MR scanning, information is being derived from multiple planes at any one time.

Cardiac and Respiratory Gating

Because of the time required for MR imaging, pulsation and respiratory motion perturb the cardiomediastinal structures and degrade the MR image. Unlike the artifacts seen with CT scanning, motion during MR imaging decreases spatial resolution and diminishes signal intensity, similar to the diminution seen with flowing blood. These motions can also cause "ghosting" artifacts that also degrade the MR image. Lanzer and colleagues (1983) showed that cardiac gating with image acquisition timed to the cardiac cycle using an electrocardiogram — ECG — does improve resolution of cardiac, mediastinal, and hilar structures. Masses within the lower mediastinum and around the heart are also better imaged. Although cardiac gating prolongs imaging time, it is used routinely in thoracic MR imaging. A problem with ECG-cardiac gating is that the heart rate determines the TR for the image. In most circumstances, the result is a TR of around 0.7 second, with a relatively T1-weighted image. A prolonged TR can be produced by gating the image to every other cardiac beat. The TR of about 1.5 seconds, if used in combination with longer TE, produces a T2-weighted image.

Respiratory gating that acquires information only during periods of apnea between breaths is feasible but does not improve MR image quality as significantly as would be expected. It also prolongs imaging time. Software improvement in MR scanners has improved image quality by suppressing some of the artifacts produced by respiratory motion without prolonging scan time. Imaging sequences can obtain slices within 15 seconds, permitting breath holding during the acquisition period. Respiratory degradation of the MR image should not be an important factor in the near future with newer imaging sequences.

Sagittal and Coronal Imaging

An advantage of MR imaging over CT scanning is its ability to acquire images in the sagittal and coronal planes, without reformating of multiple transaxial images (Fig. 13–1). With most images, the matrix size is less for

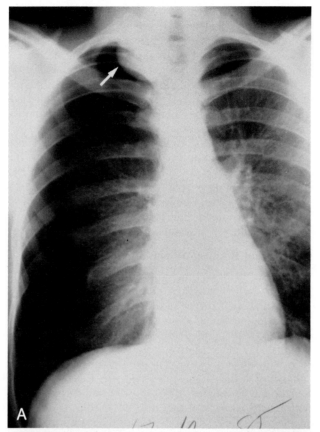

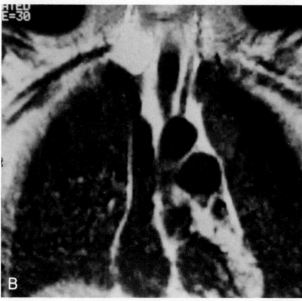

Fig. 13–1. Coronal image of an extrapleural schwannoma. *A*, Chest radiograph after a spontaneous pneumothorax shows a mass at the right apex (arrow). *B*, An ECG-gated MR (T1-weighted) scan shows the mass, which has high intensity, suggesting that it is of neurogenic origin.

coronal and sagittal images than it is for the more common transaxial images. The imaging sequences as well as cardiac gating are similar to those described for the transaxial plane. Sagittal T1-weighted SE sequences are useful for the assessment of the supraclavicular and peridiaphragmatic regions. Sagittal or coronal T2-weighted images can help evaluate abnormalities in the supraclavicular and brachial plexus areas, the superior sulcus of the lung, chest wall, and diaphragm. Webb and colleagues (1984a) reported that both sagittal and coronal images occasionally display abnormalities that are not evident on transaxial scans and help to confirm suspected abnormalities.

Cine Magnetic Resonance Imaging

Cine MR imaging is a fast process that uses rapid imaging gradient-recalled echo — GRE — sequences. Haase and co-workers (1986) described how low flip angles and GRE are used. Several versions are used, and all acquired image data with reference to the ECG. Information from about 20-msec segments of the cardiac cycle is used to create a cine-formated image with a framing rate of 20 to 40 frames per minute. The short TR allows for image acquisition in less than 12 seconds, permitting imaging during breath holding. The major thoracic application of cine MR imaging has been to evaluate cardiac and great vessel morphology, function, and blood flow. The resultant images, when displayed in a cine mode on a television monitor, have the spatial resolution of cine angiocardiograms, but less than that of conventional MR, CT, or radiographic images. A major difference between conventional MR imaging and cine MR imaging is the visibility of rapidly flowing blood with the latter technique. A signal void from the intravascular compartment at the appropriate site is an indirect measure of vascular turbulence seen with stenosis or regurgitation.

Sechtem and colleagues (1987) showed that the cardiac functions that can be evaluated with cine MR imaging are ventricular volumes and their derivations, including stroke volume; regional ventricular function, including segmental wall motion and wall thickening; valvular regurgitation through incompetent cardiac valves; and valvular stenoses. Imaging of coronary artery bypass grafts and of sites of acute myocardial infarction remains controversial. Evaluation of congenital heart disease is beyond the scope of this chapter, but a combination of SE and GRE imaging rivals angiocardiography in providing diagnostic information.

Because of the short TR and TE used in cine MR imaging, tissue contrast is low. Combined with the poor spatial resolution, the images are not useful for imaging thoracic structures apart from the cardiovascular system. Higher temporal resolution with this system does not compensate for the loss of the other imaging parameters.

Suggested Protocols

Zerhouni (1992) described a series of protocols that can be used for most thoracic lesions. Depending on the known site or nature of the suspected lesion, these protocols may be modified or changed. The suggested general protocols are as follows: 1) A survey T1-weighted SE sequence in the coronal plane to embrace the entire thorax. This series allows precise localization for the subsequent axial images. They should be 8- to 10-mm thick with a 2-mm intersection gap, 2 averages, a 256 × 192 matrix, and ECG-gated. 2) A T1-weighted SE sequence in the axial plane through the region of interest. The TR will be equal to the RR interval of the ECG, and the TE should be about 15 to 20 msec. The other parameters are similar to the coronal series. Presaturation adjacent to the imaging volume will suppress blood flow artifacts; respiratory compensation will reduce motion artifacts; oversampling in the frequency encoded direction avoids wrap-around artifacts. Lastly, 3) Optional, additional imaging sequences include: a) T1-weighted SE sequences in the sagittal plane for supraclavicular and paradiaphragmatic regions; b) tangential, T1-weighted SE sequences for chest wall invasion; c) T1-weighted SE sequences after gadolinium infusion for vascular enhancement (e.g., chest wall invasion); d) T2-weighted SE sequences in axial or coronal planes for discrimination between fat and cysts; and e) GRE sequences for enhancement of flowing blood and imaging of vascular structures.

NORMAL FINDINGS

Tissue Contrast and Characterization

The relative MR imaging intensity of thoracic tissues is completely different from their relative x-ray density as depicted on CT scans. For instance, fat is the most intense normal tissue found on MR imaging, whereas on CT scans, its density is lower than that of normal solid tissues. Alterations in the MR imaging parameters used to obtain the image can also change the relative intensity of tissues, and thus the contrast between them. On T1-weighted images, mediastinal, subcutaneous, and auxiliary fat have slightly different image signal intensities, but for practical purposes, their intensities can be considered equal.

The normal involuted thymus gland in the adult has a slightly lower MR imaging intensity than fat, and it can be distinguished from mediastinal fat within the prevascular space. Normal mediastinal lymph nodes, the esophagus, and many neoplasms have an intermediate signal intensity similar to cardiac or skeletal muscle. The normal lung and the large airways contain air and display essentially no MR signal. Cortical bone similarly has few protons susceptible to MR, and essentially no measurable MR signal. The mucosa of the trachea and esophagus can demonstrate high signal intensity on T2-weighted SE images. The tracheal and laryngeal cartilages have variable signal intensity. The mediastinum and hila have a limited variety of normal tissue and thus tissue intensities.

Generally, T2-weighted images that use long TR and TE imaging sequences eliminate most contrast between normal thoracic tissues, and between normal and ab-

normal tissues. The tissue intensities and the T1 and T2 relaxation times of abnormal thoracic tissues have been studied extensively. Abnormal tissues within the mediastinum and hila, whether inflammatory or neoplastic, generally have T1 relaxation times that are longer than those of mediastinal fat and the thymus, and they can be recognized on images with the appropriate imaging sequence, usually those with T1 weighting. Fatty masses such as lipomas or thymolipomas have specific MR imaging characteristics. Fibrous masses, such as focal mediastinitis, have low signal intensity on T1- and T2-weighted SE images. Discrimination of other benign inflammatory masses or nodes from neoplasia based on their MR signal intensity or relaxation times remains controversial. Unconfirmed studies indicate that neoplastic tissue may have slightly longer T1 and T2 relaxation times than inflammatory tissue.

Blood Flow Effects

As von Schulthess and co-workers (1985) showed, the intravascular compartment most commonly has no evident signal on SE image sequences, if blood is flowing rapidly through the vessel. MR signal can, however, be seen in vessels, depending on several factors (Table 13–1). Moving nuclei observe a disrupted imaging sequence and produce little or no signal. For instance, if the imaging plane is 8-mm thick and the imaging sequence takes 80 msec, blood with a velocity of 10 cm/sec will flow across the plane during one sequence. The velocity at which signal disappears will thus be close to 10 cm/sec. Most blood flow in large vessels exceeds 10 cm/sec, and thus on ungated images, it will not be visible. Blood flowing at lower velocities, especially less than 3 cm/sec, will be seen and may demonstrate "paradoxic enhancement," demonstrating MR signal intensity that is greater than stationary blood. Paradoxic enhancement is more apparent when TR is short and TE is long. This enhancement occurs when slowly flowing blood enters the imaging field only partially unperturbed by the RF pulses and thus more fully magnetized. The enhancement on longer echo — TE — images is caused by the longer echoes being even numbered, not because of the time involved. An artifact on MR imaging, unrelated to slow flow and producing an intravascular signal, is known as an

Table 13–1. Factors Influencing Intravascular MR Signal

Technical
    Pulse sequence
    Sectional position in multisection sequence
    Spin-echo type
    Imaging gradient
    Cardiac synchronization

Biologic
    Direction of flow
    Velocity of flow
    Acceleration/deceleration
    Velocity profile

even-echo rephrasing artifact and must be differentiated from slowly flowing blood. With GRE imaging sequences, MR can be used to image flowing blood, and both noninvasive angiography and measurement of regional blood flow and perfusion are being developed.

Normal Anatomy

In normal subjects, mediastinal and hilar structures usually seen on CT scans are readily identified on SE images. The best anatomic detail is obtained from images with a short TE and a long TR, because the signal-to-noise ratio is optimal. Cardiac gating of the images by reducing motion distortions provides even better anatomic display, even though the signal-to-noise ratio may not be optimal.

The great arteries arising from the aorta are always visible, as well as the ascending aorta, aortic arch, and descending aorta (Fig. 13–2). The walls of the aorta and great vessels, but not the contents of these vessels, are seen on SE images. The systemic venous system of the thorax, including the subclavian veins, brachiocephalic veins, and venae cavae are also demonstrated. The ascending segment and arch of the azygos vein are evident in most normal subjects. The portions of the

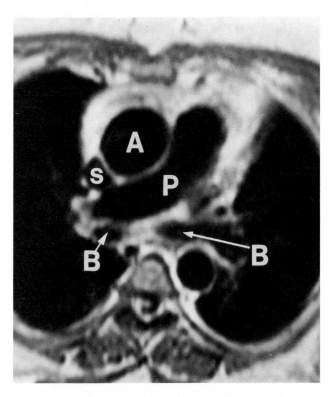

Fig. 13–2. ECG-gated SE MR image through the midthorax. The aorta (A), pulmonary arteries (P), superior vena cava (S), and bronchi (B), are all seen. The vessels appear empty because flowing blood is not seen at this portion of the cardiac cycle. *From* Lenoir S, et al: Cahiers d'IRMS, thorax. Aspects normaux et pathologiques. Paris: Masson, 1993.

airway demonstrated on spin-echo images are the trachea, main bronchi, intermediate bronchus, and lobar bronchi. The loss of signal within the lungs on MR images permits visualization of only an occasional segmental bronchus. The walls of the large mediastinal airways are often distorted by respiratory motion on MR images obtained during breathing. The vessels, trachea, and central bronchi are easily distinguished from high-intensity fat within the mediastinum. The esophagus is evident behind the trachea. On T2-weighted images, the mucosa of the esophagus and occasionally of the trachea demonstrates high intensity. On T1-weighted images, normal lymph nodes less than 10 mm in diameter are readily identified in the prevascular, pretracheal, and subcarinal regions.

The thymus, within the prevascular space, is recognized more easily by MR than by CT imaging. The shape, size, and signal intensity of the normal thymus is age dependent. In the infant and child, the thymus has intermediate intensity similar to muscle or lymph nodes. In the adult, the MR image intensity of the thymus increases with fatty replacement, although it is variable among individuals. It is considerably more intense than lymph nodes or most tumors. The thymus is more distinctive and appears larger on SE images than on CT scans.

The pericardium is shown distinctly on ECG-gated SE images through the heart, especially anteriorly and to the right of the cardiac chambers (Fig. 13–3). It appears as a thin, low-intensity line less than 4-mm thick. The superior pericardial recesses are distinctive on SE images through the base of the heart. The aorta and ventricles together with their valves, as well as segments of the coronary arteries, are routinely evident. The present resolution of MR imaging does not permit evaluation of alteration of the caliber of vessels the size of the coronary arteries.

Within the hila, the lumen of blood vessels and bronchi usually produce no signal, and are distinguished from each other by their known anatomic locations. Collections of fat are visible at three locations in the hila: lateral to the right pulmonary artery where it bifurcates in the midhilum, at the origin of the right middle lobe bronchus in the lower right hilum, and where the left pulmonary artery descends and gives origin to its left upper lobe branches in the left midlung hilum.

The main right pulmonary artery is sectioned longitudinally on transaxial images. Anterior to the pulmonary artery are the upper lobe pulmonary veins and superior vena cava, whereas the right main stem bronchus and intermediate bronchus are behind the right pulmonary artery. On the left side, the main pulmonary artery is 1 to 2 cm higher than on the right, with the superior pulmonary veins anterior, and the left main stem bronchus inferior. The top of the left atrium and the left atrial appendage are anterior to the left superior pulmonary vein. At a slightly higher level, the left pulmonary artery originates from the main pul-

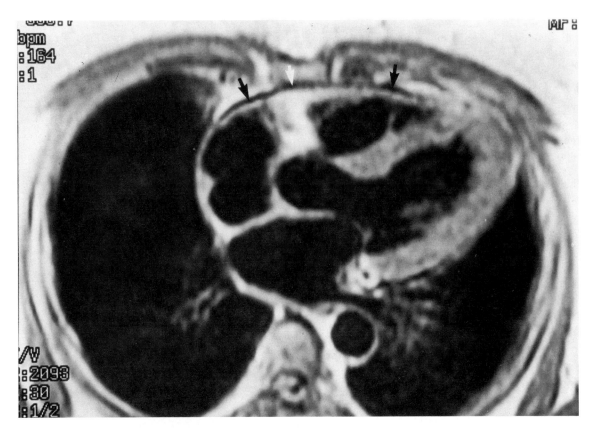

Fig. 13–3. Normal ECG-gated MR image through the heart. The cardiac chambers, myocardium, and pericardiac space (arrows) are well depicted. *From* Lenoir S, et al: Cahiers d'IRMS, thorax. Aspects normaux et pathologiques. Paris: Masson, 1993.

monary artery to course posteriorly above the left main bronchus. Medial to the left pulmonary artery is the tracheal carina.

Structures that are particularly well displayed in the sagittal and coronal projections are the venae cavae and their connections to the right atrium, the azygos veins, the central pulmonary arteries, and the descending aorta. The ascending aorta, the aortic arch, and the descending aorta can be demonstrated in continuity on oblique lateral images if the patient is positioned correctly. The central bronchi and their positions within the hila are particularly well imaged in coronal images through the midthorax.

The pulmonary circulation resembles the systemic circulation on SE images. Only the walls of the central pulmonary vessels are demonstrated. No signal is seen within the pulmonary arteries or veins unless it is caused by technical factors, gating, or slice position. Pulmonary arteries beyond the hila are not visible in normal subjects. Of the pulmonary veins, only those close to the mediastinum and left atrium are demonstrated routinely.

Loss of signal from magnetic susceptibility effects in thoracic images precludes obtaining a signal from the lungs with SE or GRE images. T1 and T2 relaxation measurements from the lungs are thus not different from background values in ungated images. With cardiac gating, measured MR image signal intensity increases during parts of the cardiac cycle. This signal represents intravascular blood imaged during vascular diastole because of pulsatile flow in the pulmonary circulation. With new intravascular contrast agents for use in MR imaging, such as gadolinium-DTPA, intravascular signal can be detected more easily, but this does not translate into useful images.

ABNORMAL FINDINGS

Mediastinum and Hila

Lymphadenopathy

Within the mediastinum, detection of normal and abnormal lymph nodes depends critically on their size and their contrast with surrounding structures. Magnetic resonance imaging can detect many normal-sized lymph nodes and most abnormal nodes. On T1-weighted images, normal nodes can be found throughout the mediastinum. Those in the lower pretracheal and subcarinal spaces tend to be slightly larger than at other sites. The contrast between high-intensity mediastinal fat and intermediate intensity lymph nodes allows for their identification. In early studies without cardiac gating, cardiac pulsation during the 10- to 15-minute image acquisition time resulted in occasional summation of several small lymph nodes into what was misinterpreted as a single large lymph node or a mediastinal mass. Magnetic resonance imaging is also of limited value in the detection of nodal calcification. Nodes less than 1 cm in transverse diameter are considered normal in size. The appearance of abnormally large lymph nodes and their changes in intensity with changes in imaging sequences cannot reliably distinguish between benign and malignant lymphadenopathy. Dooms (1984) and von Schulthess (1986) and their associates provided some provisional data indicating that the actually measured T1 and T2 relaxation times of tissues may allow discrimination between neoplastic and inflammatory tissue. This finding, however, has not been translated into a practical test in clinical imaging because of the substantial overlap between normal and abnormal tissues. In various studies, both retrospective and prospective, CT and MR imaging have shown comparable accuracies for detecting mediastinal lymphadenopathy (Fig. 13–4). In addition, MR imaging can detect hilar lymph nodes not shown with CT, especially when ECG-gated images are used.

Mediastinal Masses

The relationship between a mediastinal mass and adjacent vessels is better demonstrated with MR than with contrast-enhanced CT imaging, because of the excellent contrast between the signal void within vessels and the mass, as well as the absence of streak artifacts on SE images. On contrast-enhanced CT scans, streaking artifacts can obscure small mediastinal vessels. Similarly, MR demonstration of vascular compression or invasion by a mediastinal mass is excellent. Abnormal flow signal from a compressed vessel must, however, be differentiated from vascular invasion by the compressing mass.

Tumor is usually distinguished from normal mediastinal fat by using T1-weighted SE images (Fig. 13–5). For example, in a group of benign and malignant mediastinal masses, T1 values of the masses were about 1500 msec, whereas the T1 values of surrounding mediastinal fat averaged between 300 and 400 msec. The T2 relaxation values of inflammatory mediastinal masses can differ significantly from those of neoplastic masses. This difference, however, does not produce a characteristic difference in appearance on either T1- or T2-weighted SE images. In fact, SE images with a T2-weighted sequence produce an image in which both the tumor and mediastinal fat have similar signal intensities, and the mass may be impossible to distinguish from normal mediastinal fat.

Webb and Moore (1985) showed that volume averaging of high-intensity mediastinal fat and low-intensity flowing blood can cause an area of intermediate signal intensity that mimics a mediastinal mass. This occurs, for instance, in the aortopulmonic window with volume averaging of the left pulmonary artery. Although the

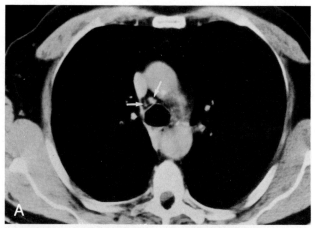

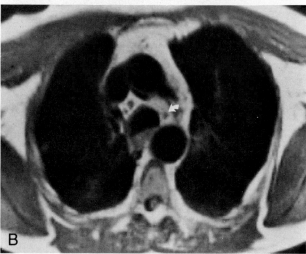

Fig. 13–4. Normal mediastinal lymph nodes, comparably seen with CT and ECG-gated MR imaging. *A,* CT scan demonstrates two small pretracheal lymph nodes (arrows). *B,* MR scan shows the same two lymph nodes and a third lymph node (curved arrow) in the aortopulmonic window.

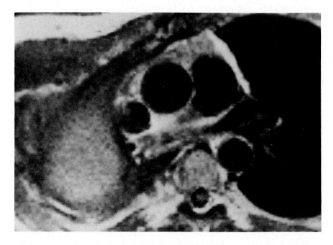

Fig. 13–5. Mediastinal metastatic tumor. A T1-weighted MR image demonstrates replacement of high-intensity mediastinal fat by low-intensity metastatic carcinoid tumor from the right lung. The patient has had a right pneumonectomy.

signal intensity of volume averaging and mass can appear the same on T1-weighted images, a mass increases in intensity relative to fat on a T2-weighted image, whereas volume averaging does not change in relative intensity.

The detection and evaluation of a mediastinal mass and its edge depends both on the contrast between the mass and surrounding tissues, and on the spatial resolution of the image. The spatial resolution of SE and GRE images is less than that of CT scans, and small masses, or the edges of larger masses, can be more difficult to evaluate with MR imaging. In comparison with CT, however, MR imaging, because of its high-contrast resolution, allows the detection of most mediastinal masses larger than 1 cm in diameter. In some instances, mediastinal masses that are not seen on CT scans are visible on MR imaging, most commonly because a small mass is mistaken for a vessel on the CT image.

Benign neoplasms of the mediastinum do not differ significantly from malignant neoplasms either in MR signal intensity or in relaxation values. Fluid-filled or necrotic masses may be diagnosed as such by MR imaging based on their longer T1 and T2 relaxation times, resulting in high signal intensity on T1- and T2-weighted images. Magnetic resonance imaging performed with T2-weighted images results in a significant increase in signal from the fluid or necrotic components of a mass, and can demonstrate heterogeneous areas not visible on T1-weighted images, as I and my co-workers (1984) showed (Fig. 13–6).

Calcification within a mediastinal mass has diagnostic significance in many circumstances. On MR images, calcifications appear as low-intensity areas, and are indistinguishable from other causes of low signal intensity.

Using both T1- and T2-weighted MR imaging, recurrent tumor has been distinguished from post-treatment radiation damage or fibrosis. Glazer and colleagues (1985) demonstrated that post-treatment fibrosis tends to have a lower signal intensity on both T1- and T2-weighted images, whereas recurrent tumor tends to have a higher signal intensity, especially on T2-weighted images. Differentiation between the two is clinically limited by the variable quantity of inflammation in areas of radiation fibrosis and by the known imprecision of MR imaging measurements. Similar reservation applies in distinguishing between a mediastinal mass resulting from fibrosing mediastinitis and other masses such as lymphomas or carcinomas.

Mediastinal hematomas can be identified with MR imaging because of their characteristic signal intensity. On T1-weighted images, fresh blood and subacute hematoma show high signal intensity because of high protein fluid in the first circumstance and methemaglobin in the second. On T2 weighting, however, the fresh hematoma shows high signal intensity while the subacute hematoma has low signal intensity. Subacute hematomas also tend to show low-intensity zones and rings of varying intensity caused by hemosiderin-laden macrophages and foci of methemaglobin.

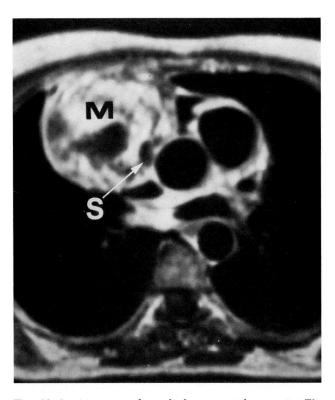

Fig. 13–6. Anterior mediastinal thymoma with necrosis. T1-weighted SE image shows a heterogeneous mass (M) encasing the superior vena cava (S). *From* Lenoir S, et al: Cahiers d'IRMS, thorax. Aspects normaux et pathologiques. Paris: Masson, 1993.

Hilar Masses

Webb and colleagues (1984b) showed that the normal pulmonary hilum consists of pulmonary arteries, pulmonary veins, small amounts of fat at specific sites, and a few inconsistent small lymph nodes. The detection of a hilar mass requires the distinction between normal structures and abnormal soft tissues. At some sites within the hilum, this differentiation can be made on anatomic grounds, but at other sites, masses and vessels are difficult to separate. Rapidly flowing blood results in little MR imaging signal and thus only the walls of the pulmonary arteries and veins are visible. Hilar masses are readily detected against the background of the walls of the bronchi and vessels (Fig. 13–7). The small amount of fat and small lymph nodes are not a significant problem in detecting hilar masses. Normal hilar lymph nodes are only 3 to 5 mm in diameter and are evident within the hilar fat. The most common causes for a hilar mass are bronchial carcinoma, lymphoma, metastatic lymphadenopathy, or inflammatory lymphadenopathy. Magnetic resonance imaging allows a confident diagnosis of hilar mass, and clearly shows the relationship of the mass to normal vessels and central bronchi. Hilar masses are considerably more conspicuous and the relationship of the mass to vessels is demonstrated at least as well with MR as with CT scanning. In several instances, hilar lymph nodes larger

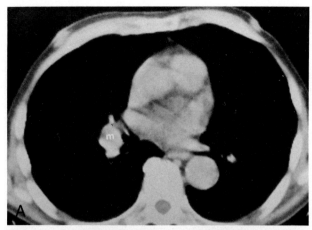

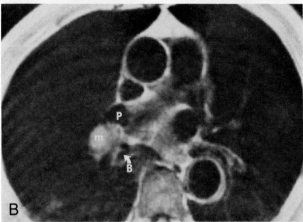

Fig. 13–7. Right hilar bronchial carcinoma. *A*, CT scan at the level of the origin of the middle lobe bronchus shows the mass (M) cannot be distinguished from the adjacent interlobar pulmonary artery. *B*, MR image at the same level demonstrated the mass (M) readily separated from the artery (P) and bronchus (B).

than 1 cm in diameter that were not seen clearly with CT have been detected by MR imaging.

In many circumstances, a radiographic evaluation of the pulmonary hilum also requires evaluation of the bronchial tree within the hilum. Bronchial narrowing is an indication of adjacent disease, and is important in guiding endoscopic evaluation of the central airways. The resolution of MR imaging at present does not permit detailed evaluation of the bronchial tree; this is better performed with CT imaging. For this reason, CT scanning is still favored for the initial evaluation of suspected hilar masses.

Thymic Hyperplasia and Thymomas

De Geer and co-workers (1986) showed that the normal thymus is readily demonstrated by MR imaging because it contrasts with anterior mediastinal fat on T1-weighted images from its longer T1 relaxation time. The average thymus-to-fat hydrogen density ratio is 0.60. Although the T1 relaxation time of the thymus is longer than that of fat in patients under 30 years of age, the difference decreases in older age groups. The

T2 relaxation time of the thymus is similar to that of fat, and does not change with age. The normal thymus is about 2.8 × 1.9 cm and is 5 to 7 cm in a craniocaudad direction. The thymus appears thicker on MR images than on CT scans in patients older than age 20 years. Magnetic resonance may be better than CT imaging in distinguishing between thymus involuted with fat and mediastinal fat.

Thymic hyperplasia, whether idiopathic, as a rebound phenomenon from steroids or chemotherapy, or associated with thyrotoxicosis, usually produces thymic enlargement without a mass effect. The signal intensity of thymic hyperplasia is the same as for the normal thymus. In patients with treated lymphoma, distinction between thymic hyperplasia and lymphomatous infiltration can be difficult. Foci of high intensity or T1- and T2-weighted images can indicate necrosis within a lymphoma. Lymphoma may also show low-intensity areas and inhomogeneity of the enlarged thymus.

Most thymomas can be detected on axial imaging studies producing a round, oval, or lobulated mass deforming the normal bilobed appearance of the thymus. With T1 weighting, they have an intermediate signal intensity similar to muscle; on T2-weighted images, they are higher in intensity and can be inhomogeneous (see Fig. 13–6). Molina and colleagues (1990) showed that ECG-gated MR is equal to or better than CT scanning for delineating the extent of local invasion of thymic tumors. The malignant potential of thymomas is closely related to their capsular invasion and mediastinal extension. Detection of mediastinal extension and transpleural spread of the tumor is important for prognosis and therapy. MR imaging for evaluation of possible thymic tumors should embrace the entire thorax to include the posterior costophrenic extent of the pleural space. In determining resectability of an invasive thymoma, the relationship of the tumor to arterial and cardiac structures is of particular importance.

From 10 to 15% of patients with myasthenia gravis have thymomas. These tumors are usually resected because up to half of them are malignant. Magnetic resonance imaging, like CT scanning, can be used as a screening method. Magnetic resonance imaging theoretically also can be useful for following the patient after treatment with radiation therapy for nonresectable thymic tumors, and MR imaging may be able to differentiate between radiation changes and recurrent or residual tumor. On T2-weighted images, thymic tumor is high in intensity, whereas radiation fibrosis remains low in intensity.

Thymolipomas are unusual benign tumors of the thymus, composed almost entirely of fat, with microscopic foci of thymic tissue. They can become large, tending to envelope the heart and pericardium and obliterating the cardiophrenic angles. Thymolipomas characteristically are well circumscribed, with high intensity on T1- and T2-weighted images. Large vessels passing through the tumor can produce low-intensity channels.

Fibrosing Mediastinitis

Fibrosing mediastinitis most commonly is caused by radiation therapy or histoplasmosis. The fibrosing process may be diffuse, or focal and masslike. The focal form is more likely to cause compression or obstruction of mediastinal veins, arteries, or bronchi. Rholl and co-workers (1985) described a focal mass that is low in intensity both on T1- and T2-weighted images. On CT scans, most cases of fibrosing mediastinitis demonstrate calcification within the mass. Unfortunately, these calcifications cannot be appreciated on the usual SE images. The collateral channels that develop with obstruction to the normal mediastinal venous pathways are evident on SE images as abnormal tubular structures without intraluminal signal or on GRE images as high-intensity structures. Obstruction of a central pulmonary artery or vein can be appreciated from narrowing and distortion of the lumen. Bronchial obstruction is more difficult to appreciate on MR imaging. The rare complication of fibrosing mediastinitis with pulmonary vein obstruction and focal pulmonary edema has been demonstrated by MR imaging.

Germ Cell Tumors

Malignant germ cell tumors of the mediastinum occur predominantly in young adult males, some of whom can show elevated levels of alpha-fetoprotein, human gonadotrophins, or both. Their MR imaging characteristics are varied with seminomatous tumors — not associated with elevated tumor markers — tending to be homogeneous and nonseminomatous germ cell tumors — always associated with marked elevations of the aforementioned tumor markers — often containing heterogeneous zones. Most anterior mediastinal masses are resected unless they are proven to be lymphomatous or malignant germ cell tumors. The initial specialized imaging study will be a CT scan. When CT does not demonstrate the relationship of the mass to vascular mediastinal structures satisfactorily, MR imaging should be considered for the additional information it may provide.

Esophageal Carcinoma

The normal esophagus is demonstrated inconsistently in the mediastinum by MR imaging as Quint and colleagues (1985) described. It can usually be seen near the thoracic inlet and the diaphragm, and can be distinguished from mediastinal fat surrounding it on T1-weighted images. The lumen of the esophagus may contain low-intensity air and the mucosal lining can be recognized by its high intensity. Neither CT nor MR imaging is accurate in showing the extent or depth of wall penetration by esophageal carcinoma. The signal intensity of tumor and muscle are not sufficiently different to show the tumor on T1-weighted SE images. Minor extraesophageal extension of tumor with obliteration of fat planes also is not an accurate or reliable finding with MR imaging especially in the middle third of the esophagus where it is flattened against the left atrium. Minor extraesophageal extension of the tumor, however, does not preclude surgery.

For determining the curative resectability of advanced esophageal carcinoma, the degree of involvement of cardiovascular and aerodigestive tract organs invaded by the tumor is of major importance. CT scanning has been shown to be accurate for this purpose. Magnetic resonance imaging can show extraesophageal extension of the tumor and mediastinal organ involvement by encasement of mediastinal vessels, distortion or compression of the trachea, or contact of the mass with more than one quarter of the circumference of the aortic wall.

Although a comparison of the relative accuracy of MR and CT imaging for staging esophageal carcinoma has not been undertaken, the multiplanar imaging capabilities of MR are attractive. Surgeons who have experience with MR staging of esophageal carcinomas appreciate the depiction of the tumor and its relationships in the coronal and sagittal planes.

Thyroid Masses

As shown by Higgins and colleagues (1986, 1988), thyroid goiters are lower in signal intensity than the normal thyroid on T1-weighted SE images, and frequently contain foci of high intensity attributable to proteinaceous cysts and subacute hemorrhage. Solid adenomas often show high signal intensity on T1-weighted images, whereas functional nodules within a goiter frequently are isointense to the normal thyroid. Zones of calcification within a goiter are seen as areas of signal void and cannot be distinguished as such. Benign goiters are well encapsulated and are diagnosed readily on MR and CT scans. Their intrathoracic extension can also be demonstrated.

Thyroid carcinoma can involve the mediastinum by direct extension or by lymph node metastases. Auffermann and co-workers (1988) showed that the MR imaging features of thyroid carcinoma are variable and do not separate benign from malignant masses. T1-weighted SE images, especially in the sagittal plane, can define the extent of mediastinal and adjacent organ invasion by a known thyroid carcinoma. T2-weighted SE images may also assist in differentiating recurrent tumor with high signal intensity from postoperative or radiation-induced fibrosis.

Parathyroid Adenomas

Imaging of the patient with hyperparathyroidism for a localized adenoma can be achieved with multiple techniques. Krubsack and colleagues (1989) compared radionuclide, sonographic, CT, and MR studies of parathyroid tumors. Magnetic resonance imaging should probably be reserved for difficult cases and for patients with persistent hyperparathyroidism after surgery. Sophisticated techniques using thin sections, a high resolution matrix, and surface coils are necessary, as described by Auffermann and colleagues (1988). Because some parathyroid adenomas may be intrathoracic — in the anterior or visceral compartment — MR imaging should include areas as far inferiorly as the base of the heart. Ectopic adenomas show low signal intensity on T1-weighted SE images and usually high signal intensity on T2 weighting, although this is variable.

Pulmonary Parenchyma

Focal Lung Disease and Pulmonary Nodules

Computed tomography and high resolution CT — HRCT — scanning remain the primary imaging techniques for focal lung masses. MR imaging has had limited clinical use for this purpose and at present is insufficient for routine use. A few applications, however, have been demonstrated. Müller and colleagues (1985) showed that neoplastic lung nodules appear as regions of substantially higher intensity than normal lung parenchyma on both T1- and T2-weighted images. Exceptions are heavily calcified or fibrotic nodules or nodular arterial venous malformations, which can be as low in intensity as the surrounding lung. For most lung lesions, T2-weighted images improve demonstration of the mass, as lung tissue remains dark and the lesion usually becomes brighter because of its longer T2 relaxation time. Primary and metastatic malignant masses tend to have long T2 relaxation times. In searching for lung nodules, MR imaging can demonstrate central nodules that may be mistaken for blood vessels on CT scans. Thus, I advocate MR in addition to CT imaging for patients being considered for resection of pulmonary metastases.

I and my colleagues (1987) have shown that distinguishing between benign and malignant pulmonary nodules is not possible based on their MR imaging characteristics. One exception to this general rule is the mass associated with early invasive aspergillosis in immunocompromised patients. Herold and co-workers (1989) showed that early invasive aspergillosis had a characteristic target-like appearance on MR images from central necrosis and surrounding subacute hemorrhage. Later hemorrhagic infarction may be a prominent feature.

Distinction between a central bronchial carcinoma and peripheral obstructive pneumonitis may be possible with MR imaging using T2-weighted images. The distal fluid-filled lung, because of its high water content, can display a higher signal intensity than the proximal tumor.

Similarly, Carrillon and colleagues (1988) showed that lipoid pneumonia has a characteristic high-signal intensity on T1-weighted images. Using analogous imaging characteristics, Herold and colleagues (1991) showed that on T2-weighted SE images of nonobstructive atelectasis, signal intensity was low, whereas with obstructive atelectasis, signal intensity was high (Fig. 13–8).

Diffuse Lung Disease

The normal lung shows no signal above background on SE or GRE images, in most adults. Bergin and colleagues (1990) presented information on MR imaging with novel sequences that allow for visualization of lung

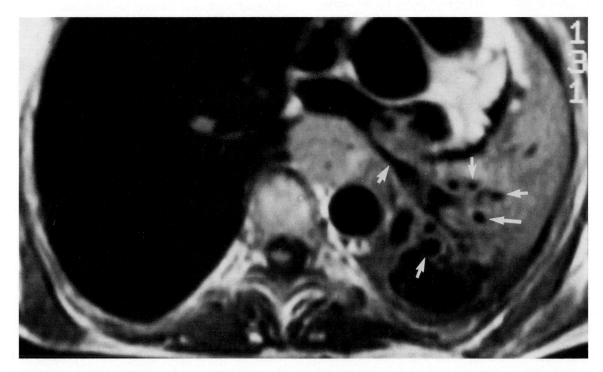

Fig. 13–8. Nonobstructive atelectasis of the left lower lobe. T2-weighted MR image shows low intensity of the consolidated lung. Round and tubular structures within the lung (arrows) are bronchi and pulmonary vessels. *From* Lenoir S, et al: Cahiers d'IRMS, thorax. Aspects normaux et pathologiques. Paris: Masson, 1993.

structures. These techniques are promising but experimental. On SE images, signal can be detected in the posterior dependent portion of the normal lung in some individuals, reflecting a combination of atelectasis, condensed lung parenchyma, and increased dependent blood flow to the lung bases in the supine position.

Pulmonary consolidation can be recognized using MR imaging, but differences in signal intensity or MR image signal characteristics among different causes of lung consolidation except for diffuse hemorrhage have not been found. The MR imaging characteristics overlap substantially in the different causes of lung consolidation, although alveolar proteinosis is notable for its low signal intensity. McFadden and colleagues (1987) studied a group of patients with interstitial lung disease. The most severely affected patients had the greatest signal intensity on MR imaging. Improvement, as indicated by a decrease in signal intensity, was seen after treatment. In this study, qualitative MR imaging was useful in predicting clinical course. Relaxation times, however, were not sufficiently precise to differentiate between active and inactive interstitial lung disease. Müller and colleagues (1992) found that consolidated areas of alveolitis in patients with infiltrative lung disease were shown equally well on CT and MR images. MR imaging was, however, not as good as CT for displaying morphologic abnormalities in the lungs.

In experimental studies in rats, Vinitski and coworkers (1986) found that MR imaging signal intensities were significantly elevated in both bleomycin-induced alveolitis and fibrosis. Both T1 and T2 values in alveolitis were the same as in controls, but were significantly decreased in fibrotic lung disease. Changes in T1 and T2 values correlated with changes in water content of the diseased lung. In practical terms, MR imaging for the diagnosis and evaluation of diffuse lung disease is an exciting area for future investigation, but at present, it cannot be considered a clinical application.

The Opacified Hemithorax

In patients with an opacified hemithorax, a combination of pleural and parenchymal abnormalities often coexists. These complex pleuroparenchymal abnormalities are often difficult to evaluate. In the absence of air and with reduced motion, the opacified hemithorax is suitable for MR imaging. Templeton and Zerhouni (1989) and Herold and colleagues (1991) showed that areas of abscess formation, tumor, compressed lung, and pleural effusion could all be readily distinguished with MR imaging (Fig. 13–9). The opacified hemithorax that is of obscure origin is a suitable indication for thoracic MR examination.

Bronchial Carcinoma

The MR image signal intensity from bronchial carcinomas varies. Most bronchial carcinomas yield low intensities on T1-weighted images, and higher intensities on T2-weighted images. Some tumors, however, show low intensities on both T1- and T2-weighted images, whereas others show high intensities on T1-

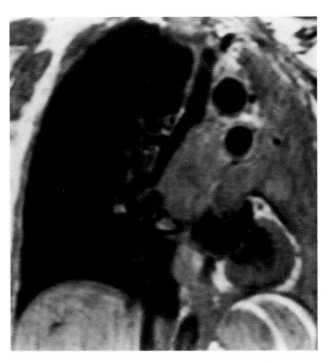

Fig. 13–9. MR image of an opacified hemithorax. Gated SE image shows the hemithorax contains a large tumor mass invading the mediastinum and encasing the aorta and pulmonary artery. *From* Lenoir S, et al: Cahiers d'IRMS, thorax. Aspects normaux et pathologiques. Paris: Masson, 1993.

weighting. The best contrast between lung carcinomas and surrounding mediastinum or hilar tissues has been with T1-weighted images. The adjacent tissues are usually fat or blood vessels, and T1-weighted imaging distinguishes between the bronchial mass or metastatic lymph nodes and fat.

The imaging of bronchial carcinoma for staging of the tumor requires a precise determination of the anatomic extent of tumor. For imaging purposes, tumors are resectable or nonresectable. Resectable tumors are confined to one hemithorax. Contiguous spread does not involve the organs of the mediastinum, spine, or sternum. Chest wall or diaphragmatic involvement is such that it can be resected. Nodal involvement is such that the metastases are intracapsular, low, and ipsilateral. Tumors that conform to the above are stage I, II, or IIIA. Tumors that are not resectable have extended beyond the confines of one hemithorax and cannot be removed. These tumors are designated IIIB or IV (see Chapters 87 and 89).

Most important in determining the resectability of the tumor is the presence and distribution of mediastinal lymph node metastases. With T1-weighted SE sequences, the lymph nodes appear less intense than surrounding fat (Fig. 13–10). With a longer TR value, the intensities of the nodes increase relative to fat, contrast decreases, and nodes may not be detected. In comparison with CT, MR imaging more often provides comparable information regarding the presence and size

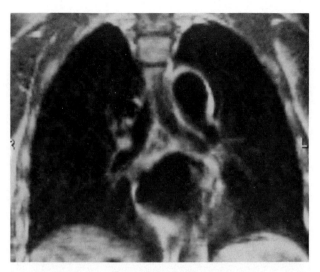

Fig. 13–10. Subcarinal metastatic lymph nodes from bronchial carcinoma. Coronal MR image demonstrates several slightly enlarged subcarinal lymph nodes not seen with CT or transaxial MR imaging and suspicious for metastasis.

of mediastinal lymph nodes. Webb and colleagues (1985) showed that CT and MR imaging usually classify nodes identically: as normal — less than 1.0 cm; suspicious — 1.0 to 1.5 cm; or abnormal — more than 1.5 cm. When MR imaging and CT interpretations differ, MR imaging may discriminate between tumors and vessels more readily.

The signal intensity of mediastinal lymph nodes and their T1 and T2 characteristics do not help distinguish lymph nodes that are involved by tumor. In the diagnosis of hilar mass or lymph node enlargement, MR imaging is superior to intravenous contrast material-enhanced CT, largely because hilar vessels and soft tissue are easily distinguished by MR scanning. Care must be taken, however, not to diagnose normal hilar tissue as abnormal. Webb and colleagues (1991), as well as others, have shown that CT and MR imaging are only about 65% accurate in determining the nodal — N — or tumor extent — T — stage of a bronchial carcinoma. In that study of over 180 patients, however, only two had lesions diagnosed as being resectable when they were found to have undetected disease that could not be removed.

With direct invasion of the mediastinum by a lung cancer, CT and MR images may both suggest invasion. Heelan and colleagues (1985) showed that direct invasion of the mediastinum adjacent to a hilar mass is usually better demonstrated on MR imaging because of the ease with which tumor and mediastinal vessels and fat can be distinguished (Fig. 13–11). The majority of paramediastinal tumors that do not have clear features of mediastinal organ invasion are resectable. Invasion of mediastinal cardiovascular and aerodigestive structures — stage IIIB — indicates nonresectable tumor, as Mountain (1985) described. Encasement or distortion of mediastinal organs is generally seen better with MR than with CT imaging.

Magnetic resonance imaging can also show tumor invasion of the chest wall. Invasion of thoracic muscle causes an increase in signal intensity that is demonstrated on T1- and T2-weighted images (Fig. 13–12). Determination of chest wall invasion, however, remains difficult. The criteria considered in the interpretation of CT may also be applicable to MR imaging. These findings include an obtuse angle of the lung mass with the chest wall; more than 3 cm of contact between the mass and the pleural surface; and thickening of the pleura adjacent to the mass. None of these signs, however, are sensitive or specific. Rib destruction by a mass involving the chest wall is specific but has little sensitivity, and rib destruction is more easily discerned on conventional radiographs or CT images.

New surgical techniques that allow resection of focal chest wall involvement by tumor may obviate the need for detection of subtle wall invasion. Proximity to the chest wall and the need for probable chest wall resection may be sufficient information prior to resection.

Bronchial carcinoma commonly metastasizes to upper abdominal organs, notably the adrenal glands and liver, and most authorities recommend scanning the upper abdomen when staging the tumor with CT. This step is not possible with MR imaging because of time constraints. With more rapid imaging sequences, however, time limits may not be a problem. In one study, the adrenal glands were the most frequent site of metastases at autopsy performed within 1 month of a "curative" resection, and were present in 38% of subjects. In a study by Falke and co-workers (1987), an adrenal mass was seen on CT scans in 21% of patients with non-small cell bronchial carcinoma. Up to two thirds of adrenal masses in patients with lung cancer are adrenal adenomas, and therefore biopsy of most enlarged glands is necessary before a diagnosis of

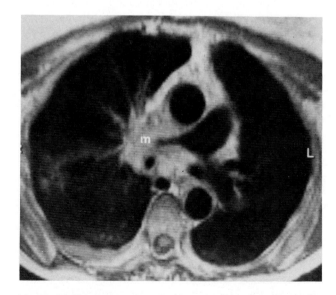

Fig. 13–11. Right hilar bronchial carcinoma invading the mediastinum. MR imaging demonstrates the lower intensity mass (M) narrowing the right pulmonary artery and surrounding the intermediate bronchus.

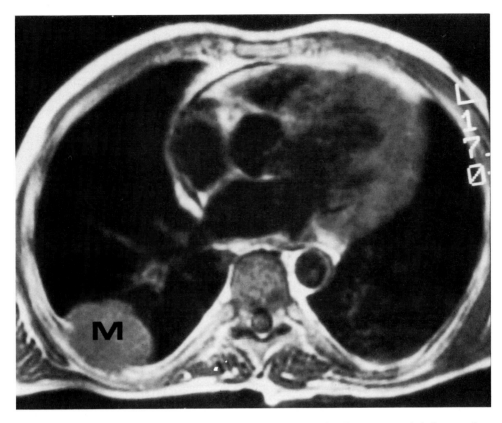

Fig. 13–12. Chest wall invasion by bronchial carcinoma. The right lower lobe peripheral tumor mass (M) disrupts the extrapleural fat and intercostal muscles. *From* Lenoir S, et al: Cahiers d'IRMS, thorax. Aspects normaux et pathologiques. Paris: Masson, 1993.

metastasis can be accepted. MR imaging with T2-weighted images can distinguish adrenal metastases and other significant neoplasms — carcinomas, pheochromocytomas — from adrenal adenomas in many patients, according to Glazer and colleagues (1986). More recent studies, however, as discussed by Reining (1992), have shown sufficient overlap between different causes of an adrenal mass for MR imaging not to be an acceptable clinical test for characterizing adrenal masses.

Bronchial abnormalities are better seen on CT than on MR imaging, primarily because of its better spatial resolution. Because not all lobar or segmental bronchi are visible on MR images in healthy subjects, a bronchus that is not seen clearly on MR imaging cannot be considered normal. The lung parenchyma and any subtle lesion within it are also poorly displayed on MR images. For these reasons, MR imaging is an adjunct in the patient with bronchial carcinoma. This technique can be of benefit for assessing the following: 1) Central tumors with equivocal mediastinal organ involvement, or penetration of the aortopulmonic window; 2) Peripheral tumors with equivocal chest wall, spine, or sternal invasion; 3) Paracardiac tumors with equivocal cardiac, pericardial, or diaphragmatic invasion; and 4) Superior sulcus tumors, as discussed subsequently.

Vascular Lesions of the Mediastinum

Magnetic resonance imaging has the capability of tomographically demonstrating large vascular structures without added contrast material and in multiple projections. With the increased experience described by many groups, MR imaging can now be accepted as the primary technique for evaluating abnormalities of the aorta, mediastinal veins, and central pulmonary arteries.

Aorta

Acute aortic rupture resulting from trauma is still best evaluated with aortography. Investigators have little experience with MR imaging in this setting, and the problems of patient monitoring and life support systems in a magnetic environment preclude the use of MR imaging in most such patients. Chronic pseudoaneurysms in survivors of aortic injury can be evaluated by MR imaging.

Congenital Anomalies. Both in children and adults, MR imaging is the most accurate method for determining the precise location and nature of aortic anomalies such as truncus arteriosis, anomalous vascular branching, coarctation, and double arches. As Rees and colleagues (1989) showed, the MR images can be oriented along the long axis of the aorta and the precise site of narrowing in lesions such as aortic coarctation are demonstrated.

Aortic Aneurysm and Aortic Rupture. White and colleagues (1986) described that both CT and MR imaging have advantages over aortography in detecting thoracic aortic aneurysms. Both can assess the thickness of the aortic wall, accurately measure the size of the aorta, and characterize the extent of the abnormality. The excellent delineation of calcifications available from CT images is advantageous in assessing the aortic wall. A contained aortic rupture can be seen on MR images as a mediastinal soft tissue density or wall thickening. The appearance of a hematoma on MR imaging is usually specific, particularly at higher magnetic field strengths. A major advantage of MR over CT imaging is the ability of cine MR imaging to detect and estimate the degree of aortic valve insufficiency. Thus, MR imaging is particularly useful in assessing aneurysms of the sinuses of Valsalva, for which CT is ill suited.

Aortic Dissection. The principal diagnostic tasks of imaging in patients suspected of having aortic dissection are to document the presence of dissection and to establish the extent of involvement if dissection is present. Both sensitivity and specificity of the primary diagnosis must be high, as false-positive and false-negative errors are unacceptable. Assignment of the type of dissection must also be accurate, because patients with type A dissections are immediate surgical candidates, whereas those with type B dissections are usually managed medically in the acute phase.

Current imaging methods in aortic dissection include angiography, CT scanning, sonography, and MR imaging. Although sonography is accurate in assessing the ascending aorta, its limited field of view precludes its use as a general diagnostic test. Angiography is still the reference standard method for patients who have dissection, although it has several limitations. It is invasive, carrying the risk of further traumatizing the vessel by the necessary catheter manipulations, and compromising the patient by the need for injection of large volumes of contrast material, with potential hemodynamic and renal toxicity. Angiography also is attended with a small incidence of both false-positive and false-negative diagnoses, and its field of view is limited to the opacified vascular lumina. CT scanning is accurate and widely used for evaluating aortic dissections; the intimal flap and the true and false lumina can be identified in many cases. The pericardium can be assessed and renal function can be roughly estimated by contrast enhancement of the kidneys. Computed tomography, however, requires a large volume of contrast material; cannot evaluate the aortic valve or reliably identify branch vessel involvement; and is limited in its ability to distinguish thrombus from slow flow in the false lumen. If any of the technical factors used with CT are suboptimal, or if artifacts are present, diagnostic accuracy is compromised.

Magnetic resonance imaging has many advantages for evaluating the hemodynamically stable patient by being able to assess the entire aorta without contrast material and noninvasively, as shown by Lois (1987) and Link (1992) and their associates.

Imaging in the axial and oblique parasagittal planes usually suffices to provide a cross-sectional view of the entire abnormality, including the intimal flap (Fig. 13–13). Because of the orientation and frequent tortuosity of the aorta and the tendency of flaps to spiral, detecting the entire extent of a dissection using only the transaxial plane occasionally is difficult. Clot and slow flow in the false lumen can usually be differentiated on GRE images. The presence of pericardial effusion or hemopericardium can also be identified. Using a GRE technique, the presence and degree of aortic insufficiency can be identified. The relationship of arch and abdominal branch vessels to the dissection often can be delineated. Mediastinal hematoma from complicating aortic rupture can be detected.

Magnetic resonance imaging has high sensitivity and specificity for detecting and typing aortic dissections. A study of MR imaging in aortic dissection by Kersting-Sommerhoff and co-workers (1988) demonstrated for an experienced reader a sensitivity of 100% and a specificity of 90%, whereas an inexperienced reader had an 83% sensitivity and a 90% specificity. About 20% of the images in this study were rated as suboptimal to inadequate. It was considered that experience is required to recognize flow artifacts and differentiate slow blood flow from thrombus. This study, however, included only standard SE images; it is likely that the addition of GRE images in potentially confusing cases would have permitted a more confident diagnosis in cases with prominent flow artifacts. A limitation of MR imaging in assessing dissections is its yet unquantified and possibly limited accuracy in determining small branch vessel involvement, such as the coronary arteries. Some surgeons, however, believe that this information is not critical in preoperative assessment.

Although most cases of dissection are readily diagnosed, some focal dissection or dissection hematoma without lumenal connection can present with focal findings or abnormalities limited to thickening of part of the circumference of the aortic wall.

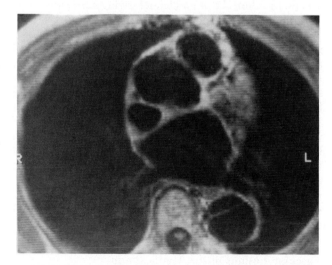

Fig. 13–13. Aortic dissection, type B. MR imaging through the descending aorta demonstrates a flap across the vessel lumen with rapid blood flow (signal void) in both the true and false lumens.

Magnetic resonance imaging can also be useful in the evaluation of patients after repair or with unrepaired chronic dissection to determine the development of complications and monitor the results of surgical treatment.

Mediastinal Veins

Magnetic resonance imaging with SE and GRE sequences has been shown by McMurdo (1986) and Weireb (1986) and colleagues to be an excellent method of displaying the mediastinal venous systems. Monitoring and positioning of long-term indwelling catheters is greatly facilitated with MR images obtained in the axial plane. Thrombosis of indwelling catheters is common and repeated positioning of catheters may be necessary. Thrombosis and slow flowing blood can be distinguished with GRE sequences or with phase-sensitive images, as shown by Tavares and co-workers (1989). In patients with thrombosis, MR images show the vein as larger than normal, frequently with perivascular haziness. Fresh thrombi are high in signal intensity, whereas older clots show reduced signal intensity.

Pulmonary Arteries

Pulmonary Hypertension

The severity of the anatomic and functional abnormalities demonstrated by MR imaging in patients with pulmonary hypertension is proportional to the severity of the hypertension. The central pulmonary arteries in the mediastinum and hila can be measured precisely on CT scans. O'Callaghan and co-workers (1982) found that the diameter of the right pulmonary artery was 16.6 to 26.6 mm in a small group of patients with pulmonary hypertension. Accurate CT measurements of the interlobar and proximal lung arteries can also be obtained. I found that the caliber of the main pulmonary artery, measured from CT scans, accurately predicts pulmonary artery pressure. Kuriyama working with me (1984) showed that pulmonary artery diameter correlated with pulmonary artery pressure with a coefficient of 0.89. The upper limit of normal for the main pulmonary artery was 28.6 mm. A diameter greater than 28.6 mm readily predicted pulmonary hypertension. Using ECG-gated MR imaging is as precise as or is more precise than CT scanning in determining caliber of the central pulmonary vessels.

Right ventricular hypertrophy, frequently with flattening or convexity of the intraventricular septum toward the left ventricular chamber, is invariably present with severe pulmonary hypertension. Magnetic resonance imaging readily demonstrates right ventricular enlargement and displacement of the intraventricular septum.

Magnetic resonance imaging can also show decreased velocity of pulmonary blood flow in pulmonary hypertension. von Schulthess and colleagues (1985) demonstrated intraluminal signal during a major part of the cardiac cycle as the MR imaging manifestation of

decreased blood velocity. In most patients with a pulmonary systolic pressure above 90 mm Hg, intraluminal signal is visible in gated MR imaging during systole. This finding is evident in only 30% of patients with a pressure below 90 mm Hg. In normotensive subjects, MR signal is evident only during late diastole when blood flow is slow. During systole and early diastole, blood flow is normally too rapid to be imaged (Fig. 13–14). In MR imaging of normal persons, the flow patterns are similar in the aorta and central

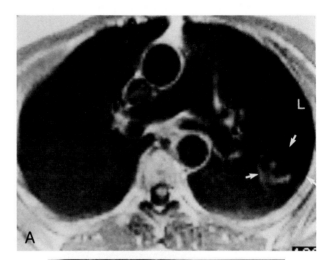

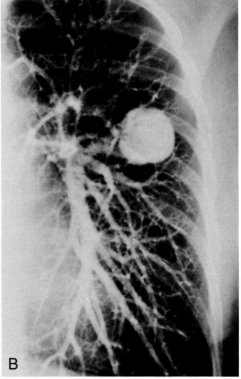

Fig. 13–14. Pulmonary arteriovenous malformation. *A*, MR imaging through the midlung demonstrates a mass (arrows) in the left lung. The mass contains a signal void, suggesting flowing blood. *B*, Pulmonary angiography demonstrates that the lesion is an arteriovenous malformation.

pulmonary arteries. Patients with pulmonary arterial hypertension also show a linear correlation between the intensity of the MR signal from the central pulmonary arteries and pulmonary vascular resistance.

Pulmonary Embolism

Blood flowing at normal velocity shows a signal void in the pulmonary arteries on ECG-gated SE images in systole. Emboli within the pulmonary arteries therefore can be suspected from these images. The intensity of pulmonary emboli varies, depending on the age of the clot. Chronic emboli produce low to medium intensity, and acute emboli have high intensity (Fig. 13–15). Intraluminal signal may also be caused by slow flow in the pulmonary arteries, as in pulmonary hypertension. Differentiation of emboli from flow signal is possible with GRE or phase-sensitive sequences.

White and colleagues (1987) made the diagnosis of central pulmonary embolism in several cases by using MR imaging, based on an intraluminal area of high signal intensity that was "fixed" during the cardiac cycle. Shad and colleagues (1989) confirmed these findings. The inconsistency with which the segmented and subsegmental pulmonary arteries are shown and the variability in signal from pulmonary emboli at this time preclude the use of MR imaging a clinically reliable technique in such an evaluation.

Pleura

Pleural effusions generally have long T1 and T2 values. The intensity of pleural effusions is low to very low on T1-weighted images, and thus small pleural effusions may go undetected when the adjacent lung is normal and thus also is very low in signal intensity. Many pleural effusions, however, become increased in intensity on T2-weighted images, and their recognition is then easier. Fluid within the lung has an intensity similar to that of fluid within the pleural space, and the recognition of pleural fluid is then based on the position

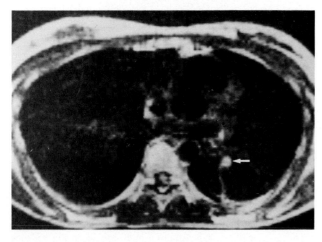

Fig. 13–15. Pulmonary embolus. MR imaging (nongated) demonstrated an intraluminal high signal lesion (arrow) in the left descending pulmonary artery. The embolus was confirmed with an angiogram.

and shape of the area of high signal intensity. Tscholakoff and colleagues (1988) showed that MR imaging has limited capability for determining the nature and type of fluid within the pleural space. In general, protein-containing exudates tend to become more intense on T2-weighted images. Thus far, investigators using MR imaging have not been able to distinguish between exudates and transudates reliably, mainly because of the degradation of the relaxation information from respiratory and fluid movement.

Hemorrhagic pleural effusions can, however, be distinguished from other pleural fluid collections. Hemothorax present for longer than a few days shows high signal intensities on both T1- and T2-weighted images. These findings have to be related to the magnetic field strength of the MR imager. Pleural hematoma presents a multicompartmented image on T1-weighted studies, with nonhomogeneous, low-intensity areas interspersed with high-intensity regions.

Thoracic Cage

Neurogenic Tumors

Siegel (1986) and Flickinger (1988) and their associates showed that MR imaging can demonstrate the region around the spine to excellent effect. The relationship of paravertebral tumors to the spine and adjacent bony structures was shown particularly well. Magnetic resonance imaging has become the method of choice for suspected paraspinal — paravertebral — mediastinal masses. Neurogenic tumors show variable intensity on T1-weighted images and tend to be heterogeneous on T2 weighting but show only high signal intensity similar to cysts. A disadvantage of MR imaging for the evaluation of paraspinal masses is its inability to detect bony destruction, and at times, both CT and MR imaging may be necessary for complete evaluation.

Chest Wall

Magnetic resonance imaging provides excellent soft-tissue contrast of the structures of the chest wall. It not only can display the morphology of chest wall lesions, but it can often provide information as to the cause of the mass or abnormality, for instance, invasion of the chest wall by a bronchial carcinoma. Recent experience has shown that gadolinium-based contrast material administered intravenously can improve the detection of chest wall invasion by a bronchial carcinoma. Haggar and colleagues (1987) showed that the finding of chest wall invasion include areas of high intensity from the invading mass, thickening of the muscle structures, disruption of the subpleural fat layer, and increased signal with otherwise normal appearing morphology (see Fig. 13–12).

Brachial Plexus

Developments in surface imaging coils and narrow-slice techniques have improved the MR demonstration

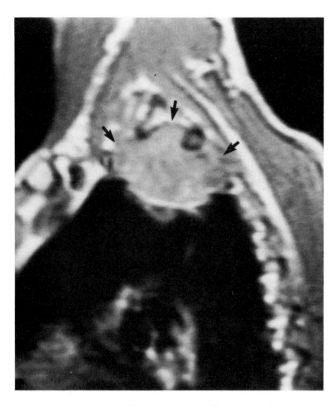

Fig. 13–16. Superior sulcus tumor. Sagittal MR image shows tumor extending from the apex of the lung into the lower neck to the region of the brachial plexus and subclavian artery (arrows).

of small superficial structures such as the organs within the neck and the brachial plexus. The contrast between soft tissues and the brachial vessels and nerves allows for detailed evaluation of anatomy and pathology in this region. Castagno and Shuman (1987) studied 47 patients with suspected brachial plexus involvement by tumor. Using multiple imaging planes and techniques, they demonstrated tumor involvement of the brachial plexus in many cases, and excluded involvement in those without disease (Fig. 13–16). On T2-weighted images, tumors tend to have higher intensity than the scalene muscles of the neck. The display of displacement and encasement of the subclavian artery by tumor is especially important. After treatment, T2-weighted SE images may differentiate residual or recurrent tumor from fibrosis.

Magnetic resonance imaging, when available, is the first choice for the evaluation of superior sulcus tumors and patients with brachial plexopathy of obscure origin.

Diaphragm

Experience with MR imaging of the diaphragm is limited. Some initial experience has shown, however, that especially in coronal and sagittal planes, it is possible to demonstrate the relationship of paradiaphragmatic masses to the diaphragm and to show transdiaphragmatic extension of these lesions.

REFERENCES

Auffermann W, et al: Diagnosis of recurrent hyperparathyroidism: Comparison of MR imaging and other imaging techniques. AJR Am J Roentgenol 150:1027, 1988.

Auffermann W, et al: Recurrent thyroid carcinoma: Characteristics of MR images. Radiology 168:753, 1988.

Bergin CJ, et al: Measuring susceptibility in the lungs (abstr). Radiology 177:313, 1990.

Carrillon Y, et al: MR diagnosis of lipoid pneumonia. J Comput Assist Tomogr 12:876, 1988.

Castagno AA, Shuman WP: MR imaging in clinically suspected brachial plexus tumor. AJR Am J Roentgenol 149:1219, 1987.

Crooks LE, et al: NMR whole body imager operating at 3.5 KGauss — 0.35T. Radiology 143:1169, 1982a.

Crooks LE, et al: Visualization of cerebral and vascular abnormalities by NMR imaging: The effects of imaging parameters on contrast. Radiology 144:843, 1982b.

de Geer G, Webb WR, Gamsu G: Normal thymus: Assessment with MR and CT. Radiology 158:313, 1986.

Dooms G, et al: Magnetic resonance imaging of lymph nodes: Comparison with CT. Radiology 153:719, 1984.

Falke THM, et al: Magnetic resonance imaging of the adrenal glands. Radiographics 7:343, 1987.

Flickinger FW, Yuh WT, Behrendt DM: Magnetic resonance imaging of mediastinal paraganglioma. Chest 94:652, 1988.

Gamsu G, et al: Nuclear magnetic resonance imaging of the thorax. Radiology 147:473, 1983.

Gamsu G, et al: Magnetic resonance imaging of benign mediastinal masses. Radiology 151:709, 1984.

Gamsu G, et al: A preliminary study of MRI quantification of simulated calcified pulmonary nodules. Invest Radiol 22:853, 1987.

Glazer HS, et al: Radiation fibrosis: Differentiation from recurrent tumor by MR imaging. Radiology 156:721, 1985.

Glazer GM, et al: Adrenal tissue characterization using MR imaging. Radiology 158:78, 1986.

Haase AA, et al: Flash imaging. Rapid NMR imaging using low flip angle pulses. J Magn Reson 67:258, 1986.

Haggar AM, et al: Chest wall invasion by carcinoma of the lung: Detection by MR imaging. AJR Am J Roentgenol 148:1075, 1987.

Heelan RT, et al: Carcinomatous involvement of the hilum and mediastinum: Computed tomographic and magnetic resonance evaluation. Radiology 156:111, 1985.

Herold CJ, Kuhlman JE, Zerhouni EA: Pulmonary atelectasis: Signal patterns with MR imaging. Radiology 178:715, 1991.

Herold CJ, et al: Invasive pulmonary aspergillosis: Evaluation with MR imaging. Radiology 173:717, 1989.

Higgins CB, Auffermann W: MR imaging of thyroid and parathyroid glands: A review of current status. AJR Am J Roentgenol 151:1095, 1988.

Higgins CB, et al: MR imaging of the thyroid. AJR Am J Roentgenol 147:1255, 1986.

Kersting-Summerhof BA, et al: Aortic dissection: Sensitivity and specificity of MR imaging. Radiology 166:651, 1988.

Krubsack AJ, et al: Prospective comparison of radionuclide, computed tomographic, sonographic, and magnetic resonance localization of parathyroid tumors. Surgery 106:639, 1989.

Kuriyama K, et al: CT-determined pulmonary artery diameters in predicting pulmonary hypertension. Invest Radiol 19:16, 1984.

Lanzer P, et al: Cardiac imaging using gated magnetic resonance. Radiology 150:121, 1983.

Link KM, Lesko NM: The role of MR in the evaluation of acquired diseases of the thoracic aorta. AJR Am J Roentgenol 158:1115, 1992.

Lois JF, et al: Magnetic resonance imaging of the thoracic aorta. Am J Cardiol 60:358, 1987.

McFadden RG, et al: Proton magnetic resonance imaging to stage activity of interstitial lung disease. Chest 92:31, 1987.

McMurdo KK, et al: Normal and occluded mediastinal veins: MR imaging. Radiology 159:33, 1986.

Molina PL, Siegel MJ, Glazer HS: Thymic masses on MR imaging. AJR Am J Roentgenol 155:495, 1990.

Mountain CF: A new international staging system for lung cancer. Chest 89:2258, 1985.

Müller NL, Gamsu G, Webb WR: Pulmonary nodules: Detection using magnetic resonance and computed tomography. Radiology *155*:687, 1985.

Müller NL, Mayo JR, Zwirewich CV: Value of MR imaging in the evaluation of chronic infiltrative lung disease: Comparison with CT. AJR Am J Roentgenol *158*:1205, 1992.

O'Callaghan JP, et al: CT evaluation of pulmonary artery size. J Comp Assist Tomogr *6*:101, 1982.

Pykett IL: NMR imaging in medicine. Sci Am *246*:78, 1982.

Quint LE, Glazer G, Orringer MB: Esophageal imaging by MR and CT: Study of normal anatomy and neoplasm. Radiology *156*:127, 1985.

Rees S, et al: Coarctation of the aorta: MR imaging in late postoperative assessment. Radiology *173*:499, 1989.

Reining JW: MR imaging differentiation of adrenal masses: Has the time finally come? Radiology *185*:339, 1992.

Rholl KS, Levitt RG, Glazer HS: Magnetic resonance imaging of fibrosing mediastinitis. AJR Am J Roentgenol *145*:255, 1985.

Schmidt HC, Tsay DG, Higgins CB: Pulmonary edema: A MR study of hydrostatic and permeability types. Radiology *158*:297, 1986.

Sechtem U, et al: Cine-MRI: Potential for the evaluation of cardiovascular function. AJR Am J Roentgenol *148*:239, 1987.

Shad HR, et al: Computed tomography and magnetic resonance imaging in the diagnosis of pulmonary thromboembolic disease. J Thorac Imaging *4*:58, 1989.

Siegel MJ, et al: MR imaging of intraspinal extension of neuroblastoma. J Comput Assist Tomogr *10*:593, 1986.

Tavares NJ, et al: Detection of thrombus by using phase-image MR scans: ROC curve analysis. AJR Am J Roentgenol *153*:173, 1989.

Templeton PA, Zerhouni EA: MR imaging of the opaque hemithorax (abstr). Radiology *173*:209, 1989.

Tscholakoff D, et al: Evaluation of pleural and pericardial effusion by magnetic resonance imaging. Eur J Radiol, In press.

Vinitski S, et al: Differentiation of parenchymal lung disorders with *in vitro* proton nuclear magnetic resonance. Magn Reson Med *3*:120, 1986.

von Schulthess GK, Fisher MR, Higgins CB: Pathologic blood flow in pulmonary vascular disease as shown by gated magnetic resonance imaging. Ann Intern Med *103*:317, 1985.

von Schulthess GK, et al: Mediastinal masses: MR imaging. Radiology *158*:289, 1986.

Webb WR, Gamsu G, Crooks LE: Multisection sagittal and coronal magnetic resonance imaging of the mediastinum and hila. Radiology *150*:475, 1984a.

Webb WR, et al: Magnetic resonance imaging of the pulmonary hila: Normal and abnormal. Radiology *152*:89, 1984b.

Webb WR, et al: Bronchogenic carcinoma: Staging with MR compared with staging with CT and surgery. Radiology *156*:117, 1985.

Webb WR, Moore EH: Differentiation of volume averaging and mass on magnetic resonance imaging of the mediastinum. Radiology *155*:413, 1985.

Webb WR, et al: CT and MR imaging in staging non-small cell bronchogenic carcinoma: Report of the Radiologic Diagnostic Oncology Group. Radiology *178*:705, 1991.

Weireb JC, Mootz A, Cohen JM: MRI evaluation of mediastinal and thoracic inlet venous obstruction. AJR Am J Roentgenol *146*:679, 1986.

Wexler HR, et al: Quantitation of lung water by nuclear magnetic resonance imaging: A preliminary study. Invest Radiol *20*:583, 1985.

White RD, Dooms GC, Higgins CB: Advances in imaging thoracic aortic disease. Invest Radiol *21*:761, 1986.

White RD, Winkler ML, Higgins CB: MR imaging of pulmonary arterial hypertension and pulmonary emboli. AJR Am J Roentgenol *149*:15, 1987.

Zerhouni EA: MR imaging in chest disease: Present status and future applications. *In* Syllabus: A Categorical Course in Diagnostic Radiology Chest Radiology. Chicago: RSNA 1992.

CHAPTER 14

RADIONUCLIDE STUDIES OF THE LUNG

William G. Spies

Ventilation/perfusion — V/Q — imaging of the lungs remains the most commonly performed radionuclide procedure of the chest in most nuclear medicine laboratories, most often performed for the detection of pulmonary thromboembolism. Since the introduction of this technique in the early 1960s, considerable refinements of the method have been developed, in terms of new radiopharmaceuticals, newer instrumentation and techniques, and more sophisticated methods of interpretation.

Ventilation/perfusion imaging has also been used for a variety of other clinical indications, such as the detection and quantification of obstructive airways disease, quantitation of right-to-left cardiac shunts, assessment of pulmonary trauma and inhalation injury, and monitoring of therapy in childhood asthma. The technique has also been used for the preoperative assessment of resectability of pulmonary neoplasms and prediction of postoperative pulmonary function. It may also be used in other clinical situations in which lung resection is contemplated in patients with compromised pulmonary function.

Gallium imaging of the chest is a sensitive but somewhat nonspecific method for the detection of neoplastic or inflammatory disorders. In the detection and staging of neoplasms such as bronchial carcinoma and lymphomas, it is used in conjunction with other techniques, including chest radiography, CT scanning, and lymphangiography. Gallium imaging has assumed an important role in the assessment of acute opportunistic infections, such as pneumocystis carinii pneumonia, and in patients with acquired immune deficiency syndrome and other entities associated with decreased immunocompetence. It can also be used for the quantification of pulmonary involvement with sarcoidosis, tuberculosis, and pneumoconioses.

Iodine-131 — ^{131}I — imaging is used to assess the presence of functioning metastases in patients with well-differentiated thyroid carcinomas. ^{131}I is also used therapeutically to ablate pulmonary metastases.

Radionuclide angiography is a useful noninvasive technique for evaluating vascular disorders of the chest, such as superior vena cava syndrome, and for assessment of the vascularity of intrathoracic masses.

Experimental methods of pulmonary radionuclide imaging have focused on the assessment of function and metabolism, such as alveolar-capillary permeability, amine receptor function, and pulmonary fluid balance. Radiolabeled monoclonal antibodies are being evaluated for the detection and treatment of a variety of intrathoracic neoplasms.

VENTILATION/PERFUSION — V/Q — IMAGING

Perfusion Imaging

Pulmonary perfusion imaging is performed by intravenously injecting radioactive particles that are large enough to be trapped in the pulmonary vasculature, specifically in the pulmonary arterioles and capillaries. The distribution of these particles is proportional to regional pulmonary blood flow. Technetium-99m — ^{99m}Tc — is the radionuclide of choice for these studies, because of its favorable gamma energy for imaging with a nuclear medicine gamma scintillation camera — 140 keV, low radiation dose to the patient, and short half-life of 6 hours.

The most commonly used radiopharmaceutical for pulmonary perfusion imaging is macroaggregated albumin — MAA — labeled with ^{99m}Tc. This agent is available commercially in kit form and provides particles in the range of approximately 10 to 60 μm in diameter. Human albumin microspheres — HAM — can also be labeled with ^{99m}Tc, resulting in a more uniform particle size, but are associated with a longer biologic half-life and greater cost, and are not widely available at present. The usual dose of ^{99m}Tc MAA given to an adult patient is 2 to 4 mCi of activity, which corresponds to approximately 200,000 to 500,000 particles injected. At this dose range, Harding and colleagues (1973) showed that less than 0.1% of the pulmonary arterioles are temporarily occluded, and therefore no physiologic effects are anticipated. In patients known to have severe pre-existing pulmonary arterial hypertension or having undergone pneumonectomy, the dose may be lowered to 1 to 1.5 mCi. Doses of more than 1 million particles are avoided, as are doses less than 100,000 particles, at which point the images may show areas of inhomogeneity on the basis of poor count statistics, in the absence of actual perfusion abnormalities. The particles are broken down and leave the pulmonary vasculature with a biologic half-life of 6 to 8 hours and are phagocytized by the reticuloendothelial system.

Adverse reactions, such as allergic responses to the radiopharmaceutical, have been reported, but are extremely rare. In addition to severe pulmonary arterial hypertension, other relative contraindications to pulmonary perfusion imaging with particulate radiopharmaceuticals include right-to-left intracardiac shunts and pregnancy. None of these is an absolute contraindication, and in fact, these agents are used clinically to quantitate known right-to-left shunts, as will be discussed. Rhodes and co-workers (1971) reported several occurrences of transient ischemic episodes after injection of radiolabeled MAA, but not with HAM. In pregnancy, a lower dose is used to minimize the radiation dose to the fetus.

One injects ^{99m}Tc-MAA intravenously while the patient is supine to minimize gravitational effects on the distribution of the particles in the pulmonary vasculature. After injection, the patient may be moved without affecting particle distribution. Imaging may be performed with the patient upright or supine. Eight views are routinely obtained: anterior, posterior, right and left posterior oblique, right and left anterior oblique, and right and left lateral. Caride and colleagues (1976) and Nielson and associates (1977) showed that the posterior oblique views are particularly important in detecting and localizing lower lobe perfusion defects, the most common site of involvement in pulmonary embolism.

Imaging is performed with a gamma scintillation camera, most often using a large field of view with a low-energy parallel hole collimator, or a smaller standard field of view camera with a low-energy diverging collimator in the case of portable examinations. Each image is generally obtained for 300,000 to 1,000,000 counts. A normal perfusion lung scan is illustrated in Figure 14–1. In some laboratories, single photon emission computed tomography — SPECT — cross-sectional tomographic images are also obtained in the transaxial, sagittal, and coronal planes, although this practice is not common and is largely limited to research applications at present.

Ventilation Imaging

Ventilation imaging is performed by having the patient inhale either a radioactive inert gas or a fine, uniform radiolabeled aerosol. The most widely used agent is xenon-133 gas — ^{133}Xe. Standard spirometric

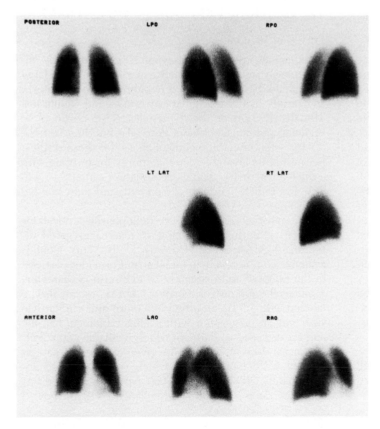

Fig. 14–1. Normal ^{99m}Tc-MAA perfusion study. Eight views. Top row, left to right: posterior, left posterior oblique, right posterior oblique. Middle row: left lateral, right lateral. Bottom row: anterior, left anterior oblique, right anterior oblique.

apparatus may be used for the study, but a system for either venting or trapping the exhaled gas must be used because of the relatively long half-life of the radionuclide — 5.3 days.

The ^{133}Xe ventilation study is usually performed in three phases. The patient first inhales deeply as 10 to 20 mCi of ^{133}Xe is injected into the intake port of the spirometer. The patient holds his or her breath as long as possible while a posterior image of the lungs is obtained for 25,000 to 250,000 counts. This single breath image reflects regional ventilatory rates. Areas of lung that are well ventilated accumulate activity, and areas that are poorly ventilated appear as photopenic — "cold" — defects. It may not be possible to obtain this image in patients who are extremely dyspneic.

The patient then breathes a mixture of ^{133}Xe and oxygen in a closed system with a carbon dioxide absorber for 3 to 5 minutes, to achieve an equilibrium in the distribution of the radioactive gas in the lungs. A 300,000 to 600,000 count equilibrium wash-in image is obtained at the conclusion of this phase. This image reflects the total ventilated lung volume, and all areas of lung that are ventilated show activity on the image. In some laboratories, serial images are also obtained during the wash-in phase.

The final and most important phase is the wash-out, during which the patient breathes room air and the exhaled ^{133}Xe is trapped in a charcoal system or vented away by an exhaust system. Serial wash-out images are obtained, typically at intervals of 30 seconds to 1 minute, for at least 5 minutes. On these images, the activity normally disappears from the lungs within 3 to 4 minutes symmetrically. Areas of obstructive airway disease appear as focal or diffuse zones of ^{133}Xe retention or asymmetric wash-out. Many nuclear medicine physicians have begun including posterior oblique images in the wash-out study to better localize ventilatory abnormalities in the anteroposterior dimension. Normal and abnormal ventilation studies are shown in Figure 14–2. Alderson and others (1974, 1976, 1980) showed that the ventilation study is nearly twice as sensitive as routine chest radiographs and at least as sensitive as spirometric pulmonary function tests for the detection of obstructive airways disease. The wash-out portion of the study is the most sensitive part of the examination, and the duration of ^{133}Xe retention is qualitatively related to the severity of obstructive airway disease, as measured by pulmonary function studies.

Imaging with ^{133}Xe has certain disadvantages. Ventilation studies with ^{133}Xe usually are performed prior to perfusion scans, because the energy of the photopeak of ^{133}Xe is lower — 81 keV — than the ^{99m}Tc photopeak — 140 keV. If the perfusion study is performed first, degradation of the ventilation images results from downscatter of ^{99m}Tc photons into the ^{133}Xe window. This effect is most detrimental to the relatively count-poor wash-out portion of the study, which is the most important phase of the ventilation scan, as previously discussed. Some advocates of postperfusion ^{133}Xe ventilation imaging argue that this approach allows

ventilation studies to be tailored to the projection best showing the greatest perfusion defect(s) and obviated in the case of a normal perfusion scan. The feasibility of this approach has been discussed by Kipper and Alazraki (1982), but it has not been widely accepted, especially because most laboratories have relatively few normal perfusion studies. The low energy of the ^{133}Xe photopeak is also not optimally suited to imaging with the gamma camera, resulting in relatively low resolution images. In addition, the long half-life requires the use of special disposal techniques, as mentioned previously, and usually precludes the performance of portable ventilation studies. Finally, because of the dynamic nature of the study, multiple projections are not routinely obtainable, with the exception of the oblique wash-out views as described.

Other ventilatory agents have been used in an attempt to overcome these shortcomings. Xenon-127 is another isotope of xenon gas that has the advantage of higher gamma energies — 172 keV, 203 keV, and 375 keV — enabling ventilation imaging to be performed after perfusion imaging. This capability allows for selection of the best projection for the ventilation study; that is, the view that best shows the perfusion abnormality on the perfusion scan. Also, because the perfusion scan is done first, the ventilation study need not be obtained in patients whose perfusion scan is normal. The longer half-life of 36.4 days allows for longer shelf-life of the radiopharmaceutical, and the radiation dose to the patient is also lower because of the absence of beta decay. The major limitations to the use of ^{127}Xe are its limited availability and greater cost, which result because it is a cyclotron-produced radionuclide.

Another gas used for ventilation imaging is krypton-81m — ^{81m}Kr — also a cyclotron-produced radionuclide. Unlike ^{127}Xe, ^{81m}Kr is available from a generator system that may be used to deliver multiple doses throughout a given day. Krypton-81m has a 190 keV photopeak, which is suitable for imaging and permits the ventilation study to be performed after the perfusion scan, or as is more often done, concurrently. The ultra-short half-life of 13 seconds eliminates disposal problems and allows portable studies to be performed without traps or exhaust systems and without undue radiation exposure to hospital personnel.

Goris (1977) and Rosen (1985) and their associates have shown how this study may be performed in conjunction with the perfusion study, obtaining multiple ventilation and perfusion views sequentially, alternately switching between the ^{99m}Tc and ^{81m}Kr photopeaks. This sequence may be performed without moving the patient, resulting in corresponding sets of ventilation and perfusion images in all eight projections. The ventilation images are obtained by having the patient breathe an ^{81m}Kr/oxygen mixture during tidal respiration. These images are nearly equivalent to single breath ^{133}Xe images, with areas of abnormal ventilation appearing as zones of decreased activity. Schor and associates (1978) and Susskind and co-workers (1980) demonstrated overall good agreement between ^{81m}Kr

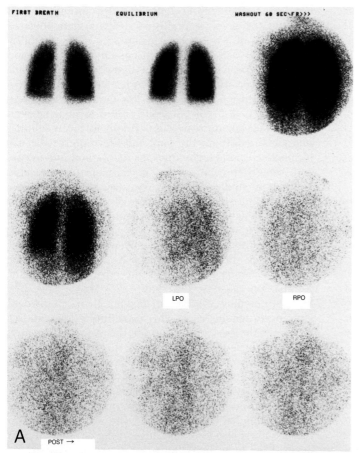

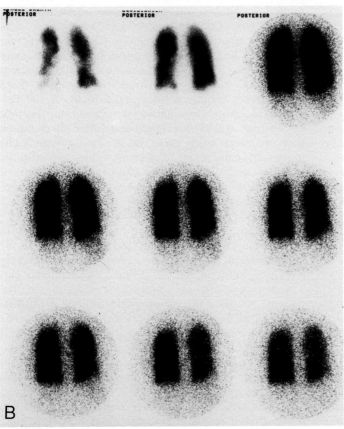

Fig. 14–2. *A,* Normal ¹³³Xe ventilation study. Top row: posterior single breath image, posterior equilibrium wash-in image, 0- to 1-minute posterior wash-out image. Middle row: 1- to 2-minute posterior wash-out image; 2- to 3-minute left posterior oblique wash-out image; 3- to 4-minute right posterior oblique wash-out image. Bottom row: 4- to 5-, 5- to 6-, and 6- to 7-minute posterior wash-out images. Uniform, symmetric ventilation is noted on the single breath and equilibrium wash-in images and normal wash-out, with complete clearance by 4 minutes. *B,* Abnormal ¹³³Xe ventilation study in a 65-year-old woman with chronic asthma and long-term ventilator dependency. Same views as *A,* except that all images are in the posterior projection. Diffusely irregular ventilation is noted on the single breath image, especially in the mid and lower lung zones, left greater than right. More uniform uptake is noted on the equilibrium wash-in image. The wash-out study demonstrates diffuse, severe ¹³³Xe retention up to the final 6- to 7-minute wash-out view.

and the xenon ventilation scans. It does appear that xenon studies are somewhat more sensitive for the detection of mild obstructive airway disease, probably because of the inability to perform a wash-out study with the ultra-short 13-second half-life of ^{81m}Kr. Other disadvantages of ^{81m}Kr include its high cost and limited availability. The parent half-life of the ^{81}Rb/^{81m}Kr generator is 4.6 hours. From a practical standpoint, the generator is only good for 1 day, and usually is no longer usable by evening nor obtainable on weekends for emergency V/Q scans.

A popular approach to ventilation imaging has been the use of ^{99m}Tc-labeled aerosols. Actually, introduced by Taplin and Poe (1965), this technique has regained popularity in recent years as a result of improved nebulizer technology, allowing for the production of a fine, uniform aerosol spray containing particles that are 1 to 2 μm or smaller. These aerosols are inhaled by the patient during tidal respiration and are deposited in the small airways. Alderson and others (1984) have shown that this technique is useable in the clinical setting, as an alternative to gas ventilation studies. Good agreement with results of ^{133}Xe and ^{81m}Kr ventilation studies was found. It is particularly useful in situations in which gases are not available or cannot be used, such as portable examinations and studies on critically ill or uncooperative patients. A potential pitfall is the deposition of the aerosol in the large central airways in patients with severe obstructive airways disease, which may lead to uninterpretable studies in approximately 6% of cases. Examples of normal and abnormal ^{99m}Tc-DTPA aerosol images are shown in Figure 14–3.

More recently, Burch (1986) and Sullivan (1988) and their associates in Australia used a ^{99m}Tc-labeled ventilation agent called "pseudogas" or "Technegas." This agent essentially consists of radioactive soot, an ultrafine, near-monodispersed aerosol — 0.12-μm diameter — produced by burning a spray of ^{99m}Tc-pertechnetate with graphite in a specialized furnace containing argon gas. The smaller particle size compared to conventional nebulizer-produced aerosols results in a more uniform distribution throughout the lungs, in normal subjects and in patients with obstructive airway disease, more closely approximating the distribution of a gas rather than an aerosol. In addition, less patient cooperation is required, because a sufficient amount of aerosol may be inhaled within one or two breaths in normal individuals and within 1 minute even in critically ill patients. Sullivan and co-workers (1988) found overall good correlation with ^{133}Xe gas and higher patient compliance when comparing the two agents in a limited pilot evaluation of patients having normal studies. This radiopharmaceutical is not yet FDA approved, and therefore it is not available for general use in the United States.

Pulmonary Embolism

By far the most common application of V/Q imaging is in the evaluation of patients with suspected pulmonary embolism — PE. Pulmonary embolism is a common cause of death in the United States, with an annual incidence of over 600,000 cases. Rosenow and others (1981) reported that more than 90% of PE originate in the deep venous system of the pelvis and thighs. Thus, the predisposing factors for deep venous thrombosis — DVT — of the lower extremities are also factors that increase the risk of PE. These factors include prolonged bed rest, congestive heart failure, recent myocardial infarction, malignancy, shock, prior thromboembolic disease, and hypercoagulable states such as pregnancy, oral contraceptives, and polycythemia vera. Recent surgery is an important risk factor, particularly pelvic, abdominal, and thoracic procedures, and orthopedic procedures such as total hip replacement. Huisman and associates (1989) reported a 51% prevalence of asymptomatic PE in patients with proven DVT undergoing V/Q scans, as compared to a prevalence of only 5% in comparable patients suspected but proven not to have DVT on subsequent objective testing. Foley and co-workers (1989) found that serial V/Q scintigraphy demonstrating new perfusion defects postoperatively after hip or knee replacement surgery was also associated with a significant number of cases of asymptomatic PE.

Dalen and Alpert (1975) estimated that approximately 89% of patients with PE survive longer than 1 hour after the initial event, but even in these patients, the correct diagnosis is made in less than one third. The mortality of untreated PE is about 30%, whereas 92% of treated patients survive. Furthermore, the signs, symptoms, and laboratory findings in PE are nonspecific. Thus, because the clinical diagnosis is difficult, and effective therapy is available but not without risk to the patient, the availability of an accurate, noninvasive diagnostic test is highly desirable.

The standard chest radiograph is neither a sensitive nor a specific test for PE. Diagnostic findings are rarely seen, and most patients demonstrate only nonspecific abnormalities such as subsegmental atelectasis, elevation of a hemidiaphragm, or small pleural effusions. Often, the chest radiograph is normal. The chest radiograph is nevertheless important, as it may reveal other causes for the patient's symptoms, and plays an important role in the interpretation of V/Q scans, as discussed subsequently. The radiograph usually is obtained immediately before or after the V/Q scan, and in no case should be more than 24 hours removed from the time of the scan.

Pulmonary angiography is considered the "definitive" test for PE, but it is an invasive, expensive procedure that may be associated with significant morbidity and mortality, especially in inexperienced hands or in critically ill patients. Furthermore, the accuracy of pulmonary angiography varies with the techniques used and method of interpretation. It is most often reserved for patients who have equivocal V/Q scans, in whom a major discrepancy exists between the prescan clinical suspicion for PE and the V/Q scan results, or those in whom heroic measures such as pulmonary embolectomy or thrombolytic therapy are contemplated. When necessary, pulmonary angiography should be performed, prefer-

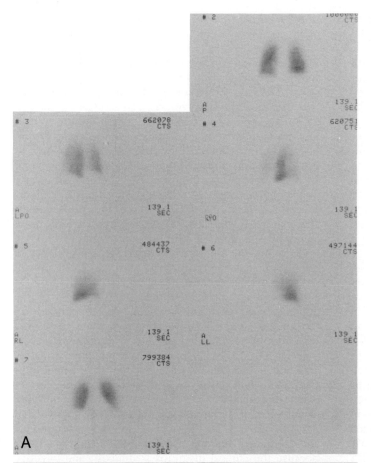

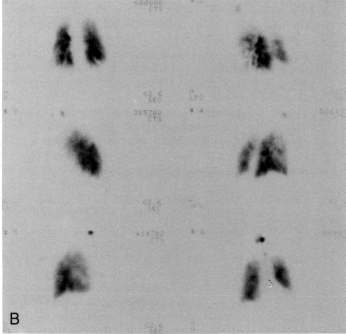

Fig. 14–3. *A,* Normal ^{99m}Tc-DTPA aerosol ventilation study. Clockwise from upper right: posterior, right posterior oblique, left lateral, anterior, right lateral, left posterior oblique. The activity inferior to the left lung represents swallowed aerosol in the stomach. *B,* Abnormal aerosol study in a 67-year-old woman with chronic congestive heart failure and obstructive airway disease. Clockwise from upper left: posterior, left posterior oblique, right posterior oblique, anterior, right lateral, left lateral. Note the central deposition of aerosol in the central airways and diffusely irregular ventilation, especially in the upper lobes. The activity superior to the lungs is aerosol adherent to the mask and tubing system.

ably within 24 hours or sooner after the lung scan, to avoid a false-negative angiogram secondary to clot lysis. In experienced hands, using the V/Q scan as a guide, pulmonary angiography is a safe and accurate procedure for the confirmation or exclusion of significant PE in selected cases.

Digital subtraction angiography has been used in some instances as a less invasive alternative to standard pulmonary angiography, as reported by Goodman and Brant-Zawadzki (1982). Advantages of this technique include the ability to obtain images in multiple projections in a short period of time and the superior contrast resolution afforded by digital image processing. On the other hand, the technique provides lower spatial resolution compared to standard radiography, and is adversely affected by artifacts from patient motion and cardiac and respiratory motion. Early proponents of this technique emphasized its noninvasive nature, using peripheral intravenous injections of contrast material, and depending on the high contrast resolution to produce adequate visualization of the pulmonary vessels. Piers and associates (1987) reported a good correlation with V/Q imaging using this technique. Musset and co-workers (1988) found the technique to be 94% sensitive for the detection of PE in the medium to large pulmonary vessels, but encountered 24% technically unsatisfactory studies, as well as an overall sensitivity in interpretable cases of only 81% when compared to conventional pulmonary angiography. Subsequently, Rosso and others (1989) from the same group concluded that in view of the inability of digital subtraction angiography to exclude PE confidently given a normal study, coupled with several false-positive examinations, that V/Q imaging should remain the screening examination of choice. Of greater interest recently has been the use of digital techniques for the recording and processing of data from conventional pulmonary angiograms as opposed to standard "cut" films, using the standard intra-arterial techniques to perform the study. In summary, although it is useful in selected cases, especially those involving intra-arterial injections, digital subtraction angiography lacks adequate spatial resolution to detect small or peripheral emboli, and clinicians may encounter significant problems related to artifacts in ill patients unable to cooperate, as well as from cardiac and respiratory motion. Its use in the detection of PE remains controversial, especially in terms of replacing conventional pulmonary angiography or V/Q imaging as noted by Alderson and Siegel (1987).

Magnetic resonance — MR — imaging has also been applied to the diagnosis of PE, as reviewed by Alderson and Martin (1987). This technique allows identification of intraluminal clots and abnormalities in pulmonary artery blood flow patterns. In addition, measurement of MR imaging T1 and T2 relaxation times associated with pulmonary infiltrates can in some cases suggest a greater likelihood of PE; an example is hemorrhagic infiltrates, which are more commonly associated with PE. More advanced methods of MR image acquisition have permitted greatly improved visualization of vascular structures. Posteraro and associates (1989) found cine MR to be superior to standard spin-echo MR imaging in detecting PE in the central pulmonary vessels. A new technique called MR angiography has permitted visualization of more peripheral vessels with significantly less artifact, as reviewed by Portman (1992). Nevertheless, to date, MR imaging has not been proven to be a clinically reliable method for

the accurate diagnosis of PE, in addition to being an expensive test not optimally suited to critically ill or uncooperative patients. Similarly, computed tomography — CT, although capable of identifying central intraluminal filling defects on contrast-enhanced studies, is not sensitive for the detection of small, peripheral clots. A new technique for rapid acquisition of CT images, called spiral volumetric CT, has been found by Remy-Jardin and co-workers (1992) to detect PE reliably in second to fourth division pulmonary vessels. Whether this technique proves to be a practical alternative method for the detection of PE remains to be seen.

Ventilation/perfusion-imaging remains the screening procedure of choice for the evaluation of suspected PE. The system of interpretation devised by Biello and co-workers (1979b) and refined by Alderson and others (1981) and by Biello (1987) has become the de facto standard for evaluating these studies. The principles on which this system is based include the overwhelming incidence of multiple emboli in patients with PE — in greater than 85% of cases — and the observation that PE usually produces perfusion defects in areas of normal ventilation; that is, V/Q mismatch. Although transient ventilatory abnormalities are demonstrated in experimental PE, such findings are fleeting, and Alderson and associates (1978) have shown that they are rarely observed clinically, except in the case of PE with infarction. Pulmonary infarction occurs in less than 10% of cases, and is usually associated with radiographic abnormalities.

Perfusion defects are categorized as to their number, size, and location. Large defects constitute 75 to 100% of a bronchopulmonary segment; moderate subsegmental defects are 25 to 75% of a segment, and small defects are less than 25% of a segment. Most authorities prefer to consider no single defect to be larger than a whole segment, and to characterize any defect larger than a single segment to constitute multiple defects. It is also a common practice to consider two moderate subsegmental defects to be essentially equivalent to a single segmental defect, although this judgment is subjective. V/Q scan findings are usually reported as high probability — greater than 90%, low probability — less than 5 to 10%, or intermediate — moderate — probability for PE.

Normal perfusion images essentially exclude PE, regardless of the findings on the chest radiograph or ventilation scan. Low probability studies demonstrate limited areas of ventilation/perfusion match or areas of mismatched perfusion abnormality that are in regions of radiographic abnormality, but are significantly less extensive. Small subsegmental perfusion defects are also not associated with angiographically demonstrable PE, even if unmatched. Less than 5% of patients with low probability scans had PE identified angiographically in the original retrospective studies of Biello and associates (1979a,b) (Fig. 14–4).

High probability scans demonstrate two or more unmatched defects in radiographically normal regions that are moderate or large in size, or unmatched defects

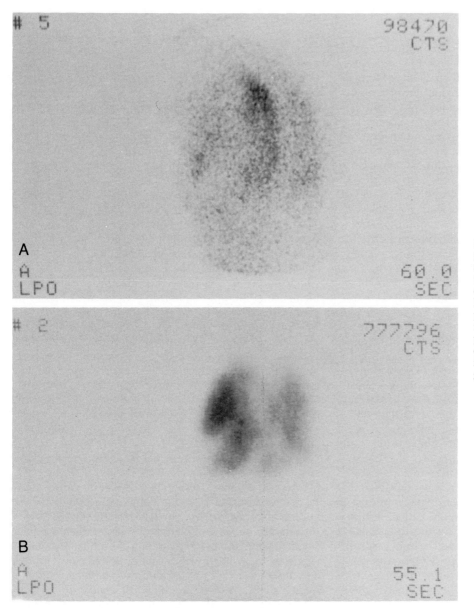

Fig. 14–4. Low probability ventilation-perfusion (V/Q) scan with matched V/Q abnormalities. *A*, 2- to 3-minute left posterior oblique ^{133}Xe wash-out image demonstrating focal areas of retention in the lingula, posterior segment of the left upper lobe, and posterior basal segment of the left lower lobe. *B*, Corresponding left posterior oblique ^{99m}Tc perfusion image demonstrates matching perfusion defects in the same segments. The chest radiograph was normal.

that correspond to radiographic abnormalities but are substantially larger. Approximately 90% of these scans are associated with PE on angiography (Fig. 14–5). The significance of a single segmental mismatch is controversial. Although originally considered to be high probability for PE, many experts have suggested that such studies be read as intermediate probability, as discussed by Biello (1987) and Catania and Caride (1990). Other entities producing perfusion abnormality out of proportion to ventilatory abnormality occasionally mimic PE, such as vasculitis, radiation therapy, pulmonary artery stenoses, and some infectious processes. The most common mimic is bronchial carcinoma, which may produce either V/Q match or mismatch, because of vascular compression or invasion, with or without bronchial obstruction. This possibility should be given strong consideration in particular in the case of a

whole-lung V/Q mismatch. Whole-lung mismatch related to pulmonary vasculitis associated with Takayasu's arteritis is illustrated in Figure 14–6. These other conditions can often be suspected on clinical grounds.

Intermediate probability is assigned to cases of extensive obstructive airway disease involving greater than 50% of the lung fields, perfusion defects corresponding to radiographic abnormalities of comparable size, when only a single unmatched defect — moderate or large — in a radiographically normal region is present, or any other cases not fitting into low or high probability categories (Fig. 14–7). In such cases, the V/Q scan provides no definitive evidence for or against the presence of PE. The post-test likelihood of PE in these patients lies somewhere between 10 and 90%, and the decision regarding further workup or therapy must be based on the level of pretest clinical suspicion and the

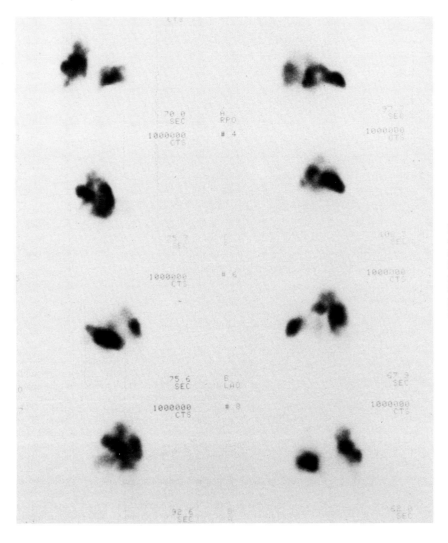

Fig. 14–5. High-probability V/Q scan in a 48-year-old male with lymphoma and acute onset of shortness of breath and hypoxia. ^{99m}Tc perfusion study demonstrating multiple segmental perfusion defects bilaterally. The ventilation study (not shown) was essentially normal, and the chest radiograph demonstrated only small bibasilar pleural effusions.

clinical status of the patient. In those patients with intermediate probability V/Q scans and high pretest suspicion for PE, treatment with anticoagulants may proceed, with a repeat V/Q scan often obtained in 10 to 14 days to assess resolution. In patients with low pretest suspicion, the V/Q results should be considered in conjunction with other clinical data, and other diagnostic possibilities should be explored. Patients with moderate clinical suspicion or relative contraindications to anticoagulation should undergo pulmonary angiography to confirm or exclude the presence of PE. In many cases, intermediate probability scans are best followed up by evaluating the patient for the presence or absence of DVT — the source of PE — by means of Doppler ultrasound, venography, or other methods.

In most centers, the majority of pulmonary angiograms are performed in patients with intermediate probability scans. Patients with high or low probability scans generally do not require angiographic confirmation, unless there is overwhelming clinical suspicion to the contrary or a contraindication to anticoagulation, in the case of a high probability scan. Angiographic proof is also usually obtained in cases of contemplated heroic

measures such as pulmonary embolectomy or thrombinolytic therapy. I and my associates (1986a) found that less than 15% of patients referred for lung scans ultimately underwent angiography over nearly a 6-year period.

The use of V/Q scintigraphy in the diagnosis of PE has not been without controversy. Robin (1977) severely criticized lung scanning, claiming that it grossly overdiagnosed PE, especially in young, previously healthy patients, leading to unnecessary and potentially dangerous overuse of anticoagulants. These remarks came at a time when lung scans were usually performed without ventilation studies and frequently comprised only two to four views. Robin also included the data from the Urokinase Pulmonary Embolism Trial — UPET — as well as from other studies as the basis for his remarks. No distinctions were made at that time regarding the size or number of perfusion defects, nor consideration given to the findings on the chest radiograph. The nonspecificity of perfusion-only lung scanning is well known; virtually all cardiopulmonary diseases may produce perfusion defects, including pneumonia, pleural effusion, congestive heart failure, and so

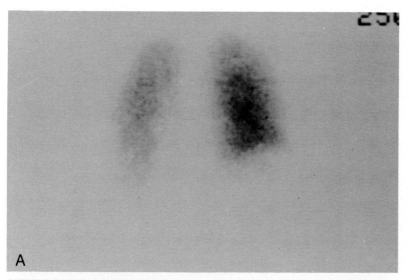

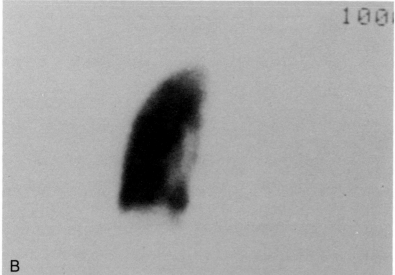

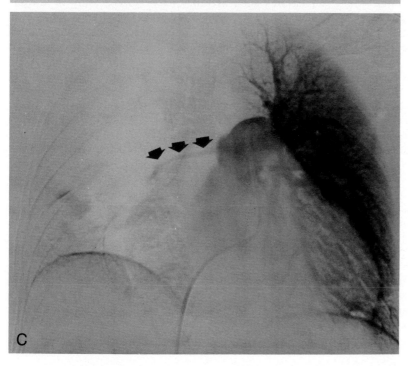

Fig. 14–6. Whole-lung V/Q mismatch in a 28-year-old female with known Takayasu's arteritis and acute chest pain and dyspnea. *A,* Posterior single breath ^{133}Xe ventilation image demonstrating ventilation to both lungs, right greater than left. *B,* Posterior ^{99m}Tc perfusion image demonstrating normal perfusion to the left lung with a prominent hilar defect and complete absence of perfusion to the right lung. *C,* Subtraction angiographic image from a main pulmonary artery injection demonstrating severe stenosis of the main right pulmonary artery (arrows) related to severe arteritis. Other views showed multiple areas of aneurysmal dilatation of the proximal left pulmonary artery branches. No pulmonary emboli were identified. *From* Spies WG, et al: Ventilation-perfusion scintigraphy in suspected pulmonary embolism: Correlation with pulmonary angiography and refinement of criteria for interpretation. Radiology *159*:383, 1986.

FIRST BREATH   **EQUILIBRIUM**

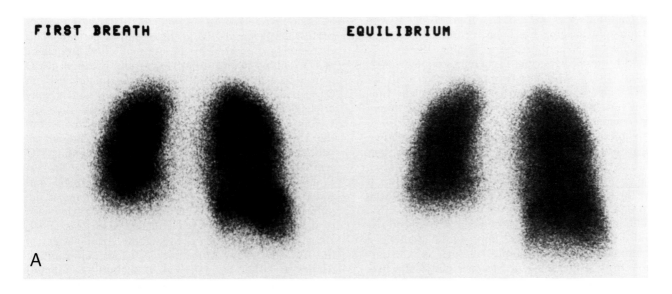

A

POSTERIOR   **LPO**

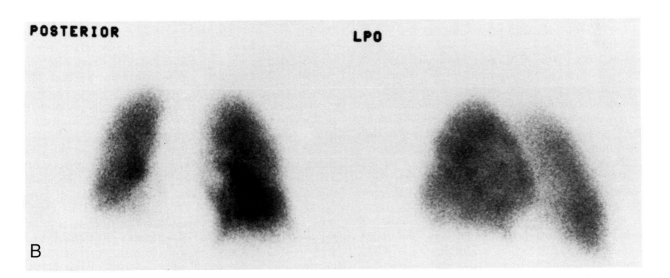

B

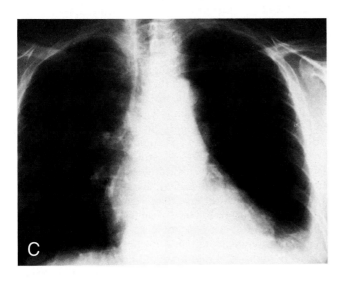

C

Fig. 14–7. Intermediate probability V/Q scan with a perfusion defect corresponding to a radiographic abnormality. The patient is a 64-year-old male with an acute left pleural effusion. *A*, Posterior single breath (left) and equilibrium wash-in ventilation images demonstrating absent ventilation at the left lung base. *B*, Posterior (left) and left posterior oblique perfusion images demonstrating a corresponding perfusion defect in the posterior basal segment of the left lower lobe. *C*, AP chest radiograph shows a corresponding left basilar pleural effusion. Even though the ventilation and perfusion defects are matched, the findings are indicative of intermediate probability of pulmonary embolism, because of the corresponding radiographic abnormality. Although pulmonary embolism is not highly likely, particularly with only one area of involvement, an embolus with associated infarction in the left lower lobe cannot totally be excluded. This type of finding (Q = CXR) is probably the most common variety of intermediate probability lung scans.

forth. The limited accuracy of the diagnosis of PE with perfusion-only imaging has been recorded by McNeil (1976) and by the author and associates (1986a).

In short, these early criticisms of lung scanning voiced by Robin (1977) and others became irrelevant with the advent of modern techniques for radionuclide lung imaging, including the routine use of ventilation imaging, comparison with chest radiographs, and use of the Biello criteria or related methods for interpretation. Comparisons between the Biello criteria and other interpretive schemes by Carter (1982), Sullivan (1983), and Webber (1990) and their associates have shown it to be the overall most accurate system for V/Q scan interpretation to date.

Additional refinements have been introduced by several investigators to further improve the accuracy of lung scanning in PE. Examples of such refinements include the "stripe sign" of Sostman and Gottschalk (1982), obtaining follow-up chest radiographs, as suggested by Vix (1983), assessing the age of radiographic abnormalities that correspond with perfusion defects, as evaluated by the author and co-workers (1986a), and comparison of V/Q scans with prior scans, as described by Alderson and others (1983) and the author and co-workers (1986a). Use of these refinements has resulted in a further slight improvement in diagnostic accuracy and decrease in the number of equivocal or intermediate probability scans. Another technique being evaluated is the use of SPECT in conjunction with lung scanning, as previously mentioned. This technique involves acquiring data using a rotating gamma camera that gradually circles the patient in a series of 64 to 128 graded steps. Tomographic images are then reconstructed in multiple planes, as in conventional transmission CT scans. This approach has met with great success in other areas of nuclear medicine, such as myocardial and cerebral perfusion imaging, and may lead to more accurate detection and localization of V/Q abnormalities, as suggested by Touya and colleagues (1986b). To date, however, SPECT lung imaging has not been widely adopted nor shown to improve diagnostic accuracy significantly.

Some criticisms of V/Q imaging have centered around the fact that the data used to validate the Biello criteria were all derived from retrospective studies. Hull and associates (1983, 1985, and 1991) conducted prospective clinical trials of the diagnosis of PE in patients referred for impedance plethysmography — IPG — for suspected DVT. This group obtained significantly poorer results with V/Q imaging. They found that 86% of high probability scans were associated with PE at angiography, but they claimed that at least 25% of "low probability" scans occurred in patients subsequently proven to have PE or DVT. These data have been the subject of considerable debate in the literature, the full extent of which is beyond the scope of the current discussion. Briefly, several factors suggest that Hull's findings are probably not representative of general clinical practice. Patient selection bias was introduced by the use of patients referred for IPG only, rather than all patients referred for V/Q imaging, suggesting higher pretest suspicion for PE in this group of patients. This suspicion is supported by the unusually high frequency of DVT found in this group, especially proximal DVT, as well as a prevalence of PE of approximately 50% in those patients who underwent pulmonary angiography or had autopsy correlation. More importantly, the techniques used for performance and interpretation of the V/Q scintigraphy were not standard, and not all patients underwent complete evaluation, including V/Q scintigraphy and angiography, as discussed by Secker-Walker (1983), Sostman and Gottschalk (1986), and Alderson and Siegel (1987). In addition, none of the publications from this group provide even a single image to illustrate their findings. Hull and associates (1990, 1991) have gone as far as to suggest abandonment of the use of the low probability category, interpreting studies as either normal, high probability or "nondiagnostic." They are to be commended for emphasizing the importance of evaluating the presence of DVT as an integral part of thromboembolic disease and providing the first major attempt to evaluate prospectively the PE diagnosis. On balance, however, it seems their results, which have not been confirmed by others, must be regarded as not representative of the consensus of opinion on this subject, and therefore not the basis for use in current practice. Such a conclusion is also supported by the results of the subsequently performed prospective trial carried out by the PIOPED investigators (1990).

The aforementioned controversies provided the impetus for the National Institutes of Health to sponsor a large, prospective multicenter trial of PE diagnosis that has come to be known as the PIOPED — Prospective Investigation of Pulmonary Embolism Diagnosis — Trial. The initial results of this study have been reported by the PIOPED investigators (1990), and data analysis from the trial is still ongoing. Although it is not feasible to discuss all of the details of this major study at present, a summary of the study and its initial conclusions provides an important understanding of the present state of the utility of V/Q scintigraphy in the diagnosis of PE.

From an initial 5587 requests for lung scans, a total of 1493 patients ultimately gave consent for entry into the PIOPED study. The most important and best evaluated group to date was the PIOPED Angiographic Pursuit arm of the study, consisting of 931 patients in whom V/Q scans were obtained, with chest radiographs and, if possible, pulmonary angiography performed within 24 hours. A total of 755 angiograms were obtained in 931 patients — 81%. All studies were performed using state of the art techniques, and studies were interpreted in blinded fashion by two central readers from different institutions than the one in which the study was performed. Third readers, and if necessary, consensus groups were used in the event of disagreements. Although overall interobserver agreement was relatively high, disagreements did occur in some cases, particularly in "borderline" V/Q scans and angiograms with questionable emboli in smaller branch vessels. The occurrence of some disagreement in the reading of the pulmonary angiograms, although not frequent, underscores the fact that angiography is not an absolute standard, and not quite the binary "positive" or "negative" test for which it is often characterized. Juni and Alavi (1991) noted that uncertainties in angiographic interpretation tended to occur in the same cases in which the V/Q scans were equivocal, namely the low to intermediate probability group.

The criteria used to interpret the V/Q scans in the PIOPED Trial, in general similar to the modified Biello criteria, had some differences. High probability scans required more extensive V/Q mismatch than the Biello criteria, with a minimum of two segmental equivalent mismatches; that is, two large, one large, and two moderate or four moderate mismatches present in radiographically normal sites. The low-probability group was subdivided into "low" and "very low" categories, the latter including cases having three or fewer small subsegmental defects in radiographically normal areas. Inclusion of a single moderate mismatch in a radiographically normal region in the low probability group proved to be an error, with roughly one third of these cases being positive for PE at angiography — note that this finding is correctly designated as intermediate probability by the Biello criteria. The PIOPED Nuclear Medicine group became aware of this oversight during the trial, but believed that altering the criteria in the midst of the study would unnecessarily complicate their data analysis (unpublished verbal communication from Alexander Gottschalk). Finally, the criteria for extensive obstructive airway disease on xenon ventilation scans varied somewhat from the modified Biello approach.

Despite these differences, the results of the PIOPED study to date, as reported by the PIOPED investigators (1990) and amplified in various presentations, tend to support the work of Biello and associates (1979a). Of patients with high probability scans and angiographic correlation, 88% had PE. Low probability cases had a prevalence of PE of 12%; in intermediate probability studies, it was 33%. The authors of the PIOPED study (1990) and others, such as Bone (1990) in an editorial accompanying the original PIOPED data summary (1990), pointed out that the sensitivity of high probability scans was only 41%, although the specificity was 97%. This result is not surprising, because it is widely known by nuclear medicine physicians that most patients with PE tend to have intermediate probability scans, often attributable either to perfusion defects corresponding to radiographic infiltrates or to areas of mismatch not sufficiently extensive to warrant a high probability designation. Bone went on to claim that the study showed that 4% of "normal or near-normal" V/Q studies proved to have PE, a conclusion that apparently is erroneous, because *none* of the actually normal studies in the PIOPED trial proved to be associated with PE (unpublished verbal communication from Alexander Gottschalk).

Further data evaluation from the PIOPED study is ongoing, including attempts to refine further the criteria for V/Q interpretation based on the enormous database acquired, but these results have not officially been promulgated at present. Available data comparing the scintigraphic and clinical assessment of patients in the study suggest that the V/Q scans were helpful in stratifying risk for thromboembolic disease in patients with equivocal clinical findings and vice versa. Preliminary results from PIOPED, in addition to prior work, suggest that a low probability scan is a good indicator of a benign long-term outcome with respect to thromboembolic disease, as discussed by Juni and Alavi (1990), Kahn (1989), Lee (1985), and Kipper (1982) and their associates. Even Hull (1990), the most outspoken critic of V/Q scintigraphy in PE, states that a normal study excludes PE. Of patients diagnosed as having PE in PIOPED, 24% died within 1 year, but only 2.5% died of PE and 8% had clinically apparent recurrent PE within 1 year. Carson and associates (1992) reported that most deaths resulted from associated conditions such as cancer, infection, and cardiac disease, and occurred most often in patients with underlying cancer, left-sided congestive heart failure, or chronic lung disease. Another entire arm of the PIOPED study, consisting of patients in whom the decision for angiography was left to the discretion of the referring physician, has yet to be analyzed and reported to date.

In summary, the PIOPED trial was an ambitious and largely successful attempt to evaluate prospectively the use of V/Q scintigraphy and pulmonary angiography in the diagnosis of PE. The results of the study to date support the continued use of the V/Q scan as the noninvasive screening test of choice for this purpose, but underscore the fact that it must be used in conjunction with other clinical data and when necessary, either followup pulmonary angiography or noninvasive or invasive studies for the detection of DVT.

Other Applications

Although V/Q scans frequently are abnormal in patients with bronchial carcinoma, the scan is rarely used for purposes of diagnosis or staging. Secker-Walker and Provan (1969) demonstrated perfusion defects associated with bronchial carcinoma, quantitated them using digital computers, and found that if the perfusion defect resulted in the abnormal lung providing less than 33% of total pulmonary perfusion, the lesion was always unresectable. Subsequent exceptions to this rule have been reported. Ventilation can also be quantitated for various lung zones, allowing calculation of regional V/Q ratios. Abnormalities in this ratio are also associated with nonresectability in most cases. It should be noted that these are indirect approaches to the assessment of tumor extent. Furthermore, these techniques are not sensitive for the detection of small or peripheral lesions. Fiberoptic bronchoscopy and CT scanning of the chest, in conjunction with the standard chest radiographs, are the procedures of choice for the staging of bronchial carcinoma. In some institutions, gallium imaging is also used for staging.

In conjunction with quantitation using digital computers, V/Q imaging can be useful in predicting postoperative pulmonary function (see Chapter 18). This determination may be of critical importance, because many patients with bronchial carcinoma have underlying chronic lung disease, and may not be able to tolerate extensive pulmonary resection. Both Kristersson (1974) and Olsen and co-workers (1974) demonstrated a good correlation between relative pulmonary perfusion assessed by prepneumonectomy perfusion lung scans, and postoperative pulmonary function, as measured by forced vital capacity and other pulmonary function indices. Kristersson (1974) and Boysen (1977) suggested pneumonectomy may be tolerated in patients with bronchial carcinoma and compromised lung function when the predicted postoperative FEV_1 is 800 ml or more. Such quantitation may also be used before resection of benign pulmonary lesions, such as bullae.

The most recent application of quantitative radionuclide lung imaging has been in the pre- and postoperative evaluation of patients undergoing unilateral pulmonary transplants, as described by the Toronto Lung Transplant Group (1986). Preoperative studies may reveal subtle asymmetry in lung perfusion that may dictate which lung is to be transplanted. More importantly, changes in perfusion, ventilation, or both to the transplanted lung may be useful in monitoring pulmonary rejection and other complications. As discussed in my review (1992), the transplanted lung usually receives significantly greater perfusion than the remaining native lung postoperatively, with relative ventilation being variable. The etiology of the chronic lung disease leading to transplantation may affect this relative pulmonary perfusion. For example, Medina and co-workers (1992) found the highest relative perfusion in the transplant in patients with primary pulmonary hypertension, compared to patients with chronic obstructive airway disease or idiopathic pulmonary fibrosis. Rejection usually produces significant reduction in perfusion to the transplant that may be reversible with successful treatment. Other complications are less likely to produce this finding, but the correlation between decreases in graft perfusion and rejection is imperfect. In the case of double lung transplants, Royal and associates (1992) found that the second lung received less relative perfusion, a finding that persisted for the first three postoperative months, than the first in proportion to increasing ischemic time.

In primary airway obstruction attributable to foreign bodies, mucous plugging, or endobronchial masses, V/Q scans show striking ventilatory abnormalities. Often noted also are corresponding but less severe reductions in perfusion, related to reflex vasoconstriction. These findings usually revert to normal when the airway obstruction is relieved, provided that irreversible lung damage has not occurred.

V/Q imaging may also be useful in the evaluation of lung injury, as reviewed by Lull and associates (1983).

Perfusion defects may be identified in patients who have undergone blunt or penetrating trauma, and in some cases may precede radiographic changes. Both perfusion and ventilation defects may be observed in patients with pneumothorax or hemothorax, although such entities are usually identified on the chest radiograph.

Xenon-133 ventilation studies are useful in the evaluation of inhalation injuries. Inhalation injuries often occur in conjunction with burns, and may result in a two- to fivefold increase in mortality, depending on the extent of the burn. In the early hours after the injury, the patient may be asymptomatic and have normal chest radiographic findings. Within several days, edema and inflammation of the airways may result in progressive airway obstruction, leading to atelectasis, infection, or the adult respiratory distress syndrome — ARDS. Intravenous administration of ^{133}Xe in saline solution during the early stages of inhalation injury will demonstrate areas of abnormal wash-out corresponding to sites of early obstructive airways involvement. In this regard, ^{133}Xe is superior to fiberoptic bronchoscopy in evaluating the distal airways, whereas bronchoscopy is better for the trachea and proximal bronchi. Agee and associates (1976) reported both proximal and distal involvement in most cases; thus, either test alone is diagnostic in about 90% of cases, and both tests together detect virtually all cases. The results of these studies are used in conjunction with clinical probability factors to help guide patient management.

A new application for ventilation imaging with radiolabeled aerosols involves the evaluation of lung disorders associated with alterations in alveolar-capillary membrane permeability. Examples of such disorders include various interstitial lung diseases, hyaline membrane disease in neonates, and ARDS. Damage to the pulmonary capillary membrane or a change in the Starling forces may result in increased alveolar-capillary permeability. Radioaerosols are normally cleared from the alveoli into the circulation and excreted by the kidneys with a pulmonary clearance half-time of approximately 90 minutes. In the presence of ARDS or other interstitial lung disease, this half-time may be substantially shortened. By measuring ^{99m}Tc-DTPA aerosol wash-out using digitally acquired images, time-activity wash-out curves can be generated. Coates and O'Brodovich (1986) have reviewed this technique. Smokers have been found to have faster aerosol clearance rates than nonsmokers. Clearance rates are normal in patients with asthma or pneumonia, but may be prolonged in patients with interstitial edema. This technique is simple and noninvasive, and has a potential role in the evaluation of patients at risk for developing ARDS or hyaline membrane disease, before the onset of clinical disease, and in the detection and monitoring of patients with other forms of interstitial lung disease or alveolitis. To date, however, it has not achieved widespread clinical use.

Whole body imaging with pulmonary perfusion agents is also used to detect and quantitate right-to-left cardiac shunts. In the presence of a shunt, some particles bypass the pulmonary vascular bed via the shunt and enter the systemic circulation, where they are trapped in end-organs in proportion to blood flow. ^{99m}Tc-HAM are frequently used for this application, when available, because they are more stable in vivo than MAA, resulting in less potentially confusing activity in the kidneys and bladder secondary to the presence of free pertechnetate. In patients with significant shunts, the images demonstrate deposition of particles in the brain, kidneys, and extremities (Fig. 14–8). The data are acquired on a computer and quantitated, expressing the shunt as a percent. Normal subjects have approximately a 4% physiologic right-to-left shunt. Gates and associates (1974) obtained a good correlation with results obtained using the Fick oxygen technique during cardiac catheterization.

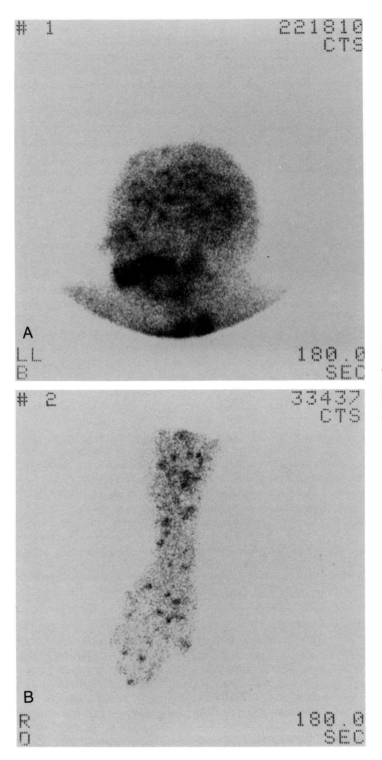

Fig. 14–8. Large right-to-left shunt. ^{99m}Tc human albumin microspheres (HAM) study. *A,* Left lateral skull image demonstrates particle deposition in the brain. Some free ^{99m}Tc-pertechnetate is present in the saliva in the mouth, salivary glands, and thyroid. *B,* Image of the right forearm and hand shows diffuse particle deposition. Quantitative analysis revealed a 49% right-to-left shunt.

GALLIUM IMAGING

Gallium-67-citrate is a radiopharmaceutical used for the evaluation of inflammatory and certain neoplastic diseases. It is a cyclotron-produced radionuclide with a half-life of 78 hours and several gamma photopeaks, of which the ones commonly used for imaging include 93, 184 and 296 keV. An iron analogue, it is largely bound to serum transferrin after intravenous injection. Gallium imaging is a sensitive but nonspecific procedure, with increased activity noted in many inflammatory and neoplastic processes. Normal sites of uptake include the liver, skeleton, salivary glands, kidneys, spleen, breasts, and large bowel. Simon and others (1980) demonstrated that faint diffuse lung uptake may be present in about 50% of normal individuals at 24 hours, which should not be confused with a diffuse pulmonary inflammatory process. For this reason, gallium imaging of the chest is usually performed 48 to 72 hours after injection, although diagnostic findings may be seen on earlier images, and earlier imaging is often performed in cases of suspected acute thoracic infection to facilitate earlier diagnosis and treatment. In children, prominent uptake may be seen in the normal thymus gland, limiting the usefulness of gallium scanning for the evaluation of mediastinal masses in the pediatric age group. During the first 24 hours after injection, 20 to 30% of the dose is excreted, primarily by the kidneys. Subsequent excretion is primarily through the colon.

Hoffer (1980) reviewed the mechanisms of gallium uptake in disease processes. Gallium accumulation in infectious processes is related to several factors, including uptake in white blood cells — primarily bound to lactoferrin in lysosomes and other cytoplasmic organelles, increased blood flow and capillary permeability at sites of inflammation, with binding to tissue lactoferrin, and direct bacterial uptake within iron-binding organelles called siderophores. Uptake in neoplastic processes is less well understood, but may involve hyperpermeability of tumor vessels, increased extracellular fluid spaces in tumors, uptake within the cytoplasm, associated with lysosomes and possibly the endoplasmic reticulum, iron-binding proteins, tumor cell surface receptors, or possibly other as yet unknown mechanisms.

Tumors with a high affinity for gallium include bronchial carcinoma, malignant mesothelioma, hepatocellular carcinoma, Hodgkin's disease, histiocytic and Burkitt's lymphoma, melanoma, and certain testicular neoplasms. Gallium scanning in the staging of Hodgkin's disease is highly sensitive in the detection of mediastinal involvement, with a sensitivity of 90% or greater, particularly in the nodular sclerosing type. Evaluation of the abdomen and pelvis is less accurate, because of interfering normal colonic activity, which may obscure sites of lymphadenopathy or simulate abnormalities. CT scanning usually is used for evaluation of abdominal or pelvic lymphadenopathy. Lymphangiography also plays a role, because it can detect involvement in lymph nodes that are not enlarged on CT scans. Hoffer (1986) reported that the detection of histiocytic and Burkitt's lymphoma by gallium imaging is at least as good as that seen in Hodgkin's disease, with virtually all metastatic foci of Burkitt's lymphoma demonstrating increased gallium uptake.

The overall sensitivity of gallium imaging in the staging of bronchial carcinoma is approximately 90%, without significant differences in the various cell types, except for a possibly slightly lower sensitivity for adenocarcinoma. In general, primary lesions as small as 2 cm in diameter can be detected by planar imaging. The utility of gallium imaging in the assessment of mediastinal spread of tumor is controversial. Although it appears that gallium imaging is superior to standard chest radiographs and plain tomography in this regard, the results of clinical trials have been variable. Alazraki and colleagues (1978) suggested that the absence of gallium uptake in the mediastinum in patients whose primary lesion concentrated gallium may obviate the need for preoperative mediastinoscopy. Other investigators, such as DeMeester and associates (1976), had less impressive results. Savage and co-workers (1976) pointed out that because gallium uptake is nonspecific, false positives related to inflammatory disorders in the mediastinum may occur. The sensitivity of gallium imaging may be improved by using tomographic techniques, such as SPECT imaging. Nevertheless, as previously discussed, CT imaging of the chest has become the primary method for the staging of bronchial carcinoma in most centers. Pitfalls in CT staging include false positives because of non-neoplastic enlargement of nodes and false negatives from tumor involvement in normal-sized nodes. The search for metastases outside of the chest is best approached using other radionuclides, such as bone and liver-spleen scanning agents, and other techniques, such as CT of the abdomen. Examples of tumor uptake on gallium scans are shown in Figure 14–9.

Gallium imaging of the chest has also assumed an important role in the evaluation of infectious and other inflammatory disorders of the chest. The standard chest radiograph remains the primary imaging tool for the detection of pulmonary inflammatory disease, yet gallium scanning plays a complementary role. It is more sensitive for the detection of early infectious processes, better delineates mediastinal involvement, and allows for better followup of the response to therapy.

Diffusely increased pulmonary uptake is seen in opportunistic infections in immunocompromised hosts, such as *Pneumocystis carinii* pneumonia — PCP — or cytomegalovirus — CMV — pneumonia, before the appearance of radiographic changes. Although previously a problem encountered mainly in patients with leukemia or lymphoma, this indication has assumed great importance with the proliferation of the acquired immune deficiency syndrome — AIDS. Barron and associates (1985) confirmed the utility of gallium imaging in AIDS patients with suspected PCP, particularly in those with normal or equivocal chest radiographs. I and

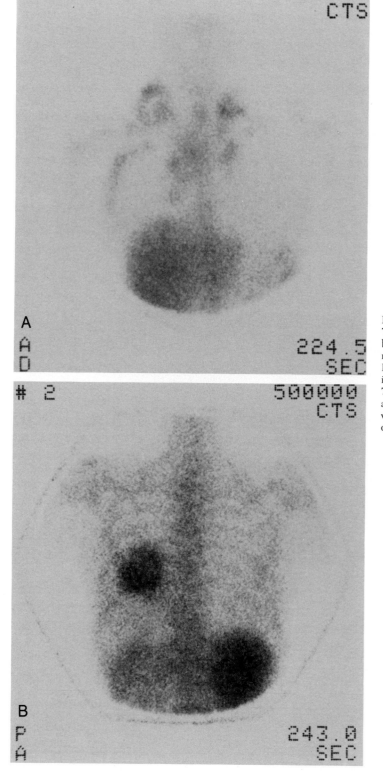

Fig. 14–9. Gallium uptake in thoracic neoplasms. *A,* A 72-hour anterior chest image demonstrates gallium uptake in bilateral supraclavicular, right hilar, superior mediastinal, and right axillary lymphadenopathy in a 39-year-old woman with Hodgkin's disease. The activity at the inferior aspect of the image is normal hepatic and splenic gallium uptake. *B,* A 72-hour posterior chest image demonstrates increased gallium activity in a left lower lobe adenocarcinoma in a 50-year-old woman. *From* Spies WG, et al.: Radionuclide imaging in diseases of the chest (part 2). Chest *83:*250, 1983.

my associates (1989a) reported a high sensitivity of 24-hour gallium images in the detection of PCP, which makes the study more valuable for rapid clinical decision-making. Kramer and associates (1986) described their experience with gallium imaging in a large series of AIDS patients presenting with acute fever or respiratory symptoms. In addition to confirming the utility of gallium imaging in the diagnosis of *Pneumocystis* and

other opportunistic pneumonias, they also pointed out the additional patterns of focal lymph node uptake, seen primarily in cases of atypical tuberculosis — *Mycobacterium avium intracellulare* — and lymphoma, and focal pulmonary uptake, often seen with acute bacterial pneumonias. Negative findings were associated with Kaposi's sarcoma or the absence of identifiable infection. Examples of normal and abnormal gallium images of the chest are shown in Figure 14–10. Hattner and co-workers (1986) emphasized the favorable economic impact of gallium scanning in this clinical setting, in which they realized a potential cost savings of 38%, as a result of obviating the need for bronchoscopy in cases of negative gallium scans. Although diffuse pulmonary uptake is highly suggestive of the presence of acute opportunistic infection in this clinical setting, the finding is nonetheless nonspecific. The differential diagnosis of diffuse pulmonary uptake of gallium includes other diffuse bacterial and viral pneumonias, such as CMV, tuberculosis, sarcoidosis, pulmonary toxicity from chemotherapeutic agents or other drugs, idiopathic pulmonary fibrosis, lymphangitic metastases, pneumoconiosis, and chemical pneumonitis following lymphangiography. Bronchoscopy and biopsy are therefore generally indicated for patients with positive findings to establish the specific diagnosis. Atypical patterns of gallium uptake in PCP may occur, as noted by Kramer and associates (1988) and by the author (1989b). Perihilar uptake may occur prior to diffuse pulmonary uptake in some patients, analogous to the progression of findings noted on chest radiographs. Upper lobe predominance may occur, possibly as the result of relative sparing of the lower lobes in patients receiving prophylactic, aerosolized pentamidine therapy, which better penetrates the lung bases.

Although not of major importance in surgical practice, gallium imaging has also been used in the diagnosis and followup of granulomatous processes, such as tuber-

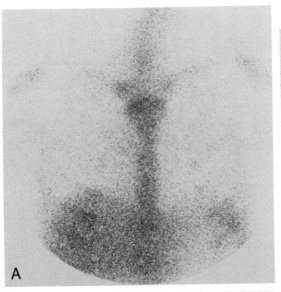
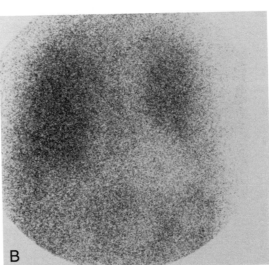
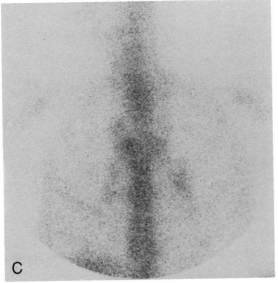

Fig. 14–10. Gallium imaging in immunocompromised patients. *A,* Normal 48-hour anterior gallium image of the chest. *B,* A 72-hour anterior chest image demonstrates diffuse bilateral increased pulmonary uptake in a 61-year-old male patient with AIDS and fever. Note the negative cardiac silhouette. The abnormality was also evident on 24-hour images. Initial chest radiographs were negative, but later images showed perihilar infiltrates. Bronchial aspirates were positive for *Pneumocystis carinii* pneumonia. *C,* A 72-hour anterior chest image shows bilateral hilar and right paratracheal lymphadenopathy in a 36-year-old male patient with AIDS who presented with nonproductive cough and fever. The patient proved to have *Mycobacterium avium intracellulare* infection, which also involved the liver and bone marrow.

culosis and sarcoidosis, and pulmonary fibrotic disorders. Increased activity correlates with the presence of histologically active disease. Pulmonary uptake can be quantitated using a computer, resulting in excellent correlation with more invasive techniques, such as bronchoalveolar lavage in sarcoidosis, as described by Fajman and co-workers (1984). Correlation with clinical symptoms and assessment of therapy, however, is weaker.

^{131}I IMAGING

Whole body imaging with ^{131}I is a standard procedure for the postoperative evaluation of patients with well-differentiated thyroid carcinoma. The whole body scan detects the presence of residual normal thyroid tissue and functioning metastases in the thyroid bed, regional lymph nodes, the lungs, or the skeleton. Uptake of ^{131}I in pulmonary metastases may be demonstrated even in the absence of identifiable lesions on the chest radiograph (Fig. 14–11). The scan findings are used to determine whether a therapeutic dose of ^{131}I should be administered for the ablation of residual thyroid tissue, as well as the dose required. Ideally, according to Beierwaltes (1978), the scan is performed approximately 6 weeks after total thyroidectomy without thyroid hormone replacement to induce maximal endogenous thyroid-stimulating hormone — TSH — stimulation of ^{131}I uptake by metastases. Followup is performed after withdrawal of synthetic thyroid (Synthroid) for 6 weeks. To minimize the duration of symptomatic hypothyroidism encountered with this approach, it is common to have the patient switch to the shorter acting triiodothyronine; that is, Cytomel, at 6 weeks, continue it until 2 to 3 weeks before the scan, and then discontinue it until after whole body ^{131}I imaging and/or therapy are completed. The usual diagnostic scan dose is 5 to 10 mCi. In some institutions, only 1 to 2 mCi are used to reduce the patient radiation dose, but some authorities believe this practice may lead to a decreased sensitivity for the detection of residual thyroid tissue and metastases. Administration of exogenous TSH to stimulate tumor uptake is not recommended; it generally results in less effective and shorter lasting stimulation than endogenous stimulation, and it may be associated with severe allergic reactions, including anaphylaxis. Typical therapeutic doses for functioning pulmonary metastases range from about 175 to 200 mCi, with followup whole body scanning performed 1 year later. Patients given doses in this range must be hospitalized until the retained dose drops below 30 mCi or 2 days after therapy, whichever occurs later. Post-therapy repeat whole body images are obtained either immediately before release from the hospital or within

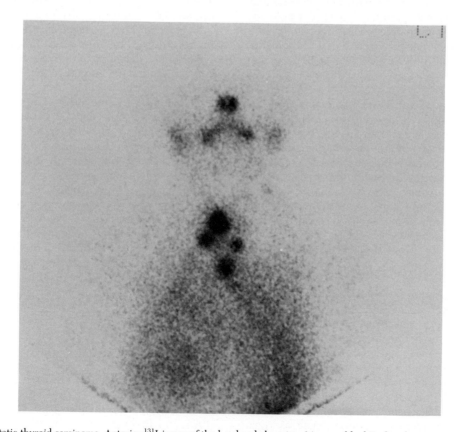

Fig. 14–11. Metastatic thyroid carcinoma. Anterior ^{131}I-image of the head and chest in a 14-year-old white female status-post total thyroidectomy for well-differentiated mixed papillary-follicular thyroid carcinoma demonstrates four foci of metastatic disease in the thyroid bed and diffuse bilateral pulmonary uptake, consistent with lung metastases. A subtle focus of activity in the left side of the neck may represent cervical lymph node metastasis. The activity in the nasal region and mouth represents normal uptake by the nasal mucosa and salivary glands.

a week of discharge in many institutions, and may provide additional diagnostic information in up to 50% of cases, as reported by the author and associates (1986). If necessary, repeat therapy may be given at yearly intervals. With this dose schedule, the incidence of toxicity related to radiation-induced pulmonary fibrosis or significant bone marrow suppression is low. On occasion, in cases of widespread, rapidly progressive metastatic disease, therapy may be repeated as frequently as 6 months apart. Followup scans may be obtained at longer intervals in patients with no evidence of recurrent disease. In some centers, use of quantitative dosimetry estimates in conjunction with diagnostic whole body ^{131}I imaging permits administration of single therapy doses larger than 200 mCi, which potentially result in superior success rates and allow for more individualized treatment plans, as reported by Maxon and associates (1992). This approach is based on calculation of the delivered radiation dose to the tumor and to normal tissues, such as the lungs and bone marrow. In earlier work, Maxon and associates (1983) estimated that doses of at least 30,000 rad to thyroid remnants and 8000 rad to metastases resulted in significantly increased rates of response to therapy. The review of Maxon and Smith (1990) indicates that approximately one half of patients with functioning pulmonary metastases show resolution after ^{131}I therapy, one quarter have some benefit, and the remaining quarter experience no appreciable effect. The highest response rate — approximately 80% complete response — occurs in patients in whom the lesions are detectable only on ^{131}I whole body scans. The 5-year mortality is significantly lower for patients whose lung metastases accumulate ^{131}I compared to those that do not — 38 versus 69% mortality. Mortality is significantly higher in cases in which the pulmonary metastases are accompanied by metastases elsewhere. Empiric use of ^{131}I therapy in patients with negative whole body scans but suspected metastases based on elevated serum thyroglobulin levels is controversial, although some patients managed in this fashion demonstrate lung uptake on followup post-therapy ^{131}I whole body scans, indicating that metastases were probably present.

RADIONUCLIDE ANGIOGRAPHY

Radionuclide angiography — RA — is a simple, safe, noninvasive method for evaluating blood flow to various organs. Muroff and Freedman (1976) suggest that it can be used to delineate vascular anatomy and patency and to evaluate the vascularity of masses. Radionuclide angiography is performed by obtaining a rapid sequence of images — 0.5 to 3 sec/image — over an area of interest, immediately after the intravenous injection of a radiopharmaceutical. It is a routine part of many nuclear medicine procedures, such as renal scans, brain scans, and bone scans performed for suspected osteomyelitis, acute fractures, or heterotopic ossification. In the chest, such studies may be obtained

alone or in conjunction with other standard nuclear medicine examinations. Almost any radiopharmaceutical may be used, with the exception of MAA or HAM, which would be trapped in the pulmonary vasculature. The examination is most often performed for evaluation of suspected vascular obstruction, as in superior vena cava syndrome (Fig. 14–12). The data may be quantitated using a digital computer. Radionuclide angiography may eliminate the need for more invasive procedures, such as contrast venography or arteriography. Other potential diagnostic uses include the noninvasive demonstration of aortic aneurysms and vascular masses, such as hemangiomas and arteriovenous malformations. The major limitation of RA relates to its relatively poor spatial resolution compared to standard radiographic techniques, such as contrast angiography and digital subtraction angiography. Technically inadequate studies occur in a small percentage of cases, because of poor bolus geometry or poor patient positioning.

FUTURE DEVELOPMENTS IN PULMONARY NUCLEAR MEDICINE

New developments in nuclear medicine have been directed toward more sophisticated evaluation of physiologic processes. Major advances usually result from the development of new radiopharmaceuticals, with the introduction of newer instrumentation then following. Pulmonary nuclear medicine has been no exception in this regard. Several approaches to improvement of the scintigraphic diagnosis of PE have already been discussed. Another technique is the use of ^{111}In-labeled autologous platelets. This technique is useful in the detection of DVT in the lower extremities, the precursor of PE. Investigations led by Davis (1980) and Moser (1980) and their associates suggested that imaging of PE in humans by this technique may be limited to emboli less than 12 hours old, and only in patients not receiving heparin. Nichols and associates (1978) reported that "hot spot" imaging of PE may be accomplished using radioactive gases labeled with positron-emitting radionuclides of carbon or oxygen. In this case, inhaled radioactive gases diffuse across the alveolar-capillary membrane and are cleared from the lungs by pulmonary blood flow. As a result of decreased blood flow, the gas is retained in areas of PE, resulting in easily identified "hot spots." Although apparently quite sensitive, this technique is not practical for widespread use at present, because it requires an expensive, specialized positron scanner — PET scanner — and an on-site cyclotron for production of these extremely short-lived radiopharmaceuticals.

Ongoing investigations involve the use of new radiopharmaceuticals for evaluation of pulmonary metabolic functions, as reviewed by Touya and associates (1986) and Budinger and colleagues (1982). In addition to its respiratory function, the lung is involved in the regulation of several circulating vasoactive substances, including the activation, deactivation, release, or re-

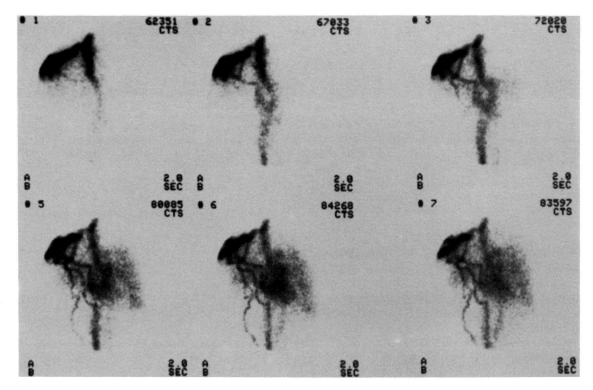

Fig. 14–12. Radionuclide angiography in superior vena cava syndrome. A 65-year-old man had poorly differentiated adenocarcinoma of the lung, brain and liver metastases, and clinical signs suggestive of superior vena cava obstruction. Selected anterior images of the chest from a radionuclide angiogram performed after injection of ^{99m}Tc-DTPA in a right antecubital vein demonstrate high-grade partial obstruction of the superior vena cava, with flow into dilated collateral veins in the right axilla and anterior chest wall. Mild reflux into the right internal jugular vein and early visualization of the inferior vena cava via collateral flow are also noted. A small amount of activity directly enters the superior vena cava and right heart.

moval of such substances as amines, hormones, drugs, and polypeptides. Examples of such substances include bradykinin, serotonin, prostaglandins, angiotensin I, histamine, and many others. One such line of research involves measuring the pulmonary uptake, extraction, and wash-out of ^{123}I-IMP, an iodoamphetamine derivative. Pulmonary uptake of this agent is a passive, saturable process, as reported by Touya and associates (1985), whereas the agent ^{123}I-MIBG — metaiodobenzylguanidine — depends on oxidative metabolism in the lung, as reported by Slosman and co-workers (1986). Metabolic functions of the lung may also be studied in a more quantitative fashion using PET imaging with ^{11}C-labeled amines. Such studies may lead to better understanding of pulmonary metabolic functions and the ability to quantitate pulmonary amine endothelial receptors. Potential clinical applications include the diagnosis and followup of treatment of such disorders as hypertension, adult and neonatal respiratory distress syndrome, cystic fibrosis, asthma, and even certain psychiatric disorders, although these approaches have not led to clinical use to date.

Slutsky and Higgins (1984) evaluated the use of thallium-201, the agent used for myocardial perfusion imaging, in the evaluation of pulmonary extracellular fluid balance, as related to the development of pulmonary edema. Lung permeability and fluid balance may also be evaluated by measuring the clearance of inhaled radiolabeled aerosols from the lungs, a process dependent on the state of alveolocapillary membrane permeability.

Imaging with radiolabeled leukocytes may allow detection of changes in kinetics and distribution of leukocytes that may occur after exposure to toxins, such as high oxygen tension, or in ARDS, as suggested by the work of Suttorp and Simon (1982) involving leukocyte-mediated lung cell cytotoxicity after sustained hyperoxia.

A final area of research not limited to pulmonary nuclear medicine is the evaluation of radiolabeled monoclonal antibodies for the detection and treatment of various neoplasms, that Keenan and associates (1985) and Schlom (1991) reported. This technique was applied by Zimmer and colleagues (1985) to the detection of small cell lung carcinoma, using an ^{131}I-labeled antibody developed in mice. Our group (1988) also performed a pilot evaluation of an ^{111}In-labeled monoclonal antibody directed against non-small cell lung carcinoma in patients with advanced primary lesions. These studies demonstrated good visualization of the primary tumors, but relative insensitivity for mediastinal involvement or other metastases in a small group of patients, in part because of high background activity in the liver and blood pool. Overall, Goldenberg (1990) reported that monoclonal antibody studies in thousands of patients with various primary tumors have proven to be safe, with detection sensitivities in the 60 to 90% range. Usually, lesions greater than 1 to 2 cm are detected, although lesions as small as 4 to 5 mm may be detected with SPECT imaging, and in some cases, lesions missed by anatomic imaging methods such as CT can be detected. Ongoing investigations in this field include attempts to develop more tumor-specific and tumor-avid antibodies, including antibody fragments, attempts to decrease immunologic responses to murine antibodies — development of human antimouse antibodies or HAMA — and the use of human rather than mouse monoclonal antibodies. In addition, newer labeling techniques allow tagging of monoclonal antibodies to ^{99m}Tc rather than ^{111}In or ^{131}I, resulting in better imaging characteristics. Labeling of monoclonal antibodies with other beta or alpha emitters may permit radionuclide ablation of the target tumor. Radiolabeling of monoclonal antibodies directed against fibrin or other constituents of thrombi are being evaluated for use in the detection of DVT and PE. The ultimate roles of radiolabeled monoclonal antibody imaging and therapy remain uncertain.

REFERENCES

Agee RN, et al: Use of 133-Xenon in early diagnosis of inhalation injury. J Trauma 16:218, 1976.

Alazraki NP, et al: Reliability of gallium scan chest radiography compared to mediastinoscopy for evaluating mediastinal spread in lung cancer. Am Rev Respir Dis 117:415, 1978.

Alderson PO, Line BR: Scintigraphic evaluation of regional pulmonary ventilation. Semin Nucl Med 10:218, 1980.

Alderson PO, Martin EC: Pulmonary embolism: Diagnosis with multiple imaging modalities. Radiology 164:297, 1987.

Alderson PO, Siegel BA: Critical Review of "Diagnostic Value of Ventilation-Perfusion Lung Scanning in Patients with Suspected Pulmonary Embolism. Invest Radiol 22:87, 1987.

Alderson PO, Secker-Walker RH, Forrest JV: Detection of obstructive pulmonary disease. Radiology 111:643, 1974.

Alderson PO, et al: The role of ^{133}Xe ventilation studies in the scintigraphic detection of pulmonary embolism. Radiology 120:633, 1976.

Alderson PO, et al: Ventilation-perfusion lung imaging and selective pulmonary angiography in dogs with experimental pulmonary embolism. J Nucl Med 19:164, 1978.

Alderson PO, et al: Comparison of ^{133}Xe single-breath and washout imaging in the scintigraphic diagnosis of pulmonary embolism. Radiology 137:481, 1980.

Alderson PO, et al: Scintigraphic detection of pulmonary embolism in patients with obstructive pulmonary disease. Radiology 138:661, 1981.

Alderson PO, et al: Serial lung scintigraphy: Utility in diagnosis of pulmonary embolism. Radiology 149:797, 1983.

Alderson PO, et al: Tc-99m-DTPA aerosol and radioactive gases compared as adjuncts to perfusion scintigraphy in patients with suspected pulmonary embolism. Radiology 153:515, 1984.

Barron TF, et al: Pneumocystis carinii pneumonia studied by gallium-67 scanning. Radiology 154:791, 1985.

Beierwaltes WH: The treatment of thyroid carcinoma with radioactive iodine. Semin Nucl Med 8:79, 1978.

Biello DR, et al: Ventilation-perfusion studies in suspected pulmonary embolism. Am J Radiol 133:1033, 1979a.

Biello DR, et al: Interpretation of indeterminate lung scintigrams. Radiology 133:189, 1979b.

Biello DR: Radiological (scintigraphic) evaluation of patients with suspected pulmonary thromboembolism. JAMA 257:3257, 1987.

Bone RC: Ventilation/perfusion scan in pulmonary embolism: 'The emperor is incompletely attired'. JAMA 263:2794, 1990.

Boysen PG, et al: Prospective evaluation for pneumonectomy using the ^{99m}technetium quantitative perfusion lung scan. Chest 72:422, 1977.

Budinger TF, McNeil BJ, Alderson PO: Perspectives in nuclear medicine: Pulmonary studies. J Nucl Med 23:60, 1982.

Burch WM, et al: Lung ventilation studies with technetium-99m pseudogas. J Nucl Med 27:842, 1986.

Caride VJ, et al: The usefulness of the posterior oblique views in perfusion lung imaging. Radiology 121:669, 1976.

Carson JL, et al: The clinical course of pulmonary embolism. N Engl J Med 326:1240, 1992.

Carter WD, et al: Relative accuracy of two diagnostic schemes for detection of pulmonary embolism by ventilation-perfusion scintigraphy. Radiology 145:447, 1982.

Catania TA, Caride VJ: Single perfusion defect and pulmonary embolism: Angiographic correlation. J Nucl Med 31:296, 1990.

Coates G, O'Brodovich H: Measurement of pulmonary epithelial permeability with ^{99m}Tc-DTPA aerosol. Semin Nucl Med 16:275, 1986.

Cooper JD, et al: Unilateral lung transplantation for pulmonary fibrosis. N Engl J Med 314:1140, 1986.

Dalen JE, Alpert JS: Natural history of pulmonary embolism. Prog Cardiovasc Dis 17:259, 1975.

Davis HH, et al: Scintigraphy with ^{111}In-labeled autologous platelets in venous thromboembolism. Radiology 136:203, 1980.

DeMeester TR, et al: Gallium-67 scanning for carcinoma of the lung. J Thorac Cardiovasc Surg 72:699, 1976.

Fajman WA, et al: Assessing the activity of sarcoidosis: Quantitative ^{67}Ga-citrate imaging. Am J Radiol 142:683, 1984.

Foley M, et al: Pulmonary embolism after hip or knee replacement: Postoperative changes on pulmonary scintigrams in asymptomatic patients. Radiology 172:481, 1989.

Gates GF, Orme HW, Dore EK: Cardiac shunt assessment in children with macroaggregated albumin technetium-99m. Radiology 112:649, 1974.

Goldenberg DM: Current status of cancer imaging with radiolabeled antibodies. Antibody, immunoconjugates, and radiopharmaceuticals 4:517, 1991.

Goodman PC, Brant-Zawadzki M: Digital subtraction pulmonary angiography. Am J Radiol 139:305, 1982.

Goris ML, et al: Applications of ventilation lung imaging with ^{81m}krypton. Radiology 122:399, 1977.

Harding LK, et al: The proportion of lung vessels blocked by albumin microspheres. J Nucl Med 14:579, 1973.

Hattner RS, Golden JA, Fugate K: Cost/benefit of real versus "ideal" management strategies of AIDS patients suspected of p. carinii pneumonia: Effect of Ga-67 pulmonary imaging. J Nucl Med 27:914, 1986.

Hoffer P: Gallium: Mechanisms. J Nucl Med 21:282, 1980.

Hoffer P: Status of gallium-67 in tumor detection. J Nucl Med 21:394, 1980.

Huisman MV, et al: Unexpected prevalence of silent pulmonary embolism in patients with deep venous thrombosis. Chest 95:498, 1989.

Hull RD, Raskob GE: Low-probability lung scan findings: A need for change. Ann Intern Med 114:142, 1991.

Hull RD, et al: Pulmonary angiography, ventilation lung scanning, and venography for clinically suspected pulmonary embolism with abnormal perfusion lung scan. Ann Intern Med 98:891, 1983.

Hull RD, et al: Diagnostic value of ventilation-perfusion lung scanning in patients with suspected pulmonary embolism. Chest 88:819, 1985.

Hull RD, et al: Clinical validity of normal perfusion lung scan in patients with suspected pulmonary embolism. Chest 97:23, 1990.

Juni JE, Alavi A: Lung scanning in the diagnosis of pulmonary embolism: The emperor redressed. Semin Nucl Med 21:281, 1991.

Kahn D, et al: Clinical outcome of patients with a 'low probability' of pulmonary embolism on ventilation-perfusion lung scan. Arch Intern Med 149:377, 1989.

Keenan AM, Harbert JC, Larson SM: Monoclonal antibodies in nuclear medicine. J Nucl Med 26:531, 1985.

Kipper MS, Alazraki N: The feasibility of performing ^{133}Xe ventilation imaging following the perfusion study. Radiology 144:581, 1982.

Kipper MS, et al: Longterm follow-up of patients with suspected pulmonary embolism and a normal lung scan. Chest 82:411, 1982.

Kramer EL, et al: Chest gallium scans in patients with ks and/or aids. J Nucl Med 27:914, 1986.

Kramer EL, et al: The variable presentation of PCP on Ga-67 scans in HIV[+] patients. J Nucl Med 29:829, 1988.

Kristersson S: Prediction of lung function after lung surgery. A ^{133}Xe-radiospirometric study of regional lung function in bronchial cancer. Scand J Thorac Cardiovasc Surg 18 (Suppl.): 5, 1974.

Lee ME, et al: "Low-probability" ventilation-perfusion scintigrams: Clinical outcomes in 99 patients. Radiology 156:497, 1985.

Lull RJ, et al: Radionuclide evaluation lung trauma. Semin Nucl Med 13:223, 1983.

Maxon HR, Smith HS: Radioiodine-131 in the diagnosis and treatment of metastatic well differentiated thyroid cancer. Endocrin Metab Clin North Am 19:685, 1990.

Maxon, HR, et al.: Relation Between Effective Radiation Dose and Outcome of Radioiodine Therapy For Thyroid Cancer. New Engl J Med 309:937, 1983.

Maxon HR, et al: I-131 Therapy for thyroid cancer: Quantitative dosimetric approach — outcome and validation in 85 patients. J Nucl Med 33:894, 1992.

McNeil BJ: A diagnostic strategy using ventilation-perfusion studies in patients suspect for pulmonary embolism. J Nucl Med 17:613, 1976.

Medina LS, et al: Postoperative evaluation of single-lung transplant patients with quantitative ventilation-perfusion imaging. Radiology 185(P):283, 1992.

Moser KM, et al: Study of factors that may condition scintigraphic detection of venous thrombi and pulmonary emboli with indium-111-labeled platelets. J Nucl Med 21:1051, 1980.

Muroff LR, Freedman GS: Radionuclide angiography. Semin Nucl Med 6:217, 1976.

Musset D, et al: Acute pulmonary embolism: Diagnostic value of digital subtraction angiography. Radiology 166:455, 1988.

Nichols AB, et al: Scintigraphic detection of pulmonary emboli by serial positron imaging of inhaled ^{15}O-labeled carbon dioxide. N Engl J Med 299:279, 1978.

Nielsen PE, Kirchner PT, Gerber FH: Oblique views in lung perfusion scanning: Clinical utility and limitations. J Nucl Med 18:967, 1977.

Olsen GN, Block AJ, Tobias JA: Prediction of postpneumonectomy pulmonary function using quantitative macroaggregate lung scanning. Chest 66:13, 1974.

Piers DB, et al: A comparative study of intravenous digital subtraction angiography and ventilation-perfusion scans in suspected pulmonary embolism. Chest 91:837, 1987.

The PIOPED Investigators: Value of the Ventilation/Perfusion Scan in Acute Pulmonary Embolism: Results of the Prospective Investigation of Pulmonary Embolism Diagnosis (PIOPED). JAMA 263:2753, 1990.

Portman MA: Cardiothoracic magnetic resonance angiography. Semin Ultrasound, CT, MRI 13:274, 1992.

Posteraro RH, et al: Cine-gradient-refocused MR imaging of central pulmonary emboli. AJR Am J Roentgenol 152:465, 1989.

Remy-Jardin M, et al: Central pulmonary thromboembolism: Diagnosis with spiral volumetric CT with the single-breath-hold technique — comparison with pulmonary angiography. Radiology 185:381, 1992.

Rhodes BA, et al: Lung scanning with ^{99m}Tc-microspheres. Radiology 99:613, 1971.

Robin ED: Overdiagnosis and overtreatment of pulmonary embolism: The emperor may have no clothes. Ann Intern Med 87:775, 1977.

Rosen JM, et al: Kr-81m ventilation imaging: Clinical utility in suspected pulmonary embolism. Radiology 154:787, 1985.

Rosenow III EC, Osmundson PJ, Brown ML: Pulmonary embolism. Mayo Clin Proc 56:161, 1981.

Rosso J, et al: Intravenous digital subtraction angiography and lung imaging: Compared value in the diagnosis of pulmonary embolism. Clin Nucl Med 14:183, 1989.

Royal HD, Trulock EP, Ettinger NA: Effects of ischemic time on relative perfusion and ventilation in double-lung transplant patients. Radiology 185(P):282, 1992.

Savage P, Carmody R, Highman J: Evaluation of gallium-67 in the diagnosis of bronchial carcinoma. Clin Radiol 27:197, 1976.

Schlom J: Monoclonal Antibodies: They're More and Less Than You Think. In Broder S: Molecular Foundations of Oncology. Baltimore: Williams & Wilkins, 1991.

Schor RA, et al: Regional ventilation studies with Kr-81m and Xe-133: A comparative analysis. J Nucl Med 19:348, 1978.

Secker-Walker RH: On purple emperors, pulmonary embolism, and venous thrombosis. Ann Intern Med 98:1006, 1983.

Secker-Walker RH, Provan JL: Scintillation scanning of lungs in preoperative assessment of carcinoma of bronchus. Br Med J 3:327, 1969.

Simon TR, Li J, Hoffer PB: The nonspecificity of diffuse pulmonary uptake of ^{67}Ga on 24-hour images. Radiology 135:445, 1980.

Slosman D, et al: Pulmonary accumulation of ^{131}I-MIBG in the isolated perfused rat lung. J Nucl Med 27:1076, 1986.

Slutsky RA, Higgins CB: Thallium scintigraphy in experimental toxic pulmonary edema: Relationship to extravascular pulmonary fluid. J Nucl Med 25:581, 1984.

Sostman HD, Gottschalk A: The stripe sign: A new sign for diagnosis of nonembolic defects on pulmonary perfusion scintigraphy. Radiology 142:737, 1982.

Sostman HD, Gottschalk A: Critical review of "pulmonary angiography, ventilation lung scanning, and venography for clinically suspected pulmonary embolism with abnormal perfusion lung scan." Invest Radiol 21:678, 1986.

Spies WG: Gallium-67 citrate imaging in acquired immunodeficiency syndrome. J Nucl Med Technol 17:23, 1989.

Spies WG: Diagnostic procedures for thoracic diseases: Nuclear techniques. Chest Surg Clin North Am 2:521, 1992.

Spies WG, Wojtowicz CH, Spies SM: Value of posttherapy whole-body scans in the evaluation of patients with thyroid carcinoma having undergone high-dose I-131 therapy. Radiology 161(P):224, 1986.

Spies WG, et al: Ventilation-perfusion scintigraphy in suspected pulmonary embolism: Correlation with pulmonary angiography and refinement of criteria for interpretation. Radiology 159:383, 1986.

Spies WG, et al: Monoclonal antibody imaging with In-111-labeled B72.3 in human non-small cell lung carcinoma. Radiology 169(P):74, 1988.

Spies WG, et al: Utility of 24 hour gallium images in the detection of acute pulmonary inflammatory processes in patients with acquired immunodeficiency syndrome. J Nucl Med 30:888, 1989.

Sullivan DC, et al: Lung scan interpretation: Effect of different observers and different criteria. Radiology 149:803, 1983.

Sullivan PJ, et al: A clinical comparison of Technegas and xenon-133 in 50 patients with suspected pulmonary embolus. Chest 94:300, 1988.

Susskind H, et al: Efficacy of Kr-81m and Xe-127 in evaluating non-embolic pulmonary disease (abstr). J Nucl Med 21:11, 1980.

Suttorp N, Simon LM: Lung cell oxidant injury: Enhancement of polymorphonuclear leukocyte-mediated cytotoxicity in lung cells exposed to sustained in vitro hyperoxia. J Clin Invest 70:342, 1982.

Taplin GV, Poe ND: A dual lung-scanning technic for evaluation of pulmonary function. Radiology 85:365, 1965.

Toronto Lung Transplant Group: Unilateral lung transplantation for pulmonary fibrosis. N Engl J Med 314:1140, 1986.

Touya JJ, et al: A noninvasive procedure for in vivo assay of a lung amine endothelial receptor. J Nucl Med 26:1302, 1985.

Touya JJ, et al: The lung as a metabolic organ. Semin Nucl Med 16:296, 1986a.

Touya JJ, et al: Single photon emission computed tomography in the diagnosis of pulmonary thromboembolism. Semin Nucl Med *16*:306, 1986b.

Vix VA: The usefulness of chest radiographs obtained after a demonstrated perfusion scan defect in the diagnosis of pulmonary emboli. Clin Nucl Med 8:497, 1983.

Webber MM, et al: Comparison of Biello, McNeil, and PIOPED criteria for the diagnosis of pulmonary emboli on lung scans. AJR Am J Roentgenol *154*:975, 1990.

Zimmer AM, et al: Radioimmunoimaging of human small cell lung carcinoma with I-131 tumor specific monoclonal antibody. Hybridoma *4*:1, 1985.

READING REFERENCES

Alderson PO, Line BR: Scintigraphic Studies of Nonembolic Lung Disease. In Gottschalk A, Hoffer PB, Potchen EJ: Diagnostic Nuclear Medicine. 2nd Ed. Baltimore: Williams & Wilkins, 1988.

Mettler FA Jr, Guiberteau MJ: Respiratory System. Essentials of Medicine Imaging. 3rd Ed. Philadelphia: WB Saunders, 1991.

Mettler FA Jr, Guiberteau MJ: Tumor and Inflammation Imaging. Essentials of Nuclear Medicine Imaging. 3rd Ed. Philadelphia: WB Saunders, 1991.

Sostman HD, Gottschalk A: Detection of pulmonary emboli. *In* Gottschalk A, Hoffer PB, Potchen EJ: Diagnostic Nuclear Medicine. 2nd Ed. Baltimore: Williams & Wilkins, 1988.

Diagnostic Procedures

CHAPTER 15

LABORATORY INVESTIGATIONS IN THE DIAGNOSIS OF PULMONARY DISEASES

Herbert M. Sommers and K. Eric Sommers

Pathology has been described as "the study of the harm that disease causes," in terms of both structure and function. The purpose of this chapter is to acquaint the surgeon with different ways of collecting this evidence, with comments on the limitations of each.

During the last decade, the role of the laboratory in the diagnosis of pulmonary diseases has greatly expanded because of the creation of several new populations of immunosuppressed patients through the human immunodeficiency virus — HIV — epidemic, the performance of organ transplantation, and the aggressive use of cytotoxic agents in the treatment of malignancy. The immunosuppressed states induced in these conditions and resultant opportunistic infections have led to a burgeoning demand for diagnostic services. Innovative diagnostic techniques have been developed and the field is evolving rapidly. As the spectrum of pathogenic microorganisms has broadened and effective treatments for many opportunistic infections have been developed, rapid and accurate diagnosis has become imperative so that appropriate treatment can be instituted.

Molecular biology has evolved to the point of transition from the research laboratory to the clinical laboratory, and no doubt the next decade will witness the emergence of the clinical molecular biology laboratory. DNA/RNA hybridization, polymerase chain reaction, and restriction fragment length analysis are proving enormously informative in the identification of pathogens as well as the epidemiology of infections.

TISSUE SPECIMENS FROM BIOPSY AND SURGICAL OPERATIONS

When selecting a site for biopsy or excision of tissue, one should consider several general principles. Benign tumors grow as an expanding mass, compressing and displacing adjacent structures. Expansion of the tumor tends to create either a real or an apparent capsule that may facilitate recognition and delineate the margin of the tumor. In contrast to benign tumors, malignant tumors invade adjacent tissue by irregular infiltration, tending to become fixed to normal structures and making the margins of the tumor irregular and difficult to define. The biopsy of a tumor should include tissue from part of the tumor as well as from adjacent tissue that may have been grossly distorted and displaced by the expanding mass. Inclusion of the tumor and adjacent tissue in the same biopsy specimen is helpful in determining whether the tumor is benign or malignant. Occasionally, primary disease processes, such as small tumors of the bronchus, can cause extensive pneumonia in lobes or in the entire lung that is far more impressive than the endobronchial tumor. All biopsy specimens should include evidence of primary disease as well as of secondary changes resulting from obstruction or other complications.

Biopsies at the time of endoscopy can present special problems. If the tumor extends into the lumen of the bronchus, the surface of the tumor may be partially necrotic. For this reason, several "bites" should be taken with the biopsy forceps to obtain enough tissue for good histologic detail. Ulcerating tumors of the bronchus may present another problem as they may excavate and spread by submucosal lymphatics. When a biopsy forceps cannot be used effectively, a direct smear taken from the ulcer may provide the diagnosis when studied by cytologic methods. Occasionally, a tumor extends under the adjacent normal mucosa, making it difficult, if not impossible, to localize. Carcinoma extending along submucosal bronchial lymphatics usually produces a slight narrowing of the bronchus despite a normal appearing mucosal surface. In such instances, random biopsy specimens from bronchi in these regions may show small collections of tumor in lymphatics (Fig. 15–1). In general, the larger the portion of tissue taken

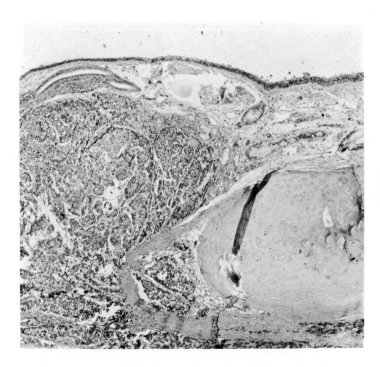

Fig. 15–1. Metastatic tumor beneath normal bronchial mucosa. Biopsy of this region would show tumor despite the intact mucosa. ×250.

for a biopsy, the more likely a correct diagnosis can be made. If biopsies do not reveal anticipated findings, the possibility of inadequate sampling should be considered and additional tissue should be obtained.

In the selection of lymph nodes for biopsy, size and firmness are usually sufficient to differentiate nodes secondarily involved with tumor from those enlarged from infection or other causes. Metastatic carcinoma in a lymph node is typically associated with varying amounts of connective tissue, resulting in an increased firmness to palpation. Occasionally, enlarged lymph nodes containing secondary tumor may be soft and appear hyperplastic owing to necrosis of the tumor from rapid growth. A normal appearing lymph node included with an abnormal node can act as a "control" for changes found in the abnormal node. The changes found in lymph nodes at different stages of a disease may be helpful in predicting the prognosis. Examination of several lymph nodes can help in differentiating generalized from focal disease.

Frozen Sections

The development of improved cryostats has made the preparation of frozen sections a more reliable procedure than it was in the past. Requests for a "frozen section" should be restricted to two situations: when it is necessary to ensure that biopsy examination has been adequate to establish a diagnosis; and when the type of operation depends on the diagnosis made on the basis of the biopsy specimen. In most instances, tissues from epithelial tumors can be diagnosed rapidly with a high degree of reliability. By contrast, tumors of the reticuloendothelial system pose a more difficult problem, as differentiation from atypical inflammatory or hyper-

plastic processes may depend on subtle changes in cellular composition or structural components, such as reticulum. Asking for a frozen section as a matter of interest when the result will not influence the operation is not warranted, because freezing the tissue induces artifacts that can make the subsequent interpretation of paraffin sections more difficult.

When taking a biopsy specimen for frozen section, include as much tissue as is prudent under the circumstances. To cut a frozen section, a certain amount of the biopsy specimen is destroyed, and, in rare instances, tumor that may have been seen in the frozen section of a small specimen may not be found in the paraffin sections. This occurrence is usually a consequence of removal of an inadequate portion of tissue for examination. If a frozen section is needed, the biopsy specimen should not be placed in a fixative solution to send to the laboratory, because coagulation by formalin and other tissue fixatives changes the water content of the tissue and lowers its freezing temperature. Most mechanically refrigerated cryostats cannot achieve temperatures low enough to freeze fixed tissue.

Consultation Between Pathologist and Surgeon

The pathologist prefers to examine the tissue and microscopic sections without being prejudiced by the clinical history and physical findings. Because this is not always practical, specimens should be accompanied by a short history along with pertinent physical findings. Even more desirable is a conference between the surgeon and the pathologist at the time the frozen section is examined. The surgeon can describe the operative findings and answer any questions the pathologist may have.

Consultation before biopsy may also be helpful for selected patients to arrange for special studies, such as immunofluorescence or electron microscopy. Collection and handling of specimens for such studies require specific reagents or prompt freezing. Advance notice of an unusual problem alerts the laboratory to be ready for the specimen and facilitates processing the tissue for any special procedure indicated. With good communication, an excellent understanding develops between the pathologist and the surgeon, with a direct reflection on the quality of patient care.

Cultures

When biopsy or excision has been completed, the specimen should be sent immediately to the laboratory in a sterile container. Unless the clinician has no question about the etiologic basis of the disease, the specimen should be cultured as well as examined histologically. Both studies can be done by giving portions of the specimen to both the microbiology and pathology laboratories, or by sending the specimen to one laboratory with explicit instructions to forward it to the other. In many instances, the recovery of infectious organisms depends on inoculation of the specimen to specific culture media. Any information concerning the clinical diagnosis or history of recent travel by the patient can be helpful in selecting media and incubation conditions for recovery of an infectious organism.

Smears

In addition to obtaining material for culture, the clinician should place three to four smears of exudate or fluid on glass slides at the time of the operation. One should be prepared with Gram's stain and the others retained, should stains for detection of tuberculosis, fungi, or parasites be necessary. It is easy to discard unneeded slides. Frequently, the diagnosis of a specific infection can be made from a stained smear long before tissue sections are ready or the organism is identified in culture; examples include nocardiosis, actinomycosis, pneumocystis, and legionnaires' disease.

CYTOLOGIC STUDIES OF BRONCHIAL SECRETIONS AND PLEURAL FLUID

Morning Sputum Specimens

Cytologic examination of sputum specimens is helpful and may provide the diagnosis of malignant pulmonary tumors. Specimens obtained immediately after arising in the morning are preferred, although they can be collected at any time. The patient should be instructed concerning the difference between sputum and saliva and given a small container of 50% alcohol so that all cells will be fixed promptly and autolytic changes stopped. Fixatives containing ether, acetone, or alcohol in concentrations greater than 50% should not be used. Precipitation of protein in such fluids produces hardening of the sediment and makes preparation of smears almost impossible. Rapid fixation of expectorated cells

is important because cells in the sputum have been completely or partially separated from their blood supply for varying periods of time and usually have undergone some autolysis in vivo. The practice of collecting sputum in fixative solutions at the bedside also decreases autolytic changes that may develop with delayed transportation of the specimen to the laboratory. Any interval between the time of collection of the specimen and the fixation of the cells decreases the quality of cellular detail and the validity of the report (Fig. 15–2).

In patients who cannot produce sputum spontaneously, the use of a heated aerosol or ultrasonic nebulizer can frequently stimulate sufficient sputum to yield satisfactory specimens. For this purpose, 10% hypertonic saline solution or 15% propylene glycol is used in the aerosol. Three specimens on three successive days should be collected to ensure maximum accuracy. Koss (1968) summarized the methods for obtaining cytologic specimens from the respiratory tract and gave recommendations for the use of heated aerosol for sputum induction. If the specimen will be used for culture as well as for cytologic studies, propylene glycol should not be used in the aerosol. Singh and Garrison (1964) found that propylene glycol inhibited or killed certain types of microorganisms. A negative culture from a specimen collected using propylene glycol as a cytologic fixative may give a false sense of security.

Pleural Fluid

Malignant tumors extending to the pleural surfaces may exfoliate varying numbers of cells (Fig. 15–3). Individual tumors vary in this respect, and the tumor occasionally incites an inflammatory reaction without shedding a significant number of malignant cells. The interpretation of cellular changes in pleural fluids can present a difficult problem to the cytologist, as the rapid proliferation of mesothelial and inflammatory cells often shows many of the changes characteristic of tumor cells, such as mitoses, large, prominent nuclei, and increased nuclear-cytoplasmic ratio. The accumulation of high protein-containing fluid within the pleural space serves as an excellent tissue culture system for free cells and consequently mitotic figures may be common. The period of time that an exfoliated cell is present within a fluid before removal by thoracentesis has a direct effect on its appearance, with older cells showing swelling and degenerative changes. Because of the accumulation of degenerating cells, the first fluid withdrawn by thoracentesis in a patient with suspected tumor in the pleural space is less satisfactory for cytologic studies than a fluid sample removed several days later. This fluid should be sent to the cytology laboratory to look for obvious malignant cells. The second thoracentesis collection should contain a younger and metabolically more active cellular population, providing a more representative sample of the different cellular elements.

Although it is preferable, centrifugation of the pleural fluid immediately to prepare smears and cell block

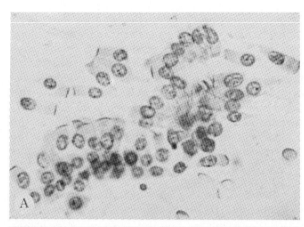

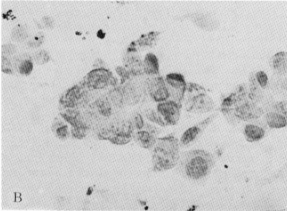

Fig. 15–2. *A,* Smear of normal cells obtained at bronchoscopy and fixed promptly in ether alcohol. Note discrete cell margins, nuclear detail, and cilia on bronchial cells. *B,* Cells from bronchoscopy allowed to dry prior to fixation in ether alcohol. Cell margins are indistinct and nuclear detail is blurred. Occasional nuclei are hyperchromatic and suggest atypical changes. Delay of fixation of bronchial smears seriously decreases the value of the specimen. ×650. Courtesy of Pacita Manalo-Estrella.

specimens may not be possible. The addition of ethyl alcohol to result in a 30 to 50% final concentration stops autolytic changes. Making a cell block as well as smears from centrifuged sediment can be helpful in identifying cellular arrangements not apparent on smears. Cell blocks are also useful for histochemical studies, such as the demonstration of intracellular mucin or the accumulation of glycogen.

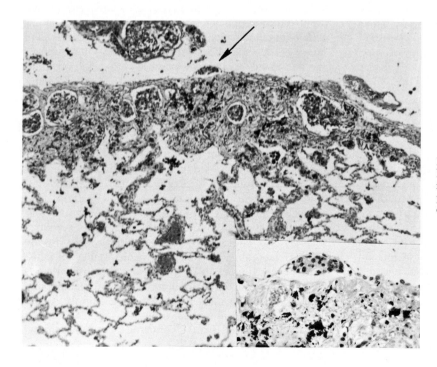

Fig. 15–3. Secondary carcinoma in subpleural lymphatics (see arrow). Groups of tumor cells shed from this surface can be identified from centrifuged pleural fluid. *Inset:* Clump of tumor cells immediately beneath pleural mesothelial membrane.

Fine Needle Aspiration

Fine needle aspiration — FNA — as noted by Frable (1983) is an easy, safe, and inexpensive diagnostic technique that is well tolerated by patients in the office or other outpatient setting. A thin — No. 21 to 23 gauge — needle is used to aspirate suspicious masses anywhere in the body, and the specimen obtained is processed for cytologic or histologic diagnosis. Although surgical biopsy offers greater likelihood of arriving at a more certain diagnosis, FNA offers less risk, less cost, and more convenience. Fine needle aspiration should be strongly considered when: 1) patients cannot tolerate major surgery; 2) the tumors are clearly unresectable; 3) new masses appear in a patient with multiple previous primary tumors; 4) metastases must be proven or unresectability of tumor must be documented; or 5) deep infections must be diagnosed. Aspiration is performed using fluoroscopy, sonography, and CT scanning for locating deep lesions. The major limitation of FNA is the risk of a negative report caused by sampling error. Multiple samples obtained by movement of the needle during aspiration produce a more uniform result and may offer an advantage over the core needle biopsy. Linsk (1986) stressed that improved localization technique increases the yield by assuring aspiration of the intended site.

LABORATORY TECHNIQUES IN THE DIAGNOSIS OF PULMONARY INFECTION

The use of sophisticated techniques in the diagnosis of pulmonary infection has grown as demand for rapid diagnosis has increased. As a consequence, many clinicians no doubt feel intimidated by the array of tests available. Without some understanding of the manner in which results are obtained, many clinicians are unsure of the value and of the limitations inherent in the performance of these examinations. A detailed presentation of the various techniques currently used in the diagnosis of pulmonary infections is clearly outside the scope of this textbook, but we will attempt an overview for the practicing physician.

Collection of Specimens For Culture

Specimens for culture may be collected in several ways. Unless due care is taken to minimize contamination from sites other than the one under study, overgrowth by organisms not associated with the infection may occur and result in inappropriate therapy.

The easiest specimen to obtain for culture is sputum. A significant disadvantage of sputum lies in contamination by oral and pharyngeal organisms. Many sputum specimens contain only salivary and oropharyngeal secretions and frequently represent an honest but ineffective effort by the patient to raise secretions from the lower respiratory tract. In one study, collection of sputum by expectoration and culture for pneumococci by standard procedures resulted in isolation of *Streptococcus pneumoniae* in only 55% of patients with both clinical pneumonia and pneumococcal bacteremia. Although all the reasons for the poor recovery of *S. pneumoniae* by culture are not known, evidence suggests that interaction with other organisms or products from organisms found in the oropharynx, such as the α-hemolytic streptococci, may suppress growth of the pneumococcus. Dilworth and associates (1975) reported that partial suppression of the endogenous flora in culture using gentamicin-containing blood agar has resulted in improved recovery of *S. pneumoniae* from sputum in patients with pneumonia.

Another method for collection of material for culture from the lower respiratory tract is the induction of sputum by ultrasonic or heated saline nebulization. Aerosolization increases the moisture content of the air going to the lower respiratory tract and improves the ability of the tracheobronchial cilia to bring up otherwise thick, viscid, or partially dehydrated secretions. Nebulization is particularly well suited for the recovery of *Mycobacterium tuberculosis* and *Pneumocystis*, but can also be used for inducing sputum in patients with other types of pulmonary infections. Properly performed sputum induction is a painstaking process, but it can save the patient an invasive procedure; Obrien and colleagues (1989) reported that induced sputum has been shown to provide the diagnosis of pneumococcal pneumonia in 66% of cases.

To determine whether a sputum specimen represents true secretions from an acutely inflamed part of the bronchopulmonary tree rather than saliva or oropharyngeal secretions, Gram's stain can be used to evaluate the quality of the specimen before it is cultured. If most are neutrophils or other types of inflammatory cells, the specimen should be inoculated to culture media, but if most of the cells appear to be from squamous epithelium, presumably from the oropharynx, the laboratory should request an additional specimen. Finding large numbers of segmented neutrophils indicates a cellular response to an acute injury, most often associated with an acute bacterial infection. Van Scoy (1977) suggested that the different types and relative numbers of bacteria should be noted also, as well as any evidence of bacterial phagocytosis.

The value of the gram stain is to determine the number and type of bacteria in the area adjacent to segmented neutrophils. If a true infection is present, most bacteria are the same type rather than mixed. Assuming the patient has a bacterial pneumonia, the bacterial morphotype seen on the gram stain should correlate with the causative agent of the pneumonia and aid the technologist in selecting the optimal isolation media. In an immunosuppressed, neutropenic patient, a gram stain showing large numbers of the same type of bacteria may be the only guide available in the early diagnosis of the infectious agent causing pneumonia.

Bronchoscopy, bronchoalveolar lavage — BAL, protected brushing, and transbronchial biopsy are now the most popular and reliable means of diagnosis in complicated lower respiratory tract infections. Each institution, indeed each clinician, no doubt follows a self-defined protocol of escalating invasiveness that takes into account the severity of the patient's illness, the clinical scenario, and the associated risk of each procedure. A potential limitation to using material collected at bronchoscopy for culture has been shown by Conte and Laforet (1962), as well as by Kleinfield and Elliss (1967), who found that local anesthetic agents used in bronchoscopy may inhibit the growth of non-acid fast and anaerobic bacteria as well as fungi. Saline used in lavage techniques must not contain bacteriostatic agents such as benzyl alcohol or methyl- or propylparaben. These agents are incorporated into saline used for injection of medication to prevent growth of contaminants and, as noted by Rein and Mandell (1973), may quickly kill the bacteria that cause acute pneumonia. Once the specimen reaches the laboratory, a wide variety of stains and cultures are performed to ensure that important pathogens are not overlooked. A representative protocol devised by Kahn and Jones (1988) for BAL specimens is presented in Figure 15–4.

Serologic Techniques

Serologic methods are classified broadly into those techniques that detect microbial antigens and those that detect the host antibody response to microbial infection. Serologic techniques depend on the use of immunoglobulins for the detection of antigens, as well as identification of circulating host antibody. Examples of an antigenic assay would be the latex agglutination assay used in the detection of cryptococcal antigen in the cerebral spinal fluid of patients with cryptococcal meningitis. Quantification of antigen assays is not imperative; in most cases, the demonstration of microbial antigen is sufficient to make a diagnosis of infection.

In contrast, quantitative serologic assay of patient antibody status is vitally important to distinguish active from past infection. Quantification is usually performed by serial dilution and reported as titers, that is, 1:4, 1:256. Active infection usually results in high titer, such as 1:256, and an increase in titer, typically fourfold or greater in a patient previously exposed to the microbe. Two time points are necessary to make this determination, and serum is taken during the active phase and the convalescence phase for this comparison. Furthermore, assay of the class of antibody can be important, because IgM class antibodies are typical of the early humoral immunologic response, whereas IgG antibody response indicates longstanding immunity from previous encounter with the microbial antigen.

A daunting number of assays are used for the evaluation of the humoral response to microbial infection. The most commonly performed include complement fixation — CF, indirect hemagglutination — IHA, direct and indirect immunofluorescence — DIF and IIF, enzyme-linked immunosorbent assay — ELISA, radioimmunoassay — RIA, and immunodiffusion — ID. The relative merits of each of these specific techniques are not particularly important to the clinician except insofar as they all represent tools to evaluate the humoral status of the patient vis a vis a specific microbe.

Histologic and Cytologic Methods

A variety of stains are available for sputum, BAL, and tissue specimens to enhance identification of pathogenic organisms. In some instances, microscopic examination is the keystone of diagnosis because growth of the organism may not be possible, such as *Pneumocystis*. Conventional staining techniques are discussed in the

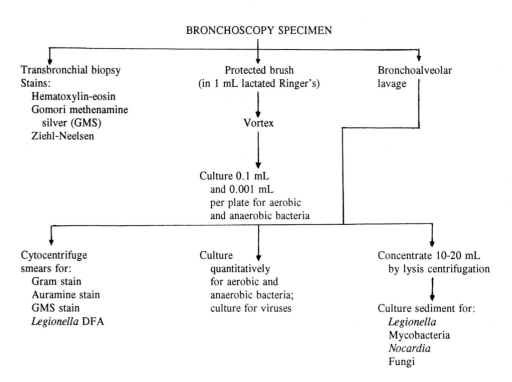

Fig. 15–4. Recommended protocol for the processing of bronchoscopy specimens.

section dealing with specific organisms. Newer staining techniques that have increased specificity and sensitivity include immunofluorescence staining and in situ DNA hybridization with probes specific to microbial genetic material.

Culture

Recovery of organisms from culture is the established standard for microbial identification. Experience and empiric experimentation have identified culture media for most pathogenic microbes. In general, laboratories plate respiratory specimens on a variety of culture media to enhance recovery of known bacterial and fungal pathogens. Viral and mycobacterial cultures usually require a separate request, and notification of the laboratory that unusual pathogens are actively under suspicion will undoubtably aid in their recovery in culture.

Different microbial species grow at different growth rates in culture, and the clinician accustomed to receiving bacterial culture results in days may be dismayed to learn that certain mycobacteria may takes months to become apparent on routine culture. A host of newer techniques that enhance identification of fastidious organisms have been, and continue to be, developed, but physicians experienced in treatment of immunocompromised patients know that in many cases, final definitive culture of many pathogens can take weeks. In addition to culture of respiratory specimens, blood culture should always be performed, because culture of organisms from blood usually denotes unequivocal evidence of invasive infection.

Molecular Biologic Methods

The application of these methods to clinical microbiology is revolutionizing the field. Some familiarity of the basic concepts behind these techniques will enhance the clinician's understanding and interpretation of test results derived from these methods. DNA hybridization is the technique whereby DNA probes consisting of genetic material complementary to that of a specific organism are annealed to the native DNA of organism of interest. Probes consist of oligonucleotides complementary to a segment in the microbe's genome and are extremely specific for each microbial species. The probe is tagged to allow detection, usually with a radioactive isotope, but attention is focusing on the development of nonradiometric probes that are more convenient and safer to use. Hybridization with DNA probes finds two primary applications in the clinical microbiology laboratory. Traditionally, hybridization has been used to speciate organisms from culture, such as mycobacteria. More recently, DNA probes have been applied with success directly to clinical specimens, including blood cultures.

The polymerase chain reaction — PCR — is the process whereby minute quantities of genetic material can be expanded literally a billion-fold. The technique of PCR is actually easy to understand in concept, if not

application. The specimen containing the organism of interest — and obviously its DNA — is incubated with: 1) a DNA primer specific to the organism; 2) the building blocks of DNA — the nucleotide bases; and 3) a heat-sensitive polymerase that will replicate DNA, given the right conditions and primer. Each cycle of PCR involves the replication of the DNA segment encoded by the primer, a process analogous to DNA replication during cell division. Because the polymerase is heat sensitive, the process can be halted and restarted simply by raising and lowering the incubation temperature. Thus, the process is easily "cycled," and with each cycle, the DNA is replicated; events quickly assume a geometric quality, hence the "chain reaction." Therein lies the enormous potential for expansion of the genetic material.

Restriction Fragment Length Polymorphism — RFLP, or DNA "fingerprinting," is another technique that is applied to the identification and speciation of organisms. In this technique, DNA is cleaved with a specific restriction endonuclease and the resulting fragments are separated by gel electrophoresis. The pattern of fragment lengths is remarkably specific between species and even between individuals — RFLP has been used in forensic medicine and has been used to identify attackers in rape cases. Molecular biology techniques and their application to infectious disease have been reviewed by Figueroa and Rasheed (1991).

Thus, molecular techniques are impressive by virtue of their remarkable sensitivity and specificity. These qualities, however, give rise to new problems relating to the interpretation of such exquisitely sensitive data. This problem is illustrated by Delgado and colleagues (1992), who prospectively studied blood samples from 24 liver transplant recipients using PCR and standard viral cultures for CMV virus. They found that PCR was able to detect CMV DNA in the blood of all 8 patients who developed symptomatic CMV illness, but PCR also detected CMV viremia in 9 of 24 patients who did *not* show evidence of virus from blood culture and did not have symptomatic disease. Thus, the sensitivity of PCR compared to culture was 100%, the specificity was 76%, but the positive predictive value only 25%. The significance of PCR-positive culture and symptom-negative result is not known, and it is likely that such interpretive problems will be encountered as PCR gains wider clinical use.

BACTERIAL INFECTIONS OF THE LUNG

Because thoracic surgeons and clinicians caring for patients with thoracic surgical problems are far more likely to be asked to provide input regarding patients with complicated or opportunistic infections of the chest, this discussion of bacterial infections will not include community-acquired pathogens. Excellent reviews, such as that of Bartlett (1991), are available for the pathogens normally associated with community-acquired infection.

Nosocomial Pneumonia

Nosocomial pneumonia is a frequent problem for patients undergoing thoracic surgical procedures, as well as for patients who undergo transplantation of thoracic organs. Many risk factors have been identified for the development of nosocomial pneumonia, but the most important are colonization of the oropharynx with gram-negative rods and *Staphylococcus*, endotracheal intubation, advanced age, poor cardiopulmonary status, immunosuppression, and prolonged mechanical ventilation. Clearly, patients who undergo thoracic surgery or transplantation either have many of these risk factors or are at risk for developing them.

The diagnosis of nosocomial pneumonia is based on four clinical features: 1) fever; 2) a new infiltrate on the chest radiograph; 3) leukocytosis; and 4) purulent tracheobroncheal secretions. The identification of a pathogenic organism is notoriously difficult in these patients, especially in the setting of mechanical ventilation. Tracheal aspirates are not specific and more invasive techniques are required to obtain reliable results. Consensus is forming in this regard. A diagnostic approach based on early bronchoscopy for BAL and protected specimen brushing — PSB — was advanced by Meduri (1990). This approach places high priority on the performance of invasive procedures to obtain a good quality specimen and avoids the use of empiric antibiotics. Use of BAL and PSB for recovery of pathogenic bacteria demands rigorous methodologic attention and guidelines for performance of these techniques, and handling of the specimens obtained by the laboratory have been established by Balselski and colleagues (1992), as well as by Meduri and Chastre (1992). Significant results are more than 10^5 cfu/ml for BAL specimens, and more than 10^3 cfu/ml for PSB cultures in patients not previously treated with antibiotics. The guidelines for the interpretation of BAL and PSB culture results in patients previously treated with antibiotics are not established.

Treatment of nosocomial pneumonia has traditionally included an aminoglycoside antibiotic and either a broad range penicillin or third generation cephalosporin. The introduction of a multitude of newer agents with broad spectrum activity against the usual pathogens of nosocomial pneumonia has expanded the options for treatment. Many clinicians now avoid the use of aminoglycoside antibiotics because of their low penetration into lung tissue and secretions, as well as the risk of nephrotoxicity. Most clinicians treat *Pseudomonas* and *Acinetobacter* isolates with two agents shown to be effective against the isolate by sensitivity testing. A review by Scheld and Mandell (1991) summarizes advances in the pathogenesis, diagnosis, and treatment of nosocomial pneumonia.

An area of intense research has been the use of decontamination regimens in the prevention of nosocomial pneumonia. The rationale for the use of these agents is based on the demonstration that organisms recovered in patients with nosocomial pneumonia are frequently demonstrated in secretions from the oropharynx and stomach, particularly in patients treated with antiulcer medication. Aspiration of these secretions is the important pathogenic mechanism. A multitude of clinical studies have demonstrated that the rates of nosocomial pneumonia can be significantly reduced using decontamination protocols, but it has been difficult to prove conclusively that this improvement has any effect on overall survival. A good review by LaForce (1992) is available.

Legionella

In July of 1976, a strange and virulent form of pneumonia struck 182 members of the Pennsylvania branch of the American Legion during their annual meeting in Philadelphia; 18 legionnaires died. During the next 6 months, an intensive investigation resulted in the isolation of a new, completely different bacterial organism, now known as *Legionella pneumophila*. This organism differs from other medically significant bacteria in that it does not stain by Gram's method and is unique in having an absolute growth requirement for cysteine. An adequate amount of this compound to grow *Legionella* is not present in blood agar, chocolate agar, or other types of primary culture media. The organism also requires an increased concentration of CO_2 for growth and may take 7 to 12 days to appear on artificial culture media. The organism grows best on buffered charcoal yeast extract supplemented with α-ketoglutarate.

Stout and co-workers (1982) showed that the isolation of *Legionella pneumophila* and related species initially from the water in air-conditioning cooling towers and subsequently from the faucets, shower heads, and hot water storage tanks in hospitals has emphasized the ubiquitousness of this group of organisms. Because the organisms are widespread, it is clear that mere exposure to contaminated water is an insufficient condition for the occurrence of legionnaire's disease; host susceptibility is undoubtedly a critical factor. Patients undergoing immunosuppression for organ transplantation or other therapeutic reasons are at high risk and should be followed carefully for the sudden onset of severe and rapidly developing pneumonia.

Clinically, the disease may occur in epidemics, such as was seen in Philadelphia, or as sporadic cases acquired in the community. As noted by Balows and Fraser (1979), it has been recognized as a major cause of serious or fatal pneumonia in immune-suppressed or immune-defective patients, many of whom develop the disease while in the hospital.

Patients with *Legionella* pneumonia have prominent constitutional symptoms including malaise, lethargy, anorexia, myalgia, and arthralgias. Fevers are typically high, unremitting, and may be accompanied with relative bradycardia. Cough is initially unproductive but can become productive of purulent or blood-streaked sputum. Associated gastrointestinal symptoms are frequent, and include abdominal pain, diarrhea, nausea, and vomiting. Elevations noted on liver function tests and hyponatremia are frequent concurrent findings on chemistry panels. The laboratory diagnosis of *Legionella* is based on rapid methods, culture, and serology. The serologic diagnosis of *Legionella* depends on development of convalescent titers and thus is not useful for diagnosis of acute disease. An exception is the demonstration of high titers; that is, 1:256 or greater, during the acute disease that is indicative of active infection, particularly because symptomatic carriage does not occur and re-infection with *Legionella* does not appear to be common. Culture is the most specific diagnostic method, but it has limited sensitivity and requires at least 2 days, and may take longer.

Thus, to guide therapy, rapid methods for the diagnosis of *Legionella* have evolved. The technique used most widely is direct fluorescence antibody — DFA — staining of sputum specimens; DFA staining is rapid but suffers from a lack of sensitivity, usually given to be around 60 to 75%. Other rapid methods include nucleic acid hybridization probes, and detection of antigen in urine, sputum, or serum. Hybridization probes are specific, and are considered by Rodgers and Pasculle (1985) as acceptable alternatives to the DFA. A nonradiometric hybridization technique has been developed by Fain and co-workers (1991). Assays for *Legionella* antigen in urine, sputum, and serum samples include ELISA, latex agglutination, and RIA techniques. These methods continue to be evaluated and may be used more widely in the future. The treatment of choice for uncomplicated *Legionella* is erythromycin. Tetracycline and rifampin are also active against this organism.

Nocardia

Nocardia is an aerobic filamentous bacterium belonging to the order *Actinomycetales*. Because they exhibit many of the morphologic characteristics of fungi in culture, such as aerial hyphae, they have been classified in the past as fungi. *Nocardia asteroides* — the predominant pathogenic species — is recognized as a significant opportunistic pathogen in immunosuppressed patients. The lung is the usual site of introduction for *Nocardia*, where it can cause a wide spectrum of histologic injury from minimal infiltration to abscess formation and necrotizing pneumonitis. Disseminated disease can follow lung infection and can progress to abscess formation in the brain. Sinus tract formation is a characteristic trait of disseminated *Nocardia* infection with tracts forming from the mediastinum or from satellite abscesses in subcutaneous tissue and skin from hematogenous spread. *Nocardia* is a relatively more common opportunistic pathogen in cardiac transplant patients in particular, but is seen rarely in patients with acquired immune deficiency syndrome — AIDS — for unknown reasons. The treatment of choice is TMP-SMX.

The diagnosis of this bacterial infection is based on demonstration of the organism in culture or by staining. Figure 15–5 illustrates a gram-stained section of material taken from a pulmonary abscess due to *Nocardia asteroides*. Because *Nocardia asteroides* is not stained by hematoxylin or eosin or the periodic acid-Schiff stain, it cannot be recognized unless Gram's stain or a methenamine silver stain is used. Although some stains of *Nocardia* may show an ability to retain an acid-fast or auramine stain, smears or sections have to be decolorized by a milder solution of acid, 1% sulfuric versus 3% hydrochloric. The ability to identify *Nocardia* in acid-fast and auramine-stained specimens varies considerably between different strains. *Nocardia* grows well on media for bacteria, fungi, and mycobacteria, and no special media are required for its recovery. Serologic assays are under development but no serologic tests are widely used for the diagnosis of *Nocardia* at present.

Mycobacteria

Before the discovery of streptomycin and other chemotherapeutic agents, the diagnosis of tuberculosis was made on the basis of the clinical picture, a radiograph of the chest compatible with that of tuberculosis, and the demonstration of acid-fast bacilli in the sputum. Isolation of the organism by culture was done in few hospitals but not routinely because the culture medium was expensive, bacterial contaminants were troublesome, and little was to be gained in treating the patients by recovery of the organism. With the development of antituberculous drugs, however, it became necessary to isolate the organism so that drug susceptibility studies could be made and resistance could be detected. As more cultures were made, variant strains from the typical type of organism — *Mycobacterium tuberculosis* — responsible for tuberculosis in human beings were found. In 1954, Timpe and Runyon described 100 such stains, proposing a grouping for "atypical" organisms. In 1959, Runyon published a more complete description of the variant mycobacteria, and for convenience, classified them into four groups, I to IV.

Inconsistencies in the grouping of many organisms under the Runyon classification, however, have led to a newly proposed classification of mycobacteria other than tuberculosis based on pathogenicity for humans. This classification, modified by Woods and Washington (1987), is illustrated in Table 15–1. This scheme obviously depends on accurate and thorough speciation of isolates.

Specimen Collection in Pulmonary Tuberculosis

Sputum is the specimen most easily collected for use in making the diagnosis of pulmonary tuberculosis. A series of three to five early-morning specimens is recommended because experience shows that the number of bacilli shed varies from day to day in patients excreting low numbers of organisms. This variation is probably related to intermittent focal ulceration of the bronchial mucosa, releasing different numbers of tubercle bacilli in the bronchi over irregular periods. Krasnow and Wayne (1969) showed that specimens collected by heated aerosol or nebulization after the patient arises in the morning produce positive cultures after shorter incubation and with fewer contaminants

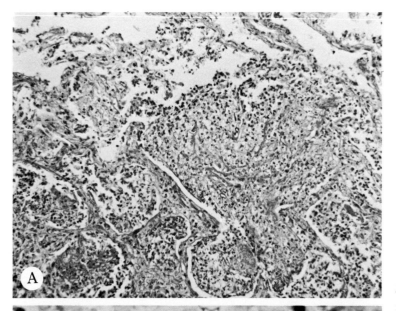

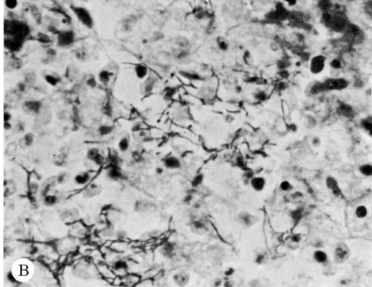

Fig. 15–5. Pulmonary abscess due to *Nocardia asteroides.* The nocardial infections cause suppuration with abscess formation. *A*, Section stained with hematoxylin and eosin or PAS does not demonstrate the organism. *B*, Gram-stained section shows thin, branching rods. ×650.

than do specimens collected over 24 hours. The 24-hour specimens yielded more positive cultures, although they required longer incubation times and were more likely to be contaminated. Both types of specimens are of value. Collection at bronchoscopy of secretions for culture is best done by using bronchial washings or bronchial lavage, but these specimens should be processed immediately if local anesthetics have been used to facilitate passage of the bronchoscope. Bronchial brushes, used in collecting specimens for cytology, provide good specimens for culture. Note that after bronchoscopy, recovery of mycobacteria increases in sputum specimens collected over the succeeding 24 to 48 hours. Early-morning gastric aspiration for organisms swallowed during the night is recommended only for infants or children or for those patients whose sputum

cannot be obtained naturally or by heated aerosol. The recovery of saprophytic, nonpathogenic species of mycobacteria from gastric aspirates can mislead the clinician until such time as identification of the organism is complete. In early stages of disseminated miliary tuberculosis, sputum specimens may not show the organism before invasion and ulceration of the bronchial tree. Demonstration or isolation of the organism in miliary tuberculosis may best be accomplished by liver biopsy, by bone marrow aspiration, or possibly by cerebrospinal fluid examination. Lung biopsy frequently is helpful.

Isolation of *M. tuberculosis* and other mycobacteria from sputum and other types of contaminated clinical specimens is facilitated by a digestion procedure to release mycobacteria from mucin, kill contaminating

Table 15–1. Mycobacteria other than *M. tuberculosis*

Group	Species
Species pathogenic in humans	*M. leprae*
Species potentially pathogenic in humans	*M. avium-intracellulare, M. kansasii, M. fortuitum-chelonae* complex, *M. scrofulaceum, M. xenopi, M. szulgai, M. malmoense, M. simiae, M. marinum, M. ulcerans, M. haemophilum*
Saprophytic mycobacteria rarely causing disease in humans	
Slow growth rate	*M. gordonae, M. asiaticum, M. terrae-triviale* complex, *M. gastri, M. nonchromogenicum, M. paratuberculosis*
Intermediate growth rate	*M. flavescens*
Rapid growth rate	*M. thermoresistible, M. smegmatis, M. vaccae, M. parafortuitum* complex, *M. phlei*

bacteria, and concentrate the number of mycobacteria to a smaller volume.

Inoculation of the concentrated specimen should be made to a minimum of two and preferably three different types of culture media, with an egg base — Lowenstein-Jensen — and an agar base — Middlebrook 7H11 agar — currently the most popular. Use of a third culture medium containing one or more antibiotics is strongly recommended to suppress nonmycobacterial organisms. Incubation of all media in 5 to 10% CO_2 results in an increased yield and rate of growth.

Stained smears of the concentrate should be made to search for the organism as well as to observe the numbers shed — an indication of the activity of the infection. Sputum smears are positive for mycobacteria in approximately 60 to 70% of specimens yielding positive cultures. Smears may be stained by one of the classic acid-fast techniques — Ziehl-Neelsen — or by a fluorochrome — auramine or a combination of auramine and rhodamine. The advantage of the fluorochrome stain is that it enables the microscopist to scan a larger field in a shorter period of time without loss of specificity. Although experienced microscopists may be able to tell different species of mycobacteria by their shape on a stained smear, identifying characteristics are subtle and usually not dependable unless the observer sees many smears from patients with different species of mycobacteria.

The complete identification of all mycobacterial isolates is almost mandatory, as the distinction between organisms known to cause disease and those not associated with disease is important in selecting proper therapy. The use of a Runyon group designation is not adequate for this purpose. Species identification can usually be accompanied by determining relatively few characteristics. Although the incidence of tuberculosis has continued to decline, the incidence of disease from

mycobacteria other than *M. tuberculosis* is becoming more common.

The proper determination of antimycobacterial drug susceptibility is a highly technical and expensive procedure. Primary drug resistance of *M. tuberculosis*, defined as resistance by an organism to one or more drugs in a previously untreated patient, was thought to be less than 5%. Kopanoff and associates (1978), however, noted that a more widely selected group of patients has shown primary drug resistance of *M. tuberculosis* in 8 to 20% of isolates, depending on geographic location and ethnic group sampled. This previously unrecognized primary drug resistance of *M. tuberculosis* has suggested the need for more frequent routine determination of susceptibility studies than was considered necessary in the past.

New Methods for Identification of Mycobacteria

Two developments have revolutionized the field of mycobacteriology: the development of radiometric procedures for the culture and identification of mycobacteria, and the application of molecular biology to identification of species. Traditional techniques of identification relied on culture of the organism — often a painstakingly slow undertaking — and then the use of a battery of biochemical tests to elucidate the species to which an isolate would be assigned. In 1977, Middlebrook and associates described a broth culture medium — 7H12 — containing 1-^{14}C palmitic acid that could be used for the detection of the growth of *M. tuberculosis*. The method relies on the measurement of ^{14}C-labeled CO_2 released during the metabolism of palmitic acid by mycobacteria in an ion chamber system (Bactec, Johnston Laboratories, Towson, MD). Initial studies with this system indicated that an inoculum of 200 viable units of *M. tuberculosis* could be detected in 12 to 14 days. The results led to further studies for the application of the technique to routine laboratory procedures to include detection, identification, and susceptibility, testing with primary antituberculosis drugs by Siddiqui and associates (1981) (Fig. 15–6). A multicenter, collaborative study reported by Snider and colleagues (1981) found that although the results of drug susceptibility tests of *M. tuberculosis* with the radiometric and standard methods were similar, agreement was better with the Bactec and the agar dilution procedure when comparing drug-susceptible strains than with drug-resistant strains. Overall, Siddiqui and associates (1981) found results with the new procedure were better when determined in a specialty laboratory for mycobacteria than in a routine clinical laboratory. Agreement for drug susceptibility testing between radiometric and standard agar dilution methods for *M. tuberculosis* was 95%. In addition, results were reportable on 98% of the tests in 5 days. Several problems were encountered with the determinations of *M. tuberculosis* susceptibility to ethambutol, which were believed to be attributable to test vials containing an inappropriate concentration of the drug.

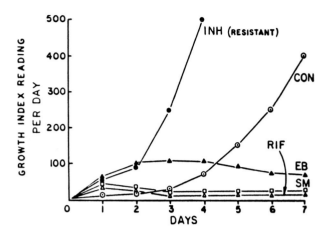

Fig. 15-6. Radiometric drug susceptibility test pattern of an INH-resistant strain of *M. tuberculosis.* CON-Control. *From* Laszlo A, Siddiqi SH: Evaluation of a rapid radiometric method for drug susceptibility testing of *Mycobacterium tuberculosis.* J Clin Microbiol 13:908, 1981.

Using the Bactec, *M. tuberculosis* usually can be detected rapidly in decontaminated clinical specimens by inoculation to a selective Middlebrook 7H12, a medium containing polymyxin B, amphotericin B, carbenicillin, and trimethoprim — PACT. Damato and colleagues (1983) showed that 70% of smear-positive specimens are culture positive in the radiometric procedure within 14 days, with or without the addition of PACT to the medium, compared with 21 days by the standard procedure. Similarly, Morgan and associates (1983) found that detection times for recovery of *M. tuberculosis* from smear-negative specimens with radiometric and conventional culture systems were 13.7 and 26.3 days, respectively. Radiometric and conventional culture procedures were approximately equivalent for the recovery of *M. tuberculosis* from 5375 clinical specimens, but Takahashi and Foster (1983) found the recovery of *M. avium* complex was better using the radiometric procedure. In another collaborative study reported by Roberts and associates (1983) involving five laboratories, recovery and drug susceptibility tests of *M. tuberculosis* were completed in 18 days using the radiometric procedure, as opposed to 38.5 days for the conventional method.

Using lysis centrifugation — Isolator — and radiometric — Bactec — blood culture procedures, it has been possible to recover mycobacteria from blood specimens in 6 to 12 days. Recovery of mycobacteria by the Isolator blood culture system is based on the principle of lysis of both the red and white blood cells in a 10-ml sample of blood followed by centrifugation and sedimentation of mycobacteria in the blood collection tube. The centrifuged pellet containing any organisms is then inoculated directly to egg-base or 7H11 mycobacterial culture media as well as 7H12A, a broth medium containing 1-^{14}C-palmitic acid for use with the radiometric growth detection ion chamber, Bactec. Macher and colleagues (1983), as well as Gill

and Stock (1987), reported that combined use of the lysis centrifugation and radiometric systems provides the most rapid recovery of mycobacteria from blood.

Speciation of cultures directly from Bactec broth cultures can now be accomplished using isotopic nucleic acid hybridization, as initially reported by Kiehn and Evans (1987). Probes are currently available for *M. tuberculosis, M. avium, M. intracellulare,* and *M. gordonae.* Probes are not available for species other than these, and speciation is done by the traditional methods. Advantages of isotopic probes are their specificity and reliability. Disadvantages include a short shelf-life for the isotopic reagents, inconvenience of dealing with radioisotopes, a high expense, and limited availability of species-specific probes. Evans and co-workers (1992) demonstrated that many of these shortcomings can be avoided with nonisotopic probes that use acridinium ester labels and chemiluminescence detection.

The pace of innovation has quickened even more with the application of PCR to clinical specimens. Kolk and colleagues (1992) used PCR to expand mycobacterial DNA in 227 patients. Specimens included cerebrospinal fluid — CSF, sputum, pleural fluid, BAL fluid, blood, pus, bone marrow, and urine samples, as well as tissue samples. Polymerase chain reaction — PCR — detected 10 of 12 culture-positive but Ziehl-Neelsen-negative samples, as well as 4 of 4 culture-negative but stain-positive samples. An even more remarkable accomplishment was reported by the group at the Centers for Disease Control, where Plikaytis and colleagues (1992) used PCR and restriction fragment length polymorphism analysis to identify and speciate isolates in a time frame that could lead to species identification within 48 hours. This technique has yet to be applied to clinical samples but shows immense promise for the near term.

Mycobacterium Avium *Complex and AIDS*

Greene and associates (1982) found that one of the most common opportunistic infections in AIDS patients is from organisms of the *Mycobacterium avium* complex — MAC. Presenting symptoms may include chronic diarrhea, associated with extensive invasion of the mucosal villi of the small and large intestine by the bacilli. Hawkins (1986) reported the possibility also of diffuse dissemination of MAC organisms to the reticuloendothelial system, including the liver, bone marrow, and spleen, as well as, but not always, to the lungs. Diagnosis of MAC infection can often be made by positive acid-fast stained smears and cultures from the stool or biopsies of the intestinal mucosa, liver, or bone marrow, or cultures of the sputum or blood. Often positive blood cultures can establish the diagnosis of MAC infection before any changes are noted on the chest radiograph. Blood cultures should be drawn from the high-risk patient on the basis of fever and malaise.

FUNGAL INFECTION OF THE LUNG

The spectrum of fungal infection of the lung is shifting from the endemic, deep-seated infection, such as *Blas-*

tomycosis, to opportunistic infection with usually low pathogenic species, like *Candida* and *Aspergillus*.

Fungal infection of the lung is best established by recovery of the infecting organism by culture. Morphologic changes in tissue biopsy specimens may be adequate to establish a diagnosis without culture. Histochemical staining, with periodic acid — PAS, methenamine silver, mucicarmine, or Gram's stain, of histologic sections is helpful and may afford specific identification of different fungi. All too often, however, it is not possible to find pathognomonic organisms in the stained specimens and only a presumptive diagnosis can be made. Perhaps the two best stains for demonstration of fungi in tissue are PAS and methenamine silver, but no one stain demonstrates all organisms.

Cultures of fungi can be made from tissues, sputum, pleural fluid, bronchial aspirates, or other clinical specimens. For optimal recovery, all specimens should be inoculated on several different types of culture media. Sabouraud's dextrose agar is an excellent general-purpose culture medium. It is able to inhibit many strains of contaminating bacteria because its high dextrose content — 4% — reduces the pH to 5.6. Specimens should also be inoculated to a second medium containing antibiotics and cycloheximide to suppress less fastidious bacteria and the contaminating molds. Because the cycloheximide and antibiotics in the second medium also inhibit certain pathogenic fungi, such as *Cryptococcus neoformans* and *Aspergillus fumigates*, use of Sabouraud's or a similar noninhibitory agar should not be omitted. Sabouraud's medium should be incubated at both 25° and 37° C, because different fungi may have varying rates of growth and different morphologic forms when grown at different temperatures. Fungi with more than one form are "dimorphic," showing a yeast-like morphology at 37° C and a mycelial growth when incubated at room temperature — 25° C. Examples of "dimorphic" fungi are *Histoplasma capsulatum*, *Blastomyces dermatitides*, and *Sporothrix schenckii*. Growth of pathogenic fungi may take from 2 to 14 days, depending on the number of organisms present in the specimens and characteristics of the individual organism. For some fungi, unique growth requirements have led to special media. Any clinical information that may indicate the most likely organism will help in selecting the medium most likely to produce growth in the minimal time.

Members of the *Candida* and *Cryptococcus* species are easily identified by fermentation and carbohydrate assimilation tests. The use of several other biochemical tests in the speciation of fungi is helpful, but most pathogenic fungi are identified by morphologic characteristics noted on culture, such as septate or nonseptate mycelia, unique macro- or microconidia, and the gross and microscopic appearance of the growth nurtured on different types of media at 37° C and at room temperatures. Identification is usually made by examining portions of the culture under the microscope and by preparing small "growing mounts," where the developing pattern of growth is followed by microscopic examination over several days. Unfortunately, some fungi lose certain of their specific features in culture, with the result that identification may take a prolonged period. Disseminated disease has been diagnosed by Musial and associated (1987) using the lysis-centrifugation procedure, confirming that the mode of spread in the acute case is similar to tuberculosis.

Skin tests to detect hypersensitivity to fungi should be restricted to persons suspected of having histoplasmosis or coccidioidomycosis. Cross reactions and lack of specificity of antigens have made skin tests for blastomycosis, candidiasis, and cryptococcosis unreliable. A positive reaction to histoplasmin or coccidioidin indicates only that the patient has had contact with the antigen at some time in the past. It may be of little value in determining whether a current illness is caused by a specific fungus unless it is known that the patient's reaction to that antigen was negative at some time in the recent past. If the reaction to the skin test becomes negative in a patient with known, active histoplasmosis or coccidioidomycosis, this change may indicate a state of anergy and a dim prognosis.

Many patients have had subclinical infections with different fungi, so a positive reaction to a serologic test for a fungal antigen in a random specimen may have little significance. To differentiate between an old and a current fungal infection on the basis of serologic tests, antibody titers are determined on serum obtained early in the course of the illness — acute phase — and at least 2 to 3 weeks later — convalescent phase. Laboratory precision in most serologic tests is seldom better than one dilution — twofold change — so that the results of most serologic tests should not be considered significant without an increase or decrease of at least two dilutions — fourfold change — such as any from 1/4 to 1/16. In some patients, fungal infections may develop during immunosuppressive therapy for tumors or organ transplants. Both humoral and cellular immune responses may then be modified by drugs so that these responses to serologic tests may not be valid. Because of the infrequent need for such tests in most hospitals, requests for fungal serologic analysis are usually forwarded to municipal or state public health laboratories, resulting in some delay in obtaining the report. Direct communication with the reference laboratory usually hastens receipt of the report.

Of serologic tests for all the so-called deep fungal infections, those for blastomycosis are the least satisfactory. Cross reactions with other antigens are most prone to occur. The immunodiffusion — ID — test for blastomycosis is specific, and a positive reaction can result in immediate treatment of the patient. The test has a sensitivity of approximately 80% and detects more blastomycosis than the complement-fixation test. Negative tests do not exclude a diagnosis. In contrast to blastomycosis, the serologic diagnosis of histoplasmosis can be made by either of two type of serologic tests, depending on the stage of the illness. In the early phase of the disease, reaction to a latex agglutination test may be positive, probably because an IgM antibody is present. As the infection progresses, the reaction to the agglutination test fades and becomes negative. Somewhat later in the infection, complement-fixing antibodies develop; these correlate well with the activity of the disease. Titers of 1:8 and 1:16 may be considered presumptive evidence of histoplasmosis, whereas titers of 1:32 are highly suggestive of this infection. Cross reactions with antigens from other fungi can occur in the complement-fixation test and be misleading. In some patients, the antigenic stimulation from a skin test with histoplasmin may be sufficient to stimulate an increase in complement-fixing antibody titer, but usually not before 15 days. For this reason, the initial or acute serum for complement-fixation studies should be obtained before skin tests are performed. Kaufman and Reiss (1985) found that if reaction to a skin test is positive in 72 hours, serum drawn for complement fixation will not reflect any change in titer at this time, although the possibility of a rise in the convalescent serum should be considered. Under these conditions, at least a fourfold or greater change in titer is needed to establish the diagnosis of active infection.

A micro-immunodiffusion procedure is also recommended for detecting infection by *Histoplasma capsulatum*. The results are qualitative. Two precipitin bands have diagnostic value. One, designated "h," is not influenced by skin testing and is consistently found in the serum of patients with active histoplasmosis. The second, designated "m," is found in both acute and chronic histoplasmosis and also appears after normal, sensitized individuals have been skin tested with histoplasmin. The "m" band has been considered presumptive evidence of infection with *H. capsulatum*. Finding only "m" antibodies in sera may be attributed to active or inactive disease or to skin testing. Therefore, if the patient has not had a recent histoplasmin skin test, detection of an "m" band may serve as an indicator of early disease, because this band appears before the "h" band and disappears more slowly. Kaufman and colleagues (1985) stated that the demonstration of both bands is highly suggestive of active histoplasmosis, regardless of other serologic results.

In coccidioidomycosis, reaction to a precipitin test may be positive in early stages of the infection. As in histoplasmosis, the complement-fixation antibody titer tends to rise as the disease becomes more advanced and falls with control of the infection. Should the infection disseminate, a state of anergy may develop with a loss of all serologic evidence of the disease. In contrast to histoplasmin, skin testing with coccidioidin does not appear to stimulate humoral antibody formation.

Cryptococcosis is one of the most common fungal infections of the lung, although in most of its subjects, it may be present in a subclinical form. The disease usually becomes apparent in patients who have some defect in their host defense mechanism, particularly those who are receiving therapy for malignant lymphomas and those who have experienced immune suppression. The causative organism may proliferate in large numbers in the lung or brain. In many instances,

the cellular reaction is minimal (Fig. 15–7), and the detection of circulating polysaccharide antigen is possible prior to the formation of circulating antibodies. When the infection appears to be controlled, either spontaneously or as a result of therapy, the polysaccharide antigen disappears, and circulating antibodies may be demonstrated by the indirect immunofluorescence antibody test or a cryptococcal yeast-cell agglutination procedure. An inverse relationship apparently exists in the time between the appearance of antigen in the serum or in the spinal fluid, during the early or acute stage of the disease, and the appearance of antibodies in the serum as the infection is brought under control. Using indirect fluorescence antibody, tube agglutination for antibody, and latex agglutination for antigen tests, Kaufman and Blumer (1968) were able to show serologic evidence of cryptococcosis in 92% of 66 patients.

With the growing number of immunosuppressed patients during the last decade, the diagnosis and treatment of invasive fungal infection has become more important. In addition to infection caused by the endemic fungi, opportunistic pathogens such as *Candida* and *Aspergillus* are important fungal pathogens in the immunosuppressed patient. The diagnosis of invasive infection with *Candida* can be challenging, because this fungus commonly colonizes mucous membranes, particularly in patients receiving broad spectrum antibiotics. For this reason, diagnosis normally requires culture of the organism from normally sterile fluids or tissues, or repeated culture from multiple sites in a predisposed patient. Serology and skin testing are not helpful in the diagnosis of invasive *Candida* infection. In the absence of a tissue diagnosis, the decision whether to treat for invasive *Candida* infection is left to the experienced clinician.

Aspergillus causes invasive infection in immunosuppressed patients and diagnosis depends on the demonstration of tissue invasion. Serologic tests exist but are not widely available. Antibody response to infection requires tests during acute and convalescent stages, and demonstration of antigen is not well studied.

PARASITIC INFECTIONS OF THE LUNG

Parasitic infections of the lungs are uncommon in the United States. When found, they usually are present in patients who are immunosuppressed or who have previously spent time in some part of the world in which echinococcosis, schistosomiasis, or amebiasis is endemic. Unfortunately, the identification of the parasite in sputum, pleural fluid, or other clinical specimens is difficult, and recovery by culture is difficult or impossible, depending on the organism. Biopsy or excision of suspected lesions may be the most rapid and definitive procedure.

Intestinal nematodes, such as *Ascaris lumbricoides*, hookworm, and *Strongyloides stercoralis*, may incite a severe inflammatory reaction in the lung during passage from the pulmonary circulation into the bronchi. Spu-

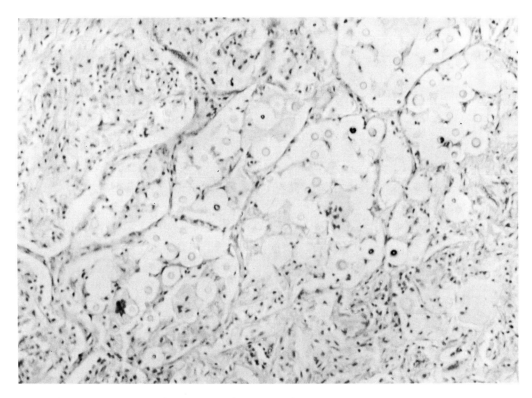

Fig. 15–7. Pneumonia from *Cryptococcus neoformans*. Note the large number of encapsulated cells filling the alveoli. The prominent capsule is well shown. In the early phase of the disease, circulating capsular polysaccharide may be demonstrated in the serum, urine, or cerebrospinal fluid before the appearance of antibodies. Periodic acid-Schiff (PAS) stain. ×450.

tum specimens may reveal filarial form of the worms. Clinically, such patients show eosinophilia, and a mottled infiltration of the lung is demonstrated in a radiograph of the chest. In some patients, nematodes become trapped in the lungs, incite an inflammatory reaction, and form hyalinized granulomas, which may persist as "coin lesions."

The development of serologic procedures to detect antibodies to different types of parasites that can be found in the lung has been of great help in both establishing and confirming the presence of active infection with different parasites. Because many of these tests were developed and standardized only recently, most are available only through public health laboratories. Walls (1985) summarized many of the tests available and methods for their performance. Several of the serologic tests are described briefly in the following paragraphs.

The indirect hemagglutination test for pleuropulmonary amebiasis is both sensitive and specific, and is particularly valuable in the detection of tissue invasion by amebae. In contrast to its sensitivity in patients with hepatic and pulmonary involvement, Healy (1968) found the test less sensitive in those with acute amebic dysentery and relatively insensitive for asymptomatic intestinal carriers.

In hydatid disease, patients with echinococcal cysts in the liver have better serologic correlation than do those with cysts in the lung. Kagan and associates (1966)

found that serologic tests for echinococcal cysts do not correlate well with pulmonary involvement. The reason for this discrepancy in the reliability of serologic tests between infection in the lungs and that in the liver is not known, but it may be that pulmonary cysts are not as closely associated with an active blood supply as are hepatic cysts.

Pulmonary schistosomiasis may develop as a further manifestation of intestinal and hepatic infection and usually is associated with pulmonary hypertension (Fig. 15–8). Although lung biopsy is a useful means of establishing the diagnosis and assessing the pulmonary vascular disease, various serologic tests are available to help establish the diagnosis. Kagan and colleagues (1962) found the cholesterol-lecithin cercarial slide flocculation test — CL — to be sensitive in 77% of patients with confirmed disease; unfortunately, the test cannot be performed on contaminated or chylous sera. A bentonite flocculation test was developed to overcome this difficulty, but Kagan (1968) found this test to be sensitive in only 70% of patients, reporting false-positive reactions in 15% of sera from patients without schistosomiasis.

Occasional instances of infection with the oriental lung fluke *Paragonimus westermani* are found in persons from the Far East. This infection may be mistaken for other types of chronic disease in the lung. Although complement fixation and other serologic tests have been described for detection of this parasite, they generally are not available in the United States owing to the

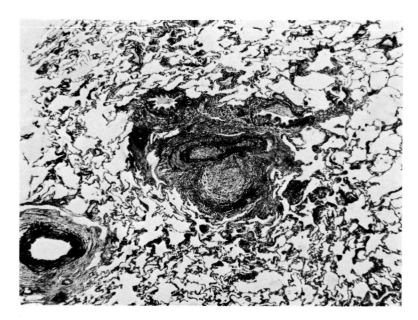

Fig. 15–8. Perivascular granuloma from *Schistosoma mansoni*. Note thickening of pulmonary vessels reflecting pulmonary hypertension. Lung biopsy is a useful means of establishing the diagnosis of schistosomal lung disease and assessing the degree of pulmonary vessel change. ×260.

infrequent need for such procedures. A more detailed discussion on the different serologic procedures that have been described for parasitic agents has been presented by Walls (1985).

PNEUMONITIS ASSOCIATED WITH PNEUMOCYSTIS CARINII

This small, unicellular organism produces a rapid, consolidating pneumonitis in debilitated patients, usually after prolonged periods of therapy with antime-

tabolites, steroids, and antibiotics (Fig. 15–9); it is a frequent complication in patients with AIDS. Attempts to isolate and culture the organism have been unsuccessful. Although the disease was first recognized in malnourished infants and children in orphanages in Europe and Korea following World War II, infection with *Pneumocystis carinii* occurs in this county in patients with AIDS, in recipients of organ transplantation, in patients with inborn immune deficiencies, or in persons with complications caused by prolonged drug therapy for malignant tumors.

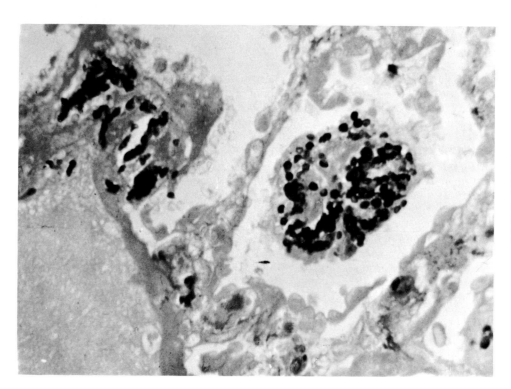

Fig. 15–9. *Pneumocystis carinii*. Large numbers of organisms are embedded in fibrin within alveoli. Tissue sections stained with hematoxylin and eosin do not show the organisms, best demonstrated with the Gomeri methenamine silver stain. ×650.

The disease is more common than it was in the past. Well over 50% of patients with AIDS present with this infection. The percentage varies depending on whether the patients are intravenous drug abusers or homosexual men; the status of the patient's T cell population also plays a role in its incidence. Perera and associates (1970) found 40 previously unrecognized instances on review of 301 consecutive autopsies performed in a children's hospital for leukemia or other types of cancer.

Hughes and colleagues (1977) showed that a combination of trimethoprim and sulfamethoxazole is effective in preventing the occurrence of pneumonia from *Pneumocystis carinii* when used for prophylaxis as well as for therapy. This combination is normally the initial treatment used in this setting. Alternative agents include Pentamidine and TMP/dapsone. These agents are used when trimethoprim/sulfamethoxazole is not tolerated or is contraindicated. The adjunctive use of corticosteroids in the treatment of *Pneumocystis carinii* is gaining favor with clinicians treating HIV-infected individuals, as well as individuals with inflammatory pneumonitis.

Because the disease may develop and progress rapidly, causing death within 4 to 6 days, the diagnosis should be made promptly so that specific therapy can begin. Although the organism has been found in sputum smears and tracheal aspirates, dependence on this finding to establish the diagnosis is unreliable because few organisms are shed and many similar appearing objects may be present on the smear. Most centers obtain an induced-sputum sample initially and then rapidly move to bronchoscopy and BAL if induced sputum is nondiagnostic. Transbronchial biopsy or even open biopsy may become necessary when BAL is nondiagnostic.

Three popular stains for cysts and trophozoite forms are methenamine silver, toluidine O, and Giemsa. According to Bartlett and co-workers (1987), the Giemsa stain should not be used exclusively. The organism is not visible on sections stained by hematoxylin and eosin. Because the methenamine stain requires special reagents, the laboratory should be alerted to the possibility of a *Pneumocystis* infection before biopsy so that sections can be stained without delay. Good results within a period of 5 to 10 minutes have been obtained with a rapid staining procedure using toluidine O, as reported by Chalvardijian and Grawe (1963). An immunofluorescence stain, using monoclonal antibody, for sputum and BAL specimens has been developed and appears to be quite sensitive, as reported by Kovacs and colleagues (1988).

Attempts to develop an immunologic test have been hampered by the inability to grow the organism in the laboratory, and still no reliable serologic assay is available. Of note, LDH levels in patients with HIV appear to be reproducibly prognostic, with LDH greater than 500 IV predictive of poor prognosis, as shown by Garay and Greene (1989).

VIRAL INFECTIONS OF THE LUNG

Although viral infections of the upper and lower respiratory tract are among the most frequent illnesses in humans, most of these infections are benign and self limited. The most common etiologic agents are the influenza, parainfluenza, adeno-, and respiratory syncytial viruses. The situation is different in the immunosuppressed patient, in whom any of these agents can cause serious life-threatening infection. Viral infections of the lung account for the majority of opportunistic viral infections in immunosuppressed patients. In patients with AIDS, Klatt and Shibata (1988) found that CMV pneumonitis was present at autopsy in about 30% of patients, and evidence of the virus was present in most lung tissue examined. Cytomegalovirus is rarely the cause of death in these patients, however, but the development of CMV in the lungs of a patient infected with another pathogen, pneumocystis for instance, portends a poor prognosis. The other herpesvirus, herpes simplex — HSV, varicella zoster virus — VZV, and the Epstein-Barr virus — EBV, are also important pathogens in the immunosuppressed host. Only the herpesviruses will be presented here.

Herpesviruses

The family of herpesviruses is unique because exposure to them is common in the general population, and these agents subsequently enter a latent state in virus-specific privileged areas within the body, that is, lymphocytes for EBV and nerve ganglia for HVZ. In the immunocompromised patient, reactivation of virus can lead to serious opportunistic infection; moreover, primary infection in the unexposed, immunosuppressed patient can manifest as overwhelming disseminated disease. CMV and EBV are also strongly immunomodulating, particularly in immunosuppressed individuals. These features of herpesviruses make them fascinating and a particular challenge in the immunosuppressed patient.

The demonstration that ganciclovir — DHPG — is an effective agent in the treatment of CMV infection in immunosuppressed patients by Kortz and Buhles (1986) and others has stressed the importance of early and accurate diagnosis. The patient with CMV infection presents with fever, leukopenia, thrombocytopenia, pneumonitis, retinitis, hepatitis, enteritis, and encephalitis. Whether or not infection in the transplant patient represents primary or secondary infection is of great importance in patients who receive organ transplant, because mortality from primary infection is far greater when compared to reactivation of latent infection. Primary infection in these patients usually represents receipt of an organ from a CMV-positive donor, or blood products contaminated with the virus. Thus, serologic status is crucial in the pretransplant evaluation of these patients. Demonstration of IgM class antibodies or an increase in antibody titers is confirmatory evidence of reactivation, but these events occur relatively late in the course of illness and are not generally helpful in the diagnosis of acute disease.

The early diagnosis of CMV infection can be made in a variety of ways. The spin amplification shell vial technique is the most widely used rapid detection method for CMV. It features concentration of the virus using centrifugation, culture, and the use of monoclonal antibody assays for viral antigens. A result can be returned within 24 hours. In situ hybridization has also been used in place of monoclonal antibodies in conjunction with the shell vial culture. The use of direct immunofluorescence monoclonal antibodies to CMV antigens is rapid but less sensitive than the shell vial assay and it has been supplanted by the shell vial technique. The polymerase chain reaction has been used successfully in the rapid detection of CMV DNA in blood and other tissues, but its use in this setting is confounded by the interpretation of positive results. Histopathologic examination of tissue specimens using Wright-Giemsa staining can demonstrate typical cytopathic appearance (Fig. 15–10), but this method is relatively insensitive and usually requires invasive procedures to obtain tissue. Routine culture of CMV is done on human fibroblast cultures that are examined for characteristic cytopathic effect — CPE; this effect usually appears within 2 weeks, depending on the inoculum, and may occur sooner if specimen titers are high.

Lung involvement with primary VZV is not common in immunocompetent persons. In immunosuppressed individuals, however, primary VZV infection and pneumonia can be life threatening. Reactivation of VZV — shingles — in recipients of organ transplants can also progress to invasive pulmonary disease. In any of these scenarios, acyclovir is the agent of choice. The diagnosis of VZV is usually not difficult because of the characteristic exanthem in primary cases and the presence of shingles in reactivation cases. Serology, however, does play an important role, especially in transplant patients, because pretransplant seronegativity should lead to administration of soon-to-be-released vaccine. In addition, postexposure varicella-zoster immune globulin — VZIG — can be administered and is effective in decreasing morbidity in immunocompromised patients, as demonstrated by Zaia and coworkers (1983). Serum titers for VZV to confirm seroconversion or the presence of IgM are done. It is important to note that cross reactivity is substantial, up to 33%, between antibody assays for herpes simplex — HSV — and VZV, and the absence of a similar titer rise to HSV may be necessary in these situations. In case of diagnostic uncertainty, materials from lesions or biopsy specimens can be submitted for routine culture, shell vial culture, and immunofluorescence staining, the latter being the most efficient method.

Epstein-Barr virus — EBV — is a ubiquitous pathogen that causes the usually self-limited clinical syndrome of infectious mononucleosis in younger patients. It only rarely causes pulmonary disease, but in transplant patients, EBV pneumonitis can be a manifestation of post-transplantation lymphoproliferative disease — PTLD. Post-transplantation lymphoproliferative disease is associated with a wide spectrum of symptoms with outcome ranging from frankly malignant lymphoma to benign expansion of lymphoid tissue that responds to reduction of immunosuppression. The virus can be cultured from throat washings, but culture of shed virus is usually not helpful diagnostically, so the diagnostic approach is based primarily on serology and examination of tissue. Although detection of heterophile antibodies is sufficient in making the diagnosis in uncomplicated infectious mononucleosis, considerably greater information can be gained from measuring the serologic status of patients to four antigens: viral capsid antigen — VCA, EBV-induced nuclear antigen — EBNA, early antigen-diffuse component — EA/D, and the early antigen-restricted component — EA/R. Five clinical states of EBV infection are recognized based on the evaluation of the humoral response to these antigens:

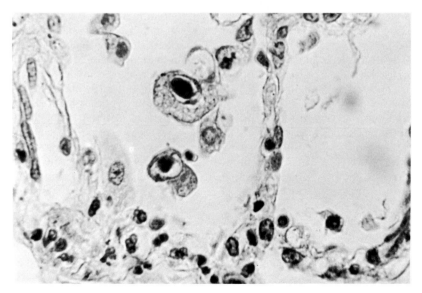

Fig. 15–10. Cytomegalovirus intranuclear inclusion body in alveolar macrophage. Not all viral diseases produce inclusion bodies, but those of the herpes-cytomegalovirus groups show well-formed intranuclear inclusions. ×650.

1) susceptible, if anti-VCA is absent; 2) current primary infection, if anti-VCA positive and anti-EBVA absent — and anti-EA components negative; 3) recent active infection, if anti-VCA is positive, anti-EBVA negative but anti-EA positive; 4) past infection, if both anti-VCA and EBVA are positive; and 5) reactivated infection shows both anti-VCA and anti-EBVA are present and positivity to one of the anti-EA components. The determination of reactivated versus primary infection can be of prognostic importance when dealing with PTLD in transplant patients, as demonstrated by Armitage and colleagues (1991). Tissue can be examined for viral antigens with an indirect immunofluorescence stain or in situ DNA hybridization.

Herpes simplex virus — HSV — usually only causes invasive infection in immunosuppressed patients with transplanted organs or malignancies under treatment with cytotoxic medications. Pulmonary disease usually manifests as tracheobronchitis, but rarely pneumonia can occur. Orolabial or genital lesions are usually present concurrently. The finding of HSV in tracheal secretions is therefore difficult to interpret, and lung tissue is usually required to render a certain diagnosis of HSV pneumonia. Tissue is cultured and, depending on the concentration of virus in the specimen, can be positive as soon as 24 hours or as late as 5 days. A variety of rapid detection techniques are available, including in situ hybridization, shell vial assay, and an immunofluorescence technique. Serology is limited in the diagnosis of HSV infection. Acyclovir is effective against HSV, and in immunosuppressed patients, it is indicated for reactivation of orolabial or genital disease, and disseminated, invasive infection.

INFECTIONS IN RECIPIENTS OF THORACIC ORGAN TRANSPLANTS AND ASSIST DEVICES

Widespread transplantation of thoracic organs resumed in the early 1980s with the introduction of the immunosuppressive agent cyclosporin A. Kriett and Kaye (1991) noted that 3054 heart, 194 heart-lung, 214 single lung, and 60 double-lung transplants were recorded in the International Society for Heart and Lung Transplantation Registry. In all groups, infection is the leading cause of death from about 2 to 4 weeks post-transplant up to 6 to 12 months, after which time rejection becomes the major source of mortality. In 1987, Hofflin and colleagues reported that the use of cyclosporin-based immunosuppression decreased the morbidity from infection compared to azathioprine/steroid regimens. The use of antilymphocyte immunoglobulins, such as antithymocyte globulin — ATG — and the monoclonal antibody agent OKT3, has been reported in many studies of extrathoracic organs to lower resistance to infection by herpesviruses, specifically CMV, and EBV with associated PTLD. In contrast, Dummer (1985) and Armitage (1991) and their co-workers, of the University of Pittsburgh, report no correlation between the use of antilymphocyte agents and the development of CMV or PTLD in recipients

of heart and heart-lung transplants. FK 506 is a new immunosuppressive agent that is more potent than cyclosporin; it is too early to evaluate its impact on infectious morbidity in thoracic organ transplant recipients.

The timing and causative organism of infections in the postoperative period are predictable in patients receiving heart transplants. In Dummer's (1989) series of 119 patients, opportunistic agents were primarily bacterial, herpesviruses, protozoan, and fungal — Aspergillosis and Candida, but not endemic mycoses. No cases of mycobacterial infection were reported. Opportunistic agents are more common in the first months after transplantation, whereas after 2 years, bacterial infections are 10 to 20 times more likely. The lung is the most common site of infection in heart and heart-lung transplant patients, with gram-negative rods the most common pathogens, but interestingly, Pneumococcus is the most common single organism. The combination of history, physical examination, chest radiograph, and gram stain of expectorated sputum can be expected to allow a presumptive diagnosis in up to 50% of cases. Bronchoscopy and lavage are used early in the evaluation of the remaining patients. Invasive tissue diagnosis occasionally is necessary. Patients who receive heart-lung transplants seem uniquely predisposed to pulmonary infections. The rate of pneumonia is approximately double that encountered in heart transplant patients, and this susceptibility is true across the spectrum of possible pathogenic organisms, as detailed by Dummer and associates (1986). Culture of the donor trachea was shown by Zenati and colleagues (1990) to be helpful in identifying patients at high risk of subsequent invasive fungal infection.

Pneumonitis and invasive infection with CMV are a source of considerable morbidity and mortality in thoracic organ transplant recipients. Up to 90% of such transplants at the University of Pittsburgh, as reported by Dummer and associates (1985), develop infection with CMV — defined as a positive viral culture, although most patients are asymptomatic. Symptomatic infection was more common in primarily infected than in reactivation infections — 69% versus 18%, and symptoms were always associated with viremia. Furthermore, seronegative patients shed virus in their urine or throat washings, and were viremic before the development of pneumonia. A large retrospective study from Stanford University by Grattan and co-workers (1989) also demonstrated that patients infected with CMV are at a significantly higher risk for developing both acute and chronic rejection, and have decreased overall survival compared with patients who do not develop CMV infection. In addition, infection with CMV predisposes heart transplant patients to superinfection with other opportunistic organisms such as Pneumocystis, Listeria, and fungi. Patients who receive heart-lung and lung transplants are likewise predisposed to infections with CMV. Primary CMV infection in these patients carries a mortality of greater than 50% as reported by Duncan and associates (1991). This figure can be reduced with recipient and organ matching, and avoidance of seropositive blood products in the seronegative recipient. In summary, CMV is a source of considerable morbidity and mortality in thoracic transplant patients, and in addition to vigilance and surveillance cultures, seronegative patients should receive organs from seronegative donors when feasible, and only receive CMV-negative blood products. Prophylaxis of heart transplant patients, by Merigan and colleagues (1992), with a short course of ganciclovir — DHPG — has been shown in a prospective, randomized study to reduce the incidence of symptomatic CMV illness as well as asymptomatic shedding of the virus. This effect, however, was limited to seropositive, but not seronegative, patients.

Epstein-Barr virus infections in transplant patients are associated with the development of PTLD. Post–transplantation lymphoproliferative disease occurs in 4% of thoracic organ transplant patients — 3.4% in heart transplant patients and 7.9% after lung transplantation — and has been classified by Armitage and associates (1991) into "early" — less than 1 year — and "late" — more than 1 year. Patients who develop early PTLD are more likely to be younger, have primary infection, are less likely to have disseminated disease, and respond to reduction of immunosuppression. Patients with late PTLD are older, are more likely to have secondary infection, have disseminated disease, and do not respond to reduction of immunosuppression. Mortality of early PTLD is 36%; in late PTLD, it is 70%. Epstein–Barr virus mRNA in liver biopsies from latently infected liver transplant patients has been detected by Randhawa and associates (1992) before the development of PTLD, using an in situ hybridization probe.

Several mechanical support devices exist for the support of patients awaiting heart transplantation — "bridge-to-transplant." The total artificial heart — TAH — was used in the early experience at the University of Pittsburgh. Review of the first 15 implants of the TAH for bridge-to-transplant by Griffith and co-workers (1988) showed that 7 patients died within 60 days of their transplant, and that 6 of these patients died of infectious complications. In most instances, patients developed pneumonia and subsequently mediastinitis. The organisms responsible were gram-negative rods — 4, mycoplasma — 2, and mixed candida/enterobacter — 1. Mechanical support techniques that leave the native heart in situ appear to be relatively free of similar infectious complications.

REFERENCES

Armitage JM, et al: Posttransplant lymphproliferative disease in thoracic organ transplant patients: Ten years of cyclosporine-based immunosuppression. J Heart Transplant 10:877, 1991.

Balows A, Fraser DWE: International Symposium on Legionnaires' Disease. Ann Intern Med 90:489, 1979.

Bartlett SG: Community acquired pneumonia. In Shelhamer J, et al: Respiratory Disease in the Immunocompromised Host. New York: Lippincott, 1991.

Bartlett JG, et al: Laboratory diagnosis of lower respiratory tract infections. In Washington JA: Cumitech 7A. Washington DC: American Society for Microbiology, 1987.

Baselski VS, et al: The standardization of criterion for processing and interpreting laboratory specimens in patients with suspected ventilator-associated pneumonia. Chest 102:571S, 1992.

Chalvardjian AM, Grawe LA: A new procedure for the identification of Pneumocystis carinii cysts in tissue sections and smears. J Clin Pathol 16:383, 1963.

Conte BA, Laforet EG: The role of the topical anaesthetic agent in modifying bacteriologic data obtained by bronchoscopy. N Engl J Med 267:957, 1962.

Damato JJ, et al: Detection of mycobacteria by radiometric and standard plate procedures. J Clin Microbiol 17:1066, 1983.

Delgado R, et al: Low predictive value of polymerase chain reaction for diagnosis of cytomegalovirus disease in liver transplant recipients. J Clin Microbiol 30:1876, 1992.

Dilworth JA, et al: Methods to improve detection of pneumococci in respiratory secretions. J Clin Microbiol 2:453, 1975.

Dummer SJ: Infectious complications of transplantation. In Thompson ME: Heart Transplantation. Philadelphia: FA Davis, 1989.

Dummer SJ, et al: Morbidity of cytomegalovirus infection in recipients of heart or heart-lung transplants who recieved cyclosporine. J Infect Dis 152:1182, 1985.

Dummer SJ, et al: Infections in heart-lung transplant recipients. Transplantation 41:725, 1986.

Duncan AJ, et al: Cytomegalovirus infection and survival in lung transplant recipients. J Heart Transplant 10:638, 1991.

Evans KD, et al: Identification of Mycobacterium tuberculosis and Mycobacterium avium-M. intracellulare directly from primary BACTEC cultures by using acridinium-ester-labeled DNA probes. J Clin Microbiol 30:2427, 1992.

Fain JS, et al: Rapid diagnosis of legionella infection by a nonisotopic in situ hybridization method. Am J Clin Pathol 95:719, 1991.

Figueroa ME, Rasheed S: Molecular pathology and diagnosis of infectious disease. Am J Clin Pathol 95:s8, 1991.

Frable WJ: Thin Needle Aspiration Biopsy. Philadelphia: WB Saunders, 1983.

Garay SM, Greene J: Prognostic indicators in the initial presentation of Pneumocystis carinii pneumonia. Chest 95:769, 1989.

Gill VJ, Stock F: Detection of Mycobacterium avium-Mycobacteria intracellulare in blood cultures using concentrated and unconcentrated blood in conjunction with a radiometric detection system. Diagn Microbiol Infect Dis 6:119, 1987.

Grattan MT, et al: Cytomegalovirus infection is associated with cardiac allograft rejection and atherosclerosis. JAMA 261:3561, 1989.

Greene JB, et al: Mycobacterium avium intracellulare: A cause of disseminated life-threatening infection in homosexuals and drug abusers. Ann Intern Med 97:539, 1982.

Griffith BP, et al: The artificial heart: Infection-related morbidity and its effect on transplantation. Ann Thorac Surg 45:409, 1988.

Hawkins CC, et al: Mycobacterium avium complex infections in patients with the acquired immunodeficiency syndrome. Ann Intern Med 105:184, 1986.

Healy GR: The use of and limitations to the indirect hemagglutination test in the diagnosis of intestinal amebiasis. Health Lab Sci 5:174, 1968.

Hofflin JM, et al: Infectious complications in heart transplant recipients receiving cyclosporine and corticosteroids. Ann Intern Med 106:209, 1987.

Hughes WT, et al: Successful chemoprophylaxis for Pneumocystis carinii pneumonitis. N Engl J Med 297:1419, 1977.

Kagan IG: Serologic diagnosis of schistosomiasis. Bull NY Acad Med 44:262, 1968.

Kagan IG, et al: A clinical, parasitologic, and immunologic study of schistosomiasis in 103 Puerto Rican males residing in the United States. Ann Intern Med 56:457, 1962.

Kagan IG, et al: Evaluation of intradermal and serologic tests for the diagnosis of hydatid disease. Am J Trop Med 15:172, 1966.

Kahn FW, Jones JM: Analysis of bronchoalveolar lavage specimens from immunocompromised patients with a protocol applicable in the microbiology laboratory. J Clin Microbiol 26:1150, 1988.

Kaufman L, Blumer S: Value and interpretation of serological tests for the diagnosis of cryptococcosis. Appl Microbiol *16*:1907, 1968.

Kaufman L, Reiss E: Serodiagnosis of fungal disease. *In* Lennette EH, et al: Manual of Clinical Microbiology. 4th Ed. Washington DC: American Society of Microbiology, 1985.

Kiehn TE, Edwards FF: Rapid identification using a specific DNA probe of *Mycobacterium avium* complex from patients with acquired immunodeficiency syndrome. J Clin Microbiol *25*:1551, 1987.

Klatt EC, Shibata D: Cytomegalovirus infection in the acquired immunodeficiency syndrome: Clinical and autopsy findings. Arch Pathol Lab Med *112*:540, 1988.

Kleinfield J, Elliss PP: Inhibition of microorganisms by topical anaesthetics. Appl Microbiol *15*:1296, 1967.

Kolk AHJ, et al: Detection of *Mycobacterium tuberculosis* in clinical samples by using polymerase chain reaction and a nonradioactive detection system. J Clin Microbiol *30*:2567, 1992.

Kopanoff DE, et al: A continuing survey of tuberculosis primary drug resistance in the United States: March 1975 to November 1977. Am Rev Respir Dis *118*:835, 1978.

Kortz SH, Buhles WC: Collaborative DHPG study group: Treatment of serious cytomegalovirus infections with DHPG in patients with AIDS and other immunodeficiencies. N Engl J Med *314*:801, 1986.

Koss LG: Diagnostic Cytology and Its Histopathologic Bases. 2nd Ed. Philadelphia: JB Lippincott, 1968.

Kovacs JA, et al: Diagnosis of *Pneumocystis carinii* pneumonia: Improved detection in sputum with use of monoclonal antibiotics. N Engl J Med *318*:589, 1988.

Krasnow I, Wayne LG: Comparison of methods for tuberculosis bacteriology. Appl Microbiol *18*:915, 1969.

Kriett JM, Kaye MP: The registry of the international society for heart and lung transplantation: Eighth official report — 1991. J Heart Transplant *10*:491, 1991.

LaForce FM: Lower respiratory tract infections. *In* Bennett JV, Brachman PS: Hospital Infections. 3rd Ed. Boston: Little Brown, 1992.

Linsk JA: Fine Needle Aspiration for the Clinician. Philadelphia: JB Lippincott, 1986.

Macher AM, et al: Bacteremia due to *Mycobacterium avium-intracellulare* in the acquired immunodeficiency syndrome. Ann Intern Med *99*:782, 1983.

Meduri UG: Ventilator-associated pneumonia in patients with respiratory failure: A diagnostic approach. Chest *97*:1208, 1990.

Meduri UG, Chastre J: The standardization of bronchoscopic techniques for ventilator-associated pneumonia. Chest *102*:557S, 1992.

Merigan TC, et al: A controlled trial of ganciclovir to prevent cytomeglovirus disease after heart transplantation. N Engl J Med *326*:1182, 1992.

Middlebrook G, Reggiardo Z, Tigert WD: Automatable radiometric detection of growth of *Mycobacterium tuberculosis* in selective media. Am Rev Respir Dis *115*:1066, 1977.

Morgan MA, et al: Comparison of a radiometric method (Bactec) and conventional culture media for recovery of mycobacteria from smear-negative specimens. J Clin Microbiol *18*:384, 1983.

Musial CE, et al: Recovery of *Blastomyces dermatitidis* from blood of a patient with disseminated blastomycosis. J Clin Microbiol *25*:1421, 1987.

Obrien RF, et al: Diagnosis of *Pneumocyctis carinii* pneumonia by induced sputum in a city with moderate incidence of AIDS. Chest *95*:136, 1989.

Perera DR, et al: *Pneumocystis carinii* pneumonia in a hospital for children: Epidemiologic aspects. JAMA *214*:1074, 1970.

Plikaytis BB, et al: Differentiation of slowly growing Mycobacterium species, including Mycobacterium tuberculosis, by gene amplification and restriction fragment length polymorphism analysis. J Clin Microbiol *30*:1815, 1992.

Randhawa PS, et al: Expression of Epstein-Barr virus-encoded small RNA (by the EBER-1 gene) in liver specimens from transplant recipients with post-transplantation lymphoproliferative disease. N Engl J Med *327*:1710, 1992.

Rein MF, Mandell GL: Bacterial killing by bacteriostatic saline solutions — potential for diagnostic error. N Engl J Med *289*:794, 1973.

Roberts GD, et al: Evaluation of the Bactec radiometric method for recovery of mycobacteria and drug susceptibility testing of *Mycobacterium tuberculosis* from acid-fast smear-positive specimens. J Clin Microbiol *18*:689, 1983.

Rodgers FG, Pasculle AW: Legionella. *In* Lennette EH, et al: Manual of Clinical Microbiology. 4th Ed. Washington DC: American Society of Microbiology, 1985.

Runyon EH: Anonymous mycobacteria in pulmonary disease. Med Clin North Am *43*:273, 1959.

Scheld WM, Mandell GL: Nosocomial pneumonia: Pathogenesis and recent advances in diagnosis and therapy. Rev Infect Dis *13*:5743, 1991.

Siddiqi SH, Libonati JP, Middlebrook G: Evaluation of a rapid radiometric method for drug susceptibility testing of *Mycobacterium tuberculosis*. J Clin Microbiol *13*:908, 1981.

Singh MD, Garrison RG: Propylene glycol aerosolization and the diagnosis of pulmonary histoplasmosis. Dis Chest *46*:82, 1964.

Snider DE Jr, et al: Rapid drug susceptibility testing of *Mycobacterium tuberculosis*. Am Rev Respir Dis *123*:402, 1981.

Stout J, et al: Ubiquitousness of *Legionella pneumophila* in the water supply of a hospital with endemic Legionnaires' disease. N Engl J Med *306*:466, 1982.

Takahashi H, Foster V: Detection and recovery of mycobacteria by a radiometric procedure. J Clin Microbiol *17*:380, 1983.

Timpe A, Runyon EH: The relationship of "atypical" acid-fast bacteria to human disease. J Lab Clin Med *44*:202, 1954.

Van Scoy RE: Bacterial sputum cultures. A clinician's viewpoint. Mayo Clin Proc *52*:39, 1977.

Walls KW: Serodiagnostic tests for parasitic diseases. *In* Lennette EH, et al: Manual of Clinical Microbiology. 4th Ed. Washington DC: American Society of Microbiology, 1985.

Woods GL, Washington JA: Mycobacteria other than Mycobacterium tuberculosis: Review of microbiologic and clinical aspects. Rev Infect Dis *9*:275, 1987.

Zaia JA, et al: Evaluation of varicella zoster immune globulin: Protection of immunosuppressed children after household exposure. J Infect Dis *147*:737, 1983.

Zenati M, et al: Influence of the donor lung on development of early infections in lung transplant recipients. J Heart Transplant *9*:502, 1990.

CHAPTER 16

BRONCHOSCOPIC EVALUATION OF THE LUNGS AND TRACHEOBRONCHIAL TREE

William H. Warren and L. Penfield Faber

The advent of fiberoptic technology has revolutionized the field of endoscopy. Nowhere is this change more evident than in bronchoscopy; the flexible bronchoscope has almost replaced the rigid bronchoscope as a diagnostic and therapeutic tool. Bronchoscopy, once dominated by a few specialists, is now performed by pulmonologists, anesthesiologists, otolaryngologists, and thoracic surgeons in a variety of clinical settings, including the hospital ward, the intensive care unit, and the operating room. The clinician must have a clear understanding of all aspects of flexible and rigid bronchoscopy, including anesthetic techniques, instrument options, and the management of complications.

FACILITIES FOR BRONCHOSCOPY

Ideally, an area of the hospital or outpatient facility should be dedicated to endoscopic procedures. Because bronchoscopy is performed routinely as an outpatient with intravenous sedation, recovery areas are also needed. The examination room must be large enough to store all equipment, supplies, and accessories.

A storage area adjacent to the endoscopic room is ideal and special holding racks and storage cases minimize breakage. A sink and storage area for cleaning solutions should be located adjacent to the endoscopy room to allow instrument cleaning and packaging while procedures are being performed. A portable cart supplied with a light source, bronchoscope, and accessories is a convenient way to perform beside examinations. It can be returned to the storage area for cleaning and may be reused several times a day. The facilities should not be crowded, allowing access to all necessary equipment to manage any complication. Ideally, such suites would allow clinicians to perform fluoroscopic studies and to administer general anesthesia.

Pulse oximetry and electrocardiogram monitoring are standard because bronchoscopy may be associated with hypoxia and cardiac irregularities, as documented by Albertini and colleagues (1975). Patients routinely have intravenous access and receive supplemental oxygen, according to a survey of North American pulmonologists reported by Prakash and associates (1991).

FLEXIBLE FIBEROPTIC BRONCHOSCOPY

Flexible bronchoscopy is a safe and reliable technique for evaluation of the tracheobronchial tree. Routinely, it is performed using intravenous sedation with little risk to the patient, providing valuable visual information and diagnostic specimens. Tracheobronchial, segmental, and subsegmental anatomy should be visualized easily. Currently available flexible bronchoscopes range from 6.2 mm in outer diameter with a 3.2-mm working channel to aspirate inspissated secretions and blood clots, to 3.5 mm in outer diameter with a 1.2-mm working channel for pediatric patients (Table 16–1). The adult bronchoscope used most often has a 5.8-mm external diameter and a 2.2-mm working channel, allowing clear visualization of the entire tracheobronchial tree down to the fourth or fifth order bronchi, and offering the capability of obtaining diagnostic specimens from them (Fig. 16–1). A forward field of view is 120°;

Table 16–1. Fiberoptic Bronchoscope Specifications

Outer Diameter (mm)	Instrument Channel (mm)	Field of View	Angle of Deflection (Up–Down)
3.5	1.2	90°	160°–100°
4.9	2.2	120°	180°–130°
5.8	2.2	120°	180°–130°
5.9	2.8	120°	180°–130°
5.9	2.0 + 1.5 (dual channel)	90°	160°–100°
6.2	3.2	90°	160°–100°

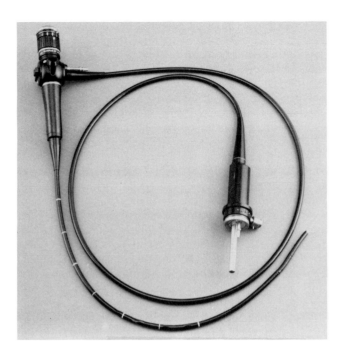

Fig. 16–1. Flexible fiberoptic bronchoscope (Olympus BF-10).

the angle of deflection is 180° upward and 130° downward. A narrower instrument with an external diameter of 4.9 mm easily passes through a bronchus narrowed by stricture or tumor, and its 180° upward deflection facilitates examination of the often difficult-to-reach apical subsegment.

Flexible bronchoscopy can be accomplished in the pediatric patient using an instrument with a 3.5 mm external diameter and a working channel of 1.2 mm. It can be passed through a small endotracheal tube or alongside a jet ventilation catheter. The active endoscopist should have a variety of flexible bronchoscopes available for diagnostic and therapeutic versatility (Fig. 16–2).

The many advantages of flexible bronchoscopy over rigid bronchoscopy are listed in Table 16–2. Diagnostic brushings and biopsies of peripheral lesions can be performed with minimal risk. Examination is usually performed using topical anesthesia and intravenous sedation, avoiding the risks of general anesthesia. Retained secretions can be aspirated at the bedside in the ward or in the intensive care unit. Patients receiving ventilator support can be examined without compromise using a side-arm adaptor (Fig. 16–3). The scope can be passed through narrowed and distorted airways, and still or videophotography is easily performed (Fig. 16–4).

Transbronchoscopic bronchial biopsies, brushing cytology, transbronchial needle aspirates — TBNA — and bronchoalveolar lavage — BAL — are readily performed, and the endoscopist should be familiar with indications and techniques for each.

RIGID BRONCHOSCOPY

The rigid, open-tube bronchoscopes commonly used in adults have an internal diameter of 6, 7, or 8 mm and are 40 cm in length (Fig. 16–5). Standard models provide only a tunnel view, but with experience, the

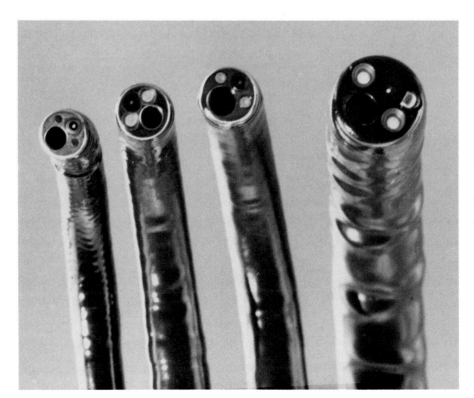

Fig. 16–2. Flexible fiberoptic bronchoscopes viewed on end. From left to right: 4.9-mm bronchoscope with 2.2-mm channel, 5.8-mm bronchoscope with 2.2-mm channel, 5.9-mm bronchoscope with 2.8-mm instrument channel.

Table 16–2. Flexible Fiberoptic Bronchoscopy

Advantages	Disadvantages
Patient comfort	Small channel
Segmental visualization	Breakdown
Segmental biopsy	Sterilization
Peripheral biopsy	
Transbronchial needle aspiration	
Bedside aspiration	
Bronchoscopy on ventilator	
Bypass distortion	
Photography	
Increased cancer diagnosis	
Brachytherapy	
Laser bronchoscopy	

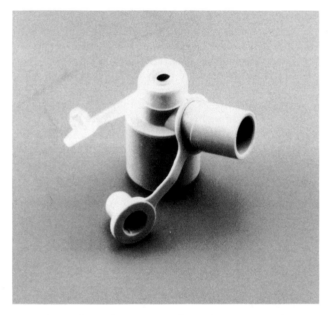

Fig. 16–3. Adaptor for the endotracheal tube to allow simultaneous ventilation and flexible fiberoptic bronchoscopy.

endoscopist becomes accustomed to this view of the bronchi. Illumination is supplied from a halogen light source; a fiberoptic cable is attached to a light carrier that passes down the side wall of the bronchoscope. A ventilating side-port permits assisted ventilation; a glass eyepiece is placed over the end to convert the bronchoscope to a nearly closed system. Visualization is significantly enhanced with 0°, 30°, and 90° telescopes. The flexible fiberoptic bronchoscope may be passed down an appropriately sized rigid bronchoscope to view fourth and fifth order bronchi, of particular advantage in assessing upper lobe and distal airways when attempting to retrieve foreign bodies in children.

More recently, rigid bronchoscopes have been designed to accept a glass Hopkins telescope, which provides optimal illumination and visualization. Using these telescopes, large but precise biopsy specimens can be obtained, in contrast to standard rigid bronchoscopy, during which visualization may be compromised by the insertion of the biopsy forceps.

The rigid bronchoscope is the instrument of choice for the removal of foreign bodies in infants and children. Although, according to Lan and co-workers (1989), foreign bodies in adult patients can be retrieved with various types of snares passed down the working channel of the fiberoptic bronchoscope; Paşaoğlu and colleagues (1991), as well as Weissberg and Schwartz (1987), reported that most foreign bodies can be removed easily and quickly with a rigid bronchoscope.

Massive hemoptysis — 600 ml in 24 hours — should be assessed with a rigid bronchoscope. Airway control with rapid and repeated suctioning is readily accomplished, and a major bronchus can be packed with an epinephrine-soaked pledget. Massive hemoptysis can be assessed using a flexible bronchoscope through a cuffed endotracheal tube, but clots are not easily

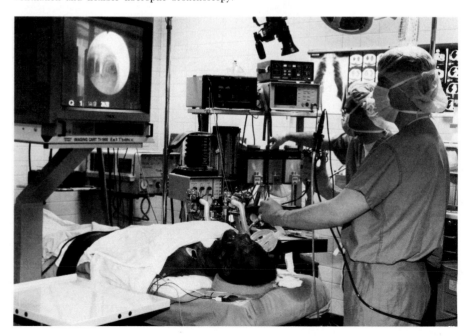

Fig. 16–4. Flexible bronchoscopy using a video-assisted technique.

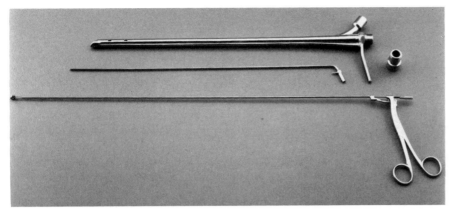

Fig. 16–5. Standard 8-mm rigid bronchoscope with light carrier, rigid biopsy forceps, and glass eyepiece.

removed and often obscure visualization. Localization of the bleeding site is compromised.

A rigid bronchoscope should always be available when tracheal lesions are examined. Bleeding from biopsy sites or tissue abrasion can obstruct a narrowed trachea, which can be forcibly dilated with a rigid instrument.

When using YAG laser photoablation, rigid bronchoscopes permit photoablation and rapid debridement of an obstructing or a bleeding lesion while simultaneously maintaining control of the airway and providing a suction channel for evacuation of clots and secretions. Clinical experience with placing endobronchial stents almost exclusively involves using the rigid bronchoscope.

A major disadvantage of rigid bronchoscopy is patient discomfort when using only topical anesthesia; rigid bronchoscopy can be easily performed using general anesthesia, but with all of its attendant risks. Despite the clearer view provided with angled telescopes, brushings and biopsies cannot be easily accomplished at the segmental level with the rigid bronchoscope. This major disadvantage can be overcome by passing a flexible bronchoscope through a rigid bronchoscope. The advantages and disadvantages of rigid bronchoscopy are listed in Table 16–3.

INDICATIONS

The diagnostic and therapeutic indications for bronchoscopy are listed in Table 16–4. The suspicion of foreign body aspiration is an indication for bronchoscopy for both diagnosis and attempted removal. Flexible bronchoscopic techniques have been described for

Table 16–3. Rigid Bronchoscopy

Advantages	Disadvantages
Foreign body removal	General anesthesia
Massive hemoptysis	Visualize segment
Infant endoscopy	Biopsy segment
Dilate strictures	Peripheral biopsy upper lobe
Tracheal obstruction	
Laser bronchoscopy	

Table 16–4. Indications for Bronchoscopy

Diagnostic	Therapeutic
Severe cough	Atelectasis
Change in cough	Lung abscess
Abnormal chest radiograph	Foreign body
Hemoptysis	Stricture
Wheeze	Laser
Unresolved pneumonia	
Abnormal sputum cytology	
Diffuse lung disease	Other Indications
Opportunistic infection	Prolonged intubation
Bacteriologic sampling	Difficult intubation
Metastatic malignancy	Bronchography
Smoke inhalation	Gastric aspiration
Pediatric airway obstruction	Lobar gas sampling
Bronchoalveolar lavage	Management of massive hemoptysis
Upper esophageal cancer	

the removal of foreign bodies using grasping and basket forceps. The endoscopist, however, must be absolutely certain that a more complicated problem does not result from either losing sight of the foreign body or impacting it distally in the tracheobronchial tree. In this regard, the rigid bronchoscope remains the instrument of choice, allowing good exposure and airway control. Inglis and Wagner (1992) reported the advantages of combining flexible and rigid bronchoscopy in such cases to improve the detection and retrieval rate, especially when fragments of the foreign body are lodged in the distal airway or in the upper lobe bronchi (Fig. 16–6).

A new and persistent cough, or a change in the cough pattern of a smoker, warrants a bronchoscopic examination. Neoplasms can be diagnosed, even in the absence of radiologic findings. Sputum can be obtained in a sterile fashion to assess for opportunistic infections, especially in the immunocompromised patient. Endoscopic lobar and segmental lavage has proved to have therapeutic benefit in patients with cystic fibrosis and in postoperative patients with persistently thick and tenacious secretions. Retained bronchial secretions are easily suctioned at the bedside with minimal patient discomfort.

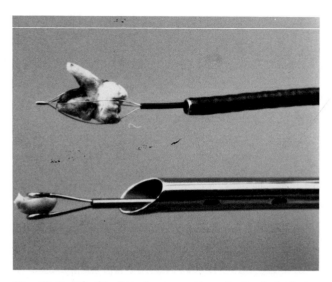

Fig. 16–6. Flexible bronchoscope with a foreign body basket retrieving a tooth, and a rigid bronchoscope with foreign body forceps grasping a peanut.

An abnormal chest radiograph suggesting carcinoma warrants a careful evaluation of the tracheobronchial tree. Clinical judgment should always be used in deciding when to use bronchoscopy, but the physician should err on the side of an endoscopic evaluation to rule out a neoplasm. An obstructing carcinoma may be the underlying cause of an unresolving pneumonia, and upper lobar pneumonia should be viewed with particular suspicion. Bronchoscopy may also be used to assess for metastatic tumors. According to a report by Mohsenifar and colleagues (1978), bronchoscopy could confirm the diagnosis 54% of the time in patients undergoing flexible bronchoscopy for the presence of metastatic disease.

Although the most common cause of hemoptysis is chronic bronchitis, carcinoma is common in patients with an abnormal radiograph of the chest. Even if the radiograph is normal, according to Jackson (1985) and Poe (1988) and their associates, malignancy should be seriously considered if the patient is 40 years of age or older, has a significant smoking history, or has repeated episodes of hemoptysis over 1 week in duration. Hemoptysis associated with a wheeze or atelectasis may be caused by a bronchial carcinoid or an inflammatory bronchial stenosis. The site of massive hemoptysis must be localized to prepare adequately for possible surgical excision, bronchial artery embolization, or endobronchial tamponade, as described by Saw and co-workers (1976).

When sputum cytology is used to screen high-risk patients for malignancy, patients with a normal chest radiograph and abnormal cytologic findings may be identified. In such cases, the mouth, pharynx, larynx, and entire tracheobronchial tree must be examined carefully to identify the site of the early carcinoma.

The bronchial mucosa must be assessed carefully for subtle changes such as irregular bronchial folds, mucosal thickening, and increased submucosal vascularity, as

illustrated by Stradling (1981). Areas in which malignancy is suspected should undergo brushing and biopsy with a diagnostic yield above 90%, according to Popovich and associates (1982). Such endobronchial findings may not be detected in peripheral lesions that should undergo biopsy using fluoroscopic guidance. Under these circumstances, the diagnostic yield by biopsy alone is 46%; the yield increases to 60%, however, when biopsy is combined with bronchial brushings, according to Cortese and McDougall (1979).

Over the last 15 years, the technique of transbronchial needle aspiration cytology, championed by Wang (1983, 1989) and Shure (1983, 1984, 1985) and their co-workers, has found increasing favor to sample subcarinal and paratracheal lymph nodes, examine widened spurs, and aspirate peripheral lung lesions. The findings must be correlated with computed tomographic findings so that the precise location of the enlarged lymph node is identified. Using an 18-gauge needle for histologic core biopsies, TBNA increased the yield of detectable submucosal or peribronchial carcinoma, according to Wang (1986).

Bronchoscopy is indicated in the early diagnosis and management of lung abscess. The passage of brushes and biopsy forceps into the abscess cavity can promote bronchial drainage, and sometimes an obstructing neoplasm or foreign body is detected. The therapeutic value of bronchoscopy to remove aspirated gastric contents remains in question, but a rapid and efficient bronchoscopy can support the diagnosis and may have therapeutic benefit. After inhalation of smoke or caustic fumes, bronchoscopy is a safe and expeditious way of assessing tracheobronchial mucosal damage. In these compromised patients, the airways frequently need to be debrided of necrotic mucosa and inspissated secretions. Patients with cystic fibrosis may also, on occasion, require aspiration of persistently thick and tenacious secretions, but this step frequently is avoided by the routine use of vigorous physiotherapy and mucolytic agents.

Bronchoalveolar lavage — BAL — is a useful technique for obtaining microbiologic specimens, especially in immunosuppressed patients. Fungal, bacterial, and viral culture specimens are easily acquired. In patients with acquired immunodeficiency syndrome — AIDS — the diagnosis of pneumocystis carinii pneumonia can also be made with a diagnostic yield exceeding 85%, according to Martin (1987), Ognibene (1984), and Pisani (1992) and their associates.

Cytologic specimens can also be obtained to establish the diagnosis in a variety of noninfectious, diffuse interstitial pulmonary diseases, including lipoid pneumonitis, histiocytosis, and berylliosis, all of which are uncommon entities. Bronchoalveolar lavage is of more limited value in the diagnosis of fibrosing alveolitis, sarcoidosis, and hypersensitivity pneumonitis, as noted by Stoller and colleagues (1987). Levy and associates (1988) reported that BAL has been used to establish the diagnosis of peripheral primary lung carcinoma. Rennard and colleagues (1990) and Pirozynski (1992) also noted this fact, but BAL has not been widely advocated as a step in the diagnosis of cancer in North America, and it should not be considered a routine diagnostic procedure. It should be performed only in those centers prepared to handle and analyze the specimens appropriately. Potential complications of BAL include bronchospasm, hypoxia, fever, and transient decline in pulmonary function. Patients must therefore be observed carefully after the procedure. The safety of BAL in patients with symptomatic asthma or with an FEV_1 less than 60% of predicted value has not been established, according to a NHLBI workshop report (1985).

The evaluation and management of the obstructed airway in infants often requires rigid bronchoscopy. Subglottic stenosis, vascular rings, webs, tracheomalacia, and cysts are some of the many conditions encountered.

TECHNIQUE

Anesthesia

Most patients are premedicated with antisialagogue — such as atropine or glycopyrrolate — to reduce secretions and inhibit vasovagal responses. Intravenous sedatives — diazepam and midazolam — are often administered for patient comfort; however, they should be used with caution, especially in elderly patients and those with limited pulmonary reserve. Midazolam has a particularly high incidence of associated sudden respiratory arrest and should be used only with appropriate precautions.

Topical anesthesia is preferred for fiberoptic bronchoscopy, but general anesthesia may be indicated, particularly for prolonged examinations required to identify an in situ carcinoma in a patient with a normal chest radiograph. General anesthesia is also the preferred technique in patients undergoing rigid bronchoscopy. The performance of rigid bronchoscopy using local anesthesia, while maintaining patient comfort, has become a lost art.

The most common agents for topical anesthesia are lidocaine — 2% and 4% — and tetracaine — 0.5%, 1% and 2%. Complications from topical anesthesia usually result from the administration of excessive amounts, as documented by Credle (1974), Suratt (1976), and Pereira (1978) and their associates. If carefully measured amounts are given and the endoscopist is always aware of the total milligram dosage instilled, reactions are minimized. Lidocaine is a safe agent with a recommended adult dose up to 400 mg, but larger amounts have been given without serious side effects. The first sign of toxicity is usually central nervous system excitation or seizure before cardiovascular collapse; the duration of action is short. Lidocaine does not provide the depth of anesthesia necessary for rigid bronchoscopy.

Tetracaine is another effective topical anesthetic, but side effects often occur when a dose of 80 mg is exceeded, and it must be used with caution. The duration of action is prolonged and the first sign of toxicity may be sudden cardiovascular collapse.

Several satisfactory methods are available to administer topical anesthesia. Using the nasotracheal route, the nasopharynx is anesthetized initially using an atomized topical agent, and the flexible bronchoscope is then passed through the nares to a level just proximal to the false cords. With the larynx in clear view, additional topical anesthetic is sprayed directly onto the vocal cords and into the trachea. The bronchoscope is then passed through the glottis and additional topical anesthesia is instilled down the tracheobronchial tree.

A second method of delivering topical anesthesia consists of initial spraying of the hypopharynx with 2% or 4% lidocaine using an atomizer (Fig. 16–7). Five milliliters of 4% lidocaine is then injected transtracheally at the level of the cricothyroid membrane using a short 21-gauge needle to minimize the risk of lacerating the posterior wall of the trachea. Slight bleeding often occurs with this technique, so it should be avoided when a patient is being examined for hemoptysis of unknown origin. Care is needed to confirm the position in the trachea by aspirating air before injecting, because it is possible to inject directly into the false cords causing respiratory compromise. Anesthesia of the larynx is achieved as the patient coughs out the medication. Supplemental 2% lidocaine is then instilled into the tracheobronchial tree while advancing the bronchoscope. Because topical anesthetic agents inhibit bacterial growth, care should be taken to minimize the amount aspirated into collection traps for microbiologic studies.

Flexible bronchoscopy is accomplished easily using general anesthesia. In the adult, a two-way swivel

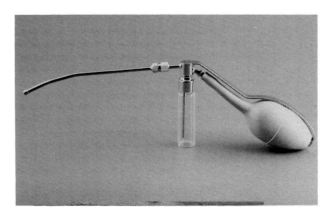

Fig. 16–7. Atomizer to administer topical anesthesia.

adaptor is attached to the endotracheal tube, and ventilation is maintained through the side arm of the adaptor. The bronchoscope is passed through a tight-fitting plastic diaphragm on the adaptor (see Fig. 16–3). As large an endotracheal tube as possible should be selected, because airflow resistance is increased significantly when a 5.8-mm bronchoscope is passed through an endotracheal tube smaller than 8.0 mm in outer diameter; use of a smaller endotracheal tube could lead to hypercapnia and respiratory distress. When bronchoscopy is performed with the patient breathing spontaneously, a cuffless endotracheal tube can be used to act as a sheath for easy access and suctioning. This technique permits the patient to breathe both through and around the endotracheal tube during the procedure.

In children, a 5.8-mm flexible bronchoscope can be passed down a 7.0-mm endotracheal tube, but the procedure must be interrupted to provide adequate ventilation. If a long procedure is anticipated, blood gas analysis or capnograph monitoring is mandatory. The pediatric 3.5-mm bronchoscope is currently the best choice among the flexible instruments for use in children.

Jet ventilation techniques may be used in children as well as adults with compromised lumina by passing small catheters either through or beside the endotracheal tube. Jet ventilation techniques, however, are not simple and the anesthesiologist must be experienced with their use.

Rigid bronchoscopy is generally performed with general anesthesia, using the ventilation port on the side of the bronchoscope and capping the end of the scope with an eyepiece to convert the procedure to a nearly closed system. The eyepiece is removed for biopsy and aspiration (Fig. 16–8). Some loss of tidal volume around the bronchoscope is inevitable, but this can be minimized by packing the hypopharynx with gauze or by compression of the supraglottic area by the fingers of

an assistant. The anesthesiologist must monitor the adequacy of the ventilation continuously; increased minute ventilation and tidal volumes are required. This method is safe for procedures lasting up to 20 minutes, but if longer periods are needed, other anesthetic techniques should be considered.

Jet ventilation through a rigid bronchoscope is a satisfactory method for delivering general anesthesia. A nitrous oxide gas and oxygen mixture can be delivered with an increased pressure that provides adequate oxygenation and a decreased arterial CO_2. Familiarity with the system is required before it can be used routinely.

Examination

The first phase of a diagnostic bronchoscopy is clear visualization of the larynx and the vocal cords. Unsuspected leukoplakia, carcinoma in situ, and invasive carcinoma may be found. Vocal cord mobility must be assessed, because recurrent laryngeal palsy secondary to carcinoma of the lung generally is considered a sign of inoperability. The larynx should also be examined before passing the rigid bronchoscope.

The flexible fiberoptic bronchoscope can be inserted through either the nose or the mouth into the hypopharynx and then through the glottis into the trachea. Passage of the instrument through the nares does not permit easy withdrawal and reinsertion for cleaning of the lens and clearing the channel of thick mucus. Biopsy and brushing cytology specimens must be withdrawn through the channel, and some of the specimen may be lost, decreasing the yield of diagnostic material.

An alternative technique involves passing an uncuffed 8.0-mm endotracheal tube through the orotracheal route as described by Sanderson and McDougall (1978) (Fig. 16–9). The patient breathes around and through the endotracheal tube with the bronchoscope in place; airway control is provided and the endotracheal tube

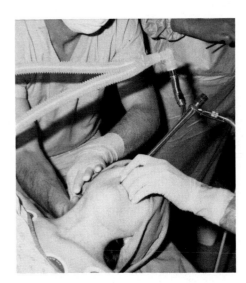

Fig. 16–8. Rigid ventilating bronchoscopy with biopsy performed using general anesthesia and open tube technique.

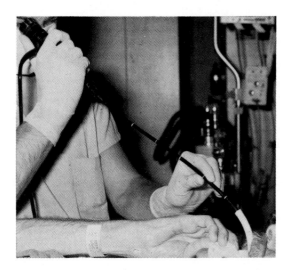

Fig. 16–9. Flexible fiberoptic bronchoscope is inserted through an oral endotracheal tube.

allows rapid insertion and withdrawal of the broncho-scope. Brushing and biopsy specimens are retrieved by leaving the brush or forceps beyond the tip of the bronchoscope, avoiding loss of the specimen in the working channel. Placement of the endotracheal tube provides the opportunity for assisted ventilation and large catheter suctioning should bleeding occur.

Rigid bronchoscopy is performed using general anesthesia. The patient is supine with an assistant positioning the head so that the neck is slightly flexed and the chin is extended. The endoscopist elevates the epiglottis with the tip of the bronchoscope, and passes the lubricated instrument through the glottis, into the upper trachea. The telescope system provides a magnified field of vision at 0°, 30°, and 90°. If angle-viewing telescopes are not available, the flexible bronchoscope can be passed through the rigid bronchoscope to view upper lobe orifices and all segmental bronchi.

Examination of the trachea is accomplished after the bronchoscope passes through the glottis, and the carina is assessed for sharpness and mobility during ventilation. Widening or fixation suggest the involvement of the subcarinal nodes by tumor or an inflammatory process. Biopsy of the carina is obtained if it is widened or if submucosal extension of malignancy is suspected.

Transbronchial needle biopsy is one of the latest innovations to sample mediastinal and submucosal central pulmonary lesions. Cytologic specimens are obtained by passing an ensheathed 21-gauge needle down the working channel of the bronchoscope within a protective outer sheath (Fig. 16–10). Ignoring this precaution has led to serious and costly repairs of flexible bronchoscopes as documented by Mehta and co-workers (1990). Once the needle is advanced beyond the tip of the scope, the needle is advanced out of the sheath and through the wall of the trachea or bronchus into the mediastinal mass or suspicious lymph nodes (Fig. 16–11). Preoperative computed tomographic or magnetic resonance scanning is imperative to define precisely the location of the area in question. The needle can be

reinserted into this region several times, applying gentle suction each time the needle is in place; suction must be avoided once the needle is completely withdrawn. Five milliliters of saline is then flushed through the needle to obtain an optimal cytologic sample, which is then immediately centrifuged; the resulting pellet is resuspended in 1 ml of saline, fixed in 95% ethanol, and prepared with Papanicolaou stain. In 1986, Wang reported that 50% of patients judged to be surgical candidates had "positive" mediastinal nodes when assessed by TBNA. Shure and colleagues (1985) described increased diagnostic accuracy when TBNA is used with bronchoscopic evidence of submucosal or parabronchial tumor. It should be noted, however, that TBNA has at least a 15% false-negative rate in assessing mediastinal nodes to stage lung carcinoma, according to Wang (1986); this number has been higher in the hands of most other investigators. Transbronchial needle aspiration should be performed before brushing or lavaging because a positive brushing or lavage could contaminate the tracheobronchial tree and theoretically lead to falsely positive specimens, according to Cropp (1984) and Schenk (1984) and their associates. Bleeding and mediastinal infection are rare complications of TBNA of the mediastinum.

All lobar and segmental bronchi must be examined carefully and systematically, because a second lesion not visible on the chest radiograph is occasionally identified. The bronchus leading to the known area of disease is then examined. The character of secretions and the bronchial mucosa are clues to the nature of the underlying pathologic condition. Subtle mucosal abnormalities associated with carcinoma include mucosal thickening, irregular bronchial folds or corrugation, and increased submucosal vascularity. Stradling (1981) reported that these findings may be associated with a loss of definition of the cartilaginous rings or circular folds, endobronchial stenosis, or extrinsic bronchial compression. The extent of the endoscopic findings must be examined carefully when anticipating a possible surgical resection.

If an endobronchial lesion is visualized, a biopsy is performed. Biopsy through the flexible bronchoscope requires persistence and practice, especially with lesions in the apical regions of the upper lobe. Biopsies should be attempted, even when the lesion is suspected to be a bronchial carcinoid, because lung-sparing resections can be accomplished with minimal resection margins with this pathologic entity. Bleeding can be controlled with topical 1/10,000 epinephrine. Small fragments of tissue are obtained with 1.5-mm biopsy forceps, and multiple biopsies are often necessary to provide diagnostic material. Biopsies of segmental lesions are easily accomplished with flexible instrumentation. Following each biopsy, the forceps is placed in saline, and concentrated formalin solution is added at the conclusion of the procedure to give a final dilution of 10%.

Kvale and associates (1976) reported that the accuracy of establishing the diagnosis of carcinoma increases with the number and types of specimens obtained. Many

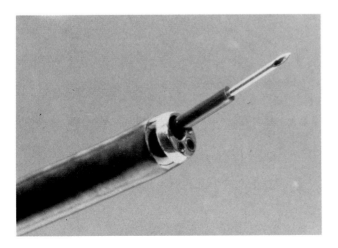

Fig. 16–10.   Transbronchial needle for aspiration of mediastinal and hilar lymph nodes and masses.

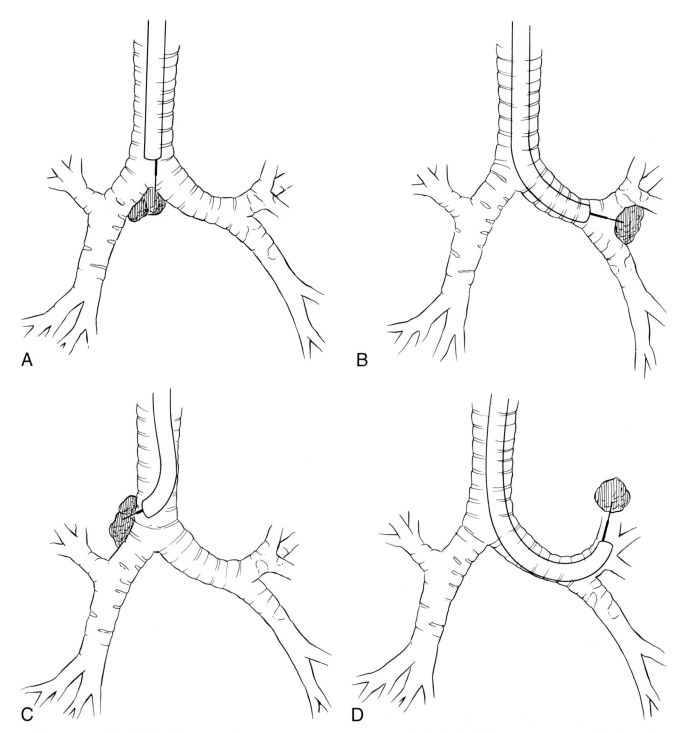

Fig. 16–11. Transbronchial needle aspirate of subcarinal lymph nodes *(A)*, a mass at the bifurcation of the left mainstem bronchus *(B)*, a nodal mass at the right tracheobronchial angle *(C)*, and a central mass in the left upper lobe *(D)*.

lesions have large necrotic areas, which do not provide diagnostic material if a biopsy is performed. Bronchial brushings are generally performed after the biopsy tissue has been obtained. A 7-mm brush is recommended for routine use because more cellular material is obtained (Fig. 16–12); 1.7-mm brushes have the advantage that they can be ensheathed and withdrawn through the working channel of the bronchoscope, but

the yield of material is smaller. The bronchial brush may be inserted into narrowed segmental bronchi to provide a positive cytologic diagnosis. The brush is passed vigorously over the surface of the lesion and is then quickly stroked onto the surface of glass slide, which is immersed immediately in 95% ethanol (Fig. 16–13). Improved results are achieved if four separate brush specimens are sent on four slides. Shure and Fedullo

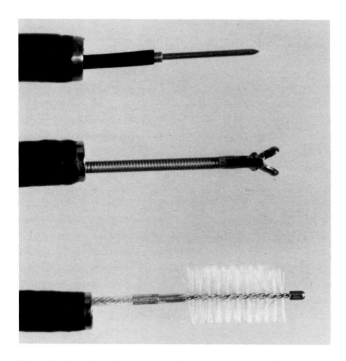

Fig. 16–12. Flexible fiberoptic bronchoscope with (from top to bottom) a 21-gauge transbronchial needle, a flexible cup biopsy forceps, and a 7-mm nylon brush.

(1983) reported use of TBNA to establish the diagnosis of peripheral primary lung carcinomas.

Specimens of peripheral lesions are obtained by brushing or biopsy under fluoroscopic control. Using this technique, the lesion should be seen to move to confirm proper placement. Transbronchial brushings and biopsies may also be used to assess pulmonary infiltrates, and may establish the diagnosis of sarcoidosis, tuberculosis, bronchioloalveolar carcinoma, or pulmonary alveolar proteinosis. The flexible bronchoscope is

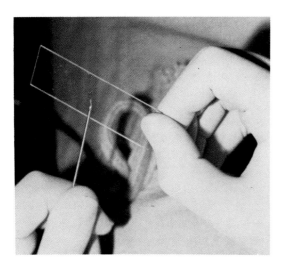

Fig. 16–13. Bronchial brush is rapidly smeared onto a glass slide, which is immediately immersed in 90% ethanol to fix the material for cytologic examination.

initially wedged in the segmental bronchus and the biopsy forceps is advanced to the periphery of the diseased region. The forceps is then drawn back 3 to 4 mm, and the jaws are opened and advanced slightly to obtain the sample of the lung. The bronchoscope is left wedged in the segmental bronchus in the event of bleeding to allow irrigation with 1/10,000 epinephrine. Five to seven transbronchial biopsies have been found to provide the optimal diagnostic yield and these samples should all be taken from the same lung to avoid the complication of bilateral pneumothorax. Visual placement of the biopsy forceps near but not at the lung surface minimizes the risk of developing a pneumothorax. Coagulation studies, platelet counts, should be obtained preoperatively to identify patients at high risk for bleeding. Uremic patients are also known to be at high risk for significant hemoptysis and precautions must be taken.

Bronchoalveolar lavage is a useful technique to diagnose opportunistic infections including cytomegalovirus, and bacterial, fungal, and *Pneumocystis carinii* pneumonia. It is performed by wedging the tip of the flexible bronchoscope into a subsegmental bronchus and irrigating and aspirating the segment with 20- to 50-ml aliquots of sterile saline. A total volume of 100 to 300 ml of saline is instilled and 40 to 70% of this volume is recovered as a specimen. In patients who have loss of elastic recoil, recovery of fluid is less, according to Helmers and Hunninghake (1989), because the subsegmental bronchiolar walls collapse when suction is applied. In addition to microbiologic studies, lavage specimens have been used to diagnose malignancies and to obtain inflammatory cells and pneumocytes for research studies.

PEDIATRIC BRONCHOSCOPY

Bronchoscopy in infants and small children requires expertise and familiarity with all available instrumentation. Examination of the infant airway using smaller Storz rigid instruments with viewing telescopes is usually performed using general anesthesia (Fig. 16–14). A 3.0 or 3.5-mm sheath permits passage of the 2.7-mm optical telescope that provides a good view of the infant's bronchi. A small suction catheter can be passed down the barrel. Secretions are readily removed for microbiologic studies, as well as for therapeutic benefit. Small biopsy and foreign-body forceps can be manipulated through this small channel with the viewing telescope in place. Muntz and associates (1992) reported their experience performing transbronchial lung biopsies in the pediatric population through a rigid bronchoscope.

Flexible fiberoptic bronchoscopy has become a practical tool in pediatrics with the development of a bronchoscope with an external diameter of 3.5 mm and a channel of 1.2 mm. It has found favor in clearing secretions, as well as aiding in localizing and retrieving foreign bodies. Examination of infants may be performed using sedation and topical anesthesia, provided it is

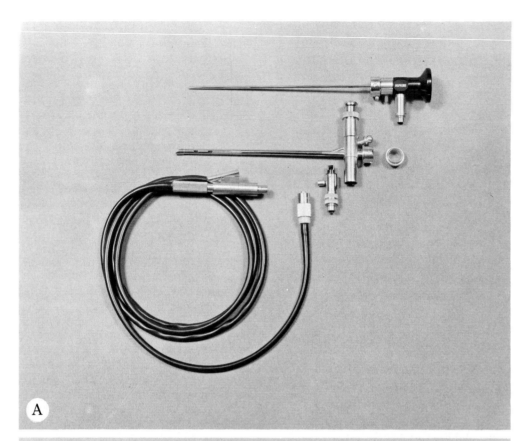

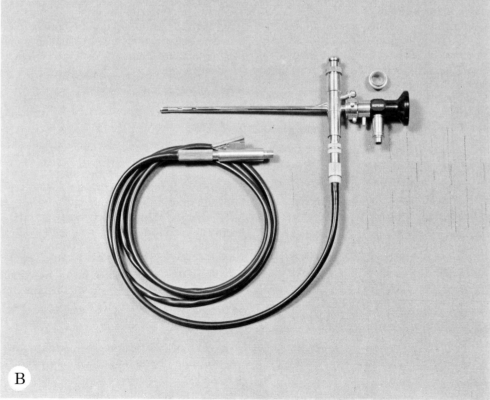

Fig. 16–14. Infant rigid bronchoscope (Storz), 3.5 mm diameter, with fiberoptic lighting. *A*, Components (from top to bottom): 1) forward-viewing endoscopic telescope (Hopkins); 2) bronchoscope with detachable window plus side channels for connection to anesthesia equipment, suctioning, and insertion of proximal light; 3) proximal prismatic light carrier; and 4) fiberoptic lighting cable. *B*, After assembly.

brief. Airway stenosis or obstruction are contraindications to flexible instrumentation.

Complications related to pediatric bronchoscopy can be life-threatening. Subglottic edema from manipulation may compromise the airway. Stridorous breathing after the procedure is an indication for humidification of supplemental oxygen and the administration of systemic steroids. A small bronchus may be perforated with resultant pneumothorax or pneumomediastinum.

CONTRAINDICATIONS AND COMPLICATIONS

There are no absolute contraindications for bronchoscopy. Even severely ill and debilitated patients can undergo bronchoscopy safely if it is performed in an appropriate facility by an experienced endoscopist. Despite the relatively low risk, the benefits of performing bronchoscopy must be weighed against the potential for complication in each patient. Credle and colleagues (1974) reported a complication rate of 0.08% and a mortality of 0.01% in over 24,000 flexible bronchoscopies. Premedication and topical anesthesia were responsible for 11 of the 22 major complications. More dilute solutions of the topical anesthetic agent provide a wider margin of safety. Intravenous diazepam counteracts the systemic effects of excessive amounts of lidocaine and should be readily available. Elderly and debilitated patients should receive minimal premedication, and topical anesthesia must be administered in carefully measured amounts. Respiratory depression can easily occur in this patient population.

Careful evaluation and preparation of the patient as well as adequate facilities to monitor the patient are required to minimize complications. Pulse oximetry, continuous electrocardiogram monitoring, and intermittent cuff blood pressure readings are all important parameters. Supplemental oxygen is supplied to minimize the risk of hypoxemia. Respiratory depression has been documented in the recovery period. According to Peacock (1989), topical anesthesia may be responsible for prolonged periods of respiratory depression. Belen (1981) and Matsushima (1984) and their associates recommend that patients should not undergo pulmonary function testing for at least 8 hours after bronchoscopy. General anesthesia may be indicated if the patient has a history of intolerance to topical anesthetic agents or of difficult endoscopies under local anesthesia.

Massive bleeding is a recognized complication of bronchoscopy, as documented by Suratt and associates (1976). Bleeding disorders must be corrected by anticoagulant reversal or by the infusion of platelets either during or immediately before the procedure. A brushing or biopsy should not be done unless the prothrombin time is over 40% and the platelet count is greater than 50,000. Patients with uremia or pulmonary hypertension also bleed easily, and, according to Zavala (1976), brushings and biopsies in these patients should be avoided. Topical epinephrine solution of 1/10,000 can be instilled into the segmental bronchus before brushing to minimize bleeding or to control established bleeding. In the event of endobronchial hemorrhage, Zavala (1976) recommended wedging the scope in the segmental bronchus to tamponade the lumen by the clot.

According to Pereira and colleagues (1978), pneumothorax can occur in up to 5% of patients undergoing a transbronchial lung biopsy. When lung biopsies are performed for diffuse lung disease, it is important to perform this procedure under fluoroscopic control to avoid perforation of the lung. Patients may complain of sharp chest pain if the parietal pleura is irritated.

Bronchoscopy should not be performed in a patient with bilateral vocal cord paralysis. The passage of the bronchoscope through the glottis can lead to edema, causing life-threatening airway obstruction and necessitating emergent intubation or tracheostomy. Patients with a tracheal obstruction should be examined cautiously, and biopsy or dilatation of the tracheal lesion should be avoided if the airway is severely compromised, unless one is prepared to proceed directly to definitive tracheal surgery.

Bronchospasm is a potential complication in patients with known asthma, but it may also occur in patients with severe chronic obstructive lung disease. Asthmatics should be premedicated with corticosteroids and bronchodilators. Laryngospasm is the direct consequence of inadequate topical anesthesia; it can be avoided if the topical agent is placed precisely onto the vocal cords and into the tracheobronchial tree.

Patients with hepatitis, human immunodeficiency virus, or suspected active tuberculosis can undergo bronchoscopy if special care is taken by all personnel in the handling of the specimens and all instruments used are appropriately sterilized. Infections transmitted after properly cleaning instruments are rare, according to Suratt and co-workers (1977). Sepsis after bronchoscopy is uncommon, but fever is occasionally seen. Patients with underlying valvular heart disease should receive prophylactic antibiotics before bronchoscopy to minimize the risk of bacterial endocarditis.

REFERENCES

Albertini RE, Harrell JH, Moser KM: Management of arterial hypoxemia induced by fiberoptic bronchoscopy. Chest 67:134, 1975.

Belen J, et al: Modification of the effect of fiberoptic bronchoscopy on pulmonary mechanics. Chest 79:516, 1981.

Cortese DA, McDougall JC: Biopsy and brushing of peripheral lung cancer with fluoroscopic guidance. Chest 75:141, 1979.

Credle WF, Smiddy JF, Elliott RC: Complications of fiberoptic bronchoscopy. Am Rev Respir Dis 109:67, 1974.

Cropp AJ, Dimarco AF, Lankerani M: False-positive transbronchial needle aspiration in bronchogenic carcinoma. Chest 85:696, 1984.

Helmers RA, Hunninghake GW: Bronchoalveolar lavage. In Wang KP (ed): Biopsy Techniques in Pulmonary Disorders. 1st Ed. New York: Raven Press, 1989.

Inglis AF, Wagner DV: Lower complication rates associated with bronchial foreign bodies over the last 25 years. Ann Otol Rhinol Laryngol 101:61, 1992.

Jackson CV, Savage PJ, Quinn DL: Role of fiberoptic bronchoscopy in patients with hemoptysis and a normal chest roentgenogram. Chest 87:142, 1985.

Kvale PA, Bode FR, Kini S: Diagnostic accuracy in lung cancer. Comparison of techniques used in association with flexible fiberoptic techniques. Chest 69:752, 1976.

Lan RS, et al: Use of fiberoptic bronchoscopy to retrieve bronchial foreign bodies in adults. Am Rev Respir Dis 140:1734, 1989.

Levy H, Horak DA, Lewis MI: The value of bronchial washings and bronchoalveolar lavage in the diagnosis of lymphangitic carcinomatosis. Chest 94:1028, 1988.

Martin WJ, et al: Role of bronchoalveolar lavage in the assessment of opportunistic pulmonary infections: Utility and complications. Mayo Clin Proc 62:549, 1987.

Matsushima Y, et al: Alterations in pulmonary mechanics and gas exchange during routine fiberoptic bronchoscopy. Chest 86:184, 1984.

Mehta AC, et al: The high price of bronchoscopy. Maintenance and repair of the flexible fiberoptic bronchoscope. Chest 98:448, 1990.

Mohsenifar Z, Chopra SK, Simmons DH: Diagnostic value of fibreoptic bronchoscopy in metastatic pulmonary tumors. Chest 74:369, 1978.

Muntz H, Wallace M, Lusk RP: Pediatric transbronchial lung biopsy. Ann Otol Rhinol Laryngol 101:135, 1992.

NHLBI Workshop Summaries: Summary and recommendations of a workshop on the investigative use of fiberoptic bronchoscopy and bronchoalveolar lavage in asthmatics. Am Rev Respir Dis 132:180, 1985.

Ognibene FP, et al: The diagnosis of *Pneumocystis carinii* pneumonia in patients with acquired immunodeficiency syndrome using subsegmental bronchoalveolar lavage. Am Rev Respir Dis 129:929, 1984.

Paşaoğlu I, et al: Bronchoscopic removal of foreign bodies in children: Retrospective analysis of 822 cases. Thorac Cardiovasc Surg 39:95, 1991.

Peacock AJ, Benson-Mitchell R, Godfrey R: Effect of fibreoptic bronchoscopy on pulmonary function. Thorax 45:38, 1990.

Pereira W, Kovnat DM, Snider GL: A prospective cooperative study of complications following flexible fiberoptic bronchoscopy. Chest 73:813, 1978.

Pisani RJ, Wright AJ: Clinical utility of bronchoalveolar lavage in immunocompromised hosts. Mayo Clin Proc 76:221, 1992.

Popovich J Jr, et al: Diagnostic accuracy of multiple biopsies from flexible bronchoscopic biopsy: A comparison of central versus peripheral carcinoma. Am Rev Respir Dis 125:521, 1982.

Prakash UBS, Stubbs SE: The bronchoscopy survey. Some reflections. Chest 100:1660, 1991.

Prakash UBS, Offord KP, Stubbs SE: Bronchoscopy in North America: The ACCP survey. Chest 100:1668, 1991.

Sanderson DR, McDougall JC: Transoral bronchoscopy. Chest 73:701, 1978.

Saw EC, et al: Flexible fiberoptic bronchoscopy and endobronchial tamponade in the management of massive hemoptysis. Chest 70:589, 1976.

Schenk DA, et al: Potential false positive mediastinal transbronchial needle aspiration in bronchogenic carcinoma. Chest 86:649, 1984.

Shure D, Fedullo PF: Transbronchial needle aspiration of peripheral masses. Am Rev Respir Dis 128:1090, 1983.

Shure D, Fedullo PF: The role of transcarinal needle aspiration in the staging of bronchogenic carcinoma. Chest 86:693, 1984.

Shure D, Fedullo PF: Transbronchial needle aspiration in the diagnosis of submucosal and peribronchial bronchogenic carcinoma. Chest 88:49, 1985.

Stradling P: Diagnostic Bronchoscopy. 4th Ed. New York: Churchill Livingstone, 1981.

Stoller JK, Rankin JA, Reynolds HY: The impact of bronchoalveolar lavage analysis on clinicians' diagnostic reasoning about interstitial lung disease. Chest 92:839, 1987.

Suratt PM, Smiddy JF, Gruber B: Deaths and complications associated with fiberoptic bronchoscopy. Chest 69:747, 1976.

Suratt PM, et al: Absence of clinical pneumonia following bronchoscopy with contaminated and clean bronchoscopes. Chest 71:52, 1977.

Wang KP: Flexible transbronchial needle aspiration biopsy for histologic specimens. Chest 88:860, 1986.

Wang KP: Flexible bronchoscopy with transbronchial needle aspiration: Biopsy for cytology specimens. *In* Wang KP: Biopsy Techniques in Pulmonary Disorders. 1st Ed. New York: Raven Press, 1989.

Wang KP, Terry PB: Transbronchial needle aspiration in the diagnosis and staging of bronchogenic carcinoma. Am Rev Respir Dis 127:344, 1983.

Weissberg D, Schwartz I: Foreign bodies in the tracheobronchial tree. Chest 91:730, 1987.

Zavala DC: Pulmonary hemorrhage in fiberoptic transbronchial biopsy. Chest 70:584, 1976.

READING REFERENCES

Fulkerson WJ: Fiberoptic bronchoscopy. N Engl J Med 311:511, 1984.

Grebski E, et al: Diagnostic value of hemosiderin-containing macrophages in bronchoalveolar lavage. Chest 102:1794, 1992.

Herf SM, Suratt PM, Arora NS: Deaths and complications associated with transbronchial lung biopsy. Am Rev Respir Dis 115:708, 1977.

Kvale PA: Flexible bronchoscopy with brush and forceps biopsy. *In* Wang KP (ed): Biopsy Techniques in Pulmonary Disorders. 1st Ed. New York: Raven Press, 1989.

Lindholm, C-E, et al: Cardiorespiratory effects of flexible fiberoptic bronchoscopy in critically ill patients. Chest 74:362, 1978.

Pirozynski M: Bronchoalveolar lavage in the diagnosis of peripheral, primary lung cancer. Chest 102:372, 1992.

Poe RH, et al: Utility of fiberoptic bronchoscopy in patients with hemoptysis and a nonlocalizing chest roentgenogram. Chest 92:70, 1988.

Rennard SI, et al: Clinical guidelines for bronchoalveolar lavage (BAL): Pulmonary malignancies. Eur Respir J 2:561, 1989.

Zavala DC: Transbronchial biopsy in diffuse lung disease. Chest 73:727, 1978.

CHAPTER 17

INVASIVE DIAGNOSTIC PROCEDURES

James W. Mackenzie and John L. Nosher

Careful physical examination of patients suspected of harboring carcinoma of the lung may disclose new lesions in the scalp or skin that may be metastatic and should undergo biopsy. As noted in Chapter 7, mediastinal lymphatic drainage is generally in ascending patterns to the scalene areas; lymphatics have also been described from the basal portions of the lung through the diaphragm.

SCALENE NODE BIOPSY

Daniels (1949) recommended excision of lymph nodes in the scalene fat pad to diagnose intrathoracic disease. Before the introduction of mediastinoscopy, this procedure was used widely for evaluation of patients with suspected bronchial carcinoma and various intraabdominal neoplasms. Certainly, palpable scalene lymph nodes require biopsy. For many of these patients, needle biopsy may be a better choice than open scalene node biopsy. Phillips and Barker (1985) reported success in 86% of 42 such patients. Rohwedder and colleagues (1990) were successful in all 55 patients with palpable supraclavicular nodes, although two required repeat needle biopsy.

Controversy still exists about the use of scalene node biopsy in patients with nonpalpable nodes. There is wide variation in the reported yield from scalene node biopsy in such patients. In the report by Brantigan and colleagues (1973), 20% of 2254 patients with carcinoma of the lung had a positive biopsy result. Bernstein and colleagues (1985) found only a 3.5% positive result. As pointed out by Leckie and colleagues (1963), partial explanation of the discrepancy between literature reports may be found in the accuracy of cervical palpation. It is, however, hard to reconcile the wide variation on this basis alone given the large size of the series reported by Brantigan. Nevertheless, as the mortality rate from mediastinoscopy is no greater than that from scalene node biopsy, the choice between the two procedures centers on the expected yield. In the report of Ashraf and associates (1980), 27% of patients with cancer of the

lung who were otherwise surgical candidates were found to have involved mediastinal lymph nodes, and Maassen (1985) found 36%. Therefore, mediastinoscopy has replaced scalene node biopsy for most patients in most centers. A notable exception, however, is the occasional patient with N2 disease who is being considered for resection. In these patients, documentation of spread outside the thorax should preclude consideration of thoracotomy.

The same reasoning applies to patients suspected of having sarcoidosis. In the report by Greschuchna and Maassen (1971), results of mediastinoscopy were positive in 98% of cases, whereas results of scalene node biopsy were positive in only 75%. The use of scalene node biopsy for nonthoracic disease has also generated controversy. It has been advocated for the staging of tumors in the pancreas, prostate, stomach, and cervix. Subsequent reports, such as that by Perez-Mesa and Spratt (1976), of patients with carcinoma of cervix with nonpalpable nodes questioned the utility of scalene node biopsy for intraabdominal disease with nonpalpable nodes. No clear-cut conclusions are to be drawn from the data available.

Procedure

Local anesthesia is used unless this operation is combined with other procedures. The incision is made on the side of palpable nodes. If they are not palpable, the incision is made on the right, except for those pulmonary lesions confined to the left upper lobe or if disease metastatic from the abdomen or pelvis is under consideration. A 5-cm incision is made in the skin crease approximately 2 cm above the clavicle extending approximately 2 cm over the lateral border of the sternocleidomastoid muscle (Fig. 17–1). The sternocleidomastoid muscle is retracted medially. Occasionally, it is necessary to divide a portion of the clavicular head of the muscle or to extend the incision between the two heads in obese or muscular patients. The omohyoid muscle is identified and retracted superiorly and laterally. The borders of the dissection are the internal

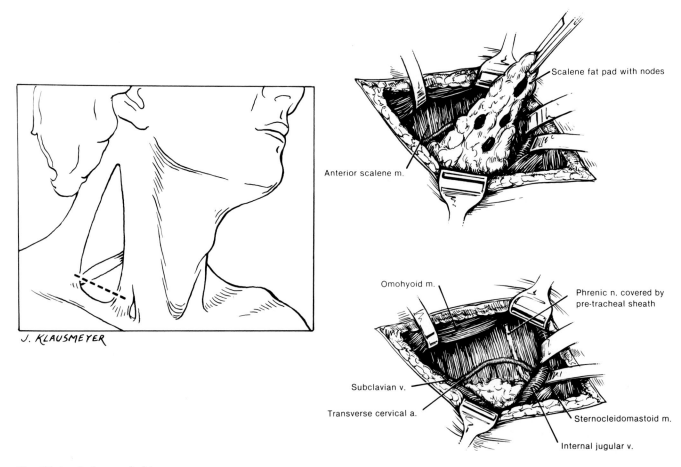

J. KLAUSMEYER

Scalene fat pad with nodes

Anterior scalene m.

Omohyoid m.

Phrenic n. covered by pre-tracheal sheath

Subclavian v.

Transverse cervical a.

Sternocleidomastoid m.

Internal jugular v.

Fig. 17–1. Scalene node biopsy.

jugular vein medially and the omohyoid superiorly and laterally. The subclavian vein at the inferior border of the dissection is often not identified clearly. The entire fat pad is excised unless obviously abnormal nodes are present, in which case it is not necessary to excise the entire fat pad. Unless frozen section confirms the presence of carcinoma, a portion of the lymph nodes should be sent for special stains and cultures.

The transverse cervical artery often requires division and the phrenic nerve should be avoided because it runs from lateral to medial in its position under the prevertebral fascia. The thoracic duct must be ligated with nonabsorbable ligature if severed, as should its counterpart on the right.

Complications

Rare complications include air embolism, pneumothorax, arteriovenous fistula, and damage to the phrenic nerve. Mortality from this procedure should be negligible.

MEDIASTINOSCOPY

Although Harken and associates (1954) suggested a way to explore the nodes in the superior mediastinum from a lateral approach after excision of the scalene fat pad, it was the development of cervical mediastinoscopy by Carlens (1959) that led to the widespread use of this procedure; first in Europe and later in North America with the strong support of Pearson (1968, 1980, 1982, 1986) and colleagues. Cervical mediastinoscopy has become an integral part of the evaluation and staging of patients with suspected lung cancer. For reasons noted previously, it has usually replaced scalene node biopsy unless cervical nodes are palpable. As demonstrated by Kirschner (1971) and Lewis and colleagues (1981), even advanced superior vena caval obstruction is not a contraindication to the operation. A report by Meersschaut and colleagues (1992) of 140 patients subjected to repeat mediastinoscopy citing no mortality, a sensitivity of 74%, and an accuracy of 94% proves mediastinoscopy is a safe and reliable procedure even in this group of patients. For the ordinary patient, the risk of mediastinoscopy is extremely small. Mortality reported by Specht (1971) in over 11,000 mediastinoscopic procedures compiled by him was 0.15%. In the prospective study of 1000 cases reported by Luke and colleagues (1986), the mortality was zero. On the Robert Wood Johnson Thoracic Surgery Service, our group has now performed over 3400 mediastinoscopic procedures with one mortality. Therefore, the safety of the procedure in experienced hands is well established.

Critics of this procedure have raised several questions about it. The first is cost. Certainly, mediastinoscopy does increase the cost of the evaluation of many patients. Nevertheless, when weighed against unnecessary thoracotomies and unnecessary mortality, the cost is insignificant. Further, the report by Vallieres and associates (1991) of 138 mediastinoscopies carried out on an ambulatory basis without one mortality and the need for admission for medical observation in only eight of these patients points the way for significant reduction in cost. The second concern is the advisability of the application of this technique to "all" patients being evaluated for carcinoma of the lung who are otherwise operable. Maassen (1985), in his experience of approximately 2000 mediastinoscopic procedures, demonstrated that even in 292 patients with peripheral T_1 lesions — less than 3 cm — the yield was 11%; the yield for central tumors in stages I and II was 23% and that for peripheral tumors in stages I and II was 19%. These data make a strong case for performing cervical mediastinoscopy in all patients suspected of having carcinoma of the lung who are otherwise operable. Other authors with smaller series advocate mediastinoscopy only in cases of central lesions, those with hilar involvement, or those with mediastinal node involvement suspected on radiographic examination. In a prospective study of 1000 patients subjected to mediastinoscopy, Luke and colleagues (1986) found tumor-bearing lymph nodes in 296 patients — 29.6%. In 72% of these patients, no abnormality was noted on review of the chest radiographs.

Early reports of the use of computed tomographic scanning suggested that it could be used to select patients for mediastinoscopy. The reports of Brion (1985) and Daly (1987) and their colleagues demonstrated a negative predictive index of about 90%.* In a prospective study of 170 patients with non-small cell disease reported by Webb and colleagues (1991), however, the sensitivity of CT imaging in detecting node metastasis was 52% and the specificity was 69%. The report by Izbicki and colleagues (1992) cast even greater doubt on the ability of CT scanning to stage carcinoma of the lung preoperatively. In this prospective study of 108 patients with carcinoma of the lung, on a patient-by-patient basis, CT scanning correctly predicted the nodal status in only 58% of patients. CT scanning apparently should not be used to exclude patients from mediastinoscopy.

Therefore, we are persuaded that mediastinoscopy is an appropriate procedure for essentially all patients before planned resection. If the likelihood is high that the cervical mediastinal exploration will be negative, it is scheduled for the same day as the proposed resection. This technique adds but 15 or 20 minutes to the operative procedure.

---

*Negative predictive index:

$$\frac{\text{No. true negative}}{\text{No. true negative} + \text{No. false negative}} \times 100$$

If one does not accept the presence of mediastinal nodes as a contraindication to operation, the procedure loses much of its appeal. Reports by Kirsh (1971), Martini (1980), and Naruke (1988) and their colleagues documented reasonable survivorship of patients with N2 disease discovered at operation. This apparently is a different set of patients than those in whom the nodes are discovered at cervical mediastinoscopy. Patterson and associates (1987) reported 34 patients who had disease in the subaortic lymph nodes — station 5 — but no metastatic disease in other mediastinal stations. The 3- and 5-year survival of the entire group was 44% and 28%, respectively. It was pointed out by Shields (1990) that, in general, a 5-year survival rate of approximately 2% can be expected in patients in whom N2 disease is clinically recognizable or is identified by standard radiographic study or is discovered at mediastinoscopy. In those patients in whom N2 disease is recognized only at thoracotomy, the 5-year survival rates are better. Nevertheless, surgical resection can be expected to salvage only 3 to 6% of patients with N2 disease. Like others, we subject patients to thoracotomy if they are good risks for operation, have N2 nodes low in the paratracheal region and no evidence of extra nodal growth at mediastinoscopy, or have isolated, mobile subaortic — station 5 — metastases.

Lesions of the left upper lobe merit special considerations. Classical anatomic studies suggest that cervical mediastinoscopy would not be productive for these lesions. Nevertheless, clinical studies reported by Maassen (1985) note that 29% of lesions of the left upper lobe were positive at cervical mediastinoscopy. It is for this reason that we use standard cervical mediastinoscopy as the initial procedure for all patients. If a lesion is in the left upper lobe and cervical mediastinoscopy is negative, one may choose to follow, while the patient is still anesthetized, with anterior mediastinoscopy or the extended mediastinoscopic procedure of Ginsberg and colleagues (1987), particularly if the CT scan suggests involvement of station 5 or station 6 — anterior mediastinal — nodes.

Increasingly, however, we terminate this procedure and schedule the patient for video-assisted thoracoscopic surgery — VATS. At that time, the subaortic and anterior mediastinal nodal areas are explored and a decision is made to deem the patient unresectable or to proceed with resection through a standard thoracotomy or with VATS.

An often contentious problem is the proper treatment of a patient with known small-cell carcinoma on the basis of results of a needle biopsy. Although most of these patients do have widespread mediastinal involvement, it is important to document metastases by needle biopsy or by mediastinoscopy. In the rare patient with small cell carcinoma without nodal involvement — N0, the 5-year survivorship is over 50%, as reported by Shah and colleagues (1992). Similar results have been reported by Karrer and Shields (personal communication, 1992).

Finally, in lesions of the anterior compartment of the mediastinum, cervical mediastinoscopy is not appropriate with the standard technique of the procedure.

Technique

The CT scans are carefully reviewed before the operation. The operating table is adjusted to decrease obvious venous distention but not enough to increase the possibility of air embolism. The patient's neck should be slightly extended; hyperextension decreases the space between the sternum and the trachea and increases the possibilities of compression of the innominate artery. The 4-cm transverse incision is centered over the trachea and made approximately 1 cm above the sternal ends of the clavicles and deepened through the platysma muscle (Fig. 17–2). The strap muscles are divided vertically in the midline, vigorous lateral traction is applied, the thyroid isthmus is retracted superiorly if in the field, and the pretracheal fascia is incised. With index finger dissection, a tunnel is created within the pretracheal fascia immediately anterior and lateral to the trachea. Approaching the lower portion of this dissection, the envelope of pretracheal fascia is opened by blunt dissection.

The index finger is withdrawn and the mediastinoscope is inserted within the tunnel created. Closed biopsy forceps or a metal suction device are used to improve exposure of the lymph nodes previously identified by palpation. If none have been identified, the nodes in the paratracheal regions, the tracheobronchial angles, and the anterior subcarinal stations are sought. As shown in Figure 17–3, the nodes of station 5 and 6 — subaortic and para-aortic — are not accessible by standard cervical mediastinoscopy. Occasionally, aspiration biopsy may be helpful. Hemostasis is obtained primarily by coagulation and packing, although application of a clip occasionally is necessary. If significant bleeding occurs, the mediastinoscope is left in place and the area is packed with gauze. After an appropriate interval of at least 10 minutes, the packing is gently removed. If the bleeding is still significant, the packing is reapplied and preparation is made for thoracotomy. If hemostasis is satisfactory, the wound is

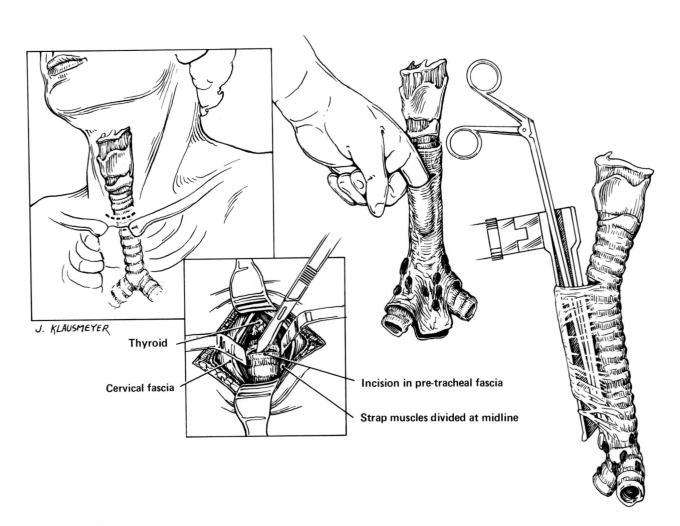

J. KLAUSMEYER

Thyroid

Cervical fascia

Incision in pre-tracheal fascia

Strap muscles divided at midline

Fig. 17–2. Mediastinoscopy.

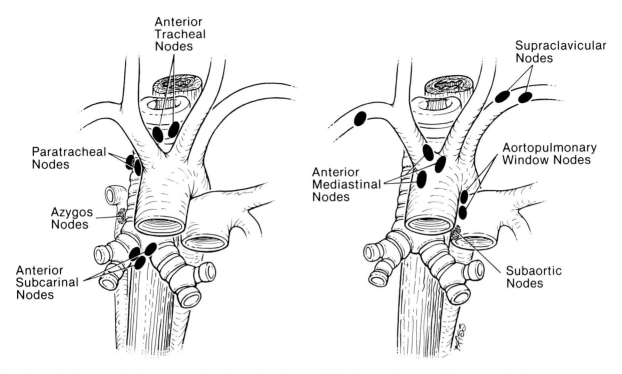

Fig. 17–3. Nodes accessible during surgical mediastinal exploration. Nodes that can be reached by the standard cervical mediastinoscopy are depicted on the left. Anterior mediastinal nodes and aortopulmonary window nodes depicted on the right require an extended mediastinoscopy, anterior mediastinotomy, video assisted thoracic surgery — VATS — or needle biopsy. *From* Shields TW: General Thoracic Surgery. 3rd Ed. Philadelphia: Lea & Febiger, 1989.

closed in layers with care to reapproximate the platysma.

Complications

The incidence of serious bleeding, as reported by Specht (1971), is between 0.1 and 0.2%; the complications of vocal cord paralysis and pneumothorax occur slightly more frequently. Very infrequent complications include damage to the esophagus, thoracic duct, bronchus and trachea. Cardiac arrhythmias may occur. Wound seeding by tumor has been an extremely rare complication.

MODIFIED MEDIASTINOSCOPY

Occasionally, standard cervical mediastinoscopy does not provide appropriate access. This situation may occur in patients with lesions of the left upper lobe in whom standard cervical mediastinoscopy is negative and in patients with lesions of the prevascular — anterior — space that is directly underneath the sternum. Ginsberg and colleagues (1987) devised a method for access to the anterior mediastinal — station 6 — and aortopulmonary — station 5 — nodes that are not accessible by standard cervical mediastinoscopy. This approach is through a tunnel created between the innominate artery and the left carotid artery (Fig. 17–4). Kirschner (1971) described a technique to provide access to this anterior space through the standard cervical

mediastinoscopy incision in which the scope is passed into the mediastinum anterior to the great vessels (Fig. 17–5). A subxiphoid approach to the anterior mediastinum was described by Arom and associates (1977). Also, Deslauriers and co-workers (1976) described a method for biopsy of the lung after digital opening of the mediastinal pleura (Fig. 17–6).

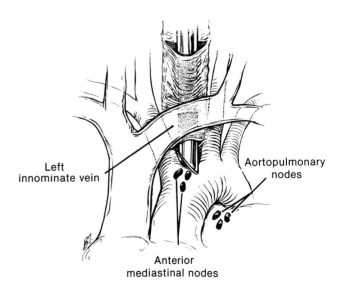

Fig. 17–4. Extended mediastinoscopy.

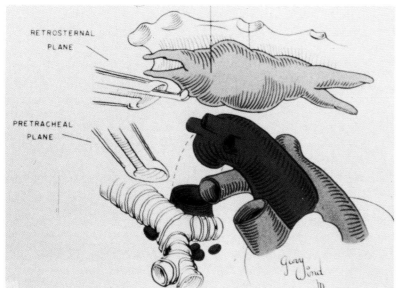

Fig. 17–5. Superior portion of the mediastinum shows the separate access with the mediastinoscope into the anterior (prevascular) and visceral (retrovascular) compartments. Note the change in angle of the mediastinoscope. *From* Shields TW: Mediastinal Surgery. Philadelphia: Lea & Febiger, 1991.

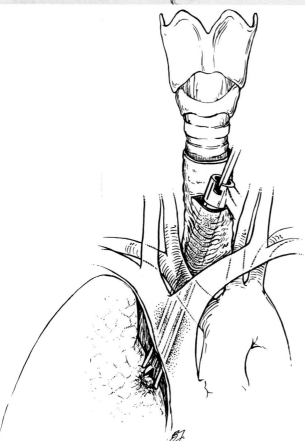

Fig. 17–6. Combined mediastinoscopy and right lung biopsy. *From* Baue AE: Glenn's Thoracic and Cardiovascular Surgery. 5th Ed. Norwalk CT: Appleton and Lange, 1991.

ANTERIOR MEDIASTINOTOMY AND ANTERIOR MEDIASTINOSCOPY

As previously noted, standard cervical mediastinoscopy does not provide access to the anterior mediastinal nodes — station 6 — or to the aortopulmonary window nodes — station 5. Many authors, therefore, advocate anterior mediastinotomy as their primary choice for left upper lobe lesions. For reasons noted previously, we prefer cervical mediastinoscopy for all lesions as the primary procedure because it is a simpler procedure, is probably safer, and does not interfere with early radiation therapy. In the past, if the results were inconclusive from cervical mediastinoscopy for lesions of the left upper lobe, an anterior mediastinotomy was performed. As noted previously, the recent development of VATS would currently make this the choice for this situation rather than anterior mediastinotomy or the extended mediastinoscopy procedure of Ginsberg.

Technique

McNeill and Chamberlain (1966) described what has become a popular approach for this operation. The second or third costal cartilage is excised subperichondrially and the posterior perichondrium is incised. The first and second intercostal bundles are divided. Alternately, an incision may be made through the second interspace without removing cartilage (Fig. 17–7). The internal mammary artery and vein are ligated individually. The pleura is mobilized laterally and the anterior mediastinal and aortopulmonary nodes are evaluated, as is the pulmonary hilum. A headlight is helpful and a mediastinoscope is often useful. Fine needle aspiration occasionally makes this operation easier and safer. Appropriate samples are obtained and frozen section is often used. If the pleural cavity is entered for lung biopsy or evaluation of the hilum, or inadvertently, it is drained with an intercostal tube brought through a separate incision and attached to underwater seal suction.

Firmly matted nodes in the aortopulmonary window — station 5 — or spread to the anterior mediastinal nodes — station 6 — preclude thoracotomy. Nodes restricted to the aortopulmonary window that are easily resectable as judged by palpation would not preclude thoracotomy as noted previously.

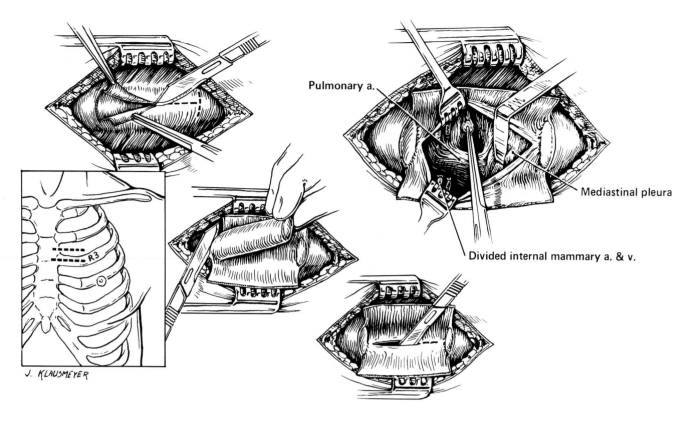

Pulmonary a.

Mediastinal pleura

Divided internal mammary a. & v.

J. KLAUSMEYER

Fig. 17–7. Mediastinotomy.

THORACENTESIS

An undiagnosed pleural effusion is the primary indication for diagnostic thoracentesis. In these circumstances, it is usually necessary to withdraw only a maximum of 100 ml of fluid. This amount provides enough sample for diagnostic studies, and withdrawal of larger amounts may be associated with higher rates of complications, as noted in a report by the Health and Public Policy Committee of the American College of Physicians (1985). Therapeutic thoracentesis for relief of symptoms requires removal of larger amounts of fluid, but Sokolowski and co-workers (1989) noted that removal of more than 1.5 liters may be associated with increased risk. If the cause of the effusion is likely to be congestive failure, it is appropriate to treat the suspected underlying cardiac disease and note the results before proceeding to thoracentesis. When performing therapeutic thoracentesis, the patient's condition should be carefully monitored, terminating the procedure if the patient complains of discomfort in the chest.

The site of aspiration is determined by radiologic localization and physical findings. Frequently, the best place is 2 inches below the superior aspect of dullness. Aspiration of small or localized effusions is aided by sonography, as reported by Harnsberger (1983) and Grogan (1990) and their colleagues. In particularly complex cases, the more expensive and time-consuming CT guidance may be helpful.

Technique

After appropriate local anesthesia is obtained, the needle is introduced close to the superior border of the rib to avoid the intercostal vessels and nerves. The needle should be placed just inside the parietal pleura, unless a catheter system is used, in which case it is threaded into the pleural cavity. This technique has many advantages, as reported by Krausz and Manny (1976). It is essential to use a needle or tube that is at least a size 18 and to ensure that air does not enter the pleural space.

A primary concern is whether one is dealing with an exudate or a transudate (see Chapter 54). Ordinarily, a specific gravity below 1.015 indicates a transudate. According to Sokolowski and associates (1989), further indication of an exudate may be noted by determining the ratio of pleural fluid protein to serum protein to be greater than 0.5, the pleural fluid LDH to serum LDH ratio to be greater than 0.6, and the pleural fluid LDH greater than two thirds of the upper limits of normal for serum LDH. Low sugar levels are suggestive of rheumatoid disease or tuberculosis. Cytologic evaluation in suspected neoplastic effusions and culture for suspected bacterial infections are clearly indicated.

PERCUTANEOUS LUNG BIOPSY

Percutaneous needle biopsy is not a new procedure, having first been described in 1851 by Leibert, with

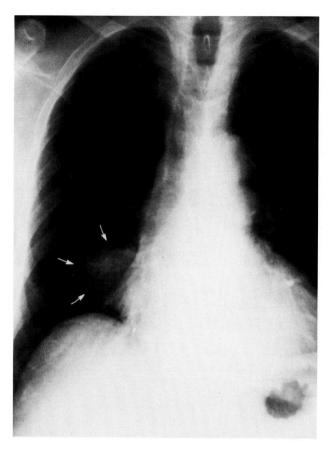

Fig. 17–8. Chest radiograph demonstrates a 5-cm mass (white arrows) in the right middle lobe.

the first percutaneous lung biopsy reported by Leyden in 1883. In the 1940s and 1950s, considerable experience in percutaneous biopsy using fine needles was gained in Europe, but only in the last two decades has this procedure gained favor in the United States.

Contributing to the growing acceptance of percutaneous fine needle aspiration biopsy — FNAB — is the accuracy of radiologic imaging techniques facilitating precise needle placement by interventional radiologists. At the same time, increased experience with cytologic interpretation complemented by the use of special stains, electron microscopy, and immunohistochemistry, assures accurate diagnoses from small tissue samples.

Fine needle aspiration biopsy of lung is performed most frequently using small diameter needles of 18 to 23 gauge. Specially designed biopsy needles with cutting edges and thin walls to increase the luminal diameter provide small cores of tissue on which cytologic and histologic diagnoses can be made. Other advances in needle design include inner stylets isolating the specimen in the lumen of the needle, slotted and toothed cutting edges to increase sample size, and automated needles designed to diminish operator dependence. Coaxial systems consisting of a 19-gauge outer needle, that is placed up to the lesion and through which 21-gauge cutting needles are passed into the lesion provide multiple biopsy samples through a single pleural

puncture. Biopsy of mediastinal, pleural, chest wall, and parenchymal masses that can be accomplished without traversing aerated lung may be performed safely with larger needle sizes ranging from 14 to 17 gauge with resultant increase in specimen size.

Planning the biopsy route to minimize the number of pleural surfaces crossed, minimize the length of the biopsy path, and avoid major vascular structures is accomplished by review of the PA and lateral chest radiographs and enhanced by a preprocedural CT scan. For parenchymal, pleural, and mediastinal lesions easily identified on standard chest radiographs, fluoroscopy provides the best biopsy guidance, particularly if biplane fluoroscopy is available. Fluoroscopic guidance is economical, minimizes the requirement for patient cooperation, and minimizes procedure time. CT guidance is used with increasing frequency because of its precise display of both needle depth and relationship to structures surrounding the lesion (Figs. 17–8, 17–9). As reported by van Sonnenberg and associates (1988), it is particularly helpful for mediastinal biopsy (Figs. 17–10, 17–11) and biopsy of nodules not readily apparent at fluoroscopy. In addition to being more costly than fluoroscopy, CT scanning increases the time required for performance of the procedure, and, in the experience of van Sonnenberg and associates (1988), results in a higher incidence of pneumothorax. Sonography may be used to guide biopsies of pleural, mediastinal, and pulmonary parenchymal masses that extend to the chest wall, as described by Yuan and colleagues (1992). Equally important in preprocedural planning is consultation between the cytopathologist and radiologist to ensure adequate handling of biopsy specimens. Review of the clinical history and differential diagnosis with the cytopathologist is particularly important with respect to the need for special stains, electron microscopy, or

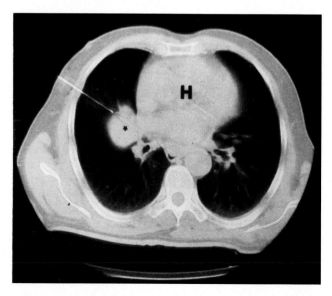

Fig. 17–9. CT-directed biopsy precisely demonstrates the needle location with respect to the mass (*) and heart (H). This biopsy could just as well have been performed using fluoroscopy. The biopsy revealed squamous carcinoma of lung.

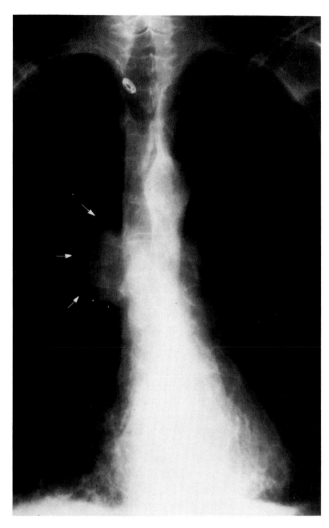

Fig. 17–10. Chest radiograph demonstrates a 6-cm mass overlying the right hilum (white arrows).

immunohistochemistry. Immediate specimen staining and slide review for tissue adequacy eliminate additional biopsy passes when sufficient material is present on the initial pass.

Indications and Contraindications

The indications for FNAB of lung include diagnosis of metastatic disease to lung in patients with known primary tumors, diagnosis of multiple pulmonary nodules, and diagnosis of solitary pulmonary nodules in patients who are either not surgical candidates or who refuse a thoracotomy without a preoperative diagnosis. As described by Weisbrod and associates (1984), pulmonary nodules and mediastinal disease can be diagnosed and staged by mediastinal FNAB. Biopsy of solitary pulmonary nodules in patients who are surgical candidates may provide a diagnosis of benign disease, identify lesions such as small cell carcinoma or lymphoma that are more appropriately treated by nonsurgical means, or provide a preoperative diagnosis of malignancy, eliminating the need for intraoperative biopsy before resection. In the experience of Yang and colleagues (1992), performed with sonographic guidance and complemented when necessary by large needle biopsy, FNAB is an accurate method of diagnosing infectious processes when bronchoscopic methods fail. Lesions suspected of being endobronchial or involving the air spaces are preferably diagnosed by transbronchial biopsy or bronchial washing.

Contraindications to FNAB are primarily uncorrectable coagulopathy or inability of the patient to cooperate during the biopsy procedure. Although emphysema increases the risk of pneumothorax, this condition does not diminish the usefulness of FNAB when the information rendered will affect patient management and less invasive diagnostic procedures have failed.

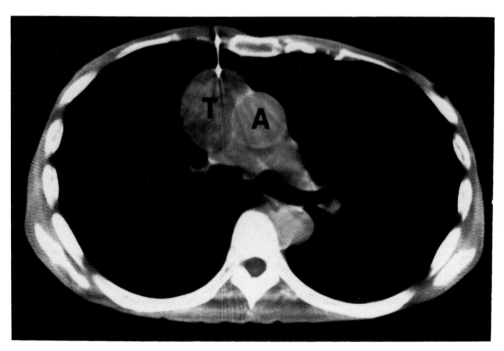

Fig. 17–11. CT-directed biopsy demonstrates this mass (T) to reside in the anterior and middle mediastinum. CT clearly demonstrates the location of the biopsy needle with respect to the mass (T) and the thoracic aorta (A). Diagnosis determined from the biopsy of this mass was thymoma.

Complications

The most common significant complication of FNAB is pneumothorax, which occurs in 8 to 61% of patients, and requires chest tube placement in as many as 20%. In the large experience of Weisbrod and co-workers (1984), pneumothorax occurred in 32% of 2421 FNAB, with chest tube placement required in 8%. This complication increases with needle size, the number of needle passes through the pleura, the use of CT guidance, and the presence of emphysema. Bleeding following FNAB occurs in 5% of patients, and in the absence of a bleeding diathesis is usually not clinically significant. Air embolism has been reported as a rare complication, as has tumor seeding of the biopsy tract. Tumor seeding occurs in less than 0.1% of FNAB; it was seen in 2 of 4000 biopsies reported by Nordenstrom and Bjork (1973) and none of almost 1500 biopsies reported by Lalli and associates (1978). Furthermore Sinner and Zajec (1976) saw no diminution in survival in patients undergoing FNAB.

Results

Fine needle aspiration biopsy is an accurate method of diagnosing bronchial carcinoma with a sensitivity of 77 to 95%, in the experience of Westcott (1981) and Lalli and associates (1978), and a specificity approaching 100%.† Sensitivity varies significantly with the skill and experience of the operator and diminishes for small and deep lesions. Characterization of cell type is less accurate than the diagnosis of malignancy. Differentiation of small cell from non-small cell carcinoma, however, is reliable and, as reported by Koss and colleagues (1984), carries a specificity of 95%. Failure to diagnose malignancy on FNAB does not exclude its presence. Sampling error, necrotic specimens, and needle misdirection account for the 5 to 25% of false-negative diagnoses of malignancy with FNAB. To exclude malignancy on FNAB reliably, a specific alternative diagnosis of benign disease, such as granuloma or hamartoma, must be rendered.

Although the sensitivity of FNAB for diagnosis of bronchial carcinoma or metastatic disease to lung is high, this is not the case for non-Hodgkin's lymphoma and Hodgkin's disease. The sensitivity for diagnosis of non-Hodgkin's lymphoma is approximately 50%, with difficulty encountered in diagnosing well-differentiated lymphomas. Fine needle aspiration biopsy is even less sensitive for the diagnosis of Hodgkin's disease. In addition, tissue typing in lymphoma and Hodgkin's disease is often inaccurate because of the small size of the biopsy specimen. In general, FNAB is best reserved for diagnosing recurrence of lymphoma or Hodgkin's disease or advancing the stage of lymphoma or Hodgkin's disease that has already been diagnosed.†

Fine needle aspiration biopsy is an excellent way to diagnose metastatic disease to mediastinal structures. As already noted, it is less accurate in diagnosing lymphoma and Hodgkin's disease involving mediastinal structures. Results of mediastinal biopsy have shown some variability. Westcott (1981) diagnosed primary or metastatic carcinoma in 94% of 72 patients with mediastinal involvement. He correctly diagnosed three thymomas, but failed to diagnose the two cases of Hodgkin's disease and only diagnosed five of nine cases of lymphoma. Herman and associates (1991) reported 143 mediastinal biopsies and correctly diagnosed 70% of metastases to the mediastinum, 91% of germ cell tumors, and 71% of thymomas, but only 42% of lymphoma and 20% of Hodgkin's disease.

With proper patient selection, FNAB is a relatively safe and highly accurate method of diagnosing benign and malignant processes involving the chest wall, pleura, lung, and mediastinum. Because the results of this procedure depend on the skills of the radiologist and cytopathologist, results may vary significantly between institutions.

LUNG BIOPSY

Transbronchoscopic biopsy with either a needle or forceps, combined with bronchoalveolar lavage and bronchial brushings, and prophylaxis or empiric treatment for *Pneumocystis carinii* have dramatically decreased the need for urgent open lung biopsy at most institutions. The newly developed VATS techniques have further decreased the need for conventional open lung biopsy. Nevertheless, open lung biopsy provides a direct way to obtain large amounts of tissue that may be needed by the pathologist, particularly in assessing chronic diffuse infiltrates as described by Carrington and Gaensler (1978). Tissue adequate for a large number of histologic, microbiologic, and special studies is readily available. In addition, the surgeon may palpate or directly inspect larger areas of the lung to obtain representative samples.

The only contradiction to open lung biopsy is the rare patient with bleeding diatheses that cannot be corrected by component therapy.

Technique

For most patients, general anesthesia with endotracheal intubation is used. The anterior intercostal incision as originally described by Klassen and associates (1949) provides adequate exposure for diffuse disease. Transaxillary thoracotomy or vertical axillary thoracotomy as described by Massimiano and associates (1988) and Baeza and Foster (1976), respectively, may provide better exposure with minimal postoperative discomfort depending on the disease process as determined by radiographic examination. The portion of the lung to be sampled is brought into the wound and excised with a stapler. Both involved and uninvolved portions of the lung should be sampled, because advanced changes in the obviously diseased portion of the lung may make them less useful diagnostically. The pleural cavity is drained with an

---

*Editor's Note: Despite the high sensitivity and specificity of FNAB in lung cancer patients, it is overused and more often than not has little effect on the management of the patient.

†Editor's Note: The use of a punch biopsy as described in Chapter 133 is successful in obtaining tissue in most patients with mediastinal lymphoma.

intercostal tube inserted through a separate stab wound and attached to underwater seal drainage. Although in most patients the wound may be closed without drainage after expansion of the lung, we believe it is safer to provide underwater seal drainage at least overnight.

Close consultation with the pathologist is needed prior to the operation. Frozen section examination is usually helpful. A small amount of tissue should be sent for gram, fungal, and acid-fast stains and cultures are sent for aerobic and anerobic bacteria, fungi, and acid-fast bacilli. Touch prints should be prepared if *Pneumocystis carinii* is suspected and, on occasion, testing for legionella immunofluorescence is required. Special handling is required if electron microscopy, heavy metal analysis, or mineral analysis are needed. Again, full preoperative consultation with the pathologist is necessary.

NEEDLE BIOPSY OF THE PLEURA

Pleural biopsy is indicated when pleural fluid analysis fails to provide the diagnosis in patients suspected of having a tuberculous or malignant effusion. Even without the presence of effusion, pleural biopsy may be helpful. In a report of 750 consecutive biopsies, Cowie and colleagues (1983) obtained adequate specimens in 79% of patients with pleural disease without pleural effusion. If empyema is suspected, pleural biopsy is contraindicated because of the risk of infection along the needle track. Also, pleural biopsy is not indicated if the effusion is thought to be associated with such diseases as pancreatitis, collagen vascular disease, or pulmonary emboli. As reported by Prakash and Reiman (1985) and Salyer and colleagues (1975), pleural biopsy may show evidence of malignant disease even when the pleural fluid cytology is not diagnostic. Similarly, the diagnosis of tuberculosis may be rendered from cultured biopsy material and from demonstration of caseating granulomas in 60 to 80% of cases of pleural tuberculosis, as documented by Feinsilver and associates (1986) and VonHoff and LiVolsi (1975). As reported by Feinsilver and colleagues (1986), a second biopsy sometimes establishes a diagnosis if the first biopsy is negative.

In general, a backward biting needle such as that designed by Cope or Abrams is preferable. If the mass is large and without fluid, a forward biting needle such as the Vim-Silverman may be used and has the advantage of providing a greater amount of tissue.

Technique

Adequate preoperative medication should be administered. Atropine is probably helpful to prevent the occasional vagal response to the procedure. After an appropriate amount of local anesthesia is given, the skin is punctured with a No. 11 blade and the needle is then inserted into the pleural space just above the selected rib. Usually, a definite popping sensation is noted. Care should be taken to prevent accidental penetration of the needle beyond the pleural space. The hook is impinged on the pleura, the cutting unit is then advanced over the hook, and the entire unit is withdrawn. The

intercostal vessels and nerves in the superior aspect of the interspace are to be avoided.

Complications

Complications are infrequent and are the expected ones of occasional hemorrhage and pneumothorax.

THORACOSCOPY

The subject of thoracoscopy is covered in Chapter 37. Open tube thoracoscopy or video-assisted thoracic surgery — VATS — are used occasionally as a primary procedure in the diagnosis of pleural disease but usually are restricted to those patients in whom thoracentesis and needle biopsy are not diagnostic.

PERICARDIAL BIOPSY

Most symptomatic cases of chronic pericardial effusions are well treated by cardiologists with pericardiocentesis directed by two-dimensional echocardiography as described by Callahan and colleagues (1985). As reported by Jansen and colleagues (1986), 87% of these patients are managed successfully with catheter decompression. Occasionally, however, surgical biopsy and drainage are required. Under these circumstances, a decision must be made whether to perform the operation using the simpler subxiphoid approach as advocated by Naunheim and colleagues (1991) or through the left anterior lateral approach, which does require general anesthesia but probably gives better long-term results, as reported by Piehler and colleagues (1985).

Technique

The subxiphoid approach is made using either local or general anesthesia. The vertical, upper abdominal midline incision extends over the xiphoid. The linea alba is divided and the xiphoid is retracted superiorly. The pericardium is identified after dissection of the diaphragm from the inner surface of the sternum. Fluid is aspirated and sent for cytologic and bacteriologic study. A window is made by excision of the pericardium as widely as can be done conveniently. The pericardial tissue is also sent for bacteriologic and histologic study. The pericardial space is drained with a soft tube connected to underwater seal.

The transthoracic approach involves an anterior lateral left thoracotomy through the fifth or sixth interspace. The pericardial window is excised anterior to the phrenic nerves. Again, the fluid and pericardium are sent for appropriate culture and histologic and cytologic study. The left pleural space is drained by two tubes brought out through separate stab wounds and attached to underwater seal.

Video-assisted thoracic surgery — VATS — may be used to perform a biopsy of the pericardium and to create a window as described by Lewis and colleagues (1992). The long-term results of this method are as yet unknown but appear promising.

Results

Most patients respond well to this procedure, although as reported by Piehler and co-workers (1985), about 10% have recurrence of symptoms from recurrent effusion or constriction. Most recurrences are noted in patients in whom the subxiphoid approach was used. In those patients, a more extensive pericardial resection should be done.

REFERENCES

Arom KV, et al: Subxiphoid anterior mediastinal exploration. Ann Thorac Surg 24:289, 1977.

Ashraf MH, Milsom PL, Walesby RK: Selection by mediastinoscopy and long-term survival in bronchial carcinoma. Ann Thorac Surg 30:208, 1980.

Baeza OR, Foster ED: Vertical axillary thoracotomy: A functional and cosmetically appealing incision. Ann Thorac Surg 22:287, 1976.

Bernstein MP, Ferrara JJ, Brown L: Effectiveness of scalene node biopsy for staging of lung cancer in the absence of palpable adenopathy. J Surg Oncol 29:46, 1985.

Brantigan JW, Brantigan CO, Brantigan OC: Biopsy of nonpalpable scalene lymph nodes in carcinoma of the lung. Am Rev Respir Dis 107:962, 1973.

Brion JP, et al: Role of computed tomography and mediastinoscopy in preoperative staging of lung carcinoma. J Comput Assist Tomogr 9:480, 1985.

Callahan JA, Seward JB, Tajik AJ: Cardiac tamponade: Pericardiocentesis directed by two-dimensional echocardiography. Mayo Clin Proc 60:344, 1985.

Carlens E: Mediastinoscopy: A method for inspection and tissue biopsy in the superior mediastinum. Dis Chest 36:343, 1959.

Carrington CB, Gaensler ED: Clinical-pathologic approach to diffuse infiltrative lung disease. In Thurlbeck WM, Abell MR (eds): The Lung. Structure, Function and Disease. Baltimore: Williams & Wilkins, 1978.

Cowie RL, et al: Pleural biopsy. A report of 750 biopsies performed using Abram's pleural biopsy punch. S Afr Med J 64:92, 1983.

Daly BDT Jr, et al: Mediastinal lymph node evaluation by computed tomography in lung cancer. An analysis of 345 patients grouped by TNM staging, tumor size, and tumor location. J Thorac Cardiovasc Surg 94:664, 1987.

Daniels AC: A method of biopsy useful in diagnosing certain intrathoracic diseases. Dis Chest 16:360, 1949.

Deslauriers J, et al: Mediastinopleuroscopy: A new approach to the diagnosis of intrathoracic diseases. Ann Thorac Surg 22:265, 1976.

Feinsilver SH, Barrows AA, Braman SS: Fiberoptic bronchoscopy and pleural effusion of known origin. Chest 90:516, 1986.

Ginsberg RJ, et al: Extended cervical mediastinoscopy. A single staging procedure for bronchogenic carcinoma of the left upper lobe. J Thorac Cardiovasc Surg 94:673, 1987.

Greschuchna D, Maassen W: Results of mediastinoscopy and other biopsies in sarcoidosis and silicosis. In Jepsen O, Sorensen HR (eds): Mediastinoscopy. Denmark: Odense University Press, 1971, pp. 79-82.

Grogan DR, et al: Complications associated with thoracentesis: A prospective, randomized study comparing three different methods. Arch Intern Med 150:873, 1990.

Harken DE, et al: A simple cervicomediastinal exploration for tissue diagnosis of intrathoracic disease. N Engl J Med 251:1041, 1954.

Harnsberger HR, Lee TG, Mukuno DH: Rapid, inexpensive real-time directed thoracentesis. Radiology 146:545, 1983.

Health & Public Policy Committee, American College of Physicians: Diagnostic thoracentesis and pleural biopsy in pleural effusions. Ann Intern Med 103:799, 1985.

Herman SJ, et al: Anterior mediastinal masses: Utility of transthoracic needle biopsy. Radiology 180:167, 1991.

Izbicki JR, et al: Accuracy of computed tomographic scan and surgical assessment for staging of bronchial carcinoma. A prospective study. J Thorac Cardiovasc Surg 104:413, 1992.

Jansen EW, et al: Treatment of pericardial effusion. J Thorac Cardiovasc Surg 90:795, 1986.

Kirschner PA: Mediastinoscopy in superior vena cava obstruction. In Jepsen O, Sorensen HR (eds): Mediastinoscopy. Denmark: Odense University Press, 1971, pp. 40-42.

Kirschner PA: "Extended" Mediastinoscopy. In Jepsen O, Sorensen HR (eds): Mediastinoscopy. Denmark: Odense University Press, 1971, p. 131.

Kirsh MM, et al: Treatment of bronchogenic carcinoma with mediastinal metastases. Ann Thorac Surg 12:11, 1971.

Klassen KP, Anlyan AJ, Curtis GM: Biopsy of diffuse pulmonary lesions. Arch Surg 59:694, 1949.

Koss LG, Woyke S, Olszewski W: Aspiration Biopsy: Cytologic Interpretation and Histologic Bases. New York: Igaku-Shoin, 1984.

Krausz M, Manny J: A safe method of thoracentesis. J Thorac Cardiovasc Surg 72:323, 1976.

Lalli AF, et al: Aspiration biopsy of chest lesions. Radiology 239:36, 1978.

Leckie WJ, McCormack RJM, Walbaum PR: The case against routine scalene node biopsy in bronchial carcinoma. Lancet 1:853, 1963.

Leibert H: Traite Practique des Maladies Cancereuse et des Affections Curable Contoundues avec le Cancer. Paris: JB Bailiere, 1851.

Lewis RJ, Sisler GE, Mackenzie JW: Mediastinoscopy in advanced superior vena cava obstruction. Ann Thorac Surg 32:458, 1981.

Lewis RJ, et al: One hundred consecutive patients undergoing video-assisted thoracic operations. Ann Thorac Surg 54:421, 1992.

Leyden H: Uber infectiose pneumonie. Dtsch Med Wochenschr 9:52, 1883.

Luke WP, et al: Prospective evaluation of mediastinoscopy for assessment of carcinoma of the lung. J Thorac Cardiovasc Surg 91:53, 1986.

Maassen W: The staging issue — problems: Accuracy of mediastinoscopy. In Delarue NC, Eschapasse H (eds): International Trends in General Thoracic Surgery. Lung Cancer, Vol. 1. Philadelphia: WB Saunders, 1985, pp. 42-53.

Martini N, et al: Prospective study of 445 lung carcinomas with mediastinal lymph node metastases. J Thorac Cardiovasc Surg 80:390, 1980.

Massimiano P, Ponn RB, Toole AL: Transaxillary thoracotomy revisited. Ann Thorac Surg 45:559, 1988.

McNeill TM, Chamberlain JM: Diagnostic anterior mediastinotomy. Ann Thorac Surg 2:532, 1966.

Meersschaut D, et al: Repeat mediastinoscopy in the assessment of new and recurrent lung neoplasm. Ann Thorac Surg 53:120, 1992.

Naruke T, et al: The importance of surgery to non-small cell carcinoma of lung with mediastinal lymph node metastasis. Ann Thorac Surg 46:603, 1988.

Naunheim KS, et al: Pericardial drainage: Subxiphoid vs. transthoracic approach. Eur J Cardiothorac Surg 5:99, 1991.

Nordenstrom B, Bjork VO: Dissemination of cancer cells by needle biopsy of the lung. J Thorac Cardiovasc Surg 65:671, 1973.

Patterson GA, et al: Significance of metastatic disease in subaortic lymph nodes. Ann Thorac Surg 43:155, 1987.

Pearson FG: An evaluation of mediastinoscopy in the management of presumably operable bronchial carcinoma. J Thorac Cardiovasc Surg 55:617, 1968.

Pearson FG: Use of mediastinoscopy in selection of patients for lung cancer operations. Ann Thorac Surg 30:205, 1980.

Pearson FG: Lung cancer. The past twenty five years. Chest 89:200S, 1986.

Pearson FG, et al: Significance of positive superior mediastinal nodes identified at mediastinoscopy in patients with resectable cancer of the lung. J Thorac Cardiovasc Surg 83:1, 1982.

Perez-Mesa C, Spratt JS Jr: Scalene node biopsy in the pretreatment of staging of carcinoma of the cervix uteri. Am J Obstet Gyncol 125:93, 1976.

Phillips MS, Barker V: Extrathoracic lymph node aspiration in bronchial carcinoma. Thorax 40:398, 1985.

Piehler JM, et al: Surgical management of effusive pericardial disease. Influence of extent of pericardial resection on clinical course. J Thorac Cardiovasc Surg 90:506, 1985.

Prakash UBS, Reiman HM: Comparison of needle biopsy with cytologic analysis for the evaluation of pleural effusion: Analysis of 414 cases. Mayo Clin Proc *60*:158, 1985.

Rohwedder JJ, Handley JA, Kerr D: Rapid diagnosis of lung cancer from palpable metastases by needle thrust. Chest *98*:1393, 1990.

Salyer WR, Eggleston JC, Erozan YS: Efficacy of pleural needle biopsy and pleural fluid cytopathology in the diagnosis of malignant neoplasm involving the pleura. Chest *67*:536, 1975.

Shah SS, Thompson J, Goldstraw P: Results of operation without adjuvant therapy in the treatment of small cell lung cancer. Ann Thorac Surg *54*:498, 1992.

Shields TW: The significance of ipsilateral mediastinal lymph node metastasis (N2 disease) in non-small cell carcinoma of the lung. J Thorac Cardiovasc Surg *99*:48, 1990.

Sinner WN, Zajec J: Implantation metastasis after percutaneous transthoracic needle aspiration biopsy. Acta Radiol *17*:473, 1976.

Sokolowski JW Jr, et al: Guidelines for thoracentesis and needle biopsy of the pleura. Am Rev Resp Dis *140*:257, 1989.

Specht G: Discussion by Carlens. *In* Jepsen O, Sorenson HR (eds): Mediastinoscopy. Denmark: Odense University Press, 1971, pp. 130.

Vallieres E, Page A, Verdant A: Ambulatory mediastinoscopy and anterior mediastinotomy. Ann Thorac Surg *52*:1122, 1991.

Van Sonnenberg E, et al: Difficult thoracic lesions: CT-guided biopsy experience in 150 cases. Radiology *167*:457, 1988.

Von Hoff DD, LiVolsi V: Diagnostic reliability of needle biopsy of the parietal pleura. A review of 272 biopsies. Am J Clin Pathol *64*:200, 1975.

Webb WR, et al: CT and MR imaging in staging non-small cell bronchogenic carcinoma: Report of the Radiologic Diagnostic Oncology Group. Radiology *178*:705, 1991.

Weisbrod G, et al: Percutaneous fine needle aspiration biopsy of mediastinal lesions. Am J Radiol *143*:525, 1984.

Westcott J: Percutaneous needle aspiration of hilar and mediastinal masses. Radiology *141*:323, 1981.

Yang P, et al: Ultrasound guided percutaneous cutting biopsy for the diagnosis of pulmonary consolidations of unknown aetiology. Thorax *47*:457, 1992.

Yuan A, et al: Ultrasound-guided aspiration biopsy of small peripheral pulmonary nodules. Chest *101*:926, 1992.

Assessment of the Thoracic Surgical Patient

CHAPTER 18

PULMONARY PHYSIOLOGIC ASSESSMENT OF OPERATIVE RISK

Gerald N. Olsen

Surgical procedures inherently carry risks as well as benefits. Identification and amelioration of the risks preoperatively will enhance postoperative outcome. In the arena of preoperative evaluation and its scientific literature, a definition is important. The definition is of the word *complication*. A complication tends to be an unplanned and unwanted second disease. This definition is important, because in the studies that purport to evaluate for, and treat, postoperative complications, investigators often report such items as mild hypoxemia, asymptomatic decrement in lung function, radiographic discoid atelectasis, or transient arrhythmia. If the "complication" does not lengthen recovery room, intensive care unit, or hospital stay, increase care costs, or increase mortality, calling the outcome a true complication may be excessive. Generally accepted postoperative complications are listed in Table 18–1. Postoperative bronchitis, which leads to lobar atelectasis, pneumonia, sepsis, respiratory failure, ventricular tachycardia, and death, constitutes a progression of abnormalities that would fit the criteria of complications by lengthening of stay, increasing hospital costs, and even causing mortality. Factors identifying those patients at increased risk are outlined in Table 18–2.

Table 18–1.   Postoperative Cardiopulmonary Complications

Atelectasis requiring specific therapy
Arrhythmias requiring therapy
Bronchitis
Death
Hypotension/shock
Myocardial infarction
Pneumonia
Pulmonary edema
Pulmonary embolism
Respiratory failure

Table 18–2.   Factors Increasing Postoperative Risk

ASA* class > 2
Advanced age?
Complicated cardiac valvular replacement
Coronary artery disease
Chronic obstructive pulmonary disease
Emergency procedure
Extensive lung resection
Immune compromise
Morbid obesity?
Prolonged operative duration
Smoking
Transplantation of major organs
Upper abdominal procedure

*American Society of Anesthesiologists classification of anesthetic risk.

Cardiopulmonary complications predominantly follow major operative procedures on the upper abdomen and thorax. This is not to say that procedures such as craniotomy, thyroidectomy, and hip replacement are free of these complications, but they tend to occur somewhat less frequently and are difficult to predict by preoperative assessment. Preoperative and postoperative anticoagulation in patients undergoing hip operations may obviate the problem of pulmonary thromboembolism. Likewise, close postoperative observation may detect post-thyroidectomy hemorrhage capable of producing tracheal and respiratory compromise.

UPPER ABDOMINAL SURGERY

Much elucidation about the upper abdomen has occurred since the rediscovery of the seminal work of Pasteur (1908). Pasteur postulated that postoperative pulmonary collapse was related to diaphragmatic dysfunction. The observations of Ford and co-workers

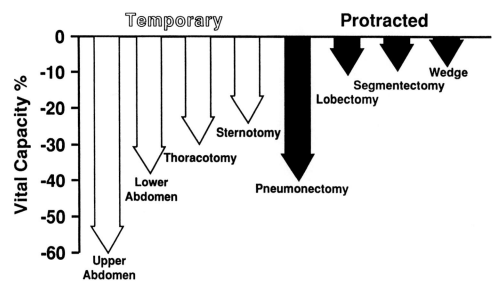

Fig. 18–1. Effect of thoracic surgical procedures on vital capacity.

(1983) tended to support this concept. The postoperative diaphragmatic dysfunction is primarily manifest in 50 to 60% reductions in vital capacity, which lasts from hours to 5 days (Fig. 18–1). The etiology of this dysfunction remains unclear, but some data suggest it is not related to pain or muscle fatigue and may be overcome by voluntary efforts of the patient. These findings have led to the hypothesis of a pathologic reflex. This phenomenon has also been seen in animals whose upper abdominal viscera have been operatively manipulated. The ability of the patient to overcome the reduced vital capacity with voluntary deep breaths has been demonstrated by Chuter and colleagues (1990). Voluntary deep breaths would appear to support the use of incentive spirometry, as first proposed by Bartlett and associates (1973). A large study by Hall and co-investigators (1991), however, showed no reduction in hospital stay or mortality associated with the routine use of postoperative incentive spirometry. Because this form of therapy is used in 95% of hospitals in the United States, it may now be as firmly entrenched as a type of postoperative therapy as was intermittent positive pressure breathing — IPPB — in the 1950s.

It appears from the meta-analyses of both Lawrence (1989) and Zibrak (1990) and their co-workers that preoperative pulmonary function testing with spirometry remains unproven as a reliable predictor of increased pulmonary risk after upper abdominal surgical intervention. These investigators, however, tend to support the use of these tests before lung resection. Perioperative respiratory management of the patient undergoing upper abdominal surgery will be a fruitful area of further investigation.

LUNG RESECTION

Thoracotomy was originally performed for drainage of empyema. The 1940s and early 1950s are viewed by some as the halcyon days of general thoracic surgery. During this time, procedures such as plombage thoracoplasty and segmentectomy were developed for the management of pulmonary tuberculosis. Although the development of isoniazid led to a reduction in surgical indications, resection is still a valuable option for management of some drug-resistant forms of tuberculosis, such as that caused by *Mycobacterium avium-intracellulare* complex. Much of the experience in dealing with the pulmonary function effects of surgery date to the benchmark study of Gaensler and associates in 1955. Current indications for thoracotomy include resection of lung cancer, diagnostic open lung biopsy, resection of bronchiectasis, management of thoracic trauma, and lung transplantation.

Approximately 10 years after the post-World War II rise in cigarette consumption came the current epidemic of bronchial carcinoma. Graham and Singer published the first complete report of a successful pneumonectomy for lung cancer in 1933. Subsequently, lobectomy became the procedure of choice and virtually the only hope for cure for those 25% of patients without obvious metastases. Complicating the surgical approach to lung cancer was the accompanying rise in cases of chronic obstructive pulmonary disease — COPD — following the rise in lung cancer by about 10 years (Fig. 18–2). Of those patients who present with bronchial carcinoma, approximately 90% have signs and symptoms of concomitant COPD. Approximately 20% of these patients have such severe pulmonary dysfunction as to compromise the safety of the resection. Complicating this fact is the knowledge that nonoperative therapy of lung cancer is rarely curative — less than 5%.

Lung resection may be curative in between 10 and 90% of patients with lung cancer. The wide difference in the ends of this spectral range is related to the presence or absence of local or distant metastases. The preoperative search for the metastases constitutes the

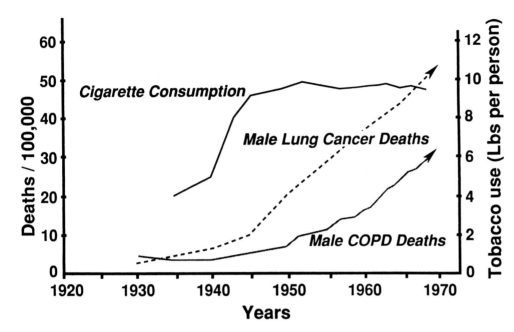

Fig. 18–2. Cigarette consumption, lung cancer, and COPD mortality. *Adapted from* Welch MH: In Guenter CA, Welch MH (eds): Pulmonary Medicine. Philadelphia: JB Lippincott, 1977.

process known as "staging." A complete discussion of this process is in Chapter 85. For the purposes of this discussion, the inability to remove, anatomically, all the tumor from the patient is called *unresectability*.

If the lung cancer is adequately staged and is presumed to be "resectable," can surgery proceed forthwith? When lung tissue is removed from a patient, several physiologic effects occur. First is the "thoracotomy effect." Even if no lung is resected, vital capacity declines approximately 25% in the early postoperative period, only normalizing after 4 to 6 weeks. Overall, the degree of pulmonary dysfunction is somewhat correlated with the volume of lung tissue removed (see Fig. 18–1). Of interest is the report of Lanier and the author (1991) showing a lesser reduction of static lung volumes — total lung capacity — by resection in patients with COPD. This blunted postoperative restriction was believed to be related to the pre-existing hyperinflation produced by COPD.

Lung tissue removal has two major consequences. The first is reduction of the pulmonary capillary bed. This reduction will have little consequence in the patient with normal lungs, even after pneumonectomy. If pulmonary dysfunction already exists, however, postoperative pulmonary hypertension may lead to cor pulmonale and death. This unfortunate outcome was a major concern early in the days of surgical treatment of tuberculosis. It seems to be a less frequent problem in lung cancer operations. The second undesirable effect of lung resection involves the removal or reduction of ventilatory capacity. In the patient with underlying COPD, this further reduction may precipitate acute and chronic respiratory failure and death. In this discussion, the inability of the patient to tolerate physiologically the loss of lung volume is called *inoperability*.

The mortality rate for pneumonectomy in the patient with normal lungs averages less than 5%. This figure climbs to as much as 25% in those with severe COPD. Producing a ventilator-dependent respiratory cripple who has had a curative resection of lung cancer is a disaster for the patient and a nightmare for the surgeon. Hence, the patient with resectable lung cancer, but who is potentially inoperable because of COPD, constitutes a frequent diagnostic and management conundrum.

PHYSIOLOGIC ASSESSMENT OF THE LUNG RESECTION CANDIDATE

Since the seminal study of Gaensler and co-workers (1955), it has been clear that a severe reduction of ventilatory function preoperatively could predict mortality postoperatively. In their study, if the maximum breathing capacity — now called maximum voluntary ventilation, MVV — was less than 50% and the FVC was less than 70% of predicted values for the patient's age, height, and sex, the mortality was 50% after pneumonectomy for tuberculosis.

In approaching these patients, a philosophic position is helpful. Each patient, no matter what the preoperative anatomic stage, should be considered a candidate for pneumonectomy. The reasoning for this position is obvious. If the patient is physiologically acceptable for pneumonectomy, then performance of a lesser resection will have an even less detrimental effect on lung function. Likewise, if, during the exploratory thoracotomy, a tumor crossing the major fissure or extending to the hilum is found and a pneumonectomy is needed, it is generally too late for an extensive physiologic evaluation. An important question, when dealing with a disease as deadly as lung cancer, is in whom is it too dangerous to attempt a curative resection?

Routine Pulmonary Function Studies

Pulmonary function studies are performed to assess airflow, lung volume, lung mechanics, and gas exchange. Most of these studies require good cooperation and are thus effort dependent. Because lung resection is primarily performed because of lung cancer, underlying severe COPD needs to be ruled out or quantified. In the distant past, these routine studies were used to "reject" patients for resection. This rejection based on routine studies is no longer tenable as knowledge about these problems has increased. These routine pulmonary function studies are now used primarily to approve a patient for resection or to indicate that further testing is advisable. Table 18–3 outlines those studies and criteria that indicate a need for further evaluation. A review of pulmonary function criteria was published by Gass and the author (1986). Many earlier studies espoused spirometric lung volume criteria, such as FEV_1 greater than 2 liters. It now appears that this is unwise. For example, an FEV_1 of 2 liters could be 50% of normal for a 6-foot-tall, 40-year-old man, but virtually normal for a 5-foot-tall, 70-year-old woman. Thus, it is preferable to think in terms of "percent of predicted" normal for the patient's age, height, and sex. Race may also be included, but normal prediction equations are based more frequently on populations of normal, nonsmoking white subjects. The MVV is an interesting test as it reflects airflow, lung mechanics, respiratory muscle strength, and endurance. It is, however, sensitive to suboptimal cooperation, pain, etc., and is thus facetiously called "the SED rate of pulmonary function studies." It is performed by having the patient breathe into and out of the spirometer as deep and fast as possible for 12 seconds. In some laboratories, this value is estimated or calculated by multiplying the FEV_1 value in liters by 40. A normal measured MVV does, however, tend to suggest good ventilatory function.

The diffusing capacity is a measure of the volume of a dilute sample of carbon monoxide that is taken up by the lungs, generally during a single breath held for 10 seconds. The test evaluates the integrity of the alveolar capillary membrane and the pulmonary capillary blood volume. The single breath-hold test is also sensitive to reduced lung volume. Thus, diffusing capacity of the lung for carbon monoxide — D_LCO — reveals a decreased surface area available for gas exchange. In a retrospective study of 237 patients Ferguson and colleagues (1988) found that the preop-

erative D_LCO was the best predictor of pulmonary complications.

The primary reason why these routine pulmonary function tests should *not* be used to reject a patient for resection is that these tests only reflect the function of both lungs working together at rest. For example, what if an adult man with lung cancer had an FEV_1 of 1.8 liters or MVV of 49% of predicted? Should he be rejected for pneumonectomy? Further testing might reveal that the lung containing the tumor was not functioning because of airway obstruction by the tumor. The patient has therefore already tolerated an "auto-pneumonectomy," and thus little further functional loss would accompany the therapeutic procedure.

Split Lung Function Studies

In the 1950s, a technique known as bronchospirometry was developed to assess unilateral lung function. In this procedure, a Carlens-type dual lumen endotracheal tube was passed to the tracheal carina. Each lumen was connected to a spirometer filled with 100% O_2. On breathing, the amount of O_2 uptake was a reflection of each lung's perfusion and the volume of air exchanged during a vital capacity or MVV maneuver was a reflection of each lung's ventilation. Neuhaus and Cherniack (1968) used this technique in 1968. They developed an equation to predict the function remaining after pneumonectomy.

Predicted postoperative function = (Total preoperative function) × (Percentage of function contributed by lung destined to remain)

Example: Postpneumonectomy FEV_1 = 2.0 L × (75% from the nontumor lung) = 1.50 L.

This simple equation achieved importance with the development and perfection of radiospirometry in the 1970s. In these less invasive studies of regional lung function, a nuclear medicine gamma camera and a radionuclide are used. Unilateral ventilation is assessed using inhalation of ^{133}Xe gas and perfusion is measured using intravenously administered ^{99m}Tc-labeled albumin macroaggregates. This methodology is available in most hospitals and is used routinely for the diagnosis of pulmonary embolism by detecting perfusion defects and areas of ventilation/perfusion mismatch. The addition of a computer to the gamma camera allows quantification of the radioactive counts emanating from

Table 18–3. Pulmonary Function Criteria for Lung Resection

Spirometric	Questionable	Operable
Forced vital capacity (FVC)	< 60% predicted	> 60%
Forced expired volume in 1 second (FEV_1)	< 60% predicted	> 60%
FEV_1/FVC ratio	< 50%	> 50%
Maximum voluntary ventilation (MVV)	< 50% predicted	> 50%
Gas Exchange		
Diffusing capacity for carbon monoxide (D_LCO)	< 60% predicted	> 60%
Arterial carbon dioxide tension (Pa_{CO_2} mm Hg)	> 45 mm Hg	< 45 mm Hg

each lung region and thus conversion into percent (Fig. 18–3). Kristersson and co-investigators (1972) from Sweden first published their experience using the assessment of unilateral ventilation to calculate postpneumonectomy function. This report was followed by that of the author and colleagues (1974) using measurements of unilateral perfusion. Subsequently, Boysen and associates (1981) also showed a good agreement was present in those patients with COPD and lung cancer between unilateral ventilation and perfusion, making measurement of both unnecessary. Using the belief that hypercapnia is often associated in COPD with an FEV_1 of less than 0.8 liters, I and my co-workers (1974) suggested this value as a lower limit of operability. We modified this position to correct for age, height, and sex by comparing the predicted value for postpneumonectomy FEV_1 to the normal value predicted for the patient. If the calculated postpneumonectomy FEV_1 was less than 35% of normal predicted for the patient, Gass and the author (1986) suggested that the patient be considered inoperable. A subsequent prospective study of Markos and colleagues (1989) confirmed the less than 35% of normal value as being associated with an unacceptably high risk.

Wernly and associates (1980) extended the radiospirometric technique to the prediction of postlobectomy pulmonary function. They developed and tested the equation:

Expected loss in FEV_1 = Preoperative FEV_1
× Percent of function of tumor containing lung
$$\times \left(\frac{\text{Number of segments of the lobe to be resected}}{\text{Total number of segments of the lung}} \right)$$

Example: Post right upper lobectomy
Preop FEV_1 = 2.0 L

$$\text{Loss in } FEV_1 = 2.0 \text{ L}$$
$$\times \text{ 40\% of perfusion from right lung}$$
$$\times \frac{3 \text{ segments in right upper lobe}}{10 \text{ segments in entire right lung}} = 0.24 \text{ L}$$

Post right upper lobectomy FEV_1 = 2.0 − 0.24 L = 1.76 L

Questions about the accuracy of lung scan prediction of postoperative lung function were raised by Ladurie and Ranson-Bitker in 1986. These investigators reported a large series of 159 pneumonectomy patients assessed by this technique. Their data showed that approximately 75% of the patients, when studied postoperatively, differed in their measured postoperative FEV_1 value by 180 to 400 ml from what had been predicted preoperatively. The error would be excessive if 0.8 liters was chosen as a "cut off" of operability. This report, however, has not been supported by other data and remains isolated in its findings.

The radionuclide lung scan remains a valuable tool to assess what might be termed regional "anatomic physiology." This technique simply allows the surgeon to assess the function of the lung to be removed, and more importantly, the ventilatory capacity the patient will probably have postoperatively.

Hemodynamic Studies

As previously stated, a concern in the 1950s was over the development of pulmonary hypertension and cor

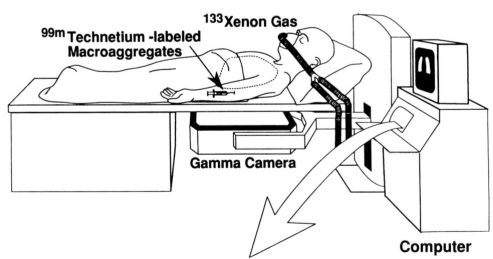

Fig. 18–3. Quantitative lung radiospirometry.

	Ventilation		Perfusion	
Right Lung	30,000 counts	55%	30,000 counts	55%
Left Lung	25,000 counts	45%	25,000 counts	45%
TOTAL	55,000 counts	100%	55,000 counts	100%

pulmonale after lung resection or thoracoplasty for tuberculosis. Carlens, Hansen, and Nordenstrom (1951) introduced a cardiac catheter that could be passed to the pulmonary artery — PA. It had an inflatable balloon like a Swan-Ganz catheter, but it was larger. Inflation of the 50-ml balloon in the main PA would occlude it and produce a "physiologic pneumonectomy." Measurements of PA pressure proximal to the balloon could be made at rest and during supine exercise to detect the presence of occult pulmonary hypertension. This technique, known as temporary unilateral pulmonary artery occlusion — TUPAO, was used effectively in a study by Uggla (1956). In this retrospective study, the author divided the patients into three groups based on postoperative outcome: "fit for work," "cardiorespiratory cripples," or "dead." The TUPAO pressure in the PA along with the systemic arterial O_2 tension — Pa_{O_2} — seem to be the best way to predict postoperative mortality. This procedure is technically demanding and had a failure rate of about 25% in a prospective study by the author and co-investigators (1975).

Fee and colleagues (1975) reported their experience using a Swan-Ganz catheter passed to the PA before treadmill exercise. The exercise is used to increase cardiac output and thus uncover pulmonary hypertension not obvious at rest. In the Fee report, the calculated pulmonary vascular resistance — PVR — seemed to be most predictive of postoperative death. A PVR of greater than 190 $dyne/sec/cm^{-5}$ seemed a predictor of postoperative mortality. These findings were not, however, supported by results of a study by the author and co-workers (1989), in which differences in PVR were not helpful in identifying patients with severe COPD who were "intolerant" of lung resection, as evidenced by death within 30 days or permanent ventilator dependency.

These hemodynamic studies are technically challenging to perform and appear to be needed rarely in preoperative assessment. They have been generally supplanted by noninvasive exercise testing.

Exercise Testing

Complications of lung resection may be "technical" as in postoperative bronchopleural fistula or hemorrhage, and "physiologic" such as cardiorespiratory failure. Few tests have the ability to predict the former, and many have been proposed to predict the latter. A brief report by Eugene and co-workers in 1982 began a new area of investigation. Previous studies used exercise and hemodynamic studies, such as cardiac catheterization, to uncover pulmonary hypertension or simply to assess the presence of unacceptable dyspnea preoperatively. The results of these studies were mixed, at best. Eugene, however, found that measurement of maximal oxygen consumption — $Vo_{2\,max}$ — on incremental cycle ergometer exercise was a strong predictor of postoperative mortality. In this study, the 75% of patients whose preoperative exercise $Vo_{2\,max}$ was less than 1.0 liters died after lung resection, and none of those with a $Vo_{2\,max}$ greater than 1.0 liters died. These

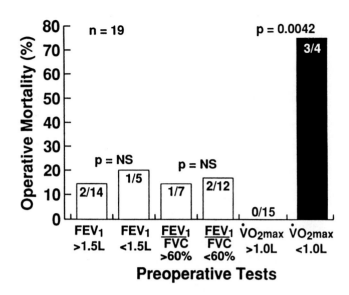

Fig. 18–4. Operative mortality and physiologic tests. *Data from* Eugene J, et al: Maximum oxygen consumption: A physiologic guide to pulmonary resection. Surg Forum 33:260, 1982.

patient groups were not significantly different from each other in their ventilatory function (Fig. 18–4).

Maximal oxygen consumption is the highest oxygen uptake measured during intense incremental workload exercise. At the point of $Vo_{2\,max}$, a further increase in work will not lead to a further increase in Vo_2, suggesting that the complete oxygen transport chain of lungs-heart-vessels-muscle are stressed to their limit (Fig. 18–5). Those patients with problems in the oxygen delivery system, such as persons with heart or lung disease, will not achieve true plateau of $Vo_{2\,max}$. Their lesser peak exercise Vo_2, however, is called "symptom-limited maximum" often confusingly abbreviated $Vo_{2\,max}$ just like the maximal Vo_2. As exercise workload is increased incrementally, at some point, usually termed the "anaerobic threshold," lactate production occurs. This lactate release signals greater muscle O_2 use by the muscles than that supplied by the cardiopulmonary-vascular transport system.

Multiple studies have been published in followup to that of Eugene and colleagues (1982). These investigators have, unfortunately, used different exercise protocols, for example, submaximal steady state versus incremental maximal exercise in diverse patient groups. Results, therefore, have been variable. The preponderance of studies thus far, however, seems to favor the measured Vo_2 as a valuable postoperative predictor. For example, Smith and co-workers (1984) found that a true $Vo_{2\,max}$ of less than 15 ml/kg/min was predictive not only of death, but also of potentially survivable complications such as cardiac arrhythmias, pneumonia, and atelectasis. They also found that the predictive value of exercise Vo_2 data was superior to that of the calculation of postoperative FEV_1 using the quantitative radionuclide lung scan previously discussed. On the other hand, Markos and colleagues (1989) found the Vo_2 on exercise

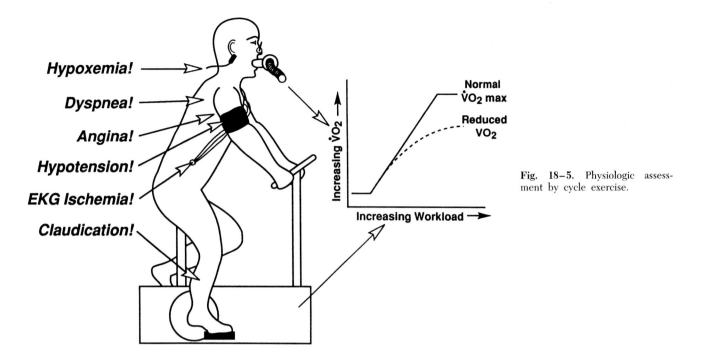

Fig. 18–5. Physiologic assessment by cycle exercise.

did *not* discriminate postoperative outcome as well as the scan prediction. A possible unifying explanation as to why those studies had such divergent results is that their patients were not preselected by any pulmonary function criteria as being at increased risk. For example, the Smith study (1984) included a patient as young as 32 years of age, and in the Markos study (1989), only one half of the patient group studied had an FEV_1 of less than 2 liters preoperatively. Perhaps, the reduced Vo_2 on exercise is best predictive of postoperative mortality in patients with severe underlying lung disease, but it does suggest an increased postoperative morbidity when used in healthier patients. This concept seems to be supported by the report of the author and co-investigators (1992) and the studies of Morice and colleagues (1992), as well as that of Nakagawa and associates (1992). The Morice study (1989) is unique in that patients with a preoperative Pa_{CO_2} greater than 45 mmHg were included and underwent successful resection. The Nakagawa study (1992) is of interest in that those investigators used flow-directed cardiac catheterization and exercised the patients to a blood lactate level of 20 mg/dl. Fatal postoperative complications were best predicted by the calculated oxygen delivery — arterial O_2 content × cardiac output — per meter of body surface area — BSA. An O_2 delivery of less than 500 ml/min/m^2 with exercise was present in all 4 patients who died postoperatively and in none of the 27 patients who survived. This study used invasive methodology to suggest the predictive value of assessing the oxygen transport system under the stress of submaximal exercise.

A "low tech" method of exercise testing has been described that is virtually free of invasive or sophisticated technologic requirements. In 1968, Van Nos-

trand and co-workers reported that those patients who were unable to climb two flights of stairs because of unacceptable dyspnea failed to survive pneumonectomy. It appears that stair climbing is a highly stressful exercise requiring a higher Vo_2 than cycle ergometry performed to the same symptom limit. Bolton and co-investigators (1987) reported acceptable correlations between steps climbed and routine pulmonary function parameters in elderly male veterans. In a followup retrospective report, the author and colleagues (1991) reported that in elderly veterans not preselected by abnormal spirometry, successful climbing of three flights — 76 steps — of stairs best separated patients after lung resection as to the length of postoperative intubation and hospital stay and the number of postoperative complications. The study was limited, however, by its retrospective design and the few postoperative deaths reported.

A patient with severe limitations of O_2 transport because of heart, lung, or vascular disease will not be able to climb stairs rapidly. The onset of chest pain, dyspnea, or claudication may signal these underlying problems. Thus, stair climbing may, after further study, prove to be a valuable preoperative screening test.

The concept is now evolving — and awaiting confirmation — that those patients who have limited cardiopulmonary transport systems preoperatively as suggested by a reduced $Vo_{2\,max}$ may not survive those complications that tend to demand a higher Vo_2 postoperatively. This concept is supported by the report of Shoemaker and colleagues (1992). In this study, high-risk surgical patients — an unknown number postthoracotomy — were stratified postoperatively by their calculated tissue oxygen debt. Oxygen debt is essentially the difference between what O_2 utilization is needed and what O_2 is delivered. Those patients with the lowest postoperative O_2 debt survived, and those with the highest debt succumbed. Those patients with intermediate values survived, but with various organ system failures. Unfortunately, none of those patients were exercised preoperatively.

SUMMARY

Patients may be evaluated preoperatively in an attempt to predict the occurrence of pulmonary complications postoperatively. This effort may be performed using a history and physical examination to detect the existence of underlying heart or lung disease. Followup physiologic tests to confirm the degree of impairment have been reported extensively. Routine pulmonary function tests appear to play a minor role in upper abdominal surgery. Their primary value appears to be highest as screening tests before lung resection. No patients, however, should be summarily rejected for a potentially curative operation for lung cancer based solely on a spirometric finding. Further testing with quantitative radionuclide "split function" lung scans will permit a prediction of pulmonary function after lung resection. Testing of exercise endurance and oxygen transport appear to be the best final arbiter of physiologic operability. An algorithmic approach to the evaluation of the lung cancer patient is illustrated in Figure 18–6.

1. Patients with FEV_1 and D_LCO that exceed 60% of their predicted normal value may undergo surgical procedures up to and including pneumonectomy without further routine testing.
2. Patients with lower FEV_1 and D_LCO results should be subjected to a quantitative ventilation or perfusion radionuclide lung scan. From these data, a predicted postpneumonectomy — or postlobectomy — FEV_1 should be calculated and compared to the predicted normal value for the patient. If the predicted postoperative FEV_1 exceeds 40% of normal for that patient, an attempt at the indicated resection is warranted.
3. For those patients whose predicted postresection FEV_1 is less than 40% of their normal value, an exercise study with measured Vo_2 may be useful. If the measured Vo_2 on the maximum tolerated exercise is greater than 15 mm/kg/min, surgical resection may be offered.
4. If the measured exercise Vo_2 value is less than 15 ml/kg/min, one need not absolutely preclude an attempt at a surgical cure. As always, however, any resection should be preceded by an earnest discussion with the patient of the risks of disability, death, and, worst of all, permanent ventilator dependency.

REFERENCES

Bartlett RH, et al: Studies on the pathogenesis and prevention of postoperative pulmonary complications. Surg Gynecol Obstet 137:925, 1973.

Bolton JWR, et al: Stair climbing as an indicator of pulmonary function. Chest 92:783, 1987.

Boysen PG, et al: Prospective evaluation for pneumonectomy using perfusion scanning. Chest 80:163, 1981.

Carlens E, Hanson HE, Nordenstrom B: Temporary unilateral occlusion of the pulmonary artery. J Thorac Surg 22:527, 1951.

Chuter TAM, et al: Diaphragmatic breathing maneuvers and movement of the diaphragm after cholecystectomy. Chest 97:1110, 1990.

Eugene J, et al: Maximum oxygen consumption: A physiologic guide to pulmonary resection. Surg Forum 33:260, 1982.

Fee JH, et al: Role of pulmonary vascular resistance measurements in preoperative evaluation of candidates for pulmonary resection. J Thorac Cardiovasc Surg 75:519, 1975.

Ferguson MK, et al: Diffusing capacity predicts morbidity and mortality after pulmonary resection. J Thorac Surg 86:894, 1988.

Ford GT, et al: Diaphragm function after upper abdominal surgery in humans. Am Rev Respir Dis 127:431, 1983.

Gaensler EA, et al: The role of pulmonary insufficiency in mortality and invalidism following surgery for pulmonary tuberculosis. J Thorac Cardiovasc Surg 29:163, 1955.

Gass GD, Olsen GN: Preoperative pulmonary function testing to predict postoperative morbidity and mortality. Chest 89:127, 1986.

Graham EA, Singer JJ: Successful removal of an entire lung for carcinoma of the bronchus. JAMA 101:1371, 1933.

Hall JC, et al: Incentive spirometry versus routine chest physiotherapy for prevention of pulmonary complications after abdominal surgery. Lancet 337:953, 1991.

Kristersson S, Lindell S, Strandberg L: Prediction of pulmonary function loss due to pneumonectomy using ^{133}Xe-radiospirometry. Chest 62:696, 1972.

Ladurie ML, Ranson-Bitker B: Uncertainties in the expected value for forced expiratory volume in one second after surgery. Chest 90:222, 1986.

Lanier RC, Olsen GN: Can concomitant restriction be detected in adult men with airflow obstruction? Chest 99:826, 1991.

Lawrence VA, Page CP, Harris GD: Preoperative spirometry before abdominal operations. Arch Intern Med 149:280, 1989.

Markos J, et al: Preoperative assessment as a predictor of mortality and morbidity after lung resection. Am Rev Respir Dis 139:902, 1989.

Morice RC, et al: Exercise testing in the evaluation of patients at high risk for complications from lung resection. Chest 101:356, 1992.

Nakagawa K, et al: Oxygen transport during incremental exercise load

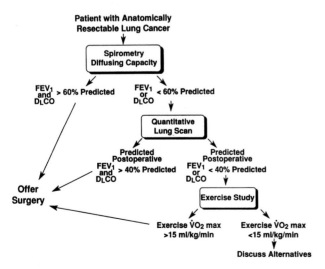

Fig. 18–6. Physiologic assessment algorithm.

as a predictor of operative risk in lung cancer patients. Chest *101*:1369, 1992.

Neuhaus H, Cherniack NS: A bronchospirometric method of estimating the effect of pneumonectomy on the maximum breathing capacity. J Thorac Cardiovasc Surg *55*:144, 1968.

Olsen GN, Block AJ, Tobias JA: Prediction of postpneumonectomy pulmonary function using quantitative macroaggregate lung scanning. Chest *66*:13, 1974.

Olsen GN, et al: Pulmonary function evaluation of the lung resection candidate: A prospective study. Am Rev Respir Dis *111*:379, 1975.

Olsen GN, et al: Submaximal invasive exercise testing and quantitative lung scanning in the evaluation for tolerance of lung resection. Chest *95*:267, 1989.

Olsen GN, et al: Stair climbing as an exercise test to predict the postoperative complications of lung resection. Chest *99*:587, 1991.

Pasteur W: Massive collapse of the lung. Lancet *2*:1351, 1908.

Shoemaker WC, Appel PL, Kram HB: Role of oxygen debt in the development of organ failure, sepsis, and death in high-risk surgical patients. Chest *102*:208, 1992.

Smith TP, et al: Exercise capacity as a predictor of post-thoracotomy morbidity. Am Rev Respir Dis *129*:730, 1984.

Uggla LG: Indications for and results of thoracic surgery with regard to respiratory and circulatory function tests. Acta Chir Scand *111*:197, 1956.

Van Nostrand D, Kjelsberg MD, Humphrey EW: Pre-resectional evaluation of risk from pneumonectomy. Surg Gynecol Obstet *127*:306, 1968.

Wernly JA, et al: Clinical value of quantitative ventilation-perfusion lung scans in the surgical management of bronchogenic carcinoma. J Thorac Cardiovasc Surg *80*:535, 1980.

Zibrak JD, O'Donnell CR, Marton K: Indications for preoperative pulmonary function testing. Ann Intern Med *112*:763, 1990.

CHAPTER 19

PREOPERATIVE CARDIAC EVALUATION OF THE THORACIC SURGICAL PATIENT AND MANAGEMENT OF PERIOPERATIVE CARDIAC EVENTS

Robert W. Anderson and John C. Alexander, Jr.

After respiratory complications, the problems associated with the highest mortality and most severe morbidity in the thoracic surgical patient are cardiovascular complications. These problems may range from benign arrhythmias to myocardial failure and death. The incidence of such complications increases with the patient's age and they occur more frequently in patients who undergo more extensive procedures such as pneumonectomy or esophageal or chest wall resection.

Thoracic surgical procedures themselves often have profound effects on the cardiovascular system. A major lung resection decreases the pulmonary vascular bed and therefore may result in a rise in right ventricular and pulmonary artery pressure and lead to right ventricular failure. Other physiologic changes associated with surgery may include a decrease in lung compliance and diffusion surface, with a resulting increase in the work of breathing. This latter change increases myocardial workload and results in a rise in myocardial oxygen consumption, which may aggravate pre-existing cardiac disease or lead to ischemia in the patient with coronary artery disease.

EVALUATION OF OPERATIVE RISK: CARDIAC FACTORS

Operative risk is defined as the probability of morbidity or mortality resulting from preoperative preparation, anesthesia, the surgical procedure, or postoperative convalescence. The decision to proceed with any therapeutic intervention, whether medical or surgical, must be determined on the basis of the potential risks and benefits of the intervention as weighed against the natural history of the disease process being considered

for treatment. The cardiac subsystem is particularly important in this evaluation, because myocardial infarction, arrhythmias, and congestive heart failure are three of the most common complications that occur in thoracic surgical patients.

The greatest cardiac risk in the patient undergoing a thoracotomy with resection is the presence of known coronary artery disease. The conclusion drawn from the data of Freeman (1989), Goldman (1977), Steen (1978), and Tarhan (1972) and their associates on 46,000 patients is that the risk of preoperative myocardial infarction is 0.15% in patients without prior evidence of clinical heart disease. In patients with a documented prior infarction, however, the incidence of re-infarction during a major noncardiac procedure has ranged from 2.8 to 17.7%, with a mean of approximately 6%. The mortality for perioperative myocardial infarction remains high, with average of approximately 50%.

Thoracic surgical procedures and upper abdominal vascular surgical procedures have the highest incidence of associated postoperative congestive heart failure, arrhythmias, and myocardial re-infarction when compared with other general surgical procedures, as noted by Detsky (1986), Goldman (1977), and Steen (1978), and their associates.

It is important to emphasize that the risk of perioperative infarction is inversely related to the time interval between the original myocardial infarction and performance of the thoracic surgical procedure. This risk follows a curvilinear, rather than a linear, relationship. Major noncardiac surgical procedures performed within 3 months of an acute myocardial infarction have been associated with a re-infarction rate of approximately 30%, whereas at 3 to 6 months after an infarction, the corresponding rate is approximately 14% and falls to 4% after 6 months. The institution of aggressive and comprehensive perioperative management guided by noninvasive hemodynamic monitoring, introduced by Rao and colleagues (1983), has been able to produce a significant decrease in re-infarction rates.

A thorough cardiovascular history is vital in the preoperative evaluation of thoracic surgical patients and the findings must then be correlated with appropriate physical findings and results of laboratory testing. The factors associated with cardiac risk in thoracic surgical patients are summarized in Table 19–1. The presence of any of the risk factors noted in Table 19–1 should arouse suspicion of significant cardiac disease and lead to a more comprehensive evaluation.

The preoperative cardiac evaluation of thoracic surgical patients requires making a series of important and reasonable decisions in a cost-effective manner. Some authors suggest that all patients over a certain age undergo an extensive noninvasive and possibly even an invasive evaluation to determine the presence of coexistent coronary artery disease. The intent of such an approach is to revascularize patients in whom disease is identified. This approach has minimal documentation to support its use and evidence that prophylactic revascularization by any technique provides protection from ischemic events more successfully than intensive medical therapy is lacking.

The cardiovascular history and physical examination are the cornerstones in the preoperative evaluation of patients being considered for thoracic surgical procedures. The clinical findings must than be correlated with a chest radiograph and an electrocardiogram. The chronology and clinical course of prior myocardial

Table 19–1. Cardiac Risk Factors in Thoracic Surgical Patients

Historical factors
  Myocardial infarction (especially within past 3 months)
  Congestive heart failure
  Angina pectoris
  Poorly controlled hypertension
  Symptomatic cardiac rhythm disturbance
  Family history of premature coronary disease
  Longstanding diabetes mellitus
  Pulmonary hypertension
Physical examination findings
  Presence of S3 gallop or venous distention
  Abnormal cardiac rhythm
  Pulmonary rales
  Significant valvular murmur
  Hypertension
Laboratory findings
  Cardiomegaly on chest radiograph
  Ischemic changes of electrocardiogram (ECG) (rest or stress)
  Ventricular ectopy on ECG
  Abnormal cardiac rhythm on ECG
  Hypotension induced by stress

infarction should be elucidated and evidence of left ventricular dysfunction as manifested by symptoms of congestive heart failure should be sought carefully. Attention should also be paid to the presence, severity, and pattern of angina pectoris and to the efficacy and appropriateness of the current medical program. Patients who are completely asymptomatic and have no significant risk factors for coronary artery disease, regardless of age, need not undergo further testing. Patients with symptomatic heart disease or baseline laboratory abnormalities suggestive of cardiac disease need further assessment. If symptoms of ischemic heart disease are present, stress testing should be considered before a major intrathoracic surgical procedure is recommended, particularly if the patient has a history of myocardial infarction, demonstrates symptomatic left ventricular dysfunction, or has had diabetes mellitus for more than 5 years.

Pharmacologic Testing

Coronary arteriography should be performed if the patient is unable to exercise to an adequate workload because of ischemic symptoms or demonstrates other abnormalities suggesting significant valvular or congenital heart disease. The demonstration of significant anatomic coronary artery disease and physiologic ischemia or valvular disease during noninvasive and invasive testing requires consideration of revascularization or valve surgery in certain instances. On the other hand, subjecting patients with advanced pulmonary disease and a limited life expectancy on the basis of their pulmonary disease to open heart surgery is not justified, from both a medical and an economic standpoint. Thoracic surgical patients must be evaluated clinically for the presence of pre-existing pulmonary hypertension that may be aggravated by extensive resection of lung tissue and lead to acute right ventricular failure. Persons thought to have pulmonary hypertension may require further noninvasive testing or a right-sided catheterization to evaluate the degree of pulmonary vascular disease.

MANAGEMENT OF SURGICAL PATIENTS WITH CARDIOVASCULAR DISEASE

During the past two decades, a substantial decrease has occurred in the mortality from cardiovascular diseases. Some authors have suggested that modifications in dietary habits and an increased awareness of physical fitness are primarily responsible for these improvements in cardiovascular health. Good evidence also exists, however, that the use of modern pharmacologic therapy to control hypertension, to modify the course of ischemic heart disease, and to alter the basic hemostatic mechanism on a chronic basis to prevent vascular events has played an important role in lowering cardiovascular disease mortality. As a consequence, many patients are surviving the ravages of cardiovascular disease and are seen by surgeons for problems, both cardiovascular and noncardiovascular, that may require surgical treatment.

Because of their older age and multiple associated illnesses, these patients present risks that must be carefully considered in the design of their overall surgical management plan. The cardiovascular diseases and the pharmacologic agents that are most frequently encountered in the thoracic surgical patient fall in five general categories: 1) hypertension, 2) chronic congestive heart failure, 3) angina pectoris secondary to ischemic heart disease, 4) low output states, and 5) arrhythmias. Considerable overlap exists between these categories, from a physiologic standpoint and in regard to the pharmacologic agents used to treat them.

Hypertension

Hypertension is a common finding in surgical patients. The number of patients treated for this disorder has increased substantially during the past two decades, and in approximately 95% of these patients, no single cause for the elevation in blood pressure can be identified. Although many popular theories exist to explain the increased peripheral vascular resistance noted in hypertension, the possibility that a single defect is responsible for all essential hypertension is unlikely.

It is well recognized from therapeutic trials that many of the vascular complications that can occur as a result of hypertension can be decreased by pharmacologic intervention. This finding has resulted in the widespread use of antihypertensive agents, some of which have a profound influence on the surgical patient.

Diuretics

The diuretic agents, including the thiazides and furosemide, are first line agents used in the treatment of mild or moderate hypertension. Because these drugs increase urinary excretion of salt and water, hypovolemia from dehydration may be of particular concern in surgical patients. This state results in tachycardia and also a predisposition to hypotension with the administration of anesthetics that interfere with sympathetic function and therefore block the reflex increase in cardiac output or peripheral vascular resistance that are normal homeostatic responses to decreasing blood pressure. As a result, trivial blood loss during an operative procedure may result in profound hypotension and a severe decrease in cardiac output if pre-existing intervascular and extracellular deficits are present as a result of dehydration associated with prolonged diuretic administration. Obtaining a full history and observation of clinical signs of volume depletion, such as orthostatic hypotension or resting tachycardia, allow the clinician to take appropriate measures to restore volume preoperatively and such problems can be avoided. The diuretics also increase delivery of sodium to the distal renal tubal. Sodium-potassium exchange occurs, resulting in potassium loss and hypokalemia following prolonged administration of the diuretic agents. In the presence of hypokalemia, the arrhythmogenic affects of digitalis or anesthetic agents that sensitize the myocardium may result in a cardiac rhythm disturbance and lead to ventricular fibrillation. Repletion of diminished total body potassium stores before major surgical procedures is essential to diminish cardiac rhythm disturbances, particularly if alkalosis or digitalis therapy coexist.

Adrenergic Blockers

A second class of agents used to manage hypertension is the adrenergic inhibitors. These drugs inhibit function of the sympathetic nervous system and are classified according to the site at which they inhibit the sympathetic reflex arc. Each class of drug exhibits different forms of potential toxicity and may produce problems in surgical patients. The peripherally acting agents, such as reserpine and guanethidine, which are not used commonly, produce profound sympathoplegia by either blocking or inhibiting biogenic amine functions in both peripheral and central neurons. The problems of depressed cardiac output and hypotension from blunted sympathetic responses in the presence of volume depletion or exposure to anesthetic agents are often seen in surgical patients receiving these agents. Therefore, it is advisable to discontinue peripherally acting adrenergic blocking agents before any elective surgical procedure. Substitution of a more rapidly acting and easily managed agent may be required.

The centrally acting adrenergic inhibitors, such as clonidine and methyldopa, reduce sympathetic outflow from vasopressor centers in the brain stem. Because they allow these centers to retain their sensitivity to baroreceptor control, these drugs do not depress normal cardiovascular reflexes and do not depress cardiac output or produce the orthostatic hypotension seen with peripherally acting agents. Abrupt withdrawal of clonidine may result in hypertensive crisis or other evidence of profound sympathetic overactivity, and this drug should therefore be continued throughout the perioperative period or gradually withdrawn while other antihypertensive therapy is substituted.

Although beta-blocking agents were used initially in the treatment of angina pectoris, it soon became apparent that they were extremely effective agents for the treatment of a variety of other disorders, such as hypertension, thyrotoxicosis, migraines, arrhythmias, and glaucoma. Most treatment programs in patients with mild or moderately severe hypertension include one of the beta blockers currently available. The beta blockers seem to be well tolerated in surgical patients and appear to offer a significant degree of protection from postoperative rhythm disturbances if continued without interruption throughout the perioperative period. Abrupt withdrawal of beta blockers has been associated with acute myocardial infarction and should be avoided.

The alpha-receptor antagonists are used rarely for the management of uncomplicated hypertension. It is preferable to discontinue their use before performing any elective surgical procedure, unless specific indications exist for continuing such therapy.

Vasodilators

Peripheral vasodilators usually are used in the management of hypertension only if a diuretic and adrenergic blocker do not control the blood pressure. Hydralazine is the only drug used routinely as an oral agent. It is usually reserved for patients with severe hypertension and is often given in combination with a diuretic and a beta blocker. Intravenous nitroprusside is the agent of choice for the control of acute hypertension in the operating room or during the postoperative period. It is rapid acting and is easily titrated under conditions of proper monitoring, which allows the prompt detection and correction of fluid deficits.

Converting Enzyme Inhibitors

Captopril was the first orally effective inhibitor of angiotensin-converting enzyme — ACE, which is the enzyme responsible for conversion of inactive angiotensin I to the pressor peptide angiotensin II. Both captopril and enalapril are potent and specific antihypertensive agents that lower total peripheral resistance, cause little change in cardiac output, heart rate, or pulmonary wedge pressure, and are particularly effective in those hypertensive patients with elevated renin levels. They do not appear to interfere with normal cardiovascular homeostatic responses even when administered simultaneously with a diuretic. If significant volume depletion occurs as a result of a concomitantly administered diuretic, however, hypotension may develop. Abrupt withdrawal of ACE inhibitors may result in severe hypertension that is difficult to manage, and these drugs should therefore be continued throughout the perioperative period.

Uncontrolled hypertension in the thoracic surgical patient is a serious problem. It is essential to formulate a rational plan for the management and control of blood pressure in the operating room and postoperatively before discontinuing any form of antihypertensive therapy. After passing the period of hemodynamic instability surrounding the immediate operative period, the patient's normal antihypertensive regimen should be reinstituted to make the perioperative management less complex. Rapidly acting agents, such as intravenous nitroprusside, are the ones of choice for severe hypertension during the intraoperative or immediate postoperative period. It is mandatory that these agents be administered only under carefully monitored conditions because of their ability to produce profound hypotension.

Congestive Heart Failure

Traditional treatment for patients with evidence of cardiac failure has consisted of salt restriction, diuretics, and the administration of a digitalis preparation for cardiac rate control and an inotropic effect. Cohn (1982) and associates (1986) recognized that an increase in impedance to left ventricular ejection is an important factor in producing the left ventricular dysfunction that characterizes cardiac failure states. This increased impedance to ejection is the result of a complex series of peripheral vascular events produced by increased activity of the sympathetic system and the renin-angiotensin system. The final result of this abnormal activity is narrowing of the arterioles, decreased arterial compliance, and a reduction in venous compliance. The concept has developed that instead of vigorously stimulating the failing heart with inotropic agents, one should attempt to reduce the cardiac load by means of vasodilator use. The concept of afterload reduction by pharmacologic means is already well established for the treatment of hypertension and has now been extended to other disease states that produce severe congestive heart failure resulting from aortic or mitral valve incompetence, ischemic heart disease, and all of the cardiomyopathic states that produce cardiac failure.

Drugs that produce vasodilation can favorably affect the performance of the heart in two ways, according to Chatterjee and Parmley (1983) and Ribner and colleagues (1982). First, by decreasing the peripheral vascular resistance through the mechanism of arteriolar relaxation, the ventricular ejection fraction improves, stroke volume improves, and end-systolic volume decreases. Second, the relaxation of venous smooth muscle shifts blood from the central circulation into the peripheral venous capacitance bed, thereby decreasing the preload or end-diastolic volume, which results in the following: 1) a reduction in myocardial wall stress and consequent lowering of myocardial oxygen requirements; 2) a decrease in end-diastolic pressure in the left ventricle with a consequent decrease in pulmonary venous pressure and relief of pulmonary congestion; and 3) improved diastolic perfusion of the myocardium as a result of the lowered transmyocardial pressure gradient between epicardial and endocardial blood vessels.

The surgical management of patients with evidence of congestive heart failure has been improved with the addition of vasodilator drugs to the therapeutic regimen. This improvement has been particularly evident in cardiovascular and thoracic surgical patients, who are treated preoperatively and then brought to the operating room in a more stable state than was previously possible. The deleterious effects of uncontrolled hypertension are well recognized, and drugs that are currently available allow precise regulation of cardiac function and blood pressure both preoperatively and during the intraoperative period.

Any patient with cardiac disease severe enough to produce symptoms or findings of congestive heart failure represents a substantial risk for any thoracic surgical operation. A comprehensive evaluation of the patient's underlying cardiac pathology, the institution or continuation of appropriate therapy, and the judicious use of intraoperative monitoring of cardiac function are mandatory to reduce surgical risk to an acceptable level. In almost all instances, drugs that have successfully controlled symptoms of cardiac failure prior to surgery should be continued or more appropriate agents used throughout the preoperative, operative, and postoperative periods.

Arrhythmias

In 1943, Bailey and Betts (1943) and Currens and associates (1943) first called attention to the incidence of both supraventricular and ventricular arrhythmias after thoracotomy for pulmonary and esophageal disease. Krosnick and Wasserman (1955) first drew attention to an association between the occurrence of postoperative arrhythmias and postoperative mortality. This argument was strengthened by Shields and Ujiki (1968) when they reported a series of 125 patients undergoing thoracotomy and on the findings of their unrandomized study suggested that prophylactic digitalization reduced mortality related to arrhythmias. Since that time, considerable controversy regarding the incidence, importance, etiology, methods for treatment, and usefulness of prophylaxis of these arrhythmias has been present in the thoracic surgical literature. Ferguson (1992) carefully reviewed and documented the relationship between cardiac arrhythmias and thoracic surgery and concluded that the etiology of these arrhythmias is clearly multifactorial and superimposed on a patient population already at high risk for arrhythmogenic complications. He concluded that despite the high incidence of arrhythmogenic complications after thoracotomy, adequate preoperative evaluation and a thorough understanding of the principles of postoperative management will suffice in almost all instances to keep the morbidity associated with this complication to a minimum.

The perioperative management of patients with cardiac arrhythmias and conduction disturbances is an important part of the care of thoracic surgical patients. Knowledge of the preoperative drug ingestion history, electrocardiographic status, and cardiovascular history is mandatory and should be combined with an understanding of the intraoperative and postoperative factors that facilitate the occurrence of cardiac rhythm disturbances. A number of factors may be encountered perioperatively that predispose to the development of arrhythmias: 1) ventilatory problems that produce hypoxia or respiratory alkalosis, 2) hypokalemia and other electrolyte abnormalities, 3) toxicity to cardioactive anesthetics and other drugs, 4) hypotension, 5) hypertension, 6) reduced cardiac output, 7) anemia, 8) myocardial infarction, and 9) the vagal irritation and sympathetic increase associated with post-thoracotomy pain that invariably are associated with thoracic surgical procedures. These factors must be considered in the evaluation of a surgical patient with cardiac rhythm disturbance, and initial treatment should always be directed toward correction of these abnormalities. Thus, the aim of modern antiarrhythmic therapy is to reduce ectopic pacemaker activity and to modify critically impaired conduction either by improving it in an area of depressed conduction or by suppressing it altogether.

The indications for the use of antiarrhythmic drugs in surgical patients must be based on a knowledge of the natural history of the rhythm disturbance and whether or not it is of physiologic significance in the overall management of the patient. Careful documentation and precise diagnosis of the type of rhythm disturbance are essential. Harrison (1985) suggested there is a limited role for the prophylactic use of drug therapy in an attempt to prevent the development of arrhythmias, because all antiarrhythmic drugs have proarrhythmic effects and therefore may precipitate a rhythm disturbance. In general, all cardiac rhythm disturbances that are potentially life-threatening, that can be shown to cause hemodynamic compromise, or that result in symptoms should be diagnosed precisely and treated specifically. Patients with no known structural heart disease usually do not require specific drug therapy for benign rhythm disturbances such as sinus tachycardia, premature atrial beats, or unifocal premature ventricular beats. The most prudent approach may be to define underlying etiologic factors such as fever, hypoxia, pain, or anxiety and attempt to eliminate them. In some patients, the presence of heart disease may complicate the use of antiarrhythmic therapy. Heart failure and conduction system disease are the most serious problems. Most of the antiarrhythmic drugs depress left ventricular function to a variable and dose-related degree, and patients with left ventricular dysfunction may tolerate these agents poorly. Drug therapy for patients with atrioventricular — AV — nodal disease or with conduction disease below the level of the AV node should be monitored carefully because of the potential for serious side effects and profound depression of cardiac conduction.

PHARMACOLOGIC MANAGEMENT OF SPECIFIC CARDIOVASCULAR PROBLEMS IN THE THORACIC SURGICAL PATIENT

Arrhythmias and Conduction Disturbances

Bradyarrhythmias

Sinus bradycardia in the surgical patient is usually caused by increased vagal tone related to direct stimulation of the carotid sinus, stimulation of the vagus nerves, or pain-induced increases in vagal tone. Myocardial ischemia should always be excluded as a cause for sudden cardiac slowing.

Bradycardia is best treated by administering atropine intravenously in 0.5-mg boluses, up to 2.0 mg over a 30-minute period. If atropine therapy is unsuccessful, a continuous infusion of isoproterenol may be administered at a rate of 1 to 10 µg/min titrated to the heart rate responses. If pharmacologic therapy is unsuccessful, a temporary pacemaker should be placed.

Ventricular Arrhythmias

This is a complex and changing area that cannot readily be simplified. The criteria for instituting therapy are not clear cut, although patients with sustained ventricular tachycardia and those with symptomatic or hemodynamically compromising ventricular dysrhythmia require treatment.

Intraoperative or postoperative ventricular ectopy is often precipitated by hypoxia, hypercarbia, hypokalemia, anxiety, fever, or drug excess, and correction of these problems often leads to cessation of the ectopy without resorting to specific drug therapy. Ventricular ectopic activity that occurs in the absence of clinical heart disease or electrocardiographic abnormalities is generally benign and well tolerated.

In patients with a history of ischemic heart disease or with electrocardiographic or clinical evidence of perioperative ischemia or infarction in whom ventricular ectopic activity in the form of frequent multifocal ventricular beats or ventricular couplets develops, lidocaine therapy should be administered as a 50 to 100-mg intravenous bolus followed by continuous infusion at a rate 1 to 3 mg/min titrated to control the ectopy. If lidocaine fails to control the rhythm, procainamide would be the second drug to administer, and bretylium may be required in cases that are particularly refractory to more conventional drugs.

Supraventricular Tachyarrhythmias

The development of new supraventricular tachyarrhythmias in the surgical patient is usually associated with certain identifiable risk factors such as myocardial infarction or ischemia, congestive heart failure, electrolyte derangements, hypoxia, pulmonary embolism, the administration of arrhythmogenic drugs such as catecholamines, or fever associated with a major infection. Correction of these problems would obviate the need for specific drug therapy in about one third of the patients.

Atrial fibrillation is the most common supraventricular arrhythmia observed in thoracic surgical patients. The first goal of treatment is to control the rapid ventricular response rate, which usually is done best by administering digoxin. For patients who have not taken digoxin or any other digitalis agent previously, a total intravenous loading dose of 1.0 mg should be administered over 6 to 12 hours, usually beginning with 0.5 mg intravenously and then repeating 0.25-mg doses at 2-hour intervals to lower the ventricular rate below 90 beats per minute. In patients with a rapid ventricular response to atrial fibrillation and no evidence of depressed ventricular function, verapamil can be given in doses of 2.5 to 5 mg intravenously every 15 minutes until a total dose of 10 mg is delivered. For severe cardiac compromise because of tachycardia, synchronized cardioversion remains the treatment of choice.

Treatment of the underlying medical problems and control of the ventricular response to atrial fibrillation usually result in conversion to normal sinus rhythm. If the patient remains in atrial fibrillation for 48 hours despite adequate control of the ventricular response, a specific antiarrhythmic drug such as quinidine or procainamide should be administered in an attempt to achieve conversion into sinus rhythm.

Control of the ventricular rate in patients with atrial flutter is often more difficult than in those individuals with atrial fibrillation. Although the treatment approach has traditionally been to administer digitalis, good clinical evidence suggests that the use of verapamil as the first drug may be more efficacious. Also, it is well known that atrial flutter is uniquely susceptible to cardioversion, and this form of treatment should be used in any patient with evidence of hemodynamic compromise.

Other forms of supraventricular tachyarrhythmia, including AV nodal re-entry tachycardia, sinus node re-entry tachycardia, intra-atrial tachycardia, automatic junctional tachycardia, or a re-entrant conduction pathway, may occur in surgical patients and may require pharmacologic treatment. In some instances, these arrhythmias may be terminated by vagotonic maneuvers, but if this effort is unsuccessful, intravenous administration of verapamil in the same dosage recommended for atrial fibrillation is the agent of choice. Verapamil should be successful in about 80% of cases, but in those patients in whom rate reduction is not achieved, the administration of propranolol is indicated.

Esmolol is an ultrashort-acting cardioselective beta blocker recently introduced in the United States. Esmolol is rapidly converted to inactive metabolites by blood esterases, and full recovery from beta blockade occurs within 30 minutes in patients with a normal cardiovascular system. The indications for esmolol are situations in which a rapid beta blockade onset and termination is desired, such as in supraventricular tachycardia, perioperative tachycardia, or perioperative hypertension. The dose range is 50 to 400 µg/kg/min intravenously.

Low Cardiac Output Syndromes

The low cardiac output syndrome in surgical patients must be recognized and treated promptly before severe cellular and organ damage occurs. The syndrome represents a state of inadequate perfusion at the tissue level and may occur for a variety of reasons. The clinical picture is characterized by evidence of decreased organ perfusion with decreasing urinary output and an altered mental state in the awake patient. Acidosis is noted because of the decreased tissue perfusion.

A low cardiac output state in a surgical patient can best be managed by a methodical and physiologic approach. Careful clinical observation and serial monitoring of hemodynamic parameters such as heart rate, arterial blood pressure, cardiac filling pressures, and cardiac output are mandatory. The metabolic status of the patient should be followed by serial arterial blood gas measurements and mixed venous oxygen content analysis. Electrolyte abnormalities should be sought and corrected as required.

The most common cause of the low cardiac output state in surgical patients is hypovolemia, which results from unreplaced blood or extracellular fluid losses that occur as a result of both the underlying disease process and the losses incurred at the time of any surgical procedure. Typical features in these patients are low cardiac output and reduced filling pressures, particularly as noted from the measurement of pulmonary capillary wedge pressure, which reflects left-sided filling pressures. Because of sympathetic compensatory efforts, the peripheral circulation is profoundly vasoconstricted and the peripheral vascular resistance is elevated.

Management of the low cardiac output state associated with hypovolemia is straightforward and involves the control of blood and fluid loss while judiciously replacing deficits with appropriate solution or blood products. Therapy should be carefully guided by the measurements of left-sided filling pressures and repeated determinations of cardiac output.

Another cause of the low cardiac output syndrome is primary myocardial dysfunction, which is the result of failure of the heart to perform as a competent pump. The usual cause of primary myocardial dysfunction in thoracic surgical patients is ischemic heart disease with regional dysfunction related to severe ischemia or infarction. This type of injury may be related to pre-existing cardiac disease, recent myocardial infarction, or the residual effects of ischemia that may occur after surgical procedures. Regardless of the etiology, the principles of diagnosis and the approach to management are the same. The filling pressures of the ventricular chambers must be carefully brought to the optimal state to take maximal advantage of the Frank-Starling mechanism without causing pulmonary edema. Cardiac rate and the normal synchrony between atrium and ventricle are important factors in the maintenance of cardiac pump function, and every attempt should be made to return them to normal, including the use of pacing devices.

The impaired myocardium functions best if the afterload or systolic wall stress against which it must function is reduced. This afterload reduction is best achieved by the use of short-acting peripheral vasodilators such as nitroprusside or nitroglycerin. Both drugs are administered intravenously under carefully monitored conditions and are titrated to maintain a systemic vascular resistance in the low-normal range. Additional support for the poorly functioning myocardium can be achieved by the use of an inotropic agent that will improve cardiac contractility without producing a pronounced increase in cardiac rate or significant increases in peripheral vascular resistance. The inotropic agents that appear to achieve these goals most ably are dopamine, dobutamine, and amrinone, used either alone or in combination. If pharmacologic and fluid therapy are unsuccessful in restoring myocardial function, revascularization or mechanical support with a device such as the intra-aortic balloon pump must be considered.

An increasingly common cause of the low cardiac output syndrome in thoracic surgical patients is the presence of systemic sepsis. A wide range of microbial agents can cause profound cardiovascular alterations leading to shock and death. The treatment of septic low flow states is more controversial than that of either hypovolemic or cardiogenic shock, and the mortality remains greater than 50% in almost all reported series.

The most important factors in the management of the septic surgical patient are prompt recognition of the problem and careful monitoring of the hemodynamic status while commencing a thorough search for the source of sepsis. Surgical drainage of sources of infection and the institution of antibiotics are crucial. In many instances, intravascular volume deficits are present and should be corrected. The hemodynamic interventions instituted in septic shock should augment cardiac output when demands for increased perfusion exist.

When perfusion cannot be improved further by expanding the intravascular volume and increasing the preload and afterload reduction, inotropic intervention with pharmacologic agents should be considered. In some forms of septic shock, the primary hemodynamic alteration appears to be intense peripheral vasoconstriction that will eventually produce tissue and organ damage unless treated. In this setting, the use of a vasodilator, such as nitroprusside or nitroglycerin, is indicated under conditions of careful monitoring. Blood pressure commonly decreases when these agents are used, despite a rise in cardiac output. Some degree of hypotension is usually well tolerated by younger patients without pre-existing coronary artery or cerebrovascular disease, but the fixed and stenotic lesions often present in the coronary and cerebral circulation of older patients place them at substantial risk for myocardial infarction or stroke.

When afterload reduction fails to improve cardiac output, the use of inotropic pharmacologic agents should be considered. The sympathomimetic agents dopamine, dobutamine, and amrinone can provide inotropic support in association with the dose-related peripheral vascular effects previously discussed.

One of us (RWA) and Visner (1990) noted that patients with hyperdynamic septic shock appear to have a unique problem and present a dilemma in management because their cardiac output is usually more than sufficient to meet the peripheral metabolic demands of the body for the delivery of oxygen and substrate. Patients in this category are often refractory to pharmacologic interventions, and by sustaining a high cardiac output, they may eventually exhaust their cardiac reserves. The use of a vasoconstricting agent would seem to be physiologically appropriate, but this type of intervention usually severely depresses cardiac output and is not recommended. Treatment in this group of patients remains controversial, but the best available evidence suggests it should be directed toward the metabolic abnormalities that appear to be the cause of this particular problem.

Acute Congestive Heart Failure and Pulmonary Edema

Current therapy for the management of acute congestive heart failure with associated pulmonary edema is a curious blend of the application of physiologic principles and the results of successful clinical trials. This situation reflects our incomplete understanding of the pathophysiology of congestive heart failure and the mechanisms by which currently accepted therapeutic agents effect improvement.

In the case of cardiac arrest, standard recommendations for cardiopulmonary resuscitation must be instituted with recovery of reasonably stable cardiac rhythm and evidence of an adequate cardiac output.

Acid-base assessment, along with determination of blood gases, serum electrolytes, and calcium and glucose levels, must be performed rapidly when congestive heart failure becomes evident. Inotropic drug infusions may be started and titrated, and associated problems such as hypothermia and rhythm disturbances must be aggressively corrected.

Acute pulmonary edema in the thoracic surgical patient is often the result of fluid overload in the presence of chronically compromised cardiac function or the occurrence of a recent myocardial infarction. Basic therapy involves the use of oxygen and a diuretic intravenously, such as furosemide, which also acts as a vasodilator. Morphine, a narcotic possessing both venodilatory and vasodilatory properties, may be of benefit and may alleviate the anxiety often seen in awake patients. In some situations, it may be necessary to aid the failing ventricle by the use of intravenous vasodilators such as nitroprusside or nitroglycerin.

In the event that a rapid diuresis occurs, aggressive replacement of potassium is necessary to prevent hypokalemia. This task is best accomplished by the intravenous route; however, care must be taken to avoid hyperkalemia, which may also result in life-threatening arrhythmias. For patients who develop pulmonary edema in association with renal insufficiency, the use of dopamine — 2 to 3 μg/kg/min — may improve renal blood flow and aid in diuresis. For those situations in which dopamine fails to work, aggressive therapy with ultrafiltration or dialysis may be needed.

Thoracic surgical patients are uniquely susceptible to acute right ventricular failure because of sudden pressure overload resulting from pulmonary artery hypertension, which may be exacerbated by intraoperative manipulation or resection of sufficient pulmonary tissue to limit the pulmonary vascular bed. This problem is best addressed by anticipating and avoiding it; however, acute pharmacologic treatment with oxygen, nitroprusside, and prostaglandin may be required.

REFERENCES

Anderson RW, Visner M: Shock and circulatory collapse. *In* Sabiston DC, Spencer FJ (eds.): Surgery of the Chest. Philadelphia: WB Saunders, 1990.

Bailey CC, Betts RH: Cardiac arrhythmias following pneumonectomy. N Engl J Med 229:356, 1943.

Chatterjee K, Parmley WW: Vasodilator therapy for acute myocardial infarction and chronic congestive heart failure. J Am Coll Cardiol 1:133, 1983.

Cohn JN: Physiologic basis of vasodilator therapy for heart failure. Am J Med 71:135, 1982.

Cohn JN, et al: Effect of vasodilator therapy on mortality and chronic congestive heart failure. N Engl J Med 314:1547, 1986.

Currens JH, White PD, Churchill ED: Cardiac arrhythmias following thoracic surgery. N Engl J Med 229:360, 1943.

Detsky AS, et al: Predicting cardiac complications in patients undergoing non-cardiac surgery. J Gen Intern Med 1:211, 1986.

Ferguson TB: Arrhythmias associated with thoracotomy. *In* Wolfe WG (ed): Complications in Thoracic Surgery. St. Louis: Mosby Year Book, 1992.

Freeman WK, Gibbons RJ, Shub C: Preoperative assessment of cardiac patients undergoing non-cardiac surgical procedures. Mayo Clin Proc 64:1105, 1989.

Goldman L, et al: Multifactorial index of cardiac risk in noncardiac surgical procedures. N Engl J Med 297:845, 1977.

Harrison DC: Antiarrhythmic drug classification: New science and practical applications. Am J Cardiol 56:185, 1985.

Krosnick A, Wasserman F: Cardiac arrhythmias in the older age group following thoracic surgery. Am J Med Sci 230:541, 1955.

Rao TLK, Jacobs KH, El-Etr AA: Reinfarction following anesthesia in patients with myocardial infarction. Anesthesiology 59:499, 1983.

Ribner HS, Bresnahan D, Hsieh AM: Acute hemodynamics responses to vasodilator therapy in congestive heart failure. Prog Cardiovasc Dis 25:1, 1982.

Shields TW, Ujiki GT: Digitalization for prevention of arrhythmias following pulmonary surgery. Surg Gynecol Obstet 126:743, 1968.

Steen PA, Tinker JH, Tarhan S: Myocardial reinfarction after anesthesia and surgery. JAMA 239:2566, 1978.

Tarhan S, et al: Myocardial infarction after general anesthesia. JAMA 220:1451, 1972.

READING REFERENCES

Opie LH: Drugs for the Heart. Philadelphia: WB Saunders, 1987.

Rose SD, Corman LC, Mason DT: Cardiac risk factors in patients undergoing noncardiac surgery. Med Clin North Am 63:1271, 1979.

Anesthetic Management of the General Thoracic Surgical Patient

CHAPTER 20

PREANESTHETIC EVALUATION AND PREPARATION

Hak Yui Wong and Edward A. Brunner

The development of modern surgery, and thoracic surgery in particular, was closely linked to the development of anesthesia and artificial ventilation. Until not too long ago, the feasibility of an operation was often limited by the patient's ability to survive the anesthesia. With advances in knowledge and techniques, this is now seldom the case. On the other hand, surgical procedures and demands are becoming increasingly complex, and patients who present for thoracic surgery are older and demonstrating greater complexity of their medical problems. The anesthesiologist's responsibility now consists not only of providing a complicated anesthetic, but also of becoming an integral part of the continuum of medical care that the patient has hitherto received and will require. To be able to discharge this function, the anesthesiologist must be thoroughly familiar with the patient's medical problems and the proposed operation.

Although a thorough history and physical examination by the primary physician provides much of the factual information sought by the anesthesiologist, it is no substitute for a preanesthetic evaluation, which, in addition to general assessment, focuses on specific areas of the patient's condition in the context of the proposed operation. Thoracic operations often interfere physically with the function of vital structures, and each operation has unique features. Thus, it is important that the person performing the evaluation knows the nature of the operation, the degree and manner by which it and the anesthetic will stress the patient intraoperatively, and the residual physiologic defects that will exist postoperatively. Current standard of care, in addition, calls for explanation of the procedure and risks to the patient and obtaining informed consent. Preanesthetic evaluation, therefore, cannot be relegated to the uninitiated.

Preanesthetic evaluation should be initiated as far in advance of the operation as possible. This plan allows time to conduct additional tests and evaluations, if unsuspected abnormalities are uncovered, for consultations between specialists, and to initiate necessary corrective therapy. In addition, the patient is allowed time to absorb and adjust to the newly acquired information and to explore any question that arises. With the current trend toward ambulatory care, this may be difficult to achieve. An anesthetic outpatient clinic may serve well in this regard for patients not requiring preoperative hospitalization.

SCOPE OF PREANESTHETIC EVALUATIONS

Included in preanesthetic evaluation are four objectives as follows: 1) detection of problems and factors in the patient's physical condition that can compromise the ability to cope with perioperative stress, or that can be aggravated by such stress; 2) appraisal of the impact of the specific pathology necessitating the surgery; 3) appraisal of several concerns peculiar to the practice of anesthesia; and 4) an assessment of risk.

General Medical Condition

It is beyond the scope of this text to describe general history-taking, physical diagnosis, and laboratory investigations. Because of their impact on surgical/anesthetic outcome — as discussed subsequently — several conditions that occur fairly commonly in thoracic surgical patients warrant special attention. These include coronary heart disease — presenting as previous myocardial infarction, angina, arrhythmia, or congestive heart failure — aortic valve stenosis, cor pulmonale, obstructive airway disease, symptomatic cerebrovascular disease, electrolyte imbalance — particularly hypokalemia — diabetes mellitus, thyroid disorder, and polycythemia. The focus in evaluating these chronic conditions should be on establishing the baseline for the particular patient and determining if optimal treatment has been achieved.

Impact of Specific Pathology

Every surgical condition poses unique stress on the body and presents a different set of problems to the anesthesia team. This situation is particularly true in thoracic surgery patients because the pathologic abnormalities often involve or impinge on the vital life-sustaining organs. From the standpoint of pathophysiology and anesthetic implications, general thoracic surgical conditions can be categorized into three groups: esophageal diseases, surgical diseases of the lungs, and diseases of the mediastinum and pleura. Table 20–1 lists such a working classification and the implications to be considered in preanesthetic evaluation.

Anesthetic Concerns

Aside from the assessment of specific medical conditions, the preanesthetic evaluation addresses a set of issues best described as of unique concern to the practice of anesthesia.

Anesthetic History

The patient's experience with anesthetics is reviewed, together with past anesthetic records when available.

Table 20–1 Anesthetic Classification of General Thoracic Surgical Pathologic Conditions

Pathologic Condition	Implications
I. Esophageal disorders	
A. Obstructive disorders	Predispose patients to preoperative dehydration and malnourishment
B. Refluxing disorders	Predispose patients to chronic or perioperative aspirations and pneumonitis
II. Surgical disorders of lungs	
A. Abnormal collection of fluid, e.g., abscess, hemoptysis	Contamination of normal lung tissues
B. Abnormal solid tissue e.g., tumor, consolidation	Right-to-left shunting
C. Obstructive lesions	Airflow obstruction, lung collapse
D. Abnormal lung tissue, e.g., bullous emphysema	Risk of barotrauma and pneumothorax
III. Disease of the mediastinum and pleura	
A. Obstruction of large airway, e.g., subcarinal tumor	Airflow obstruction unrelieved by endotracheal intubation
B. Obstruction of large vessels, e.g., superior vena cava syndrome	Hemodynamic compromise
C. Abnormal paths of communication, e.g., bronchopleural fistula	Difficult ventilation
D. Abnormal collection of fluid, e.g., empyema, pleural effusion	Contamination of lung tissue Compression of lung tissue

Taking note of previous difficulties, such as difficult endotracheal intubation, prolonged apnea, or postoperative jaundice, can avert potential disasters. Careful and pertinent family history may alert one to the possibility of malignant hyperpyrexia or pseudocholinesterase deficiency.

Drug History

Polypharmacy is an integral part of modern medicine, including modern anesthesia. It is particularly important in older patients presenting for thoracic surgery who may take up to five or six medications daily. To avoid adverse drug interaction, acquiring a drug history is mandatory (Table 20–2). This step also provides the opportunity to advise the patient on the continuation or discontinuation of medications preoperatively and to assess special precautions dictated by the intercurrent drug therapy.

Status of the Upper Airway

This evaluation includes information about the temporomandibular joints, the cervical spine, and the vertebrobasilar arteries. Because many thoracic surgical patients are at higher risk for aspiration of gastric content and many have coexisting heart and lung disease, and hence limited oxygen reserve, unexpected difficulty in maintaining airway patency or endotracheal intubation is best avoided. Many thoracic surgical procedures call for special airway instrumentation, such as endobronchial tubes, making attention to the state of the upper airway even more important. Special studies, such as tomograms or computed tomographic imaging of the airway, occasionally are necessary to achieve a complete evaluation.

Intravascular Access

The ease of intravenous access should be assessed in relation to the extent and site of the proposed operation. Patients with inadequate peripheral access should be prepared for central venous cannulation. Potential arterial cannulation sites are examined and tested for the presence of adequate collaterals.

Postoperative Ventilation

The need for mechanical ventilation after the operation is often predictable based on the nature of the operation, the anticipated impairment of the patient's respiratory reserve, the condition of the cardiovascular system, and the anesthetic technique used. In addition to advising the patient of this possibility, one may consider altering the choice of endotracheal tube — use of low pressure-high volume cuffs, the route of intubation, and the dose of respiratory depressant drugs.

Postoperative Pain Relief

A realistic assessment of the appropriate means to provide pain relief postoperatively should be made at the time of preanesthetic evaluation. Both patient-controlled analgesia — PCA — and spinal opioid ad-

Table 20–2. Drugs Associated with Significant Interaction During Anesthesia

Drug Class and Examples	Interact with	Interaction	Comment
Theophylline			
Aminophylline	Cimetidine	↑ Serum theophylline level	Substitute with ranitine
Oxtriphylline	Ketamine	Jointly reduce seizure threshold	
	Halothane and/or pancuronium	Predispose to cardiac arrhythmias when theophylline level is high	Check theophylline level before anesthesia
Alpha-adrenergic blockers			
Prazosin	Alpha-agonists	↓ Alpha-adrenergic effects	Chronic use of alpha blockers upregulates number of alpha-receptors
Phenoxybenzamine			
Labetalol			Exaggerated alpha response if alpha blockers are acutely withdrawn
Clonidine			
Beta-adrenergic blockers			
Propanolol	Beta agonists	↓ Beta-adrenergic effect	May need up to 20× usual doses of beta agonists
Timolol			
Metoprolol	Ketamine	↓ Sympathetic stabilization of circulation	Chronic use upregulates number of beta receptors
Nadolol			
Atenolol	Enflurane	↑ Cardiac depression and reduced response to hypovolemia	Do not abruptly withdraw beta-blockade perioperatively
			High dose beta blockade may be reduced to equivalent of 360 mg propranolol per day preoperatively
Calcium channel blockers			
Verapamil	Beta-blockers	Additive cardiac depression	
Diltiazem	Digitalis	↑ Blood digitalis level	
Nifedipine	Volatile anesthetics	Additive cardiac depression	
Nicardipine			
Central antihypertensives			
Reserpine	Volatile anesthetics	↓ Anesthetic requirement	
Guanabenz	Direct-acting sympathomimetics	Increased sympathomimetic response	Antihypertensives should be maintained throughout
Methyldopa		Decreased sympathomimetic response	perioperative period
	Indirect-acting sympathomimetics	May cause hypertension (due to beta$_2$- receptor blockade)	Reported with methyldopa only
	Propranolol		
Diuretics			
Furosemide	Antihypertensives	Potentiates hypotensive effect	
Bumetanide	Volatile anesthetics	Potentiates hypotensive effect	
Chlorthiazide	Digitalis	Hypokalemia ↑ toxicity	
	Muscle relaxants	Hypokalemia ↑ muscle weakness	
	Aminoglycosides	Potentiates ototoxicity	Especially with ethacrynic acid
Vasodilators and ACE inhibitors			
Captopril			
Enalapril	Volatile anesthetics	↑ Hypotensive effect	
Hydralazine			
Monoamine oxidase inhibitors (MAOI)			
Pargyline	Meperidine	Excitement, agiation, hypertension, tachycardia, rigidity, convulsion, coma	May be related to ↑ serotonin level
Isocarboxazid			
Phenelzine	Indirect-acting sympathomimetics	Hypertensive crisis	MAOI should be withdrawn for 2 weeks prior to elective surgery
Tranylcypromine	Tricyclic antidepressants	Hypertensive crisis	
	Opioids	↑ Sedation	Reported with phenelzine only
	Succinylcholine	↑ Paralysis	Reported with phenelzine only
Tricyclic antidepressants			
Amitriptyline	Barbiturates	↑ Sleeping time	
Desipramine	Anticholinergics	↑ Central and peripheral cholinergic effects	
Imipramine			
Doxepin	Direct-acting sympathomimetics	↑ Adrenergic response	
Nortriptyline			

(continued)

Table 20–2. continued

Drug Class and Examples	Interact with	Interaction	Comment
Phenothiazines and butyrophenones			
Chlorpromazine	Volatile anesthetics	↑ Hypotensive effect	Promethazine may have antianalgesic effect
Fluphenazine	Opioid drugs	↑ Sedation and respiratory depression	
Promethazine			
Haloperidol	Barbiturates	↑ Sleeping time	
	Anticholinergics	↑ Anticholinergic effects	Chronic phenothiazine therapy may cause myocardial toxicity
	Sympathomimetics	↓ Adrenergic response	
Lithium	Barbiturates	↑ Sleeping time	
	Muscle relaxants	↑ Duration of relaxation	
	Diuretics	↑ Lithium level	
Digitalis	Succinylcholine	May induce ventricular dysrhythmias	
	Volatile anesthetics	May ↓ digitalis-induced dysrhythmias	
Organophosphates			
Echothiophate	Succinylcholine	Prolonged apnea	Systemic absorption inhibits plasma cholinesterase
Isofluorophate			
Antiarrhythmics			
Quinidine	Volatile anesthetics	↑ Cardiac depression	
Procainamide	Muscle relaxants	↑ Neuromuscular blockade	
Amiodarone	Vasodilators	↑ Hypotension	May be related to alpha-blocking action
Bretylium	Direct-acting sympathomimetics	↑ Beta-adrenergic response	Only reported with bretylium

ministration are recent analgesic techniques that are superior to traditional intramuscular injections. Although PCA is simple and noninvasive, it requires a great degree of patient motivation and physical participation. Spinal opioid administration does not require patient activity, but it involves careful assessment of the patient's anatomy, ruling out contraindications, and it places high demand on the technical skill of the provider. An honest appraisal regarding postoperative discomfort and reassurance that adequate analgesia will be provided can greatly reduce the patient's apprehension at this juncture.

Assessment of Risks

Risk is defined as the chance of adverse outcome including death and serious morbidity. Pure anesthetic or surgical mishaps rarely occur, and adverse outcome after surgical procedures is multifactorial in origin. It is impossible to separate the risk of anesthesia from that of the operation or the condition that necessitates it. Thus, as summarized by Goldstein and Keats (1970), epidemiologic studies of anesthetic risk have widely varying results and severe limitations. Nonetheless, an assessment of risk before an operation is desirable to help place the potential benefits of the proposed procedure in perspective. Factors contributing to risk thus identified may also be amenable to intervention, in the hope of lowering the risk.

Events leading to adverse outcome can be divided into two groups. The first group of adverse events are mostly unrelated to the preoperative state of the patient and depend only on the nature of the surgery and the skill of the personnel. As shown by Anderson (1963), one of us (EAB) (1975), Goldman (1977), Steen (1978),

Rao (1983), and Forrest (1992) and their associates, the thoracic site of operation confers a higher risk for postoperative complication. In addition, four intraoperative threats are constantly present during thoracic surgery: sudden hemorrhage, cardiac arrhythmia, mechanical interference with the mediastinum, and ventilation/oxygenation difficulties. Other intraoperative threats not unique to thoracic surgery include adverse drug interaction and anaphylaxis, and rare occurrences such as malignant hyperpyrexia.

The second group of adverse events can reasonably be predicted from the preoperative state of the patient in the context of the proposed operation, and therefore interventions may affect the occurrence of these events. These events include pulmonary complications such as atelectasis, infection, and respiratory failure, and cardiac complications such as heart failure, myocardial ischemia or infarction, and serious arrhythmias. Identifying and modifying the factors leading to these adverse events constitute the subject of an extensive amount of literature.

One of the simplest and earliest rating scales for preoperative state is the American Society of Anesthesiologists — ASA — Physical Status classification (Table 20–3). Although it was originally conceived simply as a classification of the patient's physical status at the time of preanesthetic evaluation, Dripps (1961), Vacanti (1970), Marx (1973), one of us (EAB) (1975), and Forrest (1992) and their colleagues showed it to be a fairly good predictor of postoperative outcome. Note that this classification is not a predictor of intraoperative risks unrelated to the patient's preoperative state, such as hemorrhage and cardiac arrhythmias.

Table 20–3. American Society of Anesthesiologists (ASA) Classification of Physical Status

Status	Physical Attributes
I	Patients with no organic, physiologic, biochemical, or psychologic disturbance. The pathologic process for which the operation is to be performed is localized and not related to a systemic disturbance. Examples are the physically fit for elective inguinal herniorrhaphy or hysterectomy.
II	Patients with mild systemic disturbance caused by the condition to be treated surgically or by other pathophysiologic processes. Examples are patients with mild diabetes or mild hypertension.
III	Patients with moderate systemic disturbance from whatever cause even though it may not be possible to define the degree of disability with finality. Examples are patients with previous myocardial infarction or persistent cardiac arrhythmias.
IV	Patients with severe systemic disorder already life-threatening and not always correctable by the operative procedure. Examples are patients with cardiac insufficiency or advanced pulmonary disease.
V	Moribund patients who have little chance for survival and are subject to operation in desperation. Examples are moribund patients with a ruptured aortic aneurysm or a mesenteric thrombosis.

Pulmonary Complications

These complications are common after thoracic and abdominal surgical procedures. Respiratory insufficiency because of loss of lung tissue by surgical resection is fairly predictable based on preoperative pulmonary function and the extent of surgical intervention. This topic is discussed in detail in Chapter 18.

Pulmonary complications not directly caused by loss of lung tissue are related to the effect of surgery and anesthesia on various aspects of the respiratory system: mucociliary transport, mechanics of breathing, and decrease in the FRC and FVC. Estimation of risk of pulmonary complication is difficult. Early epidemiologic studies could be misleading: patients and case mix were often undefined, varying end points were used in morbidity measurement, the bias of preoperative treatment was ignored, and the effects of retrospective and prospective design were often not delineated in such reports. The focus of thoracic surgical literature itself has been on tuberculosis and cancer, and the risk of other types of thoracic surgical procedures therefore has to be extrapolated from data collected from these conditions.

From the existing literature, it is clear that an abnormal expiratory spirogram is a strong predictor of postoperative complication, but there is no agreement about the cut-off point for prohibitive risk. Grossly abnormal FVC, MVV of less than 50% of the predicted value and FEV_1 of less than 1 liter have been shown to be a sensitive predictor of death. Gracey and colleagues (1979) found that response to bronchodilators is another index, with good response indicating a favorable outcome. Forrest (1992) and associates in addition found that cardiac failure, myocardial ischemia,

and obesity are predictive of pulmonary complications. Based on the expiratory spirogram and findings in the cardiovascular system, central nervous system, arterial blood gas measurement, and expected postoperative course, Shapiro and associates (1985) proposed a scoring system for predicting the risks of postoperative pulmonary complications and the need for intensive postoperative support. This is a step toward quantifying the risks and providing a basis for measurement of effects of the preoperative intervention. To date, however, no data verifying the score are available.

The benefit of preoperative treatment of chronic obstructive lung disease in reducing postoperative pulmonary complications has been shown by Stein (1962), Tarhan (1972), and Gracey (1979) and their associates. Conditions amenable to such treatment include infection, acute exacerbation of bronchospasm, bronchorrhea, and cigarette smoking.

Cardiac Complications

Predicting and modifying the risk of perioperative cardiovascular morbidity and mortality have been the center of much attention in the past two decades. Reports from Topkins and Artusio (1964) and Tarhan (1972) and Steen (1976) and their associates emphasized the impact of coronary artery disease using previous myocardial infarction as a marker. The risk of sustaining a perioperative myocardial infarction after a previous infarction is about 6% — in contrast to 0.7% without previous myocardial infarction. History of a recent — less than 3 months old — myocardial infarction increases the risk five- to sixfold. Furthermore, mortality rate from perioperative reinfarction has been uniformly high — 36 to 70%. Recent reports by Wells and Kaplan (1986) and Rao (1983), Foster (1986), and Shah (1990) and their associates indicate a lower rate of reinfarction in the perioperative period. Although Rao and associates (1983) attribute this improvement to aggressive monitoring and early correction of identified physiologic abnormalities, other yet unidentified factors may be involved. Of note is the frequency of perioperative myocardial infarction during the second and third postoperative days, when many patients have already been discharged from the intensive care unit. A longer period of intensive postoperative observation may be indicated for high risk patients.

Besides previous myocardial infarction, signs of congestive heart failure and abnormal cardiac rhythm are consistent and powerful predictors of perioperative cardiovascular complications. Goldman and associates (1977) constructed a Cardiac Risk Index, which incorporates these as well as other less-weighted factors (Tables 20–4 and 20–5). Although the statistical method and universal applicability of this index have been questioned, it nevertheless highlights factors that are potentially amenable to preoperative treatment — such as congestive heart failure — and may therefore reduce morbidity and mortality.

Shields and Ujiki (1968) and Deutsch and Dalen (1969) discussed preoperative digitalization for thoracic surgery

Table 20–4. Factors Correlated with Cardiac Risk in Surgical Patients

Factor	Weighted Points
History	
Age > 70 years	5
Myocardial infarction in previous 6 months	10
Physical examination	
S_3 gallop or jugular venous distention	11
Important valvular aortic stenosis	3
Electrocardiogram	
Rhythm other than sinus rhythm or PAC	
on last preoperative electrocardiogram	7
> 5 PVC per minute at any time	7
General status	3
Pa_{O_2} <60 or Pa_{CO_2} >50 mm Hg	
K <3.0 or HCO_3^- <20 mEq/L^{-1}	
BUN >50 or creatinine >3.0 mg dl^{-1}	
Abnormal SGOT, signs of liver disease, or bedridden patient	
Operation	
Intraperitoneal, intrathoracic, or aortic	3
Emergency	4
Total Possible Points	53

From Goldman L, et al: Multifactorial index of cardiac risk in noncardiac surgical procedures. N Engl J Med 297:845, 1977.

patients. Current practice is not to use digitalization routinely to prevent cardiac arrhythmias. On the other hand, data from Mahar (1978), Hertzer (1984), Foster (1986), and Reul (1986) and their colleagues indicate that coronary artery bypass graft surgery, when otherwise indicated, confers protection against postoperative infarction in patients undergoing noncardiac surgery. Whether percutaneous transluminal angioplasty — PTCA — confers the same protection is unknown currently.

Disposition

By careful review of the medical record, patient interview, and examination, and taking into consideration the nature and demand of the proposed operation, the patient can usually be assigned to one of the following three categories: 1) the patient is in optimal condition and not at excessive risk, and anesthesia and surgery can proceed; 2) the patient's condition is questionable in some areas, and specialist consultation

and investigation are needed; and 3) the patient is obviously undertreated, and further preoperative treatment and followup evaluation are needed.

INTERDISCIPLINARY CONSULTATION

Because the anesthesiologist approaches the patient-operation complex from a perspective slightly different from that of other physicians, he or she frequently uncovers problems that may have been overlooked or ignored. The anesthesia and surgical teams must maintain open and equitable communication so that such problems can be satisfactorily resolved before an operation is performed.

In the event of a diagnostic or therapeutic uncertainty outside the defined expertise of both the surgeon and the anesthesiologist, specific specialist consultation is indicated. Examples are evaluation of chest pain and borderline electrocardiogram, diagnosis of complex arrhythmias, testing of pacemakers, and control of severe bronchospasm. Occasionally, a consultation may be needed in anticipation of a likely postoperative problem that will require specialist management, such as renal failure or total parenteral nutrition. A consultation is most rewarding when all who are involved maintain open communication and address specific questions. The traditional carte blanche "medical clearance" type of consultation is patronizing, misleading, and seldom helpful to the anesthesia and surgical teams in their patient management. Moreover, the anesthesiologist alone has to shoulder the responsibility for the stress of anesthesia and surgery on the patient, and therefore must make the final judgment, together with the surgeon, on the patient's suitability for the procedure and the anesthetic technique of choice. Del Guercio and Cohn (1980) presented data that indirectly support this position. Of 148 elderly patients who had been medically "cleared" for surgery, subsequent invasive hemodynamic data showed 23.5% to have had increased risks. All who were in this group and had surgery died. Of special interest, these patients were readily identified by experienced anesthesiologists using ASA physical status classification (see Table 20–3).

PSYCHOLOGIC PREPARATION OF THE PATIENT

Evaluation of the patient's preoperative psychologic state is an important part of the preanesthetic evalu-

Table 20–5. Correlation of Cardiac Risk with Total Points

Total Points	% Cardiac Death	% with Life-threatening Complications*	% with No or Minor Complications
0–5 (class I)	0.2 (1)[†]	0.7 (4)	99 (532)
6–12 (class II)	2.0 (5)	5.0 (16)	93 (295)
13–25 (class III)	2.0 (3)	11.0 (15)	86 (112)
>26 (class IV)	56.0 (10)	22.0 (4)	22 (4)

*Intraoperative or postoperative myocardial infarction, pulmonary edema, or ventricular tachycardia without progression to cardiac deaths.

[†]Figures in parentheses denote number of patients.

From Goldman L, et al: Multifactorial index of cardiac risk in noncardiac surgical procedures. N Engl J Med 297:845, 1977.

ation. For the patient, the impending operation is an anxiety-generating event. The anesthesiologist, because of his or her ability to modify that anxiety and to offer psychologic support, can establish close rapport in a short period. Such support and rapport have a calming effect on an otherwise anxious patient. Egbert and colleagues (1964) noted that an informative and reassuring approach from the anesthesiologist engenders patient confidence and reduces apprehension and anxiety. The patient should be encouraged to discuss fears and to explore events that will occur on the day of operation. Frank discussion of postoperative pain and assurance of the availability of adequate doses of analgesic drugs are helpful. This assurance can be augmented by appropriate drug therapy so that the patient arrives in the operating room calm, confident, and cooperative. The induction of anesthesia is safer, more controllable, and more pleasant for the calm patient than for one who is excited.

Egbert and associates (1963, 1964) emphasized that the need for strong postoperative narcotic analgesics, the incidence of postoperative complications, and the duration of hospital stay may be reduced significantly by an informative preoperative visit by the anesthesiologist.

INFORMED CONSENT

Before seeking consent to a particular course of anesthesia, the anesthesiologist has an obligation to inform the patient adequately of the potential benefits and risks of such a course, as well as of other available options. The difficulty lies in striking a balance between providing enough information and unduly alarming the patient, given the inherent risks of any anesthetic and surgery. Furthermore, the specific risks of thoracic surgery previously discussed, and possible preventive and corrective measures, must be honestly disclosed when applicable. This task may be eased in part by highlighting problems and risks that are amenable to preoperative correction, advising the patient in general terms that any anesthetic poses risks, and then inquiring if the patient wishes to know the specifics of all the possible risks. Many patients would then guide the anesthesiologist as far as their coping would allow. The essence of such discussion should be documented and forms are needed as part of the proof of informed consent. On occasion, a patient may decline any discussion of risks, or the physician may find the patient in a state unsuitable to bear such an ordeal. These also should be documented.

PREANESTHETIC MEDICATION

The aim of preanesthetic medication is to decrease anxiety without producing excessive drowsiness; facilitate a smooth, rapid induction without prolonged emergence; provide amnesia for the perioperative period while maintaining cooperation prior to loss of consciousness; and relieve preoperative pain. The classes of drugs commonly used for this purpose include: 1) sedatives, hypnotics, and tranquilizers; 2) opioids; 3) anticholinergics; and 4) antihistamines and antacids. The appropriate drugs and doses can be chosen only after the psychologic and physiologic conditions of the patient have been evaluated. The type and extent of the operation, the expected postoperative course, and the anesthetic technique to be used also need to be taken into consideration. In addition, Egbert and associates (1963) found that a good preanesthetic visit may be as effective as administration of sedatives in decreasing the level of anxiety.

Several categories of patients should only rarely receive preanesthetic medication before arriving in the operating room. These are patients with marginal cerebral function, uncorrected hypovolemia, or severe heart or lung disease, or both, whose respiratory and sympathetic drives are crucial, and those patients without informed consent.

CONCLUSION

Preanesthetic evaluation and preparation is an integral part of good anesthetic practice. It is essential for establishing physician-patient rapport and ensuring that the patient is in an optimal state for the proposed operation. By being thoroughly familiar with the patient and the operation, the anesthesiologist can take steps to minimize intraoperative risk and postoperative problems and to facilitate the performance of surgery. The choice of monitoring and anesthetic technique will follow rationally and will provide optimal safety for the patient.

REFERENCES

Anderson WH, Dossett BE, Hamilton GE: Prevention of postoperative pulmonary complications. JAMA *186*:766, 1963.
Brunner EA: Factors related to anesthesia risk. Surg Gynecol Obstet *141*:761, 1975.
Del Guercio LRM, Cohn JD: Monitoring operative risk in the elderly. JAMA *243*:1350, 1980.
Deutsch S, Dalen JE: Indications for prophylactic digitalization. Anesthesiology *30*:648, 1969.
Dripps RD, Lamont A, Eckenhoff JE: The role of anesthesia in surgical mortality. JAMA *178*:261, 1961.
Egbert LD, et al: The value of the preoperative visit by an anesthetist. JAMA *185*:553, 1963.
Egbert LD, et al: Reduction of postoperative pain by encouragement and instruction of patients. N Engl J Med *270*:825, 1964.
Forrest JB, et al: Multicenter study of general anesthesia. *III*. Predictors of Severe Perioperative Adverse Outcomes. Anesthesiology *76*:3, 1992.
Foster ED, et al: Risk of noncardiac operation in patients with defined coronary disease: The Coronary Artery Surgery Study (CASS) registry experience. Ann Thorac Surg *41*:42, 1986.
Goldman L, et al: Multifactorial index of cardiac risks in noncardiac surgical procedures. N Engl J Med *297*:845, 1977.
Goldstein A, Keats AS: The risk of anesthesia. Anesthesiology *33*:130, 1970.
Gracey DR, Divertie MB, Dider EP: Preoperative pulmonary preparation of patients with chronic obstructive pulmonary disease. Chest *76*:123, 1979.
Hertzer NR, et al: Coronary-artery disease in peripheral vascular

patients. A classification of 1,000 coronary angiograms and results of surgical management. Ann Surg *199*:223, 1984.

Mahar LJ, et al: Perioperative myocardial infarction in patients with coronary artery disease with and without aorta-coronary bypass grafts. J Thorac Cardiovasc Surg *76*:533, 1978.

Marx GF, Mateo CV, Orkin LR: Computer analysis of postanesthetic deaths. Anesthesiology *39*:54, 1973.

Reul GJ Jr, et al: The effect of coronary bypass on the outcome of peripheral vascular operations in 1,093 patients. J Vasc Surg *3*:788, 1986.

Rao TLK, Jacobs KH, El-Etr AA: Re-infarction following anesthesia in patients with myocardial infarction. Anesthesiology *59*:499, 1983.

Shah KB, et al: Reevaluation of perioperative myocardial infarction in patients with prior myocardial infarction undergoing noncardiac operations. Anesth Analg *71*:231, 1990.

Shapiro BA, et al: Clinical Application of Respiratory Care. Chicago: Year Book Medical Publishers, 1985, pp. 523–525.

Shields TW, Ujiki GT: Digitalization for prevention of arrhythmias following pulmonary surgery. Surg Gynecol Obstet *126*:743, 1968.

Steen PA, et al: Myocardial re-infarction after anesthesia and surgery. JAMA *239*:2566, 1978.

Stein M, et al: Pulmonary evaluation of surgical patients. JAMA *181*:765, 1962.

Tarhan S, et al: Risk of anesthesia and surgery in patients with chronic bronchitis and chronic obstructive disease. Surgery *74*:720, 1973.

Tarhan S, et al: Myocardial infarction after general anesthesia. JAMA *199*:318, 1972.

Topkins MJ, Artusio JF: Myocardial infarction and surgery: A five year study. Anesth Analg *43*:715, 1964.

Wells PH, Kaplan JA: Optimal management of patients with ischemic heart disease for noncardiac surgery by complementary anesthesiologist and cardiologist interaction. Am Heart J *102*:1029, 1981.

Vacanti CJ, VanHouten RT, Hill RC: A statistical analysis of the relationship of physical status to postoperative mortality in 68,388 cases. Anesth Analg *49*:564, 1970.

READING REFERENCES

Bendixen HH, et al: Respiratory Care. St Louis: CV Mosby, 1965.

Smith NT, Corbascio AN: Drug Interactions in Anesthesia. 2nd Ed. Philadelphia: Lea & Febiger, 1986.

Editorial views: The ASA classification of physical status — a recapitulation. Anesthesiology *49*:233, 1978.

Forrest WH, Brown CR, Brown BW: Subjective responses to six common preoperative medications. Anesthesiology *47*:241, 1977.

Mangano DT: Perioperative Cardiac Morbidity. Anesthesiology *72*:153, 1990.

CHAPTER 21

CONDUCT OF ANESTHESIA

Andranik Ovassapian

The anesthesiologist's responsibility begins with a careful preoperative assessment of the patient's condition. Pulmonary function tests and perfusion/ventilation studies are critical for selection of patients for intrathoracic operations and lung resection to avoid disastrous outcome. In addition to routine anesthetic problems, anesthesia for thoracic surgery is complicated by several factors: opening the chest produces a pneumothorax; manipulation of the lung, heart, and major vessels by the surgeon may interfere with ventilatory exchange and cardiovascular stability; and the lateral decubitus position changes the distribution of blood flow and pattern of ventilation and exposes the lower lung to danger of contamination by secretions from the operative lung. Thus, for safe conduct of anesthesia for thoracic surgery, the anesthesiologist should be knowledgeable about the physiology of one-lung ventilation — OLV — and be skillful in techniques for isolation of the lungs.

The introduction of double-lumen endobronchial tubes for one-lung anesthesia by Bjork and Carlens in 1950 represented a major advance in thoracic anesthesia. In 1958, Jenkins and Clark advocated the routine use of double-lumen tubes for all intrathoracic operations. Yet, the difficulty in blindly positioning these tubes and the resulting possibility of life-threatening complications discouraged their use by many anesthesiologists.

Several advances have made one-lung anesthesia safer and the double-lumen tube more popular. These include the availability of disposable, and in many ways superior, double-lumen tubes; the introduction of the bronchofiberscope — fiberscope — by Shinnick and Freedman (1982) and the author and associates (1983) for precise positioning of endobronchial tubes; and use of different treatment methods for management of hypoxemia during OLV and application of arterial blood gas or pulse oximetry for monitoring of blood oxygenation.

CHOICE OF ANESTHESIA

After thorough preoperative assessment and preparation of the patient, the anesthesiologist should choose an anesthetic plan that is both safe for the patient and suitable for the needs of the surgeon. An appropriate preoperative medication should be prescribed to make the patient relaxed and free of apprehension. Narcotics minimize patient discomfort during placement of arterial cannulae and large intravenous lines. The respiratory depression caused by narcotics in patients with advanced pulmonary disease, however, should be kept in mind. Judicious use of intravenous narcotics such as fentanyl while the patient is in the operating room and before any procedures provides the necessary analgesia. Oxygen — 2 to 3 liters — through a nasal cannula should be instituted if conscious sedation is provided for placement of various lines and an epidural catheter. Respiratory depression and hypoxemia is common with intravenous sedation.

Anticholinergic agents such as atropine or glycopyrrolate are prescribed with the premedication to decrease secretions during airway instrumentation, and to facilitate visualization of the airways when a fiberscope is used. Thornburn and colleagues (1986) showed that anticholingeric agents also improve pulmonary mechanics before general anesthesia. Because of the lower incidence of undesirable side effects, glycopyrrolate is the anticholinergic agent of choice.

General endotracheal and endobronchial anesthesia with controlled ventilation is an ideal anesthetic technique for most intrathoracic surgical procedures. A variety of high-frequency ventilation — HFV — techniques have been developed and recommended for operations performed on the airway and for intrathoracic procedures. During HFV, ventilatory excursions of the lungs are of low amplitude, which may facilitate surgical exposure and resection during intrathoracic operations. High-frequency ventilation has been used successfully in situations in which access to the airway is impaired. The success or failure of HFV and its advantages and disadvantages compared to conventional mechanical ventilation depend on the following: the type of HFV used, whether one-lung or two-lung ventilation is applied, and the type of surgical procedure. The three basic forms of HFV are high-frequency positive pressure ventilation — HFPPV, high-frequency jet ventilation — HFJV, and high-frequency oscillation — HFO. El-Baz and associates (1981, 1982) used one-lung HFPPV successfully for sleeve pneumonectomy and surgical procedures on large airways. Smith and colleagues (1981) reported successful use of HFPPV for pulmonary lobectomy. Hildebrand and co-workers (1984) applied HFJV for intrathoracic surgery, providing satisfactory operating conditions and ventilatory exchange. They indicated, however, that OLV using a double-lumen tube provides the optimal condition if the difficulties associated with placement of double-lumen tubes and related complications can be avoided. Glenski and co-workers (1986) demonstrated that HFO resulted in adequate pulmonary gas exchange and excellent surgical conditions for peripheral lung procedures; however, for procedures on the major airway or mediastinal structures, surgical conditions were unsatisfactory during HFO. They believe that the disadvantage of HFO outweighs the advantages during intrathoracic surgery.

A unique feature of thoracic anesthesia is the use of OLV. The selection of an anesthetic technique and agent will be influenced by whether OLV is used and whether a high concentration of inspired oxygen can be delivered to the patient. The volatile halogenated anesthetic agents such as isoflurane, enflurane, and halothane permit the administration of a high inspired concentration of oxygen. In addition, halogenated agents depress the airway reflexes, cause bronchodilation, and can be eliminated through the lungs. The high concentration of inhalation anesthetic agents may interfere with hypoxic vasoconstriction, however, diverting blood flow from the ventilated to the nonventilated lung, increasing intrapulmonary shunting, and decreasing Pa_{O_2}. Another disadvantage of inhalation agents is the ease with which they may depress the myocardium and decrease the cardiac output. When narcotic analgesics are added to the anesthetic regimen, the concentration of inhalation agent is lowered. This adjustment helps alleviate the aforementioned problems associated with halogenated agents.

Induction of anesthesia is achieved by the intravenous administration of 5 μg/kg fentanyl and 2 to 3 mg/kg of sodium thiopental. Anesthesia is maintained with 50% nitrous oxide and 0.4 to 0.6% of isoflurane. An additional 10 to 15 μg/kg of fentanyl is given before and during OLV when N_2O is discontinued and anesthesia is maintained with a low concentration of inhalation agent and oxygen. At the conclusion of OLV, nitrous oxide is started again and no additional narcotic is given thereafter. If necessary, higher concentrations of an inhalation agent are used to maintain adequate depth of anesthesia. Muscle relaxants are used for intubation of the trachea and preventing diaphragmatic movement during the operation.

Weinrich and associates (1980) recommended a combination of ketamine, nitrous oxide, and muscle relaxant as an anesthetic for thoracic surgery. Ketamine has sympathomimetic properties; therefore, it supports the cardiovascular system and causes bronchodilation. It is a useful drug for the induction of general anesthesia in hypovolemic patients with an unstable cardiovascular system.

The use of epidural anesthesia to supplement a "light" general anesthesia is another approach that warrants consideration. It offers the advantage of decreasing the need to use neuromuscular blocking drugs or narcotic analgesics intraoperatively. This technique may receive more attention as epidural narcotics are used increasingly for the management of postsurgical pain. Training and experience in this technique, especially when a high or midthoracic approach is used, is needed. The technique should be used regularly to help sustain the expertise needed for its safe conduct.

During thoracic operations, it may be necessary to give various additional drugs for the control of cardiac dysrythmias, systemic blood pressure, cardiac output, or acid-base balance. Their dosage is similar to that used in other types of anesthesia. Caution should be exercised, however, in the use of vasodilators and vasopressors during OLV. Vasodilators such as sodium nitroprusside and nitroglycerin interfere with hypoxic pulmonary vasoconstriction. The vasopressors exert more vasoconstriction in oxygenated vessels than in hypoxic vessels. Consequently, both groups of drugs may divert blood flow from the ventilated to the nonventilated, hypoxic lung, which may then increase shunt and hypoxemia.

MONITORING

Various devices have been introduced to improve patient monitoring during anesthesia. Monitoring requirements differ among individual patients because of their general physical conditions, the presence or absence of cardiopulmonary disease, and the nature of their operative procedures. Monitoring of patients who are healthy and undergoing minor intrathoracic operations may be limited to routine monitors used in all patients undergoing general anesthesia. For most intrathoracic operations and during OLV, monitoring of beat-to-beat arterial blood pressure and the arterial blood oxygenation is essential. Direct arterial monitoring of blood pressure not only provides beat-to-beat measurement of pressure, but also permits analysis of arterial blood gases and acid-base status during and after the operation. The pulse oximeter provides a noninvasive, continuous monitoring of the hemoglobin saturation and the heart rate. Improvement in the design of pulse oximeters, especially of the sensors, and introduction of an ear lobe oximeter probe have made the pulse oximeter a reliable, easy-to-use monitor. The pulse oximeter displays percentage of oxyhemoglobin. Over a wide range of arterial blood oxygen tension, the percentage of oxyhemoglobin does not change. Continuous monitoring of arterial blood gases and pH, which is now available, provides a better continuous monitoring method during OLV. The pulse oximeter should also be used postoperatively in postanesthesia and intensive care units.

The measurement of central venous pressure — CVP — is indicated in hypovolemic patients, when large volume shifts are anticipated, in patients with trauma and multiple injuries, and in patients with right ventricular dysfunction. Continuous or serial measurements are useful in the management of fluid and blood replacement when venous tone and myocardial function remain stable. The response of the CVP to a rapid volume infusion is a useful test of right ventricular function. The CVP is subject to mechanical interference, however, especially during thoracic surgery.

The internal jugular and subclavian veins are common sites for central venous cannulation. It is wise to use the vein ipsilateral to the thoracotomy, because pneumothorax is a known complication of deep vein cannulation. In patients with left ventricular dysfunction, the CVP may not provide accurate information about left ventricular filling pressure. Under these circumstances, a pulmonary capillary wedge pressure should be measured by using a flow-directed pulmonary artery catheter. In most patients, the pulmonary capillary wedge pressure corresponds well with the left atrial pressure. The pulmonary artery catheter allows measurements of pulmonary artery systolic, diastolic, and mean pressures, along with the pulmonary capillary wedge pressure, CVP, and cardiac output. In addition, it provides the ability to sample mixed venous blood and to calculate the shunt. Peripheral and pulmonary vascular resistance can be calculated. Serial measurements of cardiac output can help to assess the status of the circulation and guide any necessary supportive therapy. Information derived from centrally placed catheters indicates how the myocardium manages the fluid load; however, the CVP and pulmonary wedge pressure will reflect changes in blood volume when depth of anesthesia and myocardial performance are unchanged. The combination of a fall in CVP or pulmonary wedge pressure and systemic arterial pressure suggests hypovolemia, whereas a high CVP and pulmonary wedge pressure with a low arterial pressure may indicate poor myocardial performance.

New anesthesia machines are equipped with monitors and alarm systems; these include an inspired oxygen concentration monitor and a spirometer to measure expired tidal volume, a low and high airway pressure and an apnea alarm system. The use of muscle relaxants is monitored by a peripheral nerve stimulator and the body temperature is measured by an esophageal or a tympanic membrane probe. The availability of mass spectrometry or end-tidal CO_2 analysis provides additional monitoring of the patient's ventilation and confirms the proper placement of an endotracheal tube. The addition of pulse oximetry, used to monitor arterial oxygen saturation noninvasively, permits the early detection of impaired oxygenation, especially during OLV.

ONE-LUNG ANESTHESIA

One-lung anesthesia is a must under certain circumstances and provides safety for the patient and better operative conditions for surgeon. Because of its complexity, however, it adds to anesthetic difficulties. The most common indication for one-lung anesthesia providing the surgeon with a quiet operating field. A bronchopleurocutaneous fistula, communicating empyema, bronchial hemorrhage, lung abscess, and giant air cyst and operations performed through video-assisted thoracoscopy represent the absolute indications for isolating the individual lungs. This measure prevents the spread of secretions to the healthy lung and helps ensure adequate ventilation. Thoracoscopy, although not a new surgical technique, has gained popularity in recent years with the development of appropriate video equipment, and is applied for many diagnostic and therapeutic intrathoracic operations, such as drainage of empyema, evacuation of hemothorax, bleb resection, and mediastinal lymph node and lung biopsy. Deflation of the operative lung is mandatory during video-assisted thoracoscopy.

Methods of Obtaining One-Lung Ventilation

Four categories of bronchial catheters or blockers are used to achieve separation of the lungs. These are single-lumen tubes with one or two cuffs, bronchial blockers, double-lumen tubes of several types, and the Univent tube.

Single-Lumen Endotracheal Tubes

Single-lumen endobronchial tubes with one or two inflatable cuffs were the first tubes used for one-lung anesthesia. They are introduced into the bronchus of the healthy nonoperative lung. Their major disadvantage is that the operative lung cannot be inflated or suctioned without losing the separation of the lungs. These tubes are rarely used today.

Bronchial Blockers

Bronchial blockers are introduced into the bronchus of the diseased lung while the healthy nonoperative lung is ventilated through a tracheal or contralateral bronchial tube. Fogarty arterial embolectomy catheters have been used in children by Vale (1969) and Hogg and Lorhan (1970), as well as by Cay and associates (1975). They may be positioned blindly, or more usually through a conventional bronchoscope, or with the help of a bronchofiberscope under topical or general anesthesia. Ginsberg (1981) advocated the use of Fogarty catheters in adults, whereas Dalens and colleagues (1982) used Swan-Ganz pulmonary artery catheters for this purpose in children. Aspiration of secretions or temporary ventilation of the diseased lung is not possible without losing the separation of the lungs. Dislodgement of blockers is common with coughing, changing from being supine to the lateral position, or during surgical manipulation.

*Fiberscopic-Aided Placement of Balloon-Tipped
Catheters as Bronchial Blockers*

The fiberscope can be used to place a Fogarty or similar balloon-tipped catheter into the desired bronchus. As suggested by Ginsberg (1981), the distal end of the Fogarty catheter is angled to 30° to facilitate advancement into either main stem bronchus. After the patient is anesthetized and paralyzed, rigid laryngoscopy is performed and first a Fogarty catheter and then a tracheal tube are passed through the larynx into the trachea. A swivel adapter with endoscopy port is placed on the tracheal tube connector and mechanical ventilation is begun. The fiberscope is passed through the swivel adapter into the trachea to expose the catheter and the carina. The tip of the catheter is then advanced under direct vision into the desired main stem bronchus.

For left-lung blockade, the tip of the Fogarty catheter is advanced into the lower lobe bronchus so that the balloon of the catheter is positioned just above the orifice of the left upper lobe bronchus. For blockade of the right lung, the balloon is placed against the orifice of the right upper lobe bronchus. Once the catheter is positioned correctly, the balloon is inflated with air to occlude the main stem bronchus. Rao and associates (1981) placed a Fogarty catheter in the diseased lung and tracheal tube in the main stem bronchus of the healthy lung in children to achieve the same objective as double-lumen tube achieves in adults. If the Fogarty catheter fails to block the diseased bronchus, the dependent lung may still be protected by the presence of the bronchial tube. Baraka and colleagues (1982) reported a high incidence of right upper lobe collapse with blind intubation of the right main stem bronchus. This complication can be avoided by accurately positioning the tracheal tube with a fiberscope.

Double-Lumen Endobronchial Tubes

Double-lumen endobronchial tubes with two cuffs, consisting of two completely separate lumens, have their proximal ends separated into two connector limbs. A tracheal cuff is located proximal to the opening of the tracheal lumen and a bronchial cuff is located at the tip of the bronchial tube. Tubes designed for intubation of the right main stem bronchus have an opening in the bronchial cuff — bronchial cuff slit — to permit ventilation of the right upper lobe. When a double-lumen tube is positioned properly and the bronchial and tracheal cuffs are inflated, a separate airway is formed for each lung. The main advantage of double-lumen bronchial tubes is that, although isolation of the lungs is preserved, one or both lungs can be ventilated. The Carlens double-lumen tube described in 1949, which has a carinal hook, and the Robertshaw double-lumen tube described in 1962, which has no carinal hook, are used most commonly. Edwards and Hatch (1965) reviewed their clinical experience with them. Burton and associates (1983) demonstrated the advantages of the Bronchocath disposable double-lumen tubes. The advantages of these tubes include a softer and more flexible

structure, thin-walled tracheal and bronchial cuffs, a more gentle distal curve, and a greater inside-to-outside diameter ratio. These clear plastic, disposable tubes also allow observation of the humidity of exhaled air during the respiratory cycle.

After the patient is anesthetized and paralyzed, the double-lumen tube is inserted into the trachea using a rigid laryngoscope. The left-sided tube is held 90° rotated clockwise — to the right — and the right-sided tube is held 90° rotated counterclockwise — to the left — so the tip of the bronchial lumen faces anteriorly. After the tip is advanced beyond the vocal cords, the left-sided tube is rotated 90° counterclockwise and the right-sided tube is rotated 90° clockwise, to situate the tube in its normal position in the trachea, that is, the bronchial lumen facing toward the intended bronchus. With the Carlens — left-sided — and White — right-sided — double-lumen tubes with a carinal hook, as the tip of the bronchial lumen passes the vocal cords, the Carlens tube is rotated 180° counterclockwise and the White tube is rotated 180° clockwise to bring the carinal hook anteriorly to negotiate the vocal cords. After the carinal hook passes beyond the vocal cords, the Carlens tube is rotated 90° clockwise and the White tube is rotated 90° counterclockwise to have the bronchial lumen face the intended bronchus.

If rigid laryngoscopy proved difficult for tracheal intubation with a double-lumen tube, a fiberscope may be used for this purpose, as described by the author in 1990. The fiberscope is passed through the bronchial lumen of the tube. After exposure of the vocal cords, the fiberscope is advanced into the lower trachea. The double-lumen tube is maneuvered such that the tip of the tube faces posteriorly to pass beneath the epiglottis and then is rotated 180° to bring the tip anteriorly to pass through the vocal cords. After entering the trachea, the tube is rotated 90° right or left to position the tube such that the bronchial lumen faces toward the intended bronchus.

Once the double-lumen tube is placed in the trachea, the tracheal cuff is inflated. Mechanical ventilation is then initiated, with a tidal volume of 10 ml/kg and a rate of 8 breaths per minute. The rate of ventilation is adjusted to maintain a Pa_{CO_2} between 35 and 40 mm Hg. The fiberscope is then used to evaluate the bronchial tree and to position the double-lumen tube.

*Fiberscopic Positioning of Left-Sided Double-Lumen
Endobronchial Tubes*

If the double-lumen tube does not have a bronchoscopy port, a swivel adapter with a bronchoscopy port is placed on each lumen. While mechanical ventilation continues, the fiberscope is introduced into the bronchial lumen. The fiberscope is rotated 90° to the left and is advanced into the left main stem bronchus to evaluate its patency and length. Two techniques can be used for positioning the left endobronchial tube.

1. After inspection of the left main stem bronchus, the fiberscope is pulled back to position its tip 2 mm beyond the distal end of the bronchial lumen. The

fiberscope is rotated 90° to the left and the tip is angulated to view the lateral wall of the trachea. The tracheal cuff is deflated and the fiberscope and double-lumen tube are held together and advanced into the left main stem bronchus. The orifice of the left upper lobe bronchus comes into view when the fiberscope reaches 10 to 15 mm above this opening. The tube and fiberscope are advanced further until the distal end of the tube is positioned 5 mm above the opening of the left upper lobe bronchus (Fig. 21–1).

2. After evaluating the anatomy of the left main stem bronchus, the tip of the fiberscope is positioned 10 mm above the orifice of the left upper lobe bronchus. The tracheal cuff is deflated and the tube alone is advanced over the stationary fiberscope into the left main stem bronchus until it passes about 5 mm beyond the tip of the fiberscope. If the fiberscope is carefully stabilized during this maneuver, the tip of the endobronchial tube should lie 5 mm above the orifice of the left upper lobe bronchus. To confirm this positioning, the fiberscope is advanced beyond the bronchial lumen to visualize both the upper and lower lobe bronchi.

After positioning the left endobronchial tube with either technique, the fiberscope is withdrawn from the bronchial lumen and inserted into the tracheal lumen to check the position of the bronchial cuff from above and the opening of the right main stem bronchus. If the bronchial cuff is seen outside the left main stem bronchus, the tracheal cuff is deflated and the tube is advanced further until the proximal edge of the bronchial cuff lies 3 to 5 mm inside the left main stem bronchus. This placement ensures separation of the

lungs and stability of the tube, and prevents herniation of the bronchial cuff into the trachea. The bronchial and tracheal cuffs are then inflated using the minimal leak technique (Fig. 21–2).

Fiberoptic Positioning of Right-Sided Endobronchial Tubes

Proper positioning of right-sided double-lumen tubes is technically more difficult because of the short, variable-length right main stem bronchus. Rigg (1980) reported a high incidence of failure when these tubes were positioned blindly. The author and Schrader (1987) applied the following techniques successfully. The fiberscope is passed through the bronchial lumen into the right main stem bronchus. The patency, length, and anatomy of the right main stem bronchus, as well as the bronchus intermedius, are evaluated. If the right main stem bronchus is 15 mm or longer, placement of a Bronchocath right-sided double-lumen tube is possible. Either of the following two techniques can then be applied.

1. After inspection of the right main stem bronchus, the fiberscope is withdrawn inside the bronchial lumen, the fiberscope is rotated 90° to the right, and the tip is flexed anteriorly to position the tip of the fiberscope at the proximal end of the slit "Murphy eye" in the bronchial cuff. The tracheal cuff is deflated and the tube and fiberscope, while being held together, are advanced toward the right main stem bronchus. The view through the bronchial slit is the red mucosa of the tracheal and right main stem bronchial walls. The first indication of approaching the opening of the right upper lobe bron-

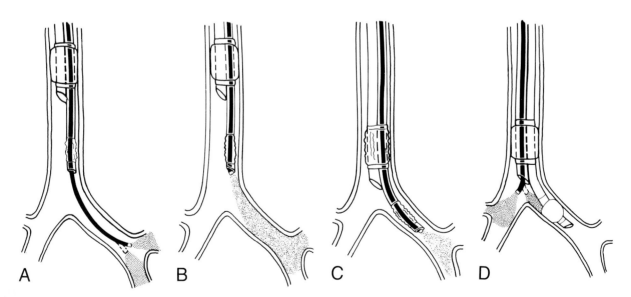

Fig. 21–1. Fiberscopic placement and positioning of left-sided, double-lumen endobronchial tube. *A*, The fiberscope is passed through the bronchial lumen into the left main stem bronchus. The patency, length, and anatomy of the left main stem bronchus and the position of the orifice of the left upper lobe bronchus are evaluated. *B*, The fiberscope is pulled back to position its tip 2 mm beyond the distal end of the bronchial lumen. The fiberscope is positioned 90° rotated to the left with the tip angulated anteriorly toward the lateral wall of the trachea. *C*, The tracheal cuff is deflated, and the tube and fiberscope are advanced together inside the left main stem bronchus until the orifice of the left upper lobe comes into view. At this point, the tip of fiberscope is 10 to 15 mm above the left upper lobe orifice. The tube is advanced further to position the distal end of the tube about 5 mm above the orifice of left upper lobe bronchus. *D*, The fiberscope is passed through the tracheal lumen to check the position of the bronchial cuff and the opening of the right main stem bronchus.

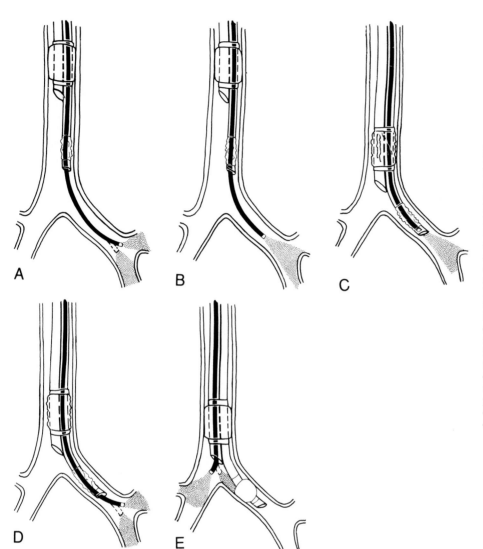

Fig. 21–2. Alternate approach to fiberscopic placement and positioning of left-sided, double-lumen endobronchial tube. *A,* The fiberscope is passed through the bronchial lumen into the left main stem bronchus. The patency, length, and anatomy of the left main stem bronchus and the position of the orifice of the left upper lobe bronchus are evaluated. *B,* The fiberscope is withdrawn, and its tip is positioned 10 mm above the origin of the left upper lobe bronchus. *C,* The tracheal cuff is deflated, and the tube is advanced over the fiberscope into the left main stem bronchus until it comes into view beyond the tip of the fiberscope. *D,* The fiberscope is advanced beyond the bronchial lumen to visualize the left upper lobe bronchus. *E,* The fiberscope is passed through the tracheal lumen to check the position of the bronchial cuff and the opening of the right main stem bronchus.

chus is a dark area at the distal end of the bronchial slit — the termination of the bronchial wall and the beginning of the orfice to the right upper lobe bronchus. This view is seen when the proximal end of the bronchial slit is about 10 to 15 mm above the opening to the right upper lobe bronchus. The tube and fiberscope are advanced further until the orifice of the right upper lobe bronchus comes into full view through the bronchial slit (Fig. 21–3). If necessary, the fiberscope can be advanced through the bronchial cuff slit into the right upper lobe bronchus to visualize the three segments of the right upper lobe. The fiberscope is then rotated 90° counterclockwise to its neutral position and is advanced beyond the tip of the endobronchial tube to check the opening of the right middle and lower lobe bronchi. The fiberscope is then withdrawn from the bronchial lumen and is passed through the tracheal lumen to check the position of the bronchial cuff and the opening of the left main stem bronchus (see Fig. 21–3).

2. After inspection of the right main stem bronchus and bronchus intermedius, the fiberscope is pulled back

and rotated 90° clockwise, and its tip is flexed anteriorly to visualize the orifice of the right upper lobe bronchus. While the fiberscope is held stationary, the tip of the fiberscope is returned to the neutral position. The tracheal cuff is deflated and the double-lumen tube is advanced over the fiberscope into the right main stem bronchus. When the distal end of the endobronchial tube comes into view through the fiberscope, advancement of the tube stops (Fig. 21–4). At this position, the bronchial cuff slit would be at the level of the orifice for the right upper lobe bronchus. It is critical that during advancement of the tube, the fiberscope is stabilized. The fiberscope is then withdrawn a few millimeters inside the bronchial lumen and its tip is flexed anteriorly to visualize the orifice of the right upper lobe bronchus through the slit in the bronchial cuff. Minor adjustments of the tube often are necessary to have a clear view of the right upper lobe orifice. The asymmetric design of the bronchial cuff in Bronchocath right-sided tubes makes it possible to position the tube correctly when the right main stem bronchus is as short

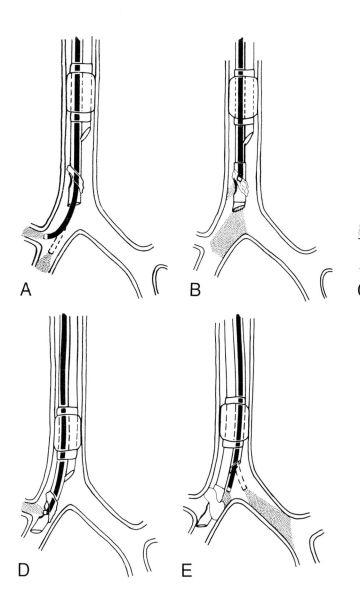

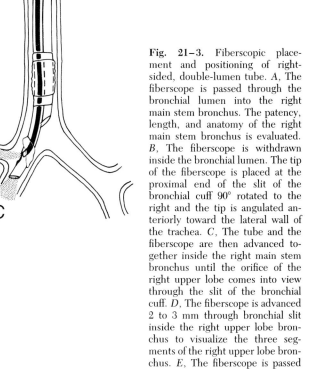

Fig. 21–3. Fiberscopic placement and positioning of right-sided, double-lumen tube. A, The fiberscope is passed through the bronchial lumen into the right main stem bronchus. The patency, length, and anatomy of the right main stem bronchus is evaluated. B, The fiberscope is withdrawn inside the bronchial lumen. The tip of the fiberscope is placed at the proximal end of the slit of the bronchial cuff 90° rotated to the right and the tip is angulated anteriorly toward the lateral wall of the trachea. C, The tube and the fiberscope are then advanced together inside the right main stem bronchus until the orifice of the right upper lobe comes into view through the slit of the bronchial cuff. D, The fiberscope is advanced 2 to 3 mm through bronchial slit inside the right upper lobe bronchus to visualize the three segments of the right upper lobe bronchus. E, The fiberscope is passed through the tracheal lumen to check the position of the bronchial cuff and the opening of the left main stem bronchus.

as 15 mm. The upper border of the bronchial cuff often is just at the level of the carina. As a result, air leak around the bronchial cuff is encountered more often with a right-sided tube than with a left-sided double-lumen tube after the patient is placed in the lateral position. Advancing the tube and fiberoptic repositioning is achieved easily while the patient is in the lateral decubitus position.

Verifying Functional Status of Double-Lumen Endobronchial Tubes

The following procedures help to determine whether the separation of the lungs has been achieved and adequate ventilation can be applied through each lung. With a mechanical ventilator set at a tidal volume of 10 ml/kg of ideal body weight and a rate of 8 breaths per minute, the exhaled tidal volume and the peak and plateau airway pressures are measured, and the expiratory flow rate on the respirometer and the humidification of both lumens by exhaled air are observed. After the tracheal connector tube is clamped, the breath sounds should only be present

on the bronchial side, and the respirometer may show a 10 to 15% decrease in the exhaled tidal volume, whereas the expiratory flow rate should remain the same. The peak airway pressure should increase by no more than 50% when compared to two-lung ventilation. The clamp is then moved to the bronchial connector tube. Breath sounds should be present on the tracheal side. Tidal volume, expiratory flow rate, and peak airway pressure should change little from one lung to another. The clamp is then removed and the tube is secured. After the patient assumes the lateral position, the measurements of tidal volume and airway pressures are repeated with each lumen occluded.

Placement is considered unsatisfactory if separation of the lungs is incomplete; if when changing from two-lung ventilation to one-lung ventilation, the tidal volume decreases by more than 15%; if the expiratory flow rate of either lung slows dramatically; or if the peak airway pressure increases by more than 50%.

If tube placement is unsatisfactory, the fiberscope is used to check the position of the bronchial cuff and to

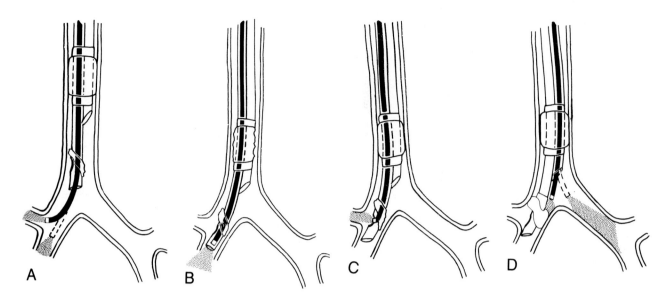

Fig. 21–4. Alternate approach to fiberscopic placement and positioning of right-sided, double-lumen endobronchial tube. *A*, The fiberscope is passed through the bronchial lumen into the right main stem bronchus. The patency, length, and anatomy of the right main stem bronchus are evaluated. The fiberscope is then rotated 90° to the right and the tip of the fiberscope is flexed anteriorly to visualize the right upper lobe bronchus. While the fiberscope is held stationary, its tip is returned to the neutral position. *B*, The tracheal cuff is deflated, and the tube is advanced over the fiberscope into the right main stem bronchus until it comes into view beyond the tip of the fiberscope. *C*, The fiberscope is withdrawn inside the bronchial lumen to visualize the orifice of the right upper lobe bronchus through the slit of the bronchial cuff. *D*, The fiberscope is passed through the tracheal lumen to check the position of the bronchial cuff and the opening of the left main stem bronchus.

ensure that the tip of the bronchial or tracheal lumen is neither pressed against the bronchial or tracheal walls nor is blocking the orifice to the left upper lobe bronchus. For right-sided tubes, the position of the slit in the bronchial cuff with respect to the orifice of the right upper lobe must be rechecked as well as the patency of the right middle and lower lobes. In the presence of advanced lung disease with loss of lung tissue, empyema, or atelectasis, more exaggerated changes in the preceding variables are expected when switching from two-lung ventilation to diseased lung ventilation. Bronchospasm may occur after bronchial intubation in lightly anesthetized patients or in patients with a reactive airway. In the presence of bronchospasm, more exaggerated changes in the variables are expected. These changes can be lessened by deepening anesthesia.

The peak airway pressure and tidal volume measurement during OLV are presented in Table 21–1.

Univent Tubes

Introduced by Inoue and associates in 1984, the Univent tube is an endotracheal tube with two lumens, a larger lumen for ventilation and a small lumen that encloses the endobronchial blocker (Fig. 21–5). The endobronchial blocker has a hollow core that may be used for insufflation of oxygen, suctioning of secretions, and possibly jet ventilation.

The bronchial blocker has a high volume cuff at its tip. A movable cap on the shaft of the bronchial blocker is incorporated to seal the leak between the shaft of the blocker and its housing lumen and to keep the blocker from moving. This cap is mounted over the blocker

Table 21–1. Tidal Volumes and Peak Airway Pressures During One-Lung Ventilation

	Supine		Lateral	
	TV	PAP	TV	PAP
Left-sided tube (N = 25)				
Two-lung ventilation	813±71	22±3	817±76	23±4
Left-lung ventilation	740±81	34±5	746±62	35±5
Right-lung ventilation	763±71	32±4	761±65	33±5
Right-sided tube (N = 8)				
Two-lung ventilation	818±81	23±4	821±90	23±4
Left-lung ventilation	750±76	36±5	759±69	35±3
Right-lung ventilation	722±69	35±7	758±58	34±4

Abbreviations: TV, Tidal volume of 10 to 12 ml/kg; PAP, peak airway pressure (cm H_2O).

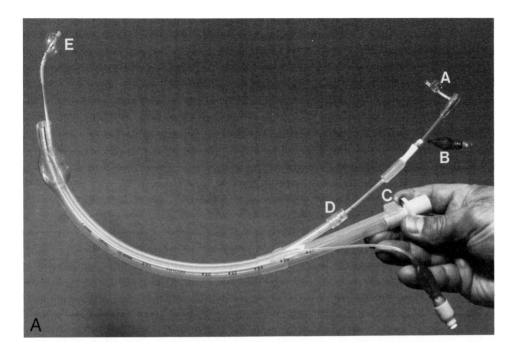

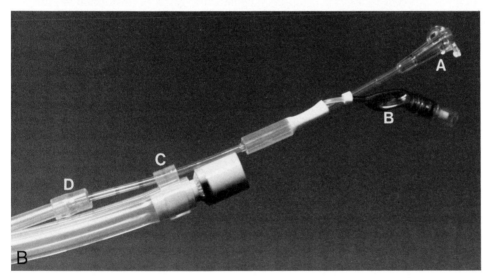

Fig. 21–5. The Univent Tube. *A*, The Univent tube with bronchial blocker is advanced outside the lumen of the tube and the balloon is inflated. A = Attached plug to close the internal lumen of the blocker when one-lung ventilation is not applied. This cap should not be engaged (bronchial blocker lumen open) during one-lung ventilation. B = Bronchial blocker inflation balloon. C = Hand stopper secures the bronchial blocker and prevents its movement. D = Moveable cap on the shaft of the bronchial blocker to seal off the leak between the blocker and its housing lumen. It also keeps blocker from moving. E = Inflated bronchial blocker cuff. *B*, Close-up of the proximal end of the Univent tube. A = Plug that closes the lumen of the blocker. B = Bronchial blocker balloon. C = Hand stopper secures the bronchial blocker. D = Movable cap on the shaft of bronchial blocker

housing lumen as soon as the blocker is placed in the bronchus. An attached plug at the proximal end of the blocker is provided to close the internal lumen of the blocker. After tracheal intubation, the endobronchial blocker may be placed in either main stem bronchus. Inflating the tracheal and bronchial cuffs provides separation of the lungs and allows OLV. The Univent tube has a relatively larger external diameter for its internal diameter relative to a standard single-lumen tracheal tube.

The tip of the blocker is hard and repeated attempts during blind placement may traumatize the tracheobronchial tree. Arari and Hatano (1987) reported dislodgement of the tip of the bronchial blocker cap. If a Univent tube is left in place for postoperative ventilation, precaution should be taken to avoid inadvertent inflation of the bronchial blocker cuff; acute airway

obstruction occurs if the blocker is moved into the trachea. One such incident was reported by Dougherty and Hannallah in 1992. MacGillivray (1988) reported that herniation of the bronchial cuff is common with the Univent tube because the Univent bronchial blocker cuff requires a larger volume of air, 6 to 8 ml, compared to double-lumen tubes, 2 to 3 ml. Herniation of the bronchial blocker cuff with the Univent tube is more likely when the blocker is placed inside the right main stem bronchus. Incomplete separation of the lungs is also encountered, although the incidence of such complications needs to be studied.

Positioning

First the bronchial blocker is lubricated and moved a few times in and out of its housing lumen to ensure free movement of the blocker. The blocker is then retracted inside the housing lumen before the Univent tube is placed inside the trachea using a conventional intubation technique. The blocker can be advanced up to 8 cm beyond the tip of the main tube. For blind placement of the endobronchial catheter — blocker, the Univent tube is rotated 90° toward the operative lung — side to be blocked — and is taped in this position. The endobronchial blocker is then advanced several centimeters to enter the intended main stem bronchus.

After proper positioning of the endobronchial blocker, the shaft of the bronchial blocker is secured to the main tube with the cap and hand stoppers. Karwande (1987) reported successful blind placement of the blocker in 45 of 50 — 90% — consecutive cases. For 5 patients, blocker placement had to be done under fiberscope guidance. In two cases, the blocker was dislodged after it was positioned. Fiberscopic positioning was possible with the patient in the lateral decubitus position. Suctioning of the operative lung is possible through the lumen of the blocker, and, if necessary, the operative lung can be ventilated with HFV. Hultgren and co-workers (1986) reported successful use of Univent tubes in 30 consecutive patients, but in 1 patient, the blocker entered the wrong side. MacGillivray (1988) reported successful seal of the intended bronchus only in 1 of 8 patients. Fiberscopic manipulation resulted in successful placement in another 4 patients, but good seal could not be obtained in 3 patients and the Univent tube was replaced by a double-lumen tube.

Fiberscopic Positioning

After the Univent tube is placed in the trachea, the tube is rotated 90° toward the operative side and taped. A bronchoscopic swivel adapter is connected to the tube. The fiberscope is passed through the Univent tube to identify the bronchial anatomy and to assist in bronchial blocker placement under fiberscopic observation. If the blocker enters the intended bronchus, the fiberscope is used for proper placement of the cuff inside the bronchus. If the blocker is not entering the intended bronchus, the fiberscope is used to guide the blocker toward the bronchus. The blocker is left in the desired position with the cuff deflated. Before going to OLV, the tube is disconnected from the anesthesia machine and the surgeon compresses the lung to collapse it. After the lung is collapsed, the blocker balloon is inflated to block the main stem bronchus. The listed advantages of the Univent tube include easier placement than occurs with double-lumen tubes, and no need to change it for fiberoptic bronchoscopy or for postoperative ventilatory support. The functional status of OLV is checked as described in the section concerning double-lumen endobronchial tubes.

One-Lung Ventilation

Larsson and associates (1987) demonstrated that functional residual capacity — FRC, compliance, and fraction of total ventilation decreases slightly in the dependent lung, when the anesthetized patient is placed in the lateral position. The FRC decreases further when the pleural cavity is opened, presumably because of further downward shift of the mediastinum. These findings are similar to that described by Froese and Bryan (1974) who attributed these changes in the lower — dependent — lung to compression of the lung by the weight of mediastinum and to the elevation of the diaphragm. General anesthesia and muscle relaxation further decrease the FRC and cause atelectasis in the dependent lung. This decrease in FRC with maldistribution of ventilation in relation to perfusion results in further decrease in Pa_{O_2}.

To avoid atelectasis of the dependent lung, tidal volume of 10 ml/kg is used. Kerr and associates (1973) showed that if minute ventilation is not decreased during OLV, the arterial carbon dioxide tension is maintained at a similar level to that of two-lung ventilation. The use of a large tidal volume to ventilate one lung results in increased peak airway pressure by approximately 50%. When airway pressure increases, Cote and colleagues (1983) showed that a larger proportion of the delivered total volume may be wasted because of the compression effect on gases or distention of the anesthesia machine breathing circuit, or both. The result may be a slight decrease in alveolar ventilation and increase in Pa_{CO_2}.

The factors contributing to hypoxemia during OLV are: shunting in the nonventilated lung, demonstrated by Kerr and associates (1973); ventilation/perfusion abnormalities in the ventilated lung; and reduction in the cardiac output. To counteract hypoxemia, the operative lung should be ventilated with 100% oxygen with large tidal volume. In a small percentage of patients, however, the Pa_{O_2} may still remain suboptimal. Various techniques have been applied to improve the arterial Pa_{O_2} under these circumstances. One such technique is insufflation of oxygen into the nonventilated lung. Results are inconclusive; Rees and Wansbrough (1982) showed improvement, whereas Capan and associates (1980) showed that it is ineffective without application of continuous positive airway pressure — CPAP. The use of CPAP to the nonventilated lung improves arterial oxygenation, but it leads to overdistention of the operative lung and suboptimal surgical conditions. Applying HFJV with low driving pressure to the operative lung, Wilks and co-workers (1985) demonstrated improved oxygenation during OLV while maintaining a good surgical field. Nakatuska and associates (1988) compared the effect of CPAP and HFJV to the nondependent lung on the cardiac output and Pa_{O_2} during OLV. The application of HFJV to the nondependent lung caused a significant increase in Pa_{O_2} compared with deflation of the lung to atmosphere pressure, and also maintained better cardiac output compared to that of CPAP. In addition, HFJV provides a quiet surgical field and satisfactory surgical exposure by delivering small tidal volumes with a low airway pressure in spite of vibratory movement of the surgical field. Malmkvist (1989) reported that intermittent re-inflation of the upper lung with 2 liters of oxygen every

5 minutes improved Pa_{O_2} during OLV. It seems logical that gentle independent ventilation of the operative lung with small tidal volumes coordinated with surgeon's movements would be a simple, inexpensive approach to improving Pa_{O_2}.

In the dependent lung, compression by the mediastinum and cephalad movement of the paralyzed diaphragm result in a decrease in FRC. This results in underventilation of well-perfused alveoli and an increase in airway closure. Trapped gas comes into equilibrium with mixed venous blood, contributing to arterial desaturation. Application of PEEP to the dependent, ventilated lung may improve the situation. Khanam and Branthwaite (1973), however, observed that application of PEEP to the ventilated lung may increase not only FRC, but also intra-alveolar pressure, shifting a higher proportion of pulmonary blood flow to the nonventilated lung, and contributing to a reduction in cardiac output.

Ashton and Cassidy (1985) showed that decreased cardiac output and systemic vascular resistance is induced by cardiac depressor reflexes as a result of stimulation of pulmonary stretch receptors. The magnitude of this cardiac depressor reflex is proportional to the magnitude of lung inflation. The effect of the reflex is antagonized by arterial baroreceptors, and a large tidal volume can reduce baroreceptor activity. This decrease in cardiac output in the face of systemic hypoxemia may lead to a significant decrease in oxygen transport. Depending on the degree of increased intra-alveolar pressure during application of PEEP and its effect on the pulmonary circulation and cardiac output, the Pa_{O_2} may increase, decrease, or remain the same, according to Katz and associates (1982). Pulmonary vascular congestion, interstitial edema of lower lung, hypovolemia, dysrhythmia, myocardial depression, and surgical manipulation can all decrease the cardiac output and contribute to arterial desaturation. Ligation of the branches of the pulmonary artery to the collapsed section of lung will reduce the shunt and improve the arterial blood oxygenation.

Kerr (1973) and Flacke (1976) and their associates have shown that the shunt through the nonventilated lung is about 20 to 25% of the cardiac output. This degree of shunt is less than one would expect from complete collapse of entire lung. Several factors are responsible. First, the effect of gravity and hydrostatic pressure in the lateral decubitus position increases the blood flow to the dependent lung. Second, the operative lung may have decreased pulmonary blood flow, because of underlying pathologic conditions. Hurford and associates (1987) showed that in many patients, the degree of preoperative perfusion and ventilation of the operative lung correlated inversely with interoperative oxygenation during OLV. Many patients with normal perfusion of the operative lung, however, did have adequate level of oxygenation during OLV. This diminishes the value of operative lung ventilation perfusion as a predictor of hypoxemia during OLV. Third, Benumof (1978) showed that hypoxic pulmonary vaso-

constriction — HPV — increases pulmonary vascular resistance in the operative lung, which diverts blood flow away from the operative lung and toward the nonoperative, dependent lung.

Anesthetic concentrations of inhalation agents may abolish hypoxic pulmonary vasoconstriction, thereby increasing the blood flow to the nonventilated lung, and consequently decreasing the Pa_{O_2}. Rogers and Benumof (1983) and Augustine and Benumof (1984) showed that halothane and isoflurane cause an insignificant change in the amount of shunted blood when used in a concentration of one minimum alveolar concentration — MAC — or less. To avoid the possible inhibition of hypoxic pulmonary vasoconstriction from higher concentrations of inhalation anesthetics and to minimize the respiratory depressant effect of high doses of narcotics, a combination of a narcotic and inhalation anesthetics may be particularly useful for intrathoracic operations.

Complications

Complications related to the isolation of lungs and application of OLV fall into two categories: technical and physiologic (Table 21-2). Because of the shape and large size of double-lumen tubes, the incidence of difficult tracheal intubation is higher than with the use of single-lumen tubes. The practical difficulties encountered with Robertshaw tubes were reviewed by Black and Harrison (1975). Complications included laceration of the tracheobronchial tree and malposition of the tube. The site of laceration is usually the posterior membranous wall of the trachea or a main stem bronchus. The diagnosis may be difficult to make, but it can be confirmed by fiberoptic bronchoscopy. Improper positioning of double-lumen endobronchial tubes reported by Read and associates (1977) includes failure to advance the tube far enough down the intended bronchus. Difficulties resulting from improperly positioned en-

Table 21-2. Complications of Bronchial Intubation and One-Lung Ventilation

Technical
Unsuccessful or difficult intubation
Trauma of the airway
Minor trauma
Rupture of tracheobronchial tree
Improper position of the bronchial tube
Tube not inserted far enough
Intubation of wrong bronchus
Tube inserted too far into the bronchus
Tube dislodgement

Physiologic
Hypoxemia
Increased venous admixture
Alteration of hypoxic pulmonary vasocontriction
Increased intra-alveolar pressure
Decreased cardiac output
Atelectasis of dependent lung

dobronchial tubes include incomplete isolation of the lungs; failure to collapse the operative lung; difficulty in ventilating one or both lungs; air entry into the wrong lung; and air trapping and unsatisfactory deflation of the lung. If not recognized, air trapping can eventually cause rupture of the lung and tension pneumothorax. If any of these circumstances arise, two-lung ventilation should be resumed, and the cause of the problem should be identified and corrected before OLV is attempted once again. The physiologic complication of OLV is hypoxemia.

BLOOD AND FLUID REPLACEMENT

Blood and fluid replacement during thoracic surgery is a delicate task and an extremely important part of the anesthetic management. Great care must be taken not to overload the circulation, especially in patients undergoing lobectomy or pneumonectomy, because the pulmonary venous capacitance is greatly reduced. Blood loss during most intrathoracic operations does not necessitate a transfusion, but major bleeding can occur at any time. A large intravenous cannula that allows blood and fluid to be administered rapidly is essential, as is the ready availability of blood. All fluids, especially blood, should be warmed during administration.

The perioperative fluid regimen recommended by Giesecke and Egbert (1986) is to replace NPO insensible loss with maintenance type solution 5% dextrose in water, 5% dextrose in 0.45% saline at a rate of 2 ml/kg/hour. During surgery, in addition to 2 ml/kg/hour of insensible loss, an additional 6 ml/kg/hour of replacement-type solution lactated Ringer's, 5% dextrose in lactated Ringer's, saline, normosal is recommended for intrathoracic surgery.

This regimen is followed only for the first hour or two of the operation to avoid overhydration. Hutchin and associates (1969) discussed the danger of overhydration of patients during pneumonectomy. Infusion of large volumes of fluids may improve the urine output and circulatory dynamics, but at the risk of developing pulmonary edema and impaired lung mechanics. Twigley and Hillman (1985) stated that crystalloid solutions given intraoperatively go to the interstitial space. Brinkmeyer (1981) and Baek (1975) and their associates noted that excessive amounts of crystalloid solutions increase interstitial fluid, which causes peripheral and pulmonary edema without correcting the plasma volume deficit. To maintain an adequate blood volume and urine output and to avoid overhydration and congestion of the tissues, including the lungs, Twigley and Hillman (1985) suggested using colloid solutions perioperatively. This suggestion is based on the fact that most intraoperative cardiovascular changes are secondary to an absolute or relative change in intravascular circulating volume, caused by bleeding and vasodilatory effects of anesthetic drugs. These changes are ideally corrected with a colloid.

Colloid solutions are useful to expand plasma volume and should be considered for replacing blood and fluid loss when the patient's blood pressure and pulse rate reflect signs of hypovolemia. The controversy of crystalloid or colloid use for blood and fluid replacement continues unresolved. In addition to monitoring of blood pressure, pulse rate, and urine output, monitoring of central venous pressure — CVP — and pulmonary artery occlusive pressure — PAOP — is helpful in guiding appropriate fluid therapy, especially in patients with poor general health and during operations with major blood and fluid losses. As indicated by Wittnich and colleagues (1986), however, care is needed in regard to technique of measurement and interpretation of PAOP. They have shown that after pneumonectomy, inflation of the balloon of the pulmonary artery catheter can result in considerable occlusion of the remaining cross-sectioned area of pulmonary circulation. This increase in right ventricular afterload results in reduced cardiac output and reduced left atrial pressure — LAP. Therefore, PAOP may reflect the correct pressure of LAP, although this is a result of acute change in cardiac output. Measuring pulmonary wedge pressure by advancing the catheter to peripheral vessels and without inflation of the balloon provides more accurate reading of the existing pressures.

Continuous measurement of CVP and pulmonary artery wedge pressures is helpful in patients with myocardial disease or advanced pulmonary disease. In a patient with a healthy heart, however, a serious overload of crystalloid solutions is possible without significant elevation of the CVP or pulmonary artery wedge pressure, particularly if infusion of fluid is constant over several hours. Soft tissue edema and increased urine output are the best signs of overload with intravenous fluids. Edema is seen most easily in the scleral conjunctiva. Congestion and edema of tissues caused by overhydration is also position dependent. In the lateral decubitus position, the nonoperative, healthy lung is dependent and accumulates more fluids. A moderate fluid overload can result in decreased Pa_{O_2} intraoperatively and moderate to severe hypoxemia in the immediate postoperative period.

The shortage of blood, together with transfusion hazards, has stimulated a search for alternatives to the use of homologous blood since the 1970s. Transmission of AIDS through blood transfusion has further increased the public's fear of accepting blood transfusion. Autologous transfusion by aspiration from the surgical field was reported by Bergman and co-workers (1974). Brewster and associates (1979) showed that intraoperative autotransfusion significantly reduced the use of homologous blood transfusion. Preoperative donation of blood by the patient and the value and importance of an autologous blood program was emphasized by Haugen and Hill (1987). Normovolemic hemodilution is possible on the day of the operation if the physical condition of the patient permits.

SPECIFIC PROCEDURES AND SUGGESTED MANAGEMENT

Bronchoscopy

During bronchoscopy, the airway is shared by the surgeon and anesthesiologist, and the patient's ventilation must be monitored carefully. Both rigid and fiberoptic bronchoscopy, under topical anesthesia and sedation, are performed by the surgeon. Patients with severe systemic or pulmonary disease or a severely compromised airway, and patients who are overly anxious, may benefit from the expertise of the anesthesiologist. Administration of atropine, 0.6 to 0.8 mg IM, or glycopyrrolate, 0.3 to 0.4 mg IM, 30 minutes before bronchoscopy is essential, as the airway must be dry for the topical anesthesia to be effective. After conscious sedation, topical anesthesia is applied as follows. Lidocaine 4% is sprayed on the base of the tongue and tonsillar fossae; after 45 seconds, lidocaine jelly is spread on the base of the tongue with a tongue blade. Lidocaine jelly is applied to an Ovassapian (1987) intubating airway (Fig. 21–6), which is then placed in the patient's mouth, and the oropharynx is suctioned. The intubating airway keeps the tongue positioned anteriorly, facilitates exposure of the larynx, and protects the bronchofiberscope from being bitten by the patient. The bronchofiberscope is advanced through the intubating airway to expose the larynx. The local anesthetic is sprayed over the laryngeal vestibule, vocal cords, arytenoids, and pyriform sinuses. After 45 seconds, the tip of the fiberscope is passed beyond the vocal cords and lidocaine is sprayed inside the trachea and carina.

General anesthesia for bronchoscopy must provide unconsciousness, sufficient relaxation for safe instrumentation of the airway, maintenance of adequate gas exchanges, and rapid recovery at the end of the procedure. Ventilation during rigid bronchoscopy in the paralyzed patient can be carried out by intermittent positive pressure ventilation — IPPV — using a ventilating bronchoscope; by manual jet ventilation using a Venturi injector device described by Sanders (1967);

by HFJV, as introduced by Erickson and Sjostrand (1977); or by positive-negative external compression or HFPPV reported by Hayek (1989). Manual jet ventilation can be achieved through a rigid bronchoscope or a fiberoptic bronchoscope, as described by Satyanarayana (1980). Vourc'h and co-workers (1983) compared manual jet ventilation with HFJV during bronchoscopy in patients with tracheobronchial stenosis. Arterial blood gas tensions were identical during both manual jet ventilation and HFJV at a rate of 150 per minute. From the endoscopist's point of view, HFJV is preferable to manual jet ventilation because the tracheobronchial wall remains immobile. During HFPPV, no air entrainment occurs, so that anesthetic gases can be delivered at known concentration. With Hayek external positive-negative internal compression, the airway is not intubated and the surgeon has access to the airway without interference. When general anesthesia is required for fiberoptic bronchoscopy, the instrument is passed through an endotracheal tube mounted with a swivel adapter with a bronchoscopic port, allowing continuation of anesthesia and IPPV. The ratio of the external diameter of the bronchofiberscope to that of the internal diameter of the endotracheal tube is critical because the instrument reduces the effective ventilatory area of the endotracheal tube lumen.

Mediastinoscopy

Mediastinoscopy can be performed using local anesthesia, but endotracheal general anesthesia is more pleasant for the patient, provides more flexibility for the surgeon, and facilitates management of a major complication that may occur during this procedure. Compression of the innominate artery by the mediastinoscope can diminish or block blood flow to the right carotid and subclavian arteries. Lee and Salvatore (1976) reported a sudden loss of pulse and blood pressure in the right arm during mediastinoscopy, which was misdiagnosed as a cardiac arrest. The right radial artery pulse should therefore be monitored by palpation or finger plethysmography to detect compression of the innominate artery. Sudden hypotension, bradycardia, or dysrhythmia may occur as a result of mechanical stimulation or compression of the trachea, vagus nerve, or great vessels. Repositioning of the mediastinoscope and intravenous administration of atropine or ephedrine may be necessary to restore the pulse rate and blood pressure. Massive bleeding caused by accidental injury to a major vessel is a distinct, but rare, possibility. The management of such bleeding necessitates thoracotomy and major surgical intervention. The anesthesiologist should be ready for massive replacement of fluids and blood. An intraoperative tension pneumothorax manifested by increased peak airway pressure, hypotension, and cyanosis is uncommon but requires immediate diagnosis and treatment, as stated by Furgang and Saidman (1972). Other reported complications associated with mediastinoscopy, reported by Ashbaugh (1970), include injury to the recurrent laryngeal nerve,

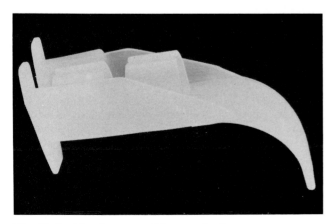

Fig. 21–6. The Ovassapian Fiberoptic Intubating Airway.

phrenic nerve, or esophagus; transient hemiparesis; and air embolism.

Cysts of the Lung

Intermittent positive pressure ventilation or vigorous coughing might result in a dangerous rise in alveolar pressure and rupture of a cyst. Ting and associates (1963) reported that the size of a cyst increases if it is in communication with the bronchus and has a valve-type action so that air may enter but not leave the cyst during IPPV. In a closed cyst, administration of nitrous oxide should be avoided, as was suggested by Isonhower and Cucchiara (1976), as it could rapidly increase the volume of and pressure within the cyst. As the size of the cyst increases, it may cause compression atelectasis and mediastinal shift and interfere with adequate gas exchange. Ventilation may also become inadequate if a significant portion of the tidal volume enters and leaves the communicating cyst without participating in gas exchange. Overinflation and rupture of the cyst may cause tension pneumothorax and cardiopulmonary insufficiency.

If the disease is confined to one lung, Isonhower and Cucchiara (1976) suggested that isolation of the lungs with a double-lumen endobronchial tube avoids IPPV to the diseased side. Bilateral air cysts represent a difficult problem because of the possible increase in their size and their interference with gas exchange in the dependent lung while the surgeon operates on the upper lung. Bilateral thoracotomy may be necessary. Normandale and Feneck (1985) successfully applied HFJV for the anesthetic management of patients with bullous cystic lung disease.

Bronchopleural Fistula

The complications associated with a large bronchopleural fistula are loss of ventilation, contamination of the contralateral lung, and development of pneumothorax when IPPV is applied. These complications are best avoided by the passage of an endobronchial tube before induction of general anesthesia. Securing the airway with a double-lumen endobronchial tube in a conscious patient is a safe, but not always easy, approach. Placing patients in a head-up lateral decubitus position with the affected side down minimizes the chance of secretions moving into the tracheobronchial tree during intubation of the trachea. Francis and Smith (1962) indicated that the double-lumen endobronchial tube permits IPPV of the healthy lung, without the loss of minute ventilation through the fistula, and prevents soiling of the healthy lung. If tracheal intubation is difficult or not desirable in the conscious patient, general anesthesia with spontaneous ventilation can be used until the airway is secured with a double-lumen endobronchial tube. If a double-lumen tube cannot be applied and a single-lumen tube is placed, Baker and co-workers (1971) suggested maintaining spontaneous ventilation until the chest is opened. During surgery, the air leak can be minimized by manually packing the

lung. Carlon and co-workers (1980) successfully applied high frequency positive pressure and carbon dioxide removal in a patient with a large bronchopleural fistula. Hildebrand and associates (1984) indicated that HFJV at 100 cycles per minute was unsuitable during lobectomy with an open bronchus and resulted in a rapid deterioration in Pa_{O_2} and a rise in Pa_{CO_2}. Their results conflict with those of Moulaert and Rolly (1983), who claimed that ventilation with an open bronchus was possible with HFJV at a rate of 250 cycles per minute.

Pneumothorax and Hemothorax

An important feature in the anesthetic management of these conditions is to drain them during local anesthesia before inducing anesthesia or administering IPPV.

Tracheal Resection

A thorough preoperative evaluation and understanding of the airway problem is essential. Good rapport must be established for the patient and heavy premedication should be avoided. Close communication between the surgeon and anesthesiologist is essential during tracheal reconstruction, and each one should be fully aware of the other's plan, approach, and readiness before induction of anesthesia.

Various methods of maintaining adequate ventilation have been applied during operations on the trachea or bronchi. Use of a single-lumen endotracheal tube placed above the tracheal lesion preoperatively and advanced inside the trachea or bronchi below the tracheal lesion during surgery has been described by Belsey (1950) and Geffin and associates (1969). It is safer to secure the airway while the patient is awake.

If an awake intubation is not possible, a slow, inhalation induction with a halogenated anesthetic agent with oxygen should be performed, with spontaneous ventilation maintained until tracheal intubation is achieved. The bronchofiberscope can be used to apply topical anesthesia to the larynx and trachea, to evaluate the site and degree of tracheal stenosis, and to intubate the trachea. The instrument enables the anesthesiologist to place the tip of the tube above the stenotic area and to avoid any trauma. After exposure of the trachea, as the surgeon starts resecting the lesion, the orotracheal tube is advanced beyond the lesion into the lower section of the trachea. The surgeon completes the resection and anastomosis in the presence of the endotracheal tube. To avoid the presence of an endotracheal tube in the surgical field, Akdikmen and Landmesser (1965) and Geffin (1969) described the use of two separate endotracheal tubes. The first endotracheal tube is placed orally above the tracheal lesion. The second sterile, armored endotracheal tube is inserted by the surgeon into the distal trachea or one of the main stem bronchi after cutting the trachea distal to the lesion. The second endotracheal tube is then connected to the anesthesia machine using sterile corrugated tubing and a Y-piece, and anesthesia is continued. After resection of the lesion and placement of sutures in the posterior tracheal wall, the surgeon removes the endotracheal tube placed in the distal trachea. The original orotracheal tube is advanced beyond the suture line into the lower trachea, or one of the main stem bronchi, until the surgeon completes the repair of the trachea.

A third approach is the use of HFJV through a small catheter, as described by Erickson (1975) and Rogers (1985) and their co-workers; manual jet ventilation, as reported by Lee and English (1974); and HFPPV as applied by El-Baz (1982). Scamman and Choi (1986) used a sterile nasogastric — NG — tube for application of low frequency jet ventilation and measurement of end-tidal CO_2 during tracheal resection. The distal end of the NG tube was cut off above the highest side hole and was placed 2 cm into the distal stump of the trachea. The larger lumen was connected to a Sander's jet apparatus and the smaller to a CO_2 analyzer. Normal arterial and end-tidal gas tensions were maintained while the surgeon completed the posterior and lateral wall anastomosis. Neuman and associates (1984) described successful use of HFJV for tracheal resection in a 7-year-old child.

To avoid contamination of the operating room from inhalation agents, intravenous anesthetics are used during HFPPV or jet ventilation. Early extubation is highly desirable to minimize the compromise of blood flow to the trachea. Woods (1961) and Coles (1976) and their associates applied extracorporal circulation for management of tracheobronchial resection.

Laser Surgery

Laser surgery of the airway presents several potential anesthetic problems. These include ventilation and oxygenation through a compromised and shared airway and hazards introduced by the laser beam. The major hazards from laser surgery are fires and destruction of normal tissues. Fire can occur when the laser strikes a rubber or plastic endotracheal tube in an oxygen-rich anesthetic mixture. Nitrous oxide, like oxygen, supports combustion, whereas halogenated anesthetic agents are not flammable and do not support combustion. To minimize the danger of fire, Brutinel and associates (1983) recommended using 50% oxygen or less in nitrogen, whereas Eisenman and Ossoff (1986) favor a mixture of oxygen and helium during general anesthesia. The use of metallic or noncombustible disposable endotracheal tubes and protection of standard rubber or plastic endotracheal tubes by wrapping them with aluminum or copper tape have been thoroughly reviewed by Hermens' co-workers (1983). Endotracheal tubes wrapped with metallic tape may cause pharyngeal and laryngeal injury because of rough edges, and pieces of tape can loosen, break off, and be aspirated. All oil-based ointments and lubricants should be avoided because they are combustible and can be ignited. In case of fire, the procedure should be stopped and the endotracheal tube should be removed immediately. The lungs as well as the trachea may be injured by either smoke inhalation or a direct thermal burn.

Using a Hayek (1989) positive and negative external compressor allows air exchange without intubation. This device is in its early stages of experimental use. If proved safe and effective, it will eliminate the need for intubation, and therefore during total intravenous anesthesia, the surgeon will have sole access to the airway.

The surgical field should be immobile to minimize the chance of laser damage of normal tissue. Choice of anesthesia for bronchoscope laser surgery depends on the surgical technique and the age and condition of the patient. Rontal and associates (1986) favor topical anesthesia with sedation whenever possible, but particularly in patients with higher grade airway obstruction. General anesthesia is the method of choice for most children and for adults who cannot tolerate local anesthesia. Dumon and associates (1984) favor spontaneous ventilation, whereas Brutinel (1983) and Vourc'h (1983) and their co-workers recommend controlled ventilation. If jet ventilation is chosen, scavenging of inhalation anesthetic agents is difficult, and total intravenous anesthesia must be provided. Prolonged respiratory depression, and the need for postoperative ventilatory support, is a potential complication of total intravenous anesthesia. Whatever the anesthetic technique, the basic principle of anesthetic management of patients with a compromised airway should be followed. Communication between the anesthesiologist and the surgical team is essential, and a plan for management of total airway obstruction must be decided before induction of anesthesia. All routine safety precautions during laser surgery, both for the patient and the operating room personnel, should be observed. A sign noting that a laser is in use should be placed on the outside of the door. Finally, postoperative care is extremely important, as respiratory depression, laryngospasm, bronchospasm, airway obstruction, and hemorrhage can all occur and require immediate treatment.

REFERENCES

Akdikmen S, Landmesser CM: Anesthesia for surgery of the intrathoracic portion of the trachea. Anesthesiology 26:117, 1965.

Arai T, Hatano Y: Yet another reason to use a fiberoptic bronchofiberscope to properly site a double-lumen tube. Anesthesiology 66:581, 1987.

Ashbaugh DG: Mediastinoscopy. Arch Surg 100:586, 1970.

Ashton JH, Cassidy SS: Reflex depression of cardiovascular function during lung inflation. J Appl Physiol 58:137, 1985.

Augustine SD, Benumof, JL: Halothane and isoflurane do not impair arterial oxygenation during one-lung ventilation in patients undergoing thoracotomy. Anesthesiology 61:A484, 1984.

Baek SM, et al: Plasma expansion in surgical patients with high central venous pressure: The relationship of blood volume to hematocrit, CVP, pulmonary wedge pressure and cardiorespiratory changes. Surgery 78:304, 1975.

Baker WL, et al: Management of bronchopleural fistulas. J Thorac Cardiovasc Surg 62:393, 1971.

Baraka A, et al: One lung ventilation of children during surgical excision of hydatid cysts. Br J Anaesthesiol 54:523, 1982.

Belsey R: Resection and reconstruction of the intrathoracic trachea. Br J Surg 38:200, 1950.

Benumof JL: Mechanism of decreased blood flow to atelectatic lung. J Appl Physiol 46:1047, 1978.

Bergman D, et al: Intraoperative autotransfusion during emergency thoracic and elective open heart surgery. Ann Thorac Surg 18:590, 1974.

Bjork VO, Carlens E: The prevention of spread during pulmonary resection by the use of a double-lumen catheter. J Thorac Cardiovasc Surg 20:151, 1950.

Black AMS, Harrison GA: Difficulties with positioning Robertshaw double-lumen tubes. Anaesth Intensive Care 3:299, 1975.

Brewster DC, et al: Intraoperative autotransfusion in major vascular surgery. Am J Surg 137:507, 1979.

Brinkmeyer S, et al: Superiority of colloid over electrolyte solution for fluid resuscitation. Crit Care Med 8:396, 1981.

Brutinel WM, et al: Bronchoscopic therapy with neodymiumyttrium-aluminum garnet laser during intravenous anesthesia. Chest 84:518, 1983.

Burton NA, et al: Advantages of a new polyvinyl chloride double lumen tube in thoracic surgery. Ann Thorac Surg 36:78, 1983.

Capan LM, et al: Optimization of arterial oxygenation during one-lung anesthesia. Anesth Analg 59:847, 1980.

Carlens E: A new flexible double-lumen catheter for bronchospirometry. J Thorac Cardiovasc Surg 18:742, 1949

Carlon GC, et al: High frequency positive pressure ventilation in management of a patient with bronchopleural fistula. Anesthesiology 52:60, 1980.

Cay DL, et al: Selective bronchial blocking in children. Anaesth Intensive Care 3:127, 1975.

Coles JC, et al: A method of anesthesia for imminent tracheal obstruction. Surgery 80:379, 1976.

Cote CJ, et al: Wasted ventilation measured in vitro with eight anesthetic circuits with and without inlet humidification. Anesthesiology 59:442, 1983.

Dalens B, et al: Selective endobrochial blocking vs selective intubation based on 10 variables. Crit Care Med 10:643, 1982.

Dougherty P, Hannallah M: A potentially serious complication that resulted from improper use of the Univent tube. Anesthesiology 77:835, 1992.

Dumon JF, et al: Principles for safety in application of neodymium-YAG laser in bronchology. Chest 86:163, 1984.

Edwards EM, Hatch DJ: Experiences with double-lumen tubes. Anaesthesia 20:461, 1965.

Eisenman TS, Ossoff RH: Anaesthesia for bronchoscopic laser surgery. Otolaryngol Head Neck Surg 94:45, 1986.

El-Baz N, et al: One-lung high frequency positive pressure ventilation for sleeve pneumonectomy: An alternative technique. Anesth Analg 60:638, 1981.

El-Baz N, et al: One-lung frequency ventilation for tracheoplasty and bronchoplasty: A new technique. Ann Thorac Surg 34:564, 1982.

Erickson I, Sjostrand I: High frequency positive pressure ventilation and the pneumatic valve principle in bronchoscopy under general anesthesia. Acta Anesth Scand (Suppl) 64:83, 1977.

Erickson I, et al: High frequency positive pressure ventilation during transthoracic resection of tracheal stenosis and during preoperative bronchoscopic examination. Acta Anaesthesiol Scand 19:13, 1975.

Flacke JW, et al: Influence of tidal volume and pulmonary artery occlusion on arterial oxygenation during endobronchial anesthesia. South Med J 69:617, 1976.

Francis JG, Smith KG: An anesthetic technique for the repair of bronchopleural fistula. Br J Anaesth 34:817, 1962.

Froese AB, Bryan AC: Effects of anesthesia and paralysis on diaphragmatic mechanics in man. Anesthesiology 41:242, 1974.

Furgang FA, Saidman LJ: Bilateral tension pneumothorax associated with mediastinoscopy. J Thorac Cardiovasc Surg 63:329, 1972.

Geffin B, et al: Anesthetic management of tracheal resection and reconstruction. Anesth Analg 48:884, 1969.

Giesecke AH, Egbert LD: Perioperative fluid therapy; crystalloids. In Miller RD: Anesthesia. 2nd Ed. New York: Churchill Livingstone, 1986, pp. 1313–1328.

Ginsberg RJ: New technique for one-lung anesthesia using an endobronchial blocker. J Thorac Cardiovasc Surg 82:542, 1981.

Glenski JA, et al: High frequency, small volume ventilation during thoracic surgery. Anesthesiology 64:211, 1986.

Haugen RK, Hill GE: A large-scale autologous blood program in a community hospital: A contribution to the community's blood supply. JAMA 275:1211, 1987.

Hayek Z, et al: External high frequency ventilation without intubation. Crit Care Med 19:406A, 1985.

Hermens JM, et al: Anesthesia for laser surgery. Anesth Analg 62:218, 1983.

Hildebrand PJ, et al: High frequency jet ventilation: A method for thoracic surgery. Anaesthesia 39:1091, 1984.

Hogg CE, Lorhan PH: Pediatric bronchial blocking. Anesthesiology 33:560, 1970.

Hultgren BL, et al: A new tube for one lung ventilation: Experience with Univent tube (abstract). Anesthesiology 65:A481, 1986.

Hurford WE, et al: The use of ventilation/perfusion lung scans to predict oxygenation during one-lung anesthesia. Anesthesiology 67:841, 1987.

Hutchin P, et al: Pulmonary congestion following infusion of large fluid loads in thoracic surgical patients. Ann Thorac Surg 8:339, 1969.

Inoue J, et al: Endotracheal tube with movable blocker to prevent aspiration of intratracheal bleeding. Ann Thorac Surg 37:497, 1984.

Isonhower N, Cucchiara RF: Anesthesia for vanishing lung syndrome report of a case. Anesth Analg 55:750, 1976.

Jenkins VA, Clark G: Endobronchial anesthesia with the Carlens catheter. Br J Anaesth 30:12, 1958.

Karwande S: A new tube for single lung ventilation. Chest 92:761, 1987.

Katz JA, et al: Pulmonary oxygen exchange during endobronchial anesthesia: Effects of tidal volume and PEEP. Anesthesiology 56:164, 1982.

Kerr JH, et al: Observations during endobronchial anesthesia. I. Ventilation and carbon dioxide clearance. Br J Anaesth 45:159, 1973.

Khanam T, Branthwaite MA: Arterial oxygenation during one-lung anesthesia. Anaesthesia 28:280, 1973.

Larsson A, et al: Variation in lung volume and compliance during pulmonary surgery. Br J Anesth 59:585, 1987.

Lee J, Salvatore A: Innominate artery compression simulating cardiac arrest during mediastinoscopy: A case report. Anesth Analg 55:748, 1976.

Lee P, English IC: Management of anesthesia during tracheal resection. Anaesthesia 29:305, 1974.

MacGillivray RG: Evaluation of a new tracheal tube with a movable bronchial blocker. Anesthesia 43:687, 1988.

Malmkvist G: Maintenance of oxygenation during one-lung ventilation effect of intermittent reinflation of the collapsed lung with oxygen. Anesth Analg 68:763, 1989.

Moulaert P, Rolly G: High frequency of jet ventilation for pulmonary resection. In Sheck PA, Sjostrand NH, Smith RB (eds): Perspectives in High Frequency Ventilation. Boston: Martinus-Nijhoff, 1983, pp. 227–32.

Nakatuska M, et al: Unilateral high-frequency jet ventilation during one-lung ventilation for thoracotomy. Ann Thorac Surg 44:654, 1988.

Neuman CG, et al: High-frequency jet ventilation for tracheal resection in a child. Anesth Analg 63:1039, 1984.

Normandale JP, Feneck, RO: Bullous cystic lung disease: its anesthetic management using high frequency jet ventilation. Anaesthesia 40:1182, 1985.

Ovassapian A: A new fiberoptic intubating airway. Anesth Analg 66:S132, 1987.

Ovassapian A: Fiberoptic aided bronchial intubation. In Fiberoptic Airway Endoscopy in Anesthesia and Critical Care. New York: Raven Press, 1990, pp. 80–104.

Ovassapian A, Schrader S: Fiberoptic-aided bronchial intubation. Semin Anesthe 6:133, 1987.

Ovassapian A, et al: Endobronchial intubation using flexible fiberoptic bronchoscope. Anesthesiology 59:A501, 1983.

Rao CC, et al: One-lung pediatric anesthesia. Anesth Analg 60:450, 1981.

Read RC, et al: Prospective study of the Robertshaw endobronchial catheter in thoracic surgery. Ann Thorac Surg 24:156, 1977.

Rees D, Wansbrough SR: One-lung anesthesia: Percent shunt and arterial oxygen tension during continuous insufflation of oxygen to the nonventilated lung. Anesth Analg 61:507, 1982.

Rigg D: A comparison of the Robertshaw and Carlens-type double-lumen tubes for thoracic anesthesia. Anaesth Intensive Care 8:460, 1980.

Robertshaw FL: Low resistance double-lumen endobronchial tubes. Br J Anaesth 34:576, 1962.

Rogers RC, et al: High frequency jet ventilation for tracheal surgery. Anaesthesia 40:32, 1985.

Rogers SN, Benumof JL: Halothane and isoflurane do not impair arterial oxygenation during one-lung ventilation to patients undergoing thoracotomy. Anesthesiology 59:A532, 1983.

Rontal M, et al: Anesthetic management for tracheobronchial laser surgery. Ann Otol Rhinol Laryngol 95:556, 1986.

Sanders RD: Two ventilating attachments for bronchoscopes. Del Med J 39:170, 1967.

Satyanarayana T, et al: Bronchofiberscope jet ventilation. Anesth Analg 59:350, 1980.

Scamman FL, Choi WW: Low frequency jet ventilation for tracheal resection. Laryngoscope 96:678, 1986.

Shinnick JP, Freedman AP: Bronchofiberoptic placement of a double-lumen endotracheal tube. Crit Care Med 10:544, 1982.

Smith RB, et al: High frequency ventilation during pulmonary lobectomy: Three cases. Respir Care 26:437, 1981.

Thornburn JR, et al: Comparison of the effects of atropine and glycopyrrolate on pulmonary mechanics in patients undergoing fiber-optic bronchoscopy. Anesth Analg 65:1285, 1986.

Ting EY, et al: Mechanical properties of pulmonary cysts and bullae. Am Rev Respir Dis 87:538, 1963.

Twigley AJ, Hillman KM: The end of the crystalloid era? Anaesthesia 40:860, 1985.

Vale R: Selective bronchial blocking in a small child. Br J Anaesth 41:453, 1969.

Vourc'h G, et al: High frequency jet ventilation versus manual jet ventilation during bronchoscopy in patients with tracheo-bronchial stenosis. Br J Anaesth 55:969, 1983.

Weinrich A, et al: Continuous ketamine infusion for one-lung anesthesia. Can J Anaesth 27:485, 1980.

Wilks D, et al: Selective high frequency jet ventilation of the operative lung improves oxygenation during thoracic surgery. Anesthesiology 63:A586, 1985.

Wittnich C, et al: Misleading "pulmonary wedge pressure" after pneumonectomy: Its importance in postoperative fluid therapy. Ann Thorac Surg 42:192, 1986.

Woods F, et al: Resection of the carina and mainstem bronchi with extracorporeal circulation. N Engl J Med 254:492, 1961.

CHAPTER 22

JET VENTILATION

Nabile M. El-Baz

Jet ventilation is based on the intermittent delivery of a narrow stream of gases at high velocity into the trachea through a small catheter or a cannula. Jet ventilation was first used by Sanders (1967) to deliver large tidal volumes at slow respiratory rates to provide gas exchange during anesthesia and bronchoscopic surgery. Jet ventilation was later used by Heijman and associates (1972) at high respiratory rates and small tidal volumes to provide alveolar ventilation during anesthesia and routine surgery. Injector jet ventilation — IJV — and high frequency jet ventilation — HFJV — achieve adequate alveolar ventilation and oxygenation by generating different gas kinetics in the airways. Both techniques, however, involve the basic principles of gas delivery for jet ventilation.

MECHANICS OF GAS DELIVERY

Jet ventilation is delivered through a noncompliant inspiratory tube and a narrow intratracheal catheter or special adaptor. Jet ventilation does not incorporate an expiratory tube, and gases are exhaled through the upper airway, which must be patent and open to the atmosphere.

Jet ventilation requires a source of gas at a relatively high pressure, such as the central oxygen supply, which is normally 50 to 60 psi. The pressure of the gas supply is regulated manually through a reducing valve and the selected pressure is referred to as the driving gas pressure — DGP. Gas flow through the inspiratory tube is interrupted by the ventilator's electromagnetic solenoid valve as shown in Figure 22–1. The function of this valve is controlled by an electric circuit, which is regulated manually through two dials to determine the number of valve openings — frequency, respiratory rate — and the duration of each opening — insufflation time, IT. The tidal volume insufflated with each valve opening is determined by the gas pressure selected — DGP — and by the duration of each opening — IT. The ventilator can deliver HFJV at a high respiratory rate and short inspiratory time or IJV at a

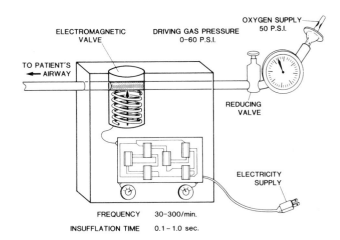

Fig. 22–1. High frequency ventilator. The reducing valve regulates the pressure of oxygen. Gas flow to the patient is interrupted by a solenoid electromagnetic valve.

low respiratory rate and long insufflation time. A spring-loaded valve, which is operated by hand for the delivery of injector jet ventilation, can be substituted for the electric circuit and solenoid valve.

GAS EXCHANGE

Injector jet ventilation delivers a large tidal volume — 500 to 1500 ml — at a slow respiratory rate of 10 to 30 breaths/minute. This method of jet ventilation achieves adequate gas exchange by convection — bulk flow — similar to conventional intermittent positive pressure ventilation — IPPV. Prolonged jet insufflation generates a negative pressure above the tip of the catheter, which causes the entrainment of air from the trachea and upper airways. As pointed out by Carden and associates (1973), this technique uses the Bernoulli principle, the venturi tube, and injector mechanics to entrain air and enlarge the insufflated tidal volume.

High frequency jet ventilation delivers a small tidal volume — 50 to 250 ml — at a high respiratory rate of 60 to 600 breaths/minute. Sjostrand (1977) noted that this method of ventilation achieves adequate gas exchange by a combination of convective flow and acceleration of gas diffusion. The repeated insufflations of small volumes at high velocity generates a turbulent flow of gases in the airways and a continuously positive airway pressure — CPAP. This increases FRC, improves gas mixing and distribution, and accelerates gas diffusion. Klain and Smith (1977) showed that the short periods of jet insufflation do not generate significant negative pressure and do not entrain air. Carbon dioxide elimination during high frequency ventilation depends on the convective flow used — tidal volume. The exact mechanism by which HFV achieves gas exchange remains unknown.

USE OF JET VENTILATION

Bronchoscopic and Laser Surgery

Sanders (1967) and Eriksson (1975), Carden (1973), and Kwok (1984) and their associates reported the use of injector and HFJV through special bronchoscopic attachments to provide an unobstructed view of airway lesions and adequate alveolar ventilation during bronchoscopic examination and laser surgery. In 1984, I and my colleagues reported the use of one-lung and two-lung HFJV through a small catheter during laser vaporization of tracheobronchial lesions. Two-lung HFJV was used in 12 patients with subglottic and tracheal stenotic lesions. After induction of anesthesia, a 2-mm ID catheter was placed in the trachea distal to the stenotic lesion. The small catheter did not interfere with the placement of the bronchoscope in the trachea alongside the catheter. The catheter's position and the tracheal lumen's size near the lesion were examined during bronchoscopy to ensure an adequate lumen for gas exit. Two-lung HFJV achieved adequate gas exchange and the small catheter provided optimal surgical conditions. The parameters of HFV used and the blood gases obtained are shown in Figure 22–2. The HFV technique was associated with continuous outflow of gases through the bronchoscope, which eliminated the smoke of tissue vaporization and prevented the contamination of the distal airways with blood and debris. In these patients, F_{IO_2} of 0.21 — air — provided adequate oxygenation and eliminated the risk of catheter ignition by laser.

Airway Surgery

The use of jet ventilation through a small catheter has been valuable during resection and reconstruction of the airways. The small size of the catheter provides optimal surgical access to the circumferences of the transected airways and facilitates the reconstruction of an airtight anastomosis. Lee and English (1974) reported that the use of IJV through a catheter during tracheal resection maintains adequate gas exchange and provides optimal surgical conditions. The use of injector jet

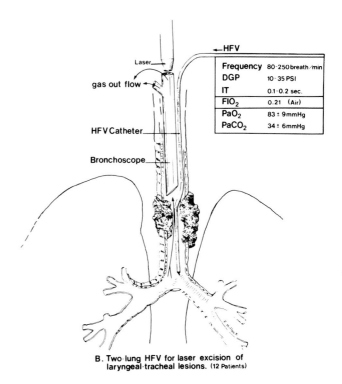

Frequency	80-250 breath/min
DGP	10-35 PSI
IT	0.1-0.2 sec.
FIO₂	0.21 (Air)
PaO₂	83 ± 9 mmHg
PaCO₂	34 ± 6 mmHg

B. Two-lung HFV for laser excision of laryngeal-tracheal lesions. (12 Patients)

Fig. 22–2. The HFV catheter is positioned distal to the airway lesion. The bronchoscope is positioned alongside the catheter. The delivered HFV gases exit through the trachea and the bronchoscope. Top table shows the parameters of HFV and blood gases.

ventilation during airway surgery, however, has been complicated, as noted by O'Sullivan and Healy (1985), by frequent displacement of the catheters and entrainment of air and blood into the airways. Chang and associates (1980) reported occasional barotrauma. Deslauriers and associates (1979) minimized these problems by using apneic oxygen insufflation supplemented with occasional jet insufflation. Eriksson and associates (1975) reported that HFJV through a catheter during tracheal resection maintains adequate gas exchange and optimal surgical conditions. I and my co-workers showed in 1982 and 1983 that one-lung HFV through a small catheter provides adequate gas exchange during tracheoplasty and bronchoplasty. We used one-lung HFV in six patients undergoing a right-sleeve pneumonectomy and tracheobronchial anastomosis. These patients initially received two-lung conventional ventilation through an endotracheal tube. After the transection of trachea and left main bronchus, a 2-mm ID catheter was advanced through the endotracheal tube and positioned inside the transected left main bronchus. Left lung HFV through the catheter was used during tracheobronchial anastomosis and maintained adequate gas exchange for periods of 1.5 to 3 hours. The parameters of HFV and blood gases obtained are shown in Figure 22–3. The small catheter provided optimal access and the small tidal volume of HFJV caused minimal movement of the catheter and the mediastinum. The continuous outflow of HFJV gases through the open bronchus prevented the contamination of the lung with the blood and debris.

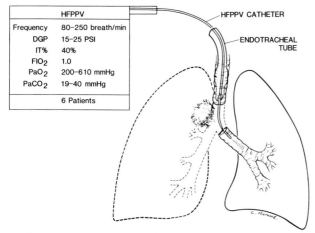

HFPPV	
Frequency	80–250 breath/min
DGP	15–25 PSI
IT%	40%
FIO$_2$	1.0
PaO$_2$	200–610 mmHg
PaCO$_2$	19–40 mmHg
	6 Patients

HFPPV CATHETER

ENDOTRACHEAL TUBE

LEFT LUNG HFPPV FOR RIGHT SLEEVE PNEUMONECTOMY

Fig. 22–3. The HFV catheter is passed through the endotracheal tube and the open trachea and then placed into the left main bronchus. HFV of the left lung achieved adequate gas exchange as shown in the top table. The delivered HFV gases exit through the open left main bronchus. After completion of the tracheobronchial anastomosis, the HFV catheter was removed and conventional ventilation was resumed through the endotracheal tube.

This technique of one-lung HFV through the small catheter, as reported by me and my colleagues (1983), was useful during the resection of tracheal and carinal lesions. In 1983, we reported that two-lung HFV provides adequate gas exchange and operative conditions during tracheal reconstruction supported with a Montgomery tracheal T-tube.

Thoracic Surgery

Kittle (1986) reviewed the use of one-lung and two-lung HFJV during intrathoracic surgery. Two-lung HFV was reported by Malina (1981) and Seki (1983) and their associates to maintain adequate gas exchange and cause minimal expansion and movement of the upper

lung during thoracic surgery. These reports were contradicted by Glenski and colleagues (1986), who found that two-lung HFJV was associated with hyperinflation of the upper lung and unacceptable surgical conditions. We reported in 1982 that one-lung HFV provided adequate gas exchange and operative conditions in 26 patients undergoing intrathoracic surgery. These patients received conventional one-lung IPPV followed by a period of isolated one-lung HFJV and then a period of modified one-lung HFJV. The isolated one-lung HFJV was associated with improvement of oxygenation as a result of an improvement of ventilation and perfusion of the dependent lung. The deflation of the endobronchial tube cuff for modified — nonisolated — one-lung HFJV was associated with further improvement of oxygenation. Modified one-lung HFJV generates a continuous gas outflow at the carina that allows the participation of the upper lung in gas exchange and causes slight inflation of upper lung. The Pa$_{O_2}$, Qs/Qt, and gas flow obtained during the use of these three methods of ventilation are shown in Figure 22–4.

TREATMENT OF BRONCHOPLEURAL FISTULA

Carlon (1981) and Turnbull (1981) and their associates reported that HFJV improves gas exchange in patients with bronchopleural-cutaneous fistula. Carlon and Howland (1985) noted that HFJV is associated with low mean and peak airway pressures, which reduces trauma and gas flow through the fistula and facilitates the healing process.

PROBLEMS

The clinical applications and value of jet ventilation have been limited because of the following problems: 1) the principle of gas delivery and the equipment for jet ventilation are completely different from those for

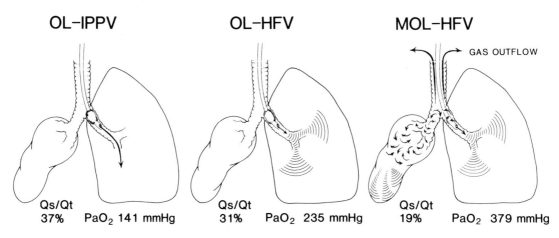

OL–IPPV   OL–HFV   MOL–HFV

GAS OUTFLOW

| Qs/Qt 37% | PaO$_2$ 141 mmHg | Qs/Qt 31% | PaO$_2$ 235 mmHg | Qs/Qt 19% | PaO$_2$ 379 mmHg |

Fig. 22–4. Three methods of one-lung ventilation (OL-IPPV, one-lung intermittent positive pressure ventilation. MOL-HFV, modified one-lung high frequency ventilation. OL-HFV, one-lung high frequency ventilation.) Deflation of the tube cuff allows for gas exit and partial ventilation of the other lung. MOL-HFV is a differential two-lung ventilation and provides effective oxygenation. The use of these three techniques in the same patients achieved different gas kinetics, Pa$_{O_2}$, and Qs/Qt, as shown under each diagram.

conventional ventilation; 2) the circuits, adapters, ventilators, and catheters are prototypes and lack standardization and expert engineering; 3) jet ventilation requires a monitoring device and an alarm system to detect mechanical malfunctions and abnormal airway pressures; 4) jet ventilation precludes the use of inhalation anesthetics, and anesthesia has to be achieved intravenously, which is associated with high incidences of awareness and delayed recovery; and 5) jet ventilation is a medicolegal liability and its use has to be justified. Despite these problems, jet ventilation through a small catheter remains the method of choice for ventilation during anesthesia for airway surgery.

REFERENCES

Carden E, et al: A comparison of venturi and side-arm ventilation in anaesthesia for bronchoscopy. Can J Anaesth *20*:569, 1973.

Carlon GC, et al: Clinical experience with high frequency jet ventilation. Crit Care Med *9*:1, 1981.

Carlon GC, Howland WS (eds.): High Frequency Ventilation in Intensive Care and During Surgery. New York: Marcel Dekker, 1985.

Chang JL, et al: Unilateral pneumothorax following jet ventilation during general anesthesia. Anesthesiology *53*:244, 1980.

Deslauriers J, et al: Sleeve pneumonectomy for bronchogenic carcinoma. Ann Thorac Surg *28*:465, 1979.

El-Baz N, et al: One-lung high frequency ventilation for tracheoplasty and bronchoplasty: A new technique. Ann Thorac Surg *34*:564, 1982a.

El-Baz N, et al: One-lung high frequency ventilation through a small uncuffed tube for lung surgery. J Cardiovasc Surg *84*:823, 1982b.

El-Baz N, et al: High frequency positive pressure ventilation for tracheal reconstruction supported by tracheal T-tube. Anesth Analg *61*:796, 1982c.

El-Baz N, et al: High frequency positive pressure ventilation for major airway surgery. *In* Scheck PA, Sjostrand UH, Smith RB: Perspectives in High Frequency Ventilation. Boston: Martinus Nijhoff, 1983, p. 216.

El-Baz N, et al: High frequency ventilation through a small catheter for laser surgery of laryngotracheal and bronchial disorders. Ann Otol Rhinol Laryngol *94*:483, 1985.

Eriksson I, et al: High frequency positive pressure ventilation (HFPPV) during transthoracic resection of tracheal stenosis and during preoperative bronchoscopic examination. Acta Anesthesiol Scand *19*:13, 1975.

Heijman K, et al: High frequency positive pressure ventilation during anaesthesia and routine surgery in man. Acta Anaesthesiol Scand *16*:176, 1972.

Kittle CF (ed.): Current Controversies in Thoracic Surgery. Philadelphia: WB Saunders, 1986, p. 183.

Klain M, Smith RB: High frequency percutaneous transtracheal jet ventilation. Crit Care Med *5*:280, 1977.

Kwok L, et al: Jet ventilation of one lung for laser resection of bronchial tumor. Anesth Analg *63*:957, 1984.

Lee P, English ICW: Management of anaesthesia during tracheal resection. Anaesthesia *29*:305, 1974.

Malina JR, et al: Clinical evaluation of high frequency positive pressure ventilation (HFPPV) in patients scheduled for open chest surgery. Anesth Analg *60*:324, 1981.

O'Sullivan TJ, Healy GB: Complications of venturi jet ventilation during microlaryngeal surgery. Arch Otolaryngol *94*:127, 1985.

Sanders RD: Two ventilating attachments for bronchoscopes. Del Med J *39*:170, 1967.

Seki S, et al: Facilitation of intrathoracic operations by means of high frequency ventilation. J Cardiovasc Surg *86*:388, 1983.

Sjostrand U: Review of physiological rationale for and development of high frequency positive pressure ventilation (HFPPV). Acta Anaesthesiol Scand *64*:7, 1977.

Turnbull AD, et al: High frequency jet ventilation in major airway or pulmonary disruption. Ann Thorac Surg *32*:468, 1981.

Vourc'h G, et al: Manual jet ventilation. V. High frequency ventilation during laser resection of tracheobroncheal lesions. Br J Anaesth *55*:973, 1983.

CHAPTER 23

ANESTHESIA FOR PEDIATRIC GENERAL THORACIC SURGERY

Babette J. Horn

Conditions requiring thoracic surgery may affect children of any age. Anesthetic considerations in the older child and adolescent are similar to those in the adult patient. It is in the newborn that the pediatric anesthesiologist encounters the greatest challenge. Besides the technical problems created by the newborn's small size, unique anatomic, physiologic, and pharmacologic differences makes neonatal anesthesia a field unto itself.

PHYSIOLOGIC CONSIDERATIONS IN THE NEONATE

Cardiovascular Adaptation

The cardiovascular system undergoes several changes during the transition to extrauterine life. Closure of the ductus venosus and foramen ovale convert the circulatory system from a parallel circuit to a series circuit (Figs. 23–1 to 23–3). Hypoxia, hypercarbia, sepsis, and hypothermia can cause undesirable right-to-left shunting of blood through the foramen ovale and ductus arteriosus, the anatomic closure of which may not be complete until 2 weeks after birth. Pulmonary resistance, elevated during fetal life and immediately after birth, falls rapidly at first and attains adult values by 2 months of age (Fig. 23–4). During this time, however, the pulmonary vascular resistance is labile, and considerable constriction and dilatation can result from physiologic, pharmacologic, and environmental manipulations. The syndrome of persistent pulmonary hypertension of the newborn — PPHN — characterized by refractory hypoxemia, hypercarbia, and acidosis, is common in patients with diaphragmatic hernias but can occur in virtually any stressed term infant.

Because it must work against increased resistance in utero, the right ventricle is hypertrophied and dominant in the newborn. Waugh and Johnson (1984) reported that both ventricles are noncompliant; their myocardial

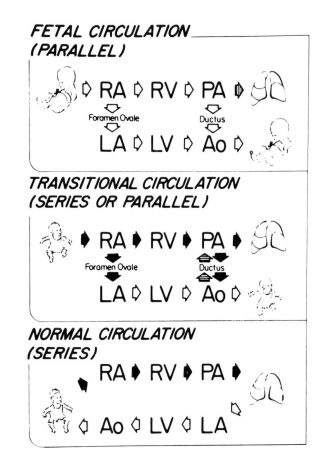

Fig. 23–1. Course of circulation during transition from fetal type circulatory pattern to adult type circulatory pattern. *From* Ryan JF, et al. (eds.): A Practice of Anesthesia for Infants and Children. Orlando, FL: Grune & Stratton, 1986, p. 176.

tissue has 30% fewer contractile elements than that of the adult.

Increases in preload cannot increase stroke volume because of the diminished contractility of the newborn

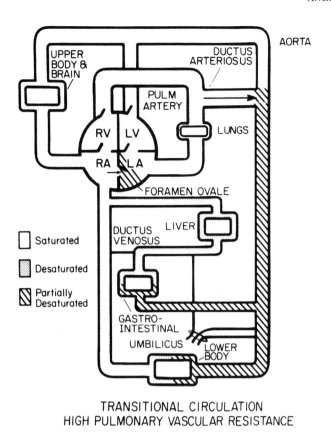

TRANSITIONAL CIRCULATION
HIGH PULMONARY VASCULAR RESISTANCE

Fig. 23–2. Transitional circulation of the neonate when pulmonary vascular resistance is high. Desaturated blood is shunted from the right atrium (RA) across the foramen ovale to partially desaturate the left atrial (LA) blood. *From* Ryan JF, et al (eds.): A Practice of Anesthesia for Infants and Children. Orlando, FL: Grune & Stratton, 1986, p. 117.

myocardium (Fig. 23–5). Thornberg and Morton (1983) suggested that the infant is functioning on an unfavorable portion of the Starling curve; only a modest rise in filling pressure can precipitate congestive heart failure. The anesthesiologist must scrupulously avoid overzealous administration of intravenous fluids.

The cardiac output of a newborn — 180 to 240 ml/kg/min, is two to three times the adult value relative to size. This difference reflects the greater oxygen consumption and metabolic rate in this age group. Increases in cardiac output are achieved primarily by increases in heart rate — normal 120 to 160 beats/minute — because the infant's myocardial contractility is relatively fixed. Sympathetic innervation of the heart is incomplete, as noted by Zaritsky and Chernow (1984), further impairing the ability to increase stroke volume. Systemic blood pressure is low in the newborn period (Table 23–1). Awareness of normal values is essential for the appropriate diagnosis and treatment of hypotension.

Respiratory Adaptation

Sarnaik and Preston (1982) reported the anatomic, mechanical, and functional peculiarities of the newborn

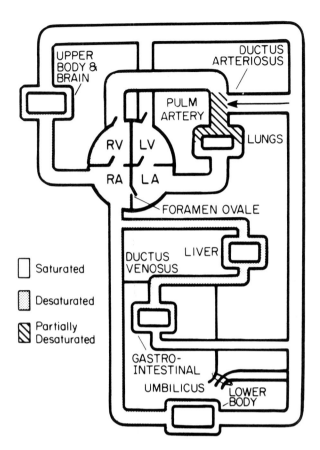

TRANSITIONAL CIRCULATION
LOW PULMONARY VASCULAR RESISTANCE

Fig. 23–3. Transitional circulation of the neonate when the pulmonary vascular resistance has fallen. Foramen ovale is closed and no intracardiac shunting can occur at that point. Left-to-right shunting of fully saturated blood from the aorta across the patent ductus arteriosus into the pulmonary artery arterializes blood flowing to the lungs. *From* Ryan JF, et al. (eds): A Practice of Anesthesia for Infants and Children. Orlando, FL: Grune & Stratton, 1986, p. 178.

respiratory system that increase the risk of arterial desaturation and hypoxemia. The trachea has an incompletely developed cartilaginous framework. Any extrathoracic obstruction, such as postextubation mucosal edema, causes tracheal collapse distally. Even a 1-mm ring of tracheal narrowing can cause severe respiratory distress because of the already small airway caliber (Fig. 23–6).

The infant has a highly compliant chest wall because of a horizontally oriented rib cage. In diseases of poor lung compliance — pulmonary edema, atelectasis — excessive lung recoil results in greater retraction of the soft chest wall and more loss of functional residual capacity than would occur in older children with stiffer chest walls.

When supine, the newborn's closing capacity impinges on tidal volume breathing. The resulting small airway collapse leads to atelectasis, ventilation/perfusion mismatch, and hypoxia. To prevent this situation from occurring intraoperatively, the anesthesiologist can use controlled ventilation and PEEP.

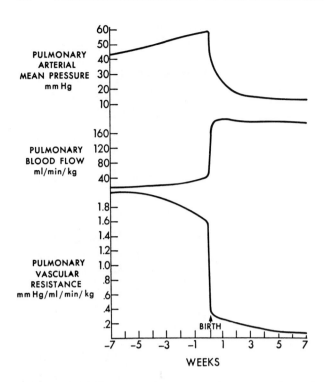

Fig. 23–4. The changes in pulmonary vascular resistance during the 7 weeks preceding birth, at birth, and in the 7 weeks postnatally. Prenatal data derived from lambs. *From* Rudolph AM: Congenital Diseases of the Heart. Chicago: Year Book, 1974, p. 31.

Table 23–1. Relationship of Age to Blood Pressure

Age	Normal Blood Pressure (mm Hg)	
	Mean Systolic	Mean Diastolic
0–12 hour (preterm)	50	35
0–12 hour (full term)	65	45
4 days	75	50
6 weeks	95	55
1 year	95	60
2 years	100	65
9 years	105	70
12 years	115	75

Because of their high oxygen consumption and increased work of breathing, infants breathe at rapid rates — 30 to 50 breaths per minute. Cook (1981) reported that the diaphragm of infants has a preponderance of fast twitch muscle fibers that are prone to early fatigue. Conditions causing increased work of breathing are therefore not tolerated for long periods of time, and hypercarbia and respiratory failure occur.

Chemical and neural control of breathing are different in the newborn. The response to hypoxia is paradoxic, characterized by a brief period of hyperpnea, followed by apnea. The central chemoreceptors have a diminished sensitivity to P_{CO_2} compared with those of adults, that is, a higher P_{CO_2} is needed to effect a similar increase in minute ventilation. Periodic breathing and apneic spells are common in the newborn, making close monitoring of respiratory function mandatory in the postoperative period.

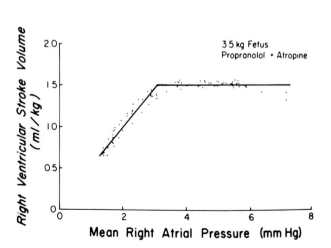

Fig. 23–5. Right ventricular stroke volume and right atrial pressure relationships in a sheep fetus. *From* Ryan JF, et al (eds): A Practice of Anesthesia for Infants and Children. Orlando, FL: Grune & Stratton, 1986, p. 180.

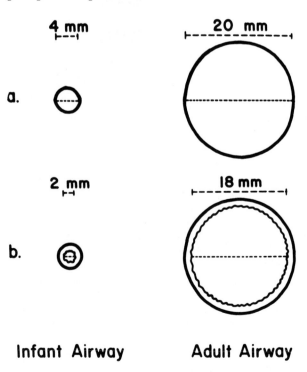

Fig. 23–6. Diagram of relative cross-sectional area of infant and adult trachea: a, no tracheal edema; b, 1 mm of edema encircling tracheal lumen.

Oxygen unloading at the tissue level is made more difficult by the high percentage of fetal hemoglobin in newborn erythrocytes. Because of its lower P_{50}, hemoglobin F "holds on" to oxygen more tenaciously than does adult hemoglobin. The generally high hemoglobin concentration at birth — 15 to 18 g/dl — is beneficial in increasing oxygen delivery to the cells (Fig. 23–7).

Metabolic Adaptation

Maintenance of normothermia is essential in the newborn. Adverse effects of hypothermia include apnea, hypoglycemia, metabolic acidosis, and increased oxygen consumption. Because of decreased subcutaneous tissue, a low surface area to volume ratio, and small body mass, the neonate has increased environmental heat losses. Nonshivering thermogenesis, mediated by catecholamine effects on brown fat deposits, is the primary heat generating process in the newborn. This process increases oxygen consumption by as much as two hundred-fold. Methods of preventing heat loss intraoperatively include increasing ambient temperature and use of radiant warmers, heating blankets, and intravenous fluid warmers. Baumgart and associates (1987) showed that covering the head and extremities with plastic wrap effectively minimizes evaporative heat losses during surgical procedures.

Hypoglycemia occurs frequently in this age group, especially in the premature or small-for-gestational-age infant, or in the infant of the diabetic mother. Causative factors in the development of neonatal hypoglycemia include diminished hepatic glycogen stores, decreased gluconeogenetic capabilities, and decreased response to glucagon secretion. Blood glucose values should be monitored frequently, adjusting the intravenous dextrose concentration accordingly. Normal blood glucose values in the newborn are listed in Table 23–2.

Table 23–2. Normal Blood Glucose Values

Age	Blood Glucose (mg/dl)
Newborn (premature)	>30
Newborn (term)	>40
Adult	60–100

PHARMACOLOGIC CONSIDERATIONS IN THE NEONATE

Virtually all drugs used in the practice of adult anesthesia have been safely used in pediatric anesthesia. Because of the physiologic characteristics of the newborn, however, drug dosages are altered and target organ responses are carefully monitored.

Muscle relaxants such as succinylcholine and the nondepolarizing agents supplement almost all newborn anesthetics. Goudsouzian (1986) noted that infants require a larger dose of succinylcholine calculated on a per kilogram basis because of their increased extracellular fluid compartment. Goudsouzian and Standaert (1986), in an excellent review of the infant myoneural junction, discussed both the pharmacodynamic — immature neuromuscular junction — and pharmacokinetic — delayed excretion, increased diaphragm fatigue — reasons behind the abnormal response of newborns to nondepolarizing agents such as pancuronium. The use of intermediate acting nondepolarizers atracurium and vecuronium in pediatric patients has been investigated extensively. Brandom (1991) summarized this research. Because of their shorter duration of action in infants, they are probably preferable to pancuronium in this group of patients.

Inhalation anesthetics such as nitrous oxide, halothane, and isoflurane are used frequently in pediatric thoracic surgical patients. Brett (1987), Friesen (1986), and Schieber (1986) and their associates reported that all these agents cause dose-dependent depression of cardiac function, and Wear (1982) and Duncan (1987) and their colleagues noted that their use impaired baroreceptor reflexes. Hypotension and bradycardia commonly occur when the potent inhalation agents are administered in high concentrations. Because halothane has a low therapeutic index in infants, it must be used sparingly, with close attention paid to blood pressure and heart rate. Waugh and Johnson (1984) and Eisele and associates (1986) reported that nitrous oxide can increase pulmonary vascular resistance, which in theory is undesirable in neonates with the potential to develop persistent pulmonary hypertension of the newborn. Clinical studies reported by Hickey and co-workers (1986), however, have shown that nitrous oxide can be used in infants without significant increase in right-to-left shunting.

Fentanyl, a synthetic short-acting potent narcotic, has been used extensively in neonatal anesthesia. Hickey and associates (1985) noted its beneficial effects in attenuating the pulmonary vasoconstrictive response to tracheal stimulation. Schieber and colleagues (1985) and Robinson and Gregory (1981) observed

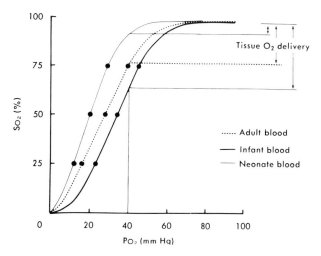

Fig. 23–7. Oxygen-hemoglobin dissociation curves with different oxygen affinities. In neonates with a lower P_{50} (20 mm Hg) and higher oxygen affinity, tissue oxygen unloading at the same tissue P_{O_2} is reduced. From Motoyama EK, Cook DR: Respiratory physiology. *In* Smith RM (ed): Anesthesia for Infants and Children. St. Louis: CV Mosby, 1980, p. 67.

cardiovascular stability with fentanyl analgesia as well. Yaster (1987) achieved a satisfactory anesthetic state in newborns presenting for a variety of surgical emergencies with doses of fentanyl in the 10 to 12.5 µg/kg range. Administration of greater than 5 µg/kg of fentanyl, a modest dose, usually precludes tracheal extubation at the conclusion of surgery, because this agent is a potent respiratory depressant. The newer, more potent narcotic sufentanil has been studied in pediatric patients undergoing cardiovascular surgical procedures. Extremely high doses in newborns were used by Hickey and colleagues (1992) with positive results. The lower doses used by Moore and associates (1985) proved unsatisfactory when sufentanil was the sole anesthetic agent. For most pediatric thoracic surgical patients, sufentanil has no clear-cut benefit over the more familiar, less expensive fentanyl.

Barbiturates such as thiopental can be used as induction agents in newborns, but low doses should be used — 2 to 3 mg/kg. Both immaturity of the blood-brain barrier and a relatively high cerebral blood flow combine to deliver a large fraction of the injected drug to the brain, thus allowing a lower dose to be used with equal efficacy. In addition, the barbiturates are myocardial depressants, and unacceptable degrees of hypotension may result from use of large doses.

Ketamine is a potent amnesic and analgesic agent that can be given intravenously — 1 to 2 mg/kg — or intramuscularly — 5 mg/kg — for the induction of general anesthesia. White and co-workers (1982) noted cardiovascular hemodynamics and spontaneous respirations are maintained because of sympathetic nervous system stimulation, accounting for the popularity of the drug for use in pediatric anesthesia. Ketamine causes copious salivation, so prior or concurrent administration of an antisialogogue — atropine 20 µg/kg intramuscularly or 10 µg/kg intravenously — is necessary.

Atropine enjoys widespread use in pediatric anesthesia because of its anticholinergic properties. In the aforementioned dose range, it counteracts undesirable bradycardia associated with halothane and succinylcholine administration, vagal stimulation during laryngoscopy, and intraoperative visceral traction. Slow heart rates can lead to a drop in cardiac output because the newborn cannot compensate by increasing this stroke volume.

MONITORING

The purpose of monitoring any variable during an operation is to identify adverse trends before they become catastrophic events. Because of their diminished cardiopulmonary and metabolic reserves, infants require close intraoperative monitoring. Confounding the goal of vigilant invasive and noninvasive monitoring is the infant's small size, which can make even the simplest of procedures, such as applying electrocardiogram leads, frustrating.

Standard Monitors

The following monitors are considered "standard of care" in pediatric anesthesia.

Temperature Probe

Rectal or esophageal temperatures most closely approximate core temperature, and are preferred over skin and axillary monitoring sites.

Electrocardiogram

Cardiac rate and rhythm are the primary data obtained from this monitor. Ischemia detection is not as important in this age group because coronary artery disease is uncommon. Smaller electrodes are available for placement on the trunk, as well as limb leads designed for use around the wrists and ankles.

Precordial or Esophageal Stethoscope

The thin chest wall of infants permits auscultation of both heart and breath sounds with a precordial stethoscope. According to Smith (1980), this monitor is one of the most useful and important in pediatric anesthesia, especially during tracheoesophageal fistula repair, when continuous use of an esophageal stethoscope is not possible.

Blood Pressure Cuff

Sizes to fit even the premature infant are now available. Usually the arm is not big enough to permit placement of a stethoscope, so only the systolic blood pressure is measured by looking for the "to and fro" movement of the sphygmomanometer needle.

Oxygen Analyzer

This device is inserted in the inspiratory limb of the anesthesia circuit. The American Academy of Pediatrics (1983), in its guidelines for perinatal care, and Lucey and Dangman (1984) emphasized that inspired oxygen concentrations must be measured carefully, because prolonged hyperoxia can lead to retinopathy in the infant whose postconceptual age is less than 46 weeks, in whom the retina has not completely matured.

Pulse Oximeter

Pulse oximetry has become an integral part of anesthesia care in the United States. The American Society of Anesthesiologists has mandated its use in all anesthetics and in the postanesthetic care unit. Excellent detailed reviews of the theory and technology behind pulse oximetry have been published by Tremper and Barker (1989), Alexander and colleagues (1989) and Severinghaus and Keller (1992). In the operating room, pulse oximetry is used primarily for detection of hypoxemia, although the plethysmographic tracing of the pulse oximeter saturation can also be used to monitor the circulation. Whether the use of pulse oximetry has resulted in improved patient outcome as a result of better detection of hypoxic events is still the subject of intense investigation, both by outcome studies, such as that of Moller and associates (1993), and closed claims analysis. One study by Coté and colleagues (1991) of pulse oximetry in pediatric patients underscores the ability of this monitor to detect clinically unrecognized hypoxemia in both the operating room and the recovery room. For operations associated with a high risk of intraoperative hypoxemia, such as tracheoesophageal fistula repair, the use of pulse oximetry, as noted by Bautista and associates (1986), has made early detection of impaired oxygenation possible.

Capnography/Capnometry

This technology makes possible the monitoring of end-tidal CO_2 concentrations in exhaled gases of an anesthetized patient. Important intraoperative applications of this noninvasive techniques, as summarized by Bhavani-Shankar and colleagues (1992), are: detection of esophageal intubation, circuit disconnect, and hypoventilation; monitoring of CO_2 production; and detection of abnormal alveolar ventilation and respiratory patterns. Presumably, the universal use of capnography will result in improved clinical outcome by virtue of earlier detection of dangerous respiratory problems.

Effective capnographic monitoring of pediatric patients is complicated by their small tidal volumes. Contamination with fresh gas flow is a problem, especially when the CO_2 sensor is placed too far from the endotracheal tube. Badgwell and associates (1991) studied the accuracy of capnography as a function of sensor location in pediatric breathing circuits. The end tidal CO_2 approximated Pa_{CO_2} most closely when the sensor was positioned within the endotracheal tube itself using a small aspirating catheter. For trending purposes, however, the sensor worked well when positioned conventionally, placed as close to the endotracheal tube as possible.

Additional Monitors

Additional monitoring devices are frequently used in pediatric thoracic surgery.

Indwelling Arterial Pressure Line

This device is an invaluable intraoperative aid. Beat-to-beat display of the blood pressure facilitates early detection of hypotension, which can result from hypovolemia or decreased venous return related to great vessel compression. Samples for blood gas, hemoglobin, and glucose analyses are obtained easily from an indwelling arterial catheter. Several sites for cannulation exist, each with its own advantages and drawbacks. The right radial artery provides access to preductal blood, but insertion of even a 22-gauge catheter may be technically difficult in a newborn. Umbilical artery catheterization is relatively easy in the first 24 hours of life but it carries the risks of lower extremity vasospasm and embolization of particulate matter to other major arterial vessels.

Doppler Ultrasonic Flow Detector

The Doppler device provides auscultatory confirmation of systolic pressures when placed over the radial or brachial artery and used in conjunction with a blood pressure cuff. Whyte and associates (1975) reported excellent agreement between Doppler readings and transduced blood pressure values.

SPECIFIC PROBLEMS REQUIRING THORACOTOMY IN NEWBORNS

Congenital Diaphragmatic Hernia

Although repair of a congenital diaphragmatic hernia is not accomplished by thoracotomy (see Chapter 47), it traditionally has been included in discussions of neonatal thoracic surgical emergencies. Based on innovative investigation, the term "emergency" may no longer be correct. Work done by Nakayama (1991) and Sakai (1987) and their associates demonstrates a deterioration in pulmonary mechanics after emergent surgery in babies with congenital diaphragmatic hernia. Both groups of authors recommend a period of stabilization before operative treatment. During this stabilization period, the infant may receive pharmacologic treatment for pulmonary hypertension — tolazoline, dobutamine — as described by Ein (1980) and Drummond (1981) and their colleagues. Nonconventional modes of ventilatory support — ECMO, high frequency ventilation — have been used successfully by Bohn (1991) and O'Rourke and associates (1991). Because of the growing realization that the degree of pulmonary hypoplasia is an important determinant of ultimate survival, Bohn and colleagues (1987) made an attempt to quantitate disease severity so that treatment may be stratified based on predictors of outcome.

Proper airway management is essential to ensure the best possible outcome. Endotracheal intubation should be preceded by oxygenation with a bag and mask. Positive pressure ventilation is contraindicated to avoid distending intrathoracic bowel and thereby increasing the infant's respiratory distress. Once an artificial airway is established, vigorous hyperventilation — Pa_{CO_2} 25 to 30 mm Hg — can be instituted.

Anesthetic management of these infants in the operating room depends on their preoperative status and level of respiratory support. Patient inhalation agents in low doses, administered with an anesthesia ventilator, have been shown to be safe and effective. Nitrous oxide is avoided because it may cause bowel distention. If the infant is receiving high frequency ventilation or ECMO support, then a total intravenous anesthetic is necessary. Fentanyl combined with neuromuscular blocking drugs has been used successfully for congenital diaphragmatic hernia repair by Vacanti (1984) and Truog (1990) and their co-workers in infants managed both with high frequency ventilation and ECMO. Because postoperative mechanical ventilation is the rule, the infant is transported from the operating room to the nursery with the endotracheal tube in place.

Tracheoesophageal Fistula

Three important problems must be addressed during the anesthetic evaluation of the infant born with a tracheoesophageal fistula. Is the patient premature, and if so, is there evidence of hyaline membrane disease? Does the patient have coexisting cardiac or gastrointestinal malformations — VATER association*? Is aspiration pneumonitis present?

The presence of any or all of these conditions may make intraoperative ventilatory management even more difficult than it usually is.

In addition to a complete blood count, a radiograph of the chest is a mandatory preoperative examination. The lung fields are examined closely, looking for infiltrates suggestive of aspiration pneumonia, or air bronchograms and reticular granular densities associated with hyaline membrane disease. In addition, the cardiac silhouette is inspected to see if cardiomegaly or a right-sided aortic arch is present. Our patients are evaluated by a neonatologist preoperatively, and a cardiologist is consulted if evidence of congenital heart disease exists.

After placement of a gastrostomy using local anesthesia, general anesthesia is administered for repair of the tracheoesophageal fistula. The relative merits and drawbacks of various induction techniques are hotly debated by pediatric anesthesiologists. Awake endotracheal intubation has the advantage of maintaining spontaneous breathing. Should intubation prove difficult or impossible, the patient will still be able to ventilate spontaneously, and, it is hoped, will not become hypoxic. In vigorous term infants, however, awake intubation can be difficult to perform. Other critics contend that the procedure is inhumane and that some anesthesia should be provided before manipulating the airway. Many advocate an intravenous rapid-sequence induction using muscle relaxants. Ideal intubating conditions exist because the patient is paralyzed. Should the endotracheal tube enter the fistula, however, oxygenation and ventilation are impossible. Buchino and associates (1986) reported severe respiratory compromise and death from persistent wedging of the endotracheal tube in the fistula. A Storz pediatric bronchoscope can be passed through the endotracheal tube to verify proper placement. Proper tube placement is above the carina and below the fistula, a distance of only several millimeters in most patients. Deliberate endobronchial intubation — verified by loss of breath sounds over the left hemithorax — is done, following which the tube is withdrawn until bilateral breath sounds are detected. If the gastrostomy tube is placed under water and bubbles with respiration, then the tube lies above the fistula and has been withdrawn too far.

---

*The VATER association is a spectrum of associated anomalies in the newborn that may consist of varying combinations of vertebral anomalies, anal malformations, tracheoesophageal fistula with esophageal atresia, renal anomalies, and radial arm malformations.

Maintenance of anesthesia is achieved with either low dose inhalational agents or intravenous narcotics. Intraoperative problems include hypotension from great vessel compression, hypoxia, and hypercarbia from lung retraction in the lateral position, and endotracheal tube obstruction from clotted blood. In the otherwise healthy term newborn without preoperative cardiopulmonary problems, extubation is usually possible at the conclusion of the operation. Premature infants, infants with serious associated anomalies, and those whose intraoperative courses have been complicated are usually brought back to the high-risk nursery with the endotracheal tube still in place.

Congenital Lobar Emphysema

Although infants with congenital lobar emphysema — CLE — may develop respiratory distress immediately after birth, most children are diagnosed after 1 month of age. Tachypnea, cyanosis, and diminished breath sounds over the affected side are the usual presenting symptoms and signs. The degree of respiratory distress is occasionally so severe that endotracheal intubation is performed before arrival in the operating room. Regardless of where the intubation is done, it is important to begin any airway manipulation with several minutes of preoxygenation with bag and mask. Positive pressure ventilation further distends the hyperinflated lobe and should be avoided if at all possible.

Thoracotomy for removal of the emphysematous lobe is the usual surgical management of this problem. If the cardiopulmonary status allows, anesthesia is induced by having the infant breathe a mixture of halothane in 100% oxygen. Nitrous oxide and positive pressure ventilation are avoided to prevent further increases in size of the affected lobe. Clinically unstable or rapidly deteriorating infants are best managed by emergent awake intubation. If possible, anesthesia is maintained with halothane, oxygen, and spontaneous ventilation. Arterial blood gas analysis, however, often shows progressive hypoventilation and respiratory acidosis after the patient is placed in the lateral position. In this case, it may be necessary to provide gentle manual positive pressure until the chest is opened and compression of the good lung is relieved. At this point, pulmonary status improves substantially. After lobectomy, most infants show complete return to normal of the arterial blood gas values. Tracheal extubation at the conclusion of the surgical procedure is routine. Goto and associates (1987) mentioned the possible role of high frequency jet ventilation in the intraoperative management of patients with congenital lobar emphysema.

THE OLDER CHILD

In general, anesthetic considerations for thoracic surgery in the older child are no different from those in the adult. One exception is the child with cystic fibrosis. Because of its early onset and chronic course, cystic fibrosis is managed primarily by pediatric subspecialists. Failure of medical therapy to control pulmonary problems such as bronchiectasis and recurrent pneumothoraces may necessitate surgery. The excellent discussion of cystic fibrosis by Maclusky and Levison (1990) provides background knowledge to ensure a safe perioperative course.

Cystic fibrosis is the most common lethal inherited disorder of whites. This autosomal recessive disease occurs in one of every 2000 live births. Generalized exocrine gland dysfunction is the hallmark of this disease. Involvement of the pulmonary, cardiovascular, and gastrointestinal systems is of greatest concern for the anesthesiologist.

The pulmonary exocrine glands of cystic fibrosis patients secrete an abnormally tenacious mucus. Impaired mucociliary clearance of this mucus plus a predisposition to chronic endobronchial bacterial colonization causes progressive pulmonary damage. Bronchiectasis develops as a result of peribronchial inflammation and leads to airway collapse and air trapping. Shunting of blood through large bronchopulmonary collateral vessels may occur, with the potential for massive hemoptysis should these vessels rupture. Repeated cycles of infection — especially with *Pseudomonas* species — and pulmonary damage leads to chronic hypoxemia and ultimately cor pulmonale. Although, as noted by FitzSimmons (1993), improved medical management in the past 20 years has resulted in doubling of the mean survival age to 28 years, most cystic fibrosis patients die of chronic pulmonary disease and secondary cardiac failure.

Gastrointestinal involvement in cystic fibrosis occurs as a result of exocrine pancreatic insufficiency. Malnutrition and malabsorption are present to a variable extent in most patients. Inadequate levels of fat-soluble vitamins, especially vitamin K, can be problematic. Hypovitaminosis K can contribute to severe bleeding problems perioperatively.

Medical management of the cystic fibrosis patient consists of the following: chest physiotherapy to aid in mobilization of secretions, antibiotic therapy for prevention and treatment of infection, bronchodilator therapy for airway hyperreactivity, and aggressive nutritional support. Situations that may require surgical intervention include severe bronchiectasis, recurrent pneumothoraces, and life-threatening hemoptysis.

Marmon and associates (1983) emphasize that preoperative optimization of the patient's medical condition is essential. This effort requires cooperation among the surgeon, pediatrician, and anesthesiologist. Cystic fibrosis patients ideally are hospitalized several days before elective thoracic surgery to institute aggressive chest physiotherapy and antibiotic coverage. Nutritional status should be made optimal as well, including hyperalimentation if necessary. Preoperative laboratory studies establish the patient's baseline pulmonary status. These include hemoglobin, chest radiograph, coagulation profile, pulmonary function tests, and arterial blood gas analysis — pulse oximetry and transcutaneous CO_2

are acceptable substitutes. If the patient has cor pulmonale or is receiving diuretics, additional information such as an echocardiogram or serum electrolytes may be indicated.

Regional anesthesia is preferable to general anesthesia in patients with cystic fibrosis, but this technique is usually not suitable for thoracic surgical procedures. Use of a general anesthetic with volatile agents such as halothane or isoflurane has been successful in these cases. Avoidance of nitrous oxide permits use of high inspired oxygen tension and prevents expansion of air-containing pulmonary bullae by the more diffusible N_2O. The use of intravenous agents such as narcotics and benzodiazepines is discouraged to minimize postoperative respiratory depression. Although a review article by Lamberty and Rubin (1985) cited a high perioperative complication rate of 10%, I think the current complication rate is lower, in part because of better patient selection, preoperative preparation, and intraoperative monitoring.

It is essential to avoid "soiling" the contralateral lung during pulmonary resection for bronchiectasis. Use of a double-lumen endotracheal tube is helpful if the patient's size permits. Experience with bronchial blockers has been limited in smaller patients.

Patients with cystic fibrosis may require intensive care after a long, difficult procedure, especially if their preoperative medical condition was poor or if unexpected intraoperative problems arose. Most patients, however, can be extubated in the operating room after thorough tracheal suctioning. They should receive oxygen therapy with pulse oximetry monitoring throughout their stay in the postanesthesia care unit and for 24 hours postoperatively.

Postoperative pain relief is an important aspect of the patient's care. Administration of narcotics is usually not recommended because of the risk of hypoventilation with subsequent hypercarbia and hypoxia. Alternative methods of postoperative analgesia include intercostal nerve block performed by the surgeon in the operating room, epidurally administered local anesthetic, or intravenous non-narcotic medications such as ketorolac. Ideally, pain control is managed by or with the assistance of a hospital-based pain service.

POSTOPERATIVE ANALGESIA

Schechter and associates (1986) noted that interest in postoperative pediatric pain control has dramatically increased in recent decades. Research in the areas of neonatal pain perception and narcotic administration in children, as reported by McGrath and Johnson (1988), has heightened physician awareness that these patients experience postoperative pain and that adequate relief of pain may improve overall outcome, especially in children undergoing thoracotomy. Coe and colleagues (1991) and Craig (1981) summarized the well-described decrease in pulmonary function after these procedures, believed to result in part from poor respiratory effort because of pain. Adequate analgesia ameliorates this problem, according to Conacher (1990) and Shulman and co-workers (1984).

Asantila and associates (1986) emphasized that a variety of options exist for the management of postoperative thoracotomy pain. Studies performed by Kambam (1989) and Ferrante (1991) and their colleagues evaluated the safety and efficacy of interpleural postoperative analgesia. Logas and associates (1987) described the use of thoracic epidural infusions for pain relief. Lumbar epidural infusions of local anesthetic alone or with morphine were used by some investigators including Guinard (1992), Salomaki (1991), Badner (1990), and Sandler (1992) and their co-workers. In general, these regional techniques provided better analgesia with fewer side effects — pruritus, nausea, urinary retention, and hypoventilation — than more traditional techniques such as parenteral narcotics. Non-narcotic parenteral agents such as ketorolac and indomethacin have been used successfully in the management of post-thoracotomy pain both in adults and children, as reported by Pavy (1990) and Watcha (1992) and their associates. Regional techniques for postoperative analgesia in children were shown by Desparmet (1987) and Dalens (1986) and their colleagues to be effective and safe after orthopedic and urologic procedures, and we have every reason to expect that children undergoing thoracotomy would derive similar benefit. Interpleural analgesia was used successfully by McIlvaine and associates (1988), but the technique has not gained widespread popularity. Use of patient-controlled analgesia — PCA — as described by Berde and colleagues (1991) has become commonplace in the postoperative pediatric population. This technique provides greater patient satisfaction with a lower incidence of side effects when compared with intramuscular injections.

Use of these less traditional, more invasive methods of analgesia requires close patient monitoring and supervision of both the family and nursing staff. Many hospitals offer an anesthesiology-based multidisciplinary pain service to implement appropriate postoperative analgesia and to ensure its safety and efficacy. Ready (1988) and Shapiro (1991) and their colleagues have reported the successes of their respective pain services.

REFERENCES

Alexander CM, Teller LE, Gross JB: Principles of pulse oximetry: Theoretical and practical considerations. Anesth Analg 68:368, 1989.

American Academy of Pediatrics and American College of Obstetrics and Gynecology: Guidelines for Perinatal Care. Evanston, IL: American Academy of Pediatrics, 1983, pp. 212-213.

Asantila R, Rosenberg PH, Scheinin B: Comparison of different methods of postoperative analgesia after thoracotomy. Acta Anaesthesiol Scand 30:421, 1986.

Badgwell JM: Oximetry and capnography monitoring. Anesth Clin North Am 9:821, 1991.

Badner NH, et al: Lumbar epidural fentanyl infusions for post-thoracotomy patients: Analgesic, respiratory, and pharmacokinetic effects. J Cardiothorac Anesth 4:543, 1990.

Baumgart S, et al: Effect of heat shielding on convective and evaporative heat losses and on radiant heat transfer in the premature infant. J Pediatr 99:948, 1987.

Bautista MJ, Kuwahara BS, Henderson CU: Transcutaneous oxygen monitoring in an infant undergoing tracheoesophageal fistula repair. Can J Anaesth 33:505, 1986.

Berde CB, et al: Patient-controlled analgesia in children and adolescents: A randomized, prospective comparison with intramuscular administration of morphine for postoperative analgesia. J Pediatr 118:460, 1991.

Bhavani-Shankar K, Moseley H, Kumar AY: Capnometry and anesthesia. Can J Anaesth 39:617, 1992.

Bohn DJ: Congenital diaphragmatic hernia. Anesth Clin North Am 9:899, 1991.

Bohn D, et al: Ventilatory predictors of pulmonary hypoplasia in congenital diaphragmatic hernia, confirmed by morphologic assessment. J Pediatr 111:423, 1987.

Brandom BW: Neuromuscular blocking drugs. Anesth Clin North Am 9:781, 1991.

Brett CM, et al: The cardiovascular effects of isoflurane in lambs. Anesthesiology 67:60, 1987.

Buchino JJ, et al: Malpositioning of the endotracheal tube in infants with tracheoesophageal fistula. J Pediatr 109:524, 1986.

Coe A, et al: Pain following thoracotomy. Anaesthesia 46:918, 1991.

Conacher ID: Pain relief after thoracotomy. Br J Anaesth 65:806, 1990.

Cook DR: Muscle relaxants and children. Anesth Analg 60:335, 1981.

Coté CJ, et al: A single-blind study of combined pulse oximetry and capnography in children. Anesthesiology 74:980, 1991.

Craig DB: Postoperative recovery of pulmonary function. Anesth Analg 60:46, 1981.

Dalens B, Tanguy A, Haberer JP: Lumbar epidural anesthesia for operative and postoperative pain relief in infants and young children. Anesth Analg 65:1069, 1986.

Desparmet J, et al: Continuous epidural infusion of bupivacaine for postoperative pain relief in children. Anesthesiology 67:108, 1987.

Drummond WH, et al: The independent effects of hyperventilation, tolazoline, and dopamine on infants with persistent pulmonary hypertension. J Pediatr 98:603, 1981.

Duncan PG, Gregory GB, Wade JG: The effect of nitrous oxide on baroreceptor function in newborn and adult rabbits. Can J Anaesth 28:339, 1987.

Ein SH, et al: The pharmacologic treatment of newborn congenital diaphragmatic hernia — a 2-year evaluation. J Pediatr Surg 15:384, 1980.

Eisele JH, Milstem MM, Goetzmann BW: Pulmonary vascular responses to nitrous oxide in newborn lambs. Anesth Analg 65:62, 1986.

Ferrante FM, et al: Interpleural analgesia after thoracotomy. Anesth Analg 72:105, 1991.

FitzSimmons SC: The changing epidemiology of cystic fibrosis. J Pediatr 122:1, 1993.

Friesen RH, Henry DB: Cardiovascular changes in preterm neonates receiving isoflurane, halothane, fentanyl and ketamine. Anesthesiology 64:238, 1986.

Goto H, et al: High-frequency jet ventilation for resection of congenital lobar emphysema. Anesth Analg 66:684, 1987.

Goudsouzian NG: Muscle relaxants in children. In Ryan JF, et al: A Practice of Anesthesia for Infants and Children. Orlando, FL: Grune & Stratton, 1986, pp. 108-109.

Goudsouzian NG, Standaert FG: The infant and the myoneural junction. Anesth Analg 65:1208, 1986.

Guinard JP, et al: A randomized comparison of intravenous versus lumbar and thoracic epidural fentanyl for analgesia after thoracotomy. Anesthesiology 77:1108, 1992.

Hickey PR, et al: Blunting of stress responses in the pulmonary circulation of infants by fentanyl. Anesth Analg 64:1137, 1985.

Hickey PR, et al: Pulmonary and systemic hemodynamic effects of nitrous oxide in infants with normal and elevated pulmonary vascular resistance. Anesthesiology 65:374, 1986.

Kambam JR, et al: Intrapleural analgesia for post-thoracotomy pain and blood levels of bupivacaine following intrapleural injection. Can J Anaesth 36:106, 1989.

Lamberty JM, Rubin BK: The management of anaesthesia for patients with cystic fibrosis. Anaesthesia 40:448, 1985.

Logas WG, et al: Continuous thoracic epidural analgesia for postoperative pain relief following thoracotomy: A randomized prospective study. Anesthesiology 67:787, 1987.

Lucey JF, Dangman B: A re-examination of the role of oxygen in retrolental fibroplasia. Pediatrics 73:82, 1984.

Maclusky I, Levison H: Disorders of the respiratory tract in children. In Chernick J (ed): Kendig's Disorders of the Respiratory Tract in Children. Fifth Edition. Philadelphia: WB Saunders, 1990, pp. 692-730.

Marmon L, et al: Pulmonary resection for complications of cystic fibrosis. J Pediatr Surg 18:811, 1983.

McIlvaine WB, et al: Continuous infusion of bupivacaine via intrapleural catheter for analgesia after thoracotomy in children. Anesthesiology 69:261, 1988.

McGrath PJ, Johnson GD: Pain management in children. Can J Anaesth 35:107, 1988.

Moller JT, et al: Randomised evaluation of pulse oximetry in 20,802 patients: I and II. Anesthesiology 78:436, 1993.

Moore RA: Hemodynamic and anesthetic effects of sufentanil as the sole anesthetic for pediatric cardiovascular surgery. Anesthesiology 62:725, 1985.

Nakayama DK, Motoyama EK, Tagge EM: Effect of preoperative stabilization on respiratory system compliance and outcome in newborn infants with congenital diaphragmatic hernia. J Pediatr 118:793, 1991.

O'Rourke PP, et al: The effect of extracorporeal membrane oxygenation on the survival of neonates with high-risk congenital diaphragmatic hernia. J Pediatr Surg 26:147, 1991.

Pavy T, Medley C, Murphy DF: Effect of indomethacin on pain relief after thoracotomy. Br J Anaesth 65:624, 1990.

Ready LB, et al: Development of an anesthesiology-based postoperative pain management service. Anesthesiology 68:100, 1988.

Robinson S, Gregory GD: Fentanyl-air-oxygen anesthesia for ligation of patent ductus arteriosus in preterm infants. Anesth Analg 60:331, 1981.

Sakai H, et al: Effect of surgical repair on respiratory mechanics in congenital diaphragmatic hernia. J Pediatr 111:432, 1987.

Salomaki TE, Laitinen JO, Nuutinen LS: A randomized double-blind comparison of epidural versus intravenous fentanyl infusion for analgesia fater thoracotomy. Anesthesiology 75:790, 1991.

Sandler AN, et al: A randomized, double-blind comparison of lumbar epidural and intravenous fentanyl infusions for post-thoracotomy pain relief. Anesthesiology 77:626, 1992.

Sarnaik BP, Preston C: Physiologic peculiarities of the respiratory system in neonates. Anesth Rev 9:31, 1982.

Schechter NL, Allen A, Hanson K: Status of pediatric pain control: A comparison of hospital analgesic usage in children and adults. Pediatrics 77:11, 1986.

Schieber RB, Stiller RL, Cook DR: Cardiovascular and pharmacodynamic effects of high-dose fentanyl in newborn piglets. Anesthesiology 63:166, 1985.

Schieber RB, et al: Hemodynamic effects of isoflurane in the newborn piglet: Comparisons with halothane. Anesth Analg 65:633, 1986.

Severinghaus JW, Keller JF: Recent developments in pulse oximetry. Anesthesiology 76:1018, 1992.

Shapiro BS, et al: Experience of an interdisciplinary pediatric pain service. Pediatrics 88:1226, 1991.

Shulman M, et al: Post-thoracotomy pain and pulmonary function following epidural and systemic morphine. Anesthesiology 61:569, 1984.

Smith RM: Anesthesia for Infants and Children. 4th Ed. St. Louis: CV Mosby, 1980, pp. 192-215.

Thornburg KL, Morton MJ: Filling and arterial pressure as determinants of RV stroke volume in the sheep fetus. Am J Physiol 244:H656, 1983.

Tremper KK, Barker SJ: Pulse oximetry. Anesthesiology 70:98, 1989.

Truog RD, et al: Repair of congenital diaphragmatic hernia during extracorporeal membrane oxygenation. Anesthesiology 72:750, 1990.

Vacanti JP, et al: The pulmonary hemodynamic response to perioperative anesthesia in the treatment of high-risk infants with congenital diaphragmatic hernia. J Pediatr Surg 19:672, 1984.

Watcha MF, et al: Comparison of ketorolac and morphine as adjuvants during pediatric surgery. Anesthesiology 76:368, 1992.

Waugh R, Johnson GG: Current considerations in neonatal anesthesia. Can J Anaesth 31:700, 1984.

Wear R, Robinson S, Gregory GB: The effect of halothane on the baroresponses of adult and baby rabbits. Anesthesiology 56:188, 1982.

White PF, Way WI, Trevor BJ: Ketamine: Its pharmacology and therapeutic uses. Anesthesiology 56:119, 1982.

Whyte RK, et al: Assessment of Doppler ultrasound to measure systolic and diastolic pressures in infants and young children. Arch Dis Child 50:542, 1975.

Yaster M: The dose response of fentanyl in neonatal anesthesia. Anesthesiology 66:433, 1987.

Zaritsky B, Chernow B: Use of catecholamines in pediatrics. J Pediatr 105:341, 1984.

READING REFERENCE

Anand KJS, Hickey PR: Halothane-morphine compared with high-dose sufentanil for anesthesia and postoperative analgesia in neonatal cardiac surgery. N Engl J Med 326:1, 1992.

Postoperative Management of the General Thoracic Surgical Patient

CHAPTER 24

GENERAL PRINCIPLES OF POSTOPERATIVE CARE

Axel W. Joob and Renee S. Hartz

The complexity and sophistication of perioperative care make thoracic surgery a uniquely challenging specialty. Surgeons must be not only thoroughly familiar with cardiac and respiratory physiology, but also well versed in current techniques of anesthetic management and intensive care technology.

Perioperative care of the thoracic surgical patient generally falls into four categories: 1) drainage and obliteration of the pleural space, 2) control of postoperative pain, 3) care of the respiratory system, and 4) care of the cardiovascular system.

DRAINAGE AND OBLITERATION OF THE PLEURAL SPACE

The unique physiology of the pleural space, with its normal negative pressure, separates thoracic surgery from other surgical disciplines. *All patients who undergo thoracotomy are left with some degree of pneumothorax and the potential for developing a residual pleural space.* Before closing the chest, the surgeon must seal all air leaks as well as possible. Large-bore thoracostomy tubes readily provide a means of evacuating air, accumulated blood, and other fluids. The types and positioning of tubes to drain the pleural space are myriad and depend on the surgeons' preferences. Both silicone and rubber catheters are commonly used after pulmonary resection and most surgeons use at least two tubes, one for air — placed at the apex of the chest — and one for fluid — placed posteroinferiorly. The pleural space is not drained after pneumonectomy unless excessive bleeding occurs or major fear of infection exists. Efforts are made to adjust the pressure in the operated hemithorax to be slightly negative, thus maintaining the mediastinum in a neutral position. Obliteration of the pleural space is normally accomplished by re-expansion of remaining lung tissue, shift of the mediastinum to the operated side, narrowing of the ipsilateral intercostal spaces, and elevation of the hemidiaphragm. Collections of air or fluid, or decreased compliance in the remaining lung tissue, may prevent the expansion necessary to obliterate the pleural space; adequate pleural drainage is therefore crucial.

Pleural drainage systems must include airtight seals to maintain an intrapleural vacuum, -3 to -5 mm Hg. The simplest form of chest drainage is the underwater seal system, which allows free egress of air and fluid from the intrapleural space. The staff must, however, be thoroughly familiar with the mechanics of the system to prevent catastrophes. The tubes should not normally be clamped — doing so may result in tension pneumo- or hydrothorax, the fluid level in the water seal bottle must be maintained at all times, and the bottles must be kept below the level of the patient to prevent siphoning of water into the chest.

For those patients with large air leaks, and for those in whom a large amount of fluid must be drained from the chest, most surgeons prefer to maintain continuous negative pressure in the pleural space. The amount of suction is variable but must exceed the intrapleural vacuum developed by the patient during inspiration. When reversal of flow occurs in the tubing during inspiration, the amount of suction is insufficient to provide obliteration of the pleural space. If intermittent bubbling occurs while the patient is on water seal, suction should also be applied.

A widely used, commercially available system for draining the pleural space is the Pleur-evac, a compact, nonbreakable, three-bottle chest drainage apparatus (Fig. 24–1). It can be used as a simple underwater seal system or attached to a vacuum line. The amount of suction is limited by the height of the column of water in the vacuum control chamber. The third component of the unit is a compartmentalized collection chamber.

The Pleur-evac drainage system is used most commonly, except when a large amount of bleeding is suspected, in which case an autotransfusion set-up is used. When more than 25 cm water suction is required to overcome an air leak, we convert to an Emerson three-bottle suction apparatus or put 2 cm of mercury in the bottom of the vacuum chamber of the Pleur-evac,

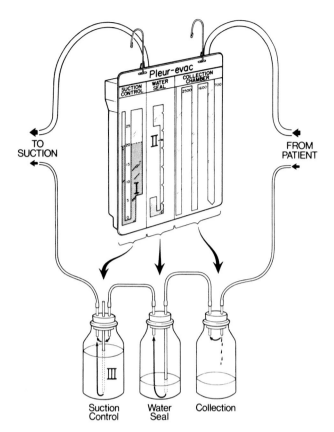

Fig. 24–1. The Pleur-evac is a compartmentalized, commercially available three-bottle suction apparatus. It can be used without suction as a simple water-seal device. The height of the column in the suction control chamber determines the amount of negative pressure applied to the pleural space (I). An additional feature of the Pleur-evac is the ability to measure the amount of negative pressure developed by the patient (II and III).

delivering, in effect, about 50 cm water of suction. The nursing staff should be instructed never to clamp chest tubes, but when a slow air leak is suspected, tubes are clamped for a few hours with the patient under close supervision. For patient comfort, we place the chest tubes at the level of the anterior/superior iliac spine. For patients who are intubated, removal of chest tubes is accomplished using an "inflate and hold" technique. One person delivers a large inspiration to the patient and holds it while a second person removes the chest tube and places the dressing. For patients who are breathing normally when the tubes are removed, they are taught to inspire and hold or to breathe quietly while the chest tubes are removed. We do not advocate that patients force exhalation while the chest tubes are removed because a large, reflex, sudden, inspiratory effort may produce a pneumothorax.

During the postoperative period, it is essential that all radiographs are obtained with the patient in the upright position. A radiograph obtained when the patient is semirecumbent or supine will fail to identify fluid or air, or both, remaining in the pleural space.

CONTROL OF POSTOPERATIVE PAIN

Significant advances in controlling postoperative pain in thoracic surgical patients have been made. A heightened awareness exists that excessive pain contributes to most postoperative complications, and control of pain is approached in a highly scientific fashion. Pain increases atelectasis because of chest wall splinting and a resulting diminution in chest excursion. Pain increases sympathetic tone so that peripheral vascular resistance and myocardial oxygen consumption are correspondingly elevated. The increase in cardiac workload may provoke arrhythmias and previously masked cardiac ischemia. Pain, as noted by Cousins and Phillips (1984), also increases vagal tone, resulting in more nausea and vomiting and elevated hormonal tone so that water retention and hyperglycemia are initiated. Failure to control postoperative pain in the elderly patient who has had a thoracotomy may result in life-threatening cardiorespiratory complications.

The techniques of pain relief used depend largely on the medical and ancillary staff. The traditional method of injecting intramuscular narcotics every few hours has serious drawbacks: the patient experiences severe pain at low narcotic levels and possible confusion and agitation at high levels. An acceptable alternative to intermittent intramuscular narcotics is continuous intravenous infusion. This method can be practiced safely in all hospitals if the physician is aware of proper loading and maintenance doses. For meperidine, the doses are clearly established; for a 70-kg patient, a 100-mg loading dose should be administered over 30 to 60 minutes and a maintenance dose of 18 to 30 mg per hour can be continuously administered. Doses are based on the volume of distribution of the drug and on the desired analgesic blood level. As emphasized by Stapleton (1979) and Cousins (1984) and their colleagues, dosage should be reduced if liver function is abnormal, if vomiting occurs, or if respirations are depressed. Although the doses for morphine sulfate are not precisely established, the usual loading dose is 7.5 mg over 1 hour followed by 2.5 mg per hour by continuous infusion.

Angle intercostal nerve block for pain relief is fairly easy to implement once the catheters have been placed by the surgeon in the operating room. The catheters are placed at the posterior rib angles at the incision and two interspaces above and below the incision. Bupivacaine 0.5% with epinephrine 1:200,000 is infused intermittently. The usual dose is 3 to 5 ml every 6 to 18 hours per interspace. Signs of local anesthetic toxicity and inadvertent vascular injection must be monitored carefully.

Epidural blockade is a highly effective method of achieving postoperative pain relief in the thoracotomy patient. Complications — nausea, vomiting, pruritis, urinary retention, and respiratory depression — reduced by careful attention to administration and proper dosage. It is crucial that those who use epidural block are well versed in catheter placement and aseptic technique, and that resuscitative equipment is readily available for patients with epidural catheters. The level of sensory block must be carefully ascertained — T10 umbilicus, T7 xiphoid, and T4–5 nipple. Subarachnoid injection may result in spinal anesthesia with hypotension, bradycardia, and apnea — motor block of T1 results in respiratory failure. In 40 postoperative thoracotomy patients treated with intermittent epidural morphine reported by Milvert and associates (1983), the mean interval between doses was 12 hours. One half of the patients required only one dose, and more than 24 hours of analgesia were produced in 13%. The authors noted a high incidence of urinary retention, but stated that most of their thoracotomy patients had urinary catheters for the procedure. Other authors prefer continuous epidural infusion of narcotics. El-Baz and colleagues (1982) compared intravenous morphine, intermittent epidural morphine, and continuous epidural morphine at 0.18 mg per hour in the relief of post-thoracotomy pain in 60 patients. Patients who received continuous epidural morphine received additional bolus injections from the nursing staff as needed. Pain scores in the continuous epidural morphine group were significantly lower than those for the other two groups. Pain control did not differ between the other two groups, but those who received intermittent epidural morphine had a high incidence of central narcosis — four patients required naloxone, one required

naloxone plus mechanical ventilation. The authors concluded that continuous morphine by the epidural route achieved "effective, segmental, and selective postoperative analgesia" (Fig. 24–2).

Brodsky and associates (1986) prefer lumbar epidural narcotics and avoid the thoracic route to lower the complication rate. The catheter is placed before the operative procedure and is used intraoperatively for injection of local anesthetics to reduce or eliminate the need for muscle relaxants. Narcotic administration begins not less than 45 minutes before the end of the operation so that "most patients awaken free of pain and are extubated in the operating room."

Our group uses epidural catheters for postoperative narcotic administration in patients who undergo major pulmonary resections and in those who are at high risk for pulmonary complications. We prefer fentanyl because its high lipid solubility lessens the possibility of ascending block and its onset of action is 15 minutes compared to approximately 1 hour for morphine. One to 1.5 µg/kg is given about 20 minutes before the incision is closed, followed by 0.5 µg/kg by continuous infusion. The catheter is left in place for 5 to 7 days after the operative procedure, during which time our patients have received almost no parenteral analgesics. The patients ambulate sooner than with conventional pain relief techniques, and it is our impression that they are discharged a day or so earlier than patients who were managed without this technique.

CARE OF THE RESPIRATORY SYSTEM

Before undertaking a pulmonary resection, the surgeon must be as confident as possible that the patient's pulmonary reserves are sufficient to tolerate the thoracotomy incision and the loss of lung volume. Once the surgeon has determined that the patient should tolerate the procedure (Table 24–1), the extent of pre-existing pulmonary disease and the extent of the resection dictate the amount of attention focused on the possibility of postoperative pulmonary complications. Dyspnea, when present, is a predictor of mortality, and its presence mandates full pulmonary function testing and blood gas determinations, as suggested by Meltman (1961). Smokers should be urged to stop smoking for as long as possible before the operation to restore bronchial ciliary action. Patients with chronic bronchitis should receive a suitable period of appropriate antibiotics — based on sputum culture results — before the planned procedure.

Preoperative education of the patient should include techniques of postoperative bronchial hygiene. *The patient must be able to generate an effective cough.* For those who cannot, instruction involves training in breathing techniques. Shapiro and colleagues (1979) recommended that the patient be taught to inspire and hold, forcefully contract the abdominal muscles, and then exhale. They also recommended teaching patients to cuddle a pillow to help their cough effort. Patients

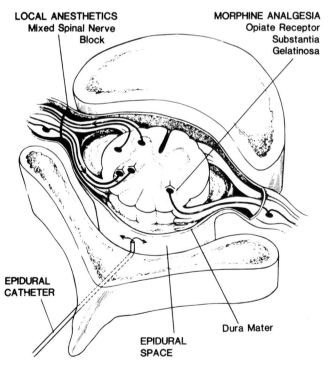

Fig. 24–2. Anatomic basis for narcotic analgesia and local anesthetic action. *From* El-Baz N, Ivankovich AD: Management of postoperative thoracotomy pain: Continuous epidural infusion of morphine. *In* Kittle CF: Current Controversies in Thoracic Surgery. Philadelphia, WB Saunders, 1986.

LOCAL ANESTHETICS
Mixed Spinal Nerve Block

MORPHINE ANALGESIA
Opiate Receptor
Substantia Gelatinosa

EPIDURAL CATHETER

EPIDURAL SPACE

Dura Mater

Table 24-1. Pulmonary Function Test Criteria for Resection

Test	Unit	Normal	Pneumonectomy	Lobectomy	Biopsy or Segmental
MBC	Liters/minute	>100	>70	40–70	40
MBC	Percent predicted		>55	40–70	35–40
FEV$_1$	Liters	>2	>2	>1	>0.6
FEV$_1$	Percent predicted		>55	40–70	$\geqq$40
FEV$_{25-75}$	Liters	2	>1.6	0.6–1.6	>0.6

From Miller J.I.: Thoracic surgery. *In* Kaplan J.A.: Thoracic Anesthesia New York; Churchill Livingstone, 1983, p. 25.

should also be taught to use an incentive spirometer during the postoperative period.

Other important factors in the postoperative care of the patient include proper positioning, chest physiotherapy, tracheal suctioning, control of pain, and possible prolonged intubation and ventilation. The role of intermittent positive pressure breathing — IPPB — remains controversial and transcatheter intratracheal injection of irritating solutions is practiced sporadically.

Proper positioning of the patient includes using gravity to assist in keeping the diaphragm depressed, the airways open, and pain at a minimum. Postural drainage is used in conjunction with positioning to assist the mucociliary action with gravity and is often accompanied with chest vibrations and percussion (see Chapter 26). Tracheal suctioning should be integral to the care of any patient who is not able to mobilize secretions spontaneously. The managing physicians and nursing staff should be familiar with tracheal suctioning and use it frequently. If tracheal suctioning does not stimulate effective coughing and clearing of secretions, bronchoscopy may be necessary. Finally, prolonged intubation and ventilation, or reintubation, may be necessary. Many surgeons prefer to extubate thoracotomy patients immediately postoperatively. After long procedures in patients with impaired pulmonary function, abnormal blood gas values, or concomitant cardiac illness, however, mechanical ventilation should be instituted as soon as any signs of respiratory insufficiency develop (see Chapter 25).

Atelectasis is always present after thoracotomy and occurs because of a decrease in functional residual capacity — FRC. The most significant cause of postoperative morbidity, it is promoted by decreased lung compliance, obstructive secretions in the airways, fluid accumulation within the operated hemithorax, and postoperative pain. Restoration of the FRC by the aforementioned measures should minimize the degree of atelectasis and prevent the development of consolidation in the atelectatic areas of the lung.

The philosophy is to encourage patient education for postoperative respiratory self-care and the implementation of such care by the thoracic surgery service. Respiratory therapy technicians are consulted liberally to assist in preoperative teaching and to administer postoperative treatments. Patients who are not believed to have pre-existing pulmonary disease can have simple screening pulmonary functions — FEV$_1$ and FVC — and room-air blood gas sampling. Patients with resting or exertional dyspnea should undergo full pulmonary function testing with and without bronchodilators.

Our group uses a simple, inexpensive, incentive spirometer and teaches its use to all patients preoperatively. We believe that blow bottles are not useful and agree with Nunn and colleagues (1965), who present evidence that they may be deleterious. We advocate vigorous nasotracheal suctioning in patients who are not maintaining good bronchial hygiene on their own, and resort early to bedside bronchoscopy. Lastly, our threshold for instituting mechanical ventilation is low, both in the immediate postoperative period and in patients who develop signs of respiratory insufficiency later in their postoperative course.

CARE OF THE CARDIOVASCULAR SYSTEM

Ischemic Heart Disease

Arrhythmia, myocardial infarction, and heart failure are common complications during and after operations on the chest, any of which may potentially lead to the death of the patient. The incidence of these complications increases in older patients, who have a higher incidence of pre-existing cardiovascular and respiratory disease and are now candidates for thoracotomy.

The most important factor in determining the presence of silent cardiovascular disease is a high index of suspicion during the preoperative evaluation. Few patients volunteer a history of angina pectoris, and each must be questioned to determine whether he or she has symptoms that suggest ischemic heart disease. Whether or not the history is positive, the preoperative electrocardiogram may yield useful information. Patients with a history that suggests ischemia and those with electrocardiographic evidence of old infarction or ongoing ischemia should undergo exercise or thallium stress testing. If the stress test is positive, the patient should undergo cardiac catheterization and coronary arteriography before undergoing thoracotomy. Some patients require myocardial revascularization. Since the introduction of balloon coronary angioplasty, it has been possible to relieve the ischemia with a less invasive procedure than coronary bypass.

In no instance should a patient with large areas of ischemic myocardium undergo elective thoracotomy, although select patients with chronic stage angina who have limited areas of ischemia may undergo thoracotomy without excessive risk. All high-risk patients should be anesthetized by skilled anesthesiologists with full knowledge of hemodynamic monitoring. An arterial line and a Swan-Ganz catheter should be placed before the induction of anesthesia so that episodes of hypotension and hypertension can be quickly detected and corrected and cardiac filling pressures can be closely monitored. During the procedure, nitroglycerin should be administered intravenously and inotropic agents should be available. Ideally, such high-risk patients should have this procedure in institutions in which an intra-aortic balloon pump is available and acute infarct intervention is practiced.

Myocardial Infarction

Arkins (1964), Driscoll (1961), and Tarhan (1972) and their associates estimated that 0.2 to 3.0% of patients undergoing thoracic surgical procedures sustain a myocardial infarction, and another 5 to 10% exhibit electrocardiographic changes. Obviously, the older the patient, the greater the likelihood of sustaining an infarct. After perioperative infarction, the patient's prognosis may be serious. In a large Mayo Clinic series, published by Tarhan and colleagues (1978), only 0.13% of patients without a history of infarction suffered a perioperative infarct. In a classic study performed later at the same institution, however, Steen and co-workers (1978) reported that of 587 patients with a history of myocardial infarction who had anesthesia and surgery, 6.1% reinfarcted, and of those patients, 69% died! When patients were operated on within 3 months of their previous infarction, 27% reinfarcted. Thus, determining not only whether but when a previous myocardial infarction occurred is crucial.

Arrhythmia

According to Beck-Nielsen and associates (1973), arrhythmias occur in approximately 20% of noncardiac thoracic operations. The incidence increases with the patient's age and the magnitude of the procedure, especially with intrapericardial ligation of the pulmonary vessels, and is higher after pneumonectomy than after lobectomy. Such rhythm disturbances contribute significantly to mortality rates: Shields and Ujiki (1968), for example, noted a 14% mortality rate in patients with postoperative arrhythmia, compared to a 4% mortality rate in its abscence. Commonly occurring arrhythmias are sinus bradycardia, premature ventricular contractions — PVCs, junctional rhythm, and atrial fibrillation and flutter. As a rule, bradycardia is more difficult to treat than tachycardia. Whenever a patient develops postoperative rhythm disturbances, hypokalemia or arterial hypoxemia should be suspected; many arrhythmias are remedied simply by correcting these abnormalities. All PVCs are ominous and should be treated aggressively with antiarrhythmic drugs even while waiting for laboratory values. Supraventricular rhythm disturbances such as atrial fibrillation, atrial flutter, and paroxysmal supraventricular tachycardia are common and are usually controlled with digitalis or with such antiarrhythmic agents as verapamil. The thoracic surgeon should be familiar with the dosages and adverse effects of all available antiarrhythmic agents and know how to institute temporary pacing for the treatment of bradycardia (see Chapters 19 and 28).

The issue of preoperative digitalis administration deserves consideration. Although the topic is controversial and the studies are not randomized, Shields and Ujiki (1968), Burman (1972), and Wheat and Buford (1961) noted that preoperative digitalis administration reduces the incidence of these complications. Some authors, such as Ellison (1979), have written that digitalis should be administered slowly over several days before the procedure and excluded when it is not considered until the night before surgery. Others, including Shields and Ujiki (1968), state that digitalis is important enough to be administered the night before surgery, especially to patients 60 years of age or older and to those for whom pneumonectomy is a possibility.

Heart Failure

Heart failure is unusual in the absence of pre-existing heart disease, but it may occur with overzealous fluid administration. If intravascular volume overload develops, the surgeon should resort immediately to the use of the Swan-Ganz catheter to monitor the reduction of the fluid overload. Management of the heart failure per se should not be difficult for any thoracic surgeon. Kaplan (1983) developed a useful table to direct the treatment of heart failure appropriately (Fig. 24–3). An early and aggressive approach to such treatment should be kept in mind; when heart failure develops, the presence of ischemic heart disease should be considered and myocardial infarction ruled out with appropriate laboratory examinations and serial electrocardiograms.

The surgeon should maintain an aggressive approach to the diagnosis and treatment of underlying heart disease before thoracotomy. The patients in our institution with suspected or proven ischemic heart disease who are to undergo thoracotomy are anesthetized with

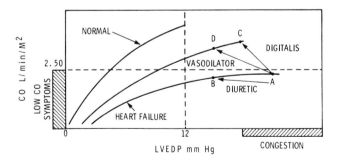

Fig. 24–3. Curves represent normal Frank-Starling mechanism, and therapeutic interventions are indicated when patients' hemodynamics fall outside the normal range. *From* Kaplan JA (ed.): Complications of Thoracic Surgery. *In* Thoracic Anesthesia. New York: Churchill Livingstone, 1983, as modified from Mason DT: Congestive Heart Failure: Mechanisms, Evaluation and Treatment. With permission of Yorke Medical Books, Technical Publishing, a division of Dun-Donnelly Publishing Corporation, a company of Dun & Bradstreet Corporation, 1976.

full monitoring — arterial lines, Swan-Ganz catheter, Foley catheter — and special attention is directed to minimizing myocardial oxygen consumption. Cardiac filling pressures, including central venous pressure and pulmonary capillary wedge pressure, are measured repeatedly, cardiac output is determined, and peripheral vascular resistance is calculated. To decrease myocardial oxygen demand, hypertension is avoided and the peripheral vascular resistance is maintained as near normal as possible. Nitroglycerin is administered continuously, and volume is given as needed to maintain the optimal filling pressures for that particular patient. The monitoring lines are kept in place for at least 24 hours postoperatively to facilitate patient management.

Routine use of pacing wire postoperatively in thoracotomy patients is not appropriate. Should bradycardia develop in the postoperative period, pacing can be instituted using the pacing port of a Swan-Ganz catheter. Digitalis should be given before major pulmonary resections, especially to patients older than age 60 years. The benefits of digitalis administration far exceed its risks. If the patient is not receiving digitalis therapy, 0.5 to 1.0 mg of digoxin is administered in the 12 to 24-hour period before the operation. This dose of digoxin should not produce toxicity in a patient with normal renal function and greatly facilitates the management of postoperative supraventricular rhythm disturbances when they occur.

REFERENCES

Arkins R, Smaessant AA, Hicks RG: Mortality and morbidity in surgical patients with coronary artery disease. JAMA *190*:458, 1964.

Beck-Nielsen J, Sorensen HR, Alstup P: Atrial fibrillation following thoracotomy for noncardiac diseases, in particular cancer of the lung. Acta Med Scand *193*:425, 1973.

Boysen PG, et al.: Prospective evaluation for pneumonectomy using the [99m] technetium quantitative perfusion lung scan. Chest 72:422, 1977.

Brodsky JB, Shulman MS, Mark BD: Management of postoperative thoracotomy pain: Lumbar epidural narcotics. *In* Kittle CF (ed): Current Controversies in Thoracic Surgery. Philadelphia: WB Saunders, 1986, pp. 228–232.

Burman SO: The prophylactic use of digitalis before thoracotomy. Ann Thorac Surg *14*:359, 1972.

Cousins MJ, Phillips GD: Sleep, pain, and sedation. *In* Shoemaker W, et al (eds): The Society of Critical Care Medicine: Textbook of Critical Care. Philadelphia: WB Saunders, 1984, pp. 787–801.

Don H: Respiratory care. *In* Roe BB (ed): Perioperative Management in Cardiothoracic Surgery. Boston: Little, Brown & Co., 1981, pp. 117–134.

Driscoll AC, et al: Clinically unrecognized myocardial infarction following surgery. N Engl J Med *264*:633, 1961.

El-Baz N, et al: Continuous epidural morphine analgesia for pain relief after thoracic surgery. Anesthesiology *57*:A205, 1982.

El-Baz N, et al: Continuous epidural morphine infusion for postoperative pain relief. Anesth Analg *62*:258, 1983.

Ellison RG: Cardiac complications of noncardiac intrathoracic surgery. *In* Complications of Intrathoracic Surgery. Boston: Little Brown & Co., 1979, pp. 93-100.

Melnert JH, Dupont TJ, Rose DH: Intermittent epidural morphine installation for control of postoperative pain. Ann Surg *146*:145, 1983.

Meltman C: Assessment of operative risk in thoracic surgery. Am Rev Respir Dis *84*:197, 1961.

Nunn JF, et al: Hypoxemia and atelectasis produced by forced expiration. Br J Anesth 37:3, 1965.

Olson GN, et al: Pulmonary function evaluation of the lung resection candidate. Am Rev Respir Dis *111*:379, 1975.

Shapiro BA, Harrison RA, Trout CA (eds.): Clinical Application of Respiratory Care. 2nd Ed. Chicago: Year Book, 1979.

Shields TW, Ujiki GT: Digitalization for prevention of arrhythmias following pulmonary surgery. Surg Gynecol Obstet *126*:713, 1968.

Stapleton JV, Austin KL, Mather LE: A pharmacokinetic approach to postoperative pain: continuous infusion of peltidine. Anaesth Intensive Care 7:25, 1979.

Steen P, Tinker J, Tarhan S: Myocardial reinfarction after anesthesia and surgery. JAMA *239*:2566, 1978.

Tarhan S, et al: Myocardial infarction after general anesthesia. JAMA *220*:1451, 1972.

Wheat MW Jr, Buford TH: Digitalis in surgery: Extension of classical indications. J Thorac Cardiovasc Surg *41*:162, 1961.

CHAPTER 25

VENTILATORY SUPPORT OF POSTOPERATIVE SURGICAL PATIENTS

Thomas R. J. Todd

POSTOPERATIVE PULMONARY PATHOPHYSIOLOGY

Pulmonary function and resultant gas exchange deteriorate after any major surgical procedure, particularly following pulmonary resections. Minute ventilation is well preserved, but its separate components are considerably altered. Churchill and McNeil (1927) reported that the vital capacity — VC — is reduced by 50 to 75% in the first 24 hours. On average, tidal volume is diminished by 20% and functional residual capacity — FRC — by 35% in thoracic and upper abdominal procedures. Normally, a return to preoperative levels is observed in 7 to 14 days. Despite the fall in tidal volume, minute ventilation is maintained by compensatory increases in respiratory rate.

Sigh, defined as a breath 3 times greater than tidal volume, normally occurs approximately 10 times per hour and helps to maintain lung volume and pulmonary compliance. This effort is greatly diminished in the postoperative period because pain limits both chest wall and diaphragmatic excursion. In addition, narcotics alter central respiratory drive. Bendixen and associates (1964), Egbert and Bendixen (1964), and Zikria and co-workers (1974) consistently reported these findings. Atelectasis may result and is often aggravated by immobility, restricted ventilation caused by pain, and retained secretions. Pulmonary defense mechanisms such as coughing and mucociliary clearance are compromised in the early postoperative period. Harris and associates (1975) reported a reduction in mucociliary clearance postoperatively from hypoxemia alone.

Latimer and associates (1971) found that the highest rates of postoperative pulmonary complications occurred with thoracic and upper abdominal procedures. Atelectasis occurs when the closing volume of the airways exceeds the expiratory reserve volume in the early postoperative period. At special risk are the elderly and smokers, whose closing volume is already elevated. In addition, obese patients already have a diminished expiratory reserve volume. Patients with chronic obstructive lung disease exhibit problems with expiratory reserve volume and closing volume.

Several other mechanisms contribute to a decrease in lung volume and compliance. A major increase in extravascular lung water may result not only in decreased compliance of the lung but also in hypoxemia. Such may occur even in the absence of the characteristic radiographic changes of pulmonary edema. Prys-Roberts and colleagues (1967) noted that alveolar-arterial oxygen gradients might increase without any abnormalities becoming apparent on standard chest radiographs. The increases in lung water may result from either fluid overload or left ventricular failure, or, alternatively, from impairment in the permeability characteristics of the pulmonary capillary membrane — so-called low pressure pulmonary edema. The latter has often been referred to as the adult respiratory distress syndrome — ARDS — and may occur following shock, sepsis, aspiration, and multiple blood transfusions, all of which may be associated with major surgical procedures. Following pulmonary surgery, these abnormalities may be exaggerated by two factors. First, the ipsilateral lung may have undergone operative trauma and contusion. In addition, its intraoperative collapse and re-expansion may result in fluid extravasation from the pulmonary capillary bed. Second, pulmonary artery pressure may increase transiently following the resection of pulmonary tissue — particularly after pneumonectomy. The major determinants of extravascular fluid movement are illustrated in Fig. 25–1. As noted, once the permeability characteristics have been unfavorably altered, the driving force becomes the hydrostatic gradient across the capillary wall. Because capillary pressure is largely determined by both left atrial pressure and pulmonary artery pressure, as noted

Starling Equation

$$\text{F.M.} = K[(Pc - Pis) - \sigma(\pi c - \pi is)]$$

F.M.	**=**	**Fluid Movement**
K	**=**	**Permeability Coefficient**
Pc	**=**	**Capillary Hydrostatic Pressure**
Pis	**=**	**Interstitial Hydrostatic Pressure**
σ	**=**	**Osmotic Reflection Coefficient**
πc	**=**	**Capillary Osmotic Pressure**
πis	**=**	**Interstitial Osmotic Pressure**

Fig. 25–1. The Starling equation with various determinants of transcapillary fluid flux separately noted.

herein: $Pc = Pla + 0.4(Ppa - Pla)$, any increase in pulmonary artery pressure — particularly if complicated by excessive fluid administration — results in additional fluid movement into the alveolar and interstitial spaces.

This accumulation of extravascular lung water may affect regional ventilation not only by subsequent alveolar flooding but also by augmenting airway closure via peribronchial cuffing. Atelectasis and decreased compliance alter regional ventilation and, in the end, adversely affect ventilation-perfusion — V/Q — matching. Hypoxemia results.

Although hypoxemia is seen early, hypercarbia is usually a late-appearing abnormality, often signifying that the patient is tiring and may soon require mechanical assistance. Indeed, unless pain is particularly severe, or the patient is oversedated, one characteristically witnesses hypocarbia following surgery, because the respiratory rate is often increased as a function of anxiety, pain, and hypoxemia.

Several postoperative cardiovascular changes may further alter V/Q matching. For example, a decrease in cardiac output resulting from hypovolemia or sepsis or an increase in left ventricular afterload may affect the degree of regional pulmonary artery perfusion and further aggravate impaired V/Q matching. Increases in right ventricular filling pressure caused by pulmonary hypertension — that may result from excision of lung tissue — may further impair left ventricular function by shifting the intraventricular septum and adversely affecting left ventricular filling. These cardiopulmonary interactions, although obvious, are frequently overlooked in the management of thoracic postoperative patients, and are emphasized further in this chapter.

PREDICTING THE NEED

Despite the pathophysiologic alterations in pulmonary function, only a few patients eventually require mechanical ventilatory support. Too often in retrospect, we can determine that the need for this support might have been predicted preoperatively. The following is an analysis of those factors that should be taken into account when assessing a patient's preoperative status and the potential need for mechanical ventilatory assistance.

Arterial Blood Gases

Arterial hypoxemia — a partial pressure of oxygen — Pa_{O_2} — less than 55 mm of mercury — Hg — on room air is insufficient by itself to predict either resectability or postoperative dysfunction. Oxygenation depends on the V/Q ratio in the remaining and the resected lung as subsequently outlined. Indeed, a high arterial Pa_{O_2} in the face of significant obstructive or restrictive lung disease is more worrisome. A patient with poor pulmonary function should not be able to sustain a Pa_{O_2} greater than 80 mmHg unless the V/Q inequalities have been maximized by obliteration of a significant portion of pulmonary vascular bed. Thus, a high Pa_{O_2} — greater than 80 mm Hg — noted when pulmonary function studies show impairment should alert the surgeon to the possibility of pre-existing pulmonary vascular hypertension.

Hypercarbia on the other hand — a Pa_{CO_2} greater than 45 mm Hg — appears to be a direct indicator of advanced lung disease and minimal pulmonary reserve. These patients often require postoperative mechanical support.

Pulmonary Function Tests and Work of Breathing

These screening tests are used to assess resectability. The sensitivity of these tests in terms of predicting respiratory failure, however, is low. Nonetheless, certain specific comments can be made. The forced expiratory volume in one second — FEV_1, the FEV_1 expressed as a percent of the forced vital capacity — FEV_1/FVC, and the maximum flow rate at 25, 50 and 75% lung capacity are reduced in obstructive lung disease. Abnormalities in these values correlate with an increased surgical risk when the values are less than 50% of the predicted norm. Mittman (1961) stated that a maximum voluntary ventilation — MVV — less than 50% of the expected value indicated a high risk. This latter measurement, however, is greatly affected by patient compliance and fatigue and should not be used as a routine means to predict either resectability or indeed the need for postoperative support.

Using a multifactorial analysis, Lockwood (1973) defined a high risk group that included patients with a VC of less than 1.85 liters, an FEV_1 of less than 1.2 liters, an FEV_1/FVC of less than 35%, and an MVV of less than 28 liters per minute. Shapiro and Walton (1982) suggested that patients in whom the percent predicted FVC plus the percent FEV_1/FVC was less than 100 had a 50% chance of developing acute ventilatory failure in the first 24 hours following a thoracic or upper abdominal procedure. This value seems excessive. The only major area of agreement concerning a predicted accuracy of postoperative pulmonary function tests is that a predicted postoperative FEV_1 of less than 800 ml is incompatible with the tasks of daily living, as Kristersson (1972) and Olson (1975) and their associates reported.

Shapiro and co-workers (1977) described the relationship between work of breathing and minute ventilation. Oxygen consumption is exponentially related to tidal volume expressed as a percentage of VC. Patients with reduced VC are at risk for two reasons. First, their ability to improve ventilation by increasing tidal volume is severely limited. Second, the relative proportion of oxygen consumption spent on the work of breathing is high and other organ systems are adversely affected postoperatively if the work of breathing must be increased. Viires and colleagues (1983) and Hussain and Roussos (1985) performed several eloquent experiments that revealed the demand the work of breathing can make on oxygen consumption and respiratory muscle blood flow. Under maximal stress, respiratory muscle

blood flow can account for 21% of the cardiac output compared to only 3% at rest. The experiments of Viires and colleagues were undertaken in animals with normal pulmonary reserve subjected to varieties of stress common in the postoperative period. That respiratory work could reach its limitation in such a situation suggests that patients with impaired respiratory function reach threshold volumes of oxygen consumption of blood flow early. As Cherniak (1959) pointed out, "increased airways resistance would exacerbate the situation."

Ventilation-Perfusion Studies

In assessing a patient for pulmonary resection, preoperative pulmonary function must be balanced against the function of the part of lung to be removed. For example, the patient with a main stem bronchial obstruction and severe chronic obstructive lung disease can, from a respiratory standpoint, withstand removal of the involved lung, barring the development of other complications. The pneumonectomy is already established functionally and removal may actually improve V/Q matching. In other cases, the functional characteristic of the part of lung to be removed may be less obvious. Under these circumstances, V/Q scans may clarify the postoperative consequences of resection. Juhl and Frost (1975) devised a formula to predict postoperative FEV_1 in which FEV_1 was equal to the preoperative FEV_1 times the percent perfusion to the uninvolved lung, that is the portion of lung remaining after resection.

When divided into lung zones, quantitative V/Q studies can be used to predict the effect of resection on VC and gas exchange. Tisi (1979) outlined four outcomes predictable from preoperative scans (Table 25–1). The need for mechanical ventilation is most likely under the third condition and somewhat less likely under the first.

Oximetry

Exercise testing is a useful adjunct to preoperative testing if combined with oximetry. High risk patients may experience a fall in arterial saturation that might be assessed with pulse oximetry. Many years ago, stair

Table 25–1. Predicted Change in Postoperative Pulmonary Function Using Quantitative Ventilation and Perfusion Scans

Function of Resected Lung	Predicted Result
V/Q (resection) equals V/Q (rest of lung)	Decline in function proportional to extent of resection
V/Q (resection) = 0/0	"Autoresection"—no loss of function
V/Q (resection) >>> V/Q (rest of lung)	Decline in function >>> extent of resection
V/Q (resection) abnormal <<< V/Q (rest of lung)	Resection of dead space—improved function

Adapted from Tisi G.M.: State of the art: Preoperative evaluation of pulmonary function. Am.Rev.Respir.Dis. *119*:293, 1979.

walking was used by surgeons to determine resectability. Data published by Bolton and colleagues (1987) support this contention. The addition of pulse oximetry has added some degree of objectivity. Johnson and co-workers (1977) did correlate the ability to perform simple exercise such as stair climbing to postoperative morbidity and mortality. In a prospective study, Miyoshi and associates (1987) concluded that whereas pulmonary function studies determine postoperative complications, exercise-induced blood lactate thresholds determined mortality.

Pulmonary Artery Pressure

Elevated pulmonary artery pressure in patients with chronic lung disease signifies extensive disease and a high operative risk. Right heart catheterization permits the use of a balloon to occlude flow to the diseased lung. Laros and Swierenga (1967) established a resting mean pulmonary artery pressure of 30 mmHg as their criterion for inoperability. Olson (1975) and Karliner (1968) and their colleagues reported similar values. Increased pulmonary vascular resistance is also a measure of vascular compliance. Fee and co-workers (1978) defined a high risk category of pulmonary vascular resistance greater than or equal to 190 dynes per second per centimeter to the fifth power. Fortunately, estimates of pulmonary vascular pressure can now be obtained from noninvasive studies, such as color echo-Doppler assessment.

Summary

Several means are available to assess the risk of respiratory failure post-thoracotomy. What tests should be routine, however, is often unclear. Patients should undergo exercise oximetry with stair climbing, arterial blood gases, and a determination of FEV_1 and the diffusing capacity for carbon monoxide — $D_{L}CO$. A normal oximetric exercise test with no history of impaired exercise tolerance, a Pa_{O_2} between 55 and 80 mmHg, and a normal Pa_{CO_2} obviate further testing, if the FEV_1 is greater than 2 liters for patients undergoing pneumonectomy or greater than 1.5 liters for those scheduled for lobectomy.

Desaturation with exercise testing, a Pa_{O_2} greater than 80 mmHg associated with a history of poor exercise tolerance or a Pa_{CO_2} greater than 45 mmHg, and an FEV_1 seemingly inappropriate to the planned extent of pulmonary resection should lead to further evaluation with V/Q scanning and pulmonary artery pressure determinations. A preoperative FEV_1 of 900 ml or less in the absence of major airway obstruction suggests a high risk of postoperative respiratory failure, particularly if a pulmonary resection is undertaken. The absolute value, however, must be taken in context with the exercise tolerance and the weight of the patient.

Persistent uncertainty at any point in this evaluation algorithm should lead to the recommendation of a 3 to 4-week respiratory rehabilitation with subsequent reassessment. Often surprising improvement in vigor, exercise tolerance, and occasionally spirometry will result from a period of abstinence from smoking and from graded exercise on a treadmill combined with intensive physiotherapy.

Concurrent Risk Factors

Serious medical or surgical problems may necessitate the use of postoperative ventilatory support independent of the degree of pulmonary dysfunction resulting from the surgical procedure.

Cardiac Function

The single most important associated medical condition is cardiac dysfunction. A careful cardiac history is a prerequisite to any major thoracic surgical procedure. A history of cardiac events, historical or physical features of cardiac dysfunction, or a history of atypical chest pain should lead to further evaluation. In particular, two-dimensional echocardiography provides an accurate noninvasive assessment of cardiac function, and thallium-persantine scanning, as suggested by Wong and Detsky (1992), can select those patients with ischemic heart disease that require either medical or surgical treatment before their planned thoracic surgery.

Cardiac risk factors outlined by Goldman and associated (1977) include age, positive cardiac history or physical examination, and electrocardiographic — ECG — abnormalities. Patients in the highest risk category have a 78% incidence of cardiac death or life-threatening complication. These patients should be ventilated prophylactically after surgical intervention to reduce the proportion of oxygen consumption consumed by the work of breathing.

In the postoperative period, the ability to maintain oxygen consumption depends on adequate oxygen delivery. From the Fick principle, oxygen consumption — V_{O_2} — is determined by cardiac output — CO — and the arteriovenous oxygen content difference — $Ca_{O_2} - Cv_{O_2}$ — such that: $V_{O_2} = CO(Ca_{O_2} - Cv_{O_2})$. With reductions in cardiac output, an increase in oxygen extraction must occur to maintain consumption. Even without a change in postoperative pulmonary function, the highly desaturated venous blood may lead to a relative arterial hypoxemia. Increases in respiratory rate then can cause a respiratory alkalosis and shift the oxyhemoglobin association curve to the left, making oxygen uptake at the tissue level more difficult. As a result, these patients may require not only fluids or inatropes, or both, to improve the cardiac output, but also prophylactic ventilation to support gas exchange.

Patients who present with atypical chest pain should be evaluated with stress testing, particularly using thallium-persantine scans. Any indication of ischemia on such preoperative evaluation necessitates further investigation with coronary angiography. In patients with significant ischemic heart disease who have recently undergone bypass or who are considered "non-bypassable" should be considered for prophylactic ventilatory support in the postoperative period to avoid the stress placed on their cardiovascular system by the increased demand for respiratory work.

Multiorgan Abnormalities

Pontoppidan and associates (1972) noted that abnormalities in other organ systems increased the chance of ventilatory failure postoperatively. A careful assessment of renal and hepatic function should be routine. An effort should be made to maximize function preoperatively to prevent further deterioration postoperatively.

Hemodynamic Instability

As noted previously, hypoperfusion and sepsis may result in an increase in extravascular lung water leading to an impairment in V/Q matching and hypoxemia. Hypotension itself may lead to a significant fall in Pa_{O_2} and even oxygen desaturation of arterial blood, depending on its affects on mixed venous oxygen saturation and the underlying pulmonary reserve and pathology. Often the resuscitation of the hemodynamically unstable patient ignores resultant changes in gas exchange, which themselves will complicate the resuscitation process. The work of breathing is increased significantly as the patient attempts to compensate for lactic acidosis resulting from poor peripheral perfusion. As a result, it is advisable to monitor oxygen saturation during resuscitation in any hemodynamic emergency and to supply oxygen to such patients routinely unless they are known retainers of carbon dioxide. One should proceed to endotracheal intubation early when signs of fatigue — as will be discussed — or arterial oxygen desaturation become evident.

Alterations in capillary permeability may occur during hypotension, postoperative aspiration, sepsis, and pneumonia. The resultant interstitial edema may cause a further narrowing of the terminal airways and alveolar collapse. Hypotension, whether from impaired cardiac function, hypovolemia, or sepsis, further reduces the transport of oxygen to the periphery.

Nature and Extent of the Surgical Plan

Postoperative ventilatory support is a useful adjunct for certain thoracic procedures. If impaired compliance of the remaining lung on the operative side can be anticipated, ventilatory support should be considered. Spontaneous ventilation in such circumstances may lead to insufficient expansion and may thus result in a pleural space problem, particularly noticeable after surgery in patients with inflammatory restrictive diseases, such as tuberculosis and pulmonary fibrosis. Patients with tuberculosis or those undergoing decortication should be considered for elective ventilatory support until postoperative compliance can be assessed.

Procedures such as esophagectomy are frequently accompanied by large third-space fluid losses and unpredictable changes in pulmonary capillary permeability. Intravenous fluid replacement may, as noted, increase interstitial edema with adverse effects on gas exchange. Additionally, these patients may have two or three incisions with significant pain and an increase work of breathing. Anesthesia is prolonged and postoperative respiratory depression is frequent. Elective ventilatory support for the first 24 hours in these patients may prevent complications, although this has never been adequately demonstrated.

POSTOPERATIVE INDICATIONS FOR SUPPORT

The decision to initiate or continue mechanical ventilation is usually based on an assessment of gas exchange, impending respiratory failure, and the ability of the patient to protect the airway. The postoperative period should then be characterized by respiratory monitoring as well as a careful clinical evaluation of the patient.

Many patients have indwelling arterial lines placed by the anesthesia staff to facilitate management of one-lung anesthesia techniques. Arterial blood can and should be sampled early to assess both Pa_{O_2} and Pa_{CO_2}. Oxygenation can, however, be adequately assessed noninvasively through pulse oximetry, as noted previously, as long as peripheral perfusion is satisfactory. The latter should be undertaken routinely in the recovery room and in the early postoperative period.

Although respiratory fatigue once established should be reflected in abnormal arterial blood gas values, it is important to recognize the clinical signs of impending respiratory muscle fatigue in order to initiate corrective measures. Such recognition requires an assessment of the patient rather than laboratory data. Mental acuity and awareness in the face of obvious freedom from pain are encouraging. The patient who is able to converse in sentences is likely to generate an adequate tidal volume. Respiratory muscle paradox is an early and reliable sign of established muscle fatigue and is an indication for mechanical ventilatory support. It is easily assessed by placing a hand on the chest and the abdomen during inspiration and expiration (Fig. 25–2). Normally, the chest and abdomen expand together when the patient inhales, because diaphragmatic descent displaces abdominal viscera. In established fatigue, the diaphragm moves paradoxically upward during inspiration, resulting in the abdominal hand moving inward while the chest expands.

In the early postoperative period, the patient's level of consciousness may be impaired from inadequate reversal of anesthesia or other complications, such as postoperative cerebral vascular accident and narcotic overdosage, which may also result in central nervous system depression sufficient to result in an inability to protect the airway. At such times, micro or macro aspiration may occur. Unless rapid reversal with naloxone hydrochloride — Narcan — is achieved, early intubation is advisable.

Postoperative respiratory failure can occur in one of three situations, as noted in Table 25–2. Most problems in the immediate postoperative period are related to pure ventilatory failure or a mixed picture. It is at this time that problems associated with inadequate reversal of anesthesia, narcotic overdosage, perioperative aspiration, or airway obstruction secondary to laryngeal

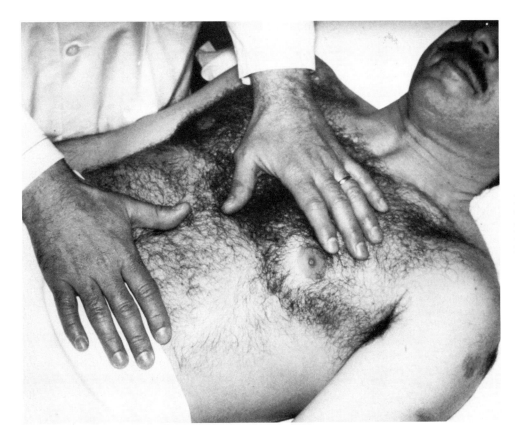

Fig. 25–2. The physical examination for paradoxic breathing. Under normal circumstances, both hands should move outward as the patient inspires.

Table 25–2. Classification of Respiratory Failure

Type	Pathophysiology	Measurement
Hypoxemic	V/Q mismatch	Pa_{O_2} Sa_{O_2}
Ventilatory	↑ V_D/V_T inadequate ventilation	$^0Pa_{CO_2} > 50$ mmHg pH < 7.30*
Mixed	As above	$Pa_{O_2} - Sa_{O_2}$ Pa_{CO_2}

*From Shapiro BA, Harrison RA, Walton JR: Clinical Application of Blood Gases. 2nd Ed. Chicago: Year Book, 1977.

edema become evident. Shapiro and associates (1977) defined acute ventilatory failure as a Pa_{CO_2} determination greater than 50 mmHg and a pH of less than 7.30. Table 25–3 is a list of other parameters. Early and quite temporary intubation is all that is required, unless the patient has developed a V/Q abnormality as well from either complicating aspiration, fluid overload, inadequate pulmonary reserve, or major atelectasis. Once

Table 25–3. Criteria of Established Ventilatory Failure*

Respiratory rate	<4 or >35
Pa_{CO_2}	>50 mmHg
V_D/V_T	>0.6
Vital capacity	<15 ml/kg
Negative inspiratory force	<−20 ml H_2O

*Note that this says nothing concerning ventilation-perfusion inequalities.

re-intubation has been accomplished, radiographic examination of the chest is necessary to ensure that none of these complications have developed.

For the patient who does well in the initial postoperative period, continued monitoring of oxygen saturation is important as long as he or she requires supplemental oxygen. This monitoring need not be continuous in the nonventilated patient, unless the FI_{O_2} is high or the saturation is marginally acceptable. The need for continued blood gas analysis depends on the following: 1) a preoperative elevation of Pa_{CO_2}; 2) a postoperative elevation of Pa_{CO_2}; and 3) unreliable or inconsistent oximetric saturation readings.

The mixed form of respiratory failure is seen in some well-defined clinical scenarios. First, it can occur when there is pre-existing carbon dioxide retention. Under such circumstances, excessive oxygen administration may remove the hypoxic drive for breathing that has become a compensatory mechanism in patients with chronic hypercarbia. Too often, the goals of oxygen administration are poorly defined and physicians assume that a high Pa_{O_2} value provides a margin of safety. A saturation of more than 95% may actually depress respiratory effort in these patients, leading to an exacerbation of the carbon dioxide retention and the onset of an acute respiratory acidosis wherein hypoxemia is a late feature. Second, in cases of mental obtundation, arterial oxygen desaturation may result in an inability to respond with an increased respiratory effort and carbon dioxide retention will complicate the hypoxia.

Third, when respiratory muscle fatigue onsets quickly because of malnutrition or associated chronic disease, both depression of oxygenation and elevation of carbon dioxide levels will occur, particularly in the patient recovering from prolonged ventilatory support after severe lung injury. Lastly, the development of a pulmonary embolus in a patient receiving mechanical ventilatory assistance is a classic example of the mixed picture. The pathophysiology of pulmonary embolism involves an increase in dead space as the vascular supply to well-ventilated alveoli is obstructed. In the spontaneously ventilated patient, reflex hyperventilation usually leads to hypocarbia. In the ventilated controlled patient, however, such a reflex increase in minute ventilation will not occur — depending on the ventilator mode and the presence or absence of paralysis — and hypercarbia will develop as a result.

Nonventilatory Management

Oxygen delivery by face mask is often all that is necessary for cases of mild hypoxemia. When concentrations greater than 50% are required, however, a tandem flow setup becomes important. As chest wall movement becomes limited by pain, the judicious use of analgesics is essential. Regional hypoventilation caused by unilateral pain may result in V/Q abnormalities on that side. Intravenous administration of narcotics tends to achieve adequate pain control with a low dosage schedule, thus reducing the risk of impaired central respiratory drive. The advent of patient-controlled analgesia has permitted fine control of pain without narcosis. Epidural anesthesia in addition is an important adjunct, particularly in the high risk patient. The latter technique makes use of the specific opiate receptors that are present on the dorsal columns of the spinal cord. Opiates can be administered using an epidural catheter into the lumbar or thoracic epidural space via an indwelling line in doses that provide adequate to complete analgesia without any systemic side effects. Nonsteroidal anti-inflammatory drugs provide important adjuvant pain relief — for reference — and may be taken orally or as a suppository.

Changes in body position may decrease hypoxemia, especially in patients with unilateral pulmonary disease. By placing the noninvolved lung in a dependent position, gravity ensures preferential flow of blood to that side. Rivara and associates (1984) demonstrated that changes from the supine to the lateral decubitus position result in significant improvement in Pa_{O_2} in mechanically ventilated patients. Similar results can be obtained during spontaneous breathing. Experimentally, Albert and colleagues (1987) showed improvement in arterial oxygenation by the reduction of intrapulmonary shunt when oleic acid lung-injured dogs were placed in the prone position.

Although no prospective randomized trials have been undertaken, aggressive chest physiotherapy, both pre- and postoperatively, definitely improves gas exchange and reduces the incidence of pulmonary complications (see Chapter 26). Mobilization of secretions and the encouragement of cough and deep breathing maintain the FRC and improve patterns of breathing. Other frequently mentioned adjunctive therapies include intermittent positive pressure breathing, incentive spirometry, and continuous positive airway pressure — CPAP. The literature describing these techniques is conflicting. Neither Celli and colleagues (1984) nor Ali and co-workers (1984) found any difference in pulmonary complications — either atelectasis or pneumonia — among patients treated with these techniques. In contrast, Stock and associates (1985) found that CPAP delivered by a tight-fitting mask prompted a more rapid return of the FRC and significantly reduced the incidence of atelectasis when compared with incentive spirometry or deep breathing. Patients in whom hypoxemia was unresponsive to spirometry or routine chest physiotherapy experienced improved Pa_{O_2} and reduced alveolar-arterial diffusion capacity of oxygen — $(A-a) D_{O_2}$ — after the use of mask CPAP, as noted by Dehaven and colleagues (1986). One must, however, be cautious in using mask CPAP in the early postoperative period because nausea and emesis may result in aspiration in patients who cannot remove the mask.

When upper airway obstruction resulting from glottic edema or tumor is suspected, a helium-oxygen mixture and racemic epinephrine can be used. At a commonly used concentration of 70% helium and 30% oxygen, the helium-oxygen mixture reduces the degree of turbulent flow in the central airways and improves laminar flow, allowing increased delivery of gas beyond the level of the obstruction. At concentrations of oxygen above 40%, the advantages of the reduced density are lost and the mixture becomes ineffective. Racemic epinephrine, administered as an aerosolized solution of 0.5 ml with 2.5 ml of saline every 4 hours, reduces inflammation and swelling of the laryngotracheal wall. These two interventions are especially useful in the patient with postextubation upper airway obstruction, whether in the recovery room or in the intensive care unit after more prolonged tracheal intubation.

The development of pulmonary infiltrates after thoracic surgery suggests a variety of diagnoses and the exact one may not be clear. It is helpful to remember that the clinical diagnosis may depend on whether the infiltrate is generalized or localized and the time of onset in the postoperative period. Localized infiltrates are likely to be infectious or represent atelectasis or localized aspiration. If occurring 3 or more days following surgery and accompanied by either fever, leukocytosis, or purulent sputum, they demand appropriate antibiotic treatment. Generalized infiltrates should alert the clinician to the presence of either ARDS, fluid overload, or aspiration. All require the judicious restriction of intravenous fluids and the addition of diuretic therapy. Although this guide to diagnosis and therapy is not specific, it remains a reliable initial approach.

When to Re-Intubate

Clinical judgment rather than plain numbers determines when conservative methods of support are inadequate. Increased work of breathing is signalled by accessory muscle recruitment. Progression to discoordinate breathing patterns in which abdominal — diaphragmatic — excursion is paradoxic to chest wall movement is a certain sign of impending respiratory failure. Tachypnea and a rising Pa_{CO_2} value should prompt action before the levels shown in Table 25–3 are reached. Hypoxemia refractory to conservative therapy indicates a continued loss of alveolar volume and FRC requiring positive pressure ventilation for correction. The combination of hypoxemia and hypercarbia should signal the need for immediate re-intubation. The fatigued patient often presents the most difficult problem. When does one decide that it is time for mechanical support? Often the patient is the best guide. The lucid patient who can speak in sentences and reports that he or she is the same or better provides a reliable index for continued conservatism. The onset of confusion, agitation, and inability to speak in sentences in the previously lucid patient indicates that re-intubation is essential. As noted, a combination of impending respiratory failure and hemodynamic instability can be lethal and warrants tracheal intubation and ventilatory support at an earlier stage. In general, ongoing and frequent re-evaluation of the patient and arterial blood gas values provides the best guide. The rapidity of change is of prognostic importance as it suggests a rapidly progressive process. Under such circumstances, early re-intubation and ventilation before overt signs are present is preferable to a respiratory or cardiopulmonary arrest.

Method of Intubation

Re-intubation for ventilatory or respiratory failure is best done with the patient awake but sedated. During awake intubation, patients must be subjected to minimal trauma and stress. The act of intubation itself can activate ventricular arrhythmias, cause aspiration, and exacerbate hypoxemia. The procedure should be explained to the patient in a reassuring manner. Intravenous diazepam, a dose of 5 to 10 mg, induces light sedation and relieves anxiety. A short-acting intravenous analgesic such as fentanyl — 50 to 100 mg — may further reduce the patient's awareness. The mouth is suctioned to remove secretions and the back of the throat is sprayed with 1% lidocaine aerosol. The laryngoscope blade is inserted and the vocal cords are visualized and sprayed with local anaesthetic. This takes time. The lidocaine should be applied to the pharynx and larynx intermittently, with 100% oxygen supplied by a tandem setup between applications. A pulse oximeter can ensure that oxygen saturation is appropriate throughout the procedure. During the application of local anaesthetic, the patient's own respiration should be assisted by an ambu bag. It is important to ensure synchrony with the patient's own efforts. Under such circumstances, oxygenation usually can be maintained and reassurance of the same obtained with continuous noninvasive saturation monitoring. In addition, the patient should not be supine, because the diaphragm is then placed in a disadvantageous position, further increasing the work of breathing. Rather, the patient should assume a high Fowler's position. Not only will it be easier to assist his or her respiratory effort, but also the intubation itself will be facilitated, particularly if a pillow remains behind the head to ensure that the oropharynx and glottis are in alignment.

Most patients can accommodate at least a 7.5-mm diameter endotracheal tube, but an 8- or 9-mm tube is preferable. Smaller tubes either do not accept the fiberoptic bronchoscope or do so only at the expense of severe limitation in air flow. Paralyzing agents are seldom required, but if used, they should be of the ultrashort-acting, nondepolarizing type, such as atracurium. The equipment required for an emergency cricothyroidotomy or tracheostomy should be at the bedside if attempts at endotracheal intubation fail.

An alternate approach is nasotracheal intubation. The nares as well as the throat must be anesthetized with lidocaine spray. A 7.5- or 8-mm tube is usually well tolerated. Successful blind intubation requires practice, although with Magill forceps and a laryngoscope, the tube can often be guided into the proper position. Once again, with the patient in a Fowler's position, the endotracheal tube is positioned through the nares into the oropharynx. By listening over the end of the tube, one can appreciate the point at which the tube lies over the vocal cords. It is imperative that the endotracheal tube has not already been cut, in which case it may be too short to reach from the anterior nares to the upper trachea.

Because flexible bronchoscopes are available to the thoracic surgeon, intubation should be neither blind nor difficult. Flexible bronchoscopy can be used for either oral or nasal routes. Pharmacologic management is the same as described. The bronchoscope is passed through the endotracheal tube and then placed into the mouth or nostril. Once the vocal cords have been visualized, 5 ml of 1% lidocaine is flushed through the suction port to anesthetize the cords. The scope is then passed between the cords into the upper trachea and into either main stem bronchus, with or without supplemental lidocaine. While in this position, the bronchoscope acts as a stent and the endotracheal tube is advanced into the airway. If advancing the endotracheal tube is difficult, a rotation of the tube usually ensures that the tip does not "hang up" on the arytenoid cartilages or the vocal cords. Proper position is confirmed by withdrawing the bronchoscope into the endotracheal tube and noting the distance of the latter above the tracheal carina.

If flexible bronchoscopy is unavailable or is unsuccessful because of anatomy, rigid bronchoscopy may be attempted, particularly as the surgeon is both familiar and adept at its passage in the face of airway obstruction. The adaptor cap for attachment to the ventilator tubing

should be removed from the endotracheal tube because this piece limits the internal diameter. A 7-mm rigid bronchoscope will pass through a 7.5-mm endotracheal tube. The principles of intubation are the same as for flexible bronchoscopy. Obviously, the nasal approach cannot be used. The rigid scope, however, can be used as a laryngoscope to lever the tongue and epiglottis out of the way for better viewing of the vocal cords. Once the scope has been passed through the cords, ventilation can be initiated with the Venturi technique to relieve hypoxemia caused by the intubation attempts. Once again, an oximeter, if available, should be used to monitor saturation during the re-intubation attempt.

Should all attempts at re-intubation fail and a surgical airway seems necessary, apneic oxygenation may provide support until proper ventilation can be established. This can be achieved with the insertion of an intracath through the cricothyroid membrane into the distal airway (Fig. 25–3). The catheter is then connected to wall oxygen at 6 to 10 liters per minute. Such endotracheal gas flow usually provides satisfactory oxygenation similar to that provided during an apnea test for brain death. Although the Pa_{CO_2} level will continue to rise, oxygen saturation can be restored and maintained.

MECHANICAL VENTILATION

The following discussion is designed as a pragmatic approach to ventilatory management. The information reflects the personal bias of the author and it is recognized that there are several means to achieve the same end. The objectives of ventilatory management are the improvement of oxygenation as assessed by Pa_{O_2} levels and the maintenance of appropriate ventilation as assessed by both the Pa_{CO_2} value and the maintenance of arterial pH in an acceptable range. Several manipulations are available for each of these objectives.

Fraction of Inspired Oxygen — FI_{O_2}

Increases in oxygen concentration may increase arterial oxygen content, but such improvement in arterial oxygen content should not delude the physician into thinking that pulmonary function has also improved. Although higher inspired levels translate into augmented Pa_{O_2}, oxygen therapy is not innocuous. Clinical experience and experimental data suggest that levels above 50% may produce irreversible lung injury within 24 hours. As Fisher and associates (1984) and Jackson (1985) described in their reviews, the current theory of oxygen-induced damage centers around the production of oxygen-derived free radicals, such as superoxide anion, hydrogen peroxide, and hydroxyl radical. These molecules damage the alveolar epithelium, causing intracellular organelle disruption and producing interstitial and then alveolar edema. Organization of the exudative alveolar fluid results in hyaline membranes similar to those found in patients with ARDS. Although no hard data exist, subclinical damage may occur with

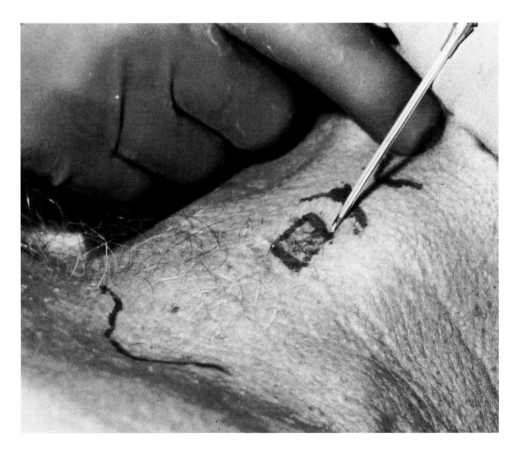

Fig. 25–3. The insertion of an intracath into the airway through the cricothyroid membrane for the purposes of apneic oxygenation.

concentrations of oxygen less than 50%. Thus, an important goal of mechanical ventilation is to achieve the lowest possible $F_{I_{O_2}}$. As a result, one should strive to maintain oxygen saturation at 90%. Levels higher than 90 to 92% are probably not necessary. A second adverse effect of high inspired concentrations of oxygen is absorption atelectasis. Normally, the nitrogen concentration of alveolar gas prevents alveolar collapse. With $F_{I_{O_2}}$ approaching 100%, persisting perfusion may lead to continued oxygen absorption and alveolar collapse with resultant decrease in functional residual capacity. As McAslan and associates (1973) demonstrated, a decrease in FRC usually results in an increase in intrapulmonary shunt.

Positive End-Expiratory Pressure — PEEP

At the end of expiration, airway pressure should equal atmospheric pressure, unless an intermediate resistance is provided that impedes the complete exhalation of inspired gas. In spontaneously breathing man, this is normally provided by the closed glottis, resulting in a positive pressure at the end of expiration. Such a positive end-expiratory pressure — PEEP — maintains a higher end-expiratory lung volume or FRC. The maintenance of an appropriate FRC decreases the work required to achieve a specific tidal breath by moving the patient to a more advantageous position on the pressure volume compliance curve (Fig. 25–4). Positive end-expiratory pressure improves arterial oxygenation by restoring FRC and by improving regional ventilation-perfusion disturbances. Functional residual capacity may be increased either through alveolar recruitment or by increasing alveolar volume. As Tyler (1983) and

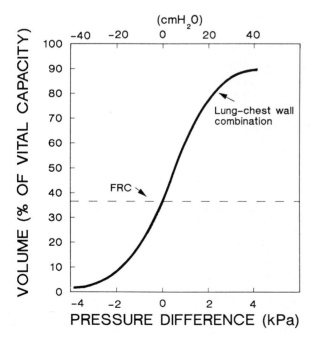

Fig. 25–4. Standard pressure-volume curve for the lungs. Note that when functional residual capacity (FRC) is reached, major increases in lung volume produce small changes in pressure or respiratory work.

Shapiro and colleagues (1984) outlined in excellent reviews, direct evidence for alveolar recruitment is lacking. Observation of immediate improvement in FRC with the application of PEEP, however, suggests that re-expansion of collapsed perfused alveoli play a major role. Increases in alveolar volume have been documented at increasing levels of PEEP. Daly and associates (1973) demonstrated that alveolar diameters in normal rats increase linearly with up to 10 cm of water PEEP. They also showed that although further increase in alveolar diameter could be measured above 10 cm of PEEP, changes in pressure rather than volume predominated.

As Hammon and colleagues (1976) showed, the addition of PEEP decreases V/Q abnormalities and thus intrapulmonary shunt by supposedly increasing ventilation to areas characterized by low V/Q ratios. Areas of low V/Q ratios are usually present in dependent lung zones. In these areas, perfusion is maximal because of the effect of gravity on the low pressure pulmonary circulation. Ventilation is impaired regionally by several factors, including retained secretions, decreased compliance — from extravascular lung water or pneumonitis — and increased pleural pressure. Hammon and colleagues (1976) demonstrated optimal levels of PEEP in normal and diseased lungs. Beyond these optimal levels, PEEP exerted a detrimental effect by over-distending nondependent alveoli and reducing perfusion to these areas, thereby contributing to increased dead space. Clinical studies by Downs (1973), Suter (1975), and Powers (1973) and their colleagues confirmed improved oxygenation under PEEP ventilation, but as Powers and associates pointed out, increased levels of PEEP may cause reduced oxygen delivery through deleterious effects on cardiac output.

In contrast to its beneficial effects on oxygenation, PEEP exerts a depressant action on the heart. Dorinski and Whitcomb (1983) and Scharfe (1992) summarized current thinking. Although the mechanisms responsible are not entirely clear, two have emerged to explain the reduction in cardiac output seen with PEEP therapy.

Decreased Venous Return

Qvist and associates (1975) found that PEEP produced a diminished cardiac output in anesthetized, paralyzed dogs. The mechanism proposed was increased intrathoracic pressure sufficient to cause a fall in right atrial and thus right ventricular filling pressure. A fluid bolus restored cardiac output and raised transluminal right-sided filling pressure. The reduction in venous return induced by PEEP does not, however, appear simple. According to Scharfe (1992), there appears to be a sympathetically mediated change in mean systemic pressure as well as an increase in the resistance to venous return. The latter may not be just a pressure-mediated phenomenon secondary to increased intrathoracic pressure; it may have a mechanical component secondary to collapse of the great veins.

In a study of patients with ARDS, Potkin and associates (1987) used radionucleotide angiography to demonstrate biventricular reductions in blood volume caused primarily by reduced ventricular preload but also by changes in ventricular configuration. This led several investigators to consider a primary effect on ventricular function.

Ventricular Dysfunction

Scharfe and colleagues (1977) proposed that increases in right ventricular afterload with PEEP could lead to right ventricular dysfunction. Haynes (1980), using two-dimensional echocardiography, demonstrated a leftward shift of the intraventricular septum, resulting in decreased left ventricular area. Correct positioning was restored by fluid re-expansion. They concluded that PEEP exerted a primary effect on the right ventricle with a secondary reduction in left ventricular function because of a septal shift. Jardin and associates (1981) support the aforementioned findings. In contrast, Cassidy and Ramanathan (1984), using similar techniques, demonstrated that lateral wall restriction rather than septal wall movement produced the reduction in left ventricular filling and left ventricular volume. This study suggested a direct impairment in left ventricular function caused by lung compression secondary to PEEP therapy.

Still other authors have cited the possibility of a neural or humeral depressant factor initiated by the application of PEEP. Liebman and colleagues (1978) found that 15 cm of water PEEP produced significant decreases in cardiac output, but the tightening of pulmonary arterial bands did not produce equivalent pulmonary vascular changes. These authors conducted several experiments wherein a depression in cardiac output was observed even when the chest wall of animals had been removed and even in dogs who were cross-circulated with other animals supported with PEEP ventilation. On the contrary, Calvin and co-workers (1981) could not demonstrate any change in the contractile state of the left ventricle in patients with acute pulmonary edema. They concluded that decreased left ventricular preload alone accounted for the observed changes in cardiac output. Robotham and associates (1983) likewise were unable to confirm a hormonally dependent decrease in left ventricular function with PEEP. As reported by Titley and colleagues (1985), Weisel's group used radionucleotide angiography in postoperative coronary bypass patients to demonstrate a reduction in cardiac index with the application of 15 cm of water PEEP. Their volume studies, however, showed no alteration in left or right ventricular performance. Metabolic studies undertaken in the same group of patients suggested only a minor role for myocardial ischemia in the cardiac response to PEEP.

With the addition of PEEP, according to Scharfe and Cassidy (1989), an increase in left ventricular transmural filling pressure apparently occurs, perhaps because of mechanical interdependence of the ventricles such that an increase in right ventricular end-diastolic volume results in a decreased left ventricular compliance. Such an effect is enhanced when the pericardium is intact.

Alternatively, Takata (1991) suggested that the same measured effect could be secondary to cardiac compression from increased lung volumes. Likely, both effects are possible and the degrees to which one or the other is operative may depend on whether venous return falls or right ventricular end-diastolic volume increases because of volume infusion.

Despite experimental evidence in animals that a neural or humeral depressant factor may exist, the overwhelming evidence to date in man suggests that the prime effect on cardiac output is a reduction in left and right ventricular preload. There is, however, an important positive effect of PEEP, and that is its decrease in left ventricular afterload. Buda (1979) noted that, depending on venous return as influenced by volume infusions, an actual increase in cardiac output may be observed with PEEP.

Monitoring PEEP

Numerous studies have identified various means of determining the best PEEP. The most accepted means are the calculation of oxygen transport — O_2 trans — and the determination of pulmonary compliance. Maximizing oxygen transport is the primary goal of PEEP therapy, as the following equation illustrates; O_2 trans = CO × (1.39 × hemoglobin × Sa_{O_2}) + 0.0031 × Pa_{O_2}). The important contributors to oxygen delivery are oxyhemoglobin saturation and cardiac output. As the equation demonstrates, Pa_{O_2} plays a minor role. Management of PEEP therapy thus requires the insertion of a Swan-Ganz catheter to obtain cardiac output. This step should be routine when levels of PEEP are above 10 cm of water.

Suter and associates (1975) documented a correlation between static compliance and oxygen transport measurements. The former can be derived from the ventilator recordings themselves with the contribution of airway pressure to compliance determined by clamping the expiratory line at end inspiration. The fall in peak airway pressure during this maneuver determines the role of airway resistance to pulmonary compliance. The equalization pressure following the clamping of the expiratory line reflects the pressure generated from pulmonary compliance. An immediate impression of the efficacy of an incremental increase of PEEP can also be obtained from an observation of the resultant increase in peak airway pressure. An increase in peak airway pressure greater than the increment in PEEP suggests that the results will be deleterious rather than efficacious. Hylkema and associates (1985) suggested optimizing the lung mechanical profile by plotting regression lines of pressure volume curves at various levels of PEEP. The value of PEEP achieving the greatest slope and smallest intersect volume was thought to represent the most efficient lung function obtainable. Despite these determinations, oxygen transport remains the standard for assessing the effectiveness of PEEP therapy.

In patients with unilateral lung disease, PEEP may prove deleterious. Kanarek and Shannon (1975) presented a case in which Pa_{O_2} decreased with the application of PEEP. They suggested that PEEP selectively increased lung volume on the normal side, secondarily raising pulmonary vascular resistance and shunting blood to the diseased lung. In an experimental study, Sanchez de Leon and colleagues (1985) showed an increased proportion of cardiac output to a collapsed lobe when PEEP was applied, thereby increasing shunting.

Adjuvant Means of Improving Oxygenation

Minimizing Lung Water

Respiratory failure is often precipitated by the accumulation of extravascular water because of permeability changes in the pulmonary capillaries, particularly after operative trauma but also in pneumonia. The determinants of transcapillary fluid movement are permeability and pressure. The pressure gradient is the result of the net difference between oncotic and hydrostatic pressure across the membrane. Clinically, the only determinant that can be manipulated is intravascular hydrostatic pressure. In the lung, this is best expressed by left ventricular preload or pulmonary capillary wedge pressure. A normal pulmonary capillary wedge pressure does not preclude diuresis when pulmonary infiltrates are believed to be secondary to increased capillary permeability. Because the amount of fluid entering the interstitium is directly proportional to the driving pressure, a lower wedge pressure is still desirable. Thus, in respiratory failure — particularly in cases of augmented permeability — the objectives should be to obtain the lowest possible wedge pressure compatible with adequate cardiac output and renal perfusion. If necessary beta-adrenergic doses of dopamine — less than 5 μg/kg/min — can be used to sustain urinary and cardiac output. Wedge pressure, however, may not always reflect left atrial filling pressures in patients with lung injury. The pulmonary circulation is a low pressure system. As such, the pressure in arterioles and venules may vary depending on their position within the lung parenchyma. Thus, arterial pressure is low in nondependent areas above the level of the main pulmonary artery and venous pressure is high in areas below the level of the left atrium. The converse is also true. Alveolar pressure, however, is relatively constant. West and colleagues (1964) described several lung zones that are defined by the relationships between pulmonary artery pressure, alveolar pressure, and left atrial pressure at various levels in the lung parenchyma (Fig. 25–5). As a result, measured wedge pressure varies depending on the zonal characteristics of the lung surrounding the catheter. The author and colleagues (1978) showed that depending on patient position, the level of PEEP, or the magnitude of left atrial pressure, catheter tips may lie in zone 2 or even in zone 1 areas. In such situations, the catheter-recorded pressures reflect alveolar and not venous pressure. Hasan and associates (1985) showed in cases of unilateral lung injury that catheters placed

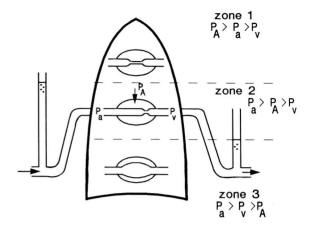

Fig. 25–5. The lung zones as defined by John West. In zone 1, alveolar pressure is greater than both arterial and venous pressure and there is little or no flow. In zone 2, the flow is determined by the gradient between arterial pressure and alveolar pressure, with a vascular waterfall existing between the alveolus and the pulmonary veins. In zone 3, both arterial and venous pressures are greater than alveolar pressure and flow is maximal. *From* Shapiro BA, et al: Clinical Application of Respiratory Care. 3rd Ed. Chicago: Year Book, 1985.

on the damaged side may actually better reflect left atrial pressure than catheters placed on the side with the normal lung. Presumably, airway pressure is better transmitted to alveolar capillaries in compliant versus noncompliant lung.

Postural Changes

As Rivara and colleagues (1984) illustrated, postural changes lead to significant improvements in oxygenation, particularly in unilateral lung disease. Frequent changes in position minimize the development of atelectasis in dependent portions. The longer a patient remains in a fixed position, the more severe the atelectasis that develops in dependent lung regions secondary to sputum retention and interstitial fluid accumulation, not to mention the effect of the pleural pressure gradient. A change in position, particularly from supine to prone, results in the best ventilated areas becoming dependent and thus exposed to maximal pulmonary arterial blood flow. Ventilation-perfusion ratios are obviously improved. Such dramatic changes in posture are difficult to achieve in ventilated patients, but they can be accomplished with a circle electric bed or a Stryker frame. Clearly, use of such devices is only indicated when the $F_{I_{O_2}}$ is excessively high or oxygenation is difficult to maintain with all other maneuvers, or both.

Airway Pressures

Improvement in gas exchange should not be made at the cost of barotrauma caused by high peak airway pressure, particularly in thoracic surgical patients with bronchial sutures lines. Patients with high peak airway pressure should be monitored closely to rule out pneumothorax. Endotracheal tube patency must be assessed bronchoscopically. The pleural spaces should be evacuated to allow full expansion of the lungs. Reducing the tidal volume reduces peak airway pressure. To maintain minute ventilation, the respiratory rate must be increased to compensate for the lower tidal volume. Thus, when peak airway pressures are high because of incremental increases in PEEP or because of additional lung pathology, airway pressure may be reduced and Pa_{CO_2} is maintained by supplying the same minute ventilation at a lower tidal volume and a higher rate. The extreme example of this principle is high frequency jet ventilation — HFJV — which is discussed subsequently.

There are, however, limits to the decrease in tidal volume. Under such conditions, permissive hypercapnia may be a viable alternative. In fact, several authors maintain that peak airway pressures in excess of 30 to 35 cm of water should always be avoided. Gattinoni (1986) and Tsuno (1990) and their colleagues provided convincing experimental evidence of unappreciated degrees of pulmonary barotrauma. Hickling and co-workers (1990) reported on the use of permissive hypercapnia in order to avoid high peak airway pressures.

Conventional Ventilators

Ventilator Settings

In initiating ventilator therapy, respiratory rate, tidal volume, inspiratory time, PEEP, and $F_{I_{O_2}}$ are adjusted on the basis of clinical knowledge of the patient. Subsequent adjustments are made by following serial arterial blood gas values. Changes in oxygenation are made by adjusting $F_{I_{O_2}}$ or PEEP while Pa_{CO_2} is altered by varying respiratory rate or tidal volume. In making subsequent adjustments, one strives to achieve the lowest $F_{I_{O_2}}$ and the lowest possible peak airway pressure. In general, only one variable should be changed at a time to avoid unpredictable interactions.

Volume Cycle Ventilation

Volume cycle ventilators are the mainstay of modern ventilatory therapy. These machines deliver a preset tidal volume at a specified respiratory rate. Generally, the inspiratory time is short — 0.5 to 1.0 second — and the gas is delivered in a sine wave pattern. Because the ventilator is designed to deliver constant volumes, high peak airway pressures may be generated during the inspiratory cycle if compliance of the lung chest wall interface is poor. All machines have built-in pressure limits to prevent excessive barotrauma. Precise adjustments of $F_{I_{O_2}}$, PEEP, inspiration/expiration ratio, tidal volume, and respiratory rate can be made on all standard ventilators. An important hidden factor must be remembered when adjusting tidal volume. Although the machine delivers constant preset volume to the system, the patient does not receive the entire amount. Changes in volume of the ventilator tubing — compression volume — account for the rest of the breath. Bartel and co-workers (1985) showed that up to 20% of the delivered tidal volume can be sequestered within the tubing in patients with low lung compliance. Most

volume cycle ventilators offer three modes of ventilator support.

Control. In this mode, ventilators initiated by the patient are not sensed by the machine. A preset tidal volume is delivered at a constant respiratory rate. This style of ventilation is generally reserved for patients who are apneic because of anesthesia, muscle relaxants, or head injury.

Assist Control. Preset respiratory rates and volumes are again delivered as in the control method. The machine also senses the patient's respiratory effort and delivers the same preset volume for all patient-driven breaths. Minute ventilation, therefore, depends on the effort of the patient, but a lower limit is assured by the preset rate. The sensitivity of the machine to a patient-initiated breath can be altered. This most common mode of ventilation is used routinely in the postoperative period as well as for patients with prolonged respiratory failure.

Intermittent Mandatory Ventilation — IMV. The ventilator is set to deliver a specific tidal volume at a predetermined rate. In the IMV mode, the ventilator also senses the patient-initiated breath as it does in the assist control mode. Unlike the latter, however, the tidal volume delivered to the patient during these breaths depends entirely on the magnitude of the patient's respiratory effort. When the machine senses an inspiration, a fresh gas flow valve opens, allowing the patient to take a breath. No preset tidal volume is delivered during the patient-initiated breath. In the IMV setting, minute ventilation is determined not only by the number of patient-initiated breaths, but also by their force. Once again, a minimum volume is assured by the preset IMV rate. Intermittent mandatory ventilation is frequently used postoperatively when extubation is expected within 24 hours, and also as a weaning strategy in prolonged respiratory failure.

Pressure-Limited Ventilation

Several forms of ventilation — permissive hypercarbia, pressure preset ventilation, pressure-limited ventilation — differ from each other in relatively minor degrees. Common to each is the desire to limit the peak inflation pressure or the mean airway pressure. Based on the work of several authors as previously noted, advocates of these modes of ventilatory support suppose that barotrauma is perhaps responsible for additive pulmonary parenchymal damage following the initiation of ventilatory support for other reasons. As a result, an effort is made to limit the airway pressure.

Marini and colleagues (1989) introduced a concept of pressure preset ventilation, a square wave form of ventilatory drive that focuses on three parameters — a preset pressure, an inspiratory time fraction, and frequency. The PEEP is usually set at 10 to 12 cm of water, and hence ventilatory pressure becomes the difference between the preset pressure and PEEP. This is a reliable means of ventilatory support that should limit or reduce barotrauma.

The inspiratory time fraction is a particularly intriguing parameter, the benefits of which were largely unappreciated until better defined by Marini and co-workers (1992). They demonstrated that extending the inspiratory time fraction results in an improvement in arterial oxygenation, unless minute ventilation was already high. It is postulated that a slowing in inspiratory time permits a better distribution of ventilation. This result is particularly appealing in ARDS, with lung units with vastly different time constants. It had been demonstrated by Pesanti (1985) that increases in inspiratory time would improve alveolar ventilation. If, however, minute ventilation is already high, such a maneuver may result in an increase in auto-PEEP — defined as the increase in end-expiratory pressure generated unintentionally by the ventilator when expiratory time is insufficient to allow for full expiration of expired gas. This circumstance rather than improving alveolar ventilation should result in an increase in dead space.

At high frequencies, therefore, pressure preset ventilation may result in hypercarbia. Such, however, should not be considered a failure of ventilatory support as long as metabolic compensation is sufficient to prevent a respiratory acidosis below a pH of 7.20. Indeed, a ventilatory mode coined "permissive hypercarbia or pressure limited ventilation" has become increasingly popular. Basically, this mode involves limiting inflation pressure irrespective of tidal volume. Initial requirements for increased ventilation can be achieved by increases in rate. If, however, Pa_{CO_2} is allowed to rise gradually, renal compensation should prevent a major deterioration in acid-base balance. Apparently, a pH of 7.2 is well tolerated without undue hematologic or hemodynamic sequelae. If gradual, the Pa_{CO_2} may rise to substantial levels. Favorable results with this form of ventilatory support have been reported in asthmatics by Darioli and Perret (1984) and in ARDS patients by Hickling and associates (1990).

High-Frequency Ventilation — HFV

High-frequency ventilation — HFV — offers an alternative when conventional ventilation fails and gas exchange is insufficient. The delivery of small tidal volumes at high frequencies may improve alveolar mixing and alleviate the gas exchange problem. Such is achieved with the maintenance of mean airway pressure but a reduction in peak airway pressure. There are several forms of HFV. High-frequency positive pressure ventilation — HFPPV — refers to conventional ventilators set to deliver small tidal volumes at rates exceeding 40 per minute. This technique is useful for bronchoscopy and some open chest procedures, as shown by Malina and colleagues (1981). To avoid overextension of the lungs, sufficient time for exhalation must be allowed.

High-frequency oscillation — HFO — delivers some volumes of fresh gas at rates of 900 to 3000 per minute. The gas flow is rapidly interrupted by a piston or ball to produce oscillations. The mechanism for gas exchange is unclear. Molecular diffusion of gas in the airways may be enhanced by the turbulence generated by the oscillations.

During high-frequency jet ventilation — HFJV, jets of gas at rates of 80 to 400 breaths per minute are delivered through a small cannula into the distal trachea. By the Venturi principle, additional gas is drawn into the airway — the biased gas flow. Traditionally, these systems have been open, wherein the biased gas is drawn from atmosphere or from an oxygen source. Because the degree of mixing of jet stream gas and biased gas remained unknown, the true $F_{I_{O_2}}$ was also uncertain. These systems have been particularly useful in the ventilatory management of patients with large bronchopleural fistulas. Table 25–4 displays the arterial blood gases on a standard volume cycle ventilator and then on HFJV in a patient with an iatrogenically created defect in the trachea and left main stem bronchus after complicated esophageal surgery, as reported by Panos and associates (1986). These systems have, however, been hampered by several difficulties. As noted, the mixing of biased gas and jet gas leads to an unknown $F_{I_{O_2}}$. In addition, humidification of the biased gas is often difficult, resulting in drying of the airways. Importantly, many of these systems lack disconnect and high pressure alarms. It is possible, however, to use a standard volume cycle ventilator set in an IMV mode — at 2 to 6 breaths per minute and a tidal volume of 200 ml — as the source of the biased gas flow. Thus, a constant $F_{I_{O_2}}$ adequate humidification, and the alarm systems of a conventional ventilator are supplied. It also allows use of PEEP to a greater extent should that be desired.

Although general agreement exists concerning the efficacy of HFJV in the management of bronchopleural fistula, controversy concerning its role in hypoxemic respiratory failure continues. MacIntyre and colleagues (1986) failed to demonstrate any advantage of HFJV over conventional ventilators in their patients with respiratory failure. Carlon and associates (1981) documented their experience in 17 patients with various abnormalities causing hypoxemia that was refractory to conventional ventilation. Of these 17 patients, 8 improved and survived with HFJV and none of the 17 individuals experienced a deterioration when switched to the high frequency technique. Experimental work by Lucking and associates (1986) demonstrated an improvement in

Table 25–4. Ventilatory Settings and Arterial Blood Gases in a Single Patient with a Large Bronchopleural Fistula*

Control-Mode Ventilation	High Frequency Jet Ventilation
Rate = 30	Rate = 20
V = 1000 ml	D/P = 10 psi
$F_{I_{O_2}}$ = 0.60	$F_{I_{O_2}}$ = 0.60
PEEP = 10	PEEP = 10
Arterial Blood Gases	
pH = 7.23	pH = 7.24
P_{CO_2} = 102	P_{CO_2} = 63
P_{O_2} = 57	P_{O_2} = 85

*Note the improvement in arterial carbon dioxide tension following the institution of high frequency jet ventilation.

cardiac output and systemic hemodynamics with maintenance in gas exchange in dogs suffering from induced right ventricular dysfunction. In my experience, the closed system alluded to has provided improved gas exchange even in cases of hypoxemic respiratory failure. Figures 25–6 and 25–7 demonstrate the rapid improvement in Pa_{O_2} and the ability to decrease FI_{O_2} to acceptable limits. Such improvement is not universal, however.

Extracorporeal Membrane Oxygenation — ECMO

Occasionally, maximum ventilatory support including HFJV is insufficient to reverse hypoxemia, hypercarbia, or both. Extracorporeal membrane oxygenation may salvage a few of these patients in terminal respiratory failure. A multicenter National Institutes of Health trial reported by Zapal and associates (1979) concluded that ECMO provided no survival advantage over continued conventional ventilatory support. The study has within its design a large beta error, that is, the risk of not demonstrating a true benefit from the therapy was high given the sample size. Several authors, including Solca (1985), Egan (1988), and Bartlett (1977) and their colleagues reported their success with varying forms of ECMO.

A technique for the rapid institution of ECMO using percutaneous catheters and a bio-medicus pump, the so-called minimembrane, has been developed. Girotti and associates (1986) described the techniques and Rice and associates (1986) presented results in five patients. Rapid percutaneous cannulation of the femoral veins provided venous drainage. Blood was returned through a cannula placed in the internal jugular vein. Oxygenation improved from 37 mm Hg pre-ECMO to 186

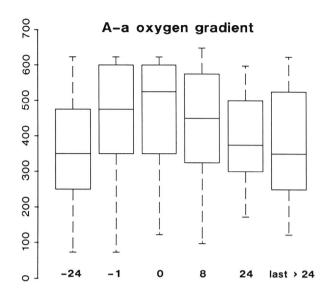

Fig. 25–7. The alveolar-arterial oxygen gradient in 67 patients with hypoxemic respiratory failure subjected to high frequency jet ventilation. The values of $(A - a)D_{O_2}$ at minus 24, minus 1, and 0 represent the progressive increases in $(A - a)D_{O_2}$ before the institution of HFJV. Note the rapid improvement in $(A - a)D_{O_2}$ following the institution of HFJV at time 0.

mm Hg post-ECMO. Carbon dioxide levels returned to normal in all cases. Three of the five patients survived their pulmonary insult and were discharged from the hospital.

Further refinement of the use of extracorporeal circuits was formalized by Gattanoni and colleagues (1986). They extended the principle of pressure-limited ventilation by removing carbon dioxide through extracorporeal circuits while still providing the support of oxygenation — at least to some degree — with a low frequency positive pressure ventilation.

SPECIFIC PROBLEMS

Fighting the Ventilator

Patients and their ventilators are out of phase when the patient attempts to initiate an inspiration during the expiratory phase of the machine cycle. This struggling leads to increased oxygen consumption, increased intrathoracic pressures, and a reduction in alveolar ventilation. The stimulus may be inadequate ventilation or oxygenation, central nervous system disturbance, acidemia, or anxiety. Under such circumstances, one must first identify and correct acid base and gas exchange abnormalities. A switch to IMV ventilation may be all that is necessary. Pain and anxiety can be relieved by narcotic sedatives. If struggling is related to central nervous system dysfunction, muscle relaxants may be required. Airway pressure should be assessed, and if it is increased, airway obstruction or pneumothorax should be suspected. If at any time the adequacy of ventilation is suspect, the patient should be disconnected from the machine and support should be pro-

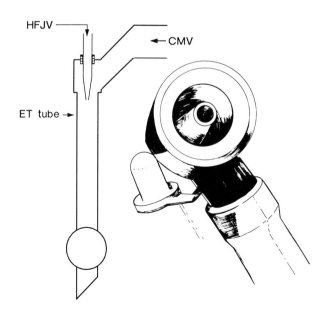

Fig. 25–6. A closed system of HFJV. A 3.5-mm cannula is inserted through the top of the swivel of the standard endotracheal tube (ET) (see insert). The biased or untrained gas flow comes from conventional mechanical ventilator (CMV) through the standard ventilatory tubing.

vided with an ambu bag delivering 100% oxygen. Manual ventilation can be synchronized with the patient's efforts and airway resistance can be assessed. A chest radiograph is required to determine the presence or absence of pneumothorax because auscultation of the ventilated patient is unreliable. Similarly, bronchospasm may not be fully appreciated if air entry is diminished. Continued agitation in the presence of poor compliance of the lung and the absence of a pneumothorax demands bronchoscopic inspection of the endotracheal tube and distal airway.

Weaning and Extubation

Methods of weaning largely reflect individual bias, as few sound data are available in support of any particular system. The only viable principle is that no one system is perfect and that failure to wean by one means does not preclude success with another.

Electively Ventilated Patients

Patients electively ventilated for reasons other than respiratory failure can be weaned and extubated quickly. The measurement of VC and negative inspiratory force — NIF — are important initial assessments. Both are easily obtained at the bedside with a standard respirometer and manometer. To evaluate VC, the patient is instructed to perform a maximal inspiration and then forcibly exhale into the respirometer. An estimate of NIF is obtained by a maximal inspiration against a closed airway. It reflects the ability to cough and clear secretions. Vital capacity indicates respiratory reserve, and because it is a voluntary maneuver, it is a measure of patient alertness and cooperation. Although no reliable data formally suggest that either measurement is foolproof, they nonetheless provide a reasonable guide. Low values are almost certainly associated with the inability to extubate, whereas normal values may not always predict successful extubation. A forced VC greater than 10 ml/kg body weight and an NIF greater than −25 cm of water are prerequisites for extubation if no trial of spontaneous ventilation with an endotracheal tube in place is attempted. When measured VC and NIF are not appropriate, a trial of weaning is undertaken, by either progressive decreases in IMV or spontaneous breathing with CPAP. The choice depends on the degree of impairment of VC and NIF and the experience and bias of the physician. Any weaning effort demands close monitoring of gas exchange, patient effort, breathing pattern, and vital signs.

Wean Following Respiratory Failure

Most patients requiring mechanical assistance for respiratory failure present a different challenge; varying degrees of continued parenchymal disease, increased bronchial reactivity, respiratory muscle debility, and cardiovascular compromise demand a more cautious approach to weaning. The initial problem is to identify that weaning is possible; this is usually signalled by an $F_{I_{O_2}}$ less than 50%, PEEP less than or equal to 7 cm of water, and a clearing of infiltrates on chest radi-

ography. Further support for the initiation of the weaning effort can be obtained in the conscious patient by the ability to generate a forced VC of at least 7 ml/kg body weight and a minimal NIF of −15 cm of water. Of the several methods of weaning, the focus of this section is on the classical method, IMV, and pressure support.

Although weaning via an open airway — T piece method — has often been quoted as a variant of a classical wean, it possesses no distinct advantage. On the contrary, potential disadvantages are that the removal of end-expiratory pressure results over time in a progressive fall in FRC and the increased probability of V/Q mismatching. Annest (1980) and Quan (1981) and their colleagues showed that this leads to an increased work of breathing.

The CPAP method — or classic method — places the entire responsibility for ventilation on the patient. It provides for intermittent stresses with periods of complete rest at levels of assisted ventilation. Theoretically, this maximal stress followed by rest should provide beneficial respiratory muscle exercise. When using the classic technique, it is important to recognize that patients initially tolerate CPAP for only a short time. Extending the interval should proceed slowly — patients should not be stressed to the point of impending failure. Cohen and associates (1982) described the clinical signs of respiratory muscle fatigue. Increased respiratory rate is followed by an alteration between rib cage and abdominal breathing, which they termed "respiratory alternans" — the paradoxic abdominal/chest wall motion described previously — and finally decreased Pa_{O_2} accompanied by a fall in minute ventilation and hypercarbia. Electromyographic recordings from their patients revealed high and low frequency discharges from the intercostal muscles. A fall in the ratio of high to low frequency power indicated fatiguing muscle and preceded the clinical signs of failure. Clinically, a simple guide to a patient's tolerance of the weaning process can be obtained by a measurement of VC and NIF at the beginning and at the end of the CPAP wean. The wean period should not be extended unless the beginning and ending values are comparable.

During the IMV technique, a patient must work constantly and may fail if he or she is not able to sustain the effort. As noted, failure occurs when fatigue results in diminishing tidal volumes, which in turn reduces FRC. Gas exchange becomes increasingly impaired. In addition, the ventilator may itself impose an increased burden on the work of breathing. Marini and associates (1986) demonstrated higher workloads during patient-triggered ventilatory breaths than during spontaneous breathing. Part of the explanation for this phenomenon lies in the resistance threshold in the ventilator itself. The resistance within the internal circuitry of respirators varies greatly. For this reason, when using CPAP, it is wise to use external circuits.

Pressure support ventilation and the use of pressure support during weaning has become popular. I have previously discussed the theory behind pressure support ventilation. When weaning, the amount of pressure support is gradually decreased until it is eliminated or until 10 cm of water has been achieved. It is a well-tolerated form of weaning. As with the classic method, however, adequate rest with maximal pressure support is a prerequisite between weaning intervals.

Nutrition

To wean successfully, a patient must be able to assume an ever-increasing workload of breathing as assisted ventilation is reduced. Importantly, the work of breathing must be efficient and coordinated or fatigue will develop and re-intubation will be required. As Roussos (1985) pointed out, respiratory muscles normally are continuously active, and when put to rest, they atrophy quickly. These muscles must be rebuilt during weaning. For this reason, adequate nutritional support is crucial to supply protein for muscle development. If necessary, total parental nutrition — TPN — should be instituted to provide sufficient calories.

Most thoracic surgical patients can tolerate enteral feeds within 24 to 48 hours, so protein depletion is not usually a problem. Esophagectomy patients often have a jejunostomy feeding tube placed intraoperatively and alimentation can begin. Total parental nutrition, however, should be instituted within 48 hours if attempts at enteral feeding fail. Nutrition requirements must be actively determined, as Dark and co-workers (1985) showed. Otherwise, increased carbohydrate calories lead to increased carbon dioxide production, which can precipitate hypercapneic respiratory failure. Unless the patient is severely catabolic, 2000 to 2500 calories are given, 50% in the form of lipids. In addition, 1 gram of protein per kilogram body weight per day should be supplied. Requirements in septic patients may be 30 to 50% higher. Fluid balance may be a problem in the thoracic surgical patient and in those with renal insufficiency. For these patients, monitoring of daily weight is a sensitive measurement of fluid accumulation, allowing judicious use of diuretics or dialysis to maintain fluid balance. Hypophosphatemia is a well-described cause of respiratory muscle fatigue that should be corrected.

The Decision to Extubate

Patients are ready for extubation when the criteria outlined in Table 25–5 are met and the patients are maintaining acceptable gas levels. Additionally, patients should be normotensive and should not have demonstrated dysrhythmia or tachycardia during the final weaning stages. Morganroth and colleagues (1984) quan-

Table 25–5. Criteria for Extubation

$F_{I_{O_2}}$	<50%
CPAP/PEEP	<7.5 cm H_2O
Respiratory rate	>8/min but <25/min
VC	10–15 ml/kg
NIF	>−20 cm H_2O

titated these factors into ventilator and adverse factor scores. Failure to achieve the aforementioned criteria predicted an unsuccessful wean in their long-term ventilated patients. These criteria are conservative and, as DeHaven and associates (1986) pointed out, may underestimate the ability of some patients to tolerate extubation. The latter report advocated gas exchange measurements of intrapulmonary shunt of less than 15% or $Pa_{O_2}/F_{I_{O_2}}$ ratios greater than 300 with room air. Using these measures, 94% of patients were extubated successfully, even though 48% did not meet the traditional standards. Many patients in this latter study, however, had not undergone prolonged ventilation. In the final analysis, the ability of the patient to sustain adequate ventilation and oxygenation with spontaneous ventilation over a fixed period of time warrants a trial of extubation. Unfortunately, no technique is fail safe nor does any system assess the ability to clear secretions after removal of an endotracheal tube. Nonetheless, trials of extubation are appropriate when patients can maintain their own support over several hours and re-intubation is not known to be difficult.

Technique of Extubation

Before extubation, it is imperative to ensure that the patient can protect the airway — gag reflects and cough — and that significant upper airway obstruction, especially glottic edema, is not present. To ensure that the airway is adequate, the cuff of the endotracheal tube is deflated and the patient is instructed to inspire. The endotracheal tube is then occluded while the patient forcibly exhales. If the patient can exhale around the tube, glottic and subglottic edema are not critical. In the absence of such a leak, the glottis and the upper airway should be examined using a flexible bronchoscope inserted transnasally. In my experience, the ability to pass the bronchoscope between the vocal cords anteriorly suggests that extubation may be attempted with caution. Postextubation stridor attributed to residual glottic edema usually responds to a helium-oxygen mixture — 30% oxygen, 70% helium — and racemic epinephrine therapy. Failure to insert the bronchoscope between the vocal cords and the tube should delay extubation for 24 to 48 hours so that edema might clear.

Tracheostomy

The timing of tracheostomy remains controversial. In many centers, endotracheal intubation — particularly transnasal — is allowed to continue indefinitely. In North America, tracheostomy is traditionally undertaken after 2 weeks. Little evidence supports this arbitrary time period, although a study by Stauffer and colleagues (1981) indicated a higher incidence of tracheal stenosis and laryngotracheal ulceration in patients undergoing tracheostomy more than 14 days after endotracheal intubation. The corollary was that no advantage was found to suggest that tracheostomy was better than prolonged endotracheal intubation. Of the many reasons given for performing tracheostomies, such as difficulty in suctioning, patient discomfort, laryngotracheal lesions, oral hygiene, and glottic edema, only the last two justify this approach. Stauffer and colleagues (1981) clearly show that difficulty in suctioning and patient discomfort were minor problems and that tracheostomy may have a higher incidence of laryngotracheal complications. Difficulty in maintaining oral hygiene is, however, a common occurrence and leads to oropharyngeal infections, sialadenitis, and mucosal ulceration. As mentioned previously, extubation is contraindicated in the presence of glottic edema, and tracheostomy maintains the airway and allows the edema to resolve. For these reasons, tracheostomy should be considered for patients intubated for 10 to 14 days and in whom it is expected that mechanical ventilatory support will be required for some time. It should be undertaken earlier when endotracheal re-intubation is indicated because of a failure to clear secretions.

Percutaneous tracheostomy at the bedside has recently gained acceptance. Hazard and colleagues (1991) have demonstrated that the technique can be performed effectively and safely. It does, however, require the ability to use a flexible bronchoscope.

Difficult Weaning

Failure to wean should prompt further investigations to reveal possible causes. A dead space to tidal volume ratio — V_D/V_T — of greater than 0.7 suggests an inability to wean, but this is a dynamic measurement and patients often show improvement over time. It becomes an accurate measurement of subtle improvement in long-term patients with severe inspiratory insult. In my experience, it may require up to 3 months of a stable respiratory situation before V_D/V_T improves and the criteria for weaning are reached. Open lung biopsy sometimes reveals unsuspected and treatable disease, but this information is less useful than in the past given the advent of protected specimen brushing and bronchoalveolar lavage. Ventilation-perfusion scanning may show areas of gross mismatch contributing to intrapulmonary shunt. Some patients fail weaning because of hemodynamic instability evident only during the weaning period. Insertion of a pulmonary artery catheter may uncover significant pulmonary arterial hypertension, which can be corrected with appropriate vasodilator therapy. Table 25-6 documents the results in a patient with left ventricular dysfunction and mitral valve replacement. The patient had failed several weaning attempts over several weeks. Once pulmonary artery pressures were controlled, weaning proceeded rapidly and successfully.

Aubier and co-workers (1987) showed that digoxin improved diaphragmatic strength by 19.5% in ventilated patients with chronic obstructive lung disease. This mechanism of action is unclear.

Hemodynamic Monitoring

Care should be taken to avoid hypervolemia in the weaning patient. The desire for fluid restriction must be weighed, however, against the need to maintain systemic perfusion. If necessary, low doses of dopamine — less than 5 µg/kg/min — can be used to maintain renal perfusion, as evidenced by urine output greater than or equal to 30 ml per hour. In the face of a diminishing urine output or an increasing inotrope requirement, a Swan-Ganz catheter should be inserted to guide therapy. Table 25-7 outlines criteria for pulmonary arterial monitoring. Information obtained can be used to estimate left ventricular filling pressures by the pulmonary capillary wedge pressure. Determination of cardiac output is necessary to monitor oxygen delivery and may be adversely affected by increasing PEEP. The decision to increase fluids, start inotropes, or institute vasodilator therapy is guided by the measurement of pulmonary arterial and systemic pressures and of cardiac output.

After pneumonectomy, pulmonary vascular resistance may rise considerably. Pulmonary arterial hypertension may lead to right and then left ventricular failure. The use of vasodilators to modify left ventricular preload or afterload or both without sacrificing oxygen delivery or systemic perfusion requires the information obtained with a pulmonary artery catheter. Acute increases in pulmonary artery pressures related to hypoxemia or pulmonary emboli may result in the development of a right to left cardiac shunt via a patent foramen ovale. Although unusual, shunting should be considered in any patient with arterial oxygen desaturation but a normal chest radiograph. This clinical scenario is always associated with either a thrombotic pulmonary embolus, a main stem bronchial obstruction with distal air trapping, or the right to left shunt noted.

Patients with a recent history of myocardial disease or with perioperative ischemic changes should be monitored to appreciate any effect that the work of breathing might have on myocardial performance.

Complications of Swan-Ganz monitoring arise primarily during insertion of the catheter. Dysrhythmias, such as premature ventricular beats and ventricular

Table 25-6. Systolic and Diastolic Pulmonary Artery Pressures Following Prolonged Mechanical Ventilatory Support*

Before Weaning	During Weaning	Day 1 Nitrates	Day 2 Weaned
60/29	80/12	47/24	35/17

*Note the major increase in systolic pressure observed during the weaning process. This was accompanied by pulmonary edema. Weaning proceeded smoothly in the face of nitrates.

Table 25-7. Indications for Swan-Ganz Catheterization

Pulmonary edema with normal central venous pressure
Hypotension with normal or high central venous pressure
PEEP >10 cm H_2O
Recent myocardial ischemia or infarction
Previous failed wean
Significant inotrope requirements

tachycardia, are treated by withdrawal of the catheter with or without intravenous lidocaine — 1 mg/kg. Recurrence of these rhythm disturbances with re-insertion demands the intravenous administration of antiarrhythmetic drugs. Patients with left bundle branch block should not be subjected to Swan-Ganz catheterization unless it is absolutely necessary. Establishment of a right bundle branch block is a complication of catheter insertion, and in these patients would result in complete heart block. If pulmonary arterial monitoring is required, a temporary transvenous pacemaker should be on standby before the catheter is inserted.

The other major complication of these catheters is pulmonary artery disruption. This complication tends to occur in elderly patients with pulmonary arterial hypertension. The most common site is the origin of the right middle lobe artery. A traumatic bronchovascular fistula is created leading to the endobronchial accumulation of blood. Important points of management are as follows. First, the bleeding is from a low pressure system and usually stops spontaneously. Second, the immediate concern is protection of the airway — management includes vigorous suctioning, rigid bronchoscopy to clear blood clot, and the insertion of an endobronchial blocker to prevent further contamination of the normal side. Figures 25–8 and 25–9 demonstrate the use of the bronchus blocker. The immediate insertion of a double lumen tube is to be condemned. Adequate suctioning is impossible and asphyxia may result. As noted, a rigid bronchoscope provides ven-

tilation and the ability to clear and control the airway. Third, the pulmonary artery balloon should not be re-inflated. It rarely occludes the artery and probably leads to further tearing of the vessel wall. Fourth, surgical resection may be necessary if a hemothorax develops, bleeding continues, or an intraparenchymal hematoma is evident. To minimize the risk of this complication, the catheter should be advanced with the balloon inflated.

COMPLICATIONS OF INTUBATION AND MECHANICAL VENTILATION

Airways

Stauffer and colleagues (1981) divided problems of achieving and maintaining airways into those that occur early and those that occur late. Insertion of an endotracheal tube requires skill and practice. The incidence of failed attempts, inadvertent esophageal intubation, mouth or lip injuries, and right main stem bronchial intubation is considerably greater in inexperienced hands. The most common early complication is an inability to maintain the airway. In the report by Stauffer and colleagues, 45% of early problems were related to self-extubation, inability to seal the airway, or excessive cuff pressures required to maintain the seal. Early complications in tracheostomy include stomal infection, hemorrhage, and a requirement for excessive cuff pressures.

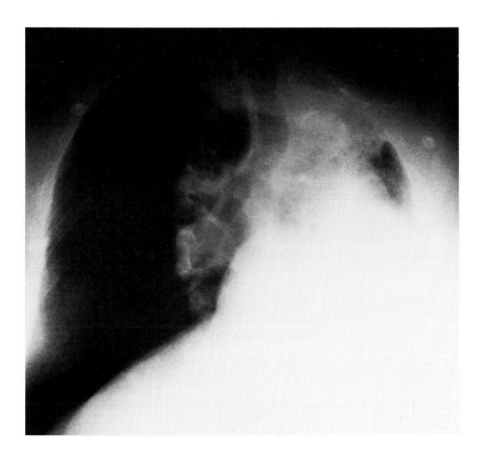

Fig. 25–8. Chest radiograph of a patient with significant hemoptysis from the left lung before the insertion of the bronchus blocker.

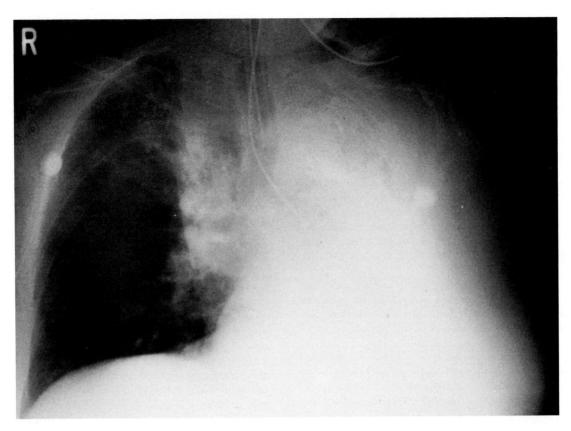

Fig. 25–9. Collapse of the left lung after inflation of the bronchus blocker.

All these problems are overcome easily. Tubes should be well secured and patients should be constantly supervised. Inadvertent extubation requires rapid re-insertion of the airway, providing high flow 100% oxygen while preparations are made. Tracheostomy tubes that fall out within 48 to 72 hours represent a particular problem. Under such circumstances, a fistulous track may not be established, suggesting that oral intubation may be safer and more expeditious. Any attempt to re-insert a tracheostomy tube should be undertaken with the patient in the operative position with the neck extended and with support under the shoulders. The requirement for a high cuff pressure to secure a seal is problematic. It suggests a capacious and dilated trachea. The insertion of a larger tube or the use of foam cuff tubes usually solves the problem.

Late complications include tracheal stenosis, at the stomal site, the cuff site, or the subglottic area. Late hemorrhage may result from tracheal ulceration, pulmonary parenchymal pathology, or tracheoinnominate artery fistula. As the latter may manifest with a herald bleed, any hemorrhage in or around a tracheostomy deserves investigation. Fiberoptic bronchoscopy by way of the tube itself clears the airway and permits examination of the distal tracheobronchial tree and assessment of the extent of hemorrhage. If the bleeding is stopped and no distal cause is apparent, the tracheostomy tube can be removed and bronchoscopy is quickly conducted through the stoma to examine the anterior tracheal wall for ulceration. If hemorrhage should continue or recur, tracheostomy tube cuffs should be hyperinflated with the tube tilted backwards, thus thrusting the cuff against the anterior tracheal wall. If this maneuver fails to control the problem, the tracheostomy tube must be removed, and the airway is secured from above with a rigid bronchoscope. The finger is inserted into the tracheal stoma and digital control of the innominate artery is obtained by compressing the artery against the right sternoclavicular joint. Cooper (1977) described the procedure in detail.

Problems following percutaneous tracheostomy are rare. I am aware anecdotally, however, of three cases of airway obstruction that resulted from the avulsion of tracheal mucosa. One of these cases was noted personally and the other two were reported in the Canadian Medical legal community. All three cases occurred when percutaneous tracheostomy was attempted after tracheal intubation and mechanical support for greater than 3 weeks.

Pulmonary Sepsis as a Major Cause of Postoperative Morbidity and Mortality

In a case review of 327 ventilated patients by Gillespie and colleagues (1986), the mortality for patients with acute lung injury was 40% and rose to 81% when accompanied by multisystem failure. Aggressive pre- and postoperative physiotherapy is important in the high-risk thoracic surgical patient. When pneumonia is suspected, accurate identification of infecting organisms is essential to guide antibiotic therapy. When the diagnosis of pneumonia is in doubt, the use of protected specimen brushings (Fig. 25–10), bronchoalveolar lavage, or protected bronchoalveolar lavage should be considered. Johansen and colleagues (1988) reported that the use of these invasive methods of diagnosis reduced the need for open lung biopsy for the diagnosis of pulmonary infection. Candidal suprainfection is a devastating complication of prolonged antibiotic usage and is seen with increasing frequency in intensive care units. Frequent assessment of culture results and the re-appraisal of antibiotic requirements reduce the incidence of this problem. Definition of the criteria of infection and the institution of appropriate therapy, as Soutter and the author (1986) indicated, results in more reasonable success.

Other Complications

Lobar atelectasis can be improved by chest physiotherapy and bronchoscopy. Absorption atelectasis, oxygen toxicity, and positional hypoxemia were discussed previously. Gastrointestinal bleeding from stress ulceration is an uncommon complication in modern intensive care units. As a result, the routine usage of an H_2 receptor antagonist is probably not justified, particularly when evidence such as that of Driks and associates (1987) suggests that cytoprotective agents such as sucralfate may avoid bacteria overgrowth and yet prevent gastrointestinal hemorrhage.

SPECIAL SITUATIONS

Flail Chest

Mechanical ventilation should not be considered a routine intervention in patients with flail chest. Indications for mechanical support are the same as for any patient with respiratory failure and include arterial hypoxemia and hypercarbia unresponsive to conventional therapy. The author and Shamji (1985) demonstrated that the unstable chest wall does lead to progressive hypoxemia even in the absence of pulmonary contusion. The V/Q abnormality appears to be secondary to decreased pleural pressure on the ipsilateral side, resulting in decreased regional ventilation. Considerable perfusion, however, is maintained, resulting in hypoxemia. European authors, including Dor

(1972) Eschapasse (1973), and Paris (1977) and their associates report a large series of patients with flail chest that was managed by operative fixation of the unstable segment. The reports are anecdotal and uncontrolled, yet the observations are convincing. In practical terms, however, the indications for operative stabilization would include the inability to wean a patient from ventilatory support once the contusion has resolved and with maximal analgesia supplied in the form of epidural narcotic administration. The requirement of a thoracotomy for other reasons should also lead one to stabilize the chest wall at the conclusion of the procedure.

Unilateral or Asymmetric Lung Disease

Reduced compliance in one lung can lead to significant barotrauma on the uninvolved side as high airway pressures and PEEP are required to overcome the restriction on the diseased side. As discussed previously, application of PEEP in these circumstances can reduce arterial oxygenation through maldistribution of ventilation and perfusion. Siegel and associates (1985) promoted independent lung ventilation through a double-lumen endotracheal tube for patients with nonhomogeneous ARDS. Simultaneous independent ventilation reduced the intrapulmonary shunt and permitted a lowering of F_{IO_2} while maintaining an acceptable Pa_{O_2}. Each ventilator is separately programmed for tidal volume, PEEP, and inspiration-expiration ratio.

Adult Respiratory Distress Syndrome — ARDS

Nothing is unique in the management of ARDS. Corticosteroids have no benefit and may actually be deleterious. Although no new specific therapies are available as yet, recent evidence suggests that breakthroughs may be imminent. Tumor necrosis factor — TNF — has long been known to be a mediator of tissue injury and sepsis, as reported by Tracey and colleagues (1987). The administration of anti-TNF monoclonal antibodies in primate models of sepsis has greatly reduced the incidence of pulmonary damage.

Bronchopleural Fistula

Large-volume bronchopleural fistulas frequently are worsened by conventional ventilation and, as discussed previously, they are amenable to closure when HFV is used. When jet ventilation does not work, alternative techniques should be attempted. Increasing the volume of saline in the chest tube drainage bottle increases the

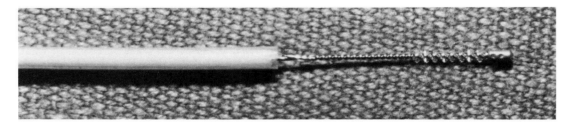

Fig. 25–10. A protected specimen brush with a double inner cannula and brush extruded.

pressure gradient against which the fistula must operate. Alternatively, ventilation to the affected segmented can be eliminated by positioning a bronchus blocker into the appropriate orifice or by reverting to one-lung ventilation, isolating the affected side. In addition, despite large losses of administered tidal volume, the continued increase in tidal volume up to 2 liters per breath may help to re-expand the lung and provide adequate ventilatory support. This technique, however, is inferior to the use of HFJV. Experience with tissue glue to seal leaking airways is anecdotal but encouraging, as McCarthy and associates (1988) noted. In post-pneumonectomy fistulas, the pleural space can be opened and packed. In these situations, the patients should be transferred to an institution where jet ventilation is available.

REFERENCES

Albert RK, et al: The prone position improves arterial oxygenation and reduces shunt in oleic-acid-induced acute lung injury. Am Rev Respir Dis 135:628, 1987.

Ali J, et al: Effect of postoperative intermittent positive pressure breathing on lung function. Chest 85:192, 1984.

Annest SJ, et al: Detrimental effects of removing end-expiratory pressure prior to extubation. Ann Surg 191:539, 1980.

Aubier M, et al: Effects of digoxin on diaphragmatic strength generation in patients with chronic obstructive pulmonary disease during acute respiratory failure. Am Rev Respir Dis 135:544, 1987.

Bartel LP, Bazik JR, Powner DJ: Compression volume during mechanical ventilation: Comparison of ventilators and tubing circuits. Crit Care Med 13:851, 1985.

Bartlett RH, et al: Extracorporeal membrane oxygenation support for cardiopulmonary failure. J Cardiovasc Thorac Surg 73:375, 1977.

Bendixen HH, Smith GM, Mead J: Pattern of ventilation in young adults. J Appl Physiol 19:195, 1964.

Bolton JWR, et al: Stair climbing as an indicator of pulmonary function. Chest 92:783, 1987.

Breivik H, et al: Normalizing low arterial CO_2 tension during mechanical ventilation. Chest 63:525, 1973.

Buda AJ, et al: Effects of intrathoracic pressure on left ventricular performance. N Engl J Med 301:453, 1979.

Calvin JE, Driedger AA, Sibbald WJ: Positive end-expiratory pressure (PEEP) does not depress left ventricular function in patients with pulmonary edema. Am Rev Respir Dis 124:121, 1981.

Carlon GC, et al: Clinical experience with high frequency jet ventilation. Crit Care Med 9:1, 1981.

Cassidy SS, Ramanathan M: Dimensional analysis of the left ventricle during PEEP: Relative septal and lateral wall displacements. Am J Physiol (Heart Circ Physiol 15) 246:H792, 1984.

Celli BR, Rodriguez KS, Snider GL: A controlled trial of intermittent positive pressure breathing, incentive spirometry and deep breathing exercise in preventing pulmonary complications after abdominal surgery. Am Rev Respir Dis 130:12, 1984.

Cherniak R: The oxygen consumption and efficiency of the respiratory muscles in health and emphysema. J Clin Invest 38:494, 1959.

Churchill ED, McNeil D: The reduction in vital capacity following operation. Surg Gynecol Obstet 44:483, 1927.

Cohen CA, et al: Clinical manifestations of inspiratory muscle fatigue. Am J Med 73:308, 1982.

Cooper JD: Tracheoinnominate artery fistula: Successful management of 3 consecutive patients. Ann Thorac Surg 24:439, 1977.

Daly BDT, Edmonds CH, Norman JC: In vivo alveolar morphometrics with positive end expiratory pressure. Surg Forum 24:217, 1973.

Darioli R, Perret C: Mechanical controlled hypertension in status asthmaticus. Am Rev Respir Dis 129:385, 1984.

Dark DS, Pingleton SK, Kerby GR: Hypercapnia during weaning: A complication of nutritional support. Chest 88:141, 1985.

DeHaven CB, Hurst JM, Branson RD: Postextubation hypoxemia treated with a continuous positive airway pressure mask. Crit Care Med 13:46, 1985.

DeHaven CB, Hurst JM, Branson RD: Evaluation of two different extubation criteria: Attributes contributing to success. Crit Care Med 14:92, 1986.

Dor V, et al: Les traumatismes graves du thorax, place de l'osteosynthese dans leur traitement — 100 cas. Nouv Presse Med 1:519, 1972.

Dorinsky PM, Whitcomb ME: The effect of PEEP on cardiac output. Chest 84:210, 1983.

Downs JB, Klein EF, Modell JH: The effects of incremental PEEP on Pa_{O_2} in patients with respiratory failure. Anesth Analg 52:210, 1973.

Driks MA, et al: Nosocomial pneumonia in intubated patients given sucralfate as compared with antacids or histamine type 2 blockers: The role of gastric colonization. N Engl J Med 317:1376, 1987.

Egan T, et al: Experience with ECMO for hypoxemic respiratory failure. Chest 94:681, 1988.

Egbert LD, Bendixen HH: Effect of morphine on breathing pattern: A possible factor in atelectasis. JAMA 188:485, 1964.

Eschapasse H, Gaillard J: Volets thoraciques: Principes de traitement. Ann Chir Thorac Cardiovasc 12:1, 1973.

Fee HJ, et al: Role of pulmonary vascular resistance measurements in preoperative evaluation of candidates for pulmonary resection. J Thorac Cardiovasc Surg 75:519, 1978.

Fisher AB, Forman HJ, Glass M: Mechanisms of pulmonary oxygen toxicity. Lung 162:255, 1984.

Gattinoni L, et al: Low frequency positive pressure ventilation with extracorporeal CO_2 removal in severe acute respiratory failure. JAMA 256:881, 1986.

Gillespie DJ, et al: Clinical outcome of respiratory failure in patients requiring prolonged (>24 hours) mechanical ventilation. Chest 90:364, 1986.

Girotti MJ, et al: Simultaneous use of membrane oxygenation and high-frequency jet ventilation in acute pulmonary failure. Crit Care Med 14:511, 1986.

Goldman L, et al: Multifactorial index of cardiac risk in noncardiac surgical procedures. N Engl J Med 297:845, 1977.

Hammon JW, et al: The effect of positive end-expiratory pressure on regional ventilation and perfusion in the normal and injured primate lung. J Thorac Cardiovasc Surg 72:680, 1976.

Harris SD, Johanson Jr WG, Pierce AK: Bacterial lung clearance in hypoxic mice. Am Rev Respir Dis 111:910, 1975.

Hazard P, Jones C, Benitone J: Comparative clinical trial of standard operative tracheostomy with percutaneous tracheostomy. Crit Care Med 19:1018, 1991.

Hasan FM, et al: Influence of lung injury on pulmonary wedge-left atrial pressure correlation during positive end-expiratory pressure ventilation. Am Rev Respir Dis 131:246, 1985.

Haynes JB: Positive end-expiratory pressure shifts left ventricular diastolic pressure-area curves. J Appl Physiol 48:670, 1980.

Hickling KG, Henderson SJ, Jackson R: Low mortality associated with permissive hypercapnia in severe ARDS. Int Care Med 16:372, 1990.

Hussain SNA, Roussos C: Distribution of respiratory muscle and organ blood flow during endotoxemic shock in dogs. J Appl Physiol 59:1802, 1985.

Hylkema BS, et al: Lung mechanical profiles in acute respiratory failure: Diagnostic and prognostic value of compliance at different tidal volumes. Crit Care Med 13:637, 1985.

Jackson RM: Pulmonary oxygen toxicity. Chest 88:900, 1985.

Jardin F, et al: Influence of positive end-expiratory pressure on left ventricular performance. N Engl J Med 304:387, 1981.

Johanson Jr WG, et al: Bacteriologic diagnosis of nosocomial pneumonia following prolonged mechanical ventilation. Am Rev Respir Dis 137:259, 1988.

Johnson AN, Cooper DF, Edwards RH: Exertion of stairclimbing in normal subjects and in patients with chronic obstructive bronchitis. Thorax 32:711, 1977.

Juhl B, Frost N: A comparison between measured and calculated changes in the lung function after operation for pulmonary cancer. Acta Anaesthesiol Scand 57(Suppl):39, 1975.

Kanarek DJ, Shannon DC: Adverse effect of positive end-expiratory pressure on pulmonary perfusion and arterial oxygenation. Am Rev Respir Dis 112:457, 1975.

Karliner JS, Coomaiaswamy R, Williams MH: Relationship between preoperative pulmonary function studies and prognosis of patients undergoing pneumonectomy for carcinoma of the lung. Dis Chest 54:32, 1968.

Kristersson S, Lindell SE, Svanberg L: Prediction of pulmonary function loss due to pneumonectomy using ^{133}Xe-radiospirometry. Chest 62:694, 1972.

Laros CD, Swierenga J: Temporary unilateral pulmonary artery occlusion in the preoperative evaluation of patients with bronchial carcinoma. Med Thorac 24:269, 1967.

Latimer RG, et al: Ventilatory patterns and pulmonary complications after upper abdominal surgery determined by preoperative and postoperative computerized spirometry and blood gas analysis. Am J Surg 122:622, 1971.

Liebman PR, et al: The mechanism of depressed cardiac output on positive end-expiratory pressure (PEEP). Surgery 83:594, 1978.

Lockwood P: The principles of predicting risk of post-thoracotomy function-related complications in bronchogenic carcinoma. Respiration 30:329, 1973.

Lucking SE, et al: High-frequency ventilation versus conventional ventilation in dogs with right ventricular dysfunction. Crit Care Med 14:798, 1986.

MacIntyre NR, et al: Jet ventilation at 100 breaths per minute in adult respiratory failure. Am Rev Respir Dis 134:897, 1986.

Malina JR, et al: Clinical evaluation of high-frequency positive pressure ventilation (HFPPV) in patients scheduled for open-chest surgery. Anesth Analg 60:324, 1981.

Marini J: New approaches to the ventilatory management of the adult respiratory distress syndrome. J Crit Care 7:256, 1992.

Marini JJ, Crooke PS, Truwit JD: Determinants and limits of pressure preset ventilation: A mathematical model of pressure control. J Appl Physiol 67:1081, 1989.

Marini JJ, Rodriguez M, Lamb V: The inspiratory workload of patient-initiated mechanical ventilation. Am Rev Respir Dis 134:902, 1986.

McAslan TC, et al: Influence of inhalation of 100% oxygen on intrapulmonary shunt in severely traumatized patients. J Trauma 13:811, 1973.

McCarthy PM, et al: The effectiveness of fibrin glue sealant for reducing experimental pulmonary air leak. Ann Thorac Surg 45:203, 1988.

Mittman C: Assessment of operative risk in thoracic surgery. Am Rev Respir Dis 84:197, 1961.

Miyoshi S, et al: Exercise tolerance tests in lung cancer patients: The relationship between exercise capacity and post-thoracotomy hospital mortality. Ann Thorac Surg 44:487, 1987.

Morganroth MJ, et al: Criteria for weaning from prolonged mechanical ventilation. Arch Intern Med 144:1012, 1984.

Olsen GN, et al: Pulmonary function evaluation of the lung resection candidate: A prospective study. Am Rev Respir Dis 111:379, 1975.

Panos A, Demajo W, Todd TR: High frequency jet ventilation in the management of bronchopleural fistula (BPF). Chest 89 (Suppl.):521S, 1986.

Paris F: Surgical fixation of traumatic flail chest. In Williams WG, Smith RE (eds): The Fourth Coventry Conference: Trauma of the Chest. Wright, 1977, p. 20.

Pesanti A, et al: Mean airway pressure vs positive end expiratory pressure during mechanical ventilation. Crit Care Med 13:34, 1985.

Pierson DJ, Horton CA, Bates PW: Persistent bronchopleural air leak during mechanical ventilation: A review of 39 cases. Chest 90:321, 1986.

Pontoppidan H, Geffin B, Lowenstein E: Medical progress: Acute respiratory failure in the adult. N Engl J Med 287:743, 1972.

Potkin RT, et al: Effect of positive end-expiratory pressure on right and left ventricular function in patients with the adult respiratory distress syndrome. Am Rev Respir Dis 135:307, 1987.

Powers SR, et al: Physiologic consequences of positive end-expiratory pressure (PEEP) ventilation. Ann Surg 178:265, 1973.

Prys-Roberts C, et al: Radiographically undetectable pulmonary collapse in the supine position. Lancet 2:399, 1967.

Quan SF, Falltrick RT, Schlobohm RM: Extubation from ambient or expiratory positive airway pressure in adults. Anesthesiology 55:53, 1981.

Qvist J, et al: Hemodynamic responses to mechanical ventilation with PEEP. Anesthesiology 42:45, 1975.

Rice TW, et al: The mini-membrane — a new method of extracorporeal membrane oxygenation (ECMO) for profound acute respiratory failure. Clin Invest Med 9:A8, 1986.

Rivara D, et al: Positional hypoxemia during artificial ventilation. Crit Care Med 12:436, 1984.

Robotham JL, Scharfe SM: Effects of positive and negative pressure ventilation on cardiac performance. Clin Chest Med 4:161, 1983.

Roussos C: Ventilatory failure and respiratory muscles. In Roussos C, Macklem PT (eds): The Thorax, Part B. New York: Marcel Dekker, 1985, p. 1253.

Sanchez de Leon R, et al: Positive end-expiratory pressure may decrease arterial oxygen tension in the presence of a collapsed lung region. Crit Care Med 13:392, 1985.

Scharfe S: Cardiovascular effects of positive pressure ventilation. J Crit Care 7:268, 1992.

Scharfe SM, Caldini P, Ingram Jr RH: Cardiovascular effects of increasing airway pressure in the dog. Am J Physiol 232:H35, 1977.

Scharfe SM, et al: Intrathoracic pressures and left ventricular configuration with respiratory manoeuvres. J Appl Physiol 66:481, 1989.

Shapiro BA, Walton JR: Ventilatory support of the postoperative patient. In Shields TW (ed): General Thoracic Surgery. Philadelphia: Lea & Febiger, 1982.

Shapiro BA, Cane RD, Harrison RA: Positive end-expiratory pressure therapy in adults with special reference to acute lung injury: A review of the literature and suggested clinical correlations. Crit Care Med 12:127, 1984.

Shapiro BA, Harrison RA, Walton JR: Clinical Application of Blood Gases. 2nd Ed. Chicago: Year Book, 1977.

Shapiro BA, et al: Clinical Application of Respiratory Care. 3rd Ed. Chicago: Year Book, 1985.

Siegel JH, et al: Quantification of asymmetric lung pathophysiology as a guide to the use of simultaneous independent lung ventilation in posttraumatic and septic adult respiratory distress syndrome. Ann Surg 202:425, 1985.

Solca M, et al: Multidisciplinary approach to extracorporeal respiratory assist for acute pulmonary failure. Int Surg 70:9, 1985.

Soutter I, Todd TRJ: Systemic candidiasis in a surgical intensive care unit. Can J Surg 29:1997, 1986.

Stauffer JL, Olson DE, Petty TL: Complications and consequences of endotracheal intubation and tracheostomy: A prospective study of 150 critically ill adult patients. Am J Med 70:65, 1981.

Stock MC, et al: Prevention of postoperative pulmonary complications with CPAP, incentive spirometry and conservative therapy. Chest 87:151, 1985.

Suter PM, Fairley HB, Isenberg MD: Optimum end-expiratory airway pressure in patients with acute pulmonary failure. N Engl J Med 292:284, 1975.

Takata M, Robotham JL: Ventricular external constraint by the lung and pericardium during positive end expiratory pressure. Am Rev Respir Dis 143:872, 1991.

Tisi GM: State of the art: Preoperative evaluation of pulmonary function. Am Rev Respir Dis 119:293, 1979.

Tittley JG, et al: Hemodynamic and myocardial metabolic consequences of PEEP. Chest 88:496, 1985.

Todd TRJ, Shamji FM: Pathophysiology of chest wall trauma. In Roussos C, Mackem PT (eds): The Thorax, Part B. New York: Marcel Dekker, 1985.

Todd TRJ, Baile EM, Hogg JC: Pulmonary artery wedge pressure in hemorrhagic shock. Am Rev Respir Dis 118:613, 1978.

Tracey KJ, et al: Anti-cachectin/TNF monoclonal antibodies prevent septic shock during lethal bacteremia. Nature 330:662, 1987.

Tsuno K, Prato PM, Kolobow T: Acute lung injury from mechanical ventilation at moderately high peak airway pressures. J Appl Physiol *69*:956, 1990.

Tyler DC: Positive end-expiratory pressure: A review. Crit Care Med *11*:300, 1983.

Viires N, et al: Regional blood flow distribution in dog during induced hypotension and low cardiac output. J Clin Invest *72*:935, 1983.

West JB, Dollery CT, Naimark A: Distribution of blood flow in isolated lung: Relation to vascular and alveolar pressures. J Appl Physiol *19*:713, 1964.

Wong T, Detsky A: Pre-operative cardiac risk assessment for patients having peripheral vascular surgery. Ann Intern Med *116*:743, 1992.

Zapal WM, et al: Extracorporeal membrane oxygenation in severe acute respiratory failure: A randomized prospective study. JAMA *242*:2193, 1979.

Zikria BA, et al: Alterations in ventilatory function and breathing patterns following surgical trauma. Ann Surg *179*:1, 1974.

READING REFERENCES

Egol A, Culpepper JA, Snyder JV: Barotrauma and hypotension resulting from jet ventilation in critically ill patients. Chest *88*:98, 1985.

Harwood SJ: Venovenous ECMO — a rapid percutaneous method for patients in severe respiratory distress. Transplant Implant Today *3*:44, 1986.

Lores ME, et al: Cardiovascular effects of positive end-expiratory pressure (PEEP) after pneumonectomy in dogs. Ann Thorac Surg *40*:464, 1985.

CHAPTER 26

PHYSICAL THERAPY FOR THE THORACIC SURGICAL PATIENT

Ralph Braunschweig

Post-thoracotomy pulmonary complications — PPC — occur frequently. O'Donohue (1985) reported an incidence of atelectasis near 30%. Post-thoracotomy pulmonary complications are presumed to be caused by decreased lung volume. The classic studies by Beecher (1933a, 1933b) showed that, after laparotomy, tidal volume, inspiratory and expiratory reserves, residual volume, and functional residual capacity — FRC — decreased. Many other authors have confirmed Beecher's findings, and Ali and associates (1974) demonstrated that the decrease in FRC after thoracic surgery is less than that after upper abdominal operations. Stock and associates (1985) suggest that shallow breathing without the normal sighing mechanism, residual anesthetic effects, pain, and assuming the recumbent position promote decreased lung volumes. In addition, narcotics given to relieve pain may depress ventilation. Shallow breaths fail to move bronchial secretions to the large airways for removal and may be another cause of PPC.

Prevention of PPC after thoracic surgery is a team responsibility, and the physical therapist is an important member of that team. The goals of chest physical therapy are to maintain or improve ventilation, reduce pain, reduce the work of breathing, mobilize and clear secretions from the bronchi and the trachea, and prevent atelectasis. Other important goals are to maintain mobility of the spine and shoulder girdle, prevent venous thrombosis by mobilization of the lower extremities, functional re-education, and improve cardiorespiratory exercise tolerance. The range of services provided by a physical therapy department for the thoracic surgical patient include preoperative patient evaluation, education and training, assistance with smoking cessation, deep breathing exercises, postural drainage of bronchial secretions, training in and assistance with forced expiration techniques, cough assistance, and patient mobilization with special attention to the shoulder girdle and the lower extremities. In addition, most departments offer chest wall percussion and vibration, the application of transcutaneous electrical nerve stimulation — TENS — to assist with control of pain, and a graduated fitness program to increase endurance in daily activities.

CRITICAL EVALUATION OF PHYSICAL THERAPY

The precise value of physical therapy to the patient is difficult to assess because other factors, such as the patient's preoperative pulmonary function, the surgeon's technique, the anesthetic management, and the intensity of nursing and surgical postoperative care, make simultaneous contributions toward the reduction in morbidity and mortality rates after a thoracic surgical procedure. Few data exist concerning the influence of physical therapy on the incidence of postoperative pulmonary complications following thoracic operations. Thoren (1954) documented a reduction in the incidence of postoperative pulmonary complications following upper abdominal operations from 42 to 12% when therapy included preoperative training; diaphragmatic, deep breathing; and coughing exercises with postural drainage. Wiklander and Norlin (1957) compared a group of patients receiving physical therapy with a control group. The incidence of moderate and severe collapse was cut in half in the treated group. Stein and Cassara (1970) reviewed the incidence of postoperative pulmonary complications in patients with normal and abnormal pulmonary function tests. They confirmed the low incidence of such complications in the group defined as "low risk." Among the "high risk" surgical patients, postoperative pulmonary complications developed in 5 of 23 — 22% — patients receiving physical therapy and 15 of 25 — 60% — controls, suggesting the effectiveness of the treatment.

Physical therapy can also be administered to patients receiving mechanical assistance to ventilation. Winning and associates (1975, 1977) reported a lower mean alveolar pressure and improved oxygenation after treatment, especially among patients with increased secretions. Mackenzie and associates (1980) demonstrated a significant increase in total lung/thorax compliance after postural drainage enhanced by percussion and vibration in mechanically ventilated patients. Ciesla and colleagues (1981) found dramatic improvement in oxygenation after bronchial drainage with percussion and vibration in patients with hypotension who were receiving mechanical ventilation with high levels of PEEP. In contrast, a decrease in the mean partial pressure of arterial oxygen during and immediately after chest physical therapy was found in studies by Newton and Stephenson (1978), Gormezano and Branthwaite (1972a, 1972b), and Holloway and co-workers (1966, 1969). This decrease was seen most often in critically ill patients or in patients after cardiac surgery with cardiovascular instability.

Because advanced age is an additional risk factor for postoperative pulmonary complications, Castillo and Haas (1985) studied, in patients older than age 65 years, the effects of pre- and postoperative chest physical therapy treatment, including bronchodilation followed by modified postural drainage, percussion and vibration, breathing exercises, and incentive spirometry. They confirmed work by Thoren (1954), Stein and Cassara (1970), and others, who found that initiating chest physical therapy before patients are in pain, highly anxious, and dulled by medication helps them learn the procedures quickly and effectively, and that post-thoracotomy atelectasis was reduced from 59% to zero. The incidence of pneumonia was not significantly affected. In the preoperative period, patients should be encouraged to stop smoking, although no hard data exist on the required time of smoking cessation for adequate reduction in sputum production and improved mucociliary function.

Other investigators have examined the benefits of individual components of chest physical therapy. The effects of deep breathing on arterial oxygenation were studied by Ward and associates (1966) with coaching by a physical therapist with and without a 5-second hold and by Hedstrand and co-workers (1978) using the incentive spirometer and two other deep-breathing devices. They found that all produced about the same improvement in oxygenation. Grimby (1974) showed that breathing exercises given to the patient postoperatively improve chest wall mobility. Vraciu and Vraciu (1977) studied the effect of adding breathing exercises taught by physical therapists to a regimen of incentive spirometry, ultrasonic nebulization, and routine instruction in deep breathing and coughing by nurses in postoperative cardiothoracic surgical patients. Although no significant difference was noted in the incidence of postoperative pulmonary complications in the low risk groups, the high risk experimental group had an incidence of only 8% compared with 46% in the "routine" treatment group.

Pain control is an essential component of all programs reducing PPC. Decline in pulmonary function following thoracotomy appears to be maximal after about 24 hours, but may persist for 5 days or more, depending on the extent of rib retraction. A major component of postoperative pain is a result of straining of the ligaments of the costovertebral and costotransverse joints as well as the posterior spinal muscles. In addition, Katz and co-workers (1992) showed that surgical incision and other noxious perioperative events may induce prolonged changes in central neural function that later contribute to postoperative pain. The mechanism has been elucidated further by Woolf (1991), Yamamoto (1992) and Abram (1993). They suggest that patients who receive pre-emptive analgesia such as alpha-2-adrenergic antagonists or pain control by epidural narcotics or intercostal nerve block before incision have less pain than those whose pain control is initiated only after the operation. At this time, it appears that optimal management should include pre-emptive analgesia — either intercostal nerve block or epidural analgesia — maintained through the first few days postoperatively. This effort will also increase effective patient mobility and the ability to deep breathe, and maintain FRC.

The effect of bronchoscopy in removing secretions from the airway and reducing atelectasis was summarized by Marini (1984). Mucus plugs of the central airways that can be visualized with the fiberoptic bronchoscope are rare to nonexistent in patients who are well hydrated and whose inspired gases during and after anesthesia are nearly saturated with humidity at body temperature. Bronchoscopy allows the instillation of 0.25% saline solution and extraction of central airway secretions; however, even when performed with supplemental ventilation through an endotracheal tube, it often produces bronchospasm, coughing, and arterial desaturation. In general, secretion retention should be treated with chest physical therapy of sufficient frequency and duration to mobilize the secretions, and bronchoscopy should be reserved for patients with persistent radiologic findings of atelectasis after 12 to 16 hours of adequate physical therapy.

DEFINING THE TREATMENT PLAN

By consulting the physical therapy department several days before the planned procedure, the surgeon can obtain maximum benefit for patients through preoperative assessment and training. The consultation request should contain the following information: the date and extent of the planned procedure, medical conditions that influence therapy, specific instructions that the surgeon may have given the patient that need to be reinforced by the therapist, e.g., smoking cessation, and the goals the surgeon seeks to achieve. To permit proper assessment, the medical record should contain a history of response to previous anesthesia and surgery, exercise tolerance, results of pulmonary function tests, chest radiographs, and arterial blood gases. If metastatic lesions are suspected, radiographs or bone scans of other areas of the body should also be available. The clinical evaluation by the physical therapist allows development of rapport between the patient and the therapist, formulation of a plan specific for that patient's condition, determination and treatment effectiveness, and preoperative patient education. After completing the assessment, the physical therapist enters the findings in the patient record and contacts the surgeon to discuss the plan for pre- and postoperative physical therapy, as well as the criteria for monitoring treatment effectiveness. At this point, the therapist may write the specific orders to be countersigned by the surgeon.

TREATMENT

Postural Drainage

Objectives

The aim of postural drainage is to use change of position and gravity to assist in mobilizing retained secretions and directing them toward the main bronchi and carina from which they may be coughed up or removed by suctioning. Knowledge of the anatomic ramifications and topographic relationships of the tracheobronchial tree (see Chapters 6 and 11) is mandatory to understand the appropriate positions for drainage of the various segments of the lung.

Technique

All the basal segments of the patient's lower lobes drain when the foot of the bed is raised; usually 18 inches is all that is required. Anterior basal segments drain when the patient is in the dorsal head-down position (Fig. 26–1). Lateral basal segments drain when the patient is in the lateral head-down position (Fig. 26–2). Posterior basal segments drain when the patient is lying prone with the head down (Fig. 26–3).

The medial basal segment of the right lower lobe drains when the patient is in the same position as that used for draining the lateral basal segment on the opposite side. The right middle lobe and lingula drain with the body rotated 45° about its long axis with the foot of the bed raised 18 inches. The lingula drains when

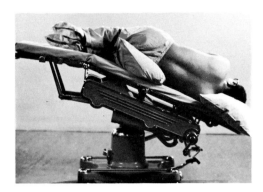

Fig. 26–2. Position for draining the lateral segments of the left lower lobe.

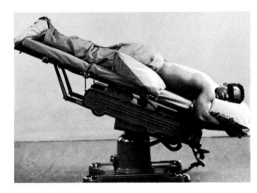

Fig. 26–3. Position for draining the posterior segments of both lower lobes.

the patient's left side is uppermost and the right middle lobe drains when the right side is uppermost. A pillow beneath one shoulder and hip helps hold the patient in position (Figs. 26–4, 26–5).

The superior segments of the lower lobes drain when the bed is horizontal and the patient is prone (Fig. 26–6). The anterior segments of both upper lobes drain when the patient lies supine with the bed horizontal (Fig. 26–7). To drain the left anterior segment, it is advantageous to raise the foot of the bed and turn the patient with slight rotation in the long axis of the body, because when the anterior segment has drained as far

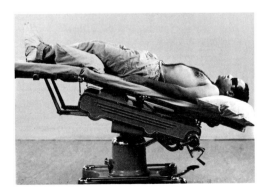

Fig. 26–1. Position for draining the anterior segments of both lower lobes.

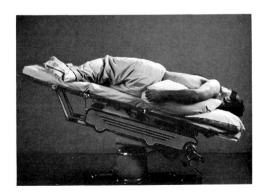

Fig. 26–4. Position for draining the lingula.

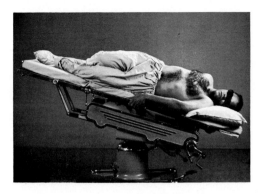

Fig. 26–5. Position for draining the middle lobe.

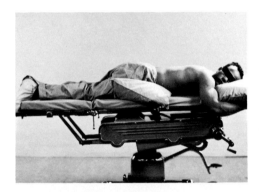

Fig. 26–6. Position for draining the superior segments of both lower lobes.

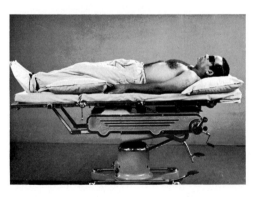

Fig. 26–7. Position for draining the anterior segments of both upper lobes.

is used for support to prevent the patient from falling forward (Fig. 26–9). The left apical-posterior segment (Fig. 26–10) drains with the patient in the opposite position, but with the head of the bed raised so that the shoulder is elevated 14 inches. The right arm lies behind the body (Fig. 26–11).

Mechanical Stimulation of the Chest Wall

Objectives

After the patient assumes the appropriate postural drainage position, mechanical stimulation of the chest

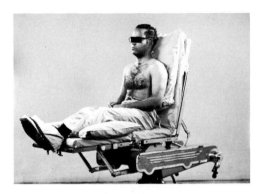

Fig. 26–8. Position for draining the right apical segment.

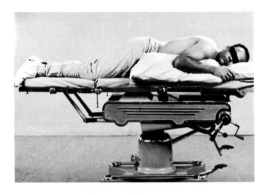

Fig. 26–9. Position for draining the posterior segment of the right upper lobe.

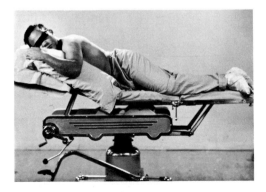

Fig. 26–10. Position for draining the apical posterior segment of the left upper lobe (view from front).

as the distal end of the left main stem bronchus, the secretions still must traverse 5 cm of this bronchus to reach the carina. If reflexes are intact, the patient will cough when secretions reach the distal end of the main stem bronchus, so raising the foot of the bed and turning the patient as described are rarely needed. On the right side, the right main stem bronchus traverses only a short distance to the carina and the basic position thus needs no modification. The right apical segment drains while the patient is sitting (Fig. 26–8). The posterior segment of the right upper lobe drains with the patient turned 45° toward the prone position with the bed horizontal. The patient's left arm is placed behind the body and the upper hip is flexed with the knee bent. A pillow

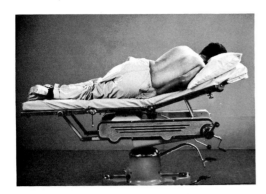

Fig. 26–11. Position for draining the apical-posterior segment of the left upper lobe (view from behind).

wall by percussion and vibration can help move secretions from the periphery toward the collecting segmental bronchi. Mackenzie and associates (1980) showed, in mechanically ventilated patients, that even in the absence of increased sputum production, atelectatic areas of the lung can be reinflated and total lung/thorax compliance can be increased following percussion and vibration.

Techniques

The physical therapist places the patient in the appropriate postural drainage position and delivers rhythmical "clapping" strokes with cupped hands to the chest wall over the affected area of the lung. The air cushion between the cupped hand and the chest wall generates the typical hollow sound, transmits the energy to the underlying lung, and helps mobilize secretions. The strokes are performed rapidly during inspiration and expiration and should not be painful to the patient. After sufficient treatment time — 3 to 5 minutes — over a given area, the physical therapist compresses the chest with vibratory movements during each expiration for several breaths and then attempts to make the patient cough or suctions the secretions derived from that area, before proceeding to the next.

Precautions

Before beginning the treatment, the therapist must ensure that ventilator tubing, endotracheal tubes, chest tubes, and other drains are secure and allow for movement without becoming dislodged. Unstable rib or thoracic spine fractures, or both, and coagulation defects, as well as increased intracranial pressure and lung abscess, are contraindications to mechanical stimulation, and the anticipated benefit must be weighed carefully against the risk of aggravating the underlying condition. Proper hand position is essential to the success of percussion and vibration. The patient's skin should be observed for evidence of erythema, soft tissue trauma, and petechiae.

Huffing and Coughing

Objectives

The rapid, forceful expulsion of air from the lungs helps remove secretions from the large airways. In coughing, the patient closes his glottis and builds up intrathoracic pressure before suddenly releasing the air. In huffing, air is expelled without closure of the glottis. Huffing is less likely to induce bronchospasm and may increase intracranial pressure less than repetitive coughing. Although huffing has not been studied in the postoperative patient, it seems to be almost as effective as coughing and it is less painful.

Technique

Adequate analgesia should be established before inducing a cough, and the physical therapist should support the patient's chest, especially in the area of the incision. The patient should be taught to support his or her own chest to allow effective coughing when the nurse or therapist is not at the bedside. The patient is instructed to take a deep breath, close the glottis, contract the muscles of expiration, and suddenly open the glottis to produce a cough. If the trachea is intubated, the patient will be unable to close the glottis, but rapid, forceful exhalation will help move secretions centrally so they can be removed by suctioning.

Precautions

Secretions must be kept thin and liquid; this can be done best by careful attention to the patient's hydration, as well as by heated humidification of inspired gases, especially for the patient with an artificial airway. Avoid repetitive coughing, as it may induce bronchospasm. If the patient cannot take an adequate breath, manual inflation with a bag-valve mask or mechanical ventilation can be used.

Suctioning

Objectives

The two specific levels of suctioning are oropharyngeal, for patients who are unable to cough effectively to expectorate secretions, and tracheobronchial, to remove secretions from the larger airways of patients who are intubated. Some practitioners believe that, even in the absence of an artificial airway, passing a catheter into the trachea is a valuable technique, provided it is done carefully. Others believe it should not be used because of the risks of laryngeal irritation, laryngospasm, and vagal stimulation. In any case, the only indication for suctioning is the presence of secretions in the airway.

Technique

Suctioning of secretions from the airway requires sterile technique and supplemental oxygen. After preoxygenating the patient by manually assisted ventilation with 100% oxygen, a sterile suction catheter is picked up with a sterile, gloved hand and attached to a vacuum source. The catheter is advanced, without applying suction, until the tip is in proper position at the carina. Suction is then applied by intermittently occluding the vent with a finger, and the catheter is withdrawn slowly with a rotating motion.

Precautions

Sterile technique must be used to reduce the risk of infection. The suction catheter should be less than half the diameter of the artificial airway to allow enough space around the catheter for air to enter and to avoid applying suction to the lung itself. Hypoxemia can be prevented by preoxygenation, avoiding suction while advancing the catheter, limiting the force of suction to less than 120 mm Hg, limiting the duration of the total suctioning process to 20 seconds, and re-expanding the lung with 100% oxygen after each procedure. For patients who become bradycardic during properly performed suctioning, a fiberoptic swivel adapter can be used to ventilate with supplemental oxygen and maintain PEEP during suctioning. During fiberoptic bronchoscopy, excessive use of the suction port to clear secretions from the tip can lead to hypoxemia. Monitoring of blood pressure and the electrocardiogram are recommended because hypotension and cardiac dysrhythmias may occur during or shortly after suctioning. They are usually caused by hypoxemia, hypercarbia, or vagal stimulation.

Breathing Exercises and Patient Mobilization

Objectives

Breathing exercises taught to patients in the preoperative period can reduce the effects of altered breathing patterns after thoracotomy and can help to obtain full expansion of the chest wall during spontaneous breathing. This ability is essential to help restore lung function and to prevent subsequent chest deformity. In addition, early upper and lower extremity exercises and early ambulation decrease the incidence of pulmonary embolism, and range-of-motion exercises and posture correction may prevent musculoskeletal dysfunction, especially frozen shoulder, following thoracotomy. Before discharge from the hospital, the patient should learn a program of graded exercises to regain a cardiorespiratory reserve.

Techniques

Relaxation Exercises. The patient is made comfortable in the supine position with pillows supporting the head, arms, and knees, with the neck and hips slightly flexed. The arms should be at the patient's sides with the palms down and the thumbs touching the body. The therapist demonstrates the difference between contraction and relaxation of individual muscles starting from the hand and working upward to the shoulders and neck. The patient should repeat these exercises many times.

Localized Breathing Exercises. Pressure is applied over the area resisting active muscular contraction to mobilize natural respiratory forces. This step helps to fix the attention of the patient to the area, suggests the direction of effort, and tends to decrease activity in previously overworked parts of the chest. Practice before surgery improves the actions of the inspiratory muscles and helps the therapist determine precisely what the patient can do, so that after surgery, when certain parts of the chest move poorly, it is easy to recognize where assistance is needed before additional function is lost. Restoration of the proper movement is begun on one side before it is applied bilaterally.

The palms of the hands are used to apply pressure on all areas except over the upper lobes, where the fingers are used as well as the palms. The pressure should be firm but not so excessive as to make the patient give up and cause movement to begin elsewhere in the chest wall. The patient should think in terms of expanding against pressure rather than inspiration. The pressure is reduced only when full inspiration has been attained. During exhalation, the hands of the therapist are relaxed, but just before inspiration, the ribs are pressed slightly inward. The therapist then uses the patient's hands to press against the active chest movements. These exercises are given with the patient lying well supported by pillows in the same position as for relaxation. Later, they can be performed while either sitting or standing. Diaphragmatic or lateral basal expansion is usually begun first, then posterior basal expansion, and finally apical pectoral expansion.

Lateral Basal Expansion. The palm of one hand is placed in the midaxillary line over the lower ribs. Pressure is applied at the end of exhalation and continues through inspiration. The patient is told to expand the ribs in the direction of the hand on that side. Pressure is relaxed at the end of inspiration. The other side of the chest should be relaxed. When expansion has increased on one side, pressure is then applied to both sides of the chest.

Upper Lateral Expansion. The technique for upper lateral expansion is the same as that for lateral basal expansion except that the hands are placed immediately below the axilla.

Apical Pectoral Expansion. For apical pectoral expansion, pressure is applied with the fingertips above the clavicles and the hands on the pectoral muscles below the clavicles. The patient expands the chest forward and upward against the pressure of the therapist's hands.

Diaphragmatic Breathing Exercises. Diaphragmatic breathing is an important exercise for all thoracic surgical patients, because the diaphragm is the most powerful muscle of ventilation. It affects the expansion of the bases of the lungs, which are prone to infection postoperatively. Of several variations of diaphragmatic exercises known for specific purposes, the one described here is adapted best for patients undergoing thoracic surgery.

The patient lies with knees bent and supported on pillows so that the hips are slightly flexed. The therapist's hands rest lightly on the anterior rib cage so the therapist is aware of anterolateral movement. During expiration, the patient contracts the abdominal muscles. These are then relaxed for inspiration. Epigastric compression may be applied at the beginning of inspiration. The patient attempts to prolong each exhalation for periods of up to 15 seconds without losing control of the next inspiration. After thoracic surgical procedures, the patient may breathe predominantly with the apices of the lungs. This should be pointed out to the patient and the therapist should demonstrate how the upper parts relax when the abdominal muscles are used during exhalation.

MODIFICATION IN PHYSICAL THERAPY TECHNIQUES FOR SPECIFIC THORACIC OPERATIONS

Empyema

Localized breathing exercises should not be used for patients in the acute stage of empyema. They may be used later to help the lung expand.

Pneumonectomy

Localized and diaphragmatic breathing exercises should be performed mainly on the normal side. Postural drainage is contraindicated postoperatively if the pericardium has been opened. These patients should be taught to "huff." Arm movements should be encouraged and the patients should be ambulatory within 24 hours of the operation.

Lobectomy or Thoracotomy

In lobectomy or thoracotomy, localized breathing exercises should be performed, particularly on the side of operation. When bronchiectasis is present, diaphragmatic breathing exercises, coughing, and postural drainage with percussion and vibration are especially valuable. Percussion should not be used when hemoptysis is present.

Decortication

After decortication, lung expansion should be encouraged by having the patient perform the localized breathing exercises that were practiced preoperatively. After the operation, these exercises should be performed as soon as the patient is able to cooperate. Percussion and vibration are contraindicated in the early postoperative period.

TRANSCUTANEOUS ELECTRICAL NERVE STIMULATION

Objectives

Transcutaneous electrical nerve stimulation — TENS — is the application of an electric current to peripheral nerves by externally applied electrodes to produce analgesia without respiratory depression or cardiovascular side effects. Warfield and associates (1985) delivered TENS by peri-incisional electrodes in the immediate postoperative period and demonstrated shorter recovery room stays and better tolerance of chest physical therapy for bronchial hygiene. Using similar techniques, Navarathnam and co-workers (1984) showed significant improvement in forced vital capacity among the patients receiving TENS, whereas Rooney and associates (1983) also confirmed decreased narcotic requirements in a similar group of patients following thoracotomy. Pain control with TENS also allows the patient to cooperate more fully with the therapist during deep breathing, coughing, and range-of-motion exercises.

Techniques

Sterile electrodes are applied in the operating room to the skin adjacent to the incision before the dressing is applied, and connecting cables are attached and secured. When the patient regains consciousness, the cables are attached to the stimulator and the pulse width, frequency, and amplitude are adjusted for maximum patient comfort.

Precautions

Although no clear contraindications to TENS have been established, use caution in applying electrical stimuli to patients who depend on a demand cardiac pacemaker. The pulse and electrocardiogram should be monitored when initiating treatment to determine if the output of the pacemaker is inhibited by the TENS unit.

REFERENCES

Abram SE: Morphine, but not inhalation anesthesia, blocks post injury facilitation: The role of preemptive suppression of afferent transmission. Submitted for publication.

Ali J, et al: Consequences of postoperative alteration in respiratory mechanics. Am J Surg 128:376, 1974.

Bartlett R, et al: Respiratory maneuvers to prevent postoperative pulmonary complications: A critical review. JAMA 224:7, 1973.

Beecher HK: The measured effect of laparotomy on respiration. J Clin Invest 12:639, 1933a.

Beecher HK: Effect of laparotomy on lung volume: Demonstration of a new type of pulmonary collapse. J Clin Invest 12:651, 1933b.

Castillo R, Haas A: Chest physical therapy: Comparative efficacy of preoperative and postoperative in the elderly. Arch Phys Med Rehabil 66:376, 1985.

Ciesla N, et al: Chest physical therapy to the patient with multiple trauma: Two case studies. Phys Ther 61:202, 1981.

de la Rocha AG, Chambers K: Pain amelioration after thoracotomy: A prospective, randomized study. Ann Thorac Surg 37:239, 1984.

Gormezano J, Branthwaite MA: Pulmonary physiotherapy with assisted ventilation. Anaesthesia 27:249, 1972a.

Gormezano J, Branthwaite MA: Effects of physiotherapy during intermittent positive pressure ventilation. Anaesthesia 27:258, 1972b.

Grimby G: Aspects of lung expansion in relation to pulmonary physiotherapy. Am Rev Respir Dis 110:145, 1974.

Hedstrand U, et al: Effects of respiratory physiotherapy of arterial oxygen tension. Acta Anaesthesiol Scand 22:349, 1978.

Holloway R, et al: The effect of chest physiotherapy on the arterial oxygenation of neonates during treatment of tetanus by intermittent positive-pressure respiration. S Afr Med J 40:445, 1966.

Holloway R, et al: Effect of chest physiotherapy on blood gases of neonates treated by intermittent positive pressure respiration. Thorax 24:421, 1969.

Katz J, et al: Preemptive analgesia. Clinical evidence of neuroplasticity contributing to postoperative pain. Anesthesiology 77:76, 1992.

Mackenzie CF, et al: Changes in total lung/thorax compliance following chest physiotherapy. Anesth Analg 59:207, 1980.

Marini JJ, et al: Acute lobar atelectasis: A prospective comparison of fiberoptic bronchoscopy and respiratory therapy. Am Rev Respir Dis 54:542, 1979.

Marini JJ: Postoperative atelectasis: Pathophysiology, clinical importance, and principles of management. Respir Care 29:516, 1984.

Navarathnam RG, et al: Evaluation of the transcutaneous electrical nerve stimulator for postoperative analgesia following cardiac surgery. Anaesth Intensive Care 12:345, 1984.

Newton DA, Stephenson A: Effect of physiotherapy on pulmonary functions: A laboratory study. Lancet 2:228, 1978.

O'Donohue Jr. W: National survey of the usage of lung expansion modalities for the prevention and treatment of postoperative atelectasis following abdominal and thoracic surgery. Chest 87:76, 1985.

Rooney SM, et al: Effect of transcutaneous nerve stimulation on postoperative pain after thoracotomy. Anesth Analg 62:1010, 1983.

Stein M, Cassara EL: Preoperative pulmonary evaluation and therapy for surgery patients. JAMA 211:787, 1970.

Stock M, et al: Prevention of postoperative pulmonary complications with CPAP, incentive spirometry, and conservative therapy. Chest 87:151, 1985.

Thoren L: Postoperative pulmonary complications: Observations on their prevention by means of physiotherapy. Acta Chir Scand 107:193, 1954.

Vraciu JK, Vraciu RA: Effectiveness of breathing exercises in preventing pulmonary complications following open heart surgery. Phys Ther 57:1367, 1977.

Ward RH, et al: An evaluation of postoperative respiratory maneuvers. Surg Gynecol Obstet 123:51, 1966.

Warfield CA, et al: The effect of transcutaneous electrical nerve stimulation on pain after thoracotomy. Ann Thorac Surg 39:462, 1985.

Wiklander O, Norlin U: Effect of physiotherapy on postoperative pulmonary complications: A clinical and roentgenographic study of 200 cases. Acta Chir Scand 112:246, 1957.

Winning TJ, et al: A simple clinical method of quantitating the effects of chest physiotherapy in mechanically ventilated patients. Anaesth Intensive Care 3:237, 1975.

Winning TJ, et al: Bronchodilators and physiotherapy during longterm mechanical ventilation of the lungs. Anaesth Intensive Care 5:48, 1977.

Woolf CJ: The induction and maintenance of central sensitization is dependent on N-methyl-b-aspartic acid receptor activation; Implications for the treatment of post injury pain hypersensitivity states. Pain 44:293, 1991.

Yamamoto T: Comparison of the antinociceptive effects of pre- and post-treatment with intrathecal morphine and MK 801, and NMDA antagonist, on the formalin test in the rat. Anesthesiology 77:757, 1992.

READING REFERENCES

Frownfelter DL: Chest Physical Therapy and Pulmonary Rehabilitation. An Interdisciplinary Approach. 2nd Ed. Chicago: Year Book, 1987.

Hough A: Physiotherapy in Respiratory Care. A Problem-Solving Approach. San Diego: Singular Publishing, 1991.

Mackenzie CF, et al (ed): Chest Physiotherapy in the Intensive Care Unit. Baltimore: Williams & Wilkins, 1981.

Pulmonary and Tracheal Resections

CHAPTER 27

THORACIC INCISIONS

Willard A. Fry

The most popular incision for open general thoracic surgical procedures is the lateral thoracotomy, sometimes also called the axillary thoracotomy. For years, the posterolateral thoracotomy was considered the incision of choice for most operations involving the lung and esophagus. With increased use of double-lumen endotracheal tubes and refinement of instrumentation, particularly the stapling devices, however, the traditional posterolateral incision is reserved for difficult operations in which wide exposure is mandatory. Likewise, interest in using median sternotomy for operations on the lung has waned, although median sternotomy is still considered the operation of choice for most anterior mediastinal lesions. With increasing use of video-assisted thoracic surgical procedures — VATS, small accessory incisions, as suggested by Lewis and colleagues (1992), are becoming more popular (see Chapter 37).

When the patient is positioned for thoracotomy, especially in the lateral decubitus position, pad pressure points about the elbows with foam pads, place an axillary roll under the dependent axilla — to take pressure off of the brachial plexus, and place one or two pillows between the legs. Consider measures to discourage venous thrombosis in the lower extremities, such as tight elastic hose and a sequential compression device. These measures, if used, should be in effect at the beginning of the operation. Salzman (1985) and Scurr (1987) suggested that external pneumatic compression with sequential compression sleeves connected to a sequential compression device is the safest and most cost-effective prophylaxis against venous thromboembolic disease.

The use of prophylactically antibiotics for general thoracic surgical procedures remains controversial. Cameron (1981) and Ilves (1981) and their associates reported conflicting results in controlled trials. In general, a first or second generation cephalosporin is used, and the main emphasis is on prophylaxis of the wound from *Staphylococcus aureus* infections. On the basis of the work of Olak and associates (1991), I cannot

recommend giving more than a single intravenous dose before making the skin incision. This recommendation is supported by Meakins (1993) writing on behalf of the American College of Surgeons.

POSTEROLATERAL THORACOTOMY

The posterolateral thoracotomy incision is made with the patient in the lateral decubitus position, with proper padding to the elbows, knees, and dependent axilla. Various maneuvers are available to hold the patient in an appropriate lateral position, including placing a sandbag under the operating table mattress, rolled sheets front and back, and bean bags. Two straps of 2-inch adhesive tape are used as well. The dependent arm is flexed at the elbow. The superior arm can be flexed similarly and appropriately padded — obtaining the so-called "praying position," or it can be extended on a padded Mayo stand (Fig. 27–1A).

Only hairy portions of the skin that will be directly in the line of the incision or the chest tubes or their taping should be shaved, and if shaving is necessary, it should be done immediately prior to the operation, as recommended by Cruse and Foord (1973). My colleagues and I often find shaving is not necessary at all.

It is helpful to outline the proposed incision with a felt-tipped marking pen. Most pulmonary operations are best performed through a fifth interspace incision.

As shown in Figure 27–1B, the incision starts in front of the anterior axillary line, curves 4 cm under the tip of the scapula, and then takes a vertical direction between the posterior midline over the vertebral column and the medial edge of the scapula. It is usually not necessary to go farther than the level of the spine of the scapula.

The electrosurgical unit is used for hemostasis and for musculofascial dissection. It is not recommended for incisions in the skin or subcutaneous tissues, based on the extensive wound healing studies of Cruse and Foord (1973). Glover and associates (1978) emphasized that use of the cutting current destroys less tissue than constant

381

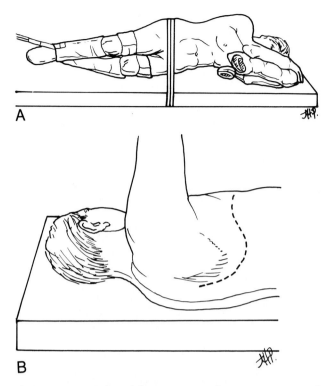

Fig. 27–1. Posterolateral thoracotomy. *A,* The patient is positioned in "praying position" with pillows between the knees and padding under the elbows. Wide adhesive tape secures the position. Note the axillary roll and the sequential compression device. *B,* The incision curves in an "S-shape" passing 4 cm under the tip of the scapula over in the fifth interspace anterior.

use of the coagulation current. On the other hand, my colleagues and I use the electrosurgical unit more frequently when operating on patients who are HIV or hepatitis positive. The lower portion of the trapezius muscle is divided, and, in the same plane more anteriorly, the latissimus dorsi muscle is also divided. Next, the lower portion of the rhomboid muscle, if the thoracotomy is high, and the continuous plane with the serratus anterior muscle are divided.

The desired interspace is located by placing a large right-angle retractor beneath the scapula and passing the hand up paraspinally. Sometimes, the first rib is obscured to easy palpation, but attachments of the serratus posterior superior muscle to the second rib serve as an added guide.

Rib section at the costovertebral angle level is recommended for patients over 40 years of age to decrease the incidence of rib fracture (Fig. 27–2). Generally, small portions of the superior and inferior rib are excised subperiosteally to prevent the cut edges from overriding in the postoperative period. Although some recommend section over clips or ligatures of the neurovascular bundle, it is not necessary. It is unusual to resect a long segment of rib for a routine thoracotomy, although that was usually done in the past. For repeat thoracotomies, however, it is often advisable to

resect a long rib segment subperiosteally and to approach the pleural space through the bed of the resected rib, as extensive adhesions are often encountered on such reoperations, and the wider entry into the pleural space through the bed of a resected rib can be beneficial (Fig. 27–3).

The intercostal muscle incision down to the parietal pleura is made carefully in the lower portion of the interspace to avoid injury to the neurovascular bundle. The surgeon pauses to see if the lung moves freely under the pleura. If it does move freely, then few adhesions in the area of the interspace can be expected. If the lung does not move freely, the surgeon must anticipate a significant number of adhesions and the need to divide them with care, particularly when the operation is a repeat thoracotomy. A large Finochietto-type rib spreader is inserted with attention to place the large superior blade behind the scapula. If desired, a smaller, Tuffier-type rib spreader can be placed more anteriorly to ensure a wide surgical field. The rib spreader is opened slowly and in stages to minimize the chance for rib fracture.

Closure of the incision is begun by inserting one or two chest tubes through a separate stab incision inferior to the skin incision in the anterior and midaxillary lines. The tract for the tube is tunneled for several centimeters to direct the tube — low and posterior for the back tube to drain fluid and high and anterior for the front tube to remove air. Tunneling the tube tract also reduces the chance for a pleurocutaneous fistula in the event that the tubes must remain in place for a long time, as in the case of a prolonged postoperative air leak. Generally, two tubes are used if a significant resection has been performed, as the operator can expect both air and fluid accumulation. In selected cases, such as a local excision of a lung lesion or an esophageal operation in which the lung has not been cut, a single tube suffices. The size of the chest tube to be used depends on the preference of the operating surgeon, the size of the patient, and the nature of the particular operation. In general, it is not necessary to use a posterior tube larger than 32F or an anterior tube larger than 28F. Tubes smaller than 24F tend to kink. Plastic tubes are preferred over rubber, as they are less likely to clot. The chest tubes should be secured, when inserted, with a heavy suture; our preference is for No. 1 nylon, to prevent slippage. The tubes are attached to a Y-tube connector, which is in turn affixed to an appropriate chest drainage system.

My colleagues and I (1990) prefer continuous epidural analgesia — CEA — for our posterolateral and axillary thoracotomy patients. In the event that CEA is not feasible, we perform an intercostal nerve block with a long-acting local anesthetic such as 0.5% bupivacaine with epinephrine at the time of chest wall closure. Gallo and colleagues (1983) emphasized that an intercostal vascular injection must be avoided, as the intravascular injection of such compounds can have dire cardiovascular consequences. Generally, we block from the

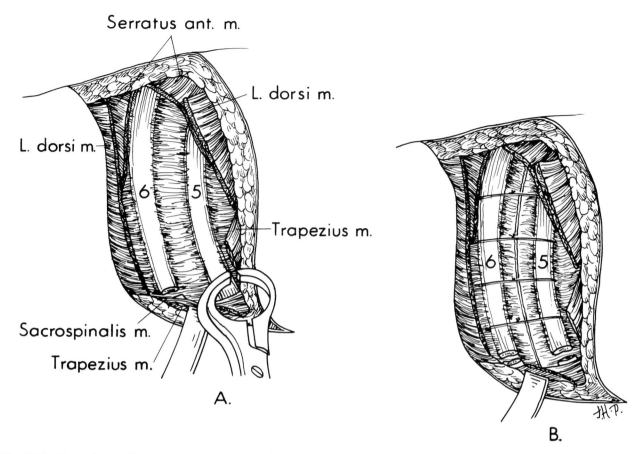

Fig. 27–2. Posterolateral thoracotomy. *A,* One or two ribs are sectioned at the costovertebral angle. A small portion of bone is removed to prevent overriding of the fragments at the time of closure. *B,* Four or more sutures of heavy absorbable suture are placed as pericostal sutures. The interspace distance is maintained. It is not necessary to suture the divided intercostal muscles except when a tight seal is desired for pneumonectomy.

second to the seventh interspace. Inject at least 8 cm off the midline to avoid a subdural injection that would produce spinal anesthesia.

Pericostal sutures, usually four, of heavy absorbable material such as No. 2 polyglycolic acid are then placed. Each of the two musculofascial planes is closed with running suture of a similar material, usually size 1 or 0, the subcutaneous tissues with a size 2-0 running suture of the same material and the skin with the surgeon's preferred material.

The main advantage of the posterolateral thoracotomy is the superb exposure for most general thoracic procedures. The main disadvantages are the time expended because of the length of the incision and the amount of muscle and soft tissue transected.

AXILLARY THORACOTOMY

The axillary thoracotomy was originally developed for operations on the upper thoracic sympathetic nerve system. It was modified for first rib resection for thoracic outlet syndromes. Jensik (1993) used it preferentially for many years for pulmonary resections. Siegel and Steiger

(1982) described how it has been rediscovered for more extensive general thoracic surgical procedures. Mitchell (1990) and Ponn and associates (1992) report several large series of axillary or lateral incisions with excellent results, although the largest series with which I am familiar comes from Noirclerc's group (1973). Some groups refer to it as a lateral thoracotomy to avoid confusion with small, high axillary incisions for first rib resections or apical bleb resections. Other groups refer to it as a "mini-thoracotomy" or "muscle-sparing thoracotomy," but such nonspecific terminology should be discouraged. I prefer this incision for uncomplicated and straightforward pulmonary operations. It is not recommended for bulky tumors, sleeve resections, radical pneumonectomies, or repeat thoracotomies. This incision is particularly useful when a double-lumen endotracheal tube can be used, as the controlled atelectasis combined with the ability of the anesthesiologist to elevate the mediastinum toward the operative field provides favorable operating conditions. The chief advantages are the speed of opening and closing, the reduced blood loss from minimal muscle transection, and the resulting reduced postoperative discomfort. As

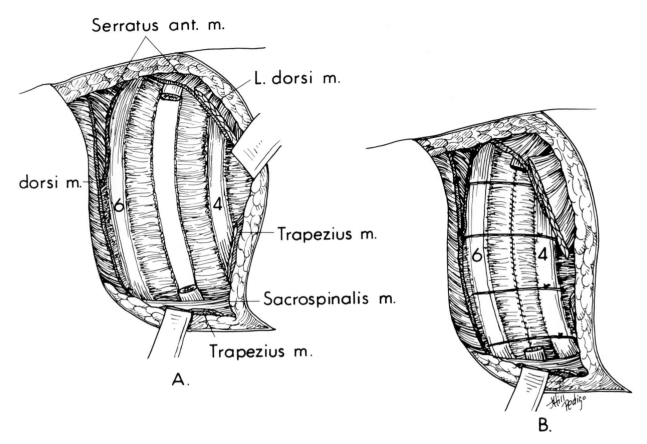

Fig. 27–3. Posterolateral thoracotomy. *A,* The fifth rib is resected subperiosteally and the pleural cavity is entered through an incision in the rib bed. Long rib resection is recommended for repeat thoracotomy. *B,* The rib bed is closed with running absorbable suture. The retained periosteum will regenerate rudimentary bone. The interspace distance is maintained.

shown in Figure 27–4, the only muscle group that is actually transected is the intercostals.

Upper lobe lesions are best approached through the fourth interspace. Middle and lower lobe lesions are easily handled through the fifth interspace. The patient is placed in a lateral decubitus position with the arm abducted at 90° and positioned on an arm rest. The antecubital fossa over the arm rest is padded. The skin incision is made over the desired interspace, the latissimus dorsi muscle is elevated bluntly for a short distance and retracted posteriorly, and the serratus anterior muscle is split in the direction of its fibers. The surgeon should not divide the muscle too far posteriorly to avoid injuring the long thoracic nerve to serratus anterior muscle. The intercostal muscles are divided in a way similar to that described for a posterolateral thoracotomy, and the pleural space is entered. The incision is so limited that wound towels and intercostal towels are not used. The intercostal muscle incision is carried forward to the anterior curve of the ribs and posteriorly to the level of the sacrospinalis muscle group. A Finochietto rib spreader is placed between the ribs, and a Tuffier rib spreader is placed in the opposite direction to retract the skin and latissimus dorsi muscle.

Closure of the axillary thoracotomy is accomplished with three pericostal sutures of No. 2 polyglycolic acid

after the placement of one or two chest tubes and consideration of an intercostal nerve block. Generally, traction on the pericostal sutures suffices to close the chest wall, as it is difficult to use a ratchet-type rib approximator through the small axillary thoracotomy incision. If a problem with rib approximation develops, a towel clip can be used to bring the ribs together. The serratus anterior muscle is closed with a running absorbable suture, as is the subcutaneous fascial layer. Skin closure technique is again at the surgeon's discretion.

The axillary thoracotomy is not recommended for the occasional thoracic surgeon or for a difficult operation, as the exposure is more limited than that of a posterolateral thoracotomy. In my opinion, however, it is a useful incision that deserves wider application than it has received in recent years. I believe the axillary thoracotomy is associated with less postoperative discomfort than is noted with either the posterolateral thoracotomy or the median sternotomy.

MEDIAN STERNOTOMY

The development of cardiac surgery has made median sternotomy the most common thoracic incision. It is the incision of choice for most cardiac operations and is used

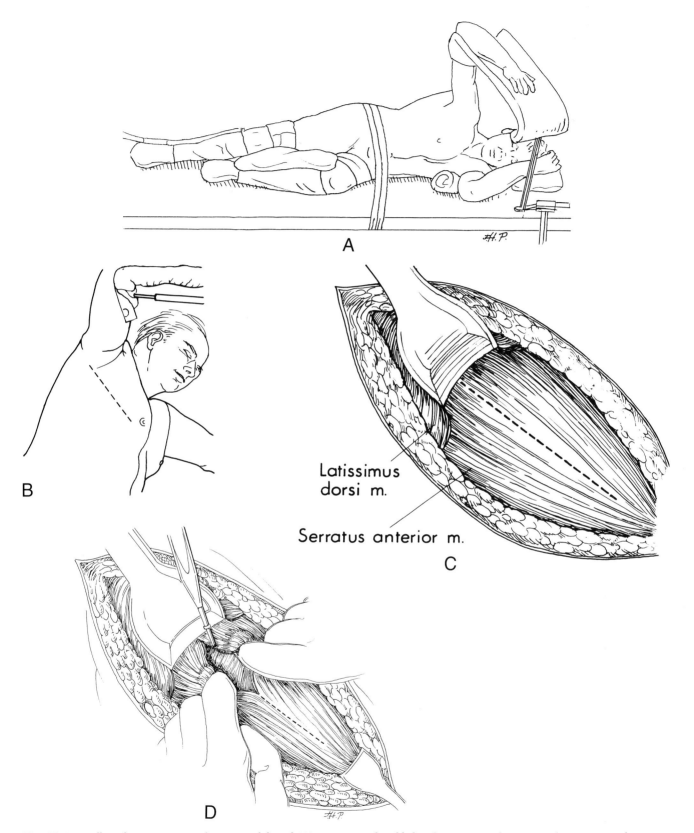

Fig. 27–4. Axillary thoracotomy. *A,* The arm is abducted 90° on a rest and padded with care. Note the sequential compression device on the legs and the axillary roll. *B,* An incision is made in line with the desired interspace. It is not necessary to raise skin flaps. *C,* The latissimus dorsi muscle is retracted posteriorly to expose the serratus anterior muscle. *D,* The serratus is spread in the direction of its fibers, using the electrosurgical unit with care, being careful to avoid injury to the long thoracic nerve to the serratus anterior muscle.

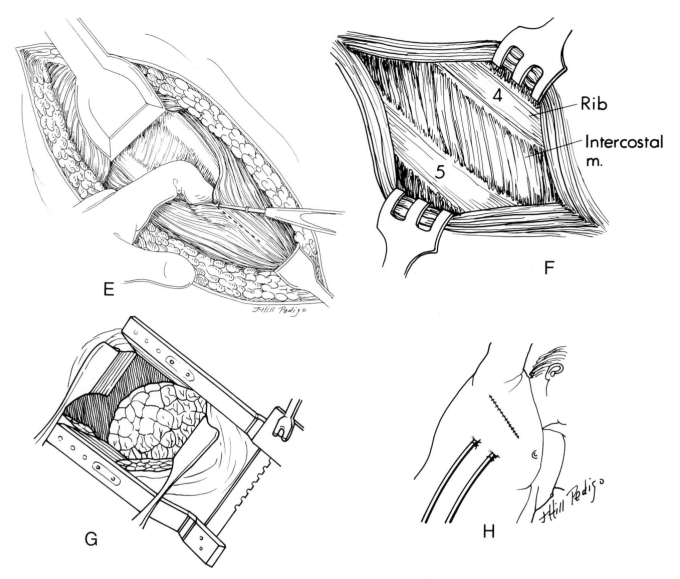

Fig. 27–4. (continued) *E*, The anterior portion of the serratus is divided with the cutting current to expose the intercostal muscles. *F*, The intercostal muscle is divided in its inferior attachment to the rib. *G*, Two rib spreaders facilitate exposure. *H*, Generally two chest tubes are used, and they are brought out near each other, so that a single maneuver will suffice at the time of tube removal. *From* Landreneau RJ, et al: General Thoracic Surgery — Current Trends. Norwalk CT: Appleton-Lange, 1993.

by preference by many thoracic surgeons for anterior mediastinal lesions, bilateral procedures such as the surgical treatment of bilateral spontaneous pneumothorax, and resection of multiple pulmonary lesions. Urschel and Razzuk (1986) wrote that they prefer it for many elective pulmonary resections, except for left lower lobe pulmonary resections. Cooper and colleagues (1978) demonstrated less alteration in pulmonary function by median sternotomy than by posterolateral thoracotomy. Median sternotomy was recommended by Baldwin and Mark (1985) and Perelman (1987) for anterior transpericardial repair of postpneumonectomy bronchopleural fistula. Orringer (1984) described a partial median sternotomy for exposure of the lower cervical and upper thoracic esophagus.

The patient is positioned supine, with one or both arms extended, at the preference of the surgeon and the anesthesiologist. Both arms are often placed at the patient's side. The vertical skin incision is made from just below the suprasternal notch to a point between the xiphoid process and the umbilicus (Fig. 27–5). The pectoral fascia is divided and the periosteum is scored with the electrosurgical unit. Care is needed when mobilizing tissues off of the area of the manubrium and dividing the tough interclavicular ligament. The tissues just to one side of the xiphoid process are mobilized and the sternum is divided with a power saw, from the top down or from the bottom up. The anesthesiologist should reduce ventilatory efforts as the sternum is being cut to lessen the chance of injury to the lung. Once

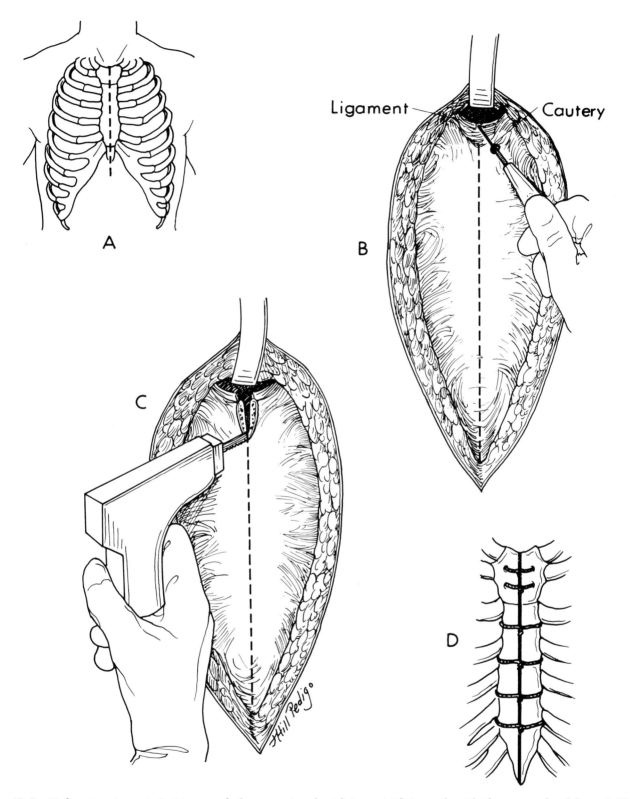

Fig. 27–5. Median sternotomy. *A*, Incision is made from suprasternal notch to a point between the xiphoid process and umbilicus. *B*, The interclavicular ligament is divided with care. *C*, The sternal saw can be used in either direction. The anesthesiologist should not ventilate the lungs while the sternum is being divided. *D*, The upper two wires of No. 5 monofilament steel are passed through the manubrium.

the sternum is split, the two edges are gently but firmly retracted, and periosteal bleeding points are controlled with the electrosurgical unit. Bone wax is often not necessary in general thoracic surgical procedures, because the patient is not anticoagulated, as is usual for patients undergoing cardiac procedures. Robiscek and colleagues (1981) suggested that the foreign body effect of bone wax can have a deleterious effect on wound healing. A sternal spreader is placed low in the incision to minimize excessive traction on the upper ribs, with attendant occult fracture and neurologic insult, as described by Van der Salm (1980). The use of the Lebsche sternal blade should be familiar to the thoracic surgeon so that sternotomy can be performed if the power saw fails or is unavailable.

Chest tubes or mediastinal drains, if the pleural space has not been entered, are passed through separate stab incisions. Sternotomy closure is accomplished with four to seven parasternal sutures of No. 5 stainless steel wire, ends of which are securely twisted and buried in the sternal tissues. The pectoral fascia is closed with a running polyglycolic acid suture, as is the linea alba. The subcutaneous tissues are closed with running absorbable suture and the skin is closed with the surgeon's preferred material.

The scar from the usual vertical median sternotomy incision is a source of concern to some patients, especially young females. Various alternatives have been proposed, and the transverse submammary skin incision described by Laks and Hammond (1980) appears to have definite cosmetic advantages for certain patients. Those authors do caution about skin flap viability for prolonged operations, as rather extensive undermining of the skin flaps is required.

The main advantages of median sternotomy for general thoracic surgical procedures are its speed in opening and closing, its familiarity to many surgeons, and its outstanding exposure for anterior mediastinal lesions. The major disadvantage is poor exposure of posterior hilar structures, especially those of the left lower lobe. My colleagues and I think that a median sternotomy is more painful in the postoperative period than an axillary thoracotomy and that it is similar in the degree of postoperative discomfort to a posterolateral thoracotomy.

ANTERIOR THORACOTOMY

The anterior thoracotomy has the distinct advantage of allowing the patient to remain supine, with a resulting improvement in cardiopulmonary function. It has been used with decreasing frequency because of improvement of anesthetic techniques and management, the option of median sternotomy, the development of mediastinal staging procedures such as mediastinoscopy and mediastinotomy and the rapid development of video-assisted thoracic surgery for lung biopsy. It remains the incision of choice of some surgeons for open lung biopsy. It is occasionally used in the Ivor Lewis procedure for carcinoma of the esophagus to eliminate the need for repositioning the patient after the intra-abdominal portion of the operation. Its main disadvantage is the limited exposure it provides.

The patient is positioned with a roll under the back and hips to elevate the operated side. The ipsilateral arm is placed under the back, on an elevated arm board, or on an overarm rest at the preference of the surgeon. An incision is made over the fourth or fifth interspace from the midaxillary line to curve parasternally (Fig. 27–6). In women, the incision is made in the inframammary crease. The pectoral muscles are divided with an electrosurgical unit, and the intercostal incision is made in the usual fashion. If a major resection is expected, one or two costal cartilages may be divided parasternally to facilitate exposure of the surgical field. If the cartilages are divided, the neurovascular bundles are divided over clamps and ligated to avoid tearing and excessive stretching of the blood vessels.

Closure of the anterior thoracotomy is similar to that of the other thoracotomy incisions. A heavy absorbable suture is placed through each end of the cartilage parasternally, if it has been divided.

TRANSVERSE THORACOSTERNOTOMY

Cooper (1991) and Pasque and associates (1990) redescribed the transverse thoracosternotomy and sometimes refer to it as the "cross-bow" or "clam shell" incision. Its primary role has been for bilateral lung transplantation. I, however, recommend it as an alternative to median sternotomy for bilateral general thoracic surgical procedures, such as the resection of bilateral metastatic lesions to the lungs and bilateral simultaneous treatment of spontaneous pneumothorax.

THORACOABDOMINAL INCISION

The thoracoabdominal incision provides extended exposure, particularly for operations in the lower thorax and upper abdomen. It has been used less frequently in the past and has been maligned more by hearsay perhaps than by actual fact. It can be particularly useful for difficult operations involving the lower esophagus. A seventh or eighth interspace incision is extended on the same oblique line into the upper quadrant over toward the midline. The costal margin is cut with a knife. Ginsberg (1993) recommended not excising a segment of cartilage and placing pericostal closure sutures securely on either side of the transected costal margin but not through the cartilage. He suggested that the incision results in a stable thorax with no significant increase in discomfort or dysfunction over a standard posterolateral thoracotomy. A curvilinear or radial incision can be made in the diaphragm to facilitate exposure. The diaphragm is closed with a running nonabsorbable suture such as No. 0 prolene. Costochondritis has been reported in some series. Its incidence is low, but if it

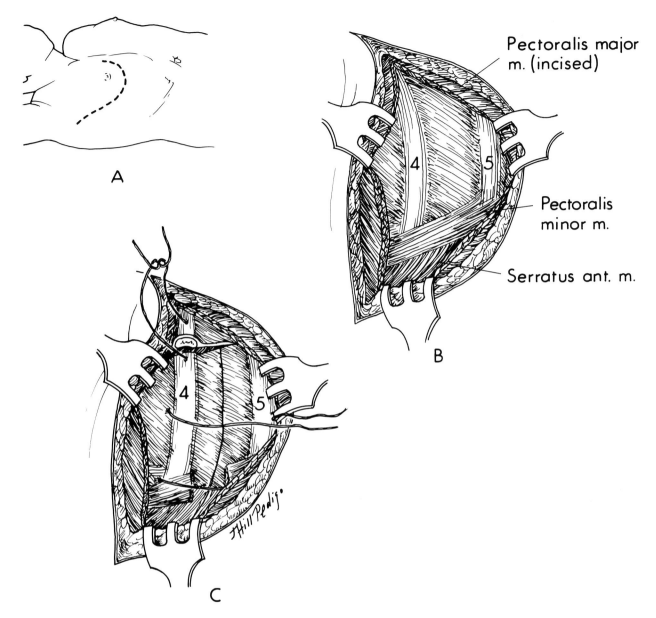

Fig. 27–6. Anterior thoracotomy. *A*, Outline of skin incision. *B*, Pectoralis major muscle divided over the fourth interspace. *C*, Closure of the intercostal incision by placement of pericostal sutures of heavy polyglycolic acid as well as sutures of the same material through the sectioned costal cartilage.

occurs, it is a troublesome complication. Heitmiller (1988) gave an excellent review of the incision.

REFERENCES

American College of Surgeons Manual of Preoperative and Postoperative Care. Philadelphia: WB Saunders, 1983, pp. 365-366.

Baldwin JC, Mark JBD: Treatment of bronchopleural fistula after pneumonectomy. J Thorac Cardiovasc Surg *90*:813, 1985.

Cameron JL, et al: Prospective clinical trial of antibiotics for pulmonary resections. Surg Gynecol Obstet *152*:156, 1981.

Cooper JD, in discussion of Patterson GA, et al: Comparisons of outcomes of double and single lung transplantation for obstructive lung disease. J Thorac Cardiovasc Surg *101*:623, 1991.

Cooper JD, Nelems JF, Pearson FG: Extended indications for median

sternotomy in patients requiring pulmonary resection. Ann Thorac Surg *26*:413, 1978.

Cruse PJE, Foord R: A five-year prospective study of 23,649 surgical wounds. Arch Surg *107*:206, 1973.

Fry WA, Kehoe TJ, McGee JP: Axillary thoracotomy. Am Surg *56*:40, 1990.

Gallo, Jr JA et al: Complications of intercostal nerve blocks performed under direct vision during thoracotomy J Thorac Cardiovasc Surg *86*:628, 1983.

Ginsberg R: Personal communication, 1993.

Glover JL, Bendick PJ, Link WJ: The use of thermal knives in surgery: Electrosurgery, lasers, plasma scalpel. Curr Probl Surg *15*:(1):26, 1978.

Heitmiller RF: The left thoracoabdominal incision. Ann Thorac Surg *46*:250, 1988.

Ilves R, et al: Prospective, randomized, double-blind study using prophylactic cephalothin for major, elective general thoracic operations. J Thorac Cardiovasc Surg *81*:813, 1981.

Jensik RJ: Personal communication, 1993.

Laks H, Hammond GL: A cosmetically acceptable incision for the median sternotomy. J Thorac Cardiovasc Surg 79:146, 1980.

Lewis RJ, et al: One hundred consecutive patients undergoing video-assisted thoracic operations. Ann Thorac Surg *54*:421, 1992.

Meakins JL: American College of Surgeons. Care of the surgical patient. VI. Perioperative Care, 3 Prophylactic antibiotics. Sci Am, 1993, pp. 1-3.

Mitchell RL: The lateral limited thoracotomy incision: Standard for pulmonary operations. J Thorac Cardiovasc 99:590, 1990.

Noirclerc M, et al: Les thoracotomies. *In* Encyclopédie médico-chirurgicale. Paris: Techniques Chirurgicales Thorax, pp. 1-16.

Noiclerc M, et al: La thoracotomie latérale large sans section musculaire. Ann Chir Thorac Cardiovasc *12*:181, 1973.

Olak J, et al: Randomized trial of one dose versus six-dose cefazolin prophylaxis in elective general thoracic surgery. Ann Thorac Surg *51*:956, 1991.

Orringer MB: Partial median sternotomy: Anterior approach to the upper thoracic esophagus. J Thorac Cardiovasc Surg 87:124, 1984.

Pasque MK, et al: Improved technique for bilateral lung transplantation rationale and initial clinical experience. Ann Thorac Surg *49*:785, 1990.

Perelman MI: Late treatment of chronic bronchopleural fistula with long stump after pneumonectomy. International Trends in General Thoracic Surgery. Vol. 2. Philadelphia: WB Saunders, 1987.

Ponn RB, et al: Comparison of late pulmonary function after posterolateral and muscle sparing thoracotomy. Ann Thorac Surg 53:675, 1992.

Robicsek F, et al: The embolization of bone was from sternotomy incision. Ann Thorac Surg *31*:357, 1981.

Salzman EW: Physical techniques for prevention of venous thrombosis. *In* Bergan JJ, Yao JST (eds): Surgery of the Veins. Orlando: Grune & Stratton, 1985, pp. 519-528.

Scurr JH, Coleridge-Smith PD, Hasty JH: Regimen for improved effectiveness of intermittent pneumatic compression in deep venous thrombosis prophylaxis. Surgery *102*:816, 1987.

Siegel T, Steiger Z: Axillary thoracotomy. Surg Gynecol Obstet *155*:725, 1982.

Urschel H, Razzuk M: Median sternotomy as the standard approach for pulmonary resection. Ann Thorac Surg *41*:130, 1986.

Van der Salm TJ, Cereda JM, Cutler BS: Brachial plexus injury following median sternotomy. J Thorac Cardiovasc Surg *80*:447, 1980.

READING REFERENCES

Ashour M: Modified muscle sparing posterolateral thoracotomy. Thorax *45*:1935, 1990.

Bethencourt DM, Holmes EC: Muscle-sparing posterolateral thoracotomy. Ann Thorac Surg *45*:337, 1988.

Dart CH, Braitman HE, Larab S: Supraclavicular thoracotomy for diagnosis of apical lung and superior mediastinal lesions. Ann Thorac Surg *28*:90, 1979.

Dartevelle P, et al: L'intérêt de la voie combinée cervicale et thoracique dans la chirurgie des syndromes de Pancoast et Tobias d'origine tumorale. Chirurgie *109*:399, 1983.

Dartevelle P, et al: L'intérêt de la cervicotomie ´elargie dans les syndromes de Pancoast-Tobias. Ann Chir *38*:80, 1984.

Lemmer JH, et al: Limited lateral thoracotomy. Arch Surg *125*:873, 1990.

Mathey J, Aigueperse J, Lalardrie JP: La voie axillaire rétro-péctorale en chirurgie thoracique: Technique et indications. Ann Chir *15*:1115, 1961.

Murray KD, et al: A limited axillary thoracotomy as primary treatment for recurrent spontaneous pneumothorax. Chest *103*:137, 1993.

Ravitch MM, Steichen FM: Atlas of General Thoracic Surgery. Philadelphia: WB Saunders, 1988, pp. 111-146.

CHAPTER 28

GENERAL FEATURES AND COMPLICATIONS OF PULMONARY RESECTIONS

Thomas W. Shields

Resections of the lungs may vary from a minimal incision of the visceral pleura and enucleation of a hamartoma to a pneumonectomy. Most resections are unilateral, but synchronous bilateral excisions may be carried out. The standard procedures (Table 28–1) may be extended to include excision of a part of the chest wall; one of the thoracic parietes — pleura, pericardium, or diaphragm; an adjacent vascular structure — portion of the atrium or vena cava; and rarely part of the esophagus. Some pulmonary resections may be accomplished using local anesthesia — open lung biopsy — but most are performed with general, endotracheal anesthetic management (see Chapter 21).

OPERATIVE POSITIONS AND THORACIC INCISIONS

Although each operative procedure has its own unique features, the standard operations are performed with the patient in the lateral decubitus, the supine, or the prone position. The selection of which position in which to place the patient is determined by the operation planned and, in part, the patient's physiologic condition. The

Table 28–1. **Pulmonary Resections**

Pneumonectomy
  Pleuropneumonectomy
  Tracheal sleeve pneumonectomy

Lobectomy
  Bilobectomy
  Sleeve lobectomy

Segmentectomy

Lesser resections
  Wedge excision
  Precision excision
  Bleb- or bullectomy
  Enucleation

supine position is associated with fewer physiologic changes in the patient's cardiopulmonary function than are noted with the other positions.

Lateral Decubitus Position

The lateral position permits the best access to the hilus of the lung. The structures contained within the hilus may be approached from either the anterior or posterior aspect, and thus the operator has greater control of the various structures than is afforded by the other approaches. The major disadvantage of the lateral position is that ventilation of the dependent lung is more difficult than in the posterior or supine position; however, perfusion of the dependent lung is increased as a result of the gravitational changes.

The Prone Patient

The posterior approach while the patient is prone has a major advantage in that the bronchial secretions will not flood the trachea because of the superior position of the main stem bronchus. Also, the main stem bronchus is the most accessible structure and may be isolated and divided as the initial stage in the dissection of the hilar structures. The major disadvantages are that the access to the entire hilus is limited initially and that the vascular structures are the most distant from the operator.

The Supine Patient

The anterior approach is now used commonly. The anterior thoracotomy approach, except for the more minor operative procedures, is used infrequently in North America. The disadvantage of poor access to the hilus and to contained structures generally outweighs the physiologic considerations. In many European clinics, however, this incision is still used for lobectomies and even occasionally for pneumonectomies. On the other hand, a median sternotomy incision for various types of pulmonary resection has become popular throughout the world. With controlled deflation of the lung and appropriate packing to elevate the lung anteriorly, the hilar structures are readily accessible on the right side. A left pneumonectomy, a left lower lobectomy, or other procedures on this lobe are difficult because of the position of the hilar structures, particularly that of the inferior pulmonary vein, behind the heart. As a consequence, a median sternotomy approach is not recommended for these procedures.

The multiple incisions and modifications thereof for the various intrathoracic operations have been described in Chapter 27. The trend is to use shorter posterolateral incisions and to spare the division of the major thoracic muscles as much as is compatible with appropriate operative exposure. The subperiosteal resection of a rib is done infrequently, although I believe better and tighter closure of the thoracic wall and pleural space can be accomplished and is indicated when a pneumonectomy is to be performed. Division or excision of a small posterior portion of a rib or ribs adjacent to the intercostal incision to improve exposure and to prevent a possible fracture of the rib as the intercostal space is retracted is practiced on an individual basis. If a fracture of one or more ribs occurs, control of any bleeding is mandatory and fixation of the fracture site by sutures is indicated to prevent overriding of the fractured ends to prevent further vascular injury or the occurrence of severe postoperative pain on chest wall movement.

GENERAL TECHNIQUES

The specific techniques of the various standard pulmonary resections are discussed in their respective chapters. The new technique of video-assisted thoracoscopic resection is discussed in detail in Chapter 37. As an introduction, however, a discussion of the general features of the dissection and management of the bronchi, large vessels, and lung surfaces is appropriate.

Dissection and Control of the Major Arteries

Dissection of a major pulmonary artery is carried out with care. The vessel is thin walled and is easily injured. Simultaneous traction and countertraction on the vessel wall once the proper plane has been established is to be avoided, although the fascial envelope can be retracted as the vessel wall is dissected away from it (Fig. 28–1). Pulling on a branch of the artery is also best avoided because the branch may easily be partially or completely avulsed from the main vessel wall. Both sharp and blunt dissection should be used, and finger mobilization of the posterior aspect of the larger vessels is helpful. In dissecting the main pulmonary artery on the right side, the truncus anterior of the artery may be isolated and divided to obtain greater length of the main stem vessel. On the left side, the pulmonary artery may be isolated up to, or even proximal to, the ligamentum arteriosum, although one must guard against injury to the recurrent laryngeal nerve as it passes underneath the aortic arch from the front to the back of the aorta at this point.

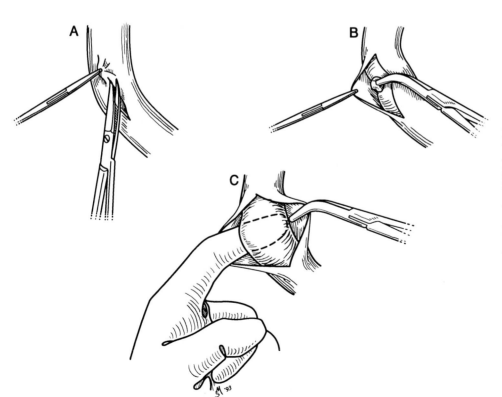

Fig. 28–1. Technique of dissection of a major pulmonary artery. *A,* Fascial envelope is elevated and incised longitudinally. *B,* Fascial layer is grasped and the vessel is bluntly dissected from it in the opposite direction. *C,* After freeing the vessel, the index finger is passed beneath the vessel between the fascial layer and the arterial wall, and a clamp is passed beneath the vessel using the finger as a guide.

The ligation of a major artery is accomplished in several ways. If it is long enough, the vessel may be doubly ligated with No. 00 or No. 0 nonabsorbable suture and the proximal end suture is ligated to prevent rolling off of the proximal ligature. A simple transfixation suture is not sufficient, but a figure of 8 suture through the center of the vessel and tied around it is satisfactory. Peterffy and Henze (1983) recommend the use of a purse-string suture. The vessel is then divided. If the vessel is too short to ligate safely in this manner, the artery may be held with two vascular clamps and divided, and the proximal cut end is closed with a continuous suture of No. 4-0 or No. 5-0 nonabsorbable suture. Some surgeons prefer to treat the pulmonary artery in this manner as a routine procedure. A third method of controlling the vessel is the use of a mechanical stapling device such as a TA 30 instrument using 3.5-mm or V staples.

The smaller branches of the artery may be satisfactorily controlled by triple ligation and division between the two most distal ligatures. With moderate-sized vessels, a transfixation suture is appropriate. Tension on any of these ligatures should be avoided, for even back bleeding from the lung side, if a ligature is pulled off, is troublesome.

If injury to the vessel occurs, the bleeding should be controlled initially by pressure with a gauze sponge, guarding against any maneuver that might further tear the vessel. Next, adequate exposure is ensured and proximal and distal control beyond the injury is obtained, or, when possible, a fine vascular clamp is applied directly to control the injured site. Repair is accomplished with an over and over fine vascular suture material.

Dissection and Control of the Major Veins

The major pulmonary veins and their branches are managed in a manner not dissimilar to that described for the pulmonary artery. The walls of the veins are stronger than those of the arteries, and injuries to them are less likely to occur. Occasionally, it is necessary to enter the pericardium to obtain sufficient length of the superior or inferior pulmonary vein. Once the vessel is free of the pericardial reflections (see Chapter 6), the vein is usually divided between vascular clamps and closed with a fine continuous vascular suture. Even a portion of the left atrial wall may be included in the excision and the atrial incision is closed in the standard manner. The pericardial defect, if small, is closed. If the opening is too large to close without compromise of the pericardial space, one of two maneuvers must be done to prevent postoperative herniation of the heart through the pericardial defect, with potential strangulation of the vessels and subsequent cardiac arrest. On the left side, the pericardium is opened down to the diaphragm; on the right side, because this maneuver does not prevent herniation, the cut edges of the pericardium are tacked to the surface of the heart or the defect is closed with a prosthetic "soft tissue" patch.

Piccione and Faber (1991) suggest closing all large defects, either right or left sided, routinely with a "soft tissue" patch.

Ligation of the veins as the initial step in a pneumonectomy for carcinoma has been advocated to lessen the possibility of spilling tumor cells into the circulation. The routine use of this maneuver, however, has not been shown to be beneficial, and the maneuver probably is not important. It has been suggested that initial ligation of the veins leads to overfilling of the vascular bed, resulting in an overdistended lung, which would be difficult to manipulate during the operative procedure, as well as resulting in a loss of an excessive amount of blood when the lung is removed. Miller and associates (1968) showed experimentally, however, that with initial ligation of the veins, reflex shunting of the blood from the lung occurs promptly, and thus distention of the vascular bed does not occur.

Dissection and Closure of the Bronchus

Main Stem Bronchus

The main stem bronchus is usually the last hilar structure isolated in a pulmonary resection. On the right side, the dissection can be carried up to the tracheal carina without difficulty, but care is taken, even during lymph node dissection, not to completely denude the bronchus of its investing adventitial tissue and the contained blood supply. On the left side, the main bronchus should likewise be freed to the tracheal bifurcation, but this effort is more tedious because of its position within the aortic window. The proximal site of division of a main stem bronchus should be close to the bifurcation and the line of division should be placed across the bronchus to avoid a blind pocket on its lateral side. Moreover, the residual stump should be as short as possible. As a general rule, a clamp should not be placed proximal to the proposed line of division when attempting a suture closure of the stump. Similarly, it is unnecessary if a stapling device is to be used to secure closure.

Takaro (1987) summarized the use and advantages of the mechanical stapler in bronchial closure. Hood (1985) recommended the TA 35 device with a staple size of 4.8 mm if a mechanical stapler is used. Both authors, among others, believe that the use of the stapler has reduced the incidence of breakdown of the bronchial closure. Peterffy and Calabrese (1979) reported the decreased incidence of a bronchopleural fistula with the use of a stapler versus the use of a chromic catgut suture closure. Such a comparison is not germane, because few would recommend catgut as the suture material of choice — a nonabsorbable suture such as silk, a fine monofilament stainless steel wire suture, or synthetic suture such as Vicryl or Dexon are the presently acceptable suture materials for closure of a bronchus. Furthermore, the recently noted decrease in incidence of a bronchial stump breakdown is more likely the result of a different selection of patients undergoing operations. In a discussion of Takaro's report, Vanetti and Bazelly (1987) reported better results with manual closure of the bronchial stump than with the use of a mechanical device. In fact, they were critical of the use of the new Premium TA 55 clip with which Hakim and Milstein (1985) recorded an alarming 15% incidence of bronchial fistula. With the use of the standard stapler, however, Vester and associates (1991) report only a 1.6% incidence of bronchial leak.

In the manual closure of the bronchus, an occluding clamp is placed distal to the line of division to prevent soilage of the operative field from any contained material within the distal bronchial tree. A suture is placed in each lateral side of the bronchus just proximal to the line of excision and the bronchus is divided, either completely before closure or in sequence to avoid a completely open stump. With either method, the posterior membranous wall is approximated to the anterior cartilaginous wall with interrupted single or mattress 00 or 000 sutures of the operator's choice. Before complete closure, the proximal stump and trachea should be aspirated by means of a sterile catheter. Once the closure is complete, the stump is tested for any persistent air leaks by covering the stump with a sterile solution and having the anesthesiologist apply or increase inspiratory pressure to that side of the tracheobronchial tree. Any areas of leakage are controlled by additional sutures as necessary. Fibrin sealant has been used successfully by many surgeons to seal small leaks of the suture or staple line, as reported by Jensen and Sharma (1985) and Matthew and associates (1990). The technique of application of the glue is discussed in detail by the latter authors. Mouritzen (1990) suggested the use of the sealant routinely on all bronchial closures.

Occasionally, a small tear in the membranous wall of the closed stump is identified. A buttress of adjacent tissue or a pledget of synthetic material should then be incorporated into a mattress suture closure of the area.

Frequently, one or two bronchial arteries need to be ligated after the bronchus has been divided. If bleeding is not controlled, these vessels may serve as a significant source of postoperative blood loss; the bronchial arterial system carries approximately 1% of the cardiac output.

After closure of the proximal end, the bronchial stump is covered with adjacent tissue, such as a pleural flap, the azygos vein, a pedicle graft of pericardial fat, or adjacent pericardium to provide the stump with a viable tissue cover to help prevent the possible development of a leak from the stump, which normally heals by secondary intention. This cover is particularly important on the right side, because no natural coverage for the stump is available. On the left side, the short proximal stump recedes into the depth of the aortic window and is surrounded by the adjacent tissues.

Further precautions to protect the stump to ensure healing are indicated in the patient who has received preoperative irradiation; who has an active inflammatory process — such as tuberculous endobronchitis or positive acid fast organisms in the sputum; who is un-

dergoing a completion pneumonectomy for a recurrent or continuing inflammatory process after a previous lesser resection; or in whom a bronchopleural fistula is being closed. In all these situations, the risk of bronchial dehiscence is increased. McGovern and associates (1988) have stressed the increased morbidity and problems with the bronchial stump in patients undergoing a completion pneumonectomy for an inflammatory disease. As prophylaxis against bronchial dehiscence, coverage of the stump is recommended using a transplanted muscle flap, as described by Pairolero and Payne (1983), or a pericardial fat pad, as described by Brewer and colleagues (1953, 1955).

Lobar and Segmental Bronchi

The surgical closure of the divided lobar or segmental bronchi entails the same principles and techniques of management as for the main stem bronchi. As a general rule, however, it is unnecessary to cover these bronchial stumps with additional tissue when sufficient pulmonary parenchymal tissue is present, which on inflation surrounds the bronchial stump. If one is unsure that this will occur, simple coverage with a freed pleural flap is sufficient.

Lesser Bronchi

The small subsegmental branches of the bronchial tree need only be ligated to obtain adequate and satisfactory closure of the stump. It is important to stress that when an incomplete fissure has been dissected or a segmentectomy has been done, small bronchial openings should be sought carefully and ligated to prevent any major postoperative air leak.

Raw Surface of the Lung

Any parenchymal raw surfaces that are present after a resection should be thoroughly inspected, and any significant bleeding should be controlled. A moist sponge is applied to the surface and the lung is expanded. After 5 to 10 minutes, the sponge is removed and the lung surface is reinspected. If the dissection of the intersegmental plane has been done carefully, only small alveolar air leaks will be present. These tend to seal over promptly with re-expansion of the lung during the postoperative period. Any leakage from small bronchi, however, must be recognized and controlled; otherwise, the leak will persist and predispose to serious postoperative difficulties. Jensik (1986) advocated covering the raw surfaces with pleural flaps or reconstituting the lung by bringing the adjacent segments together. Such a step is generally unnecessary and may even lead to increased postoperative problems.

Matthew and associates (1990) suggested the use of fibrin glue to control air leaks and bleeding from parenchymal raw surfaces, but no data were given as to its efficacy in this particular situation. In a study by Mouritzen (1990), the use of fibrin glue applied to the raw lung surfaces reduced the incidence and the persistence of postoperative air leakage as compared to a control group in which the glue was not applied.

INTRAOPERATIVE COMPLICATIONS

The three major life-threatening complications during the operation, other than those associated with the anesthetic management of the patient, are injury to a major vessel with massive hemorrhage, cardiac arrhythmias, and the development of a contralateral pneumothorax. The avoidance and management of the first has been discussed previously. The second — cardiac arrhythmias — may indicate underlying cardiac disease with or without the occurrence of an acute myocardial infarction or may result from excessive manipulation of the heart. The incidence of the first type should be reduced by an appropriate cardiac evaluation preoperatively; minimal manipulation of the heart during the resection reduces the incidence of arrhythmias related to excessive manipulation. According to the report of Ritchie and associates (1990), the prophylactic use of digitalis has no effect on reducing the occurrence of perioperative arrhythmias.

The incidence of the development of a contralateral pneumothorax is low. Vogt-Moykopf (1990) reported an incidence of 0.8%. It is thought to be a greater potential threat in patients undergoing an operation for bullous or bleb disease of the lung. It may occur, however, during any thoracotomy. Vogt-Moykopf (1990) stated that it may occur during an ultraradical lymph node dissection with perforation of the mediastinal pleura, but the few I have seen have occurred as a result of the spontaneous rupture of an unsuspected contralateral bleb. As a result of positive pressure anesthesia, an increasing amount of air accumulates in the contralateral pleural space, the lung on the affected side becomes increasingly difficult to ventilate, and effects of insufficient gas exchange become evident. With recognition of the complication, prompt evacuation of the air from the contralateral space becomes mandatory. This evacuation may be accomplished by placement of a closed thoracotomy tube via the mediastinum or by a transcutaneous route.

A catastrophic, although rare, complication that can occur during the operation is injury to the spinal cord with resultant paraplegia, usually resulting from attempts to control persistent bleeding from an intercostal vessel or to stop continued oozing at the posterior angle of the intercostal incision or at the site of removal of a portion of a vertebra. The use of unipolar cautery is to be avoided in these areas, as is forceful packing of the area with hemostatic substances. The fragile dural covering of the intervertebral foramen is easily disrupted. Either continued bleeding with egress of blood into the spinal canal or migration and swelling of the hemostatic material within the canal as reported by Short (1990) may compromise the space and result in pressure on the spinal cord. Compression of the spinal cord is poorly tolerated and paraplegia readily develops. The avoidance, prophylactic management, and early

recognition of this complication during the operative procedure were discussed by Walker (1990) and Benfield (1990). Unfortunately, recognition of the complication, even early in the postoperative period, and prompt neurosurgical decompression of the spinal cord frequently fail to reverse the process.

MANAGEMENT OF THE PLEURAL SPACE

The management of the pleural space is fundamentally different after a pneumonectomy than after a lobectomy or a lesser resectional procedure. After a pneumonectomy, the major concern is to have the space slowly obliterated by the subsequent anatomic changes in the position of the heart, mediastinal structures, the diaphragm, the contraction of the intercostal spaces, and the accumulation of fluid, without the occurrence of infection. After a lobectomy or a lesser resection, re-expansion of the remaining lung tissue to obliterate the pleural space without any major fluid collections is the desired clinical goal.

The Postpneumonectomy Pleural Space

After removal of the specimen, the pleural space is irrigated and the chest wall is inspected for any sites of continued bleeding. When present, these are controlled with cautery or suture ligation as necessary. Special care, as previously noted, is required in the event of persistent bleeding from an intercostal vessel or continued oozing at the posterior angle of the intercostal incision.

It is of major importance that the pleural space be dry — absence of continued bleeding — because the development of an acute massive hemothorax that necessitates re-exploration is associated with a higher mortality rate and an increased incidence of a bronchopleural fistula, as noted by Peterffy and Henze (1983). After control of any bleeding sites, the pleural space is irrigated once again. Many surgeons instill a broad-spectrum antibiotic in a small amount of sterile solution into the space just before closure. No prospective data support this practice, but its use is reassuring in that the fluid that accumulates within the space is an excellent culture medium.

The postpneumonectomy pleural space usually is closed without drainage. If the development of an infection within the space is likely, a drainage tube may be placed in the space. The tube is then opened periodically to drain the accumulated fluid. Some surgeons (personal communication, Pellett, 1992) routinely drain the space for 24 hours to prevent too rapid accumulation of fluid in the space and to enable the detection of excessive postoperative bleeding if it occurs. Balanced pleural drainage to maintain the mediastinum in a normal midline position as suggested by Laforet and Boyd (1964) is not recommended.

After closure of the incision, the pressure within the space is adjusted as necessary to approximate a negative pressure of 2 to 4 cm of water on inspiration and a positive pressure of 2 to 4 cm of water on exhalation.

Adjustment may be made simply by thoracentesis and removal of air until the trachea is in the midline at the sternal notch, or the actual pressures may be measured using a manometer.

Some authors advocate daily adjustment of the intrapleural pressure within the pneumonectomy space for 4 to 5 days after the pneumonectomy. When this is done, antibiotics may be placed within the cavity. Others, including myself, have found this procedure unnecessary and meddlesome, preferring to check the pressure only if clinical signs indicate its need.

Fate of the Pleural Space

After pneumonectomy, elevation of the ipsilateral leaf of the diaphragm, shift of the mediastinum toward the operated side, and narrowing of the intercostal spaces of the ipsilateral side occur. In addition, serosanguinous fluid accumulates in the empty pleural space to fill the residual volume. The rate of accumulation of the fluid and the complete absorption of the air from the space are variable. Generally, the process is completed within 3 to 4 weeks, but it may take as long as 7 months (Fig. 28-2).

In the past, the phrenic nerve on the side of the pneumonectomy was crushed to obtain a more prompt and higher elevation of the diaphragmatic leaf to reduce the residual volume of the postpneumonectomy space. The resultant paralysis of the ipsilateral leaf of the diaphragm, however, permits paradoxic motion of this portion of the thoracic cage. Although this effect is of no real consequence during normal breathing, the paradoxic motion of this paralyzed leaf does interfere with the efficacy of the cough mechanism. Thus, it is not recommended as a routine procedure.

Also, a thoracoplasty often was performed postoperatively to obliterate the residual pleural space, thereby preventing the overdistention of the remaining contralateral lung and reducing the incidence of infection of the space. Overdistention of the contralateral lung, however, is in itself not detrimental to lung function, and a standard thoracoplasty does adversely affect the function of the contralateral lung. Gaensler and Strieder (1951) showed a loss of approximately 25 to 30% of the preoperative vital capacity and approximately 20% of the maximum voluntary ventilation in the contralateral lung after a standard thoracoplasty was performed over a nonfunctioning lung. A plombage type of thoracoplasty is followed by less functional loss, but the foreign body frequently becomes associated with infection and consequently its use is not advised.

The fluid within the pleural space is gradually absorbed so that only a potential space remains. As absorption takes place, the heart and mediastinum shift farther toward the ipsilateral side and the remaining contralateral lung herniates anteriorly and partially into the postpneumonectomy space to fill this residual thoracic volume (Fig. 28-3). Spirn (1988) has noted that this anterior herniation occurs after either a left or right pneumonectomy to a variable degree in all cases. Posteroprevertebral lung herniation occurs only after a left pneumonectomy and in only 50% of cases; its occurrence is not observed after a right pneumonectomy.

Complete absorption of the fluid is uncommon. Suarez and colleagues (1969) found complete absorption occurred in only 10 of 37 patients who died at varying time intervals after pneumonectomy. In the other 27 individuals, variable amounts of air or fluid remained in simple or loculated spaces. This early observation, that in only one third of postpneumonectomy patients does the space become obliterated completely, was confirmed by the computed tomographic — CT — evaluation of the postpneumonectomy space by Biondetti and

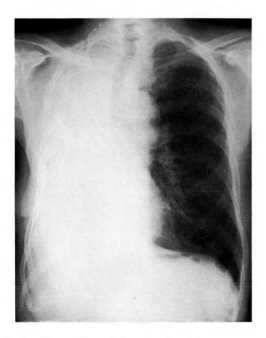

Fig. 28–2. Chest radiograph 2 weeks after right pneumonectomy.

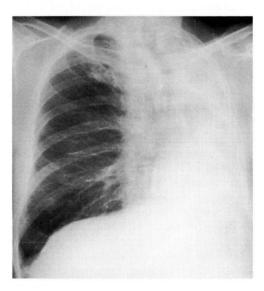

Fig. 28–3. Chest radiograph 3 years after pneumonectomy.

associates (1982). In the latter study, two thirds of the postpneumonectomy spaces contained a unilocular fluid-filled space of varying size surrounded by thick fibrous margins.

The Postlobectomy Pleural Space

After a lobectomy, the pleural space is drained routinely. Two thoracostomy tubes are used, one near the apex and one at the base, along the costal margin of the hemidiaphragm. These tubes are connected to an underwater seal drainage system. Supplemental negative suction may be used according to the preference of the operator. The tubes are kept in the pleural space until no air leak is present and the drainage is less than 50 ml per 24 hours. Care is needed to maintain patency of the drainage system as long as the thoracostomy tubes are in place.

With the re-expansion of the remaining lung, elevation of the diaphragmatic leaf, and shift of the mediastinum toward the ipsilateral side, the pleural space is usually obliterated within several days to a week. An asymptomatic persistent air space may remain, however, for a longer period.

Approximately 10% of persistent spaces become complicated, and Conlan (1990) reported that in 3%, the complication is of serious import — empyema or bronchopleural fistula. In patients in whom insufficient lung to fill the pleural space is anticipated, especially those with inflammatory disease processes, Lynn (1960) and Tamimi and colleagues (1976) recommend a preresection apical tailoring thoracoplasty to reduce the size of the pleural space and thus prevent the high incidence of serious morbidity seen in these patients. This procedure is rarely done at present, however, and is not recommended. If such a problem is anticipated, the chest wall incision should be performed so that the chest wall muscles are preserved for a possible transplant if one becomes necessary. Intraoperatively, if it is recognized that insufficient lung tissue is present to fill the pleural space, Brewer (1956) and Miscall (1956) and their associates suggested the use of a pleural partition or construction of a pleural tent to reduce the size of the space. Conlan (1990) discussed the technique of constructing the tent and its fate. Although this procedure was believed to have had advantages in reducing space complications when resections for inflammatory diseases were more common, there appear to be few indications for its use at present. Deslauriers (personal communication, 1992), however, is a strong advocate for its use when it appears that insufficient lung volume remains to fill the pleural space after an upper lobectomy. He reports the value of a postoperative pneumoperitoneum to reduce the volume of the ipsilateral hemithorax, particularly if a basilar space is anticipated. He also suggests temporary paralysis of the ipsilateral leaf of the diaphragm, which I believe is contraindicated, however, because of the adverse effects of paradoxic motion of this leaf on the diaphragm, especially with coughing.

Adjunctive or concomitant tailoring thoracoplasty has also been suggested to reduce the size of the pleural spaces, but its use has been abandoned because of the deranged chest wall physiology postoperatively. Conlan (1990) suggested the use of an osteoplastic thoracoplasty to prevent the chest wall instability. Talamonti and colleagues (1989) favored a modified plombage thoracoplasty using an inflatable prosthesis to fill the space. Most surgeons, however, recommend a muscle transplant to fill a potentially hazardous residual pleural space (see Chapter 56).

The Postsegmentectomy Pleural Space

The pleural space after a segmentectomy or other lesser resectional procedure should be managed in a fashion similar to that described for the postlobectomy space. Air leaks for a greater or lesser period of time are the major problem in these patients.

Management after Minimal Resections

In most situations, even if minimal or no pulmonary tissue is resected, it is best to drain the pleural space as is done for a lobectomy or a segmentectomy. An exception may be the patient who has had only a lung biopsy or in whom the pleural space was entered by a limited anterior or occasionally a small axillary thoracotomy. In these instances, simple aspiration of the pleural space by use of a small catheter just before complete closure of the incision is all that is necessary. On the other hand, in patients with a standard posterolateral thoracotomy in whom only an exploratory procedure was performed, adequate postoperative thoracostomy tube drainage is indicated; usually, only one lower thoracostomy tube is necessary. Significant amounts of fluid may collect, necessitating subsequent thoracentesis if proper drainage has not been effected.

PHYSIOLOGIC EFFECTS

Ventilatory Changes

Postpneumonectomy. Early after a pneumonectomy, the ventilation of the remaining lung may be improved by a compensatory increase in the depth and rate of breathing. The lung becomes stiffer, however, and the elastic recoil pressure at total lung capacity increases. As a result, the work of breathing is increased. Diffusion capacity — $D_{L}CO$ — is also decreased. As the remaining lung adjusts to the changes in the thoracic volume available to it, the lung becomes hyperinflated. The result is an increase of 10 to 30% in its vital and total capacities.

Van Mieghem and Demedts (1989) found an overall 35 to 40% reduction of the preoperative FVC, FEV, and $D_{L}CO$ after pneumonectomy. These observations are similar to those of Ladurie and Ranson-Bitker (1985), who found that the vital capacity was over 50% of the predicted value 5 years after pneumonectomy in 98 patients.

In children, the late functional loss after pneumonectomy is less than that observed in the adult. Gas exchange is normal when the child is at rest. The total lung capacity and vital capacity are increased well above that predicted for one lung, and the maximum voluntary ventilation — maximum breathing capacity — is generally normal. Diffusion capacity is normal if the pneumonectomy is performed before puberty; this is probably the result of growth of the remaining lung in the young child. Cagle and Thurlbeck (1988) presented a thorough review of the experimental and clinical observations relative to postpneumonectomy compensatory lung growth. Many facets of the mechanisms stimulating this occurrence remain to be elicited, but stretch of the remaining lung is thought to be the initial stimulus for the compensatory growth of the remaining lung tissue.

If pneumonectomy is performed after puberty, reduction of the diffusion capacity occurs, as is noted in the adult. After pneumonectomy in children, pulmonary hypertension is not a significant development.

Postlobectomy. With resection of a lobe of the lung, a part of the total alveolar, bronchial, and vascular masses is removed. Overinflation of the contralateral as well as of the remaining ipsilateral lung tissue results.

The remaining lung parenchyma is subjected to increased perfusion, despite an absolute reduction in the diffusion surface. The ratio of the dead space to the total lung volume increases, but a decrease of the dead space with respect to the tidal volume occurs. As a result, ventilatory efficiency, is actually improved.

Ali and associates (1980) reported an early disproportionate functional loss after lobectomy that was greater than the predicted loss. They reported a mean fall of approximately 30% in the FVC and FEV_1 when only a 25% reduction was predicted. Markos and colleagues (1989), however, did not observe this disproportionate loss; in fact, the observed mean losses in FVC and FEV_1 were less than had been predicted. The reasons for these discrepancies are unresolved. Van Mieghem and Demedts (1989) reported only a 15% decrease in the FVC after lobectomy. Berend and associates (1980) noted similar findings — a decrease of 12 and 10%, respectively, in the TLC and VC after lobectomy. They observed only a slight reduction of the FEV_1 and no change in the D_LCO.

The loss may vary in the individual patient, however, and is influenced by the degree of functional loss present preoperatively and the presence or absence of postoperative complications. The occurrence of hemorrhage, effusion, air leak, empyema, fibrothorax, or bronchopleural fistula exerts a serious adverse effect on postoperative pulmonary function.

Postsegmentectomy and Lesser Procedures. The physiologic changes after a segmentectomy are the same as those noted after a lobectomy. The late functional loss is related to the number of segments removed as well as to the occurrence of postoperative complications. The functional gain by the preservation of a segment of lobe is generally less than expected from its volume. The parenchymal tissue saved, however, may play a valuable role in helping to fill the pleural space. Unfortunately, even this is relative, because the incidence of postoperative complications occasionally is greater after segmentectomy than after a lobectomy. In the prospective study of the North American Lung Cancer Groups reported by Ginsberg (1991), those patients who underwent a segmentectomy or a lesser resection exhibited an initial ventilating functional advantage over those who underwent a lobectomy. This functional advantage was lost, however, after the first year of observation.

The physiologic changes subsequent to a wedge resection in the absence of postoperative pleural complications are minimal. Those seen are more directly related to the thoracotomy incision than to the removal of the small part of lung. Early in the postoperative period, the lung volume is restricted. Inspiratory capacity and the expiratory reserve volume are decreased. The end expiratory position is depressed as the result of pain in the chest wall. Alveolar hypoventilation with carbon dioxide retention and some degree of respiratory acidosis occurs. Oxyhemoglobin desaturation occurs and is greatest on the second and third postoperative days; it may persist for as long as 10 days. Compliance is reduced, resulting in an increased work of breathing. This reduction is most remarkable the first few hours after the operation and returns gradually to near normal within the first postoperative week.

Hemodynamic Changes

After a pneumonectomy, the pulmonary artery pressure is usually normal at rest. As noted by van Mieghem and Demedts (1989), however, maximum effort tolerance decreases after pneumonectomy and an increase in both the pulmonary artery pressure and pulmonary vascular resistance occur with effort. Cardiac output and stroke volume decrease during effort. These changes are accompanied with an increase in the peripheral arterial blood pressure as well as in the peripheral vascular resistance. Oxygen saturation decreases on effort, possibly because of an absolute decrease in the D_LCO. After a lobectomy, similar hemodynamic changes are seen, but to a lesser degree.

Van Mieghem and Demedts (1989) suggested that the cardiovascular changes can be explained by the hypothesis that the removal of a substantial part of the vascular bed may result in an increase in the afterload of the right ventricle, which may interfere with the emptying of this ventricle. The increased afterload increases both the end-systolic and end-diastolic volumes of the right ventricle, which may in turn cause a shift of the interventricular septum to the left with resultant changes that result in a decreased cardiac output. Speculative changes in metabolic function of the lungs also may lead to increased systemic vascular resistance with resultant increased left ventricular afterload and decrease in both stroke volume and cardiac output.

Of clinical interest is that, according to Ladurie and Ranson-Bitker (1985), sinoauricular tachycardia is present in over 75% of the late survivors of a pneumonectomy; in one fourth of the patients, over 100 beats per minute were recorded. A functional, persistent systolic murmur at the right heart base was observed in 12% of the patients. Right heart overload, determined electrocardiographically, was present in 6% of the patients in their study.

The older the patient at the time of pneumonectomy or the greater the degree of pre-existent chronic obstructive airway disease in the remaining lung, the greater the likelihood of functional incapacity. In evaluating the functional capacity, a direct relationship to the pulmonary artery pressure apparently exists; as the functional reserve decreases, the pulmonary artery pressure increases. The reduction in the functional capacity appears to be related more directly to the pulmonary artery pressure and pulmonary blood flow relationships in the remaining lung than to arterial saturation per se. The functional capacity appears to be governed and limited by the expansibility of the remaining vascular bed. When the limit of the bed is reached or exceeded, persistent pulmonary hypertension occurs and cor pulmonale results.

MORBIDITY AND MORTALITY

Morbidity

Multiple factors influence the incidence and types of nonfatal complications seen after pulmonary resections. These include the physical status of the patient, the nature of the pathologic process, the extent of the procedure, and the addition of various preoperative or postoperative adjuvant therapeutic modalities.

Nonfatal complications may be classified as those either unique to, or directly related to, the procedure: technical, pleural, pulmonary, cardiac, or septic, and as those related to the performance of any major operative procedure: cardiovascular, genitourinary, peripheral vascular, neurologic, thromboembolic, hematologic, or others.

Of the complications related to the procedure per se, more than one etiologic factor, that is, technical, septic, or failure of healing, may play a role in the development of the complication.

After a pneumonectomy, the nonfatal morbidity rate varies greatly; the usual rates are reported to be as low as 15 to as high as 51%. The major, significant complications are atelectasis, cardiac arrhythmias, pneumonia, respiratory insufficiency, empyema, bronchopleural fistula, and hemothorax. Patel and associates (1992) reported 232 complications in 197 patients who had undergone a pneumonectomy. Respiratory complications and cardiac problems were encountered most often, but interestingly, renal failure was observed in 15% of the patients. The high incidence of this particular complication was related to an age greater than 70 years and was found to be an important factor for in-hospital mortality.

After lobectomy, the nonfatal complication rate frequently is higher, particularly after resection in patients

with inflammatory disease processes. Keagy and associates (1985), however, reported that postlobectomy morbidity is more common in patients with carcinoma. Complications are also more common in men than in women. The number of complications increases in the elderly and in patients undergoing extended resections, extensive radical lymphatic node dissections, or bronchoplastic procedures.

As with pneumonectomy, the nonfatal complications after a lobectomy may result from technical errors, may be common to any extensive operative procedure, or may be caused primarily by the removal of one of the lobes of the lung. In a series of 369 lobectomies reported by Keagy and associates (1985), 41% had nonfatal complications: 224 complications occurred in 151 patients. The respiratory system was involved in one third — 50 patients required prolonged ventilation and 27 had atelectasis or excessive secretions. The incidence of pneumonia per se was not documented. Cardiac complications also occurred in one third, arrhythmias being the most common. In the remaining one third, air leaks, pleural effusions, pneumothoraces, empyema — 2.4%, postoperative hemorrhage, bronchial stump leaks — 1.3%, pulmonary emboli, wound infections, and one instance of lung gangrene occurred. Postoperative massive atelectasis (Fig. 28–4), persistent residual air space (Fig. 28–5), and prolonged air leaks present problems not seen after a pneumonectomy.

After a segmentectomy, the nonfatal complications are similar to those occurring after a lobectomy. The major complications are prolonged air leak, either peripheral alveolar pleural fistula or true bronchopleural fistula, empyema, and persistent pleural air space. All are interrelated, and the incidence of any one alone, or in combination, varies most directly with the disease process and the difficulty experienced in the dissection of the intersegmental planes.

The morbidity rate after a wedge resection is minimal. When present, the complication is most often the result of either retention of secretions or pleural problems. Persistent air spaces occur, but with an incidence of less than 10%. Most of these spaces produce no symptoms and required no treatment.

The morbidity after bronchoplastic and tracheoplastic procedures is discussed in Chapters 31 and 35, respectively.

Postoperative Mortality

The mortality rates after pulmonary resection should be computed on a 30-day basis. In some situations, as in those involving pulmonary tuberculosis, this time should be extended to at least 60 days. All in-hospital deaths should be considered as an operative mortality.

After pneumonectomy, the mortality rates vary from as low as 3% to as high as 30%. In patients undergoing a pneumonectomy for the treatment of tuberculosis, the average mortality rate has often been between 8 and 10%. In a report by Pomerantz and associates (1991), however, the mortality rate in 40 pneumonectomies for tuberculosis was only 2.5%. In patients with carcinoma

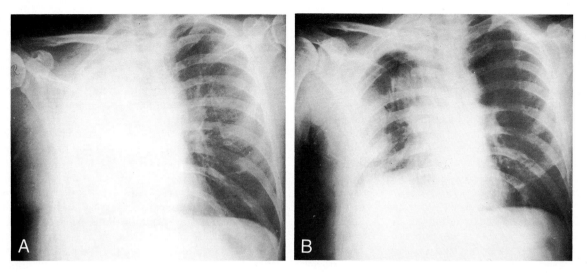

Fig. 28–4. *A,* Chest radiograph reveals massive atelectasis of remaining right lung 24 hours after right upper lobectomy. *B,* Re-expansion of remaining right lung after bronchoscopy.

of the lung, the rates vary but are in the range of 5 to 15%. Ginsberg and associates in the North American Lung Cancer Study Group (1983) reported an overall 30-day postoperative mortality rate of only 6%, as did Nagasaki and colleagues (1982) from the Sloan-Kettering Cancer Center. In patients 70 years of age or older, the mortality rate may be as high as 30%; however, with proper preoperative selection and meticulous postoperative care, the mortality rate in patients over age 70 years may be kept as low as 6%, as reported by Ginsberg and associates (1983). Waki (1989) and Patel (1992) and co-workers reported a mortality rate of 13% in this older

age group, whereas Ishida and associates (1990) recorded no deaths after pneumonectomy in 11 patients in this age group. Roxburgh and associates (1991) noted a higher mortality rate after pneumonectomy in the elderly, but the difference was not significant. In patients who have undergone an extended pneumonectomy — a pleuropneumonectomy or a tracheal-sleeve pneumonectomy — the 30-day postoperative mortality rate is higher than that associated with a standard pneumonectomy. Rates as high as 25 to 30% have been recorded, but Faber (1986) recorded a rate of approximately 10% after pleuropneumonectomy, and

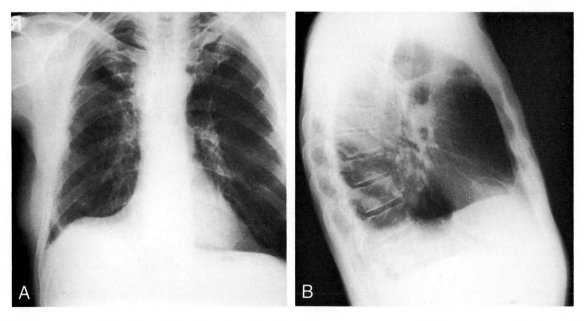

Fig. 28–5. Posteroanterior *(A)* and lateral *(B)* radiographs of the chest show an asymptomatic residual air space 4 weeks after a right upper lobectomy for carcinoma of the lung.

Dartevelle and associates (1988) and Mathisen and Grillo (1991) recorded rates of approximately 10% after tracheal-sleeve pneumonectomy.

The major causes of death after a pneumonectomy are pulmonary insufficiency, septic complications — for example, postoperative pneumonia or an empyema that may or may not be associated with a bronchopleural fistula — cardiac arrhythmias, myocardial infarction, and pulmonary embolus. As noted, renal failure may be a major factor in older patients. Concomitant medical disease has also been suggested by Patel and associates (1992) to be a significant factor. Interestingly, most postoperative deaths occur after a right pneumonectomy, as noted by Nagasaki (1982), Washi (1989) and Cybulsky (1992) and their colleagues, among others.

Postpneumonectomy pulmonary edema is an unusual complication that is lethal when unrecognized. Peters (1987) reported that it usually follows a right pneumonectomy in a patient whose preoperative pulmonary function was good and whose first 12 to 24 hours postoperatively were uneventful. Progressive dyspnea and apprehension appear first. Hypoxemia develops, and when the condition is unrecognized and untreated, death occurs. Peters postulated from clinical observations and studies in the laboratory by Zeldin and associates (1984) that perioperative excessive fluid is the etiologic factor. The single remaining lung must remove a large fluid load, and the fluid filtered in the lung exceeds the capacity of lymphatics. Fluid accumulates in the peribronchial spaces initially, which makes the lung stiffer, increasing the work of breathing. When the peribronchial space is filled, the alveoli fill rapidly with fluid, hypoxemia occurs, and death ensues. Treatment consists of morphine, diuretics, and ventilatory support. The best treatment, of course, is prevention of fluid overload during and immediately following the procedure.

Patel and colleagues (1992) reported that the 24-hour perioperative fluid infusion of greater than 3 liters of fluid was significantly related to postoperative morbidity and mortality. Verheijen-Breemharr and associates (1988) reported 11 cases of severe postpneumonectomy edema in 243 patients; the majority were observed after a right pneumonectomy — 8 in 113 patients, 7% , and only 3 after a left pneumonectomy, 2%. Overhydration was the common denominator, and of note, was that edema was found in 3 of 7 patients who required reoperation for control of postoperative hemorrhage. Patel and associates (1992) recorded 30 cases of varying magnitude of postpneumonectomy edema in 197 patients. Thirteen of these 30 patients died — a mortality rate of 43%. Postpneumonectomy pulmonary edema also occurs as one of the major fatal complications after a tracheal sleeve pneumonectomy. The pulmonary edema can develop even when strict attention is paid to the amount of perioperative fluid used. Mathisen and Grillo (1991), as well as Deslauriers (personal communication, 1992) suggest that the extensive interruption of the major lymphatic channels to the remaining lung as the

result of the operative procedure may play a major role in the occurrence of the edema, but this theory remains unproven. Nonetheless, when the process becomes clinically evident, usually 24 to 48 hours after the operation, the attendant ventilatory dysfunction progresses relentlessly, despite aggressive therapeutic intervention to reverse the process, and results in the death of the patient.

Another infrequent complication after pneumonectomy is embolization from pulmonary arterial stump thrombosis. Chuang and colleagues (1966) reported that this condition occurred in 1% of patients after a pneumonectomy. It is said to occur twice as often after a right than after a left pneumonectomy. Because a ligature of the arterial stump produces puckering and infolding of the vessel wall, which theoretically could increase in the likelihood of thrombosis, vascular closure by suture technique or by the use of a stapler may lessen the minimal risk of this complication.

Pulmonary embolism from other sites also may cause death, as reported by Abbey Smith (1970) and Nagasaki and associates (1982). The latter authors noted that one half of the patients who suffer an embolus die as a result. The occurrence of myocardial infarction is fortunately infrequent, because it may result in death in three fourths of the patients in whom it occurs. Massive gastrointestinal hemorrhage, cerebrovascular accidents, and technical accidents at operation account for a few deaths.

The mortality rates are lower after lobectomy than after pneumonectomy. Patient selection and disease process are the major factors influencing the occurrence of postoperative death. In patients with pulmonary tuberculosis, the mortality rate is in the range of 1 to 2%; in patients with carcinoma of the lung, it may be as high as 8 to 10%, but as reported by Ginsberg (1983) and Keagy (1985) and their colleagues, it should be no greater than 3%.

The major causes of death after lobectomy are septic complications and cardiopulmonary insufficiency. Fatal pulmonary embolism occurs infrequently. Fatal cardiac and other nonpulmonary complications, such as upper gastrointestinal hemorrhage, occur occasionally.

Segmentectomy is essentially a benign procedure, and mortality rates of approximately 1% are reported when the procedure is done electively in patients with satisfactory pulmonary function. Jensik (1986) and Martini and associates (1986) reported it may, however, be as high as 4 to 6% in patients with poor pulmonary function, when more extensive tumor is present, or in those patients with a previous pulmonary resection.

SPECIFIC COMPLICATIONS

Postoperative Hemorrhage

Major hemorrhage after thoracotomy and resection is most commonly the result of inadequate hemostasis of a bronchial artery or a systemic vessel in the chest wall;

infrequently, the slipping of a ligature from a major pulmonary vessel or an unrecognized injury to a systemic vein is the cause. Bleeding related to a coagulation abnormality is rare, and when present is often associated with the use of a large number of units of stored blood transfusions — usually greater than 10 — during the operative procedure. When a coagulopathy is suspected, coagulation studies are indicated and the appropriate therapy — fresh frozen plasma, cryoprecipitate, or platelet transfusion — is given as indicated.

When inadequate hemostasis is the cause, prompt re-exploration and identification and control of the site of bleeding is necessary. Generally, the continued bleeding is accompanied by hypotension, tachycardia, and pallor, but any one or all of these may be absent initially. In the patient in whom the slipping of a ligature from a major pulmonary vessel is the cause, sudden syncope with failure to respond to fluid replacement is the initial manifestation.

When chest tubes are in place, an output of blood of more than 200 ml per hour for 4 to 6 hours indicates massive bleeding, but lesser output may occur because of clot formation within the pleural space or in the drainage system. The reliance on the amount of drainage to determine the blood loss can be misleading. When massive bleeding is the suspected cause of the patient's hypotension, radiographs of the chest to determine the degree of opacification of the ipsilateral hemothorax are indicated. Any one of the following — failure to respond to adequate blood replacement, a large amount of blood in the hemithorax, or continued excessive bleeding from the chest tubes — is an indication for re-exploration.

In a series of 1428 resections, Peterffy and Henze (1983) reported 113 hemorrhagic episodes — 30% occurred after a pneumonectomy, 66% after a lobectomy, and 4% after a segmentectomy. Emergency thoracotomy was required in 37 patients — an incidence of 2.6%. Six of the patients died — 4 as the result of hemorrhage and 2 because of a subsequent bronchopleural fistula. In another 3 patients, massive bleeding — 2 from the pulmonary artery and 1 from a systemic vessel — was found to be the cause of death at autopsy. Thus, the overall incidence of mortality related to uncontrolled bleeding was less than 0.1%.

Hypotension in the Absence of Bleeding

Hypotension associated with an elevated central venous pressure may be attributable to cardiac tamponade — occasionally seen when the pericardium has been opened — or to heart failure. The former may be identified by a chest radiograph or an echocardiogram and requires surgical treatment. Heart failure is managed medically with digitalis or inotropic agents — dopamine — or both.

Pulmonary Edema

Pulmonary edema, as noted, is manifested by respiratory failure with tachypnea, cyanosis, and restlessness. The most common cause is overhydration resulting from excessive fluid replacement during the operative procedure, and this situation should be avoided. Other causes are acute myocardial infarction with left heart failure and, infrequently, decreased serum protein concentration, capillary injury from sepsis, or prolonged inspiration of high oxygen concentration in the inspired gases. The lethality of postpneumonectomy pulmonary edema has been discussed.

Respiratory Insufficiency

Respiratory insufficiency after a pneumonectomy may manifest clinically as dyspnea, tachypnea, rapid pulse, anxiety, and, not infrequently, mental confusion. The latter, particularly in elderly persons, may be a prominent and early sign of hypoxia. Results of blood gas studies reveal a fall in both Po_2 and Pco_2 values, although if the situation deteriorates, Pco_2 levels may become elevated. A shift in the mediastinum toward the remaining lung, elevation of the left leaf of the diaphragm caused by gastric distention after a right pneumonectomy, retention of secretions with areas of atelectasis in the remaining lung, and restriction of chest wall movement because of severe postoperative pain are the major mechanical factors that may initiate the problem, and they should be corrected by appropriate therapeutic intervention. In a patient who has undergone a lobectomy or a lesser procedure, shallow breathing, reflex splinting of the chest wall, and impaired cough lead to retention of secretions in the ipsilateral lung. If the airway is not kept clear, atelectasis of the remaining lobe or lobes occurs on the ipsilateral side. If massive atelectasis does develop, the patient becomes acutely short of breath and a variable degree of cyanosis ensues. Along with the tachypnea, a rapid pulse and a sharp temperature elevation occur. Physical findings and, if necessary, radiographic examination of the chest confirm the diagnosis. Prompt tracheobronchial suction, which may include bronchoscopic aspiration of the retained secretions, is indicated. If retention of secretions continues to be troublesome, a tracheostomy may be necessary.

The remaining lung tissue itself may be the underlying element in the causation of respiratory insufficiency. The functional capacity of the residual lung tissue may be insufficient for adequate gas exchange. Impaired ventilatory function preoperatively as determined by the reduction of FEV_1 or MVV from the predicted normal value suggests that respiratory insufficiency may occur postoperatively. Ali (1976) and associates (1980) noted that when the FEV_1 is equal to 2.5 liters or more — >85% of predicted normal — the patient can tolerate a pneumonectomy. When the FEV_1 is between 1 and 2.4 liters — 40 to 80% of predicted normal — the patient has mild to moderate ventilatory impairment. When the FEV_1 is less than 1 liter — <40% of predicted normal — severe impairment is present and pneumonectomy is contraindicated. When an MVV has been performed, a result of less than 45 to 50% of predicted normal contraindicates pneumonectomy.

In patients with borderline pulmonary function, Kristersson (1972), as well as Olsen (1974a,b) and Boysen (1977) and their colleagues, reported that when the predicted postoperative FEV_1 determined by radionuclide studies (see Chapter 18) exceeds 800 ml, the patient should be able to tolerate a pneumonectomy. Nonetheless, the mortality in patients with such compromised pulmonary function exceeds 15%. Ali and associates (1983) showed that patients with reduced perfusion of the tumor-bearing lung — Q <33%, usually in the presence of large T2 or centrally located tumors — may tolerate a pneumonectomy. In 13 such patients, the 30-day postoperative mortality rate was 15%. Additional studies on the effect of pulmonary function on postoperative pneumonectomy mortality rates have been published by Putnam and associates (1990) and are discussed in Chapter 89.

Postoperatively, reduced functional capacity may be exacerbated by varying degrees of inadequate ventilation, diffusion, or perfusion. Retained secretions, patchy areas of atelectasis, and pulmonary edema with resultant functional arteriovenous shunting may further contribute to the problem. Oxygen therapy, tracheobronchial toilet, tracheostomy, and assisted or controlled ventilation may be indicated to sustain the patient over the acute phase.

Pulmonary insufficiency, although less common than after pneumonectomy, may occur after a lobectomy, even in the absence of other complications, and is most often related to the preoperative selection of the patients. The management of postoperative respiratory insufficiency is discussed in Chapter 25.

Pulmonary Atelectasis and Pneumonia

Atelectasis, primarily as the result of retained secretions with the subsequent lack of aeration of variable parts of the remaining pulmonary parenchyma, can be observed in many patients after pulmonary resection. The events leading to the retention of secretions and the management of atelectasis were discussed in the section concerning respiratory insufficiency.

In some patients, infection may be superimposed on unresolved atelectatic areas or may also result from unrecognized episodes of aspiration. The true incidence of postoperative pneumonia is difficult to establish; in most reviews, this complication is considered together with atelectasis and major problems associated with retention of secretions. Keagy and associates (1985) noted this conglomerate group of complications in 7% of 369 patients who had undergone lobectomy, and Waki and colleagues (1989) reported an incidence of 6.6% in 197 patients who had undergone a pneumonectomy. Although the overall incidence of pneumonia was not recorded, Von Knorring and associates (1992) reported it was the cause of death in 1.3% of 598 patients undergoing resection for lung cancer. Tedder and associates (1992), in a review of bronchoplastic procedures, noted that postoperative pneumonia per se occurred in 6.6% of the reported patients and was

responsible for 15.4% of the postoperative deaths observed.

Although data are sparse, it is likely that postoperative pneumonia is most often seen in patients who require prolonged ventilatory support or who have continued inordinate difficulty in clearing their tracheobronchial secretions. Aerobic, anaerobic, and mixed infections occur, and proper collection — bronchoscopic aspiration — and cultural procedures for identification of the offending organism(s) are mandatory (see Chapter 15). Appropriate antibiotics, nutritional support, and good tracheobronchial toilet are essential for recovery. Pseudomonas and Serratia infections, as in other clinical settings, are the most difficult with which to deal.

Lobar Torsion and Gangrene

A 180° rotation of a lobe on its bronchovascular pedicle occasionally is observed intraoperatively with excessive traction and manipulation of the lung during a pulmonary resection. It may also occur spontaneously postoperatively. Rotation is seen most commonly with a freely mobile — complete major and minor fissures — middle lobe on the right, as recorded in a survey of Wong and Goldstraw (1992), but it may occur with either the upper or lower lobe of the left lung as well. If unrecognized and not corrected, vascular occlusion with resultant infarction and gangrene of the involved lobe occurs.

Obviously, the remaining lung after a lobectomy should be inspected to assure its proper position and lack of torsion before closure of the chest incision. Also, a freely mobile middle lobe after either an upper — most commonly associated with torsion of the middle lobe — or lower lobectomy should be stabilized by a number of interrupted sutures to the other remaining lobe to prevent the occurrence of torsion of the middle lobe postoperatively. Such fixation or stabilization is rarely if ever warranted on the left side despite reports of a few isolated cases by Kelly (1977), Linaudais (1980), and Kucich (1989) and their associates.

When this rare event does occur postoperatively, failure of complete expansion and opacification of the lobe — often in an unusual anatomic position — can be observed on the postoperative radiographs. Failure of expansion after the usual tracheobronchial suction requires prompt bronchoscopy. Piccione and Faber (1991) report that bronchoscopy will reveal a compressed bronchus that has a fishmouth appearance and, although the scope may be passed through the obstruction, the involved bronchus will collapse as the scope is withdrawn. Other studies — perfusion scans or angiograms — may be done, but add little to the diagnostic differentiation from a simple atelectatic process.

When torsion of the lobe is suggested by the radiographic and bronchoscopic findings, immediate reoperation is indicated to release the torsion and to stabilize the involved lobe, if viable, in the correct anatomic position. If the lobe is not viable, a lobectomy of the involved middle lobe on the right or a completion pneumonectomy on the left side becomes necessary.

When the torsion remains unrecognized, infarction and gangrene of the involved lobe will occur with the resultant local thoracic and systemic findings of infection. Gangrene of a lobe also may occur in the absence of torsion, as noted by Piccione and Faber (1991), the underlying cause being an unrecognized ligature or compromise of either the venous outflow or of the pulmonary arterial supply of the lobe. In either instance, reoperation and resection of the involved lobe is mandatory. The rarity of the occurrence of lobar gangrene is supported by the data reported by Keagy and associates (1985) in which only one instance of this complication was noted in 224 complications — 0.4% — in 369 patients — 0.27% — who had undergone a lobectomy.

Right Pneumonectomy Syndrome

In infants and young children, and infrequently in adults, excessive mediastinal shift after a right pneumonectomy may cause severe functional problems. The displacement of the heart — counterclockwise rotation — of the great vessels and of the trachea may lead to stretching and narrowing of the left main stem bronchus between the aorta and pulmonary artery, and to compression of the left pulmonary vessels resulting in severe respiratory failure — the right pneumonectomy syndrome. Adams (1972), Szarnicki (1978), and Wasserman (1979) and their associates were among the first to describe this catastrophic event, although Maier and Gould (1953) were the first to describe the pathophysiology resulting in the syndrome in a patient with agenesis of the right lung. The syndrome does not occur after a left pneumonectomy when the intrathoracic vascular anatomy is normal. Quillin and Shackelford (1991), as well as Shepard (1986) and Grillo (1992) and their colleagues, however, have described its occurrence after a left pneumonectomy in patients with a right-sided aortic arch. Bronchoscopic examination and the findings on CT examination of the chest, as described by Shephard and colleagues (1986), are diagnostic (Fig. 28–6). Numerous procedures to fill the right pleural space with various prosthetic materials to prevent the excessive shift have been described by Wasserman (1979), Powell (1979), Riveron (1987), Rasch (1990), and Grillo (1992) and their associates with fair to good results. Direct approach to correct the left main stem

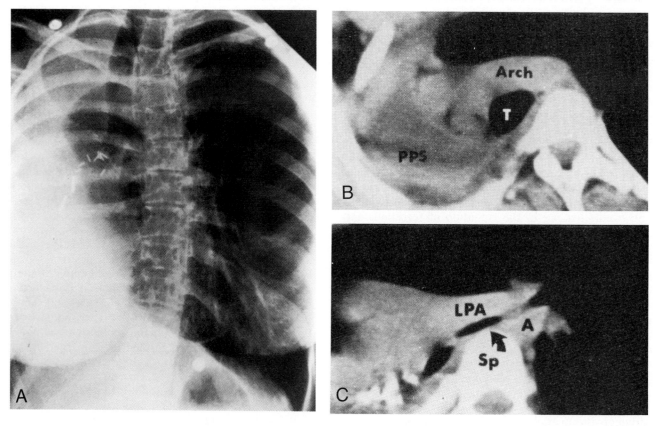

Fig. 28–6. The right postpneumonectomy syndrome. A, PA chest radiograph with shift of the left lung into the right hemithorax. CT scans reveal compression of the left main stem bronchus by the adjacent vessels. Soft tissue windows at the level of the aortic arch (B) and the left pulmonary artery (C) demonstrate a small postpneumonectomy space (PPS). The aortic arch (Arch) and pulmonary artery are rotated counterclockwise. The trachea (T) is to the right of the spine (Sp), and the left main bronchus (arrow) crosses anterior to the thoracic spine and posterior to the left pulmonary artery (LPA). *From* Grillo HC, et al: Postpneumonectomy syndrome: Diagnosis, management, and results. Ann Thorac Surg 54:638, 1992.

bronchial narrowing by use of silastic implants reported by Wasserman and associates (1979) and support of the elongated posterior wall suggested by Nissen (1954) and Herzog and colleagues (1987) also has been used with varying success. Correction of the tracheo- or bronchiomalacia was emphasized by Sheperd and colleagues (1986). As noted subsequently by Grillo and associates (1992), however, the management of concurrent severely malacic airways is difficult. Two of their three patients died despite repair of the airway and they concluded the optimal treatment is unclear.

Cardiac Dysrhythmias

Cardiac arrhythmias after pulmonary resection occur most frequently in patients age 60 years or older and only rarely in anyone under the age of 50 years, as noted by the author and Ujiki (1968). The incidence after pneumonectomy in the older age group is approximately 20 to 30%. After lobectomy, the incidence is lower, but it may be as high as 15 to 20%. This complication is seen only infrequently after lesser resections.

The arrhythmia may be sinus tachycardia, runs of premature ventricular contractions, a nodal rhythm, bradyrhythmia, bigeminy, or auricular fibrillation or flutter or both. Infrequently occurring arrhythmias include paroxysmal atrial tachycardia with block, multifocal atrial tachycardia, ventricular tachycardia, the sick sinus syndrome, and torsades de pointes — atypical ventricular tachycardia. Auricular fibrillation and flutter are the most common.

Abnormal rhythms usually arise during the first postoperative week. Ritchie and associates (1990) showed that with continuous monitoring initiated at the induction of anesthesia, over one half of the arrhythmias are recognized within the first 24 hours of the beginning of the operative procedure — perioperative and early postoperative period. In their experience, this was more often the case after pneumonectomy then after lobectomy.

The duration is variable, and at times, the heart may spontaneously revert to a normal rhythm. This change occurs most often in patients who develop atrial fibrillation. A variable number of patients require therapy with antifibrillatory medication. Those with supraventricular tachycardia and bradyrhythmia usually require treatment. All potentially lethal arrhythmias require urgent therapy.

The cause of the abnormal rhythms is unknown, although mediastinal shift, hypoxia, and abnormal pH of the blood, as well as other factors, have been implicated but unproved. What is known is that the occurrence of an arrhythmia is more common with advanced age of the patient, those with coronary artery disease, and with a more extensive operative procedure, the incidence being highest after intrapericardial ligation of the pulmonary vessels. Krowka and colleagues (1987) also noted that it occurred frequently in the postpneumonectomy patient who develops postoperative interstitial pulmonary edema or perihilar edema. Previous cardiac arrhythmia, frequent premature atrial or ventricular contractions preoperatively, and a complete or incomplete right bundle branch block on the preoperative electrocardiogram have also been associated with increased incidence of this complication. Von Knorring and associates (1992) also recorded that an abnormal response to exercise and intraoperative hypotension were strong predictors of the possible postoperative occurrence of cardiac arrhythmias.

As a result of the high incidence and the potential seriousness of postoperative arrhythmias, particularly if persistent or recurrent, many clinicians use prophylactic digitalization in the older patient undergoing pneumonectomy or lobectomy. The potential danger of digitalis toxicity must be considered, but the advantages of its prophylactic use in reducing the incidence of arrhythmias, as shown by Wheat and Burford (1961) as well as by the author and Ujiki (1968), seem to outweigh this possible danger. Many in our group use this prophylaxis in all patients 60 years of age or older when contemplating a pulmonary resection. The aforementioned clinical trials, however, were retrospective and uncontrolled. Many surgeons, therefore, question the prophylactic use of digitalis. Krowka and associates (1987) from the Mayo Clinic are opposed to its use, but one must cite the high incidence of arrhythmias their patients experienced as well as the 25% incidence of mortality associated with these complications. In a nonrandomized study, Patel and colleagues (1992) also found the use of prophylactic digitalization to be of no benefit in the reduction of the occurrence of postpneumonectomy arrhythmias. These authors reported a 26% mortality rate with this complication. In a prospective, controlled, randomized study, Ritchie and associates (1990, 1992) reported that prophylactic digitalization was of no benefit, but the design of their study was different than that of the previous clinical trials.

Borgeat and associates (1989) suggested the use of flecainide as a prophylactic measure to prevent the development of postoperative arrhythmias. They recommended a loading dose of 2 mg/kg in 1 hour after admission to the postoperative unit, followed by a maintenance infusion at a rate of 0.15 mg/kg/hour up to 72 hours postoperatively. A significant reduction in the number of arrhythmias was noted as compared to a randomized control group that received only a placebo. In a subsequent report by Borgeat and colleagues (1991), a similar decrease in the incidence of postsurgical arrhythmias was observed in a flecainide-treated group as compared to a control group of patients who received digoxin prophylactically. In both studies, the incidence of arrhythmias was essentially the same in the placebo- and the digoxin-treated patients. The authors concluded that the use of flecainide was a safe and effective prophylactic measure to reduce the high incidence of cardiac arrhythmias seen after noncardiac general thoracic surgical procedures. This conclusion must be confirmed by additional studies.

When prophylactic digitalization has not been used and an atrial arrhythmia occurs postoperatively that does not revert spontaneously to a normal rhythm, intravenous administration of digoxin is begun and repeated at 4-hour intervals up to a loading dose of 1 mg. If the rhythm fails to convert back to normal — typically, 80% of patients respond to this regimen — verapamil may be given — 5 mg intravenously over 2 to 3 minutes and may be repeated in 10 minutes if necessary. Pairolero and Payne (1983) suggested the use of oral quinidine sulfate — 200 mg 3 times per day — to control the dysrhythmia. Electrical cardioversion is rarely necessary.

Ventricular tachycardia should be treated promptly with an intravenous bolus of lidocaine hydrochloride, 50 to 100 mg. Once controlled, a lidocaine drip — 1 to 3 mg/minute — should be continued.

Bradyrhythmia should be managed by the use of atropine or intravenous isoproterenol. Cardiac pacing may be required when a third-degree atrioventricular block or a sick sinus syndrome is present.

Myocardial Ischemia and Myocardial Infarction

Transient myocardial ischemia is uncommon, but von Knorring and associates (1992) reported this finding in 3.8% of 598 patients undergoing resection for lung cancer. It has been suggested that patients with coronary heart disease and previous myocardial infarction may be more prone to develop this complication. Silent ischemia may be identified by postoperative monitoring and is usually seen on the second to fourth postoperative day. Khan (1992) suggested that such patients receive enteric-coated aspirin, 160 to 325 mg daily, as well as an appropriate beta blocker, although this therapy has not been proven in clinical trials to protect the patient from infarction and death.

Myocardial infarction was recorded in 1.2% of patients reported by the aforementioned authors, but of more significance was that the event was fatal in 57% of the patients in whom it occurred. The presence of coronary artery disease may be a predictor of the possible occurrence of a postoperative myocardial infarction, but the significance of preoperative ST-, T-changes on the electrocardiogram as predictors of the possibility of a postoperative myocardial infarct is controversial. The appropriate cardiac evaluation of the cardiac status of a prospective thoracic surgical patient is discussed in Chapters 19 and 89.

Subcutaneous Emphysema

Air trapped within the pleural space after a pneumonectomy, or air from a leak that is not being removed effectively by the chest tube drainage system after a lobectomy or lesser resection, may be forced out through the incision in the rib cage into the soft tissues of the chest wall on change of position or coughing. This subcutaneous air may be localized only to the wound area, but when excessive amounts of air are forced into the adjacent tissue planes, it may extend up into the face and down to the groin and into the scrotum. No specific therapy other than to improve and ensure patency of the drainage system is required. On occasion, a sudden massive air leak may be indicative of the occurrence of a bronchopleural fistula, but in most instances, subcutaneous emphysema is a benign, self-limiting situation. Upper airway obstruction as the result of the emphysema is a rare complication and the use of cervical incisions to decompress the area is not indicated. If airway obstruction is suggested clinically, endotracheal intubation should be done.

Residual Pleural Air Space

A persistent residual air space frequently occurs after a lobectomy. It is more common in older persons and in those who have undergone resection for pulmonary tuberculosis than in other lobectomy patients. After resection for pulmonary tuberculosis, the incidence is as high as 21%. Approximately two thirds to four fifths of these persistent spaces do not cause symptoms, and the clinical course of the patient is unaffected by their presence. An asymptomatic space gradually disappears over a period of months, by absorption of the gases within the space and further expansion of the remaining lung or by the deposition of a pleural peel in the area. The other one fifth to one third of the air spaces, however, do cause symptoms and require surgical intervention of varying magnitude for their eventual control. The symptoms may consist of pain, dyspnea, hemoptysis, fever, or signs of continued air leak. The persistent air leak may be caused by seepage from the alveoli — a small peripheral parenchymal fistula — or from a frank bronchopleural fistula. With alveolar seepage, the composition of the gas in the space is the same as that of the gas in the alveolar spaces rather than the gas in the venous blood. Although it is impossible to maintain a negative pressure within the space because of this seepage, the space may remain sterile. In the presence of frank bronchopleural fistula, however, not only is a major air leak present, but also an empyema ultimately develops. Such a space is controlled by drainage and obliteration of the space, as discussed in Chapter 56.

The incidence of persistent pleural air space after a segmentectomy is as high as 33% in patients with pulmonary tuberculosis (Fig. 28–7), but it is less after one for the removal of a lung tumor. Compared with the pleural air spaces occurring after a lobectomy, however, a smaller percentage of those occurring after segmentectomy become symptomatic. When serious complications develop as a result of the space, they are most likely septic.

Persistent air spaces after a wedge resection occur infrequently. The incidence is less than 10%. Almost all are benign and resolve without treatment.

Persistent Air Leak

After pulmonary resections of lesser magnitude than a pneumonectomy, an air leak from a residual raw parenchymal surface is a common occurrence. With complete re-expansion of the lung and obliteration of

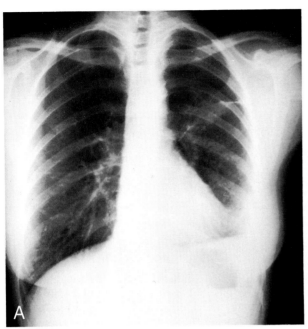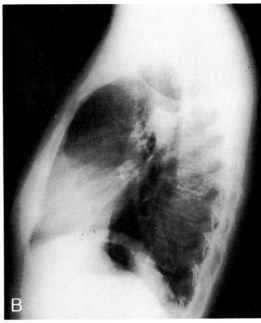

Fig. 28–7. Posteroanterior (A) and lateral (B) chest radiographs reveal an asymptomatic air space 6 weeks after a left apical posterior segmentectomy was performed for treatment of pulmonary tuberculosis.

pleural space, the leak usually stops in 2 to 3 days; the persistence of the leak beyond 7 days is considered abnormal. Various maneuvers — increasing or decreasing the suction applied to the water seal system, conversion to water seal drainage only, placement of additional chest tubes — may be tried empirically. In most instances, the air leak will stop even if the space persists.

There is no one correct way to manage a persistent air leak. The ingenuity and experience of the surgeon greatly affect the approach in the individual patient in whom infection of any accompanying air space is absent. Identification and embolization of the subsegmental bronchus supplying the leaking site may be attempted. It is possible that a thoracoscopic approach and the use of fibrin glue may be useful. Undue haste for re-exploration is to be avoided. If sepsis develops, however, the presence of a frank bronchopleural fistula must be assumed and appropriate management to resolve the issue is warranted.

Bronchopleural Fistula

A bronchopleural fistula is observed in approximately 1 to 4% of patients after a pneumonectomy or a lobectomy and less often after a segmentectomy or lesser procedure. Vester and associates (1991) reported an incidence of 3.9% after 503 pneumonectomies — 3.7% after stapled closure of the bronchus and 12.5% after manual closure; 1.1% incidence after 1083 lobectomies; and 0.3% after 650 segmentectomies. Asamura and associates (1992) reported an incidence of 2.1% after 2359 pulmonary resections for lung cancer. Of interest is the report of Sarsam and Moussali (1989), who recorded no fistulas after the use of a bronchoplastic

method of closure of the bronchial stump — using a membranous flap from the posterior bronchial wall described by Jack (1965) — in a series of 332 pneumonectomies despite the use of chronic catgut as the suture material.

A bronchopleural fistula is more common after resections for inflammatory disease of the lung, especially in patients with active tuberculosis and positive sputum culture — Pomerantz and colleagues (1991) noted a 10.5% incidence after resection in 85 patients with resistant mycobacterial infections; in patients who received a full course of preoperative mediastinal and hilar irradiation — Yashar and associates (1991) reported an incidence of 9.6% after resection in 31 patients who had received preoperative chemotherapy and irradiation; and in patients undergoing a completion pneumonectomy for persistent or recurrent inflammatory disease. In a multivariate analysis of the 1360 most recent lung cancer resections reported by Asamura and associates (1992), the significant risk factors for the occurrence of a bronchopleural fistula were: pneumonectomy, residual tumor at the bronchial stump, preoperative irradiation, and the presence of diabetes. These authors also noted that most bronchopleural fistulae occur after resections of the right lung, particularly a right pneumonectomy (Table 28–2), as have most surgeons.

Early, 1 to 2 days, even up to 7 days, after a resection, a bronchopleural fistula may occur because of a technically poor closure of the bronchial stump. After a pneumonectomy, an early bronchopleural fistula manifests by a massive air leak with the development of a progressive increase in clinically evident subcutaneous emphysema; a small amount of subcutaneous emphysema is normally seen, as some of the air in the

Table 28-2. **Prevalence of Bronchopleural Fistula According to Side of Resection**

Resection	Percent of Operations Performed	
	Right Side	Left Side
Segmentectomy	0	0
Lobectomy	1.7	0.3
Pneumonectomy	8.6	2.3
Bronchoplasty	6.9	0
Pleuropneumonectomy	25.0	0
All resections	3.0	0.9

Adapted from Asamura H, et al: Bronchopleural fistulas associated with lung cancer operations. Univariate and multivariate analysis of risk factors, management and outcome. J Thorac Cardiovasc Surg *104*:1456, 1992.

postpneumonectomy space at the time of closure is expelled into the tissue of the chest wall with coughing or is forced out with a rapid accumulation of fluid within the space. Along with the development of the massive subcutaneous emphysema, the patient may exhibit varying degrees of respiratory insufficiency, because the bronchopleural fistula physiologically represents a modified open pneumothorax. Ventilatory support, often best accomplished by the use of intubation and jet ventilation, may be necessary at this stage.

When the bronchial leak occurs later in the postoperative course, usually postoperative day 8 or 10, it may be caused by failure of healing because of inadequate viable tissue coverage of the stump or as the result of infection of the fluid within the space and rupture of the empyema through the suture line of the bronchial stump. At this stage, the patient coughs up variable quantities of serosanguinous, frothy fluid from the respiratory tract. Danger of flooding of the remaining lung is present. The patient should be placed with the affected side down and the head elevated. Prompt, emergent drainage of the affected pleural space is indicated.

When a bronchopleural fistula occurs later than 2 weeks after pneumonectomy, it is most likely the result of rupture of a frank empyema through the bronchial stump, although at times, failure of healing of the bronchial stump may be the underlying cause. Clinically, the patient is most likely febrile and has a cough productive of purulent sputum. Hemoptysis may or may not occur.

An occult bronchopleural fistula — without expectoration of pleural fluid — occasionally occurs. A fall of more than 1.5 cm in the height of the fluid level should arouse suspicion. Whether or not the fluid escapes through the bronchus and is swallowed unnoticed by the patient or is lost by absorption through the parietal pleura as the result of the increased intrapleural pressure, which becomes potentially greater than atmospheric pressure, is unresolved. Nonetheless, confirmation of the diagnosis can be sought by instilling methylene blue into the postpneumonectomy space and watching for its appearance in the sputum. The management of an occult bronchopleural fistula poses a vexing clinical problem. When the patient remains asymptomatic and no signs of clinical infection are present, expectant treatment with systemic antibiotics and close observation is acceptable, as suggested by O'Meara and Slade (1974). More often than not, there will be no further difficulty. If any finding of clinical infection occurs, however, prompt drainage of the pleural space is mandatory.

The management of a clinically evident bronchopleural fistula depends on the time of its development postoperatively and its underlying cause. Early in the postoperative period, reoperation and repair of the bronchial stump may be indicated. With operative repair, coverage of the new bronchial suture line is mandatory. A transposed muscle flap, the pericardial fat pad, or an omental pedicle flap may be used (see Chapter 56). Otherwise, initial evacuation of the fluid in the affected pleural space and institution of proper drainage are indicated. Jensen and Sharma (1985) suggested using fibrin glue to occlude the opening when the fistula is small. Moritz (personal communication, 1986) had success with this method for closing small bronchopleural fistulas that developed from a technical failure with the use of a mechanical stapling device. Glover and associates (1987) also reported successful use of fibrin glue for the closure of small bronchopleural fistulas after similar suture line failures. In most situations, however, in the presence of a major bronchopleural fistula, additional measures to achieve closure of the fistula and control of the associated empyema are necessary. The various methods of drainage of the pleural space, obliteration of the pleural space, and ultimate closure of the fistula are discussed in detail in Chapter 56.

Trans-sternal transpericardial exposure and division of a long bronchial stump associated with a bronchopleural fistula has become popular. The bronchus must be divided and each end is closed by the appropriate suture technique. When the distal stump cannot be removed, a tissue flap, preferably muscle, should be transposed between the two divided ends. Simple stapling of the long stump proximal to the leak is not to be done; failure with refistulization inevitably occurs. Abruzzini (1961) was one of the first to report the division of the stump to control a fistula. Maassen (1975), Bruni (1987), Perelman (1987), and Perelman and Ambatiello (1970) also recorded the use of this procedure in Europe. In the United States, Baldwin and Mark (1985) and Cosgrove (1985), and in Canada, Ginsberg and associates (1989) also have reported its use. The technique and indications for the trans-sternal approach for the closure of a bronchopleural fistula are presented in Chapter 36. Perelman and associates (1987) also described a right posterior approach to the left main bronchial stump (Fig. 28-8) that was accomplished in 25 patients, with good results in 20 patients. Four late deaths occurred, two related to bronchial recanalization and two related to progressive empyema.

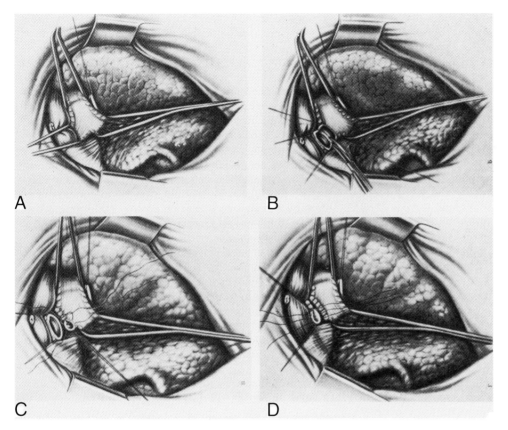

Fig. 28–8. Right posterior approach to the left main stem bronchus. *A*, The trachea and both main stem bronchi have been isolated and tapes placed about them. *B*, The left main stem bronchial stump is dissected off the trachea. *C*, The trachea is closed with interrupted sutures. *D*, The remaining distal stump is closed in a similar manner. *From* Perelman MI, et al: Bronchopleural fistula: Surgery after pneumonectomy. *In* Grillo HC, Eschapasse H: Major Challenges: International Trends In General Thoracic Surgery. Vol. 2. Philadelphia: WB Saunders, 1987.

Bronchopleural fistula also may occur after a lobectomy; at present, the incidence is low. The management of the open bronchial stump and the usually associated empyema space is like that following a pneumonectomy except that the presence of pulmonary tissue in the hemithorax modifies their management to a variable extent (see Chapter 56). Occasionally, it is advisable to perform a completion pneumonectomy, although as noted by McGovern and colleagues (1988), the complication rate is high — over 50%. Deslauriers (1988) emphasized the hazard of previous irradiation when a completion pneumonectomy is contemplated. He also noted that when a bronchial dehiscence is the indication for the completion pneumonectomy accompanying a "benign" inflammatory process, other therapeutic options deserve serious consideration whenever possible before resorting to this procedure because of its high morbidity and mortality rates in this situation. Bronchial dehiscence and fistula formation also occur after broncho- or tracheoplastic procedures. In a survey of 1562 such procedures performed in Japan, Maeda and associates (1989) reported this complication to have occurred in 5.6% of cases and to have resulted in death in 47.7% of the patients in whom it occurred, for an overall mortality rate of 2.7%. This complication is discussed in more detail in the specific chapters related to these procedures (see Chapters 31 and 35).

The overall mortality rate after the development of a bronchopleural fistula is variable. Rates as low as 16% to as high as 71% have been recorded. Most of the series reported have not comprised comparable patients, disease states, or operations, so that it is impossible to state categorically which patients are most likely to succumb as a result of the complication. Apparently, however, those who have undergone an extensive peribronchial dissection or a right-sided pneumonectomy or who received preoperative irradiation are at the greatest risk. Others at high risk are those who have undergone a tracheo- or bronchoplastic procedure, have borderline pulmonary function, have a serious comorbid disease, or are elderly.

Bronchovascular Fistula

The occurrence of a bronchovascular fistula with fatal hemorrhage is a rare event after a standard pulmonary resection, but it may develop in approximately 3% of patients who have undergone a bronchoplastic procedure, according to the review of Tedder and associates (1992). In most instances, the fistula is the result of a small, clinically asymptomatic abscess from a minor leak of the bronchial suture line that erodes into an adjacent ligated pulmonary artery or one of its branches or through the suture line of an adjacent angioplastic repair. It is best avoided by interposition of a viable tissue flap between the bronchial and vascular suture lines at the time of operation.

Empyema

Empyema occurs less often than it once did, but it still is seen after a pneumonectomy in 1 to 3% of patients. It may or may not be associated with a bronchopleural fistula. At operation, most surgeons instill antibiotic solutions into the pneumonectomy space, and systemic antibiotics are given postoperatively to lessen the likelihood of the development of this septic complication. If gross contamination occurs at operation or if reoperation is necessary for control of the postoperative hemothorax or early bronchial leak, the risk of developing empyema increases. Gaud (1987) noted that mechanical ventilation postoperatively also increases the risk of empyema.

When empyema occurs, the patient shows a greater or lesser degree of systemic toxicity, the white blood count is elevated, appetite is poor, and general deterioration occurs. Drainage of the space is indicated, bacterial cultures and sensitivity studies of the fluid are obtained, and definitive management of the empyema is carried out as discussed in Chapter 56.

As after pneumonectomy, empyema with or without a bronchopleural fistula is one of the major postoperative complications of lobectomy. It is more common after resections for inflammatory disease than after those for tumor. Interestingly, a residual basal space seems to be associated more commonly with subsequent infection than the more frequent apical residual spaces. The initial treatment consists of adequate drainage. The space must be obliterated subsequently, but this is less of a problem after a lobectomy than after pneumonectomy because lung tissue remains. It is noteworthy, however, that pulmonary function on the involved side generally is reduced by the development and the subsequent treatment of the empyema.

Wound Infections

Infection of a thoracotomy or sternotomy incision after a pulmonary resection is rare. When present, the usual signs and symptoms of infection are present. Open drainage and antibiotics are indicated in its management.

Wound Dehiscence

Complete breakdown of a thoracic incision after a pulmonary resection is even less common than a wound infection. Early dehiscence requires prompt reclosure, but late dehiscence, most often the result of wound infection, may be managed initially by local debridement and pleural drainage with subsequent reclosure when the infection has been controlled.

Postresection Chylothorax

Injury to the thoracic duct with subsequent chylothorax is rare after pulmonary resection. Simpson (1990) stated that the incidence of such injury was less than 0.05%; however, Brie and associates (1990) recorded an incidence of 0.3% in their experience. Several decades ago — 1950 to 1970 — most injuries followed resections for benign diseases — pulmonary tuberculosis — but at present, they are more common after

resections for the management of carcinoma of the lung, particularly during aggressive resection of the local tumor or mediastinal lymph nodes involved by extensive metastatic disease. The injury to the duct may occur anywhere along its course or to one of the small lymphatic channels from the lung or mediastinal lymph nodes that enter directly into the thoracic duct, which were demonstrated by the anatomic study of Riquet and associates (1989). Such injuries have occurred after lobectomies — upper and lower — or after pneumonectomies on either side. The injury is not generally recognized until the patient resumes oral alimentation. In the postlobectomy patient, the chylothorax is manifest by the change in the character of the drainage to a milky fluid and an increase in the amount of drainage. In the postpneumonectomy patient, as noted by Karwande (1986) and Brie (1990) and their colleagues, a rapid accumulation of fluid within the postpneumonectomy space may result in a shift of the mediastinum and heart toward the contralateral hemithorax with resultant compression of the remaining lung and subsequent respiratory compromise — a tension chylothorax. Thoracentesis will reveal the characteristic milky fluid, and immediate closed tube thoracostomy is indicated.

Ngan and colleagues (1988) suggested that lymphangiography be performed soon after the diagnosis is made. Standard lipiodol lymphangiography, despite the risk of an occasional pulmonary complication, may demonstrate the site of the leak or the lack of one at best. Nuclear lymphangiography, although used by Rice and associates (1987), may not be successful in this regard. Lipiodol lymphangiography is both diagnostic and prognostic. When no major leak is seen and the contrast material appears at the terminus of the thoracic duct, certain investigators believe that conservative management is more likely to be successful.

Definitive therapy in either situation — postlobectomy or postpneumonectomy — consists of an initial trial period of expectant therapy with continued drainage and total parenteral nutrition for 7 to 14 days. With re-expansion of the remaining lung in the postlobectomy patient, the leak frequently seals over — approximately 50% or more of patients, but closure of the leak from the thoracic duct injury is less likely to occur in the postpneumonectomy patient. In a postpneumonectomy patient, a continued leak of more than 300 ml per day is an indication for surgical intervention with ligation of the thoracic duct as described in Chapter 59. In the series reported by Brie and associates (1990), this step was necessary in all four patients who had undergone a pneumonectomy. In the postlobectomy patient, a persistent leak of 500 ml per day is an indication of failure of conservative management. Operative intervention — ligation of either the leak or the proximal thoracic duct — is then required. Stenzl (1983) and Akaogi (1989) and their associates reported successful closure of the leak with the use of fibrin glue applied through tube thoracostomies. Morita and colleagues

(1990) have also been successful in using a thoracoscopic approach.

Esophageal Injury

Injury to the esophagus may occur during a difficult dissection for a pneumonectomy performed because of either inflammatory or extensive neoplastic disease. Shama and Odell (1985) reported an incidence of 0.5% in a series of 869 pneumonectomies for inflammatory disease. Van den Bosch and associates (1980) noted that most occurred on the right — 92% — and after resection of inflammatory disease in two thirds of all cases. Benjamin and colleagues (1969) reported its occurrence during resection for carcinoma. Most esophagopleural fistulae after resection for cancer occur late postoperatively. Evans (1972) believes most are the result of rupture of a peribronchial abscess into the esophagus. He noted that seven of the eight cases he reported were associated with a bronchopleural fistula. The events, however, could just as well be reversed — an unrecognized esophageal leak resulting in an empyema that subsequently erodes through the bronchial stump. This explanation seems more reasonable because rupture of an abscess through an uninjured esophageal wall is unlikely.

When recognized at operation, immediate repair usually is successful, but if the injury is overlooked, mediastinitis and thoracic empyema occur. Recognition of the source of the infection may be elusive until oral feedings are observed in the thoracic drainage. The injury may be confirmed by a barium swallow. Treatment is use of one of the many options for any late recognized esophageal injury, as described in Chapter 117.

Peripheral Tumor Embolus

A tumor embolus may be dislodged from an involved pulmonary vein during the isolation and ligation of the vessel during the operative procedure. Whyte and associates (1992) reported 2 cases and reviewed an additional 18 cases of embolization in patients with bronchial carcinoma; an additional 5 patients had a sarcomatous lesion. The site of embolization was the aortic bifurcation or femoral vessels in 50% of patients. Other sites included vessels of the upper extremities, cerebral circulation, and the mesenteric arteries. Fifty percent of the patients died as a result of the embolic episode. Removal of the embolus is indicated when possible. Those who survive such an episode, according to Heitmiller (1992), die as a result of the metastatic spread of the original tumor — all have stage IIIb disease — and not of the effects of the embolic episode per se. Prevention of embolization when a major pulmonary vein is involved is primarily by proximal intrapericardial ligation of the vessel, including excision of a portion of the adjacent atrium if necessary. The use of a cardiopulmonary bypass, as suggested by Mansour and colleagues (1988), to remove tumor from the atrium, except in patients with a low grade sarcoma,

would appear to be an inappropriate procedure in patients with lung cancer.

Injury to Intrathoracic Nerves

Phrenic Nerve. Unsuspected injury to the phrenic nerve rarely occurs during pulmonary resection. Occasionally, it can occur when dense mediastinal adhesions need to be divided for hilar exposure, but more often the nerve is knowingly sacrificed in the removal of a tumor invading the mediastinum or in the excision of metastatic nodes anterior to the superior pulmonary vein. Purposeful injury or division of the nerve to paralyze the hemidiaphragm to reduce the volume of the ipsilateral hemithorax is to be avoided as previously noted, except in unusual circumstances.

Left Recurrent Nerve. Injury to this nerve results in hoarseness, which initially may be disturbing to the patient. Dissection of mediastinal lymph nodes in the aortopulmonary window at the ligamentum arteriosum should be done carefully and exposure of the nerve at this site may be helpful in avoiding its injury. In a series of complete mediastinal lymph node dissections in patients with lung cancer, unintentional injury was observed in 3 of 62 patients by Bollen and associates (1992). The number of left-sided dissections was not recorded, so the actual incidence of this injury remains unknown. It should be noted that this injury usually is not recorded by the many advocates of systematic lymph node dissection in lung cancer patients.

In patients who have received neoadjuvant therapy for locally advanced lesions, injury to or the necessary removal of either the vagus or phrenic nerves because of the extent of the disease process, as noted by Yashar and colleagues (1992), may increase the number of these injuries in the future.

REFERENCES

Abbey Smith R: Long-term follow-up after operation for lung carcinoma. Thorax 25:62, 1970.

Abruzzini P: Trattenento chirurgico della fistule del broncho principale consecutive a pneumonectomia per tubercolosi. Chir Torac 14:165, 1961.

Adams HP, et al: Severe airway obstruction caused by mediastinal displacement after right pneumonectomy in a child. A case report. J Thorac Cardiovasc Surg 63:534, 1972.

Akaogi E, et al: Treatment of postoperative chylothorax with intrapleural fibrin glue. Ann Thorac Surg 48:116, 1989.

Ali MK: Preoperative pulmonary function evaluation for the lung cancer patient. In Clark RL, Howe CD (eds): Cancer Patients Care at M.D. Anderson Hospital and Tumor Institute. Chicago: Year Book, 1976.

Ali MK, et al: Predicting loss of pulmonary function after pulmonary resection for bronchogenic carcinoma. Chest 77:337, 1980.

Ali MK, et al: Regional and overall pulmonary function changes in lung cancer. J Thorac Cardiovasc Surg 86:1, 1983.

Asamura H, et al: Bronchopleural fistulas associated with lung cancer operations. Univariate and multivariate analysis of risk factors, management and outcome. J Thorac Cardiovasc Surg 104:1456, 1992.

Baldwin JC, Mark JBD: Treatment of bronchopleural fistula after pneumonectomy. J Thorac Cardiovasc Surg 90:813, 1985.

Benfield JR: Invited commentary of Short HD: Paraplegia associated with the use of oxidized cellulose in posterolateral thoracotomy incisions. Ann Thorac Surg 50:290, 1990.

Benjamin I, Olsen AM, Ellis FH, Jr: Esophagopleural fistula: A rare postpneumonectomy complication. Ann Thorac Surg 7:139, 1969.

Berend N, Woolcock AJ, Marlin GE: Effects of lobectomy on lung function. Thorax 35:145, 1980.

Biondetti PR, et al: Evaluation of post-pneumonectomy space by computed tomography. J Comput Assist Tomogr 6:238, 1982.

Bollen ECM, et al: Mediastinal lymph node dissection in resected lung cancer. Morbidity and accuracy of staging. Ann Thorac Surg 55:961, 1993.

Borgeat A, et al: Prevention of arrhythmias by flecainide after noncardiac thoracic surgery. Ann Thorac Surg 48:232, 1989.

Borgeat A, et al: Prevention of arrhythmias after noncardiac thoracic surgery: Flecainide versus digoxin. Ann Thorac Surg 51:964, 1991.

Boysen PG, et al: Prospective evaluation for pneumonectomy using the 99m technetium quantitative perfusion lung scan. Chest 72:422, 1977.

Brewer LA III, Bai AF: Surgery of the bronchi and trachea. Experience with the pedicled pericardial fat graft reinforcement. Am J Surg 89:331, 1955.

Brewer LA, Bai AF, Jones WM: The development of the pleural partition to prevent overexpansion of the lung following partial pulmonary resection. J Thorac Surg 31:165, 1956.

Brewer LA III, et al: Bronchial closure in pulmonary resection. A clinical and experimental study using a pedicled pericardial fat graft reinforcement. J Thorac Surg 26:507, 1953.

Brie M, et al: Chylothorax complicating pulmonary resection. In Deslauriers J, Lacquet LK (eds): Thoracic Surgery: Surgical Management of Pleural Diseases. St. Louis: CV Mosby, 1990.

Bruni F: Bronchopleural fistula: Treatment of lung stump after pneumonectomy. In Eschapasse H, Grillo H (eds): International Trends in General Thoracic Surgery. Vol. 2. Philadelphia: WB Saunders, 1987.

Cagle PT, Thurlbeck WM: Postpneumonectomy compensatory lung growth. Am Rev Respir Dis 138:1314, 1988.

Chuang TH, et al: Pulmonary embolization from vascular stump thrombosis following pneumonectomy. Ann Thorac Surg 2:290, 1966.

Conlan AA: Prophylaxis and management of postlobectomy infected spaces. In Deslauriers J, Lacquet LK (eds): Thoracic Surgery: Surgical Management of Pleural Diseases. St. Louis: CV Mosby, 1990, p 279.

Cosgrove DM III: Closure of postpneumonectomy bronchopleural fistula. Presented at the Clinical Congress, American College of Surgeons. Thoracic Surgery Postgraduate Course, Chicago. October 15, 1985.

Cybulsky IJ, et al: Prognostic significance of computed tomography in resected N_2 lung cancer. Ann Thorac Surg 54:533, 1992.

Dartevelle PG, et al: Tracheal–sleeve pneumonectomy for bronchogenic carcinoma: report of 55 cases. Ann Thorac Surg 46:68, 1988.

Deslauriers J: Indications for completion pneumonectomy. Ann Thorac Surg 46:133, 1988.

Evans JP: Post-pneumonectomy oesophageal fistula. Thorax 27:674, 1972.

Faber LP: Malignant pleural mesothelioma: Operative treatment by extrapleural pneumonectomy. In Kittle CF (ed): Current Controversies in Thoracic Surgery. Philadelphia: WB Saunders, 1986.

Gaensler EA, Strieder JW: Progressive changes in pulmonary function after pneumonectomy. J Thorac Surg 22:1, 1951.

Gaud C: Role of mechanical ventilation in the genesis of empyema and bronchopleural fistula. In Grillo HC, Eschapasse H (eds): International Trends in General Thoracic Surgery. Vol 2. Philadelphia: WB Saunders, 1987, p 447.

Ginsberg RJ, et al: Modern thirty-day operative mortality for surgical resections in lung cancer. J Thorac Cardiovasc Surg 86:654, 1983.

Ginsberg RJ, et al: Closure of chronic postpneumonectomy bronchopleural fistula using the transsternal transpericardial approach. Ann Thorac Surg 47:231, 1989.

Ginsberg RJ, Rubinstein L, for the Lung Cancer Study Group: Patients with T_1N_0 non-SCLC lung cancer. Lung Cancer 7(Suppl):83 (Abstract 304), 1991.

Glover W, et al: Fibrin glue applications through the fiberoptic bronchoscope: Closure of bronchopleural fistulas. J Thorac Cardiovasc Surg 93:470, 1987.

Grillo HC: Notes on the windpipe. Ann Thorac Surg 47:9, 1989.

Grillo HC, et al: Postpneumonectomy syndrome: Diagnosis, management and results. Ann Thorac Surg 54:638, 1992.

Hakim M, Milstein BB: Role of automatic staplers in the etiology of bronchopleural fistula. Thorax 40:27, 1985.

Heitmiller RF: Prognostic significance of massive bronchogenic tumor embolus. Ann Thorac Surg 53:153, 1992.

Herzog H, et al: Surgical therapy for expiratory collapse of the trachea and large bronchi. In Grillo HC, Eschapasse H (eds): International Trends in General Thoracic Surgery. Vol 2. Philadelphia: WB Saunders, 1987, p 74.

Hood RM: Operations involving the lungs. In Hood RM (ed): Techniques in General Thoracic Surgery. Philadelphia: WB Saunders, 1985.

Ishida T, et al: Long-term results of operation for non-small cell lung cancer in the elderly. Ann Thorac Surg 50:919, 1990.

Jack GD: Bronchial closure. Thorax 20:8, 1965.

Jensen C, Sharma P: Use of fibrin glue in thoracic surgery. Ann Thorac Surg 39:521, 1985.

Jensik RJ: The extent of resection for localized lung cancer: Segmental resection. In Kittle CF (ed): Current Controversies in Thoracic Surgery. Philadelphia, WB Saunders, 1986.

Karwande SV, Wlocoot MW, Guy WA: Postpneumonectomy tension chylothorax. Ann Thorac Surg 42:585, 1986.

Keagy BA, et al: Elective pulmonary lobectomy: Factors associated with morbidity and operative mortality. Ann Thorac Surg 40:349, 1985.

Kelly MV, Kygere R, Miller WC: Postoperative lobar torsion and gangrene. Thorax 32:501, 1977.

Khan MG: Angina. In Khan MG: Cardiac and Pulmonary Management. Philadelphia: Lea & Febiger, 1993, p 57.

Kristersson S, et al: Prediction of pulmonary function loss due to pneumonectomy using I_{33}Xe-radiospirometry. Chest 62:649, 1972.

Krowka MJ, et al: Cardiac dysrhythmia following pneumonectomy. Chest 91:490, 1987.

Kucich VA, Villarreal JR, Schwartz DB: Left upper lobe torsion following lower lobe resection. Early recognition of a rare complication. Chest 95:1146, 1989.

Ladurie M L, Ranson-Bitker B: Quality of life following resection for lung cancer. In Delarue NC, Eschapasse H (eds): Lung Cancer. International Trends in General Thoracic Surgery. Vol. I. Philadelphia: WB Saunders, 1985, p 296.

Laforet EG, Boyd TF: Balanced drainage of the pneumonectomy space. Surg Gynecol Obstet 118:1051, 1964.

Linaudais W, Cavanaugh DG, Greer TM: Rapid postoperative thoracotomy for torsion of the left lower lobe: Case report. Milit Med 145:698, 1980.

Lynn RB: The prevention of postresection spaces following resection for pulmonary tuberculosis. Surg Gynecol Obstet 111:647, 1960.

Maassen W: The transsternal and transpericardial approach for surgical treatment of fistulas of the main bronchus after pneumonectomy. Thoraxchirurgie 23:257, 1975.

Maeda M, et al: Statistical survey of tracheobronchoplasty in Japan. J Thorac Cardiovasc Surg 97:402, 1989.

Maier HC, Gould WI: Agenesis of the lung with vascular compression of the tracheobronchial tree. J Pediatr 43:38, 1953.

Mansour KA, Malone Ce, Craver JM: Left atrial tumor embolization during pulmonary resection: Review of the literature and report of two cases. Ann Thorac Surg 46:455, 1988.

Markos J, et al: Preoperative assessment as a predictor of mortality and morbidity after lung resection. Am Rev Respir Dis 139:902, 1989.

Martini N, et al: The extent of resection for localized lung cancer: lobectomy. In CF Kittle (ed): Current Controversies in Thoracic Surgery. Philadelphia: WB Saunders, 1986.

Mathisen DJ, Grillo HC: Carinal resection for lung cancer. J Thorac Cardiovasc Surg 102:16, 1991.

Matthew TL, et al: Four years' experience with fibrin sealant in thoracic and cardiovascular surgery. Ann Thorac Cardiovasc Surg 50:40, 1990.

McGovern EM, et al: Completion pneumonectomy: Indications, complications, and results. Ann Thorac Surg 46:141, 1988.

Miller GE, Aberg, THJ, Gerbode, F: Effect of pulmonary vein ligation on pulmonary artery flow in dogs. J Thorac Cardiovasc Surg 55:668, 1968.

Milson JW, et al: Chylothorax: An assessment of current surgical management. J Thorac Cardiovasc Surg 89:221, 1985.

Miscall LD, Duffy RW, Nolan RB: The pleural tent as a simultaneous tailoring procedure in combination with pulmonary resection. Am Rev Respir Dis 73:831, 1956.

Morita R, et al: A case of postoperative chylothorax successfully treated by thoracoscopic fibrin gluing. Nippon Kyobu Geka Gakkai Zasshi 38:2465, 1990.

Mouritzen, C: Sealing of bronchial-alveolar leaks with Beriplast after pulmonary resections and decortications. Presented at the 39th Annual Meeting of the Scandinavian Association for Thoracic and Cardiovascular Surgery, Reykjavik, Iceland, August 29, 1990.

Nagasaki F, Flehinger BJ, Martini N: Complications of surgery in the treatment of carcinoma of the lung. Chest 82:25, 1982.

Ngan H, Fok M, Wong J: The role of lymphangiography in chylothorax following thoracic surgery. Br J Radiol 61:1032, 1988.

Nissen R: Tracheoplastic zur Beseitigung der Erschalffung des membranosen Teils der Intrathorakalen. Luftrohre Schweiz Med Wochenschr 84:219, 1954.

Olsen GN, Block AJ, Tobias LA: Prediction of postpneumonectomy function using quantitative macroaggregate lung scanning. Chest 66:13, 1974a.

Olsen GN, et al: Pulmonary function evaluation of the lung resection candidate: A prospective study. Am Rev Respir Dis 111:379, 1974b.

O'Meara JB, Slade PR: Disappearance of fluid from the postpneumonectomy space. J Thorac Cardiovasc Surg 67:621, 1974.

Pairolero PC, Payne WS: Postoperative care and complications in the thoracic surgical patient. In Glenn WWL, et al (eds): Thoracic and Cardiovascular Surgery. 4th Ed. Norwalk, CT: Appleton-Century-Crofts, 1983, p 338.

Patel RL, Townsend ER, Fountain SW: Elective pneumonectomy: Factors associated with morbidity and operative mortality. Ann Thorac Surg 54:84, 1992.

Perelman MI: Late treatment of chronic bronchopleural fistula with long stump after pneumonectomy. In Eschapasse H, Grillo H (eds): International Trends in General Thoracic Surgery. Vol. 2. Philadelphia: WB Saunders, 1987.

Perelman MI, Ambatiello GP: Transpleuraler, transsternaler und kontralateraler Zugang bei Operationen wegen Bronchial fistel nach Pneumonectomie. Thorax Chir Vaskul Chir 18:45, 1970.

Perelman MI, Rymko LP, Ambatiello GP: Bronchopleural fistula: Surgery after pneumonectomy. In Eschapasse H, Grillo H (eds): International Trends in General Thoracic Surgery. Vol. 2. Philadelphia: WB Saunders, 1987.

Peterffy A, Calabrese E: Mechanical and conventional manual sutures of the bronchial stump. Scand J Thorac Cardiovasc Surg 13:87, 1979.

Peterffy A, Henze A: Haemorrhagic complications during pulmonary resection. A retrospective review of 1428 resections with 113 haemorrhagic episodes. Scand J Thorac Cardiovasc Surg 17:283, 1983.

Peters RM: Postpneumonectomy pulmonary edema. In Eschapasse H, Grillo H (eds): International Trends in General Thoracic Surgery. Vol. 2. Philadelphia: WB Saunders, 1987.

Piccione W Jr, Faber LP: Management of complications related to pulmonary resection. In Waldhausen JA, Orringer MB (eds): Complications in Cardiothoracic Surgery. St. Louis: Mosby-Year Book, 1991, p 336.

Pomerantz M, et al: Surgical management of resistant mycobacterial tuberculosis and other mycobacterial pulmonary infections. Ann Thorac Surg 52:1108, 1991.

Powell RW, Luck SR, Raffensperger JG: Pneumonectomy in infants and children: The use of a prosthesis to prevent mediastinal shift and its complications. J Pediatr Surg 14:231, 1979.

Putnam JB Jr, et al: Predicted pulmonary function and survival after pneumonectomy for primary lung carcinoma. Ann Thorac Surg 49:909, 1990.

Quillin SP, Shackelford GD: Postpneumonectomy syndrome after left lung resection. Radiology 179:100, 1991.

Rasch DK, et al: Right pneumonectomy syndrome in infancy treated with an expandable prosthesis. Ann Thorac Surg 50:127, 1990.

Rice TW, et al: Simultaneous occurrence of chylothorax and subarachnoid pleural fistula after thoracotomy. Can J Surg 30:256, 1987.

Riquet M, Hidden G, Debesse B: Les collaterales dur canal thoracique d'origine ganglio-pulmonaire etude anatomique et chylothorax apres chirurgie pulmonaire. Ann Chir Thorac Cardiovasc 43:646, 1989.

Ritchie AJ, Gibbons JRP: Prophylactic digitalization in pulmonary surgery. Thorax 47:41, 1992.

Ritchie AJ, Bowe P, Gibbons JRP: Prophylactic digitalization for thoracotomy: A reassessment. Ann Thorac Surg 50:86, 1990.

Riveron FA, et al: Silastic prosthesis plombage for right postpneumonectomy syndrome. Ann Thorac Surg 50:465, 1990.

Roxburgh JC, Thompson J, Goldstraw P: Hospital mortality and long-term survival after pulmonary resection in the elderly. Ann Thorac Surg 51:800, 1991.

Sarsam MA, Moussali H: Technique of bronchial closure after pneumonectomy. J Thorac Cardiovasc Surg 98:220, 1989.

Shama DM, Odell JA: Esophageal fistula after pneumonectomy for inflammatory disease. J Thorac Cardiovasc Surg 89:77, 1985.

Shephard JO, et al: Right-pneumonectomy syndrome: Radiographic findings, and CT correlation. Radiology 161:661, 1986.

Shields TW, Ujiki G: Digitalization for the prevention of cardiac arrhythmia following pulmonary surgery. Surg Gynecol Obstet 126:743, 1968.

Short HD: Paraplegia associated with the use of oxidized cellulose in posterolateral thoracotomy incisions. Ann Thorac Surg 50:288, 1990.

Simpson L: Chylothorax in adults: Pathophysiology and management. In Deslauriers J, Lacquet LK (eds): Thoracic Surgery: Surgical Management of Pleural Diseases. St. Louis: CV Mosby, 1990.

Spirn PW, et al: Radiology of the chest after thoracic surgery. Semin Roentgenol 23:9, 1988.

Stenzl W, et al: Treatment of postsurgical chylothorax with fibrin glue. Thorac Cardiovasc Surg 31:35, 1983.

Suarez J, Clagett OT, Brown AL, Jr.: The postpneumonectomy space. J Thorac Cardiovasc Surg 57:539, 1969.

Szarnicki R, et al: Tracheal compression by the aortic arch following right pneumonectomy in infancy. Ann Thorac Surg 25:231, 1978.

Takaro T: Use of staplers in bronchial closure. In Grillo HC, Eschapasse H (eds): International Trends in General Thoracic Surgery. Vol 2. Philadelphia: WB Saunders, 1987.

Talamonti MS, et al: A new method of extraperiosteal plombage for atypical pulmonary tuberculosis. Chest 96:237S, 1989.

Tamimi TM, et al: The value of thoracoplasty before extensive unilateral resection for pulmonary tuberculosis. Am Surg 42:71, 1976.

Tedder M, et al: Current morbidity, mortality, and survival after bronchpolastic procedures for malignancy. Ann Thorac Surg 54:387, 1992.

Van den Bosch JM, et al: Postpneumonectomy oesophagopleural fistula. Thorax 35:865, 1980.

Van Mieghem W, Demedts M: Cardiopulmonary function after lobectomy or pneumonectomy for pulmonary neoplasm. Respir Med 83:199, 1989.

Vanetti A, Bazelly B: Discussion of use of staples in bronchial closure. In Grillo HC, Eschapasse H (eds): International Trends in General Thoracic Surgery. Vol. 2, Philadelphia, WB Saunders, 1987.

Verheijen-Breemhaar L, et al: Postpneumonectomy pulmonary oedema. Thorax 43:323, 1988.

Vester SR, et al: Bronchopleural fistula after stapled closure of the bronchus. Ann Thorac Surg 52:1253, 1991.

Vogt-Moykopf I: Contralateral pneumothorax occurring after pulmonary surgery. *In* Deslauriers J, Lacquet LK (eds): Thoracic Surgery: Surgical Management of Pleural Diseases. St. Louis: CV Mosby, 1990, p. 158.

Von Knorring J, et al: Cardiac arrhythmias and myocardial ischemia after thoracotomy for lung cancer. Ann Thorac Surg 53:642, 1992.

Waki R, et al: Determinants of perioperative morbidity and mortality after pneumonectomy. Ann Thorac Surg 48:33, 1989.

Walker WE: Paraplegia associated with thoracotomy. Ann Thorac Surg 50:178, 1990.

Washi R, et al: Determinants of perioperative morbidity and mortality after pneumonectomy. Ann Thorac Surg 48:33, 1989.

Wasserman K, et al: Postpneumonectomy syndrome: Surgical correction using silastic implants. Chest 75:78, 1979.

Wheat MW, Jr, Burford TH: Digitalis in surgery. J Thorac Cardiovasc Surg 41:162, 1961.

Whyte RI, Starkey TD, Orringer MB: Tumor emboli from lung neoplasms involving the pulmonary vein. J Thorac Cardiovasc Surg 104:421, 1992.

Wong PS, Goldstraw P: Pulmonary torsion: A questionnaire survey and a survey of the literature. Ann Thorac Surg 54:286, 1992.

Yashar J, et al: Preoperative chemotherapy and radiation therapy for stage IIIa carcinoma of the lung. Ann Thorac Surg 53:445, 1992.

Zeldin RA, et al: Postpneumonectomy pulmonary edema. J Thorac Cardiovasc Surg 87:359, 1984.

CHAPTER 29

PNEUMONECTOMY AND ITS MODIFICATIONS

Peter Goldstraw

As necessity is the mother of invention, the rising epidemic of lung cancer in the first half of this century, as noted by Holmes Sellors (1955) and Rigdon and Kirchoff (1958), among others, demanded the development of surgical methods for its treatment. In 1912, but reported in 1913, Morriston Davies, then at University College Hospital in London, undertook the first dissection lobectomy for lung cancer. The patient died on the eighth postoperative day, leaving Tudor Edwards at the Brompton Hospital with the credit of performing the first successful lobectomy for lung cancer in 1928, which was then subsequently reported in 1932. Graham and Singer, in St Louis, reported the first successful removal of the entire lung for cancer in 1933. As noted by Bave (1984), Graham preferred the term "pneumectomy" to describe this operation. He did not dissect the hilar structures, preferring to transfix the hilar vessels and bronchus as they emerged from the mediastinum. Important as this landmark operation was, our modern technique of pneumonectomy owes more to the dissection method first undertaken in 1930 by Churchill in Boston, as recorded by him and associates in 1950. Once more, necessity spurred progress, and when attempting pneumonectomy by mass ligation of the hilar structures, he found the tumor too close to the hilum and was forced to dissect out each structure and ligate them separately. Unfortunately, his failure to close a bronchus led to the patient's death, and it fell to Reinhoff (1936) in Baltimore to undertake the first successful dissection pneumonectomy for cancer in 1933.

Pneumonectomy then became established, as pioneers in many countries benefited from these early experiences and the scientific community witnessed parallel progress in radiology, anesthesia, and the development of blood transfusion and antibiotics. The publications of Meade (1961), Smith (1982), Burford (1958), Churchill (1958), and their colleagues in the United Kingdom and the United States attest to this progress. Indeed, pneumonectomy became so routine

that many surgeons, such as Johnson and associates (1958), considered it the only proper operation for lung cancer. Ochsner (1978) recalled the debate, quoting the strong condemnation of lesser resections by leading authorities in the 1940s. In the succeeding decades, most surgeons came to appreciate that the best operation was the least resection that removed the primary tumor and its involved lymphatics. Each more conservative resection was introduced as a compromise for the patient unable to tolerate more extensive resection, and each — lobectomy, sleeve resection, and segmentectomy — has been shown to be an adequate cancer operation, with survival as least as good as with more extensive resections, as long as the basic oncologic principal of resecting all of the primary tumor and its involved lymphatics can be achieved. Still in many cases, however, this is only possible by pneumonectomy.

INDICATIONS FOR PNEUMONECTOMY

The majority of pneumonectomies are still performed for lung cancer. Occasionally, one may perform pneumonectomy for bronchiectasis or for a lung destroyed by chronic suppuration. Although these are common indications in the Third World, they are rare in developed countries. Pneumonectomy occasionally is performed for pulmonary metastases and rare thoracic tumors. These problems are discussed no further in favor of concentrating on pneumonectomy for lung cancer.

As the extent of resection is rarely known before surgery, all patients to undergo thoracotomy for lung cancer should be assessed for their suitability for pneumonectomy. This is essentially a cost-benefit assessment. The "cost" of operation includes many factors other than the financial cost and the time off work, but uppermost in the patient's mind is the risk of death postoperatively and the likely reduction in exercise capacity. These risks depend on the assessment of patient fitness, which is covered in Chapters 18 and 19. The "benefit" offered by pneumonectomy is the possibilities for cure or of extended survival, which depend on preoperative staging, covered in Chapter 87. The author has come to appreciate that no matter how carefully the preoperative staging is undertaken, intraoperative staging is essential to review the situation before proceeding with resection, as Gaer and I (1990) and Fry (1984), Gephardt and Rice (1990), Albertucci (1992), Izbicki (1992), and their colleagues have stated. I (1991) think of thoracotomy as the final investigation before undertaking treatment by resection. Fernando and I (1990) showed that preoperative staging of lung cancer underestimates the extent of disease in almost one half of the patients coming to thoracotomy. Although resection is still reasonable in 95% of patients, in some groups, who can only be identified by intrathoracic staging, complete resection is not possible or resection is not likely to offer survival advantages. In these cases, it is preferable to withdraw, causing as little damage as possible, rather than to compound the error by futile resection.

If the tumor is found at thoracotomy to be resectable only by pneumonectomy, the surgeon must weigh this added risk against the reduced prospects of cure for the tumor now known to have a more advanced stage. Although in most cases the decision will be to proceed with resection, situations will arise in which resection by lobectomy would have been reasonable, yet pneumonectomy is undesirable. One can reliably assess that pneumonectomy, once begun, can be accomplished, as all the hilar structures can be identified and confirmed to be free of tumor prior to commencing resection. Unfortunately, this does not apply to lesser resections, and one can only be sure of being able to complete lobectomy, or other conservative resections, after dividing segmental vessels and moving on to inspect the underlying lymph nodes around the bronchus. It is best to avoid this "resection cascade," especially if the surgical options are restricted by physiologic considerations.

Bronchoscopy is an important component of preoperative staging, as Spiro and I noted (1984). Increasingly, the diagnosis is established by one's medical colleagues with fiberbronchoscopy. The surgeon should, however, repeat the bronchoscopy immediately before thoracotomy. Anatomic features, of little import to the physician, may affect decisions at thoracotomy. A tumor may lie in the intermediate bronchus, but the surgeon knows that if the origin of this bronchus is invaded, only pneumonectomy will suffice, whereas if the tumor lies at the termination of the same bronchus, middle and lower lobectomy may be adequate. Similarly, some abnormalities of bronchial anatomy, particularly with the right upper lobe as noted by Le Roux (1962) and discussed in Chapter 6, may create difficulties if lobectomy is attempted. The wise anaesthetist looks for distortion of the bronchial tree to aid placement of double-lumen tubes.

Although pulmonary resection is possible through a wide variety of incisions, the lateral thoracotomy approach allows a fuller assessment of the tumor and the mediastinum than the anterior, posterior, or median sternotomy incisions. It has therefore become the standard approach used by me. It matters less whether one has been trained to use a thoracotomy through the interspace, or through the bed of a rib, and the fifth or sixth rib allows adequate access for pneumonectomy. The details of these incisions are covered in Chapter 27.

At thoracotomy, the surgeon should commence with a careful intraoperative evaluation to provide answers to four key questions.

Question 1. What is the Diagnosis?

It may seem facile to pose this question, but many legal cases hinge on the basis for the diagnosis. Surgeons often urge patients to proceed with thoracotomy on the basis of a highly suspicious chest radiograph, perhaps supported by suspicious cytologic findings. Although it is right that we recommend this procedure, we have a responsibility to obtain a firm histologic diagnosis before resecting lung tissue. Rapid section histology must be on hand, and the surgeon must carefully select the tissue to biopsy. This sampling is often straightforward, but surrounding inflammatory changes occasionally obscure the underlying malignant process. It may not prove possible to get accurate biopsy samples without risk of damage to segmental bronchi or vessels. At the final analysis, the surgeon must proceed on the basis of all available evidence; the biopsy findings, the radiographic appearances, and the clinical features. One may have to perform lobectomy on the suspicion that an underlying malignancy cannot be excluded. Usually, this is proven to be the case when the resection specimen is subsequently sectioned. In any event, for this to be necessary, the lobe is sufficiently damaged by such an extensive inflammatory process as to have little function. Rarely, during the course of lobectomy, tumor is encountered. The surgeon then can obtain histologic confirmation at this point, and proceed with pneumonectomy if necessary. It has never proved necessary in the author's experience to perform pneumonectomy without a diagnosis justifying such an extensive resection.

Question 2. Can the Proven Malignancy now be Resected by Pneumonectomy?

To answer this question, the surgeon must carefully and systematically circumnavigate the hilum, checking that each structure to be divided can be controlled at a point free of tumor. The details of this step are discussed subsequently. If the hilar structures have to be exposed intrapericardially, the pericardiotomy should be limited at this stage to preserve the phrenic nerve. One is always able to confirm that complete resection is possible before dividing any vital structures, and if resection is not possible, the minimum amount of damage has been inflicted.

Question 3. Does the Intrathoracic Staging Indicate that the Consequences of Pneumonectomy are Justified by the Prospects for Cure?

By now, the local extent of the tumor, its T stage, has been more fully defined. Pleural metastases have been excluded, invasion into the chest wall, diaphragm, or mediastinum confirmed or refuted. Critically, by now the mediastinal lymph nodes have been dissected out and examined, as will be described in detail, and a more accurate N stage has been determined.

Question 4. Can This Proven Malignancy be Resected by More Conservative Resection Without Compromising Prospects for Cure?

It is at this point that attention is focused on the hilum, and the prospects for lobectomy, sleeve resection, or segmentectomy are evaluated. I prefer to proceed in this order because, as already mentioned, one may not be able to complete the lesser resection if tumor is encountered after dividing segmental structures; one is committed to resection, and it is better to make the decision regarding resection on the cost-benefit assumption of pneumonectomy.

TECHNIQUE

Let us assume that the patient comes to surgery with a firm histologic diagnosis or that we have, with rapid section analysis, answered question 1. Let us follow the routine steps to evaluate the hilum, dissect the mediastinal lymph nodes, provide the answers to questions 2 and 3, and undertake pneumonectomy. The detailed steps for right pneumonectomy through a right lateral thoracotomy incision are described subsequently. All lymph node station references relate to the nodal chart of Naruke and associates (1978).

Right Pneumonectomy

Once intrapleural dissection has freed any adhesions, the operative lung can be collapsed using the double-lumen endobronchial tube. The lung is retracted posteriorly and inferiorly to gain access to the area of the pulmonary artery, superior pulmonary vein, and azygos arch (Fig. 29-1). The sheath of the pulmonary artery is opened on its superior aspect, as the upper lobe branches are arising. The nodes in this position — station 10 on the Naruke chart — are reflected upwards, off the superior surface of the right main bronchus, to the undersurface of the azygos arch. As for all other nodal groups cleared while encircling the hilum, these are put on one side on a swab for more detailed evaluation before resection. It is convenient at this point to continue the dissection of the right paratracheal nodes (stations 2, 3 and 4). This maneuver is described in more detail in Chapter 33, but it is my practice to conserve the azygos vein, dissecting the nodes from beneath it, and completing the dissection of the higher nodes

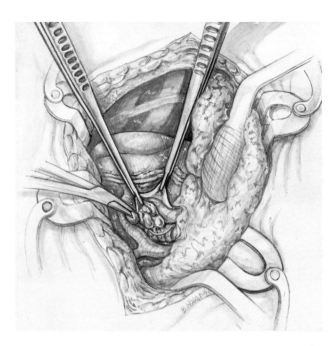

Fig. 29-1. Lung is retracted posteriorly and inferiorly to access the pulmonary artery, superior pulmonary vein, and azygos arch. The superior aspect of the pulmonary artery is opened as the upper lobe branches arise. Station 10 nodes are reflected upwards, off the superior surface of the right main bronchus to the undersurface of the azygos arch.

through a small incision in the mediastinal pleura above the arch.

The lung is then retracted anteriorly. Dissection continues posteriorly along the undersurface of the azygos arch, mobilizing the superior margin of the main bronchus. By dividing the vagal branches and bronchial arteries that lie on the posterior wall of the right main bronchus, the esophagus can be retracted (Fig. 29-2) to provide access to the main carinal nodes — station 7. The fascia enveloping these nodes is incised, and the nodes are removed to clear the inferior aspect of the carina. The surgeon should now be able to pass a finger around the main bronchus, ensuring resectability at this point.

Dissection can continue inferiorly along the anterior aspect of the esophagus, removing nodes in station 8, freeing the inferior pulmonary ligament with its small nodes — station 9 — and identifying the inferior pulmonary vein (Fig. 29-3). Dissection should clear this vein so that a finger can be passed around it. Small vessels bleeding on the esophagus require cautery, and one must exercise great care to avoid injury to the esophagus with resultant fistula. It may be preferable to see what natural hemostasis can achieve while the operation continues.

The dissection continues around the undersurface of the inferior pulmonary vein, moving onto the anterior aspect of the hilum and moving the retractor to depress the lung posteriorly. The superior pulmonary vein is mobilized and its middle and upper lobe tributaries are

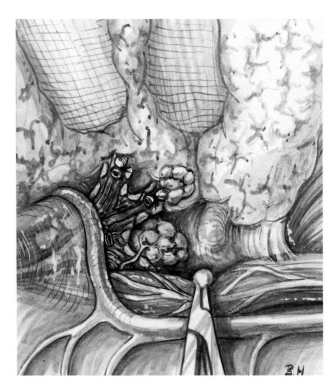

Fig. 29–2. Retraction of the esophagus gives access to the main carinal nodes.

identified. Anomalies of pulmonary venous anatomy occur! A pericardial reflection extends anteriorly as a ligament between the superior pulmonary vein and the pulmonary artery. This structure is incised to clear the superior margin of the superior vein and the anterior and inferior aspects of the pulmonary artery (Fig. 29–4). The surgeon should be able to encircle both these

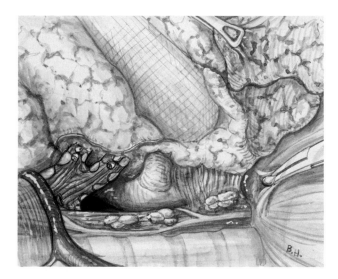

Fig. 29–3. Dissection along the anterior aspect of the esophagus allows removal of station 8 nodes, freeing of the inferior pulmonary ligament, and identification of the inferior pulmonary vein.

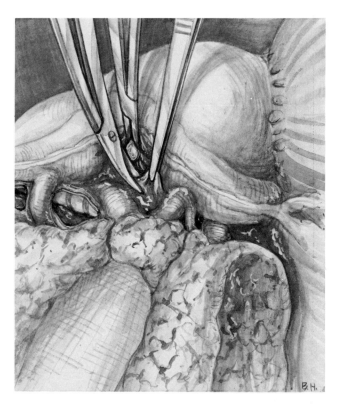

Fig. 29–4. Dissection around the undersurface of the inferior pulmonary vein, moving onto the anterior aspect of the hilum and moving the retractor to depress the lung.

structures with a finger, confirming resectability at this point.

The surgeon has now completed the circumnavigation of the hilum. All the structures that have to be divided to permit pneumonectomy have been identified at a point free of tumor. If detailed examination of the resected mediastinal lymph nodes confirms that pneumonectomy could offer survival advantages to compensate for the loss of the lung parenchyma, and if lesser resection has been considered but pronounced oncologically inadequate, the surgeon proceeds with pneumonectomy.

There is no merit to dividing the hilar structures in any order; I divide them in order of ease and convenience. I shall begin with the pulmonary artery. The index finger is looped around the vessel (Fig. 29–5A) to devolve it from the mediastinum, separate it from adjacent structures, and guide the passage of a crushing clamp. A Ronald Edwards clamp, which looks like a right-angled Roberts clamp, is ideal. Two clamps are applied at least 1 cm apart and the vessel is divided (Fig. 29–5B), taking care to leave a generous flange distal to the proximal clamp. Each end is transfixed with a braided 2-0 suture. It is important to transfix each margin of the vessel close to the edge (Fig. 29–5C). Only a single throw of the knot is performed at this stage. The suture then encircles the vessel, and the suture is tied, on the other side of the vessel (Fig. 29–5D). This transfixition suture is tied tight as the

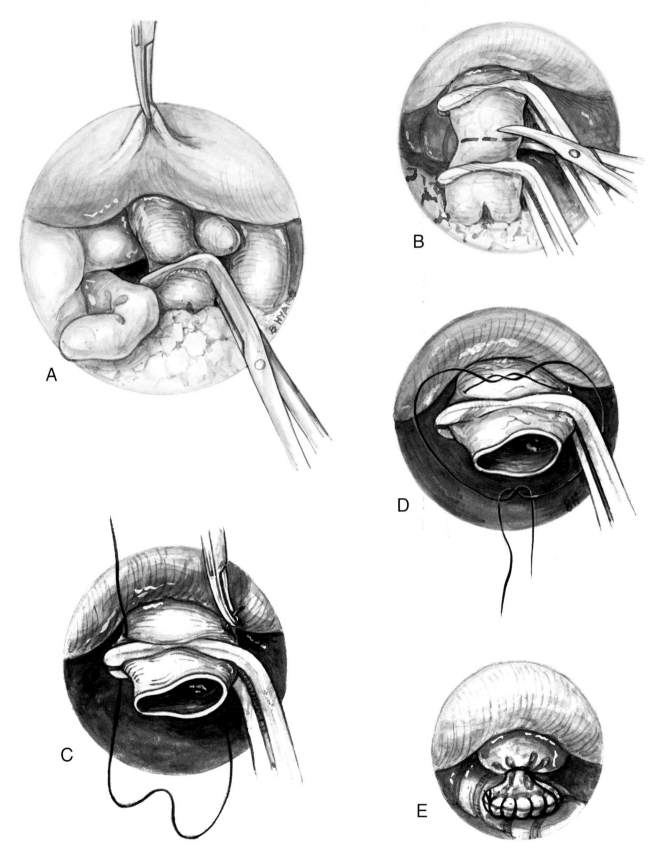

Fig. 29–5. Dividing hilar structures. *A*, The index finger devolves the pulmonary artery from the mediastinum, and guides the passage of a crushing clamp. *B*, Two clamps are applied and the vessel is divided. *C*, Margins are transfixed with a braided suture. *D*, The suture circles the vessel and is tied on the other side. *E*, Reinforcing throws are used over the proximal stump.

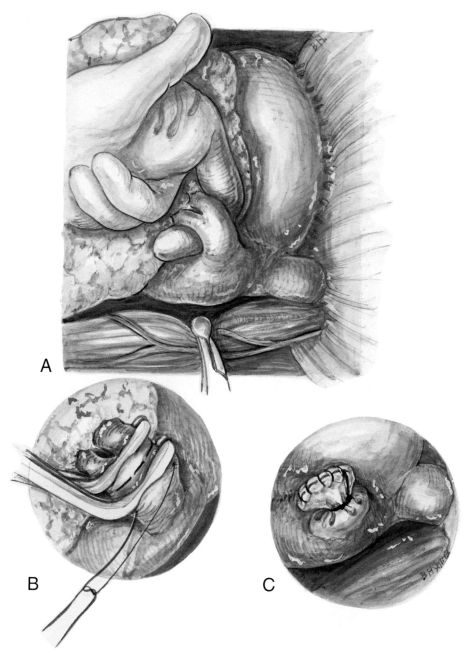

Fig. 29–6. Division of the pulmonary veins, as described in Figure 29–5. The lung is retracted superiorly to control the inferior vein.

clamp is released, and the knot is then completed. Further reinforcing throws are used over the proximal stump (Fig. 29–5E).

The pulmonary veins are dealt with similarly. The inferior vein is best controlled by retracting the lung superiorly (Fig. 29–6).

At this stage, only the bronchus is left. Many surgeons have been trained to staple the bronchus, but it is my practice to suture the bronchial stump. The method includes a crushing clamp, but if length does not permit, the same suture technique can be used in an open method. The technique is thus applicable in all situ-

ations. Cattelani and associates (1993) reviewed the results of this technique in 476 consecutive pneumonectomies, of which 23 (4.8%) were for benign conditions such as tuberculosis, and 27 (5.7%) were completion pneumonectomies. Working in a postgraduate institution, this method has been taught to many surgeons in training with safe results. The overall fistula rate for these pneumonectomy cases is 1.5%. In the 359 pneumonectomies performed by the author, only 2 bronchopleural fistulae were noted, for an incidence of 0.55%. When pneumonectomy was performed by a surgeon in training, the risk of fistula rose to 4.3%, but many trainees had no failures. No evidence exists that stapling is safer, even in the restricted situations in which it is applicable. Each surgeon, however, uses the technique that they were taught and that they find safe and effective.

The lung is lifted to expose the carina (Fig. 29–7A). A crushing clamp is applied flush with the exterior landmark of the carina. If length permits, and especially if infected secretions are dammed within the lung, a second, distal clamp is applied. The bronchus is divided, leaving a flange of 2 to 3 mm distal to the proximal clamp, and the lung is removed. The stump is sutured with a 2-0 monofilament suture; I prefer using non-absorbable material. A continuous, horizontal mattress suture runs the length of the stump, immediately proximal to the clamp, around the edge of the bronchus, and back to the standing end of the suture (Fig. 29–7B). The flange of the bronchus is then excised along the distal edge of the clamp (Fig. 29–7C) and sent for histologic evaluation. The clamp is released as the suture is tied, usually causing the stump to corrugate slightly. Closure is completed with a second suture running over and over the crushed flange distal to the previous suture (Fig. 29–7D).

The pleural space is irrigated and the bronchial stump is tested as airtight by the anesthetist, with inflation to 40 cm of water pressure while the stump is immersed. Hemostasis is checked.

The bronchial stump is buried by apposing mediastinal tissues over it (Fig. 29–8). A continuous suture repairs the incision in the mediastinal pleura above the azygos arch, and runs across the azygos vein to pull it over the stump. The azygos vein is occluded, but its sacrifice provides a good pledget of tissue to cover the bronchial stump. This suture continues inferiorly, drawing the esophagus to the posterior aspect of the sheath of the pulmonary artery and the pericardium, to the lower limit of the mediastinal dissection at the inferior pulmonary vein.

The thoracotomy is closed without drainage. A drain is only necessary if continued bleeding is a concern, as may be the case after extensive chest wall resection or with pleuropneumonectomy. The patient is turned supine and excess air is aspirated from the pneumonectomy space (Fig. 29–9) to bring the mediastinum to the side of surgery. Usually 1.5 to 2 liters of air are removed. The final assessment of the mediastinal position is made by judging the tracheal position once the endobronchial tube has been removed, and on postoperative chest radiographs.

Left Pneumonectomy

The dissection for left pneumonectomy differs only in the area of the aortic arch (Fig. 29–10). The lung is retracted inferiorly and the vagus and phrenic nerves are identified as they lie beneath the mediastinal pleura over the aortic arch. The former lies deep to the superior intercostal vein, a useful landmark in difficult dissec-

tions. Nodes anterior to the vagus nerve — station 5 — and over the anterior aspect of the arch beneath the phrenic — station 6 — are removed to expose the pulmonary artery. The recurrent laryngeal branch of the vagus must be clearly identified and preserved before removing the glands at station 4 lying on the upper aspect of the main bronchus beneath the aorta.

As on the right side, dissection continues over the superior and posterior aspects of the main bronchus to gain access to the nodes at the main carina (Fig. 29–11). All hilar structures are encircled as nodes are resected to complete the intrathoracic staging and to confirm resectability. The transection and closure of these structures is as described for right pneumonectomy.

The bronchial stump is buried (Fig. 29–12) by approximating the esophagus to the posterior aspect of the sheath of the pulmonary artery and pericardium, taking care not to damage the recurrent laryngeal nerve.

Intrapericardial Ligation of the Pulmonary Vessels

More advanced tumors may require the intrapericardial division of the pulmonary vessels to achieve complete clearance. Again, one should limit damage until complete resection is assured and until intrathoracic staging has shown pneumonectomy is desirable. The pericardium is therefore opened at a point clear of the phrenic nerve. This area may be immediately adjacent to the entry of the vessels, or if invasion of the pericardium is more widespread, anterior to the phrenic nerve. If resection proceeds, the steps are as already described.

On the right side, the pulmonary artery is seen superiorly and the pericardial reflection usually passes obliquely across the artery. The vessel may be readily encircled just proximal to this point. On occasion, the pericardial reflection is more medial and the artery must then be exposed medial to the superior vena cava between this latter vessel and the aorta. The superior and inferior pulmonary veins are usually covered with the serous pericardium for approximately three fourths of their circumference. Therefore, it is necessary to open this pericardial serous layer above and below each vessel in order to pass a finger about the vessel.

On the left side, the pulmonary artery is prominent and the fold of Marshall is a readily recognized landmark. Relative to the veins, approximately 75% of the superior pulmonary vein is covered with serous pericardium as it is on the right side; however, the inferior vein is almost completely covered, so only a small part of its wall is not free within the pericardial sac.

On occasion, a clamp is applied to the left atrium and both pulmonary veins are divided simultaneously. The tumor may be too close to the point of division of artery or veins to allow a second, distal clamp. The security of the proximal clamp must not be endangered by trying to insert the distal clamp or by transection of the vessel

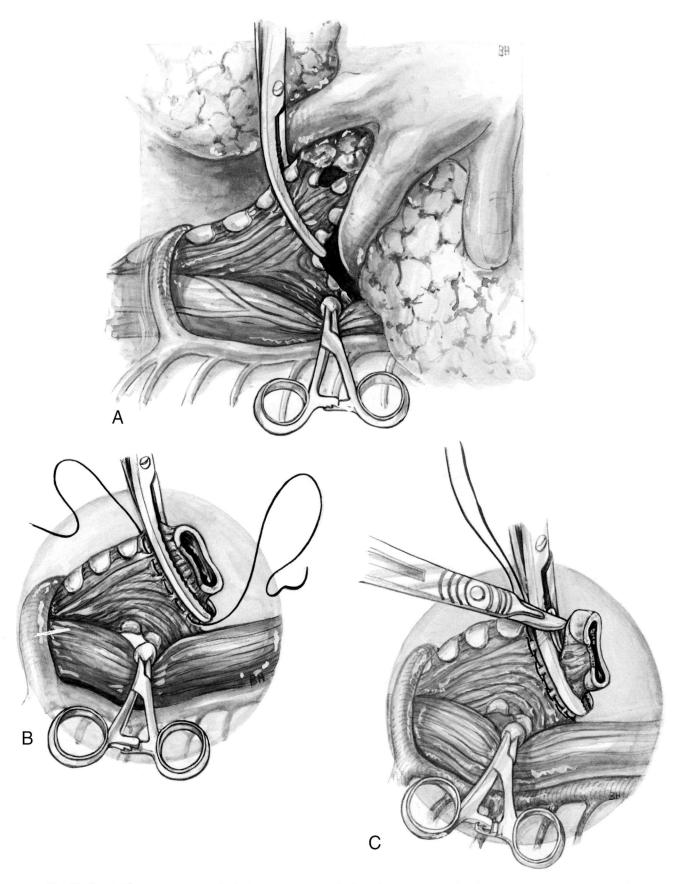

Fig. 29–7. *A,* The carina is exposed. *B,* Suture pattern on the bronchus stump. *C,* The flange of the bronchus is excised.

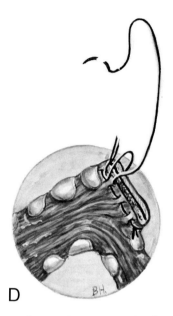

D

Fig. 29–7. (continued) *D*, Closure is completed with sutures over the crushed flange distal to the previous suture.

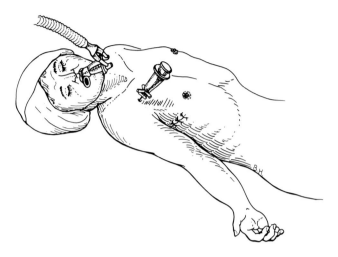

Fig. 29–9. Patient positioning after thoracotomy.

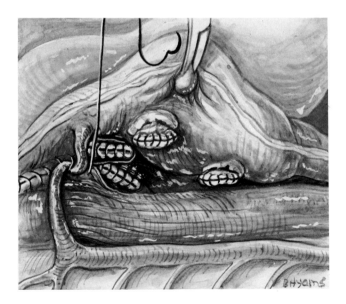

Fig. 29–8. Bronchial stump is buried by apposing mediastinal tissues.

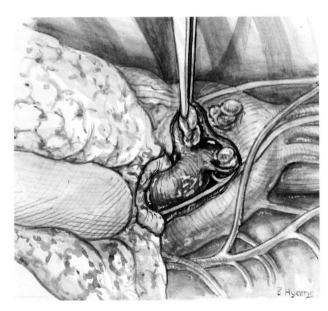

Fig. 29–10. Dissection for left pneumonectomy.

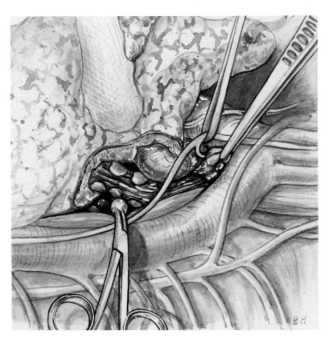

Fig. 29–11. Dissection over the superior and posterior aspects of the main bronchus allows access to the nodes at the main carina.

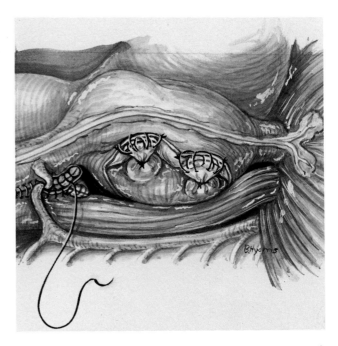

Fig. 29–13. Anterior margins of small pericardial defects are sutured to the stumps of the pulmonary veins.

too close to leave a safe flange distal to this clamp. If this happens, the tissues may squeeze from between the clamp, with resultant severe hemorrhage. It is preferable in these circumstances to deal with the other hilar structures first, and then divide the final vessel without a distal clamp. In my experience, bleeding from the distal lumen is usually minimal because the tumor has occluded the vessel, but it is easy to suture the distal stump if any sequestrated blood threatens to obscure the operative field.

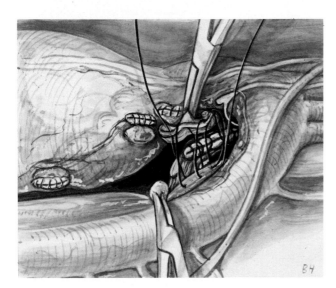

Fig. 29–12. The bronchial stump is buried by approximating the esophagus to the posterior aspect of the sheath of the pulmonary artery and the pericardium.

Any pericardial defect after pneumonectomy deserves attention. The options, however, differ on the right or left side, as the consequences of cardiac herniation differ in these circumstances. After right pneumonectomy, cardiac herniation is associated with torsion and rotation on the vena cavae, which leads to venous inflow occlusion with rapid and dramatic fatality. All pericardial defects after right pneumonectomy must therefore be closed. After left pneumonectomy, however, the heart may freely prolapse into the pneumonectomy space without any physiologic upset, unless constriction occurs. After left pneumonectomy, therefore, the surgeon may close the defect in the pericardium or enlarge it sufficiently to allow free herniation. Small pericardial defects, on either side, may be closed by suturing the stumps of the pulmonary veins to the anterior margins of the defect (Fig. 29–13). The left atrium is adherent to the posterior pericardium, and rotation and herniation cannot occur posteriorly because the heart is fixed by the contralateral pulmonary veins.

Large pericardial defects on the right side usually are associated with resection of the phrenic nerve. One can therefore use a pedicled vascular patch of the diaphragm to repair the pericardial defect and at the same time plicate the diaphragm (Fig. 29–14). The diaphragmatic patch is mobilized from the periphery of this structure, close to the costal attachment. If this step is not possible through the original thoracotomy incision, a second intercostal incision can be made three ribs lower. Once mobilization begins, the patch is reflected superiorly to visualize the inferior phrenic vessels. The diaphragmatic closure proceeds as one

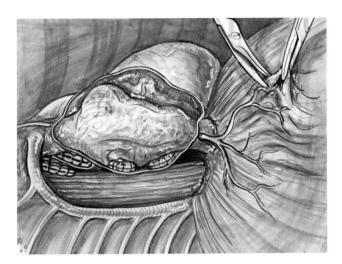

Fig. 29–14. Pedicled vascular patch of the diaphragm is used to repair a large pericardial defect.

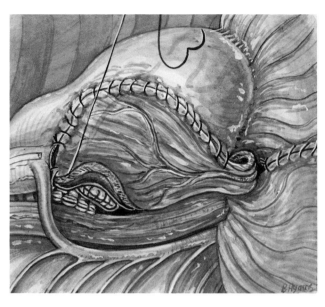

Fig. 29–16. The patch is turned over and sutured to the margins of the pericardial defect with the peritoneal aspect facing outward.

develops the patch (Fig. 29–15). Be bold, a large patch is needed and the diaphragm always comes together! The patch is hinged upward on a narrow pedicle near the inferior vena cava that contains the inferior phrenic vessels. The diaphragmatic defect is closed completely but for a tiny foramen around these vessels, near the inferior vena cava. The patch is then turned over and sutured to the margins of the pericardial defect with the peritoneal aspect facing outward

(Fig. 29–16). It is preferable to leave a gap in this closure over the superior vena cava to avoid compression of this vessel, but small enough to prevent herniation. The bronchial stump may then be buried by suturing theesophagus to the posterior margin of the pericardial defect or to the patch (Fig. 29–17). Although this method is preferred by the author, the pericardial defect may be closed by using other adja-

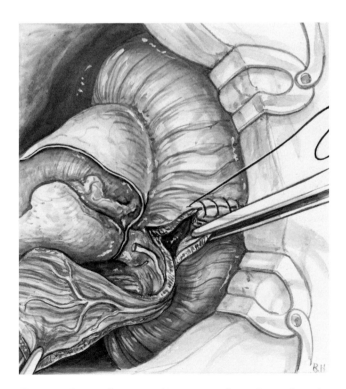

Fig. 29–15. Diaphragmatic closure proceeds as the patch is developed.

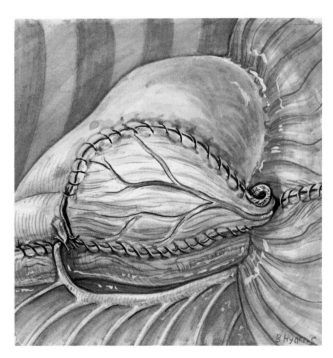

Fig. 29–17. Bronchial stump is buried by suturing the esophagus to the posterior margin of the pericardial defect or the patch.

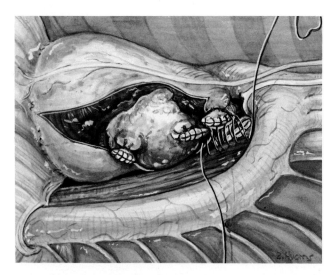

Fig. 29–18. Large pericardial defect is repaired while preserving the phrenic nerve.

cent tissue flaps or a prosthetic soft tissue patch, as noted in Chapter 28.

After left pneumonectomy, small pericardial defects may be closed, but large ones are enlarged down to the diaphragm, preserving the phrenic nerve (Fig. 29–18). If the phrenic nerve has been sacrificed, the diaphragm should be plicated, through a second intercostal incision if necessary.

Other Modifications

Other modifications of pneumonectomy are rare. Pleuropneumonectomy is undertaken for chronic suppuration, and involves only the extrapleural mobilization of the chronically inflamed cortex adherent to the lung. This procedure is bloody, but dissection around the hilum proceeds as described. The surgeon may encounter difficulty if adherent and calcified nodes hinder access to the vessels. The supra-aortic pneumonectomy described by Smith and Nigam (1979) has been abandoned by most surgeons. Sleeve pneumonectomy, resecting the carina and lower trachea with the lung, is rarely indicated in lung cancer. It is described in detail in Chapter 35.

REFERENCES

Albertucci M, et al: Surgery and the management of peripheral lung tumors adherent to the parietal pleura. J Thorac Cardiovasc Surg 103:8, 1992.

Baue AE: Evarts A. Graham and the first pneumonectomy. JAMA 251:257, 1984.

Burford TH, et al: Results in the treatment of bronchogenic carcinoma: An analysis of 1008 cases. J Thorac Surg 36:316, 1958.

Cattelani L, et al: Bronchopleural fistula after pneumonectomy: A twelve-year experience with manual suturing techniques. Eur J Cardiothorac Surg, In press.

Churchill, ED, et al: Further studies in the surgical management of carcinoma of the lung: A further study of the cases treated at the Massachusetts General Hospital from 1950 to 1957. J Thorac Surg 36:301, 1958.

Churchill ED, et al: The surgical management of carcinoma of the lung. J Thorac Surg 20:349, 1950.

Davies HM: Recent advances in surgery of the lung and pleura. Br J Surg 1:228, 1913.

Edwards AT: The surgical treatment of intrathoracic new growths. Br Med 1:827, 1932.

Fernando HC, Goldstraw P: The accuracy of clinical evaluative intrathoracic staging in lung cancer as assessed by postsurgical pathologic staging. Cancer 65:2503, 1990.

Fry WA: Decision making at the time of exploratory thoracotomy (editorial). Ann Thorac Surg 38:310, 1984.

Gaer JA, Goldstraw P: Intraoperative assessment of nodal staging at thoracotomy for carcinoma of the bronchus. Eur J Cardiothorac Surg 4:207, 1990.

Gephardt GN, Rice TW: Utility of frozen-section evaluation of lymph nodes in the staging of bronchogenic carcinoma at mediastinoscopy and thoracotomy. J Thorac Cardiovasc Surg 100:853, 1990.

Goldstraw P: Consensus report of the IASLC working party on pretreatment minimal staging. Lung Cancer 7:7, 1991.

Graham EA, Singer JJ: Successful removal of an entire lung for carcinoma of the bronchus. JAMA 101:1371, 1933.

Holmes Sellors T: Results of surgical treatment of carcinoma of the lung. Br Med J 1:445, 1955.

Izbicki JR, et al: Accuracy of computed tomographic scan and surgical assessment for staging of bronchial carcinoma: A prospective study. J Thorac Cardiovasc Surg 104:413, 1992.

Johnson J, Kirby CK, Blakemore WS: Should we insist on "radical pneumonectomy" as a routine, procedure in the treatment of carcinoma of the lung? J Thorac Surg 36:309, 1958.

Le Roux BT: Anatomical abnormalities of the right upper bronchus. J Thorac Cardiovasc Surg 44:225, 1962.

Meade RH: The evolution of pulmonary surgery. In Meade RH (ed): A History of Thoracic Surgery. Springfield, IL: Charles C Thomas, 1961, pp. 28–97.

Naruke T, Suemasu K, Ishikawa S: Lymph node mapping and curability at various levels of metastasis in resected lung cancer. J Thorac Cardiovasc Surg 76:832, 1978.

Ochsner A: The development of pulmonary surgery, with special emphasis on carcinoma and bronchiectasis. Am J Surg 135:732, 1978.

Reinhoff WF: The surgical technique of total pneumonectomy. Arch Surg 32:218, 1936.

Rigdon RH, Kirchoff H: Cancer of the lung from 1900 to 1930. Int Abstracts Surg 107:105, 1958.

Smith RA: Development of lung surgery in the United Kingdom. Thorax 37:161, 1982.

Smith RA, Nigam BK: Resection of proximal left main bronchus carcinoma. Thorax 34:616, 1979.

Spiro SG, Goldstraw P: The staging of lung cancer (editorial). Thorax 39:401, 1984.

READING REFERENCES

Berend N, Woodcock AJ, Marlin GE: Effects of lobectomy on lung function. Thorax 35:145, 1980.

Bignall JR, Martin M, Smither DW: Survival in 6086 cases of bronchial carcinoma. Lancet 1:1067, 1967.

Firmin RK, et al: Sleeve lobectomy (lobectomy and bronchoplasty) for bronchial carcinoma. Ann Thorac Surg 35:442, 1983.

Ginsberg RJ, et al: Modern thirty-day operative mortality for surgical resections in lung cancer. J Thorac Cardiovasc Surg 86:654, 1983.

Jensik RJ, Faber LP, Kittle CF: Segmental resection for bronchogenic carcinoma. Ann Thorac Surg 28:475, 1979.

Jensik RJ, et al: Sleeve lobectomy for carcinoma; a ten-year experience. J Thorac Cardiovasc Surg 64:400, 1972.

Kirsh MM, et al: Carcinoma of the lung: Results of treatment over ten years. Ann Thorac Surg 21:371, 1976a.

Kirsh MM, et al: Major pulmonary resection for bronchogenic carcinoma in the elderly. Ann Thorac Surg 22:369, 1976b.

Roxburgh JC, Thompson JC, Goldstraw P: Hospital mortality and long-term survival after pulmonary resection in the elderly. Ann Thorac Surg 51:800, 1991.

Van Mieghem W, Demedts M: Cardiopulmonary function after lobectomy or pneumonectomy for pulmonary neoplasm. Respir Med 83:199, 1989.

Wilkins EW, Scannell JG, Craver JG: Four decades of experience with resections for bronchogenic carcinoma at the Massachusetts General Hospital. J Thorac Cardiovasc Surg 76:364, 1978.

Williams DE, et al: Survival of patients surgically treated for stage 1 lung cancer. J Thorac Cardiovasc Surg 82:70, 1981.

CHAPTER 30

TECHNICAL ASPECTS OF LOBECTOMY

Stanley C. Fell and Thomas J. Kirby

OVERVIEW

Lobectomy by hilar dissection, first reported by Blades and Kent in 1940 for the surgical treatment of bronchiectasis, is now performed most commonly for the definitive treatment of lung cancer. The incision for lobectomy is usually a posterolateral thoracotomy, because it allows greater exposure and maneuverability for the surgeon. Anterolateral thoracotomy, median sternotomy — except for the left lower lobe, and muscle sparing lateral thoracotomy are also used. Posterior thoracotomy, developed during the era of surgery for pulmonary tuberculosis and bronchiectasis, as described by Overholt and Langer (1951), and generally performed on a special operating table with the patient prone, is now of historical interest. Video-assisted thoracoscopic lobectomy, as reported by Lewis and associates (1992), is currently in the investigational stage and is not yet recommended as an acceptable alternative. Key points in performance of lobectomy are: mobilization of the lobe, fissure dissection, and management of the vessels and bronchus.

Mobilization of the Lobe

The pleural cavity is entered through the fifth intercostal space or through the bed of the fifth rib, often subperiosteally resected. If adhesive pleuritis is anticipated, entrance through the bed of the resected fifth rib allows for more expeditious mobilization of the lung, either in the intrapleural or the extrapleural plane. Weblike avascular adhesions are managed by finger dissection and a sponge stick; cautery is applied for vascular adhesions. Inflammatory and cavitary lesions adherent to the parietal pleura are mobilized in the extrapleural plane.

The authors gratefully acknowledge the support of the Feldesman Fund for Thoracic Surgery at Montefiore Medical Center.

Controversy exists regarding the need for chest wall resection for tumors adherent to the parietal pleura. Trastek and associates (1984) advocate en bloc resection of lung and chest wall in this situation. McCaughan and colleagues (1985) recommend attempting extrapleural dissection if extrapleural extension is not documented preoperatively. If an extrapleural plane is readily achieved, chest wall resection is not performed, because these tumors often involve only visceral pleura. If determination of tumor fixation to the chest wall is made intraoperatively, the extrapleural approach is abandoned and en bloc resection is performed. This approach did not adversely influence the survival rate.

After mobilization of the lung, the mediastinal pleura is incised about the hilum, the pathology is evaluated, and node sampling is performed as indicated.

Fissure Dissection

Incomplete fissures result from congenital fusion of lung substance, inflammation, or extension of the pathologic process to the adjacent lobe. Combined sharp and blunt dissection along the interlobar plane is generally sufficient to separate the lobes. Application of a stapling device, or dividing lung parenchyma by clamp and suture, may be required. The interlobar arterial branches must be visualized during these efforts. Fused lobes may also be separated by retrograde dissection and traction on the divided bronchus using the intersegmental vein as a guide. Small blood vessels and air leaks require suture; if clamps or stapler are used, diminution of lung volume and distortion of the remaining lobes should be kept to a minimum.

Single lung anesthesia and stapling devices have facilitated lobectomy, but total reliance on these methods is to be decried. The double-lumen endotracheal tube may be unavailable, unable to be properly placed, or become displaced. The surgeon must be able to dissect the lobar hilum and the fissures of a partially inflated lung, preferably manually ventilated.

Management of Lobar Vessels

The key to an orderly lobectomy is thorough knowledge of the anatomy of the pulmonary artery, variations in its branching, and its proper dissection (see Chapter 6). In contrast to the fragile pulmonary segmental arteries, located deep within the fissures and intimately related to the segmental bronchi, the pulmonary veins and their tributary trunks have relatively strong walls, and are easily accessible at the anterosuperior and posteroinferior aspects of the hilum. Occasionally, a common extra pericardial pulmonary vein is encountered.

The pulmonary arteries are best dissected from their fibrous sheath using scissors in the long axis of the vessel. Once a sufficient length of the vessel has been exposed, the sheath is grasped on either side and the artery is then rolled out of its sheath, allowing the passage of a right angle clamp to encircle the vessel and to draw a ligature beneath it. Dissection of the artery with a clamp without prior sharp dissection invites hemorrhage. If segmental branches are short, additional length may be obtained by dissecting into lung parenchyma and dividing the lung substance with cautery.

Bronchial closure is generally performed with a 3.5 or 4.8-mm stapling device, depending on the compliance of the bronchus. Manual sewing of the bronchus may be indicated in some circumstances, an example being to ensure that the bronchial resection is proximal to an endobronchial tumor. Suture materials currently used include silk, polyglactin, and polypropylene. Manual closure proceeds as follows. A suitably sized toothed bronchus clamp is applied to the specimen side of the bronchus, and stay sutures are inserted in the upper and lower borders of the bronchus. With the underlying vascular structures protected by a Semb clamp, the bronchus is transected. Bronchial sutures are placed approximately 3 mm apart and 3 mm from the cut edge. In the absence of single lung ventilation, placing the first suture at the midpoint of the bronchus reduces air leak. Surgeons' knots reduce tension on the cartilage, the knots being placed over the suture hole in the membranous portion to seal possible air leak from this area. The traction sutures may be tied in place or over the cut end. Repleuralization of the bronchial stump is of dubious value after a lobectomy, the stump being readily covered by the remaining parenchymal tissue within the hemithorax.

After removal of the specimen, the integrity of the bronchial closure is tested by the application of positive pressure to the endotracheal tube with a saline-filled hemothorax. Parenchymal air leaks are also localized and repaired. Two thoracostomy tubes are placed through stab wounds in the anterior axillary line. The lower tube extends posteriorly on the diaphragm and the upper tube lies anteriorly to reach the apex of the pleura. An absorbable suture from the tip of the anterior tube to the apical pleura ensures its proper position. After closure of the chest, negative suction from 10 to 20 cm of water is applied to the drainage systems. The tubes are removed serially, once drainage is less the 60 ml in 24 hours and air leak has ceased.

RIGHT UPPER LOBECTOMY

The anatomy of the hilar structures of the right upper lobe is more complex than that of any other lobe, and arterial anomalies are more common. In approximately 80% of individuals, the anterior segment of the right upper lobe is partially or completely fused to the middle lobe, and a segmental dissection of this area is required.

The mediastinal pleural is incised about the hilum of the right lung, lateral to the superior vena cava, inferior to the azygos vein, continuing posteriorly over the bronchus, anterior to the vagus nerve that is visible subpleurally, to the level of the bronchus intermedius. Anteriorly, the incision is carried to the level of the superior pulmonary vein, posterior to the phrenic nerve (Fig. 30–1A). A pledget dissector is used to push the azygos vein superiorly, demonstrating the upper border of the right main bronchus and the upper lobe bronchus originating from it. Inferior to the azygocaval junction, a lymph node is found. Just below this lymph node is the upper border of the pulmonary artery. The areolar tissue overlying the pulmonary artery is dissected and the superior arterial trunk is visualized. This artery and its apical and anterior segmental branches are dissected. The apical segmental vein crosses the anterior segmental artery and it is often convenient to ligate and divide this vein before dealing with the artery (see Fig. 30–1B). The superior arterial trunk is doubly tied with 0 silk; the apical and segmental branches are tied and then divided. If the segmental arteries are short, additional length may be obtained by dissecting with a right angle clamp into the pulmonary parenchyma overlying the branches, dividing the parenchyma with cautery. Suture ligatures or clips are then applied, and the segmental arteries are divided.

After division of the superior trunk of the pulmonary artery, the common stem of the apical and anterior segmental veins is dissected and divided. The interlobar trunk of the pulmonary artery lies directly beneath the upper and middle stems of the superior pulmonary vein and this dissection must be performed cautiously.

The remaining arterial supply to the right upper lobe is the posterior ascending artery, present in 90% of patients. Dissection of this artery can be the most formidable task in the procedure. Three approaches have been described: an anterior approach, approach through the oblique fissure, and a retrograde approach.

The anterior approach requires prior division of the posterior and inferior venous tributaries of the middle stem of the superior vein, which is closely applied to the anterior surface of the inferior trunk of the pulmonary artery. Further dissection of the interlobar artery is required, because the posterior segmental artery arises from the anterior aspect of the interlobar

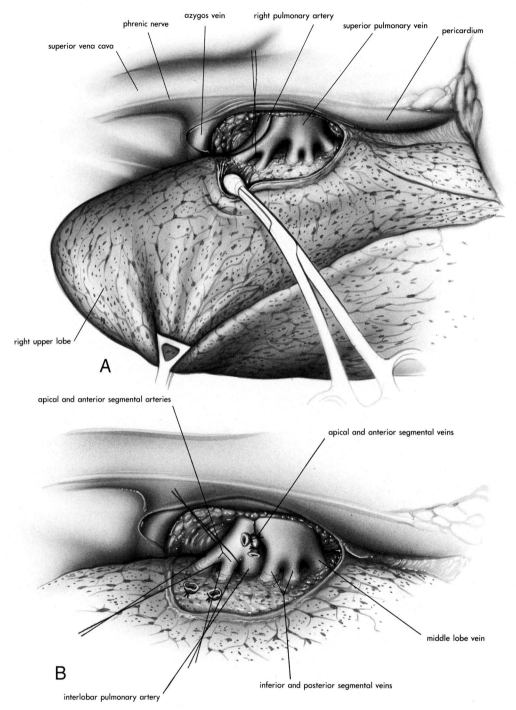

Fig. 30–1. *A*, Anterior aspect of the right hilum. Division of the apical segmental vein facilitates dissection of the superior trunk of the pulmonary artery. *B*, The superior arterial trunk before ligation. The anterior as well as the apical segmental vein has been divided to demonstrate the interlobar trunk of the pulmonary artery.

artery just above the superior segmental artery. Isolation of the right pulmonary artery may be required because laceration of the posterior ascending artery or the interlobar artery from which it arises may occur during this dissection.

Approach to the posterior segmental artery via the oblique fissure is acceptable provided the oblique fissure is virtually complete. Otherwise, the artery is again at

risk of injury. The retrograde method for completion of the dissection is both safe and expeditious.

Retrograde exposure of the posterior ascending artery proceeds as follows. Attention is directed to the posterior aspect of the hilum. The vagus nerve is grasped with an Allis clamp and retracted, thus demonstrating its branches to the right upper lobe. The branches are divided (Fig. 30–2A). Deep to the vagal branches, the

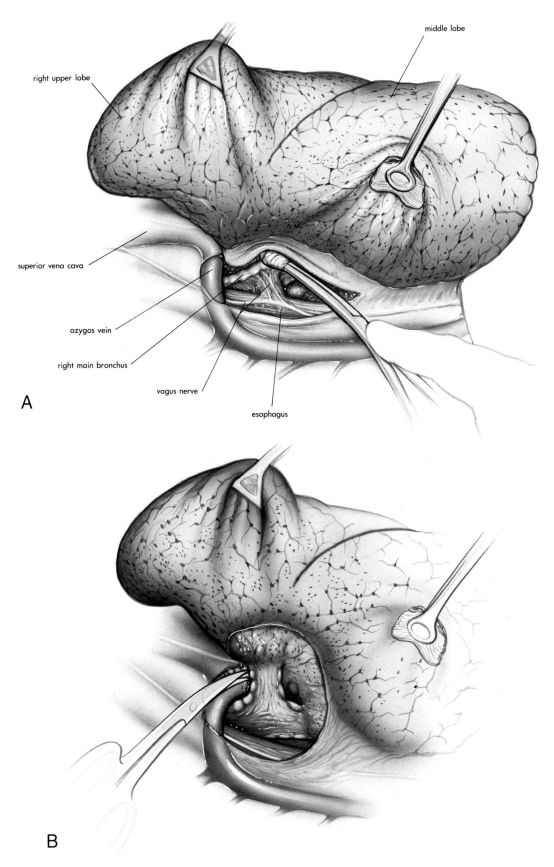

right upper lobe

middle lobe

superior vena cava

azygos vein

right main bronchus

vagus nerve

esophagus

A

B

Fig. 30–2. *A*, Posterior aspect of the right upper lobe hilum after division of the mediastinal pleura. Vagal branches posterior to the bronchus are not yet divided. *B*, The right upper lobe bronchus is dissected.

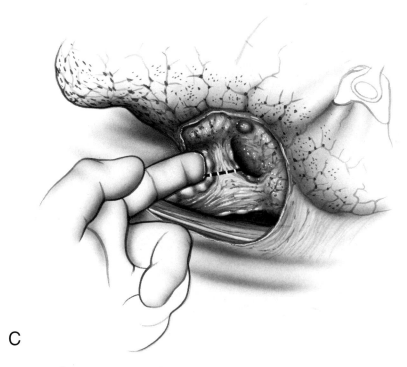

C

Fig. 30–2. (continued) *C*, Finger dissection separates the bronchus from the interlobar pulmonary artery.

bronchial artery may be observed; it is clipped and divided. The lower border of the upper lobe bronchus is dissected. In the crotch between the upper lobe bronchus and the intermediate bronchus is a constant lymph node. This node is dissected toward the specimen, clearing the inferior border of the right upper lobe bronchus. It is not advisable to pass a clamp from the lower border of the right upper lobe bronchus medially to encircle the bronchus, because the posterior ascending artery may be lacerated. Rather, scissor dissection of the medial surface of the bronchus is performed, sweeping areolar tissue and nodes toward the specimen (see Fig. 30–2*B*). The bronchus is not denuded of its fascia, which supplies the vascularity required for healing. An index finger can then be inserted along the anterior aspect of the bronchus to reach its lower border (see Fig. 30–2*C*). A right angle clamp may then be passed safely about the right upper lobe bronchus. A Semb clamp is used to widen the peribronchial space, allowing for the passage of a 4.8-mm stapling device. The bronchus is either stapled and divided, or manually sutured. If stapled, the staple line generally includes the bronchial artery to the right upper lobe. The cut edge of the specimen side of the bronchus is grasped with an Allis clamp. Traction is placed on the Allis clamp, a toothed bronchus clamp is applied, and the Allis clamp is removed. By turning the handle of the bronchus clamp medially, thus elevating the cut bronchus, the fissure dissection is facilitated. With gentle medial traction on the bronchus clamp, the areolar tissue and nodes are readily dissected off the interlobar pulmonary artery and the posterior ascending artery is identified, ligated, and divided (Fig. 30–3). Occasionally, an additional arterial branch to the anterior segment originates from the interlobar artery. Rarely, the posterior segmental artery originates from the superior segmental artery.

Attention is next directed to the fissures, which may be managed by sharp dissection along the intersegmental vein using partial inflation of the middle and lower lobes against the now airless upper lobe; by stapled division; or by a combination of both methods (Fig. 30–4). With the bronchus divided and the posterior segmental artery transected, it is safe to pass a stapling device to divide the posterior aspect of the oblique fissure. The minor fissure is similarly completed. We emphasize that attempts to divide fissures without prior identification of the segmental arteries may lead to hemorrhage. Medial traction of the bronchus clamp and further dissection with the interlobar artery under direct vision lead immediately to the middle trunk of the superior pulmonary vein and its posterior and inferior tributaries. At this point, the operator can appreciate the intimate relationship of these branches to the inferior trunk of the pulmonary artery (Fig. 30–5*A*). The common stem of the posterior and inferior veins is identified and the site of insertion of the middle lobe vein into the superior pulmonary vein is identified and preserved. The venous stem is doubly ligated, as are the posterior and inferior veins, which are then divided. The stapling device generally is not useful for managing the right superior pulmonary vein. The importance of minimizing air leak from the middle lobe cannot be overemphasized. The intersegmental vein defines the proper plane of dissection.

After the specimen is removed, the pleural cavity is irrigated and the bronchial closure is tested. The inferior

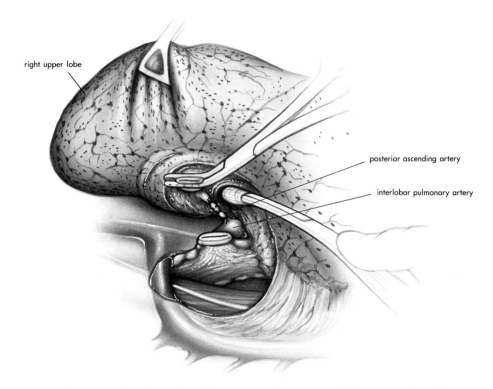

Fig. 30–3. The bronchus has been stapled and divided. Medial traction on the specimen facilitates dissection of the posterior ascending artery.

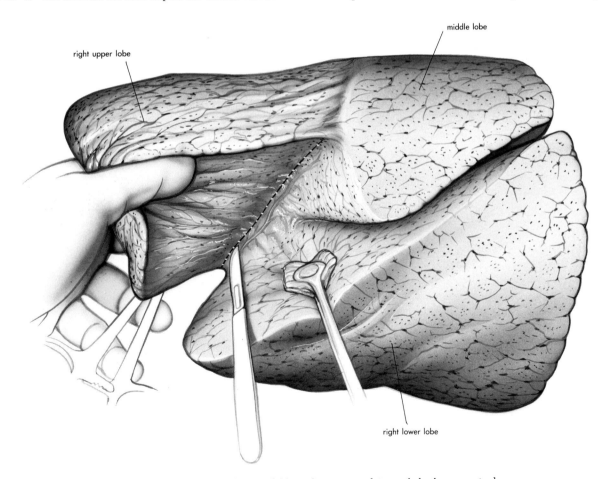

Fig. 30–4. The oblique fissure is completed by a sharp and blunt dissection and is stapled where required.

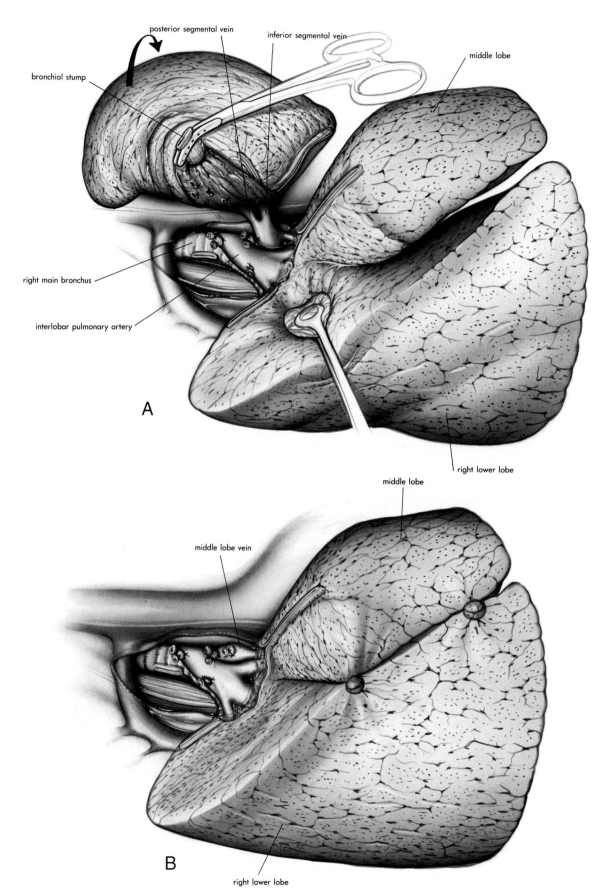

Fig. 30–5. *A*, Retracting the lobe medially and stapling the minor fissure exposes the middle trunk of the superior pulmonary vein. Note the relationship of this trunk to the underlying interlobar pulmonary artery. The middle lobe vein has been identified and preserved. *B*, Edges of the middle and lower lobes are approximated with silk ties to prevent middle lobe torsion.

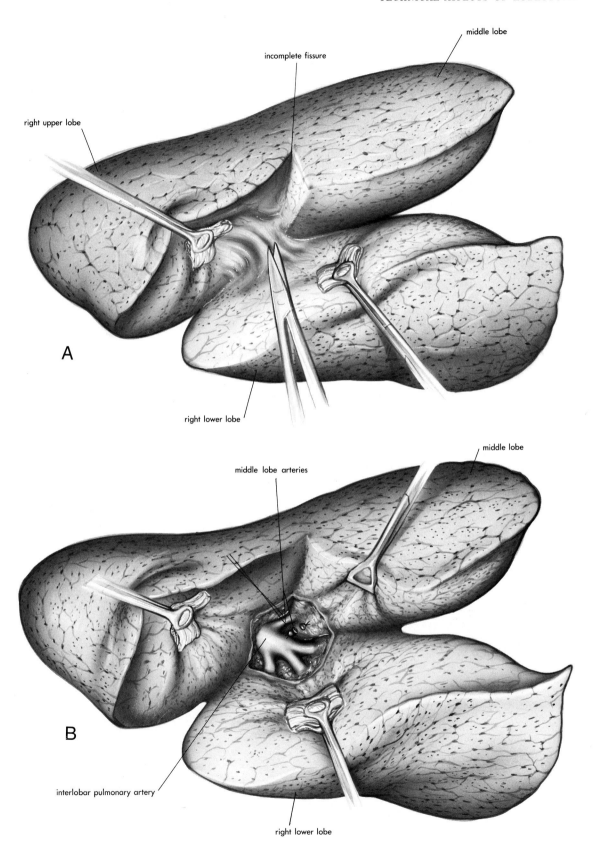

Fig. 30–6. *A* and *B*, Dissection of the oblique fissure at its junction with the horizontal fissure demonstrates the interlobar pulmonary artery and its branches. One middle lobe artery is divided.

pulmonary ligament is divided, allowing rotation of the lower lobe to facilitate complete filling of the pleural space. Because the fissure between the middle and lower lobes is generally complete, torsion of the middle lobe is possible. To prevent such torsion, the edges of the partially expanded middle and lower lobes are grasped with an Allis clamp and a silk tie is used to approximate these edges along the course of the fissure (see Fig. 30–5B). A single application of a TA 30 stapling device accomplishes the same results, at much greater cost.

MIDDLE LOBECTOMY

Middle lobectomy is not commonly performed as an isolated procedure. In years past, it was performed for "middle lobe syndrome." Incomplete fissure and hyperplastic or calcified lymph nodes, adherent to segmented arteries and the middle lobe bronchus, made it a formidable procedure, generally requiring proximal control of the right pulmonary artery.

Most often, middle lobectomy is performed in association with either upper or lower lobectomy for tumors that cross fissures. Combined middle and lower lobectomy was often required for the treatment of bronchiectasis.

If upper and middle lobes are resected, the bronchi are closed separately; for middle and lower lobectomy, the bronchus intermedius is divided just distal to the right upper lobe bronchus. The major fissure is opened and the lower lobe is retracted posteriorly (Fig. 30–6A). By following the posterior edge of the middle lobe as it joins the major fissure, and dissecting deep within the fissure, lymph nodes are noted, indicating the site of the interlobar pulmonary artery. The artery is dissected proximally in the subadventitial plane and the middle lobe artery is identified (see Fig. 30–6B). Generally, there are two middle lobe arteries; the first one identified arises from the interlobar artery anteriorly more or less opposite to the superior segmental artery arising posteriorly. Further proximal dissection of the interlobar artery demonstrates a second, and rarely a third, artery to the middle lobe. Occasionally, an anomalous branch of the middle artery to the upper lobe is identified. After ligation and division of the middle lobe arteries, the table is rotated posteriorly and the anterior aspect of the hilum is dissected, isolating and ligating the middle lobe vein that enters the lower portion of the superior pulmonary vein (Fig. 30–7). After division of the middle lobe vein, the bronchus is readily accessible (Fig. 30–8A). In difficult dissections, it may be more expeditious to divide the middle lobe vein, isolate and divide the bronchus, and then ligate and divide the middle lobe arteries. Manual suturing is generally easier than inserting a stapling device.

The closed middle lobe bronchus is deep with the parenchyma and disruption of this bronchial closure is virtually unknown. The distal portion of the transected middle lobe bronchus is grasped with a bronchus clamp. Using differential inflation and traction on the bronchus

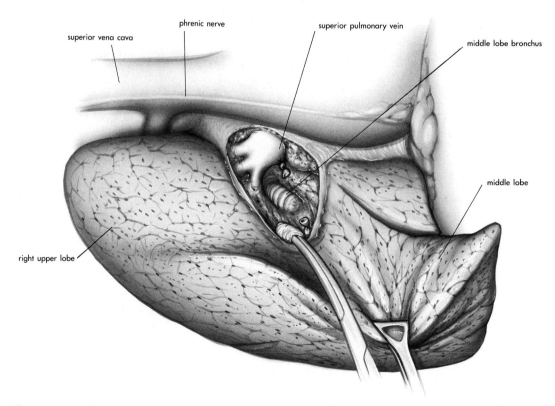

Fig. 30–7. The anterior mediastinal pleura is incised. The middle lobe vein is isolated and divided.

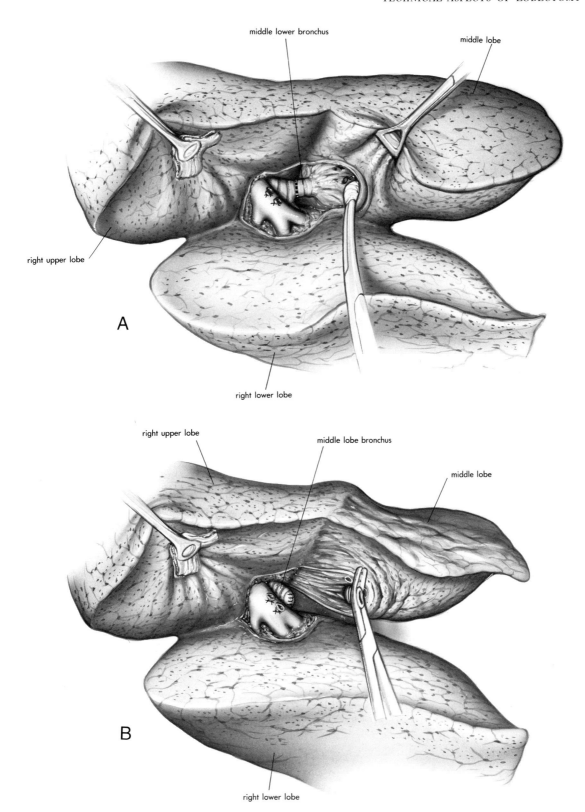

Fig. 30–8. *A*, The middle lobe bronchus is identified. The line of bronchial transection is illustrated. *B*, Traction on the specimen bronchus and differential inflation facilitate completion of the horizontal fissure.

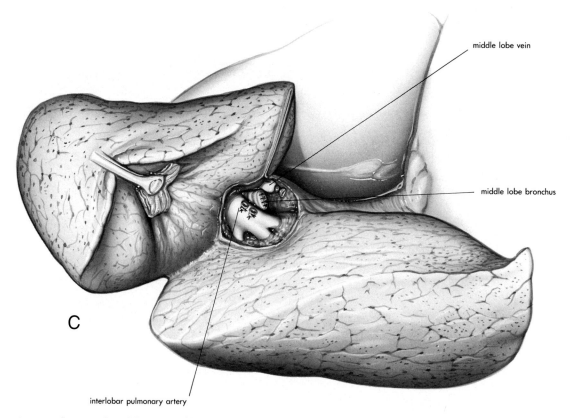

middle lobe vein

middle lobe bronchus

interlobar pulmonary artery

Fig. 30–8. (continued) *C*, Hilum following middle lobectomy.

clamp, the fissure may then be completed along the lines of the intersegmental veins, by a combination of sharp and blunt dissection and stapling (see Fig. 30–8*B*). After completion of the fissure and removal of the specimen, the raw surfaces of the upper lobe are approximated to the lower lobe by several ties to help seal air leak.

RIGHT LOWER LOBECTOMY

The oblique fissure is opened while retracting the right upper and middle lobes anteriorly and the lower lobe posteriorly. The interlobar pulmonary artery is deeply situated in the region where the oblique and horizontal fissures meet (see Fig. 30–6*B*). The temptation to staple and divide areas of fusion between the posterior segment of the right upper lobe and the superior segment of the lower lobe before demonstrating the interlobar pulmonary artery and its branches must be avoided. The visceral pleura overlying the interlobar artery is opened and the pulmonary artery is dissected. The middle lobe artery, originating from the antero-medial surface of the interlobar artery, must be demonstrated. Directly opposite and posterolaterally lies the superior segmental artery. Rarely, the posterior ascending artery to the upper lobe originates from the superior segmental artery. Occasionally, the superior segment of the right lower lobe has two branches. Often,

it is best to isolate and divide the basal arteries first, distal to the middle lobe and superior segmental arteries (Fig. 30–9). The basal arteries may have a short common trunk from which two branches originate: one supplying the anterior and medial segments and the other supplying the posterior and lateral segments. Occasionally, the four basal segmental arteries originate separately distal to the middle lobe artery, and dissection into the lung parenchyma is required to obtain adequate length for ligation and division. Attention is then directed to securing the superior segmental artery, taking care to preserve the posterior segmental artery to the right upper lobe.

The lobe is retracted anteriorly and superiorly. The inferior pulmonary ligament is divided up to the lymph node at the lower border of the inferior pulmonary vein (Fig. 30–10*A*). The posterior mediastinal pleura is incised over the posterior surface of the inferior pulmonary vein, which is cleared of areolar tissue, and the pleural incision is carried superiorly to above the level of the bronchus intermedius. The interval between the lower border of the bronchus and the superior pulmonary vein is dissected. The anterior surface of the inferior pulmonary vein is then cleared. With an index finger serving as a guide, the inferior pulmonary vein is then isolated, using a Semb clamp (see Fig. 30–10*B*). The interval between the lower lobe bronchus and the inferior vein is widened so that a vascular stapler may be inserted to occlude the cardiac end of

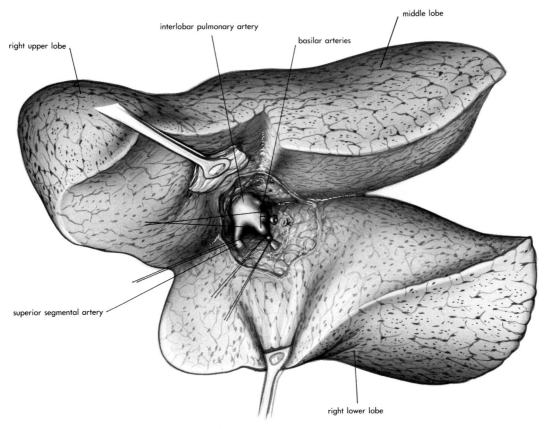

Fig. 30–9. Arterial supply of the right lower lobe. The origin of the middle lobe artery is visualized. Stapling the posterior portion of the oblique fissure facilitates the dissection of the superior segmental artery.

the vein. The extrapericardial portion of the right inferior pulmonary vein is short. It is not advisable to ligate the vein because the tie may spring off the fibrous pericardium. Rather than sacrifice length, application of a Sarot clamp to the specimen side of the vein and cutting on the clamp ensures sufficient length of the vein to be clamped and closed by a vascular suture or divided after application of a vascular stapler (see Fig. 30–10C). Alternatively, the superior and basilar segmental veins are ligated individually. The lower lobe bronchus is then dissected. Because the middle lobe bronchus and the superior segmental bronchus originate from the intermediate bronchus at almost the same level, it may be necessary to close the basal segmental bronchus and the superior segmental bronchus separately to avoid obstructing the middle lobe bronchus. Usually, an oblique application of the 4.8-mm stapling device does not occlude the middle lobe bronchus (Fig. 30–11A). It is advisable to apply the stapler, close it without firing, and then re-aerate the right lung to ensure the patency of the middle lobe bronchus. Although a similar anatomic situation exists in regard to left lower lobe bronchus and the lingular bronchus, the risk of occluding the middle lobe bronchus is far greater than that of occluding the lingular bronchus. Alternatively, the lower lobe bronchus may be sutured as previously described.

LEFT UPPER LOBECTOMY

The most common anatomic variation encountered during left upper lobectomy is the number of segmental arterial branches, which vary from three to eight. The procedure is straightforward, provided the apical and anterior arteries are not injured during their isolation and division. To best accomplish this safely, proximal control of the left pulmonary artery is recommended, and these proximal branches are the last to be dissected and divided.

The left lung is retracted inferiorly, and the mediastinal pleura overlying the pulmonary artery is incised (Fig. 30–12A). Following identification of the course of the phrenic nerve, the pleural incision is carried over the medial portion of the superior pulmonary vein just lateral to the pericardium (see Fig. 30–12B). Posteriorly, the incision is made to a point below the level of the bronchus. The vagus nerve is visible subpleurally, marking the posterior limit of the hilar dissection (Fig. 30–13). Areolar tissue overlying the convex surface of the pulmonary artery is cleared. The upper border of the left main bronchus is defined after division of vagal branches. A pledget dissector is used to roll the pulmonary artery away from the left main bronchus. Anteriorly, the interval between the pulmonary artery and the superior pulmonary vein is

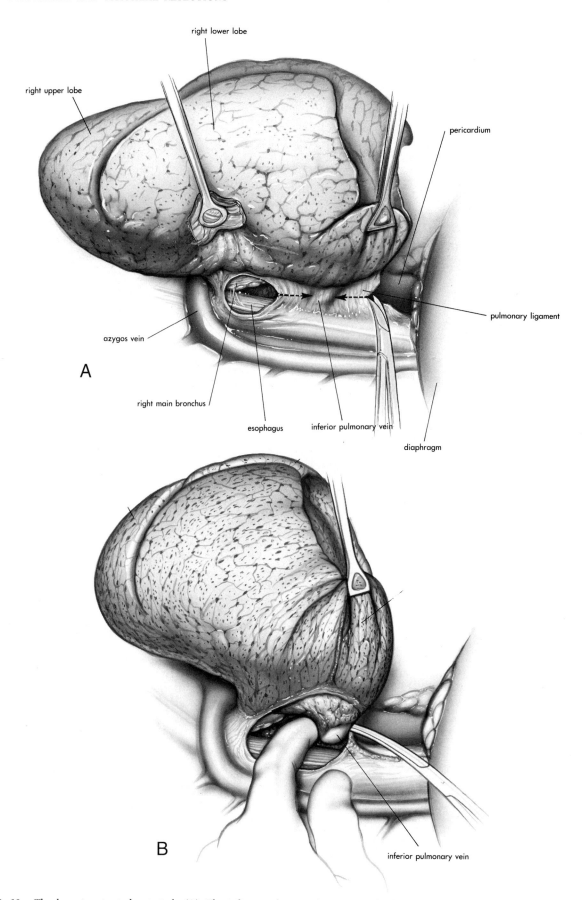

right lower lobe

right upper lobe

pericardium

pulmonary ligament

azygos vein

right main bronchus

esophagus

inferior pulmonary vein

diaphragm

A

B

inferior pulmonary vein

Fig. 30–10. The lung is retracted anteriorly *(A)*. The inferior pulmonary ligament is divided *(B)*,

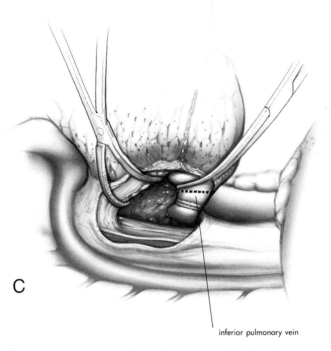

inferior pulmonary vein

Fig. 30–10. (continued) and the inferior pulmonary vein is dissected, stapled, and divided *(C)*.

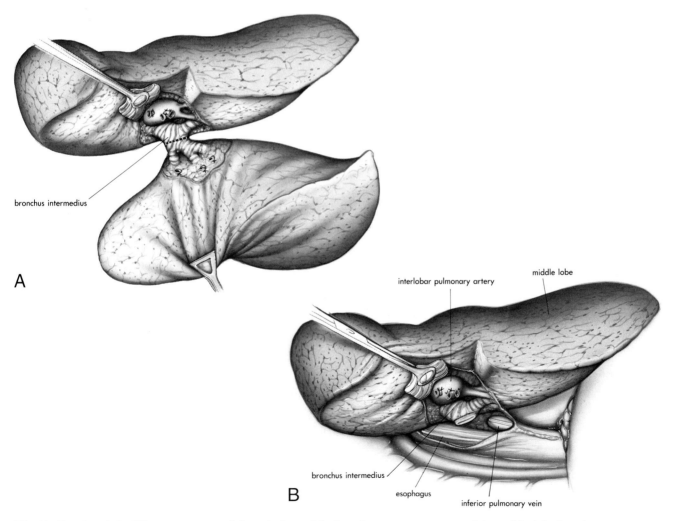

bronchus intermedius

A

interlobar pulmonary artery

middle lobe

bronchus intermedius

esophagus

inferior pulmonary vein

B

Fig. 30–11. *A* and *B*, Oblique transection of the right lower lobe bronchus preserves patency of the middle lobe bronchus.

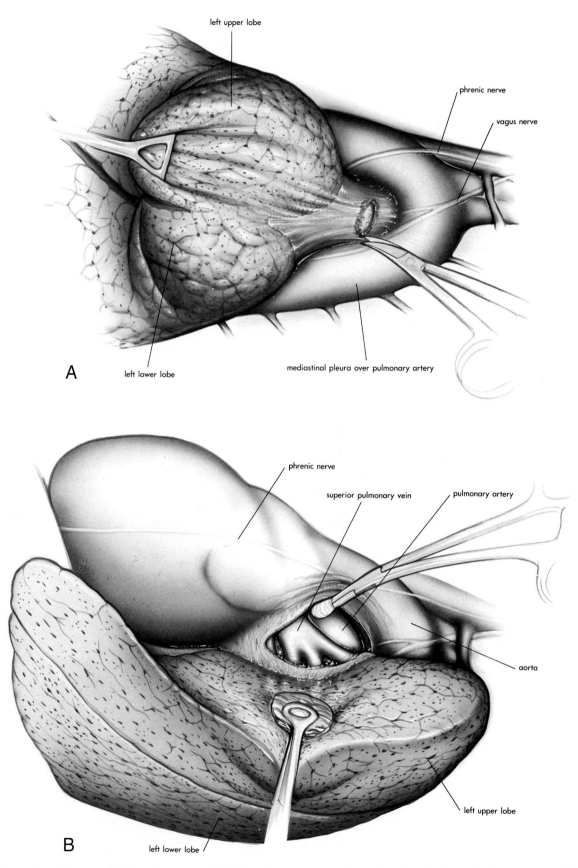

Fig. 30–12. *A* and *B*, The mediastinal pleura is incised and the pulmonary artery is dissected in the subadventitial plane. The interval between the pulmonary artery and the superior pulmonary vein is defined.

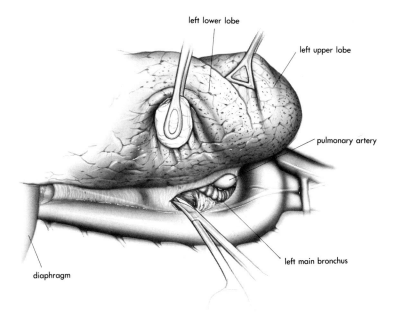

left lower lobe

left upper lobe

pulmonary artery

left main bronchus

diaphragm

Fig. 30–13. Dissection of the posterior aspect of the left upper lobe hilum medial to the vagus nerve.

defined, and again the pulmonary artery is rolled out of its sheath, allowing an index finger to encircle the artery (Fig. 30–14). A Semb clamp may then be used to draw a silastic vessel loop about the artery. The ends of the loop are tied with a heavy silk suture and the loop is allowed to lie in the chest, readily accessible in the event of pulmonary artery injury.

The lung is retracted anteriorly and the pulmonary artery is dissected into the oblique fissure (Fig. 30–15A). If necessary, the posterior part of the fissure is completed with clamps or a stapler with the pulmonary artery visualized. The pulmonary artery is dissected over the middle point of its presenting surface as it curves around the left upper lobe bronchus. As the fissure dissection proceeds, the posterior segmental arteries are noted opposite the superior segmental artery (see Fig. 30–15B). Further distal dissection demonstrates one or two lingular arteries; the arterial dissection is complete when the basilar segmental branches are identified. With the lower lobe retracted inferiorly and the upper lobe retracted superiorly, the lingular branches are isolated and divided. The upper lobe is then rotated clockwise and the posterior segmental branches are ligated and divided. Proceeding in this fashion, from the lingular arteries proximally, and rotating the lobe make each subsequent arterial isolation easier. The apical and anterior branches arise from the convex surface of the pulmonary artery often as a short trunk, slightly anterior to the middle point of the artery. These branches are the last to be divided (Fig. 30–16). Ligation and division of the apical segmental vein may enhance the visualization of the apical and anterior segmental arteries. The now completely mobilized pulmonary artery is rolled away from the upper lobe bronchus, and is inspected for

anomalous branches originating from its medial surface. This maneuver facilitates the later transection of the bronchus.

The lobe is retracted posteriorly and the anterior surface of the superior pulmonary vein is cleared of areolar tissue. The posterior surface of the pulmonary vein is freed by carrying the dissection on the anterior surface of the bronchus just external to the peribronchial connective tissue. Three or four branches enter the superior pulmonary vein and are encircled with ligatures. The extrapericardial length of pulmonary vein is often inadequate for safe ligation; therefore, it is an ideal place for the use of a vascular stapler. In the absence of a stapling device, the branches are tied, a vascular clamp is applied proximally, and the vein is divided and then closed with a vascular suture. It is often easier to divide the bronchus first. To divide the bronchus at the appropriate level, the interval between the lingular bronchus and the lower lobe bronchus is defined by rolling the pulmonary artery posteriorly, thus exposing the bifurcation of the left main bronchus (Fig. 30–17A). The upper lobe bronchus is occluded with a stapling device. Differential inflation ensures that the lower lobe bronchus is not compromised; the stapler is fired and the bronchus is transected with a Semb clamp positioned between the bronchus and the vein to protect the vein. After closure of the bronchus, the specimen end of the bronchus is grasped with a bronchus clamp. Elevation of the clamp exposes the deep surface of the superior pulmonary vein (Fig. 30–17B). The superior pulmonary vein is then managed as previously described. The inferior pulmonary ligament is divided to allow the left lower lobe to advance upward to better fill the thoracic cavity.

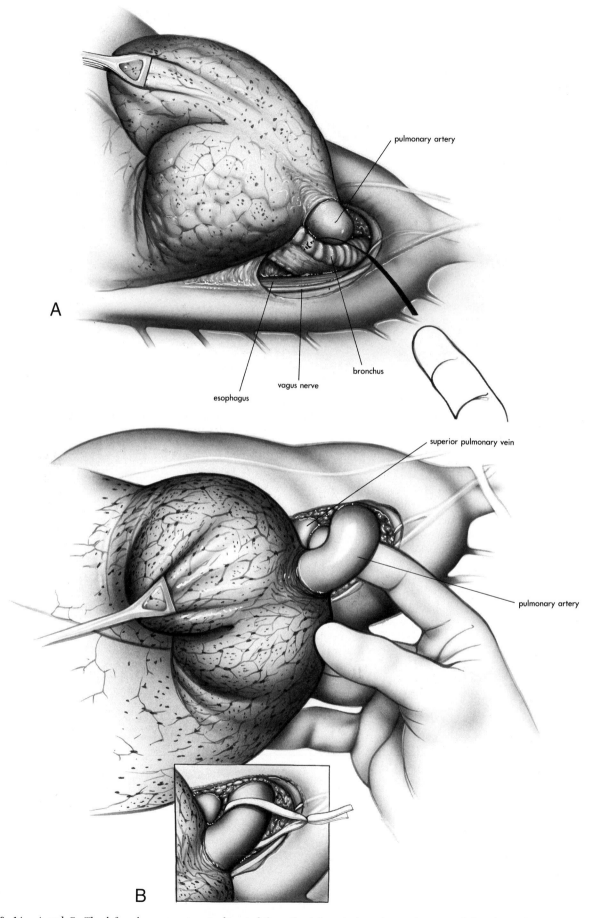

pulmonary artery

esophagus

vagus nerve

bronchus

A

superior pulmonary vein

pulmonary artery

B

Fig. 30–14. *A* and *B*, The left pulmonary artery is dissected from the left main bronchus and is encircled with a Silastic loop.

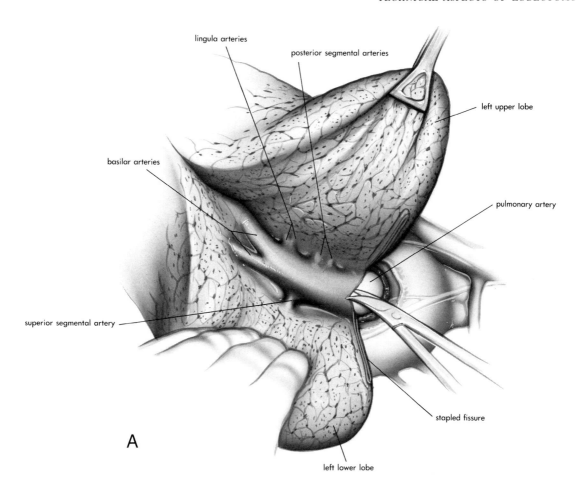

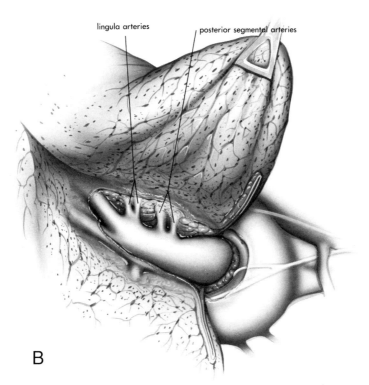

Fig. 30–15. *A* and *B*, The posterior portion of the fissure is completed by stapling and the segmental arteries are demonstrated.

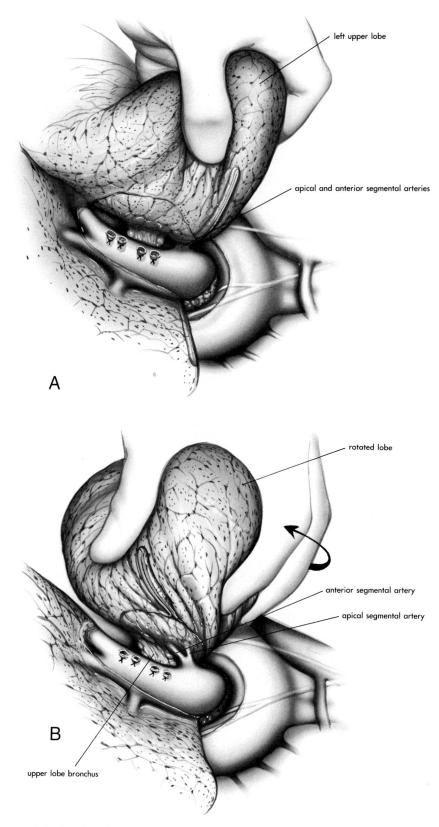

left upper lobe

apical and anterior segmental arteries

A

rotated lobe

anterior segmental artery

apical segmental artery

upper lobe bronchus

B

Fig. 30–16. After division of the lingula and posterior segmental arteries *(A)*, rotation of the lobe aids dissection of the apical and anterior segmental arteries *(B)*.

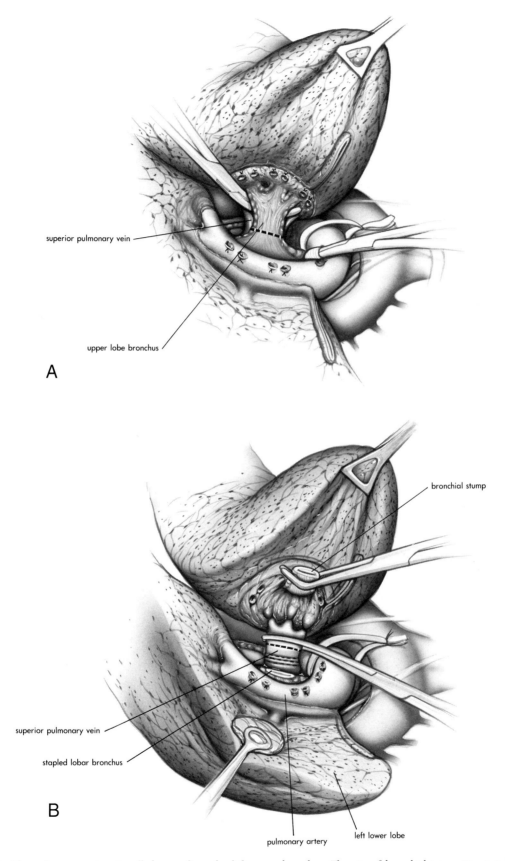

Fig. 30–17. *A*, The pulmonary artery is rolled away from the left upper bronchus. The site of bronchial transection is indicated. *B*, The left upper lobe bronchus is stapled and divided. The superior pulmonary vein is stapled and occluded distally by a Sarot clamp.

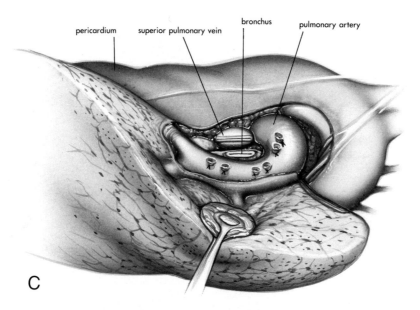

pericardium   superior pulmonary vein   bronchus   pulmonary artery

C

Fig. 30–17. (continued) *C*, Left upper lobe hilum after lobectomy.

LEFT LOWER LOBECTOMY

Provided that the oblique fissure is complete, left lower lobectomy is the simplest of all to perform; vascular anomalies are not commonly noted. The lung is retracted anteriorly and the posterior mediastinal pleura is incised from the level of the bronchus to the inferior pulmonary ligament, which should be divided at this time. The upper lobe is retracted anteriorly and superiorly and the lower lobe is moved posteriorly and inferiorly, exposing the pulmonary artery in the fissure (Fig. 30–18A). It is best to commence dissection of the pulmonary artery from its sheath at the posterior aspect of the fissure. If the fissure is obliterated by adhesions, dissection of the posterior segment of the upper lobe from the superior segment of the lower lobe is accomplished by pledget dissection of the interlobar pulmonary artery from the overlying parenchyma, as well as by the creation of a tunnel so that a stapling device or clamps may be inserted to complete enough of the fissure to allow further exposure of the interlobar artery. The anteromedial portion of the fissure is easily completed after bronchial closure. The superior segmental artery arises from the posterolateral surface of the interlobar pulmonary artery at a slightly lower level than the posterior segmental artery to the left upper lobe. Dissection of the interlobar artery along its midpoint is continued to delineate the origin of the lingular arteries, which must not be sacrificed. The basal trunk is then dissected, exposing the basal segmental branches. Occasionally, it is possible to double ligate the basal trunk distal to the lingular arteries and have one distal tie, but usually the basal branches must be ligated separately to ensure adequate length of the proximal stump (see Fig. 30–18B).

The inferior pulmonary vein is then cleared of areolar tissue, demonstrating its superior segmental and basal tributaries, and the interval between the bronchus and the vein is defined (Fig. 30–19A). The extrapericardial portion of the left inferior pulmonary vein is longer than the right; double proximal ligation is acceptable. The prefered management, however, is stapling the cardiac end of the vein, or application of a vascular clamp and suture. Additional length may be obtained by occluding the specimen side with a Sarot or other nonslipping clamp (see Fig. 30–19B).

The bronchus is cleared of areolar tissue and the crotch below the upper lobe bronchus is dissected. The stapling device is applied just distal to the upper lobe bronchus to avoid creating a cul de sac, or the bronchus is closed manually as described previously (Fig. 30–20).

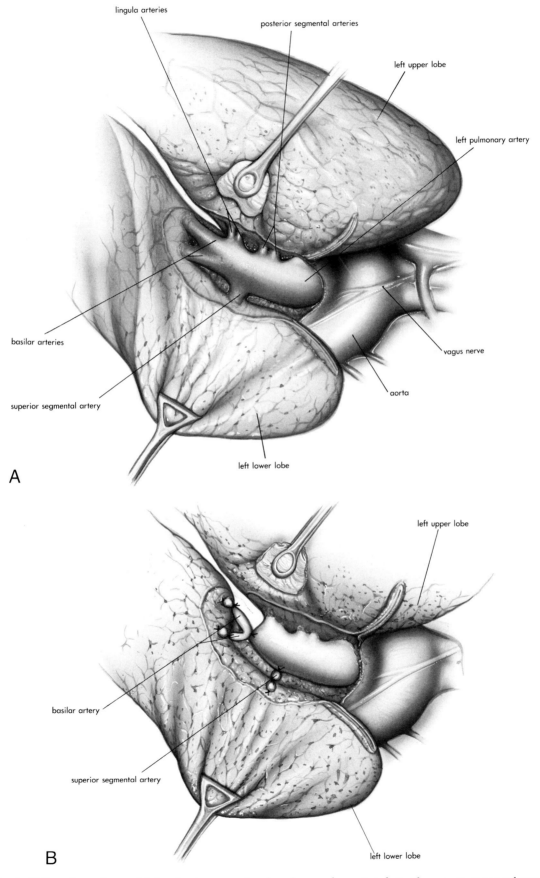

lingula arteries

posterior segmental arteries

left upper lobe

left pulmonary artery

basilar arteries

vagus nerve

superior segmental artery

aorta

left lower lobe

A

left upper lobe

basilar artery

superior segmental artery

left lower lobe

B

Fig. 30–18. *A*, Oblique fissure is completed and pulmonary artery branches are demonstrated. *B*, The superior segmental artery is ligated. Basal arteries are ligated and divided after the lingula arterial branches are demonstrated.

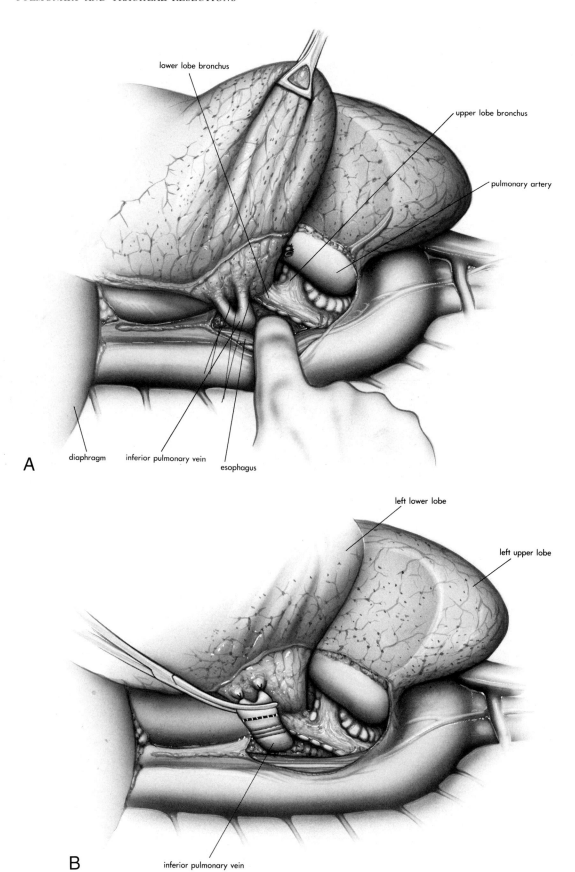

lower lobe bronchus

upper lobe bronchus

pulmonary artery

diaphragm   inferior pulmonary vein   esophagus

A

left lower lobe

left upper lobe

inferior pulmonary vein

B

Fig. 30–19. *A,* The interval between the pulmonary vein and the lower lobe bronchus is defined. *B,* The inferior pulmonary vein has been stapled. A Sarot clamp is applied to the specimen side prior to transection.

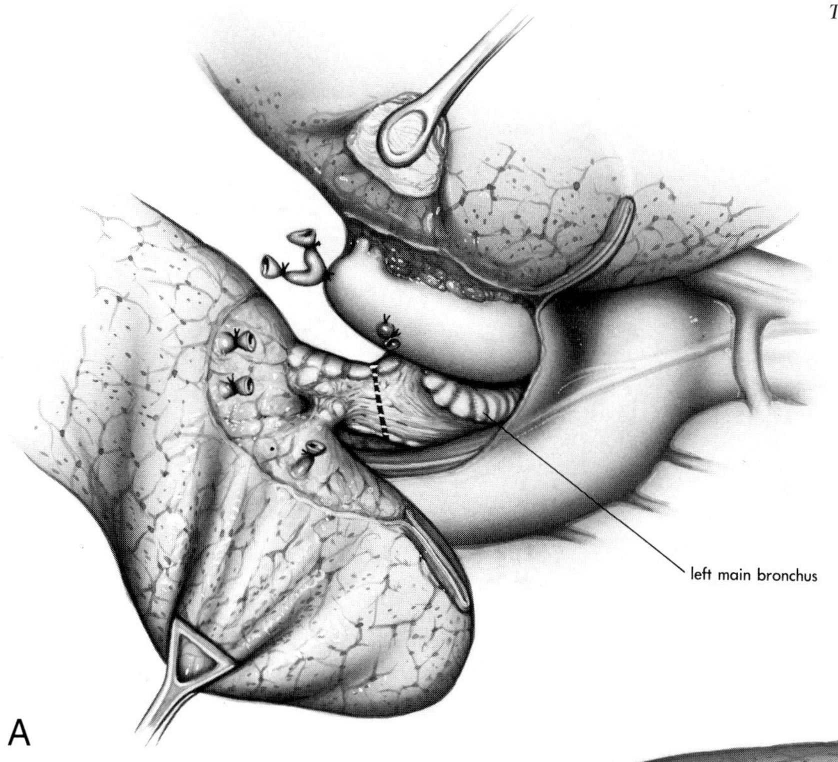

Fig. 30–20. *A,* Oblique transection of the bronchus prevents formation of a cul de sac. *B,* View of the hilum after left lower lobectomy.

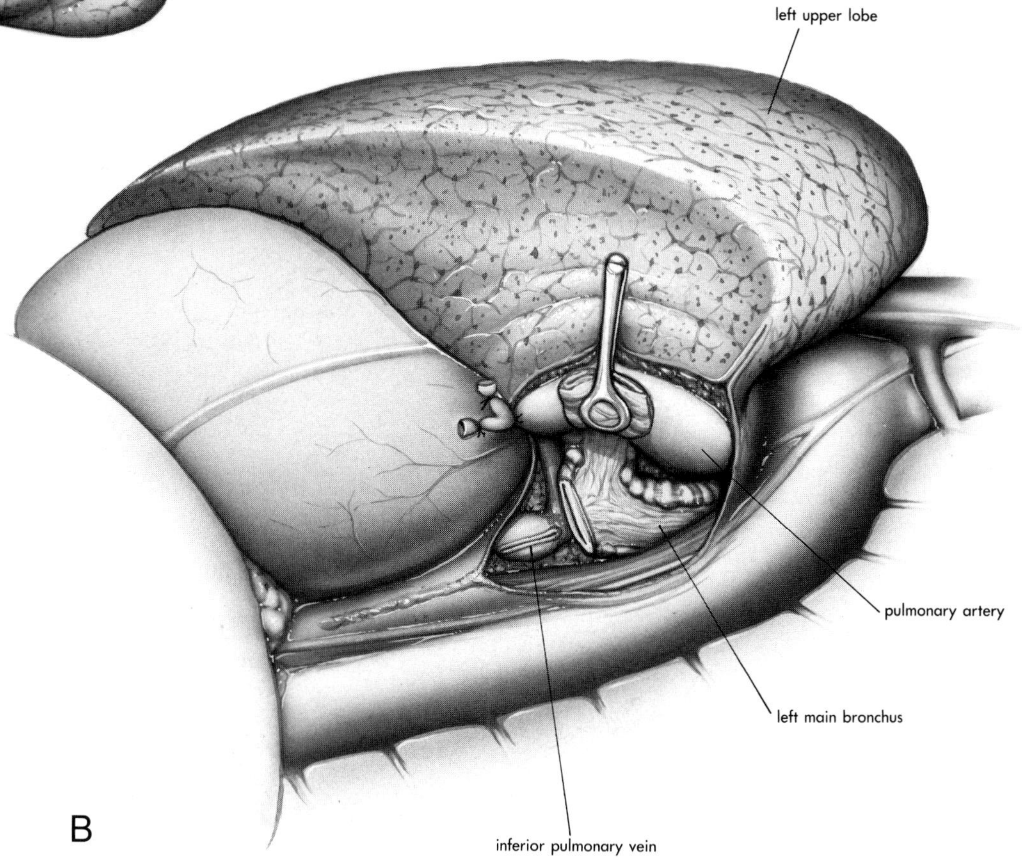

REFERENCES

Blades B, Kent EM: Individual ligation technique for lower lobectomy. J Thorac Surg *10*:84, 1940.

Lewis RJ, Sisler GE, Caccavale RJ: Imaged thoracic lobectomy: Should it be done? Ann Thorac Surg *54*:80, 1992.

McCaughan BC, et al: Chest wall invasion in carcinoma of the lung. J Thorac Cardiovasc Surg *89*:836, 1985.

Overholt RH, Langer L: The Technique of Pulmonary Resection. Springfield IL: Charles C Thomas, 1951.

Trastek VF, et al: En bloc (non-chest wall) resection for bronchogenic carcinoma with parietal fixation. Factors affecting survival. J Thorac Cardiovasc Surg *87*:352, 1984.

READING REFERENCES

Edmunds JH Jr, Norwood WI, Low DW: Atlas of Cardiothoracic Surgery. Philadelphia: Lea & Febiger, 1990.

Waldhausen JA, Pierce WS (eds): Johnson's Surgery of the Chest. 5th Ed. Chicago: Year Book, 1985.

CHAPTER 31

SLEEVE LOBECTOMY

I. Vogt-Moykopf, Stephen Trainer, Joadiim Schirren

HISTORY

The specific operative technique of bronchial sleeve resection is used to treat both benign and malignant disorders. It avoids the need for pneumonectomy and spares healthy lung tissue distal to the pathologic lesion. This type of operation may be performed as a single procedure or in combination with a segmental or tangential resection of the pulmonary artery.

Price Thomas (1956) reported the first sleeve lobectomy, which was performed in 1947 for a bronchial adenoma. Also treating bronchial adenoma, D'Abreau and McHale (1952) carried out an isolated resection of the left main bronchus. Gebauer (1953) removed a long tuberculous bronchial stenosis using the sleeve resection technique. Allison (1954) described the use of this technique to treat bronchial carcinoma.

Numerous authors have since reported their experiences with this surgical procedure. Among the early reports were those of Björk (1952) and Paulson (1955, 1970) and their associates, as well as Matthes (1956) and Johnston and Jones (1959). Many other studies have been reported and are listed in the Reading References.

The first author to mention angioplastic procedures in the dissection was Allison (1954). Wurning (1967) described tangential resection of the pulmonary artery. Pichlmaier and Spelsberg (1971) were the first to report four successful combined sleeve resections performed on the bronchus and pulmonary artery; Toomes and one of us (I. V-M.) (1985) described the first transposition of a complete lobe with a combined sleeve resection of the bronchus and the pulmonary artery and the transposition of the inferior pulmonary vein to the stump of the resected superior pulmonary vein.

INDICATIONS AND PREOPERATIVE DIAGNOSIS

The aim of sleeve resections of the bronchus and the pulmonary artery is to avoid pneumonectomy in centrally located pathologic lesions. Particular benefit is derived from this technique by elderly patients or those individuals with limited respiratory or general functional reserves. These patients would frequently not be in a condition to undergo any more extended surgery. In recent years, sleeve resections have been performed more often in young patients as well in order to avoid the detrimental effects of pneumonectomy, which reduces both the capacity for work and quality of life. Although sleeve resections involve technically more demanding procedures, they do not result in any increased operative risk.

Basically, the indications can be subdivided as follows: 1) a benign or malignant tumor or 2) a non–neoplastic bronchial stenosis as the result of precious trauma — post-traumatic — or subsequent to an inflammatory — infectious — disease process. Among the group with a neoplasm, bronchial carcinoma is most often the basic disorder, because it has been established that parenchyma-sparing procedures can achieve satisfactory radical removal of the tumor and its spread. Other less frequent indications are centrally located bronchial carcinoids, lung metastases with endobronchial infiltration, pulmonary sarcomas, mucoepidermoid tumors, bronchial adenomas, and even more rare types.

Most of the stenoses that are resected using bronchoplastic methods are caused by infections, most frequently after tuberculosis. An isolated resection without the removal of lung parenchyma is frequently possible when the stenoses are located in the left main bronchus.

In planning the surgical strategy, an exact preoperative diagnosis is absolutely indispensable. Beside the analysis of lung function and gas exchange, an exact bronchoscopic assessment of the pathologic lesion is required. Perfusion scans and, in certain cases, ventilation scintigraphy are indicated to assess each side separately.

In lung cancer patients, computed tomography must be performed, and in cases of mediastinal lymph node involvement, mediastinoscopy might be required to exclude N3 tumors. In our clinic, N2 tumors are radically resected as a matter of routine. Angiography of the pulmonary artery can indicate that angioplastic surgery is required. Hemodynamic studies of the pulmonary artery pressure in patients with restricted function may further assess the surgical risk.

In the management of bronchial carcinoma, we distinguish four basic groups of indication: 1) central tumor growth limited to the main bronchus, mostly left sided; 2) a tumor growing outward from or at the level of any lobar bronchial orifice — even the middle lobe — 3) extrabronchial tumor growth proximal to the lobe bronchus and infiltrating the peribronchial tissue; and 4) a peripheral tumor with involved hilar or bronchial lymph nodes and infiltrating the central bronchus or the peribronchial tissue. The same indications based on infiltration by the primary tumor or its hilar lymph node metastases apply to segmental resections of the pulmonary artery or — rarely — the pulmonary veins.

SPECIFIC ANESTHESIA REQUIREMENTS

In addition to the routine requirements for major surgery — continuous pulse oximetry, continuous measurement of blood pressure via a peripheral artery — sleeve resections of the bronchus require double-lumen intubation with the bronchial tube placed into the main bronchus of the contralateral side. The correct positioning of the tube is controlled using bronchoscopy. The single-lumen technique with intubation of the left main bronchus for resections on the right side, as described by several authors, can jeopardize the continuous gas exchange until the pulmonary artery has been clamped. This causes problems, particularly in patients with reduced functional reserves but with the perfusion being equally balanced. We no longer use this technique. High-frequency jet ventilation may be required when the bronchial anastomosis has to be carried out close to the carina, or when problems arise with the placement of the bronchial tube on the right side.

SURGICAL TECHNIQUE AND THE VARIOUS FORMS OF BRONCHO- AND ANGIOPLASTIC PROCEDURES

The most common approach in broncho- and angioplastic operations is the standard posterolateral thoracotomy. More rarely, a median sternotomy is used. Urschel and Razzuk (1986) found that bronchoplastic procedures could be performed with the latter approach without any problems. We have confirmed this finding for resections on the right side, but not for those on the left. In the resection of carcinomas, radical dissection of the mediastinal lymph nodes may turn out to be difficult in the lower mediastinum, particularly in the paraesophageal region. In elderly patients and those with heart disorders, hemodynamics may be severely affected by the manipulation of the heart. For the isolation of the anterior and posterior hilar structures and for dissection of the mediastinal lymph nodes, we find the posterolateral thoracotomy is the most convenient approach.

The range of bronchoplastic procedures includes all single bronchial resections without removal of parenchyma, anatomic segmental sleeve resections — superior segment of either lower lobe, sleeve lobectomies, and bilobectomies. Beside the "classic" bronchial resections of tumors in the right or left upper lobe or after upper and middle bilobectomies, specific techniques are being performed: the upper lobe bronchus is reanastomosed after removing the lower lobe, and middle-lobe sleeve resections and bronchial sleeves are performed after lower and middle bilobectomies, as are Y-sleeves on the left side (Fig. 31–1).

In recent years, when a lesion cannot be resected in patients with reduced functional reserves, treatment has also included extracorporeal resection* with reimplantation of the parts of the lung that can be preserved. Another procedure used more frequently that is performed together with extensive lung resections, mostly with upper right-sided — double — sleeve bilobectomies, is the transposition lobectomy. This procedure involves transplanting the lower lobar vein into the proximal stump of the upper lobe vein to ensure the tension-free anastomoses of both the bronchus and the artery.

The range of angioplastic procedures includes tangential resections of the pulmonary artery, complete segmental sleeve resections, and reanastomoses of segmental arteries (Fig. 31–2). This type of angioplastic

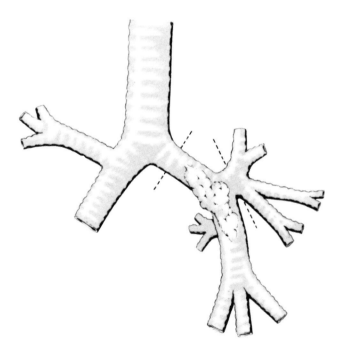

Fig. 31–1. Resection lines in a left lower sleeve lobectomy with anastomosis of the upper lobe bronchus to the left main bronchus (Y-sleeve).

---

*Extracorporeal resection is a descriptive term for a special surgical technique. We first perform a pneumonectomy if we are not able to remove the tumor by a standard sleeve lobectomy with the lung in situ. We then resect the tumorous parts of the lung at a separate table under sterile conditions, and replant the preservable part of the lung into the patient's chest.

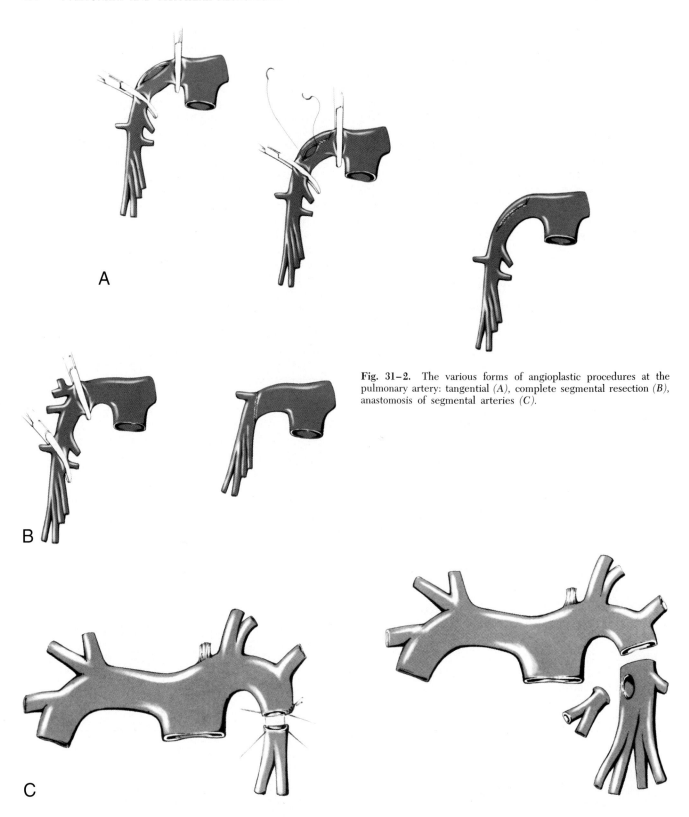

Fig. 31–2. The various forms of angioplastic procedures at the pulmonary artery: tangential *(A)*, complete segmental resection *(B)*, anastomosis of segmental arteries *(C)*.

resection is required most often in combination with bronchoplastic resections and is used almost exclusively to treat malignant tumors.

The technical approach for the different kinds of sleeve resections is as follows.

Bronchial Sleeve Resection

The success of the operation depends essentially on the observation of the following fundamental rules. Sufficient blood supply to the cut edges is indispensable. This provision may be particularly difficult at the distal incision line. The surgeon should avoid overly extensive skeletization of the tracheobronchial tree, which may be difficult when N2 involvement requires extensive dissection of the mediastinal lymph nodes. Frequently, it is impossible to preserve the subcarinal bronchial arteries. The lymph node dissection must be carried out before the anastomosis of the bronchus to avoid unnecessary mechanical strain. The extent of the resection must be controlled intraoperatively by frozen section examinations of the resection lines. The margins of resection should show fine petechial bleeding, and no severed — exposed — cartilage can be left in situ.

Where potential circulatory problems exist in the anastomosed parts, such as, after extensive lymph node dissection, or if the anastomosis is performed in a previously irradiated area, viable tissue can be used to cover the anastomosis. The most suitable covering material is the greater omentum, which should be prepared via transdiaphragmatic laparotomy and drawn up into the thorax as a pedicle flap. Neither closing the diaphragm nor mobilizing the omentum should put the blood supply of the latter at risk. Care must be taken when using an omental flap that it is not too voluminous, and one must take into account that its preparation means additional time that must be tolerated by the patient. Alternative material described in the literature, such as pedicles from intercostal muscles, diaphragm, the serratus muscle, or other muscles, often prove too thick. Thinner tissue can be obtained from the pericardium or a fat-free pleural patch. We have been able to operate without recourse to these procedures in most cases, because we perform the anastomoses without any

tension. The same approach has been described by Deslauriers and associates (1986).

The ends of the bronchus are anastomosed end-to-end, either edge-to-edge or as a "telescope anastomosis," in which the narrower distal part protrudes slightly into the proximal end. The latter method is used in cases of large differences in lumen size. In our experience, all types of atypical wedge-shaped excisions or similar methods to adapt different lumen sizes have been unsatisfactory. The resection of the bronchus must be carried out as vertically to its course as possible. Generally, wedge-shaped resections easily result in kinking at the anastomosis. Discrepancies in lumen size at the bronchial ends are adapted by gathering the membranous part of the larger segment. The membranous anastomosis is therefore completed last. Irregular sections of cartilage must be excised thoroughly, so as not to impair the exact juxtaposition of the resection margins.

The anastomosis must be performed absolutely free of tension, as emphasized. We used to assume that a slight amount of tension would prevent bronchial kinking, but we have revised our earlier opinions. No kinking occurs after anastomostic procedures that are technically correct.

To achieve a tension-free anastomosis in "classical" sleeve resections of the upper lobe, sufficient mobilization of the distal bronchus is obtained by detaching the pulmonary ligament. These resections are used when the defect is no larger than 1.5 to 2 cm. For more extended defects of up to 5 cm (Fig. 31–3), the following procedures are performed. In most cases on the right side, to ensure mobilization of the tracheal

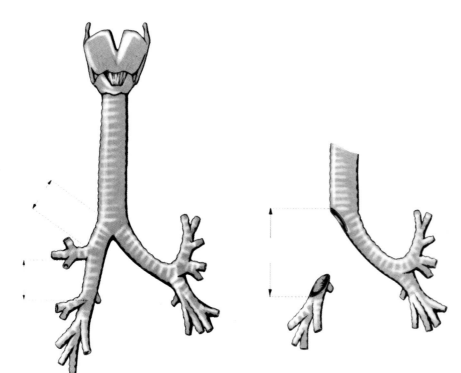

Fig. 31–3. The extent of bronchial defect depends on the kind of resection (right-sided): 1.5 to 2 cm in upper sleeve lobectomies, up to 5 to 5.5. cm in upper bilobectomies with wide bronchial resection.

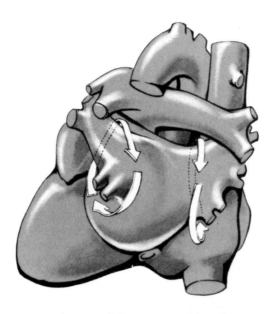

Fig. 31–4. Circular pericardial incision around the pulmonary veins.

bifurcation, the azygos vein must be divided. On the left side, by dividing the ligament of Botallo and Marshall's fold, the aortic arch can be mobilized. The pulmonary artery is drawn ventrally after performing a circular pericardiotomy specifically around the opening of the lower pulmonary vein into the left atrium. This step is indispensable for further mobilization of the lower and, if necessary, the middle lobe, and is practically mandatory to achieve tension-free anastomoses in bronchial sleeves combined with segmental arterial resections (Fig. 31–4). When even more extensive defects must be bridged, lobe transposition might be required. This technique requires transfering the lower lobe vein to the opening of the upper lobe vein (Fig. 31–5).

The bronchial anastomotic suture is carried out pericartilaginously through all layers using an interrupted

suture technique. We use monofilament, absorbable suture material, 4-0 and 5-0 poly dioxanone suture — PDS. The extramucous row of sutures mentioned repeatedly in the literature is practically impossible to perform. The bronchial ends must be apposed exactly, with strict attention paid to their lumen sizes and topographic position — beware of contorsion! Granulomas occur only rarely if this procedure is performed correctly. The distance between sutures must be appropriate to ensure that the blood supply to the edges of the anastomosis is not impaired.

After completing the anastomosis, its airtightness is checked by means of water test under ventilation — $P_{max} = 40$ cm H_2O. Before the thorax is closed, flexible bronchoscopy is performed to also ensure correct conditions at the anastomosis. This step allows us to clean the respiratory tract adequately.

A summary of the most important requirements in performing bronchial anastomosis is as follows: 1) petechial bleeding at the resection margins, 2) leave no severed cartilage in situ, and 3) tension-free anastomosis.

Sleeve Resection of the Pulmonary Artery

The extent of tumor growth, lymph node involvement, or both, and technical requirements, such as kinking that occurs in the bronchial anastomoses when the extent of the bronchial excision is too large or after injuries or trauma, are indications for arterial sleeve resection. More than 90% of vascular sleeve resections are performed in association with an upper lobectomy or bilobectomy, and most often in combination with a bronchial sleeve.

The most simple reconstructive technique of the pulmonary artery is a tangential suture to cut off segmental arteries, if tumor extension makes it impossible to perform the usual suture ligation. After clamping the vessel, excision and a continuous suture repair with monofilament nonabsorbable suture material 5-0 or 6-0 follow. The tumor growth often lies adjacent

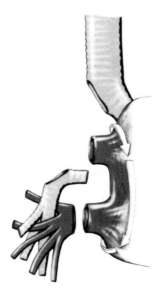

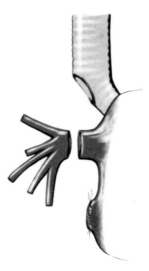

Fig. 31–5. Transposition lobectomy. Beside the double-sleeve resection of the pulmonary artery and the bronchus, the lower lobe vein is transferred to the site of the upper vein at the left vestibule.

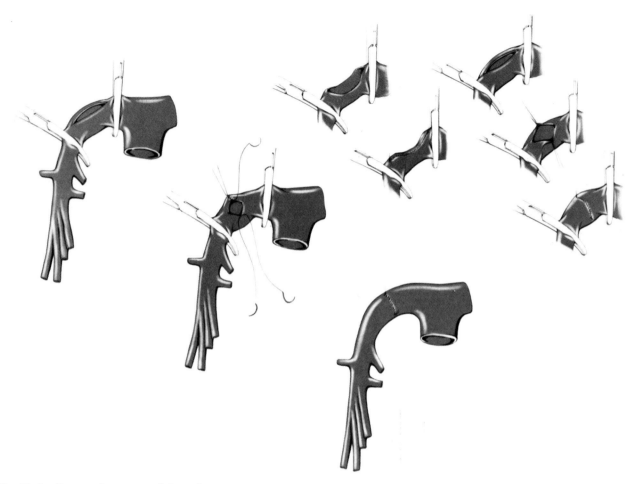

Fig. 31–6. Tangential resection of the pulmonary artery: transverse suturing to prevent artificial stenosis in larger defects.

to the adventitia, requiring a partial resection of the arterial wall. It has to be decided whether a sleeve resection is the more appropriate procedure or whether a part of the arterial wall tissue can be preserved by a transverse repair (Fig. 31–6). For sleeve resections, the pulmonary artery must be exposed proximally to its origin. This step creates the necessary space to apply a central atraumatic clamp. Concurrently, the azygos vein must be severed on the right side to be able to retract the vena cava medially. On the left side, the ligament of Botallo — beware of the recurrent nerve! — and the pericardial fold are divided. Pericardiotomy is necessary in both cases. To guarantee a bloodless field, either a second clamp is applied at the distal interlobar site or the remaining pulmonary veins are temporarily clamped. In this way, the blood remaining runs out of the lung after the resection of the involved portion of the artery. We administer 5000 to 7500 International Units of heparin systemically in advance — the exact amount depends on the patient's weight — to prevent any intravascular coagulation.

The anastomosis is accomplished with a continuous suture of monofilament, nonabsorbable material 5-0 or 6-0 PDS. Different calibers can be adjusted using oblique incisions or by additionally incising the distal end of the vessel. In exceptional cases, for example, when the vessels of the middle lobe or of the lingula are to be reanastomosed with the main trunk of the pulmonary artery, an interrupted suture technique is required.

Combined Sleeve Resections of the Bronchus and the Pulmonary Artery

The majority of so-called double-sleeve resections are performed together with upper lobectomies (Fig. 31–7). The bronchial anastomosis is carried out first to avoid mechanical damage to the vulnerable vascular anastomosis. For technical reasons, it is not always possible to keep to this order. Where the bronchial and arterial anastomotic lines are apposed, a thin layer of adjacent viable tissue may be placed between the bronchial and the arterial sutures; such as, from the pericardium or a fat-free pleural flap. A greater omental patch is usually too thick and compromises the vascular anastomosis. The more tension-free these anastomoses, the lower the complication rate in these sleeve resections. Both extracorporeal resection and lobe transposition require an additional venous anastomosis. The suture technique for anastomosis of the vein corresponds with that used for the pulmonary artery.

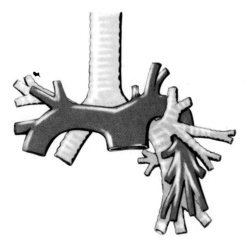
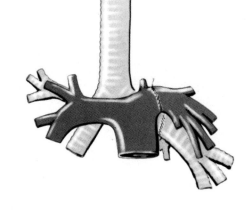

Fig. 31–7. Double sleeve resection of the left upper lobe.

POSTOPERATIVE CARE

The postoperative care is basically the same as after standard resections. It is essential to perform the extubation as early as possible to prevent adverse effects of ventilation under positive pressure. Extubation occurs under bronchoscopic guidance, combined with concomitant bronchial toilet. It may be necessary to flush the airway system to free it of encrustations and viscous mucus. We recommend bacteriologic examination of the aspirated bronchial secretion. The further course depends on sufficient bronchial toilet by intensive respiration training, broncholytics, incentive spirometry, vibratory massage, postural drainage, and possibly applying bronchodilators, as the ciliary function in the anastomosed bronchus is affected. The patient should therefore learn the appropriate respiratory techniques preoperatively. If the patient has retained secretions, atelectasis, or both, bronchoscopy is required. After bronchial sleeve resections, we do not use blind nasotracheal aspiration, because it might cause damage to the bronchial anastomosis. We perform a tracheostomy with a plastic tube — in patients with persisting mucus retention or who have developed atelectasis and pneumonia. This measure enables us to perform bronchoscopy under visual control as often as required, without putting any strain on the patient.

At the end of the first postoperative week, the anastomosis is examined bronchoscopically. Before the patient is discharged, we record the functional result using perfusion and ventilation scintigraphy. Further bronchoscopy performed 6 weeks later principally serves to recognize any stenosis at an early stage. This complication can then be treated by endoscopic procedures such as dilation, laser removal, or stenting in severe cases. Further followup management depends on each individual situation. Pulmonary angiography to assess the arterial blood flow and the venous drainage is only necessary if, for example, intravascular coagulation is suspected.

COMPLICATIONS

Impairment of the healing process at the bronchial anastomosis is the most typical complication after reconstructive surgery. Limited shallow necrosis of the mucosa normally heals without problems. Small fistulae manifest clinically in a wheezing sound during respiration or in partial collapse of the lung. Most heal spontaneously. In patients being artificially ventilated, the small fistulae most often progress to total necrosis, which can result in complete dehiscence of the suture line.

Total necrosis at the anastomosis, followed by suture line dehiscence, can be recognized by regularly performing bronchoscopy. It is sometimes difficult to differentiate between limited shallow necrosis of the mucosa and complete bronchial wall necrosis. In those cases, the clinical condition of the patient — fever, leukocytosis, poorer general condition, infected pleural effusion, air leakage — is the decisive factor. A great deal of experience is required in any case in deciding whether to perform a completion — secondary — pneumonectomy or to continue with observation. If the patient's functional reserves permit, secondary pneumonectomy must be performed promptly if complete dehiscence is seen. This procedure is mandatory if dark-red hemoptysis appears; this is a sign of bleeding as a consequence of erosion of the pulmonary artery.

Bronchial kinking will not occur when the procedure has been performed correctly. Because we no longer do partial bronchial sleeve resections, we do not see this complication any more. Cicatricial stenosis after secondary healing is treated endoscopically, that is, by applying a stent. In rare cases, when no treatment is possible, cicatricial stenosis can result in a destroyed lobe. This situation makes secondary — completion — pneumonectomy unavoidable, if the patient's general condition is good enough to tolerate this procedure.

Both acute and chronic thrombotic occlusions are typical complications after sleeve resections of the pulmonary artery. The former occurs as an acute syndrome within the early postoperative period, manifesting as a rapid deterioration in the patient's general condition and severely impaired gas exchange, similar to the symptoms of pulmonary embolism. Diagnosis can be confirmed instantaneously by angiography. Completion pneumonectomy is the treatment of choice. Chronic thrombosis is not associated with any relevant clinical symptoms. It is detected in a discrepancy between scintigraphic ventilation and perfusion. No therapeutic management is required in most cases. The lung can be left as a kind of "plug."

The use of extracorporeal resection and lobe transpositions may cause a specific form of vascular complication, namely thrombotic occlusion of the venous anastomosis. It results in hemorrhagic infarction of the lung. Its clinical manifestations are similar to those of acute thrombosis of the pulmonary artery although with a greater degree of infiltration seen on the chest radiograph. Diagnosis is confirmed angiographically. Completion pneumonectomy is required for treatment.

RESULTS

In our clinic, we have performed 771 broncho- and angioplastic procedures to treat bronchial carcinomas between 1973 and 1991. From October 1986 onward, we were able to analyze 502 of these patients prospectively. In this group, we carried out 121 "classical" bronchial sleeve resections and 42 bronchial sleeve resections with reanastomosing of the upper lobe — Y sleeves. A total of 65 "classical" double sleeves plus 6 Y-double sleeves were performed, including 14 extracorporeal resections and lobe transpositions with triple anastomosis. In 13 patients, arterial segmental resections were performed as an isolated procedure, as were partial vascular resections in 237 patients. In exceptional cases, moreover, we performed 18 partial bronchial anastomoses (Table 31–1).

The 30-day mortality rate after sleeve resections is reported to be between 0 and 12%. We found a rate

Table 31–1. Broncho- and Angioplastic Procedures to Treat Bronchial Carcinoma*

Surgical Technique	Number of Patients
"Classic" bronchial sleeve resection	121
"Y"-bronchial sleeve resection	41
"Classic" double-sleeve resection	65
"Y"-double sleeve resection	6
Arterial sleeve resection	13
Partial bronchial sleeve resection	18
Partial vascular sleeve resection	237
	501

*Prospective analysis in our series, 1984 to 1991. Fourteen extracorporeal resections and lobe transpositions are included in the double sleeve resections.

of 8% in patients with carcinoma. No deaths were recorded in our patients aged 30 years or younger regardless of the underlying disease. A few reports cite larger series of the aforementioned combined procedures. The mortality rate in our patients varied between 7.6 and 10%, depending on the combination of techniques used. The higher rate is found after combining complete bronchial sleeves with complete vascular anastomosis in patients with high functional risks. One typical cause of death is the bleeding after erosion of the anastomoses. In 9 of 22 patients with this complication, we prevented fatal hemorrhaging by reoperating promptly. All other causes of death, such as respiratory failure, empyema, sepsis, and heart failure, do not differ from those found after standard resection.

The incidence of bronchopleural fistulae reported in the literature is between 1 and 11.4%. Our data show a rate of 9.4%. Empyema occurs in 3.4% of all cases.

The 5-year survival rates after those specific bronchoplastic procedures on bronchial carcinoma vary in the literature from 17 to 50%. Correlated to the respective stages, we found rates of 40% in stage I patients and 17% in patients with stage II and III disease after all angio- and bronchoplastic procedures.

Local recurrence was caused mainly by undetected carcinoma in the lymphatics associated with hilar lymph node metastasis. This situation is described in the literature with an incidence of 2 to 51%. In our patients, we observed recurrences in 16% of stage I and II patients. Local recurrence is treated with secondary resections, if possible, or with irradiation.

Analyses of the functional results must be based on a comparison of the values found after pneumonectomy of the involved lung. Using perfusion and ventilation scintigraphy, one of us (I. V-M.) and associates reported that a significant amount of functionally active lung tissue had been maintained as early as 3 weeks after surgery (1985). No systematic prospective analyses are available. In two thirds of our patients, the proportion was on average 20%, regardless of the type of anastomosis, compared with the contralateral lung. Long-term followup of lung function by Deslauriers and associates (1986) showed only minor restrictions in 19 patients compared with normal findings for their age.

Because the surgical risk is not higher than that for pneumonectomies, and a significantly better postoperative quality of life and physical capacity is ensured by preservation of functioning and intact lung tissue, broncho- and angioplastic procedures should be chosen over pneumonectomy, if technically possible, in the treatment of bronchial carcinoma. Use of simple pneumonectomy to treat this condition should be the exception rather than the rule. In patients with benign diseases, such as bronchial stenosis requiring surgical intervention, bronchoplastic methods represent the only means of corrective surgical management that can improve lung function.

REFERENCES

Allison PR: Course of Thoracic Surgery in Groningen 1954.

Björk VO, Carlens E, Craford C: The open closure of the bronchus and the resection of the carina and of the tracheal wall. J Thorac Surg 23:419, 1952.

D'Abreau AL, McHale SJ: Bronchial "adenoma" treated by local resection and reconstruction of the left main bronchus. Br J Surg 39:355, 1952.

Deslauriers J, et al: Long-term clinical and functional results of sleeve lobectomy for primary lung cancer. J Thorac Cardiovasc Surg 92:871, 1986.

Gebauer PW: Bronchial resection and anastomosis. J Thorac Surg 26:241, 1953.

Jensik RJ, Faber LP, Kittle CF: Sleeve lobectomy for bronchogenic carcinoma: The Rush-Presbyterian-St. Luke's Medical Center experience. Int Surg 71:207, 1986.

Johnston JB, Jones PH: The treatment of bronchial carcinoma by lobectomy and sleeve resection of the main bronchus. Thorax 14:48, 1959.

Matthes TH: Über Möglichkeiten von Lungenteil- und Bronchus-resektionen mit End-zu-End-Anastomose bei ausgewählten Fällen von Bronchialkarzinomen. Thoraxchirurgie 4:106, 1956.

Naruke T, Suemasu K: Bronchoplastic surgery for lung cancer and the results. Jpn J Surg 13:165, 1983.

Paulson DL, Shaw RR: Preservation of lung tissue by means of bronchoplastic procedures. Am J Surg 89:347, 1955.

Paulson DL, et al: Bronchoplastic procedures for bronchogenic carcinoma. J Thorac Cardiovasc Surg 59:38, 1970.

Pichlmayer H, Spelsberg F: Organerhaltende Operation des Bron-chialkarzinoms. Langenbecks Arch Chir 328:221, 1971.

Price Thomas C: Conservative resection of the bronchial tree. J R Coll Surg Edinb 1:169, 1956.

Toomes H, Vogt-Moykopf I: Conservative resection for lung cancer. *In* Delarue NC, Eschapasse H (eds): International Trends in General Thoracic Surgery. Vol. I. Philadelphia: WB Saunders, 1985, p. 88.

Urschel HC Jr, Razzuk MA: Median sternotomy as a standard approach for pulmonary resection. Ann Thorac Surg 41:130, 1986.

Vogt-Moykopf I, Toomes H, Fritz I: Manschettenresektion des Bronchus und der Pulmonalarterie. Prax Klin Pneumol 39:574, 1985.

Vogt-Moykopf I, et al: Bronchoplastic techniques for lung resection. *In* Baue AE, Naunheim KS (eds): Glenn's Thoracic and Car-diovascular Surgery. Fifth Edition. Vol. 1. Norwalk: Appleton and Lange, 1990, p. 403.

Wurning P: Technische Vorteile bei der Hauptbronchusresektion rechts und links. Thoraxchir Vask Chir 15:16, 1967.

READING REFERENCES

Ayabe H, et al: Bronchoplasty for bronchogenic carcinoma. World J Surg 6:433, 1982.

Bennett FW, Smith AR: A twenty-year analysis of the results of sleeve resection for primary bronchogenic carcinoma. J Thorac Car-diovasc Surg 76:840, 1978.

Dortenmann I: Indikation und Technik der parenchym-erhaltenden Bronchusresektion. Thoraxchir Vask Chir 11:554, 1964.

Faber LP, Jensik RJ, Kittle CF: Results of sleeve lobectomy for bronchogenic carcinoma in 101 patients. Ann. Thorac. Surg. 37:279, 1984.

Fujimura S, et al: Prognostic evaluation of tracheobronchial recon-struction for bronchogenic carcinoma. J Thorac Cardiovasc Surg 90:161, 1985.

Jensik RJ, et al: Sleeve lobectomy for carcinoma, a ten-year expe-rience. J Thorac Cardiovasc Surg 64:400, 1972.

Naruke T, et al: Bronchoplastic procedure for lung cancer. J Thorac Cardiovasc Surg 73:927, 1977.

Rees GM, Paneth M: Lobectomy with sleeve resection in the treatment of bronchial tumors. Thorax 25:160, 1970.

Van Den Bosch JMM, et al: Lobectomy with sleeve resection in the treatment of tumors of the bronchus. Chest 80:154, 1981.

Vogt-Moykopf I, et al: Organsparende Operationsverfahren beim Bronchialkarzinom, Ergebnisse. Langenbecks Arch Chir 355:117, 1981.

Weisel RD, et al: Sleeve lobectomy for carcinoma of the lung. J Thorac Cardiovasc Surg 78:839, 1979.

CHAPTER 32

SEGMENTECTOMY AND LESSER PULMONARY RESECTIONS

Joseph LoCicero, III

Parenchyma-sparing pulmonary resections are important procedures for many patients. Although lobectomy and pneumonectomy remain standard operations for patients with primary lung cancer, many authors advocate less than lobectomy as an equal operation, particularly in the patient with limited pulmonary reserve. When resection of a pulmonary metastasis may provide prolonged survival, a lesser resection is an ideal procedure. These techniques are also applied for diagnosis of the indeterminate pulmonary nodule prior to consideration for lobectomy.

SEGMENTECTOMY

This form of resection, popularized in midcentury, is considered an anatomic operation because it removes the segmental bronchus back to its primary branch along with all of the lung parenchyma and lymph node groupings supplied by the bronchus and its associated segmental pulmonary artery. This technique was used in the treatment of pulmonary tuberculosis, bronchiectasis, and other suppurative pulmonary lesions. As these infections became less common, after development of effective antituberculous chemotherapy and broad spectrum antibiotics for suppurative diseases, the operation became less common. Many authors over the last two decades, however, such as Jensik and associates (1973, 1979, 1987), Shields and Higgins (1974), and Crabbe and colleagues (1989, 1991), suggested its use in early lung cancer. However, Ginsberg (personal communication, 1993) and Warren and Faber (1993) suggest that lobectomy, in those who can tolerate it, should remain the treatment of choice. With the resurgence of *Mycobacterium tuberculosis* in urban areas and the development of drug-resistant atypical strains, this technique may find considerably more usefulness in the coming decades.

Technique

Standard lateral thoracotomy position using double-lumen endotracheal tube anesthesia is the most popular approach at present. A posterior approach in the prone position may be used, particularly when one expects copious secretions from a suppurative process. This approach has limited application today and should be undertaken only by those familiar with the special positioning required to avoid brachial plexus injury.

The initial steps in segmentectomy are all the same as for any standard resection of the lung. The hilar structures are identified and the major fissure is opened. The surgeon must be familiar with intraparenchymal anatomy of the bronchus and pulmonary artery to accomplish a segmentectomy successfully.

On the right side, the bronchus is the most posterior hilar structure. The upper lobe branches of the pulmonary artery are the most superior hilar structures in the chest (Fig. 32–1). In the major fissure, the pulmonary artery can be exposed, demonstrating the continuation of the main pulmonary artery into the lower lobe. Anterior and posterior branches originate opposite one another and go, respectively, to the middle lobe and the superior segment of the lower lobe forming a cross. Often, a posterior ascending branch arises from the posterior segmental artery and supplies part of the posterior segment of the upper lobe (Fig. 32–2).

On the left side, the pulmonary artery crosses superiorly above the left main stem bronchus to become the most posterior structure in the hilus. The apical-posterior and anterior and segmental branches are located anteriorly and superiorly. A separate posterior segmental branch is often found posteriorly on the main pulmonary artery, just at or above the major fissure (Fig. 32–3). In the major fissure, the lingular branches anteriorly and the superior segment branch posteriorly form a cross on the continuation of the pulmonary artery

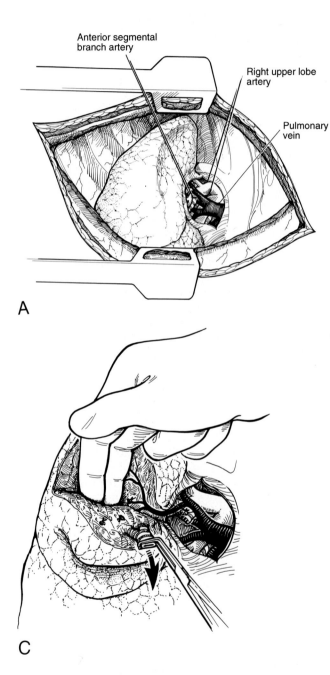

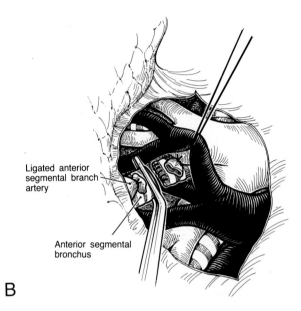

Fig. 32–1. A right anterior segmentectomy. *A*, Isolation of the right upper lobe artery and ligation of the anterior segmental branch. *B*, Division of the anterior segmental bronchus. *C*, Traction and finger fracture of the pulmonary parenchyma visualizing the pulmonary vein in the intersegmental plane.

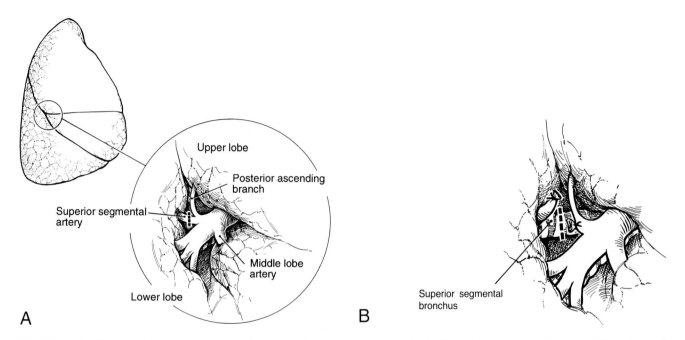

Fig. 32–2. A right superior segmentectomy. *A,* Exposure of the pulmonary artery in the fissure demonstrating the middle lobe artery and the superior segmental artery opposite one other with identification and preservation of the posterior ascending arterial branch. *B,* Division of the superior segmental bronchus.

(Fig. 32–4). The surgeon must be mindful of the high degree of variability of the branches of the pulmonary artery and carefully identify each branch before ligation (see Chapter 6).

The artery and bronchus are ligated and divided. The order of division depends on the segment to be removed. For the apical and anterior segment of the upper lobe on the right side, the artery is ligated first and elevated to locate the segmental bronchus. For the posterior right upper lobe segment, it may be easier to divide the bronchus first and then the artery, which may be deep in the parenchyma and not easily isolated anteriorly because of the other segmental branches. On the left side, the arterial branches are more easily isolated first because the bronchus is the middle structure on that side.

Before dividing the bronchus, differential deflation and inflation of the segment to be removed should be done to help delineate the intersegmental planes, keeping in mind that filling of the deflated segment may occur from adjacent segments by means of collateral ventilation. With the advent of the double lumen tube, it is often easier to inflate the entire lung, clamp the bronchus, and allow the rest of the lung to deflate. The segment will remain inflated for a longer period of time, even with some loss from collateral ventilation. Once the appropriate segmental bronchus is identified, it is divided. The proximal stump may be closed either with a mechanical stapler or with interrupted fine absorbable sutures. Additional coverage of the stump is usually not necessary.

After the bronchus and artery are ligated, traction is placed on the bronchus and the segment is removed

in a retrograde manner. The plane is developed using digital blunt dissection with division of the pleura by scissors or cautery. The pulmonary veins course through the intersegmental planes and provide an excellent anatomic guide. Individual branches of the vein emanating from the segment into the fissure are sequentially divided.

After removal of the specimen, the raw surfaces of the adjacent segments are inspected and any significant bleeding is controlled. A sponge is applied to the expanded lung. After 5 to 10 minutes, the sponge is removed and the lung surface is again inspected. If the dissection of the intersegmental plan has been done carefully, only a few alveolar air leaks will be present. These tend to seal over promptly with re-expansion of the lung during the postoperative period. Any leaking from small bronchi, however, must be recognized and controlled; this type of leak may cause persistent problems and predispose to postoperative space problems and infections. Jensik (1986) advocated covering the raw surfaces with pleural flaps or reconstituting the lung by bringing the adjacent segments together. Such a step generally is unnecessary and may lead to increased postoperative problems.

Management of the Pleural Space

Two thoracostomy tubes usually are placed into the space before the wound is closed — one anteriorly and one posteriorly. These tubes are connected to an underwater drainage system. When negative suction is applied to the tubes, significant air leak may result, particularly on positive pressure ventilation. It may be best to withhold suction until the patient is in the

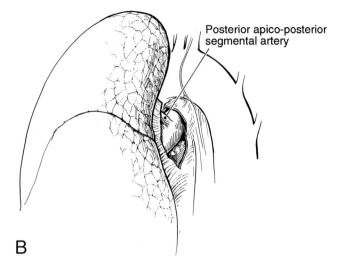

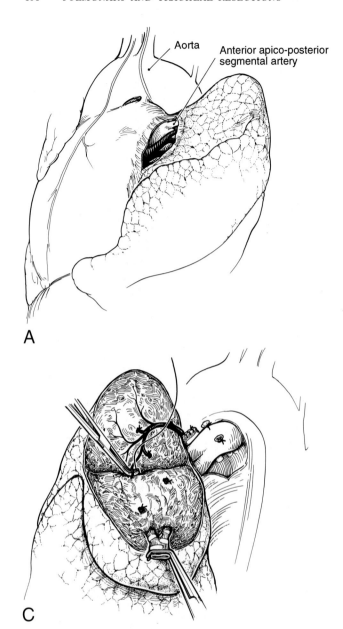

Fig. 32–3. A left apicoposterior segmentectomy. *A*, Identification and ligation of the anterior artery. *B*, Identification and ligation of the posterior artery. *C*, Parenchymal dissection of the segment exposing the vein in the intersegmental plane.

postanesthesia care unit. When a patient is breathing spontaneously, suction may be applied cautiously. Once the lung is re-expanded, suction may be used to maintain this expansion. Subsequent management of the pleural tubes is the same as that described for lobectomy.

Physiologic Effects

The physiologic changes after segmentectomy are the same as those noted after a lobectomy. The patient reacts in the same way as after a lobectomy because of the significant dysfunction following handling of the lobe during the operation. Late functional results are related to the number of segments removed. Over the next several months, the patient regains function of the remaining segments, although functional gain by the

preservation of a segment of a lobe is generally less than expected from its volume.

Morbidity and Mortality

The nonfatal complications are similar to those occurring after a lobectomy. The major ones are prolonged air leak, either peripheral alveolar pleural fistula or a true bronchopleural fistula; empyema; and persistent pleural airspace. All are interrelated and the incidence of any one alone or in combination varies most directly with the disease process and the difficulty experienced in the dissection of the intersegmental planes.

The incidence of persistent pleural airspace is as high as 33% in patients with pulmonary tuberculosis. Compared with pleural airspaces occurring after lobectomy, however, only a small percentage of those noted after

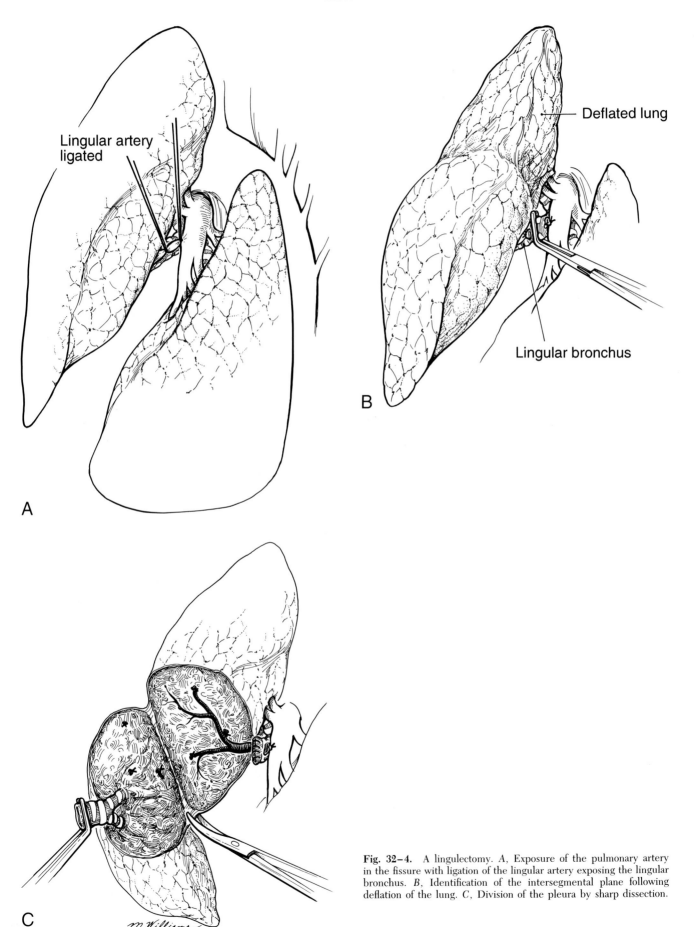

Lingular artery
ligated

A

Deflated lung

Lingular bronchus

B

C

m Williams

Fig. 32–4. A lingulectomy. *A*, Exposure of the pulmonary artery in the fissure with ligation of the lingular artery exposing the lingular bronchus. *B*, Identification of the intersegmental plane following deflation of the lung. *C*, Division of the pleura by sharp dissection.

segmentectomy produce symptoms. When serious complications develop as a result of the space, they are most likely to be septic. The empyema with or without bronchopleural fistula must be treated in the usual manner.

Segmentectomy is essentially a benign procedure and the mortality rate should approximate 1%. It may, however, be as high as 4 to 6% in patients with poor pulmonary function or in those with previous pulmonary resection, as reported by Jensik (1986).

NONANATOMIC PARENCHYMA-SPARING RESECTIONS

Patients with metastatic lesions from sites such as the gastrointestinal tract, head and neck, breast, and genitourinary tract are ideal candidates for metastatectomy using nonanatomic resections. These patients may have multiple lesions or may present with additional lesions on subsequent occasions. Anatomic resections may remove a considerable amount of unaffected normal functioning lung, which might render these individuals pulmonary cripples and severely affect their quality of life. Mountain and colleagues (1984) reported an overall survival rate of 35% in large collected series of patients. McAfee and co-workers (1992) found a 5-year survival rate of 35% for colon carcinoma. Lanza and associates (1992) reported a 35% 5-year survival for breast carcinoma. Progrebniak and colleagues (1992) were able to

extend median survivals of patients with renal cell carcinoma to 43 months. Patients who may also benefit from such an approach are those with marginal function who have an early stage I or stage II lung cancer. In a small series of collected patients with marginal lung function and early cancers, Miller and Hatcher (1987) showed a 5-year survival rate of 35%. Errett and associates (1985), Peters (1982), and Lewis and colleagues (1992) advocated similar approaches for the patient with marginal lung function.

Several methods are available for performing nonanatomic resections of the lung, including stapling devices, electrocautery, and laser. The techniques for each of these are all similar.

Technique

Patients undergoing limited lung resection using any one of the variety of the aforementioned methods may have one of a variety of incisions ranging from a standard posterolateral incision or sternotomy for bilateral disease to the minimally invasive video-assisted thoracic surgical techniques. Most patients are placed in the lateral thoracotomy position with double-lumen tube anesthesia. After entry into the chest, thorough inspection is made to assure that all areas of disease are identified. If the patient has multiple metastatic lesions, each should be addressed separately.

Several stapling devices are now available that are helpful in performing a nonanatomic wedge resection.

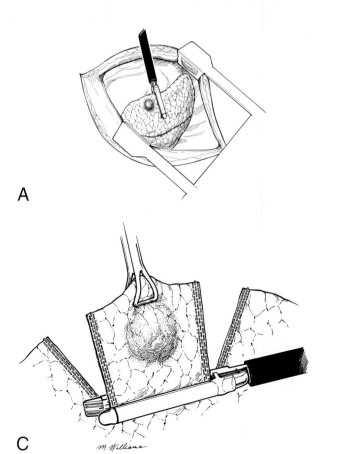

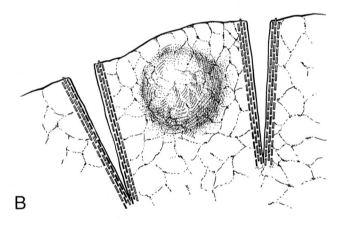

A

B

C

m Williams

Fig. 32–5. A wedge resection. *A*, Exposure of the lesion, collapse of the lung, and stapling with an endoscopic stapler. *B*, Placement of the two parallel staple lines. *C*, Placement of the final staple line with traction on the parenchyma.

The wedge is best performed by using a U-type rather than a V-type resection. The new GIA staples, which cut and divide at the same time, are excellent for this procedure (Fig. 32–5). Two parallel lines are placed into the lungs, several centimeters separated from the lesion. The lesion is then elevated and one or two additional staple lines are placed at the proximal margin. This technique allows more complete removal without compromise of the proximal margin as occurs when one performs a V-type incision.

Electrocautery may be used to remove a lesion. This device can cut and coagulate simultaneously; the technique for its use was described by Urschel (1986). A linear incision is made over the lesion in the parenchyma and the lesion is exposed. By using traction and countertraction and applying cautery just beneath the lesion, it can be excised, leaving essentially all normal lung tissue. To accomplish this excision, a setting of at least 70 watts must be applied to coagulate the tissue. At this power, resection proceeds with adequate coagulation of small and medium blood vessels. The major disadvantage is that the hot cautery blade may stick to the parenchyma.

An alternative to this approach was described by Cooper and colleagues (1986). They described the use of a bipolar cautery. When traction and countertraction is applied, small amounts of tissue are grabbed with the bipolar forceps and coagulated. All larger vessels and bronchi are ligated individually. This technique produces good results with minimal air leak or injury to the remaining parenchyma. It is laborious and time consuming, however, and any vessel greater than 1 mm must be ligated individually.

Another tool for resection is the Neodymium: YAG laser, an excellent cutting and coagulating tool for the surgeon. One major advantage of the YAG laser is that it does not have to touch the tissue, and thus no sticking occurs. At a power setting of 80 watts, it can coagulate vessels up to 2 mm in diameter and seal air leaks from bronchi up to 1 mm in diameter. It produces a considerable smoke plume, which must be evacuated through filtered suction. The technique for removing a lesion is again similar to that described by Urschel (1986) but modified by me and my colleagues (1989) (Fig. 32–6). Traction and countertraction are applied and the laser is used to excise the entire lesion. Because

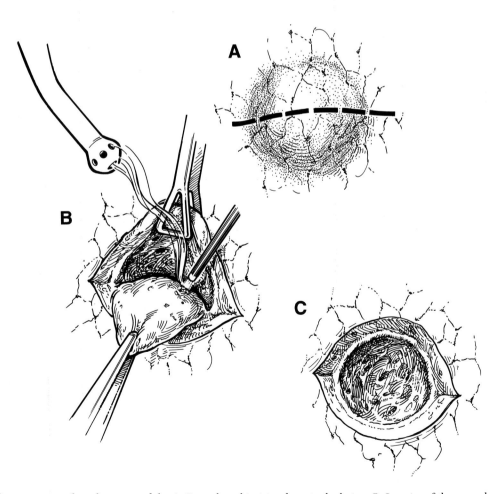

Fig. 32–6. A laser resection of a pulmonary nodule. *A*, Parenchymal incision down to the lesion. *B*, Lasering of the parenchyma using traction and countertraction. *C*, Open crater following laser excision.

the laser produces considerable shrinkage of tissue, one must aim approximately 1 to 2 cm from the lesion. Larger blood vessels not coagulated by the laser should be individually ligated. One theoretic advantage of the laser is that because of its depth of penetration, it may be destroying additional small micrometastasis up to 4 mm away from the lesion.

Postoperative care is similar to that of lobectomy and segmentectomy. During the early postoperative period, chest radiographs frequently show a halo around the site where the laser or cautery is used. This area eventually collapses and disappears, a process that occurs over several months. Such a scar may be difficult to evaluate radiographically, and the followup of malignant lesions, even by computed tomographic scans is difficult. It is necessary to obtain a scan in the early postoperative period so that this area may be evaluated in comparison to later postoperative studies.

Physiologic Effects

The physiologic changes subsequent to a wedge resection in the absence of postoperative pleural complications are minimal. Those seen are related more directly to the thoracotomy incision than to the removal of a small portion of lung. Early in the postoperative period, the lung volume is restricted. Inspiratory capacity and expiratory reserve volume are decreased. Alveolar hypoventilation, with carbon dioxide retention and some degree of respiratory acidosis, sometimes occurs. Again, because of pain, compliance may be reduced and the chest wall may be stiff, resulting in an increased work of breathing. This situation is usually noted within the first few hours of operation, but returns gradually to normal within 1 to 2 weeks following surgery.

Morbidity and Mortality

The morbidity rate after a wedge resection is minimal. When present, complications are most often the result of either retention of secretions or pleural problems. Persistent airspaces occur with an incidence of 10%. Most of these spaces produce no symptoms and require no treatment.

The mortality rate for wedge resection is near zero for patients with benign inflammatory disease and no more than 0.5% for those with malignant disease or pulmonary tuberculosis.

REFERENCES

Cooper JD, et al: Precision cautery excision of pulmonary lesions. Ann Thorac Surg *41*:51, 1986.

Crabbe MM, Patrisi GA, Fontenelle LJ: Minimal resection for bronchogenic carcinoma: Should this be standard therapy? Chest *95*:968, 1989.

Crabbe MM, Patrisi GA, Fontenelle LJ: Minimal resection for bronchogenic carcinoma: An update. Chest *99*:1421, 1991.

Errett LE, et al: Wedge resection as an alternative procedure for peripheral bronchogenic carcinoma in poor risk patients. J Thorac Cardiothorac Surg *90*:656, 1985.

Jensik RJ: The extent of resection for localized lung cancer: Segmental resection. *In* Kittle CF (ed): Current Controversies in Thoracic Surgery. Philadelphia: WB Saunders, 1986.

Jensik RJ: Mini resection of small peripheral carcinomas of the lung. Surg Clin North Am *66*:951, 1987.

Jensik RJ, Faber LP, Kittle CF: Segmental resection for bronchogenic carcinoma. Ann Thorac Surg *28*:475, 1979.

Jensik RJ, et al: Segmental resection for a lung cancer: A fifteen year experience. J Thorac Cardiothorac Surg *66*:563, 1973.

Lanza LA, et al: Long-term survival after resection of pulmonary metastasis of the breast. Ann Thorac Surg *54*:244, 1992.

Lewis R, et al: Video-assisted thoracic surgery resection of malignant lung tumors. J Thorac Cardiothorac Surg *104*:1679, 1992.

LoCicero J, et al: Laser-assisted parenchyma-sparing resection. J Thorac Cardiothorac Surg *97*:732, 1989.

McAfee MK, et al: Colorectal lung metastasis: Results of surgical excision. Ann Thorac Surg *53*:780, 1992.

Miller JI, Hatcher CR: Limited resection of bronchogenic carcinoma in the patient with marked impairment of pulmonary function. Ann Thorac Surg *44*:340, 1987.

Mountain CF, McMutery MJ, Hermes KE: Surgery for pulmonary metastasis: A twenty year experience. Ann Thorac Surg *38*:323, 1984.

Peters RM: The role of limited resection in carcinoma of the lung. Am J Surg *143*:706, 1982.

Progrebniak HW, et al: Renal cell carcinoma: Resection of solitary and multiple metastasis. Ann Thorac Surg *54*:33, 1992.

Shields TW, Higgins GA: Minimal pulmonary resection in treatment of carcinoma of the lung. Arch Surg *108*:420, 1974.

Urschel HC: Discussion of Cooper et al: Precision cautery excision of pulmonary lesions. Ann Thorac Surg *41*:53, 1986.

Warren WH, Faber LP: Segmentectomy vs. lobectomy in patients with stage I pulmonary carcinoma. Presented at the 73rd Annual Meeting of the AATS, Chicago, April, 1993.

CHAPTER 33

MEDIASTINAL LYMPH NODE DISSECTION

Tsuguo Naruke

The basic controversy surrounding the necessity of complete mediastinal lymph node dissection for lung cancer is similar to the controversy related to the need and efficacy of lymph node dissection in tumors of other organ systems. The resection of the primary lesion, including the regional lymph nodes en bloc, is the universally accepted surgical treatment of lung cancer in Japan and in many other countries.

The four major arguments against complete mediastinal lymph node dissection are as follows: 1) systemic nature of the cancer; cancer has spread outside of the thoracic cavity; 2) "complete" dissection; difficulty of 100% removal of all lymph nodes; 3) effect on the immune system; removal of normal lymph nodes may reduce normal immunologic resistance; and 4) surgical risk; increased surgical risk has not been justified by improved patient prognosis.

The four basic arguments supporting complete dissection are as follows: 1) microscopic identification; the only method to verify the true stage of the lung cancer; 2) postoperative treatment plan; reliable staging information will produce a more effective treatment plan; 3) surgical risk; complete lymph node dissection does not increase operative risk, operative mortality, or postoperative quality of life; and 4) survival rates; many surgeons report increased survival rates when complete dissection is performed. Among these surgeons are Smith (1978), Rubinstein and colleagues (1979), Kirschner (1981), Kirsh and Sloan (1982), Martini and associates (1983), Levasseur and Regnard (1990), Watanabe and co-workers (1991a,b), and the author (1967), as well as with my associates (1976, 1988). Other surgical reports are noted in the Reading References.

The standard surgical procedure for patients with lung cancer in Japan is either lobectomy or pneumonectomy combined with mediastinal lymph node dissection. Cases in which the lobe or lung containing the primary lesion has been resected and mediastinal lymph nodes have been dissected are termed by the author as "radical" — complete — operations. Cases in which mediastinal lymph node resection has been performed incompletely are termed "palliative" — noncurative — operations.*

With a complete mediastinal lymph node dissection, not only ipsilateral mediastinal lymph nodes, but also the contralateral lymph nodes, are dissected on the right side by a standard right posterolateral thoracotomy. A bilateral lymph node resection cannot be performed on the left side by standard left thoracotomy; it is necessary, depending on the site and presence of ipsilateral mediastinal lymph node metastases, to perform a contralateral lymph node dissection by mobilization of the aortic arch or with an additional median sternotomy.

The following basic operative procedures, including operative steps to take, are presented as the author's method of complete — systematic — mediastinal lymph node dissection.

SITES AND NOMENCLATURE OF LYMPH NODES

Although many reports have been presented in the past on the topography of the mediastinal lymph nodes and on the usual routes of lymphatic spread, no standard terminology was available for the location of mediastinal and bronchopulmonary lymph nodes in order to record the sites of nodal metastases clinically. The author (1967), based on a large number of lymph node dissections combined with lung resection for lung cancer and using the many basic studies of Rouviere (1932), Borrie (1952), Nohl (1956, 1962), and Cahan (1960), among others, suggested a nomenclature for the mapping of the sites of the intrathoracic lymph nodes (see Chapter 7). This system of lymph node mapping was

---

*Editors Note: This terminology is used widely in Japan for complete and noncurative — incomplete — resections. As I have noted (1989), however, a resection should be termed "incomplete" only if histologic proof has been obtained that residual disease remains in the hemithorax.

subsequently recommended by the American Joint Committee (1976) and its use has been supported by the reports of Mountain (1976) and Martini (1976). These reports of the classification of lung cancer were in agreement for the graphic representation of the operative findings with the suggested TNM classification of malignant tumors by Union Internationale Contre le Cancer — UICC. Although some classifications have been published with modifications such as those by the American Thoracic Society (1983), by Glazer and associates (1985), and, most recently, by the International Union Against Cancer (1989), the mediastinal lymph node map used here has been authorized and used by The Committee of the Japan Lung Cancer Society in accordance with the General Rule for Clinical and Pathological Record of Lung Cancer (1987) since 1980 and continuously and consistently to the present (Fig. 33–1).

The site of mediastinal lymph node stations and their designation as used in this chapter are as follows:

#1. The superior mediastinal lymph nodes present along the upper one third of the trachea within the thorax. These nodes include those located about the trachea, the location of which is defined by the horizontal line at the level of the upper edge of the subclavian artery and the horizontal line at the center point of the trachea, where the upper edge of the

brachiocephalic vein crosses the front of the trachea as the vein ascends to the left.

#2. The paratracheal lymph nodes are those nodes located between stations #1 and #4, and are present at the lateral sides of the trachea.

#3. These nodes are classified into pretracheal — #3, retrotracheal — #3p, and anterior mediastinal — #3a — lymph nodes; the nodes located posterior to the trachea are called retrotracheal lymph nodes — #3p, and those present in the prevascular compartment on the anterior aspect of the brachiocephalic vein and the upper portion of the superior vena cava are called #3a.

#4. The tracheobronchial lymph nodes are located at or close to the obtuse angle between the trachea and either main stem bronchus. The nodes on the right side are in the obtuse angle level with and beneath the azygos vein. Those on the left side are located on the medial aspect of the subaortic lymph nodes.

#5. The subaortic lymph nodes are those adjacent to the ligamentum arteriosum.

#6. The paraaortic lymph nodes are located on the anterolateral wall of the ascending aorta and aortic arch and anterior to the vagus nerve.

#7. The subcarinal lymph nodes are the nodes located just beneath the point where the trachea is divided into the two main stem bronchi.

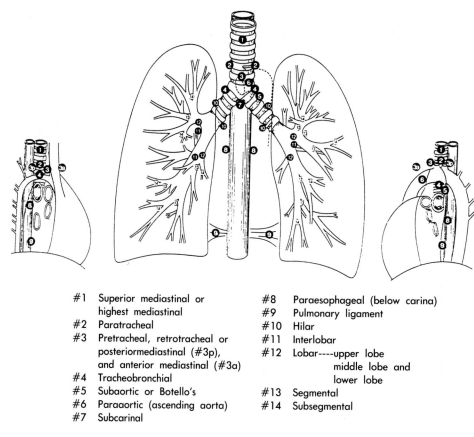

#1	Superior mediastinal or highest mediastinal	#8	Paraesophageal (below carina)
#2	Paratracheal	#9	Pulmonary ligament
#3	Pretracheal, retrotracheal or posteriormediastinal (#3p), and anterior mediastinal (#3a)	#10	Hilar
		#11	Interlobar
		#12	Lobar----upper lobe middle lobe and lower lobe
#4	Tracheobronchial		
#5	Subaortic or Botello's	#13	Segmental
#6	Paraaortic (ascending aorta)	#14	Subsegmental
#7	Subcarinal		

Fig. 33–1. Lymph node map and numeric designations for the mediastinal and bronchopulmonary stations.

#8. The paraesophageal lymph nodes are caudad to the level of the bifurcation of the trachea and are adjacent to the esophagus.

#9. The pulmonary ligament lymph nodes are those within the ligament. The lymph nodes that are present on the posterior wall and the lower edge of the inferior pulmonary vein are included in this designation.

#10. Lymph nodes just distal to the trachea and extending along the length of the main stem bronchi — these are also referred to as hilar lymph nodes.

#11. Interlobar lymph nodes and those present in-between the lobar bronchi. On the right side, when these nodes have to be specified, these nodes are classified as lymph nodes existing between the upper and middle lobes — 11s — and as the nodes existing between the middle and lower lobes — 11i.

#12. Lymph nodes present around a lobar bronchus.

#13. Lymph nodes located along a segmental bronchus.

#14. Lymph nodes present around a subsegmental bronchus or distal to this site.

ANESTHESIA

General anesthesia using a double-lumen endobronchial tube is the standard procedure for pulmonary resections with mediastinal lymph node dissection. After the endotracheal tube has been inserted into the trachea, the position of the tube is confirmed by visualization with the bronchofiberscope — 3.0-mm diameter Olympus Bf type 3C, and the tube is then fixed in place. Whenever the patient's position is changed, the location of the endotracheal tube is rechecked for proper positioning.

POSITION OF PATIENT

The patient is placed in the appropriate complete lateral decubitus position and a standard posterolateral thoracotomy is carried out. The skin incision is started at the midpoint between the thoracic vertebral column and the medial edge of the scapula at the level of the third rib. It is extended to the point at the inferior angle of the scapula in a loose arc, continued as far as the fifth costal cartilage, and is extended to a site 3 cm beyond the mamillary — nipple — line. The chest wall muscles are incised by electroknife in the same line as the skin incision. The pleural space is entered through the fourth intercostal space. The fourth and fifth ribs are partially dissected for a length of 1.5 to 2.0 cm just proximal to the vertebrae, and a section of each rib is excised. The fifth rib is also cut at its junction with the anterior cartilage.

In patients with cancer in the right lung, it is possible to perform a dissection of the potentially involved left contralateral mediastinal lymph nodes combined with a complete dissection of the right ipsilateral mediastinal lymph nodes with the standard right posterolateral thoracotomy. In patients with cancer in the left lung, however, a contralateral lymph node dissection cannot be performed by the standard left thoracotomy for anatomic reasons.

As a standard approach in patients with cancer in the left lung, a left posterolateral thoracotomy may be used if only an ipsilateral mediastinal lymph node dissection is contemplated. A median sternotomy may also be used but it has disadvantages, as will be noted. If a bilateral lymph node dissection is indicated, a median sternotomy with a left anterior intercostal incision may be used or the sternotomy may be combined with a standard left posterolateral thoracotomy.

When a left lung resection is combined with mediastinal lymph node dissection by a median sternotomy only, the disadvantage is that a complete dissection of the subcarinal lymph nodes and of the posterior mediastinal lymph nodes can be difficult to perform because of the location of the heart. Likewise, a left lower lobectomy is difficult to accomplish readily. Therefore, this incision alone is not recommended.

In patients with cancer in the left lung, frequent metastases are found in the subaortic — #5 — and the paraaortic — #6 — lymph nodes. Therefore, in my opinion, the initial procedure to perform for the mediastinal lymph node dissection is a standard left posterolateral thoracotomy with the patient in the right lateral decubitus position. In patients with metastases present in either the tracheobronchial — #4 — or the subcarinal — #7 — lymph nodes, or both, however, it is logical to assume the potential presence of metastases in the lymph nodes in the contralateral mediastinum. Because squamous cell carcinomas have a tendency toward localized locoregional growth only, in some cases, the lymphatic route is the major source of spread of disease. Therefore, it is essential to identify possible metastases to the tracheobronchial — #4 — and the subcarinal — #7 — lymph nodes by frozen section diagnosis during the operation. When metastases have been identified in these areas, it is then possible to perform a more complete contralateral lymph node dissection via a sequential median sternotomy with the patient in the supine position.

MEDIASTINAL LYMPH NODE DISSECTION

Timing

A principle of lung cancer surgery should be the ligation of the pulmonary vein first, followed by en bloc dissection of the mediastinum and hilum together with the lung, without interrupting lymphatic channels during the dissection. Particularly in cases when nodal enlargement suggests metastases extending from the hilar lymph nodes to mediastinal lymph nodes, the lymphatic channels should not be incised during the dissection. The order of the operative procedure should be changed appropriately during the operation, however, depending on the site and size of the tumor as well as its extent. When the pulmonary lobes in the diseased lung obscure the visual field, the accuracy of dissection is lowered. The basic rule is to vary the standard procedure as necessary, but nonetheless perform a complete dissection even though it may take a longer time to complete the operation than is usually required.

Technique

Dissection of the mediastinal lymph nodes is carried out with scissors and electroknife to excise en bloc the fatty tissues of the hilum and mediastinum that contain the lymph nodes while completely exposing all structures and walls of the organs present within the hilum and mediastinum. As noted, the lung, including the fatty alveolar tissues and lymph nodes, are to be dissected en bloc.

Before starting the mediastinal dissection, the pulmonary ligament is separated from the mediastinal pleura adjacent anteriorly and posteriorly to it. The mediastinal pleura inferior to the hilum is then separated from the fatty tissue adjacent to the esophagus. For the dissection of the superior mediastinum, the mediastinal pleura is incised vertically from the upper edge of the hilar pleura — just below the azygos vein — to the apex of the thorax and opened and retracted away from the mediastinal structures by retraction sutures. The vagus and phrenic nerves are identified, taped, and preserved carefully.

Fatty tissues including the lymph nodes, held by a lymph node forceps or Allis' intestinal forceps, are separated gently to expose the arteries, veins, trachea, bronchi, esophagus, and the aforementioned nerves. At all times, it is necessary to be careful not to damage the lymph nodes but to dissect free the adipose tissue enclosing the lymph nodes. The adipose tissues are grasped by the forceps without grasping the lymph nodes. When lymph nodes are squeezed, cancer cells can spread into the operated field; therefore, the nodes should not be grasped during the procedure. It is necessary to ligate any small blood vessels and to cauterize small lymphatic channels by electroknife to prevent postoperative bleeding and exudation of lymphatic fluid into the hemithorax postoperatively.

Patients with Carcinoma of the Right Lung

Right Upper Lobectomy

When a right upper lobectomy is performed, I prefer initially to stand at the back of the patient and to move to the front after the thoracotomy incision has been completed. The hilar pleura is opened anteriorly just posterior to the phrenic nerve and the phrenic nerve is then isolated, taped, and retracted to prevent any injury to it. Next, the fatty tissues and contained lymph nodes are dissected off of the pericardium from the site of the pleural incision toward the hilum to expose the superior pulmonary vein. The superior pulmonary vein, except for its branch from the middle lobe, is isolated, ligated, and divided. Following this maneuver, the azygos vein can be divided, or this step

can be done after the upper mediastinal dissection has been completed, depending on feasibility at the respective times.

The tracheobronchial lymph nodes — #4 — are present on the medial side — undersurface — of the azygos vein, and when the cancer is located in the right upper lobe, these # 4 nodes, as well as the pretracheal lymph nodes — #3, are frequently involved by metastatic disease. When it is suspected by the gross appearance of these nodes that they are involved, the azygos vein is not divided at its middle but is divided proximally as it enters the superior vena cava and distally as it turns anteriorly from its location on the vertebral bodies. That portion of the azygos vein overlying the tracheobronchial lymph nodes — #4 — is thus left attached to this nodal group, and a combined excision of the azygos vein and tracheobronchial lymph nodes is performed.

The lung is next retracted anteriorly to expose the posterior aspect of the hilum and the pleura is incised posterior to the hilar structures. The vagus nerve is exposed and taped. The pulmonary branch or branches of the vagus nerve are divided. Next, an intestinal flexible ribbon retractor is placed beneath the bifurcation of the trachea and the area is exposed, taking care to avoid injury to the descending aorta. The contralateral left main stem bronchial lymph nodes — #10 (left) — are brought to the midline by the use of a lymph node forceps and dissection of the subcarinal lymph nodes — #7 — is started. A branch of the bronchial artery, which runs from the tracheal bifurcation to the posterior wall of the right main bronchus, is ligated and divided. The medial side of the left main stem bronchus is exposed as it ascends toward the tracheal bifurcation. Along with the contralateral left main stem bronchial lymph nodes — #10 (left), the subcarinal lymph nodes — #7, the right main stem bronchial lymph nodes — #10 (right), and the right upper lobe bronchial lymph nodes — #12 — are dissected en bloc from the surrounding structures. It is readily seen during the dissection that these lymph nodes are in direct continuity with each other (Figs. 33–2, 33–3).

The next step is separation of the interlobar fissure, and then the posterior ascending artery is isolated, ligated, and divided. The lymph nodes present between the lobes are dissected free from the pulmonary artery in continuity with the upper lobe. The lymphatic sump area, described in Chapter 7, located in the area between the upper lobe bronchus, middle lobe bronchus, and the superior segmental branch of the lower lobe bronchus, contains regional lymph nodes — #11s — that receive lymphatic drainage from the upper lobe. It is necessary to dissect and to remove these nodes as completely as possible together with the peribronchial lymph nodes — #12 — of the upper lobe bronchus.

When it is suspected that the dissection of superior interlobar lymph nodes — #11s — might be incom-

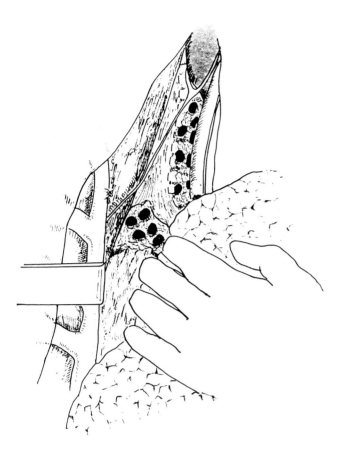

Fig. 33–2. Exposure of the subcarinal area during a right upper lobectomy by retraction of lung toward the operator at the front of the patient.

The mediastinal pleura is then opened from the upper edge of the hilar pleura upward toward the apex of the thorax. Sutures are placed through either edge of the opened upper mediastinal pleura at four points and the pleural incision is held open by traction on these sutures to expose the superior aspect of mediastinum above the hilum.

The pleura is incised further cephalad to the level of the upper edge of the subclavian artery. The right recurrent nerve is identified and protected from injury. The wall of the subclavian artery is exposed and the superior mediastinal lymph nodes — #1 — and the adjacent fatty tissue are dissected free from the mediastinal structures. The right brachiocephalic vein is retracted anteriorly with an intestinal flexible ribbon retractor. The adipose tissues located at the highest level of the anterior and the right lateral surfaces of the trachea are grasped with lymph node forceps or Allis' intestinal forceps and retracted toward the operator, and

plete when only a right lobectomy is carried out in some cases of a right upper lobe tumor, a more complete dissection of these nodes, as well as of the peribronchial lymph nodes — #12, may be accomplished by a right upper and middle bilobectomy. Furthermore, if the sump area contains large, involved lymph nodes and the bronchus or pulmonary artery, or both, have been infiltrated by metastatic disease from the involved lymph nodes or by the tumor itself, a pneumonectomy is indicated.

When the dissection of the subcarinal, hilar, and peribronchial lymph nodes is completed, the surgeon should move to the opposite — back — side of the patient. When division of the azygos vein has not been performed previously, it is now exposed and ligated. The vein is then transfixed and divided. As noted previously, a part of the azygos vein may be left attached to underlying tracheobronchial lymph nodes — #4 — and removed together with the lymph nodes at the completion of the dissection.

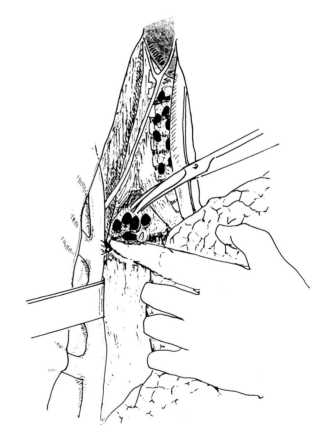

Fig. 33–3. Sharp scissors dissection of the subcarinal fat pad containing the subcarinal — #7 — lymph nodes.

sharp dissection is performed to free this tissue and any contained lymph nodes from this portion of the trachea (Figs. 33–4, 33–5). To prevent postoperative lymphatic leaks or bleeding, ligation or electrocauterization of all cut vascular or lymphatic vessels is done as completely as possible. The right vagus nerve is exposed starting at the level of the takeoff of the recurrent nerve. Then, the right lateral wall of the esophagus and right lateral wall of the trachea are exposed. The adipose tissue, including the contained lymph nodes existing at the highest site — #1, are held by lymph node forceps and the dissection is continued downward toward the hilum. A few thin venous branches from the right brachiocephalic vein and superior vena cava are usually present; these branches are ligated and divided. The intestinal flexible ribbon retractor is slid downward a little and inserted between the trachea and the right brachiocephalic vein near its junction with the superior vena cava. At the bottom of this site, the ascending brachiocephalic artery is identified. Because the right wall of the ascending aorta is further caudal, the dissection is carried down along the aforementioned arterial branch until the wall of the aorta is exposed.

The pretracheal lymph nodes — #3, which, as noted, are located where the upper edge of the left

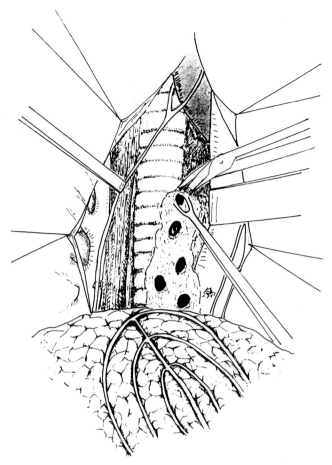

Fig. 33–5. Continued downward dissection along the anterolateral wall of the trachea with the retraction of the superior vena cava anteriorly to free the paratracheal — #2 — lymph nodes.

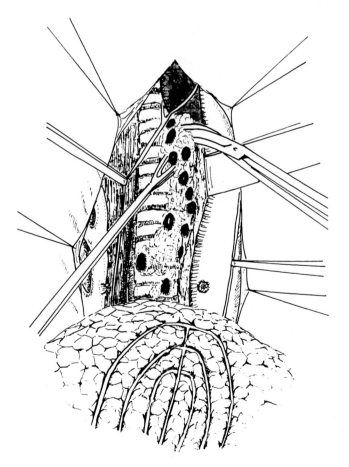

Fig. 33–4. Beginning dissection of the superior mediastinal lymph nodes at the level of the right subclavian artery.

brachiocephalic vein crosses the anterior aspect of the trachea, are then dissected in continuity with the tissues already freed from above. The lymph nodes at this site are numerous and metastasis to these nodes in patients with cancer in the right upper lobe occurs frequently; only the tracheobronchial lymph nodes — #4 — and the paratracheal lymph nodes — #2 — are more prone to metastatic involvement.

The retrotracheal — #3p — lymph nodes are then freed and the paratracheal — #2 — nodes along with previously dissected fatty tissue and lymph nodes from above are dissected away from the tracheal wall and the posterior wall of the lower portion of the superior vena cava. The dissection is continued down to and including the superior tracheobronchial — #4 — lymph nodes and attached section of the azygos vein when these latter lymph nodes are enlarged, thus completing the superior mediastinal lymph node dissection.

Next, the right pulmonary artery is exposed and the upper lobectomy combined with dissection of the mediastinal lymph nodes is completed by the following procedure. The right upper lobe artery — the truncus anterior — is isolated, ligated, and divided. The lymph nodes attached to the anterior aspect of the upper lobe bronchus are dissected in continuity with the tracheo-bronchial lymph nodes — #4, which have been freed previously (Fig. 33–6). The dissection is completed by isolation, division, and closure of the right upper lobe bronchus. In patients with cancer in the upper lobe, it is not necessary to perform a dissection of the paraesophageal — #8 — lymph nodes, but the pulmonary ligament lymph nodes — #9 — are removed with the specimen.

Middle Lobectomy

In patients with a cancer in the middle lobe, a bilobectomy of the middle and upper lobes or of the middle and lower lobes is performed, depending on the extent of metastasis to the interlobar lymph nodes — #11s or #11i. Pneumonectomy is carried out as necessitated by the extent of the spread of metastasis to the lymph nodes or the direct extent of the primary tumor. The mediastinal lymph node dissection is essentially the same as that carried out for upper lobe tumors.

Right Lower Lobectomy

For excision of the right lower lobe, I stand at the back of the patient. After opening the right side of the

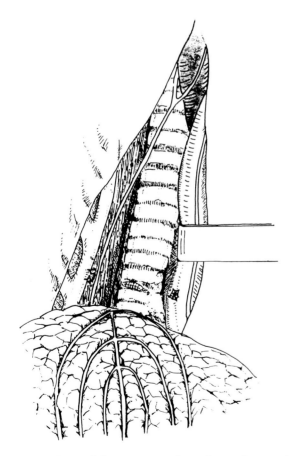

Fig. 33–6. Status of the superior mediastinal area after complete dissection and removal of the right upper lobe. Proximal and distal ligated ends of the azygos vein are clearly seen.

chest and freeing any adhesions as necessary, the mediastinal pleura is incised just anterior to the pulmonary ligament, as well as posterior to it. The esophagus is exposed from the diaphragm up to the inferior pulmonary vein. Dissection continues in a superior direction and the pulmonary ligament and paraesophageal — #9 and #8 — lymph nodes are dissected en bloc with the adjacent fatty tissue up to the inferior pulmonary vein. The pleura behind the vein is incised and the inferior pulmonary vein is exposed, ligated, and divided.

The surgeon now moves to the front of the patient and the esophagus is retracted posteriorly by an intestinal flexible ribbon retractor placed at the level of the bifurcation of the trachea. The lung is retracted anteriorly toward the surgeon's side and the bifurcation of the trachea is exposed. Dissection of lymph nodes at the bifurcation of the trachea — #7 — is performed first and then the nodes present along the right main stem bronchus — #10 (right) — are dissected down to the lower lobe. Next, the major interlobar fissure is opened using an electroknife to expose the bronchovascular structures. The interlobar lymph nodes — #11s and #11i — and the lymph nodes clustered around the lower lobe bronchus are dissected free along with the previously dissected lymph nodes at the bifurcation of the trachea and the peribronchial lymph nodes of the right main bronchus. The pulmonary artery branch or branches to the lower lobe are isolated, ligated, and divided. Next, the lower lobe bronchus is divided and the proximal stump is closed. Then, the lymph node dissection of the upper mediastinum is performed as previously described.

Right Pneumonectomy

The technical steps of a right pneumonectomy are taken in the order of the dissection of the inferior mediastinum, ligation and division of the inferior and superior pulmonary veins, dissection of the bifurcation of the trachea, dissection of the upper mediastinum, ligation and division of the pulmonary artery, and finally the division and closure of the right main stem bronchus. The area of dissection of the lymph nodes present in the hilum and mediastinum when a right pneumonectomy is performed is shown in Figure 33–7.

Patients with Carcinoma of the Left Lung

Left Upper Lobectomy

For a left upper lobectomy, the surgeon moves to the front side of the patient after performing the thoracotomy incision into the pleural space. The mediastinal pleura is incised anterior to the hilum. The phrenic nerve is identified and taped. Lymph nodes in the region of the pulmonary vein are dissected from the anterior aspect of the pericardium toward the pulmonary side of the superior pulmonary vein. The superior pulmonary vein is isolated, ligated, and divided.

The lung is retracted anteriorly toward the surgeon, and dissection of subcarinal lymph nodes — #7 — is

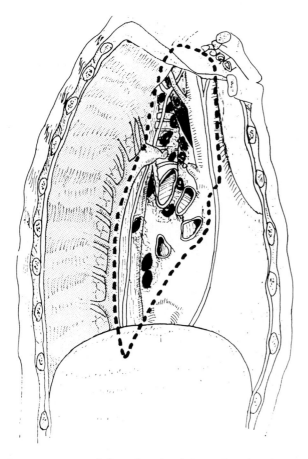

Fig. 33–7. View of the right side of the mediastinum. Outline denotes the region of dissection of the right hilum and mediastinum with contained hilar and mediastinal structures exposed during right pneumonectomy.

separated. The branches of the pulmonary artery are ligated and divided from below upward, but all of the arterial branches may not be divided at this stage.

Next, the upper mediastinal pleura is incised as far as the apex of the thorax, and the phrenic and vagus nerves are identified and taped. Four retraction sutures are placed in the cut edges of the mediastinal pleura. The hemiazygos vein is identified, isolated, ligated, and divided. Anteriorly, the thymic fatty tissue is identified and the pericardium is reached when this adipose tissue is dissected free. The ascending aorta is exposed and the paraaortic — #6 — lymph nodes are dissected from the aortic wall. The dissection is carried toward the main pulmonary artery in the hilum. The left brachiocephalic vein is also exposed. Now, a portion of the anterior mediastinal fat pad containing the anterior mediastinal — #3a — lymph nodes can be dissected.

The left common carotid and the left subclavian arteries are exposed at the apex of the thorax and caudad dissection of the fatty tissue containing the lymph nodes is carried out. The superior mediastinal — #1 — and paratracheal — #2 — lymph nodes are dissected as shown in Figure 33–9. The left superior mediastinal lymph nodes — #1, as on the right, are the nodes present at the apex to the level where the upper edge of the brachiocephalic vein crosses the midline of the trachea; the lymph nodes present below this level on the side of the trachea are the paratracheal lymph nodes — #2. The lymph nodes located on the frontal aspect of the left common carotid artery are pretracheal — #3 — and are also dissected at this time.

The thoracic duct is in the deepest area between the left common carotid artery and the left subclavian artery;

started. First, the vagus nerve is isolated and taped. The descending aorta and esophagus are retracted posteriorly by an intestinal flexible ribbon retractor and the bifurcation of the trachea is exposed (Fig. 33–8). The bronchus is exposed from the inferior border of the upper lobar bronchus toward the main bronchus. Lymph nodes about the left upper lobar bronchus are mobilized and the dissection is continued distally on the bronchus to the area of the bifurcation of the bronchus between the upper and lower lobes — the left lymphatic sump. The pulmonary branches of the vagus nerve are ligated and divided. With completion of these steps, the visual field of the tracheal bifurcation is increased by further retraction of the left lung toward the surgeon by use of the left hand or a lung retractor. Lymph nodes are dissected away from the inferior surface of the right main bronchus — #10 (right), then the subcarinal lymph nodes — #7 — are dissected free, and lastly, the left bronchial — hilar — lymph nodes — #10 (left) — are mobilized. It is necessary at the site of the bifurcation of the trachea to ligate and divide the branch of the left bronchial artery. The dissection of the sump lymph nodes between the upper lobe and lower lobe bronchus is completed after division of the interlobar fissure and the lobes have been

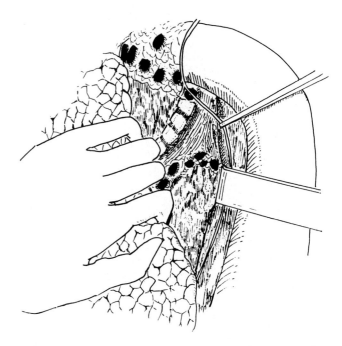

Fig. 33–8. Exposure of the subcarinal area from the left side after division of the inferior pulmonary vein. Retraction of the left lung anteriorly and the esophagus posteriorly permits the operative exposure of the carina and both the right and left main stem bronchi.

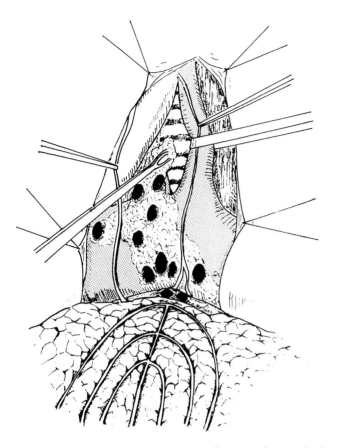

Fig. 33–9. Exposure of the left superior mediastinal and paratracheal lymph nodes during a standard left thoracotomy by retraction of the left common carotid artery posteriorly and the left brachiocephalic vein anteriorly.

The remaining — ordinarily the more proximal — pulmonary arteries of the upper lobe are now isolated, ligated, and divided. After exposing the left upper lobe bronchus together with the dissected nodes, the bronchus is divided. By this procedure, left upper lobectomy combined with mediastinal lymph node dissection has been completed.

When metastases are identified in the subcarinal lymph nodes — #7 — or the tracheobronchial lymph nodes — #4, or both, it is necessary to perform a complete dissection of the superior mediastinal — #1, paratracheal — #2, pretracheal — #3, and posterior mediastinal — 3p — lymph nodes. This may be accomplished by one of two procedures. The steps of one of the procedures are to tape the subclavian artery, incise the pleura at the posterior side of the aorta, ligate and divide a few intercostal arteries, and tape the descending aorta. The left subclavian artery and aorta are retracted anteriorly and the left wall of the trachea and esophagus are exposed. The superior mediastinal — #1, paratracheal — #2, pretracheal — #3, and retrotracheal — #3p — lymph nodes are more readily dissected with this maneuver (Fig. 33–10). At

however, the thoracic duct, as a rule, cannot be identified. Damage to mediastinal branches of the thoracic duct can result in a postoperative chylothorax. Therefore, all lymphatic channels and fine blood vessels should be ligated and divided. When the left subclavian artery is taped, paratracheal lymph nodes — #2 — can be dissected more easily. Lymph nodes in the deeper area between the left brachiocephalic vein and left common carotid artery are pretracheal lymph nodes — #3. It is impossible to dissect all the nodes on the anterior surface of the trachea with the standard operative procedure of a left thoracotomy; therefore, when dissection in this area is necessary, the aorta should be mobilized and retracted (Fig. 33–10) or the dissection of the superior mediastinum should be performed through a median sternotomy. After dissection of the paratracheal and pretracheal nodes, attention is turned to the dissection of the remaining paraaortic and subaortic nodes

In patients with cancer in the left upper lobe, it is most important to dissect the paraaortic lymph nodes — #6 — as well as the subaortic lymph nodes — #5. The tracheobronchial lymph nodes — #4 — are located at the median side of the subaortic lymph nodes, and these nodes can be dissected easily after Botallo's ligament has been ligated and divided.

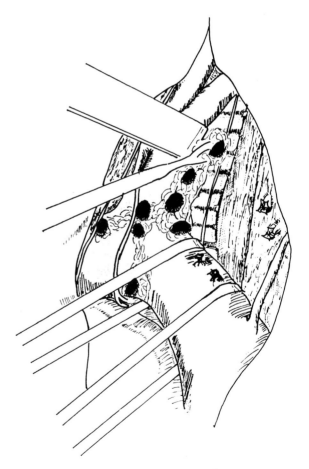

Fig. 33–10. Upper intercostal arteries have been divided and the aorta and the left subclavian and common carotid arteries have been retracted anteriorly to give more complete access to the superior mediastinal — #1, the left paratracheal — #2, the pretracheal — #3, and the retrotracheal — #3p — lymph nodes during a standard left thoracotomy incision.

this time, it is necessary to pay careful attention to avoid damaging the recurrent nerve, which runs upward along the left lateral wall of the trachea. By incision of Botallo's ligament, the tracheobronchial — #4 — lymph nodes can be dissected easily as previously described. The other option is to move the patient to a supine position and to perform a median sternotomy to carry out a more complete mediastinal lymph node dissection. This operative approach is described subsequently.

Left Lower Lobectomy

When a left lower lobectomy is performed in patients with the primary lesion in the left lower lobe, the surgeon moves to the front of the patient. The pulmonary ligament lymph nodes — #9 — are freed and the paraesophageal — #8 — lymph nodes are dissected from about the esophagus from the anterior surface of the descending aorta posteriorly to the pericardial surface anteriorly. These nodes are dissected upward and the inferior pulmonary vein is exposed. The inferior pulmonary vein is then isolated, ligated, and divided. The lung is further retracted anteriorly toward the surgeon and dissection of the contralateral hilar lymph nodes — #10 (right), the subcarinal lymph nodes — #7, and the ipsilateral hilar lymph nodes — #10 (left) — is performed. After opening the interlobar fissure, the dissection of the interlobar lymph nodes — #11 — is accomplished. The lower lobectomy is completed by ligation and division of the pulmonary arterial branches to the lobe and division and closure of the bronchus. In patients with cancer in the left lower lobe, as well as in those patients with metastases to subaortic lymph nodes — #5, the subcarinal lymph nodes — #7 — are frequently involved and must be included in the dissection.

Left Pneumonectomy

When a left pneumonectomy is indicated, the operative steps for dissection of mediastinal lymph nodes are started by the surgeon moving to the front side of the patient after the pleural space is entered. The area of dissection of the hilar and the mediastinal lymph nodes during a left pneumonectomy is shown in Figure 33–11. The pulmonary ligament lymph nodes — #9 — and the paraesophageal — #8 — lymph nodes, as for a lower lobectomy, are dissected and the dissection is continued superiorly as far as the inferior pulmonary vein. This vein is ligated and divided. Next, the superior pulmonary vein is ligated and divided. The mediastinal dissection is then continued as described for a left upper lobectomy. As noted previously, the area of the left upper mediastinum is narrow and its borders are not defined as clearly as are the borders of the right upper mediastinum. The superior mediastinal — #1, pretracheal — #3, and paratracheal — #2 — lymph nodes are covered by the aorta and its branches. Therefore, it is not possible to perform a complete dissection of these nodes unless the brachiocephalic vein, aorta, and carotid arteries are retracted. With the nodal dissection completed, the main pulmonary artery is exposed, ligated, and divided. By dividing the left main bronchus,

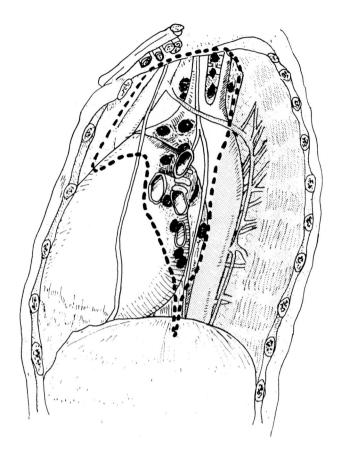

Fig. 33–11. The mediastinum as viewed during a standard left thoracotomy. Outline denotes the region of hilar and mediastinal dissection with contained exposed hilar and mediastinal structures during a left pneumonectomy.

the left pneumonectomy has been accomplished with dissection of the mediastinal lymph nodes en bloc. Of course, the mediastinal lymph node dissection can be performed after the pulmonary resection has been performed. As a rule, however, the lung can usually be collapsed easily, and therefore the operation is not difficult with the lung in place and is recommended as the procedure of choice.

Upper Mediastinal Dissection Via a Median Sternotomy

In patients with cancer of the left lung and metastases in the subcarinal lymph nodes — #7 — or in the tracheobronchial lymph nodes — #4, particularly those persons with squamous cell carcinoma, a more complete dissection of the mediastinum is indicated. This may be performed by accomplishing the dissection via a median sternotomy. The patient is placed supine and a median sternotomy is carried out to improve the dissection of the upper mediastinal lymph nodes. The left brachiocephalic vein is exposed and taped. The right brachiocephalic artery and common carotid artery are taped. Care is needed to avoid damaging the recurrent nerve that is present at the left side of the trachea. Dissection is started precisely underneath the thyroid gland, and the superior mediastinal lymph nodes —

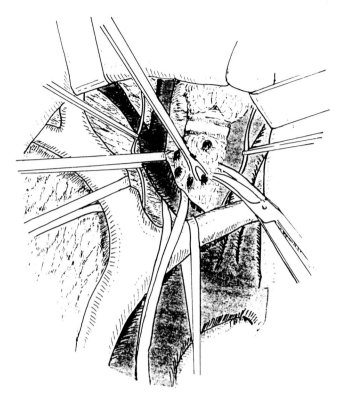

Fig. 33–12. Upper mediastinal lymph node dissection through a median sternotomy. The superior portion of the trachea is exposed by downward retraction of the innominate artery and left brachiocephalic vein.

#1, the paratracheal lymph nodes — #2 — bilaterally, and any pretracheal lymph nodes — #3 — are dissected en bloc (Fig. 33–12). To expose lymph nodes in the inferior portion of the trachea, the pericardium between the superior vena cava and ascending aorta is incised. The aorta is retracted out of the way by using an intestinal flexible ribbon retractor, and the posterior wall of the pericardium is incised medial to the superior vena cava and as far inferiorly as the lower edge of the pulmonary artery. The superior vena cava is retracted to the right side and the brachiocephalic artery is retracted upwards. The superior mediastinal lymph nodes — #1, which already have been dissected, the left and right paratracheal lymph nodes — #2, and the pretracheal lymph nodes — #3 — are dissected downward, going underneath the brachiocephalic artery. The dissection is then carried downward to the level of the tracheal bifurcation by retraction of the superior vena cava to the right and the ascending aorta to the left (Figs. 33–13, 33–14). The superior tracheobronchial — #4 — lymph nodes on the right, as well as any tissue on the left that remains despite the previous dissection of the area during the initial standard left thoracotomy, are removed. During the left-sided dissection, care is needed to protect the left recurrent nerve. The subcarinal — #7 — area is further inspected, although this area should be clear as a result of the dissection accomplished during the left thoracotomy.

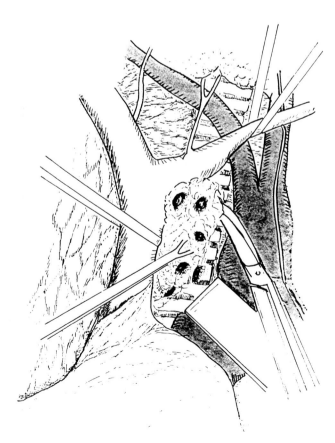

Fig. 33–13. Dissection of the pretracheal — #3 — and paratracheal — #2 — lymph nodes through a median sternotomy. The superior vena cava is retracted to the right and the aorta to the left after division of the upper anterior and posterior layers of the pericardial sac.

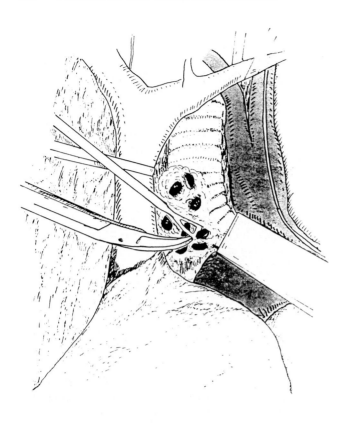

Fig. 33–14. Continued dissection of pretracheal — #3 — and subcarinal — #7 — lymph nodes through the median sternotomy incision described in Figure 33–13.

REFERENCES

American Thoracic Surgery Clinical Staging of Primary Lung Cancer. Am Rev Respir Dis 127:1, 1983.

Borrie J: Primary carcinoma of the bronchus: Prognosis following surgical resection. Ann R Coll Surg Engl 10:165, 1952.

Cahan WG: Radical lobectomy. J Thorac Cardiovasc Surg 39:555, 1960.

Carr DT: Staging of Lung Cancer. Chicago: American Joint Committee for Cancer Staging and End-Results Reporting: Task Force on Lung. 1979.

Glazer GM, et al: Normal mediastinal lymph nodes: Number and size according to American Thoracic Society mapping. AJR Am J Roentgenol 144:261, 1985.

International Union Against Cancer — Union Internationale Contre le Cancer TNM: Atlas Illustrated Guide to the TNM/pTNM-Classification of Malignant Tumors. 3rd Ed. Genera: Union internationale contre le cancer, 1989, p. 134.

Kirschner PA: Lung cancer. Preoperative radiation therapy and surgery. NY State Med J 198:339, 1981.

Kirsh MM, Sloan H: Mediastinal metastases in bronchogenic carcinoma: Influence of postoperative irradiation, cell type, and location. Ann Thorac Surg 33:459, 1982.

Levasseur PH, Regnard JF: Long-term results after surgery for N2 non-small cell lung cancer. Presented at the IASLC workshop, June 17–21, 1990, Bruges, Belgium.

Martini N: Improved methods of recording data in lung cancer. Clin Bull Memorial Sloan-Kettering Cancer Center 6:93, 1976.

Martini N, et al: Results of resection in non-oat cell carcinoma of the lung with mediastinal lymph node metastases. Ann Surg 198:386, 1983.

Mountain F: "Cancer of the Lung" Classification and Staging of Cancer by Site. Chicago: American Joint Committee on Cancer, 1976, p. 95.

Naruke T: The spread of lung cancer and its relevance to surgery. J Jpn Surg Soc 68:1607, 1967.

Naruke T, Suemasu, Ishikawa S: Surgical treatment for lung cancer with metastasis to mediastinal lymph nodes. J Thorac Cardiovasc Surg 71:2, 1976.

Nohl HC: An investigation into the lymphatic and vascular spread of carcinoma of the bronchus. Thorax 11:172, 1956.

Nohl HC: The Spread of Carcinoma of the Bronchus. London: Lloid-Luke Ltd, 1962, p. 37.

Rouviere H: Anatomie der Lymphatiques de l'Homme. Paris: Masson et Cie, 1932.

Rubinstein I, et al: Resectional Surgery in the treatment of primary carcinoma of the lung with mediastinal lymph node metastases. Thorax 34:33, 1979.

Sellers AH: A Brochure of Checklists. Geneva, UICC, 1980.

Smith PA: The importance of mediastinal lymph node invasion by pulmonary carcinoma in selection of patients for resection. Ann Thorac Surg 25:5, 1978.

Shields TW: The incomplete resection. Ann Thorac Surg 47:487, 1989.

The Japan Lung Cancer Society: General Rule for Clinical and Pathological Record of Lung Cancer. 3rd Ed. Tokyo: Kanehara Syuppann, 1987, p. 69.

Watanabe Y, et al: Aggressive surgical intervention in N2 non-small cell cancer of the lung. Ann Thorac Surg 51:253, 1991a.

Watanabe Y, et al: Mediastinal nodal involvement and the prognosis of non-small cell lung cancer. Chest 100:422, 1991b.

READING REFERENCES

Fossella FV, et al: Omtero, report of a prospective randomized trial of neoadjuvant chemotherapy plus surgery versus surgery alone for stage IIIa non-small cell lung cancer (NSCLC) (abstract). Proc Am Soc Clin Oncol 10:240, 1991.

Gozzetti G, et al: Surgical management of N2 lung cancer (abstract). Lung Cancer 2:96, 1986.

Hirono T, et al: Surgical treatment of N2 non-small cell lung cancer. Lung Cancer 4(Suppl):A90, 1988.

Mountain CF: A new international staging system for lung cancer. Chest 89(Suppl):225S, 1986.

Pearson FG, et al: Significance of positive superior mediastinal nodes identified at mediastinoscopy in patients with resectable cancer of the lung. J Thorac Cardiovasc Surg 83:1, 1982.

Skarin A, et al: Neoadjuvant chemotherapy in marginally resectable stage IIIMO non-small cell lung cancer: Long-term follow-up in 41 patients. J Surg Oncol 40:266, 1989.

Takita H, et al: Chemotherapy followed by lung resection in inoperable non-small cell lung carcinomas due to locally far-advanced disease. Cancer 57:630, 1986.

CHAPTER 34

SURGICAL ANATOMY OF THE TRACHEA AND TECHNIQUES OF RESECTION

Hermes C. Grillo

ANATOMY

Functionally, the trachea serves principally as a conduit for ventilation. Viewed in this way, it would seem to be an ideal structure for replacement or reconstruction when involved by surgical disease. Anatomically, however, it presents several unique features that partially account for the difficulty in its surgical management. These are its unpaired nature, its unique structural rigidity, its short length, its relative lack of longitudinal elasticity, its proximity to major cardiovascular structures, and its blood supply.

My colleagues and I (1964) reported that the adult human trachea averages 11.8 cm in length — range: 10 to 13 cm — from the infracricoid level to the top of the carinal spur. There are usually from 18 to 22 cartilaginous rings within this length, approximately 2 rings per centimeter. Occasionally, rings are incomplete or bifid. In an adult man, the internal diameter of the trachea measures about 2.3 cm laterally and 1.8 cm anteroposteriorly. These measurements vary roughly in proportion to the size of the individual and are usually smaller in women. The cross-sectional shape in the adult is approximately elliptic. In infants and children, it is more nearly circular. The configuration may change with disease. Thus, the lower two thirds may be flattened in tracheomalacia or rigidly narrowed from side to side to produce "saber-sheath" trachea.

The surgeon usually visualizes the trachea as he or she learned to see it in the "thyroidectomy" position, with the neck extended, as a structure that is half cervical and half thoracic. Mulliken and I (1968) pointed out that the trachea becomes almost entirely mediastinal when the neck is flexed, for the cricoid cartilage drops to the level of the thoracic inlet. This may be the permanent position in the aged because of cervical kyphosis. These simple observations contributed to the

development of surgical reconstructive techniques that obviate the requirement for prostheses.

The trachea, when viewed laterally in the upright individual, courses backward and downward at an angle from a nearly subcutaneous position at the infracricoid level to rest against the esophagus and vertebral column at the carina. The larynx and the origin of the esophagus are intimately related anatomically at the cricopharyngeal level. Below this point, the posterior membranous wall of the trachea maintains a close spatial relationship to the esophagus. A distinct, easily separable plane is present below the cricoid level, but a common blood supply is shared. Anteriorly, the thyroid isthmus passes over the trachea in the region of the second ring. The lateral lobes of the thyroid are closely applied to the trachea, and common blood supply is obtained from the branches of the inferior thyroid artery. Lying in the groove between trachea and esophagus are the recurrent nerves, coursing from beneath the arch of the aorta on the left side and, therefore, having a longer course in proximity to the trachea there than on the right side, where the nerve has looped around the subclavian artery and then approached the groove. A nonrecurrent nerve rarely is present on the right in conjunction with an anomalous subclavian artery. These nerves enter the larynx between the cricoid and thyroid cartilages just anterior to the inferior cornua of the thyroid cartilage.

The anterior pretracheal plane may be developed easily in the cervical region. Fibrofatty tissue, lymph nodes, and fine branches of the anterior jugular vein are present in front of this plane. The innominate vein lies anteriorly, away from the trachea. The innominate artery, however, crosses over the midtrachea obliquely from its point of origin from the aortic arch to the right side of the neck. In children, the innominate artery is higher and is encountered in the lower part of the neck. In some adults, the artery is unusually high and crosses the trachea at the base of the neck when slight extension is present. Occasionally, a tiny branch of this artery may be encountered in the segment of the artery that crosses the trachea. At the level of the carina, the left main bronchus passes beneath the aortic arch, and the right beneath the azygos vein. The pulmonary artery lies just in front of the carina. On either side of the trachea lies fibrofatty tissue containing lymph nodes chains; a large packet of nodes lies just beneath the carina (see Chapter 7).

The course of the trachea from the anterior cervical position to the posterior mediastinal position with close relationships to major vascular structures makes access to the entire trachea through a single incision difficult. I (1969) emphasized that these anatomic facts demand precise definition of the extent and nature of the tracheal lesions in planning surgical procedures.

The cartilaginous rings give the human trachea its lateral rigidity. The rings extend approximately two thirds of the circumference. The posterior wall is membranous. The trachea is lined with respiratory mucosa, which is tightly applied to the inner surface of the cartilages, grossly. The normal epithelium is columnar and ciliated. The cilia clear particulate matter and secretions. Mucous glands are liberally present. In chronic smokers and in persons with other chronic irritation, squamous metaplasia frequently occurs; in extreme instances, few ciliated cells remain. Such individuals must clear secretions by coughing vigorously. This observation, plus the demonstrated feasibility of cutaneous reconstructions and occasional successes with prosthetic interpositions, makes it clear that ciliated epithelium, although highly desirable, is not essential for tracheal reconstruction. Between the cartilaginous rings and in the membranous wall, the submucosa is fibromuscular.

Considerable contraction of the muscular membranous wall can occur with coughing and with spasm, the tips of the cartilages being drawn inward. Such transient narrowing of the airway may be observed fluoroscopically and during bronchoscopy in normal individuals. Some longitudinal flexibility exists; a degree of elasticity is present that appears to be greater in youth and to decrease with age. Calcification of the rings is seen most often with advancing age, although to lesser degree than in the cricoid cartilage. Local trauma or operation may lead to calcification. The normal trachea slides easily in its layer of fibrofatty areolar tissue from neck to mediastinum.

The blood supply of the human trachea is segmental, largely shared with the esophagus, and derived principally from multiple branches of the inferior thyroid artery above and the bronchial arteries below. The arteries approach laterally and fine branches pass anteriorly to the trachea and posteriorly to the esophagus. Miura and I (1966) noted that the inferior thyroid artery nourishes the upper trachea, usually through a pattern of three principal branches with fine subdivisions and very fine collateral vessels, but with many variations, as noted by Salassa and colleagues (1977). The bronchial vessels nourish the lower trachea. Sometimes, the

internal mammary artery contributes (Fig. 34–1). Excessive circumferential dissection with division of the lateral pedicles during an operative procedure can easily devascularize the trachea.

METHODS OF RECONSTRUCTION OF THE TRACHEA

Surgical approach to the trachea developed more slowly than other areas of thoracic surgery, because of the rarity of tracheal tumors, the anatomic complexities of reconstruction, and the biologic incompatibilities that met efforts at prosthetic reconstruction. Earlier hesitations because of problems of physiologic management during reconstruction proved to be less formidable. The growth in frequency of postintubation benign lesions, as a result of the success of modern respiratory therapy, increased the urgency of developmental work.

The concept of direct end-to-end anastomosis of trachea to trachea was generally accepted as the ideal method of tracheal repair following reconstruction. It was long believed, however, as stated by Belsey (1950), that no more than 2 cm — about four tracheal rings — could be removed and anastomosis consistently made. As a result, lateral resection was done when possible, with attempts made to patch the defect in various ways, using fascia, skin, pericardium, other tissues, and foreign materials. When such technique was applied to malignant neoplasms, inadequate removal of tumor resulted, with early recurrence. Failure of healing of such patches also occurred. Partial cicatrization was an additional factor. Attention was directed early to the development of an artificial trachea.

Prosthetic Replacement

Many materials have been used for prosthetic replacement of the trachea. Most work has been done in animals, but a scattered experience in man has been reported. Replacements have consisted of tubes made of glass or metal; stainless steal mesh in either tubes or coils and tantalum mesh; lucite, polyethylene, and other plastic cylinders; tubes of Ivalon or Marlex mesh; Teflon with combinations of Ivalon or Dacron; more recently polytetrafluoroethylene — PTFE — and Silastic tubes, often with stainless steel wire or plastic rings to supply rigidity. Early prostheses were usually solid tubes that bridged defects between the two ends of the trachea. Their failure led to use of rigid meshwork cylinders that were intended to allow incorporation into the surrounding connective tissue. More recently, flexible meshwork has been supported by splinting plastic rings. These meshwork prostheses were based on the theory that they would be incorporated by connective tissue and that epithelium would then grow down over this bed of new connective tissue; the rigid rings would maintain an open airway. In most experiments, only short prosthetic bridges have been incorporated to any extent. Some of the longer prostheses maintain an open airway, but firm healing with full tissue encasement and epithelialization has not occurred. This basically un-

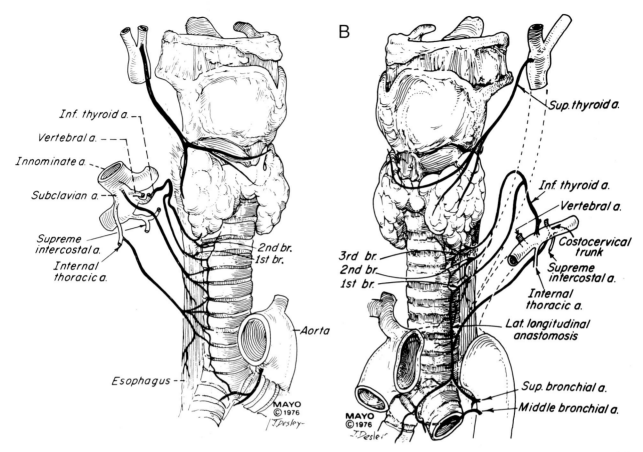

Fig. 34–1. Blood supply of the trachea. *A.* Right anterior view; *B.* Left anterior view. The right side varies in some respects. *From* Salassa JR, Pearson BW, Payne WS: Gross and microscopical blood supply of the trachea. Ann Thorac Surg 24:100, 1977.

healed state might be acceptable as an airway, but these longer prostheses have been subject, in a high percentage of instances, to occlusion by formation of granulation tissue at the nonhealing ends, strictures at these ends, sepsis causing rejection of the prosthesis, or erosion of major vessels with fatal hemorrhage. An occasional long-term success has occurred, largely as an exception rather than as the rule. The problem is the biologic instability caused by placing a foreign body in a bed of connective tissue adjacent to an epithelium that necessarily is contaminated with bacteria. With a foreign body in place, a chronic abscess is presented to the mediastinum, with the described results. Borrie and Redshaw (1970) attempted to solve these problems by accepting a foreign tube as a permanent airway but making it with suturable cuffs that they hoped would become incorporated by connective tissue. Neville and associates (1990) reported successes with a similar prosthesis. Vogt-Moykopf and Mickisch (1987) noted the many complications that occur.

Anatomic Mobilization

Perhaps most crucial to the evolution of mobilization techniques for tracheal reconstruction was recognition that the cervical trachea — as seen in the hyperextended surgical "thyroid" position — may be delivered into the mediastinum by cervical flexion. A few reports of clinical resections greater than 2 cm appeared, but few systematic studies of the anatomic potential are recorded. Michelson and associates (1961) noted that careful mobilization of the entire trachea in eight cadavers allowed for anastomosis with 1 pound of tension, after resection of 4 to 6 cm, with an additional 2.5 to 5.0 cm obtained by division of the left main bronchus.

Our detailed anatomic studies in cadavers attempted to answer the surgical questions of how much trachea could be resected and primary anastomosis made when the trachea was approached in progressive fashion from either a cervical or a transthoracic approach, depending on the location of the lesion. In one study, Mulliken and I (1968) mobilized the trachea through a cervicomediastinal approach, carefully preserving the lateral tissue that bears the blood supply. Using a standard tension of 1000 to 1200 g for approximation, it was possible, with the neck in 15 to 35° of flexion, to resect an average length of 4.5 cm — about 7 rings — and to increase this by 1.4 cm by entering the pleural space and mobilizing the right hilus (Fig. 34–2A). With greater degrees of cervical flexion, even longer resections are possible. Suprahyoid laryngeal release, described by Montgomery (1974), adds 1.0 to 1.5 cm while

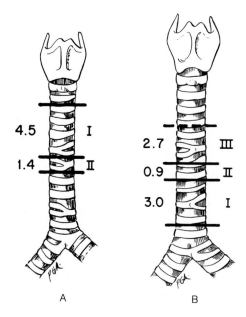

Fig. 34–2. The amounts of trachea that can be removed and yet permit primary anastomosis. *A,* Cervicomediastinal mobilization permitted removal of 4.5 cm under 1000 g tension, with cervical flexion. Intrathoracic dissection permitted removal of an additional 1.4 cm. *B,* Transthoracic hilar dissection and division of the pulmonary ligament, with the cervical spine in the neutral position, permitted removal of 3 cm, intrapericardial dissection an additional 0.9 cm, and division of the left main bronchus with reimplantation in the bronchus intermedius an additional 2.7 cm. The use of cervical flexion has demonstrated that the area designated I may be significantly greater than 3 cm. *From* Grillo HC: Surgical approaches to the trachea. Surg Gynecol Obstet *129:347, 1969.*

minimizing the difficulties in swallowing that attended earlier techniques for release. Alternating lateral division of the intercartilaginous ligaments of the trachea to obtain extension has been proposed experimentally, but not applied clinically to any extent. This technique has the disadvantages of probable interference with tracheal blood supply and the need for extensive tracheal exposure to obtain a rather limited extension of length.

In approaching the lower half of the trachea, my colleagues and I (1964) accomplished mobilization progressively by first, freeing the hilus of the right lung and dividing the pulmonary ligament; second, freeing the pulmonary vessels from their pericardial attachments; and third, transplanting the left main bronchus, which is held in place by the arch of the aorta, to the bronchus intermedius. In these earlier studies, we did not use cervical flexion but instead held the neck in the neutral position. At tensions under 1000 g, the first maneuver allowed for resection of 3 cm and the second for 0.9 cm additional; the radical measure of bronchial implantation permitted an additional 2.7 cm (see Fig. 34–2*B*). It has since become clear that cervical flexion combined with hilar and pericardial mobilization plus division of the pulmonary ligament allows lengths of 5 to 6 cm to be removed by the transthoracic approach. These figures represent only guidelines. The length of

trachea that may be resected safely in an individual varies widely with age, posture, bodily habitus, extent of disease and prior tracheal surgery. Bronchial implantation has been reserved for carinal excision or similar complex maneuvers in order to avoid adding another unnecessary risk to operation. Reimplantation of the left main bronchus into the bronchus intermedius was first used clinically by Barclay and associates (1957).

The limits of safety with varying anastomotic tensions have not been established in man. Cantrell and Folse (1961) found in dogs that tensions below 1700 g permitted safety from disruption after anastomosis. In anatomic studies in the cadaver, we found that an average tension of 675 g only was required for approximation — maximum 1000 g — after a 7-cm resection. Such clinical measurements as we have made show tensions of about 600 g in resections of 4 to 5 cm in length.

Anatomic and clinical observations show that great attention must be paid to the lateral blood supply in tracheal mobilization. This fine segmental supply cannot be disrupted safely, particularly for anastomosis of a long distal segment to a short proximal segment; the distal segment must not be freed circumferentially.

Another peculiarity of tracheal reconstruction depends on the relative rigidity of the anterolateral walls. Transverse wedging of the anterior wall of the trachea may buckle the posterior wall into a partially obstructing valve. Circumferential resection — which may, however, be beveled — is most often preferable.

SURGERY OF THE TRACHEA

Anesthesia

The airway must be under full control at all times during reconstructive surgery of the trachea, so that hasty maneuvers are unnecessary and hypoxia does not occur. The patient should breathe spontaneously during the operation and at its conclusion so that ventilatory support is not necessary. Cardiopulmonary bypass has been used for tracheal surgery, but it is not necessary for relatively simple resection and, as noted by Geffin and colleagues (1969), presents real hazards for more complex procedures requiring extensive manipulation of the lung. Procedures are carefully explained to the patients before the operation. Induction is carried out slowly and gently, especially in a patient with a highly obstructed trachea. If a benign stenosis presents an airway diameter of less than 5 mm, dilatation is performed and an endotracheal tube is passed beyond the lesion, to prevent arrhythmia caused by CO_2 buildup during the early stages of operation. Occasionally, a nearly obstructing tumor has required prompt bronchoscopy — with a ventilating bronchoscope — shortly after induction, with subsequent intubation. Frequent monitoring of blood gases and an electrocardiogram are essential. Bronchoscopic examination should be done by both the surgeon and the anesthetist who must deal with this airway until surgical access distal to the lesion has been obtained. If tracheostomy is already present, induction is simplified. Initial dissection is always done carefully to avoid increasing the degree of obstruction by roughness or pressure. The area below the obstruction is isolated first, so that a transection of the trachea can be performed at any point and an airway can be introduced across the operative field, should the degree of obstruction increase. Sterile anesthesia tubing, connectors, and endotracheal tubes are available in the operative field. I have not found it necessary to make distal incisions in the tracheobronchial tree for insertion of ventilatory catheters but, rather, have proceeded as described. If transthoracic resection is performed close to the carina, the endotracheal tube is passed into the left main bronchus and that lung alone is ventilated; if the Po_2 falls toward unsatisfactory levels, a previously isolated right pulmonary artery is temporarily clamped to eliminate the shunt through the right lung. This is rarely required. Slow increase in shunting may occur during prolonged operation owing to low tidal ventilation, increasing atelectasis, and aspiration of secretions, and must be

guarded against, as noted by Wilson (1987). High frequency ventilation is a useful adjunct, especially in complex carinal reconstruction, as reported by El-Baz and associates (1982).

Surgical Approaches

Lesions in the upper half of the trachea that are known to be benign are best approached cervically (Fig. 34–3A). If a malignant lesion is present, be prepared for the cervicomediastinal and, possibly, thoracic approach. Placement of the cervical incision depends on the pathologic state, the presence of existing stomas, and the possible need for sternotomy. If a postoperative temporary tracheostomy stoma may be required after a difficult laryngotracheal anastomosis, then the incision must be planned so that a stoma can be made away from the incision. If the initial dissection through the neck indicates need for further exposure, the upper sternum is split to a point just beyond the angle of Louis; horizontal division of the sternum into an intercostal space is not necessary. Because the great vessels present anteriorly, division of more than the upper sternum is not helpful; division simply allows room to maneuver

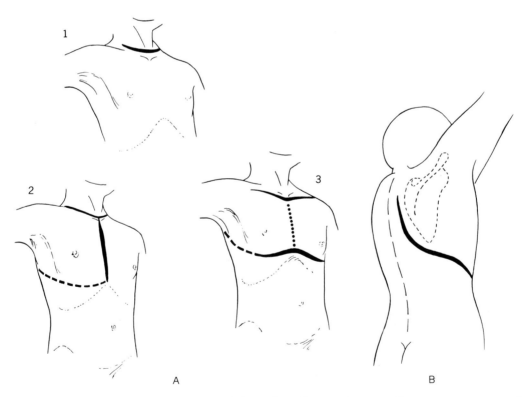

Fig. 34–3. *A*, Incisions for approach to the upper portion of the trachea. (1) Cervical incision allows access to upper trachea and to the mediastinum with somewhat limited exposure. (2) Median sternotomy, usually carried only through the upper two thirds of the sternum, allows more extended dissection into the mediastinum. Extension of the incision to the right fourth intercostal space (dotted line) allows exposure of the entire trachea from cricoid to carina and permits mobilization of the hilus. (3) Cervicomediastinal approach is here carried out beneath a bipedicled anterior skin flap. The flap is kept intact in case it is necessary to fashion a mediastinal tracheostomy. Such an incision is rarely needed. *B*, Incision for approach to the lower trachea and carina. The thorax is entered through the fourth intercostal space or the bed of the resected fourth rib. The high incision shown permits the scapula to be drawn out of the way. *From* Grillo HC: Surgical approaches to the trachea. Surg Gynecol Obstet *129*:347, 1969.

in managing the more distal trachea. Innominate vein division also adds nothing.

Rarely, this incision must be extended through the fourth intercostal space on the right to permit additional mobilization of the intrathoracic trachea by freeing the hilus of the right lung. Such an incision permits wide exposure of the entire trachea from cricoid to carina. This is almost never necessary in benign stenosis. If extirpative surgery and terminal tracheostomy are expected, the incision should avoid a vertical limb even if sternal division is needed. A large bipedicled flap is prepared through two horizontal incisions, as I suggested in 1966. A long-segment cutaneous tracheal replacement may also be so fashioned. Such circumstances are unusual but should be kept in mind in planning extensive procedures.

Neoplastic lesions of the lower half of the trachea are most easily approached directly through a high right thoracotomy incision (see Fig. 34–3B). It is possible to excise even very low benign lesions from the anterior approach described. Cervical flexion devolves sufficient trachea into the mediastinum so that lower tracheal tumors are usually approachable completely through the right side of the chest without a sternal component. Fourth intercostal space or fifth rib resection is used. Median sternotomy with dissection between the superior vena cava and aorta, and anterior and posterior pericardial division, provides access to the lower trachea and carina, but the exposure is poor for extensive dissection or complex reconstruction.

Reconstruction of the Upper Trachea

The upper flap is raised with or without circumcising an existing tracheostomy incision or including it in the original incision; individualization is required in each patient. Many existing tracheostomy stomas, even if they are to be allowed to close spontaneously later, usually have to be remade in another opening in the skin because of changed postoperative relationships between trachea and overlying skin. If the lesion is high, benign, and short, only a limited field is required. Dissection is confined chiefly to the midline, the upper flap being raised to the level of the cricoid and the lower to the sternal notch to allow dissection in the pretracheal plane as needed. Dense scar is often present in association with benign stenosis and dissection is done close to the trachea to avoid damage to the recurrent nerves, especially near the cricoid. Isolation of the nerves is avoided because this would increase the danger of injury. Freeing the trachea below the lesion early allows easy establishment of airway control and expedites dissection of a cicatrized segment from the esophagus or prevertebral fascia. Mobilization is made as required before and behind the trachea both proximally and distally. Tentative approximation with traction sutures, while the neck is flexed by the anesthetist, demonstrates whether approximation may be accomplished or whether further dissection is needed. A single layer of anastomotic sutures is placed in interrupted fashion so that the knots are tied on the outside.

Fine — No. 4-0 — absorbable polymeric sutures are preferred. I prefer Vicryl. In many instances, the sutures become inaccessible to direct vision during typing and must not break (Fig. 34–4). The anterior approach may also be used for tumor, but in this situation, sternotomy is often required for adequate removal of paratracheal tissue. In this instance, the recurrent nerves are usually identified and preserved, if they are not involved by tumor.

When benign stenosis of the upper trachea also involves the subglottic larynx, one-stage reconstruction is possible. As I (1982) reported, the technique is complex. The anterior subglottic larynx is resected and, where the stenosis is circumferential, the posterior cricoid lamina is bared but preserved in order to protect the recurrent laryngeal nerves (Fig. 34–5). The distal tailored trachea is advanced to replace the anterior subglottic laryngeal wall with cartilages and to resurface the posterior cricoid plate with membranous tracheal wall. I and Mathisen (1992) have had generally good results.

Reconstruction of the Lower Trachea

After confirmation of the extent of a tumor, anatomic mobilization is usually accomplished prior to severing the trachea. If obstruction appears to be imminent during mobilization, the trachea is transected and distally intubated. If the line of transection is supracarinal, the left main bronchus is intubated. The need for elimination of an arterial shunt through the right lung has been discussed. Access to the subcarinal lymph nodes and lower paratracheal nodes is excellent. The recurrent nerves reach a point adjacent to the trachea promptly and should be sacrificed only deliberately as required. Cervical flexion by the anesthetist devolves a fair segment of trachea into the chest even in the lateral position and this, in combination with the mobilization maneuvers earlier noted, permits end-to-end anastomosis (Fig. 34–6). Complex maneuvers may be necessary for excision and reconstruction of carinal lesions or lesions involving the right main stem bronchus or upper lobe bronchus (Fig. 34–7). In general, my principle is to excise the tumor with a satisfactory margin and then use a suitable reconstruction for the specific situation. As I have described (1965, 1970), a second layer flap is always placed around intrathoracic anastomoses, usually a carefully pedicled pericardial fat pad. I described specific techniques of carinal reconstruction in detail. Laryngeal release is not helpful in carinal resection.

Tracheostomy is avoided after tracheal reconstruction to avoid drying of secretions or injury to the anastomosis. On rare occasions, it may be necessary, temporarily, after laryngotracheal anastomosis.

Complex Methods

One sees few benign lesions or potentially curable malignant lesions that require resection of lengths of trachea and still leave a functional larynx, in which end-to-end reconstruction may not be done by present

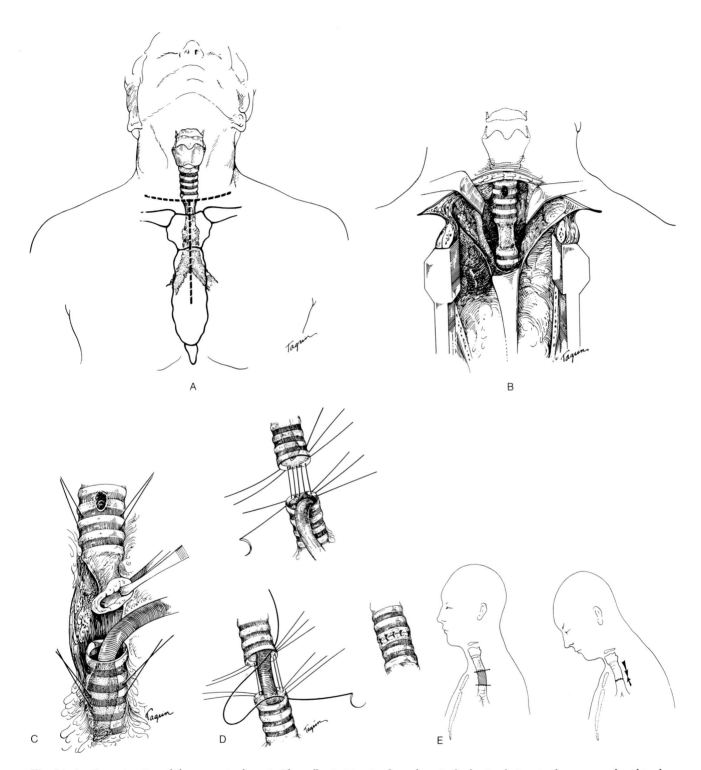

Fig. 34–4. Reconstruction of the upper trachea. *A,* The collar incision is often adequate for benign lesions in the upper and mid-trachea. Partial division of sternum allows access to the mediastinum over the great vessels. *B,* The innominate vein is retracted but not divided because greater exposure will not be so obtained owing to the posterior position of the lower trachea. The pleura is intact. *C,* Direct intubation has been performed following division of the trachea below an adherent stenotic lesion. Dissection is now simplified. Traction sutures are shown and also the scar of the prior tracheostomy. *D,* Details of placement of sutures. Interrupted sutures passing through the cartilage and membranous wall are used. Knots are tied on the outside. *E,* Diagram to indicate that the majority of mobilization in the approach to the upper trachea is obtained by cervical flexion with downward devolvement of the trachea and a lesser amount by upward movement of the distal trachea. *A* to *D, From* Grillo HC: Surgery of the trachea. Curr Probl Surg, July 1970.

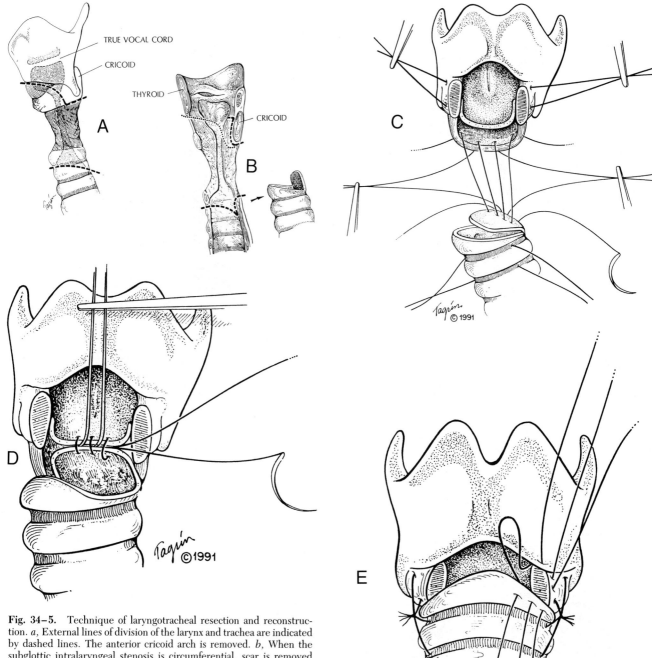

Fig. 34–5. Technique of laryngotracheal resection and reconstruction. *a,* External lines of division of the larynx and trachea are indicated by dashed lines. The anterior cricoid arch is removed. *b,* When the subglottic intralaryngeal stenosis is circumferential, scar is removed from the front of the posterior cricoid lamina, baring the cartilage. The residual posterior cricoid lamina protects the recurrent laryngeal nerves. Distally, the trachea is beveled over the length of one cartilage to fit the anterolateral subglottic defect that has been created. A broad-based flap of membranous tracheal wall is fashioned to resurface the bared cricoid plate. *c,* The posterior flap is fixed to the lower margin of the cricoid plate with four extraluminal sutures (4-0 Tevdek). The lateral traction sutures (2-0 Vicryl) are also shown in the larynx proximally and in the trachea distally. *d,* Posterior mucosal anastomotic sutures (4-0 Vicryl) are placed with knots to lie behind the mucosa. Traction sutures are omitted in this diagram for simplicity. *e,* After placement of all the posterior and posterolateral anastomotic sutures as far anteriorly as the lateral stay sutures, the patient's neck is flexed, the stay sutures are tied, the sternal fixing Tevdek sutures are tied, and then the posterior mucosal sutures are tied. The anterior and anterolateral anastomotic sutures are then placed and finally tied serially. *a* and *b, From* Grillo HC: Primary reconstruction of airway after resection of subglottic laryngeal and upper tracheal stenosis. Ann Thorac Surg 33:3, 1982. *c–e, From* Grillo HC, Mathisen DJ, Wain JC: Laryngotracheal resection and reconstruction for subglottic stenosis. Ann Thorac Surg 53:54, 1992.

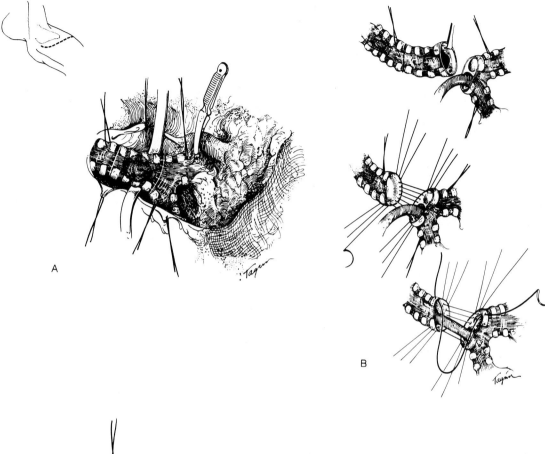

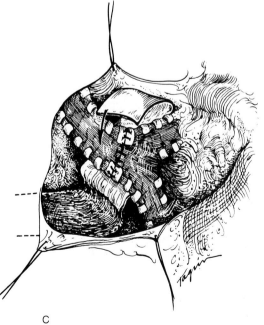

Fig. 34–6. Reconstruction of the lower trachea. *A*, Exposure through a thoracotomy. Hilar mobilization has been accomplished and also circumferential dissection of the trachea. When a tumor is present, paratracheal nodal tissue is excised with the specimen. Traction sutures have been placed proximally and distally. The lines of resection are shown. A clamp may be placed on the pulmonary artery later if the patient fails to maintain adequate oxygenation on intubation of the left main bronchus alone. This step has been necessary in lesions close to the carina as well as in carinal resections. *B*, Details of management of resection and suturing. Intubation has been carried out across the operative field and the specimen is then removed. After placement of sutures on the anterior and lateral walls of the trachea, an elongated endotracheal tube is passed from above into the left main bronchus and the balance of the posterior sutures are placed prior to their being tied. *C*, Following completion of the anastomosis, which is facilitated by flexion of the patient's neck, a second layer of pedicled pleural flap is placed about the anastomosis. *From* Grillo HC: Surgery of the trachea. Curr Probl Surg, July 1970.

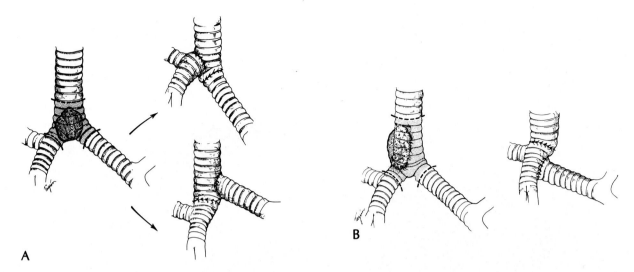

Fig. 34–7. Tracheal reconstruction after carinal resection. *A,* When the lesion is of limited extent, a neo-carina may be fashioned. *B,* Following carinal resection without removal of a long segment of trachea, reconstruction is most frequently performed by implanting the left main bronchus into the stump of the devolved lower trachea. The right main bronchus is then implanted preferentially in a side opening fashioned in the lower portion of the trachea. *C,* When a longer segment of trachea has been resected, it frequently is necessary to mobilize the right lung and elevate the right main bronchus to reach the trachea, which has also been devolved as far distally as it will go. In such cases, the left main bronchus may have to be anastomosed to the bronchus intermedius. Preservation of some blood supply for all of these segments of airway is essential for the repair to heal successfully. *From* Grillo HC: Tracheal tumors: Surgical management. Ann Thorac Surg 26:112, 1978.

methods. In a rare instance, I (1965) applied an extension of an earlier method developed experimentally and clinically for replacement of cervical trachea by fashioning an invaginated, horizontally bipedicled tube of full-thickness skin supported by fully buried polypropylene rings. Results have been no more dependable than the use of prostheses. At present, I believe both should be avoided. The alternatives are T-tubes for benign lesions and irradiation for malignant lesions nonresectable because of length.

Mediastinal Tracheostomy

Rarely, when a lesion involves a large portion of trachea and larynx but seems to be within possible bounds of cure, resection of both larynx and trachea may be indicated, either for palliation of severe airway obstruction or for potential cure. The cervical esophagus may also have to be removed en bloc. Attempts to pull the deeply situated distal tracheal stump to the surface place excess tension on the suture line; attempts to carry complex skin tubes down to the trachea led to separation at the suture lines, sepsis, and osteomyelitis of the sternum. Massive hemorrhages from the innominate artery and aortic arch have been frequent complications of such methods. Muscle flaps have not fully protected these vessels. A technique that I devised (1966) attempted to eliminate these problems by bringing the anterior skin down to the stump of the trachea by removing the heads of the clavicles, the upper portion of sternum, and the medial ends of the first two ribs (Fig. 34–8). This procedure is done extrapleurally. Excellent blood supply is present in the flap, and the anastomosis is made to a circular opening in the middle

point of the flap so that the suture line is simple. Hazards of bleeding do attend such procedures, however, if primary healing is not obtained. Elective division of the innominate artery, with appropriate preoperative angiography and intraoperative EEG monitoring, plus advancement of pedicled omental flaps to the upper mediastinum as recorded by the author and Mathisen (1990), have avoided such incidents. Waddell and Cannon (1959) and Orringer (1992) recommended transposition of the tracheostome to the right of the innominate artery.

TRACHEOSTOMY AND ITS PROBLEMS

Immediate complications of tracheostomy, such as intra- and early postoperative hemorrhage, incorrect placement, injury to adjacent structures, and hypoxia during the procedure, essentially have been eliminated by the deliberate performance of tracheostomy over an emergency airway established by endotracheal intubation or rigid bronchoscopy. Later complications, such as plugging of the tube, valve-like obstruction at the tip caused by dry secretions, slippage of cuffs or of the tube, and local sepsis, have been reduced in incidence by meticulous care of the tracheostomy, and their consequences have been minimized by early recognition and correction. In addition to the late obstructive complications to be discussed in Chapter 69, erosion of the innominate artery and tracheoesophageal fistula must be remembered, as pointed out by Mulder and Rubush (1969) as well as others. I and my colleagues (1976) described a single-stage method for repair of postintubation tracheoesophageal fistula, which has given excellent results.

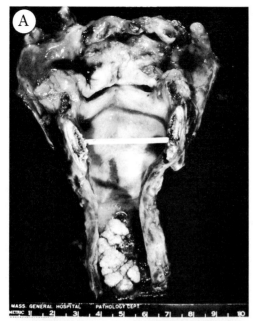

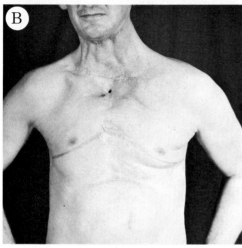

Fig. 34–8. Mediastinal tracheostomy. *A*, Laryngotracheal specimen to remove two obstructing lesions — mucoepidermoid carcinoma of the larynx and squamous cell carcinoma of the trachea, concurrently. Regional node dissections were done later. *From* Grillo HC: Surgery of the trachea. Curr Probl Surg, July 1970. *B*, Photograph of a patient 18 months after initial resection shows the anatomic features of a low mediastinal tracheostomy. The procedure was carried out between two horizontal incisions, one across the base of the neck and the other beneath the nipples. The upper chest wall defect is the result of the removal of the upper sternum and medial ends of clavicles and upper two ribs. The stoma sits just above the aortic arch. The short horizontal incision just below the stoma was necessary for control of bleeding in the innominate artery postoperatively. The horizontal incision below the xiphoid was initially placed as a relaxing incision to allow advancement of flaps upward.

I prefer to perform a tracheostomy through a short horizontal incision about 1 cm below the cricoid, and to identify the cricoid precisely so that the correct level of second and third rings may be selected. The thyroid isthmus usually must be divided. A vertical incision in the trachea is used. Extreme care should be exercised to avoid injuring the first ring, because subsequent erosion may damage the cricoid and produce a subglottic stricture that is extremely difficult to repair. If necessary, the tracheal opening should include the fourth ring also. A tube with an inner cannula is preferable. Initially, it is held not only by tapes but also by skin sutures passed through the flanges and tied.

Another rare complication of tracheostomy is a persistent stoma that does not close even after many months. This situation usually results from a long, persistent tracheostomy, a large stoma caused by the operative procedure or sepsis, healing of skin to tracheal epithelium, and debilitating systemic states that depressed the healing response. Lawson and I (1970) devised a technique for closure that circumscribes the stoma, using the healed skin as a first-stage circular flap (Fig. 34–9). When this skin is inverted with a subcuticular suture, a healed epithelial surface is presented to the tracheal lumen. The strap muscles are approximated and the skin and platysma are closed horizontally over this area. Results of repair by this method have been excellent.

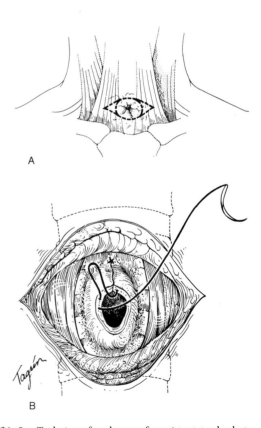

Fig. 34–9. Technique for closure of persistent tracheal stoma. *A*, The skin around the margin of the stoma is elevated with a circumferential incision. The lateral extensions create an ellipse to provide access and permit plastic closure. *B*, After dissection of the skin and platysma above and below, and mobilization of the strap muscles laterally, the central circular flap is created, with great care not to destroy its basal blood supply. It is now closed with a subcuticular suture. The epithelial surface faces the lumen. The strap muscles are next approximated and the skin and platysma are closed above in a horizontal layer. *From* Lawson DW, Grillo HC: Closure of a persistent tracheal stoma. Surg Gynecol Obstet *130*:995, 1970.

REFERENCES

Barclay RS, McSwan N, Welsh TM: Tracheal reconstruction without the use of grafts. Thorax 12:177, 1957.

Belsey R: Resection and reconstruction of the intrathroacic trachea. Br J Surg 38:200, 1950.

Borrie J, Redshaw NR: Cervical tracheal reconstruction in sheep, using silastic prostheses with subterminal suture cuffs. Proc Univ Otago Med School 48:32, 1970.

Cantrell JR, Folse JR: The repair of circumferential defects of the trachea by direct anastomosis: Experimental evaluation. J Thorac Cardiovasc Surg 42:589, 1961.

El-Baz N, et al: One-lung high-frequency ventilation for tracheoplasty and bronchoplasty. Ann Thorac Surg 34:564, 1982.

Geffin B, Bland J, Grillo HC: Anesthetic management of tracheal resection and reconstruction. Anesth Analg 48:884, 1969.

Grillo HC: Circumferential resection and reconstruction of mediastinal and cervical trachea. Ann Surg 162:374, 1965.

Grillo HC: Terminal or mural tracheostomy in the anterior mediastinum. J Thorac Cardiovasc Surg 51:422, 1966.

Grillo HC: Surgical approaches to the trachea. Surg Gynecol Obstet 129:374, 1969.

Grillo HC: Surgery of the trachea. Curr Probl Surg, July 1970, p. 1.

Grillo HC: Primary reconstruction of airway resection of subglottic laryngeal and upper tracheal stenosis. Ann Thorac Surg 33:3, 1982a.

Grillo HC: Carinal reconstruction. Ann Thorac Surg 34:356, 1982b.

Grillo HC, Mathisen DJ: Cervical exenteration. Ann Thorac Surg 49:401, 1990.

Grillo HC, Dignan EF, Miura T: Extensive resection and reconstruction of mediastinal trachea without prosthesis or graft: An anatomical study in man. J Thorac Cardiovasc Surg 48:741, 1964.

Grillo HC, Mathisen DJ, Wain JC: Laryngotracheal resection and reconstruction for subglottic stenosis. Ann Thorac Surg 53:54, 1992.

Grillo HC, Moncure AC, McEnany MT: Repair of inflammatory tracheo-esophageal fistula. Ann Thorac Surg 22:112, 1976.

Lawson DW, Grillo HC: Closure of a persistent tracheal stoma. Surg Gynecol Obstet 130:995, 1970.

Michelson E, et al: Experiments in tracheal reconstruction. J Thorac Cardiovasc Surg 41:784, 1961.

Miura T, Grillo HC: The contribution of the inferior thyroid artery to the blood supply of the human trachea. Surg Gynecol Obstet 123:99, 1966.

Montgomery WW: Suprahyoid release for tracheal anastomosis. Arch Otolaryngol 99:255, 1974.

Mulder DS, Rubush JL: Complications of tracheostomy: Relationship to long-term ventilatory assistance. J Trauma 9:389, 1969.

Mulliken J, Grillo HC: The limits of tracheal resection with primary anastomosis. Further anatomical studies in man. J Thorac Cardiovasc Surg 55:418, 1968.

Neville WE, Bolandowski PJ, Kotia GG: Clinical experience with silicone tracheal prothesis. J Thorac Cardiovasc Surg 99:604, 1990.

Orringer M: Anterior mediastinal tracheostomy with and without cervical exenteration. Ann Thorac Surg 54:628, 1992.

Salassa JR, Pearson B, Payne WS: Growth and microscopic blood supply of the trachea. Ann Thorac Surg 23:100, 1977.

Vogt-Moykopf I, Mickisch GH: Prosthetic replacement of the trachea: Discussion. *In* Grillo HC, Eschapasse H (eds): International Trends in General Thoracic Surgery. Vol. 2. Philadelphia: WB Saunders, 1987, p. 147.

Waddell W, Cannon B: A technique for subtotal excision of the trachea and establishment of a sternal tracheostomy. Ann Surg 149:1, 1959.

Wilson RS: Anesthetic management for tracheal reconstruction. *In* Grillo HC, Eschapasse H (eds): International Trends in General Thoracic Surgery. Vol. 2. Philadelphia: WB Saunders, 1987, p. 3.

CHAPTER 35

TRACHEAL SLEEVE PNEUMONECTOMY

Yoh Watanabe

Tracheal sleeve pneumonectomy is an aggressive procedure for resection of bronchial carcinoma involving the tracheobronchial angle, carina, or lower trachea and lung. The airway is reconstructed by anastomosis of the opposite main stem bronchus to the lower trachea. This procedure is a type of extended resection, a term suggested by Chamberlain and associates (1959).

In 1950, Abbott first reported experience with the surgical resection of the carina, tracheal wall, and contralateral bronchial wall in patients undergoing right pneumonectomy. He also detailed the technical difficulties encountered in that procedure. In 1959, Gibbon also described a patient who underwent resection of the distal trachea during right pneumonectomy and anastomosis of the left bronchus to the residual trachea and survived for 6 months. After that, however, only a few reports of tracheal sleeve pneumonectomy were published for some years. Mathey and colleagues (1966) reported two patients with epidermoid carcinoma who had undergone right tracheal sleeve pneumonectomy and survived for 1.5 and 4.5 years, respectively, and Thompson (1966) reported a patient undergoing right tracheal sleeve pneumonectomy.

In 1972, Jensik and associates reported 17 cases of tracheal sleeve pneumonectomy. Since then, the results of tracheal sleeve pneumonectomy in a moderate number of patients have been reported subsequently by Jensik (1982), Deslauriers (1979, 1985, 1989), and Dartevelle (1988) and their associates. The operative mortality described in these reports was 11 to 29%, and the 5-year survival rates was only 13 to 23%.

More recently, the results of tracheal sleeve pneumonectomy were reported by Fujimura (1985), Tsuchiya (1990), Watanabe (1990a), Muscolino (1992) and their associates. Their series had fewer patients, but a lower operative mortality. The results with respect to long-term survival, however, remained unsatisfactory.

Because of unfavorable results of tracheal sleeve pneumonectomy, Grillo (1982) expressed concern about the validity of using this procedure for treating bronchial carcinoma involving the carina. He has done a large number of carinal resections for tracheal tumor, but has performed few tracheal sleeve pneumonectomies for bronchial carcinoma, because he believes that the procedure should be reserved for patients who are potentially curable on the basis of preoperative mediastinoscopy — absence of mediastinal lymph node involvement and the exclusion of remote metastases. Few central lesions fulfill these criteria in his opinion.

SELECTION OF PATIENTS

Tracheal sleeve pneumonectomy may be considered in a patient in whom bronchial carcinoma is centrally located at the hilus of the lung with extension to involve the orifice of the main stem bronchus or the lateral aspect of the lower trachea. The most favorable histologic type is squamous cell carcinoma, and the best results are achieved in patients with this type of lesions.

The initial step in identifying a possible candidate for this procedure is bronchoscopy. Random samples for biopsy must be taken proximal to determine the possible line of dissection in the tracheobronchial tree. According to Deslauriers and associates (1985, 1989), tissue should be taken from any doubtful area and also in the trachea at 3 cm above the carina. Local invasion up to that level by lung cancer indicates an aggressive tumor and would make a curative procedure virtually impossible. Faber (1987) reported that involvement of the carina or tracheobronchial angle was indicated by mucosal thickening, widening of the carina, or erythema and corrugation of the mucosa at the tracheobronchial angle.

Tomography, computed tomography — CT, and magnetic resonance imaging — MRI — are also helpful in defining the extrabronchial extent of the lesions (Fig. 35–1). With the aid of these examinations, precise delineation of pulmonary artery and main bronchial involvement can be obtained along with detection of enlarged mediastinal lymph nodes. Correlation of the

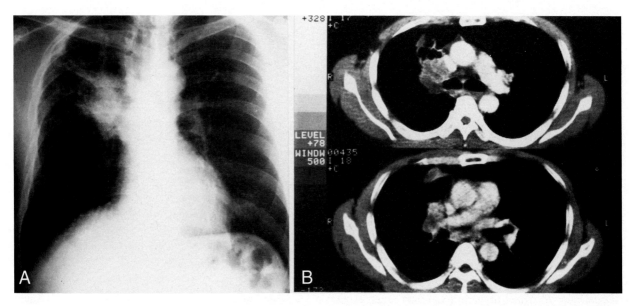

Fig. 35–1. Preoperative chest radiograph *(A)* and CT scan *(B)* of a 49-year-old male who underwent right tracheal sleeve pneumonectomy.

bronchoscopic and CT findings is important in determining the appropriate type of resection.

Deslauriers and colleagues (1979, 1985, 1989) recommended mediastinoscopy as part of the preoperative staging, because neoplastic involvement of the superior mediastinal nodes (N2 disease) generally represents an absolute contraindication to tracheal sleeve pneumonectomy. Faber (1987) also recommended mediastinoscopy when the mediastinal lymph nodes were greater than 1.0 cm in diameter. Both these authors believe that contraindications to resection were positive superior mediastinal nodes and positive contralateral tracheal nodes. If mediastinal nodes are positive at the midtracheal level or at the azygos vein, a difference of opinion exists as to whether or not resection should be carried out. I believe that although long-term survival may be low, some patients benefit from resection of the primary tumor and positive mediastinal nodes; this opinion is not shared by all (see Chapter 89). Dartevelle and co-workers (1989) concluded from their results that lymph node involvement in the upper mediastinum and tumors involving more than 2 cm of the distal trachea are contraindications for this operation. Deslauriers and associates (1989) reported that a tension-free or tumor-free reconstruction was unlikely if the tumor extended more than 4 cm above the carina.

Carinal resection in patients with tumor recurrence in the bronchial stump after prior pneumonectomy is another possible surgical indication for tracheal sleeve resection. In these patients, either the right or left main stem bronchus is anastomosed to the trachea after resection of the carina. We have performed such an operation in only one patient, but the carinal resection series reported by Grillo (1982a), Jensik (1972, 1982), Deslauriers (1979, 1985, 1989), and their colleagues include a few cases of carinal resection after previous pneumonectomy.

PREOPERATIVE ADJUVANT THERAPY IN PATIENTS WITH BRONCHIAL CARCINOMA

As preoperative adjuvant therapy, radiation therapy, bronchial arterial infusion therapy — BAI, and neoadjuvant chemotherapy are applicable. Jensik and colleagues (1972, 1982) recommended preoperative radiation therapy for sterilization of the mediastinal lymph nodes and the primary lesion. Twenty-five of the 30 patients in their group received radiation therapy administered from either a cobalt or linear accelerator source. The dose varied from 3200 to 5000 rads, but most individuals received 4000 rad administered over a 4-week period. They experienced 8 perioperative deaths, most of them being related to the development of bronchial fistulas. It was difficult, they claimed, to incriminate the preoperative radiation as a causative factor for fistula. They also stated that the benefits resulting from reduction in tumor volume and the improvement of the lesion on bronchoscopic examination justify its use. On the other hand, Dartevelle (1988), Deslauriers (1979, 1985, 1989) and their associates emphasized that preoperative irradiation increases the risk of bronchopleural fistula.

In our series (1990b) of 18 patients, no one underwent preoperative irradiation, although five patients underwent BAI therapy as a preoperative adjuvant treatment. These patients received mitomycin C — 8 mg, Esquinone — Carbazilquinone, 6 mg, and ACNU — Nimustine, 50 mg. Figure 35–2 shows the disappearance of atelectasis related to tumor shrinkage after two courses of BAI therapy. The patient subsequently underwent left tracheal sleeve pneumonectomy. Among the five patients undergoing preoperative BAI therapy, one developed bronchopleural fistula 20 days after right tracheal sleeve pneumonectomy, but it was not clear that the preoperative therapy was related to this anastomotic dehiscence.

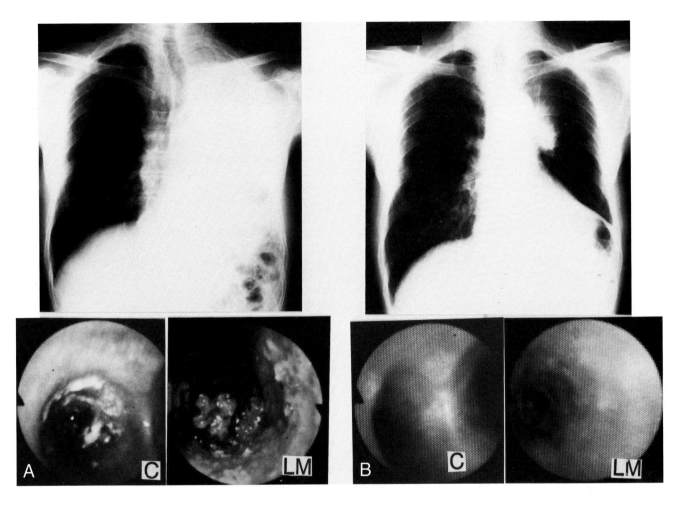

Fig. 35–2. Effect of bronchial arterial infusion (BAI) as preoperative adjuvant therapy. *A*, Chest radiograph and bronchoscopic findings in a 66-year-old male with epidermoid carcinoma of the left hilum that caused complete atelectasis of the left lung. *B*, Chest radiograph and bronchoscopic view taken 11 days after the second course of BAI therapy. The patient underwent left tracheal sleeve pneumonectomy 20 days after the second course of BAI therapy. C = carina; LM = left main bronchus.

The effects of neoadjuvant therapy for advanced lung cancer are still under evaluation. It may be considered that neoadjuvant therapy can be applied in patients who are candidates for sleeve pneumonectomy. In no reports yet, however, was neoadjuvant therapy routinely used before tracheal sleeve pneumonectomy.

SURGICAL APPROACH

For right tracheal sleeve pneumonectomy, I have always used posterolateral thoracotomy and believe it is the best approach. Muscolino and associates (1992), however, performed right tracheal sleeve pneumonectomy by an anterior thoracotomy through the fourth intercostal space in seven patients without any surgical mortality. They concluded that anterior thoracotomy might be considered as improving the surgical management of these patients. Pearson and colleagues (1984) preferred to use median sternotomy in patients requiring carinal resection. They point out that this technique has several advantages over a right posterolateral thoracotomy in selected cases, because any type

of pulmonary resection is possible through a median sternotomy. In addition, a cervical collar incision combined with median sternotomy provides easy access for a superior laryngeal or suprahyoid release procedure when required. This incision also provides adequate exposure for an intrapericardial mobilization of the right pulmonary hilum, which may also be necessary to minimize tension on a tracheal or tracheobronchial anastomosis.

With regard to left tracheal sleeve pneumonectomy, controversy exists regarding the best surgical approach, and it is also controversial whether this should be a one-stage or two-stage operation.

Abbott (1955), Grillo (1982), and Salzer and co-workers (1987) reported a one-stage operation using a left posterolateral thoracotomy, but this approach is seldom used because proper exposure of the carina underneath the aortic arch is difficult. In fact, Grillo (1982) mentioned that if the left main stem bronchus is divided close to its bifurcation into upper and lower lobe bronchi, the trachea cannot be brought down to this point; no method is available to advance the residual left main stem bronchus. Perelman and Koroleva (1980) solved this problem, however, by stapling the left main stem bronchus distal to the tumor and reanastomosing the trachea to the right main stem bronchus. In a series of 10 patients, they noted no difficulty with shunting or infection in the left lung. In contrast, when Grillo (1982) used this technique, the patient experienced tachycardia and tachypnea for 8 months postoperatively because of massive vascular shunting through the non-aerated left lung, and left pneumonectomy was required for relief. In another patient, Grillo performed a left pneumonectomy through a separate incision after completion of the resection and anastomosis of the trachea to the right main stem bronchus; the patient developed pneumonia in the right lung postoperatively and died.

Deslauriers (1985, 1989) and Gilbert and associates (1988) recommend a two-stage procedure. In the first stage, left proximal pneumonectomy is carried out, and the carina is resected from the right side 3 to 5 weeks later. They emphasize caution, however, in using this operative method. Because of the local inflammatory reaction and mediastinal shift that follows pneumonectomy, mobilization of the left main stem bronchus stump is potentially dangerous and one must be aware of the proximity of the left pulmonary artery stump and left recurrent laryngeal nerve.

I have done one-stage operations by median sternotomy combined with anterolateral thoracotomy in one patient undergoing left tracheal sleeve pneumonectomy and one receiving carinal resection after prior left pneumonectomy. This approach provides excellent exposure and access for lung resection as well as reconstruction procedures, which ultimately facilitates performance of the operation. Thus, I suggest and strongly recommend the median sternotomy approach combined with anterolateral thoracotomy for the performance of left tracheal sleeve pneumonectomy.

MAINTENANCE OF VENTILATION

Maintenance of adequate ventilation and oxygenation is of crucial importance in tracheobronchial surgery. In general, provision of ventilation is incompatible with an unobstructed operative field; a bulky endotracheal tube permits adequate ventilation, but impedes access to the operative field for anastomosis.

A tube ventilation system coming from above or across the operative field is the most conventional method. Abbott (1950) described the use of a long tube directed into the left main stem bronchus to maintain ventilation with left endobronchial anesthesia during the operative procedure. Jensik and co-workers (1972, 1985) used this method in the majority of their patients, although it was modified in some instances with a supplementary sterile tube and connector, which is placed into the left main stem bronchus after it is divided. The other end of the connecting tube is directed outward through the incision and over the anesthetic screen. After the first portion

of the anastomosis is completed, the tube is withdrawn and the original endobronchial tube is directed beyond the suture line into the left main stem bronchus. The anastomosis is then completed over the tube. Geffin and associates (1969) showed that this method can be adapted to all types of carinal reconstruction. This system has the disadvantage, however, of requiring repeated tube manipulations with frequent interruption of airway suturing. If the tube runs across the operative field — for example, an armored tube into the left main stem bronchus, it further restricts surgical access to the carina.

Frumin (1959), Heller (1964), and their colleagues described the technique of prolonged apneic oxygenation for carinal reconstruction. After hyperventilating the patient with 100% oxygen, 10 to 12 minutes of total apnea can often be tolerated. Deslauriers and associates (1979) used this technique in a few cases of tracheal sleeve pneumonectomy, but they commonly noted arrhythmias, acidosis, and hypercapnia for 15 minutes after the initiation of the prolonged apneic oxygenation. Thus, this technique is used rarely because the duration of safe apnea and the cardiovascular response are unpredictable in any individual patient.

McClish and colleagues (1985) described the value of the high-flow catheter technique after using it in 18 patients undergoing tracheobronchial reconstruction. This method has specific advantages with regard to the simplicity of the equipment and anesthetic technique. It involves positive pressure ventilation with a high flow of gas and without air entrainment. Oxygen is applied from a high-pressure source capable of delivering it at a pressure of 50 psi and a flow of 100 L/min. Depending on the airway resistance and lung compliance, the inflation flow can be adjusted through a reducing valve to generate an airway pressure of 25 to 40 cm H_2O. Deslauriers and associates (1985, 1989) now use this method preferentially.

High-frequency jet ventilation — HFJV — can also be used to provide good ventilation and oxygenation. Our group (1988) uses this ventilatory method in all our patients undergoing tracheobronchial reconstructive surgery (Fig. 35–3). El-Baz and colleagues (1981) first reported the use of HFJV in six patients undergoing tracheobronchoplastic surgery. I and my colleagues (1988) analyzed arterial blood gas values during HFJV in 21 patients receiving major airway reconstructive surgery, including 9 who underwent tracheal sleeve pneumonectomy. I would like to emphasize the advantages of HFJV over classic intermittent positive pressure ventilation using an endotracheal tube. In tracheal sleeve pneumonectomy, a relatively high driving gas pressure — 1.5 to 2.5 kg/cm^2 — at 360 to 480 cycles per minute provides optimum ventilation and oxygenation. This method permits greater accuracy in placing and tying sutures and eliminates the need for intermittent withdrawal and reinsertion of the endotracheal tube into the contralateral main bronchus. Use of HFJV delivered through a small-bore catheter can facilitate

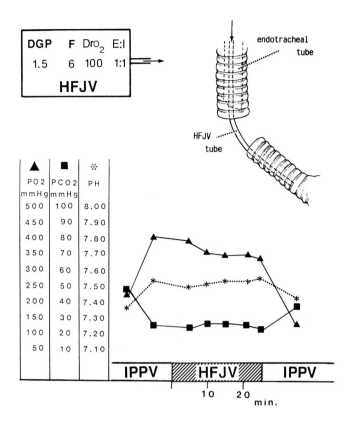

DGP	F	DrO$_2$	E:I
1.5	6	100	1:1

HFJV

endotracheal tube

HFJV tube

▲	■	※
PO2 mmHg	PCO2 mmHg	PH
500	100	8.00
450	90	7.90
400	80	7.80
350	70	7.70
300	60	7.60
250	50	7.50
200	40	7.40
150	30	7.30
100	20	7.20
50	10	7.10

IPPV HFJV IPPV

10 20 min.

Fig. 35–3. The ventilatory method and blood gas analyses in a patient (75-year-old male) who underwent right tracheal sleeve pneumonectomy. IPPV = intermittent positive pressure ventilation; HFJV = high-frequency jet ventilation; DGP = driving gas pressure; F = frequency; DrO$_2$ = O$_2$ content of driving gas; EI = expiratory/inspiratory ratio.

performance of the anastomosis, and thus directly contribute to the elimination of complication along the suture line and ultimately to improving the surgical outcome.

Perelman and Koroleva (1980) reported the use of hyperbaric oxygenation. They performed the first four operations on the trachea that were ever done in a hyperbaric chamber. Compression was begun 10 to 15 minutes before entering the tracheobronchial tree. The air pressure in the operating room was raised to 2.5 to 3 atmospheres, and it was possible to discontinue lung ventilation intermittently for 8 to 10 minutes.

OPERATIVE PROCEDURE

Right Tracheal Sleeve Pneumonectomy

The patient is placed in the left lateral position and posterolateral thoracotomy is the approach. The thoracic cavity is entered through the fifth intercostal space. At thoracotomy, the posterior mediastinal pleura is longitudinally incised along the trachea, the right main stem bronchus, and the esophagus from the apex to the base of the right hemithorax to expose the tracheo-

bronchial tree. It is mandatory to ligate the azygos vein and to mobilize the trachea; the pericardium may be opened at this time. After careful observation from outside the tracheobronchial tree to detect tumor extension, the feasibility of tracheal sleeve pneumonectomy is finally determined in combination with the findings obtained by preoperative endoscopic examination. Once the decision to use tracheal sleeve pneumonectomy is made, the pericardium is opened along the phrenic nerve to expose the right main pulmonary artery and veins. These vessels are interrupted intrapericardially. The carina is then fully mobilized from its mediastinal bed and tapes are passed around the lower trachea and the left and right main stem bronchi.

Both trachea and main stem bronchus are transected at the intercartilaginous ligament (Fig. 35–4A). The trachea is transected 1.0 cm proximal to the tumor, usually at the first or second distal tracheal ring, but sometimes transection must extend as high as 3.0 cm above the carina. The left main stem bronchus is also divided at a level free of tumor, but it is seldom necessary to make the division more than one ring below the carina. Frozen sections are examined to confirm that the site of transection is free of tumor.

Before starting the reconstruction procedure, mobilization of the trachea and left main stem bronchus is accomplished to lessen the tension at the anastomosis. The left main stem bronchus is relatively fixed by the aortic arch. Gentle blunt dissection of this bronchus from the aortic arch and surrounding tissue is done, excluding the posterior, membraneous portion. This maneuver is continued down to the left upper lobe bronchus. The trachea is pulled down in the same way, and maximal flexion of the neck fully reduces the tension at the anastomosis.

The suture material used in all patients is absorbable 3-0 Vicryl. The anastomosis is commenced at the farthest point from the operator (see Fig. 35–4B). Cartilage-to-cartilage apposition of the left lateral wall of the trachea to the lateral wall of the left main stem bronchus with the placement and tying of two sutures forms the basis of the anastomosis, and more sutures are then added to the cartilaginous part of the bronchus. Sutures are placed through the full thickness of the trachea and bronchus, making certain that the knots are tied outside of the lumen (see Fig. 35–4C). The membranous part of the bronchus is anastomosed as the last part of the procedure. Luminal disparity is equalized by expanding the membranous portion of the smaller bronchus and crimping that of the larger trachea (Fig. 35–4D). Once the anastomotic procedures are completed, the suture line should be checked for air leaks and the endotracheal tube should be located at sufficient distance above the suture line.

The anastomotic site is covered routinely by a circumferential pleural flap to prevent suture leaks or dehiscence (see Fig. 35–4E). In tracheal sleeve pneumonectomy for bronchial carcinoma, lymph node dissection of the hilar and mediastinal nodes is also

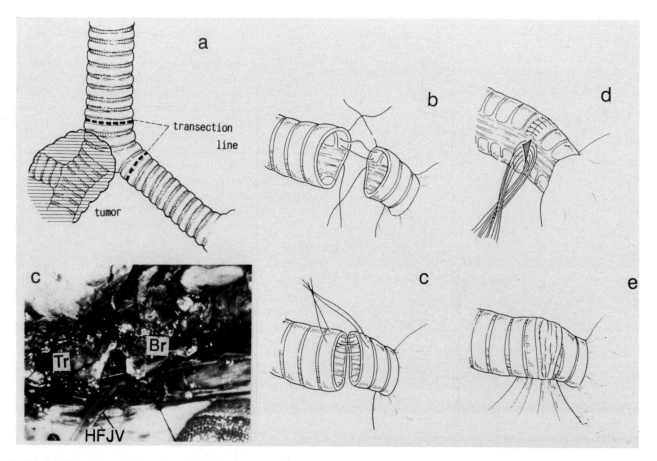

Fig. 35–4. Operative procedure for right sleeve pneumonectomy. *a,* Transection lines for the trachea and bronchus. *b,* The first two stitches of the anastomotic procedure. *c-right,* Anastomosis of the cartilaginous portion. *c-left,* Operative view of anastomosis. HFJV, which has been maintained through a small-bore catheter inserted from the operative field, is being switched to IPPV through an endotracheal tube for a completion of anastomosis at the anterior part of the cartilaginous and membraneous portions. Tr = trachea; Br = bronchus. *d,* Equalization of luminal disparity by crimping the membranous part. *e,* Covering of the suture line with a circumferential pleural flap.

performed as in routine lobectomy or pneumonectomy for malignant lung tumors.

Left Tracheal Sleeve Pneumonectomy

Left tracheal sleeve pneumonectomy is a relatively rare procedure in every series reported. As mentioned previously, controversy still exists regarding the best surgical approach and whether a one- or two-stage operation should be performed. Our group uses a one-stage operation involving median sternotomy combined with left anterolateral thoracotomy. The operation starts with median sternotomy. Exposure of the carina and main bronchus requires a transpericardial approach. The anterior pericardium is opened vertically — from the level of the innominate vein to the bottom of the pericardium — to permit circumferential mobilization of the ascending aortic arch, which is then retracted leftward. The posterior pericardium is incised vertically. The superior vena cava is displaced laterally and to the right. The right main pulmonary artery is exposed and displaced inferiorly. By these maneuvers, the entire mediastinal trachea and carina are clearly exposed (Fig. 35–5). Then, anterolateral thoracotomy at the fourth

intercostal space is added to allow lung resection. By this approach, transection of the trachea and left main stem bronchus for pneumonectomy and anastomosis of the trachea and right main stem bronchus can be done easily in the same fashion as already described for right tracheal sleeve pneumonectomy. Division of the trachea at a point 1.5 cm above its bifurcation is sufficient for most tumors, but it is also possible to resect an additional length of distal trachea and elevate the right main stem bronchus for primary anastomosis, if necessary.

PERIOPERATIVE AND POSTOPERATIVE MANAGEMENT

As soon as the anastomosis is completed, intraoperative bronchoscopy is performed through an adaptor while ventilation is maintained. The anastomotic site is observed and blood clots or mucus are aspirated from the distal bronchus. Most patients are extubated within 4 to 5 hours after the operation. In my experience, almost all patients suffer from transient bronchorrhea, which is probably related to denervation, the interruption of lymphatics, and damage to the ciliary ep-

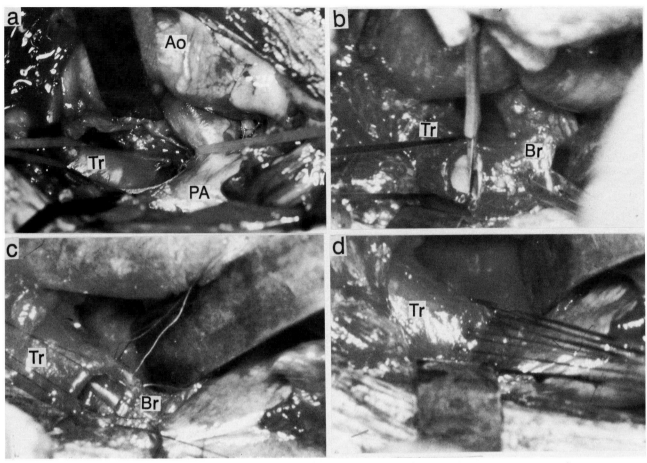

Fig. 35–5. Intraoperative view of left tracheal sleeve pneumonectomy through median stenotomy. Ao = aorta; PA = pulmonary artery. *a,* Exposure of trachea and bronchus via pericardium. *b,* Transection of distal trachea. *c,* Anastomotic procedure of cartilaginous part. *d,* Completion of anastomosis.

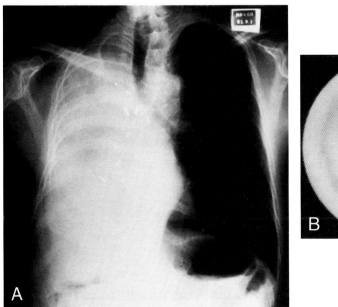

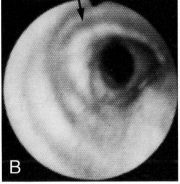

Fig. 35–6. *A,* Chest radiograph taken 19 months after right tracheal sleeve pneumonectomy in a 54-year-old male shows the normal caliber of the airway at the anastomotic site. *B,* Bronchoscopic view of the anastomotic site 2 years after left sleeve pneumonectomy in a 66-year-old male shows a clear anastomotic line (arrow).

Table 35–1. Results of Tracheal Sleeve Pneumonectomy

Authors	Number of Patients	Operative Mortality (%)	5-year Survival Rate (%)
Mathey et al. (1966)	2	0	—
Jensik et al. (1972)	17	12	—
Deslauriers et al. (1979)	16	31	—
Grillo (1982)	5	0	—
Jensik et al. (1982)	34	29	15
Deslaurier et al. (1985)	27	27	23
Fujimura et al. (1985)	7	0	—
Deslauriers et al. (1989)	38	29	13
Dartevelle et al. (1989)	55	11	23*
Watanabe et al. (1990)	12	17	—
Tsuchiya et al. (1990)	15	13	—
Muscolino et al. (1992)	7	0	—
Watanabe et al. (1992)	18	17	—

*Excluding six operative deaths.

ithelium. It is recommended that patients are placed in the lateral decubitus position — resected-side down — for postural drainage of bronchial secretions. Pernasal bronchoscopy is performed at the bedside on the first postoperative day to remove any secretions at the anastomosis and for infusion of antibiotics into the reconstructed lung. This procedure is repeated for several days, if necessary. Neck flexion is recommended for 7 days after the operation. During that time, oral intake is totally avoided and nutrition is maintained by intravenous hyperalimentation. Figure 35–6 shows a chest radiograph and bronchoscopic findings after tracheal sleeve pneumonectomy.

MORTALITY AND PROGNOSIS

The surgical outcomes after tracheal sleeve pneumonectomy is shown in Table 35–1. In 1982, Jensik and associates reported survival in 34 patients — 30 right and 4 stump recurrence after prior pneumonectomy — undergoing tracheal sleeve pneumonectomy. The perioperative mortality rate was 29% and the 5-year survival rate of the entire group was 15%. Dartevelle and colleagues (1988) reported 55 tracheal sleeve pneumonectomies — 53 right and 2 left. The overall operative death rate was 11% and actuarial 5-year survival rate — excluding 6 operative deaths — was 23%. Deslauriers and associates (1989) reported 38 patients undergoing tracheal sleeve pneumonectomy — 33 right, 3 left, and 2 stump recurrence. The operative mortality rate was 29% and the 5-year survival rate was 13%. Fujimura and co-workers (1985) reported 7 tracheal sleeve resections with no operative mortality. Two of the patients were still alive at 2 years, 9 months, and 4 months, respectively. Tsuchiya and colleagues (1990) reported 15 tracheal sleeve pneumonectomies with 2 operative deaths — 13%. Seven patients were alive with no evidence of disease after 1 to 30 months at the time of reporting. So far, our group has done 18 tracheal sleeve pneumonectomies with 3 operative deaths — 17%. To date, we have no 5-year survivors,

with 54 months being the longest survival from surgery. Muscolino and associates (1992) reported 7 right tracheal sleeve pneumonectomies without operative mortality. The median disease-free interval was 12 months, and 2 patients were alive with no evidence of disease at 46 and 47 months, respectively, after surgery.

It is true that only a few patients can survive for long among the group in which a curative operation is accomplished. In fact, some controversy exists as to whether or not tracheal sleeve pneumonectomy is an appropriate procedure for bronchial carcinoma, because the number of patients who die postoperatively is similar to the number of long-term survivors. Faber reported that they have not performed a tracheal sleeve pneumonectomy in the past 3 years, probably because they have undertaken a more aggressive preoperative treatment program consisting of combination chemotherapy and radiation. He confessed that the mortality and survival data have also tempered their earlier enthusiasm for this type of resection.

REFERENCES

Abbott OA, et al: Experiences with the surgical resection of the human carina, tracheal wall and contralateral bronchial wall in cases of the right total pneumonectomy. J Thorac Surg 19:906, 1950.

Chamberlain JM, et al: Bronchogenic carcinoma. An aggressive surgical attitude. J Thorac Cardiovasc Surg 38:727, 1959.

Dartevelle PG, et al: Tracheal sleeve pneumonectomy for bronchogenic carcinoma: Report of 55 cases. Ann Thorac Surg 46:68, 1989.

Deslauriers J, et al: Sleeve pneumonectomy for bronchogenic carcinoma. Ann Thorac Surg 28:465, 1979.

Deslauriers J: Involvement of the main carina. In Delarue NC, Eschapasse H (eds): International Trends in General Thoracic Surgery. Vol. 1. Philadelphia: WB Saunders, 1985, p. 136.

Deslauriers J, Beaulieu M, McClish A: Tracheal-sleeve pneumonectomy. In Shields TW (ed): General Thoracic Surgery. 3rd Ed. Philadelphia: Lea & Febiger, 1989, pp. 382.

El-Baz NM, et al: One-lung high frequency positive-pressure ventilation for sleeve pneumonectomy. An alternative technique. Anesth Analg 60:683, 1981.

Faber LP, et al: Results of surgical treatment of stage III lung carcinoma with carinal proximity. Surg Clin North Am 67:1001, 1987.

Frumin JM, Epstein RM, Cohen C: Apneic oxygenation in man. Anesthesiology *20*:789, 1959.

Fujimura S, et al: Prognostic evaluation of tracheobronchial reconstruction for bronchogenic carcinoma. J Thorac Cardiovasc Surg *90*:161, 1985.

Geffin B, et al: Anesthetic management of tracheal resection and reconstruction. Anesth Analg *48*:884, 1969.

Gibbon JH: In discussion to Chamberlain M, et al: Bronchogenic carcinoma. An aggressive surgical attitude. J Thorac Cardiovasc Surg *38*:727, 1959.

Gilbert A, et al: Tracheal sleeve pneumonectomy for carcinoma of the proximal left main bronchus. Can J Surg *27*:583, 1984.

Grillo HC: Carinal reconstruction. Ann Thorac Surg *34*:356, 1982.

Heller ML, Watson TR, Imredy DS: Apneic oxygenation in man. Polarographic arterial oxygen tension study. Anesthesiology *25*:25, 1964.

Jensik RJ, et al: Tracheal sleeve pneumonectomy for advanced carcinoma of the lung. Surg Gynecol Obstet *134*:231, 1972.

Jensik RJ, et al: Survival in patients undergoing tracheal sleeve pneumonectomy for bronchogenic carcinoma. J Thorac Cardiovasc Surg *84*:489, 1982.

Mathey J, et al: Tracheal and tracheobronchial resections. Technique and results in 20 cases. J Thorac Cardiovasc Surg *51*:1, 1966.

McClish A, et al: High-flow catheter ventilation during major tracheobronchial reconstruction. J Thorac Cardiovasc Surg *89*:508, 1985.

Muscolino G, et al: Anterior thoracotomy for right pneumonectomy and carinal reconstruction in lung cancer. Eur J Cardiothorac Surg *6*:11, 1992.

Pearson FG, Todd LC, Cooper JD: Experience with primary neoplasms of the trachea and carina. J Thorac Cardiovasc Surg *88*:511, 1984.

Perelman M, Koroleva N: Surgery of the trachea. World J Surg *4*:583, 1980.

Salzer GM, Muller LC, Kroesen G: Resection of the tracheal bifurcation through a left thoracotomy. Eur J Cardiothorac Surg *1*:125, 1987.

Thompson DT: Tracheal resection with left lung anastomosis following right pneumonectomy. Thorax *21*:560, 1966.

Tsuchiya R, et al: Resection of tracheal carina for lung cancer. J Thorac Cardiovasc Surg *99*:779, 1990.

Watanabe Y, et al: The clinical value of high-frequency jet ventilation in major airway reconstructive surgery. Scand J Thorac Cardiovasc Surg *22*:227, 1988.

Watanabe Y, et al: Results in 104 patients undergoing bronchoplastic procedures for bronchial lesions. Ann Thorac Surg *50*:607, 1990a.

Watanabe Y, et al: Reappraisal of bronchial arterial infusion therapy for advanced lung cancer. Jpn J Surg *20*:27, 1990b.

CHAPTER 36

MEDIAN STERNOTOMY AND PARASTERNAL APPROACHES TO THE LOWER TRACHEA AND MAIN STEM BRONCHI

Michail I. Perelman

The transmediastinal approach to the lower trachea and main stem bronchi is indicated chiefly for postpneumonectomy patients with bronchial fistulas. Other conditions for which this approach is indicated are rare and include selected cases of tracheal bifurcation tumors, a lung with multiple bronchial fistulas and empyema, and pulmonary hemorrhage in a severely ill patient who has previously undergone pulmonary surgery. In the latter condition, preliminary transmediastinal transection and occlusion of the pulmonary artery and bronchus may be the first stage of a two-stage pneumonectomy. In patients with empyema, the advantage of transmediastinal approach over the conventional transpleural route is that it affords aseptic access to the trachea and main bronchi through the mediastinal tissue and pericardium.

In 1960, Padhi and Lynn advocated the use of median sternotomy preceded by intrapericardial ligation of the pulmonary artery and superior pulmonary vein for operations to amputate a main bronchial stump that is closely adherent to pulmonary vessel stumps.

In 1963, Boguslavskaya and I reported the first two operations, performed in 1961, for fistulas of the right and left main bronchi, respectively, from a transsternal approach. On the right, a small incision of the pericardium was made over the right pulmonary artery stump, while on the left, the transpericardial route of approach was used with ligation and transection of the left pulmonary artery stump; we also presented results of topographic studies undertaken to validate the use of transsternal access to bronchial fistulas. Also in 1963, Abruzzini described a technique of operation on main bronchial stumps from a transsternal approach without opening the pericardium. He recommended, regardless of the side of intervention, gaining access to the stump through the space between the aorta and the superior vena cava. Bogush and associates (1972) examined in detail various transsternal approaches to main bronchial stumps and recommended the transpericardial approach in all instances; this approach is now used fairly often. These authors showed that the best spatial relations are created by approaching the right main bronchial stump through the aortocaval space and the left stump through the aortovenous space.

STERNOTOMY

I always performed a complete median sternotomy, as did other authors, until I found that dissection of the sternum longitudinally from the jugular notch to the level of the third intercostal space is sufficient in many patients with a long sternum. Dissecting the sternum transversely at this level and bringing the right and left halves of the dissected sternum apart with a single retractor provides an adequate operative field.

MEDIASTINAL APPROACH

Lower Trachea and Bronchi

The transitional pleural fold over the — usually — dilated left lung is dissected off to the left, and to the right of the ascending aorta, a tetragonal space is entered, the sides of which are the right margin of the ascending aorta and the initial portion of brachiocephalic trunk on the left, the superior vena cava on the right, the left brachiocephalic vein cranially, and the transitional pericardial fold — which corresponds to the margin of the right pulmonary artery — caudally. Once the superior vena cava and the ascending aorta with brachiocephalic trunk have been drawn apart, this tetragon is generally 5 to 7 cm in height and width.

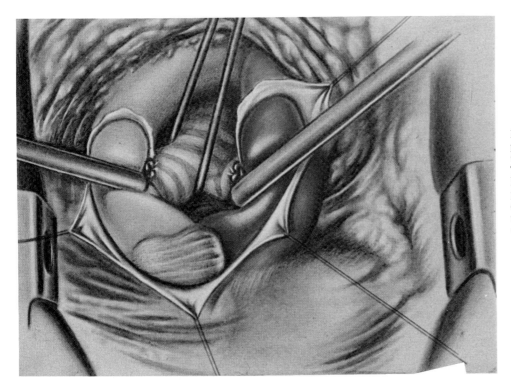

Fig. 36–1. Mediastinal-transpericardial approach to the lower trachea and right main bronchus. The aorta and superior vena cava have been drawn part. The dorsal pericardial wall has been dissected over the right pulmonary artery, which is held with a rubber catheter.

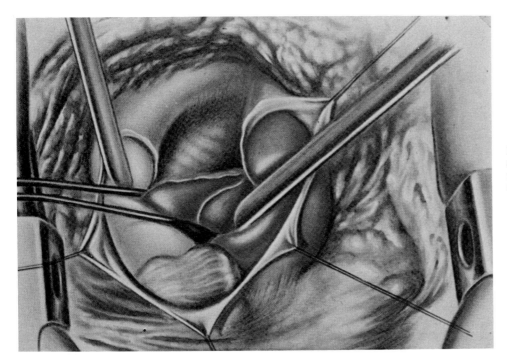

Fig. 36–2. The right pulmonary artery has been transected. The right main bronchus is held with a rubber catheter.

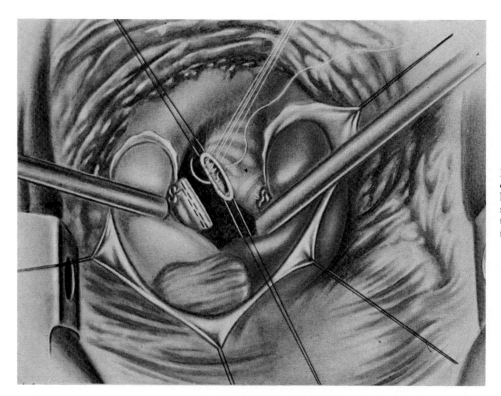

Fig. 36–3. The right main bronchial stump has been sutured with linear mechanical suture and dissected off from the trachea. The tracheal opening is closed with interrupted sutures.

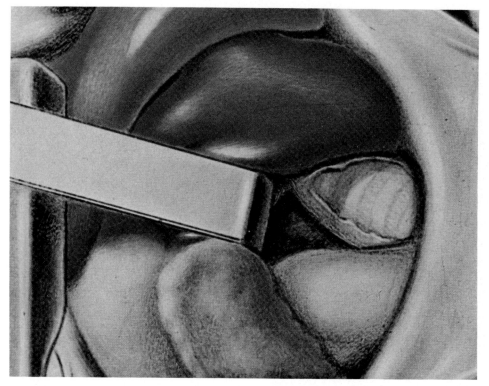

Fig. 36–4. Mediastinal-transpericardial approach to the left main bronchus. The pericardium has been opened and the dorsal pericardial wall dissected over the left main bronchus.

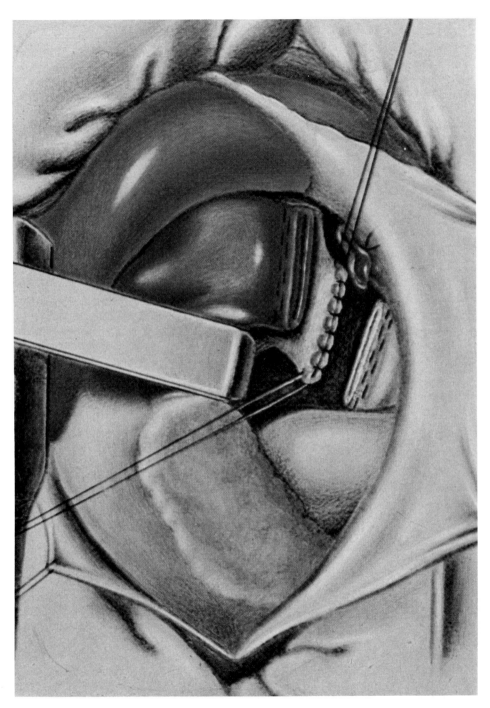

Fig. 36–5. The left pulmonary artery has been sutured with linear mechanical suture and transected, and a ligature has been applied to the distal end of the artery. The left main bronchial stump has been transected near the trachea. Interrupted sutures have been placed on the proximal end of the stump and a linear mechanical suture, on its distal end.

The trachea and its bifurcation are now palpable on the bottom of the space formed between the vessels and filled with fatty tissue and lymph nodes. The portion of the trachea above the bifurcation can be separated from the esophagus, after inserting a thick tube into the latter, and held on a rubber catheter or stay suture. The right main bronchus and the initial portion of the left main bronchus can also be mobilized.

Such a purely mediastinal access to the trachea and main bronchi has limited exposure. It is therefore advisable, as a rule, to open the pericardium after

sternotomy. The transpericardial approach affords a broader scope for surgical manipulations.

MEDIASTINAL-TRANSPERICARDIAL APPROACH

Trachea and Right Main Bronchial Stump

After the sternotomy and after the transitional pleural fold has been moved to the left, the pericardium is opened by a vertical incision slightly to the right of the

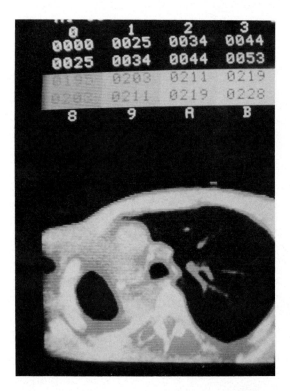

Fig. 36–6. CT scan after left pneumonectomy reveals the mediastinum is grossly displaced to the left.

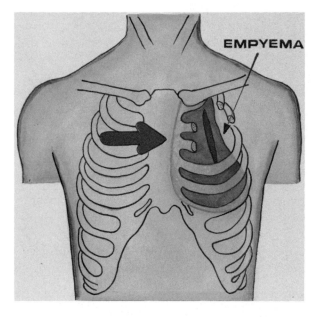

Fig. 36–7. Parasternal mediastinal-transpericardial approach to the left main bronchus after pneumonectomy, with resection of cartilages of the second and third ribs.

midline. The edges of the pericardium are sutured with stay sutures. The aorta and the superior vena cava are drawn apart. In right postpneumonectomy patients, the right pulmonary artery stump is ligated and transected for better operative exposure. The dorsal pericardial wall is dissected over the artery, which is then held in place with a rubber catheter (Fig. 36–1). The proximal end of the artery is sutured with a linear mechanical suture using a stapler with branches 30 mm long, and a ligature is applied to the distal end. Distal to the applied stapler, the artery is divided and an additional ligature is applied proximal to the staple line, bypassing the stapler. The opening in the dorsal pericardial wall is widened, thereby obtaining access to the lower trachea and the right main bronchus; only the proximal part of the left main bronchus is accessible (Figs. 36–2, 36–3).

If a bronchopleural fistula is present, it is best to reamputate and remove the bronchial stump, if it is feasible. A linear mechanical suture — UO or TA stapler — is applied to the lateral tracheal wall, or the tracheal opening is closed with interrupted Vicryl 3-0 or 4-0 sutures. A bronchial stump that has been separated from the trachea and sutured may be the source of longlasting mucous discharge into the residual pleural cavity or of a retention cyst. If removal of the stump is impractical or hazardous, it is advisable to destroy its mucosa chemically — with silver nitrate or trichloroacetic acid — or by electrocoagulation and then suturing it with interrupted absorbable — Vicryl or PDS — sutures.

Left Main Bronchial Stump

After sternotomy, the transitional pleural fold is moved to the right and the pericardium is opened by a vertical incision 10 to 11 cm long to the left of the midline, 2 to 3 cm anterior to the left phrenic nerve. The pericardial edges are brought apart by stay sutures. The operating table is then tilted sideways and to the right, the heart is moved somewhat to the right, and the dorsal pericardial wall is opened (Fig. 36–4). As far proximally as possible, the left pulmonary artery stump and, in some cases, the superior pulmonary vein stump are ligated and transected. Bogush and colleagues (1972) considered that ligation and division of only the superior pulmonary vein are often sufficient. Vessels are mobilized after dissection of the dorsal pericardial wall, and their proximal ends are sutured with a linear mechanical suture and ligated additionally; the distal ends are ligated after transection. The opening in the dorsal pericardial wall is widened, gaining access to the left main bronchial stump (Fig. 36–5). In operations for bronchial fistula, the same procedure is followed as on the right side.

PARASTERNAL MEDIASTINAL-TRANSPERICARDIAL APPROACH

Left Main Bronchial Stump

After a left pneumonectomy, the mediastinum usually shifts to the left; in many patients, it is grossly displaced

(Fig. 36–6). In such instances, I perform thoracotomy not transsternally but parasternally on the left, resecting cartilages of the second and third ribs (Fig. 36–7). Then, the — usually — thick and dense transitional pleural fold must be separated from the pericardium by sharp and blunt dissection and drawn to the left. This maneuver provides more convenient access to the pericardium anterior to the left phrenic nerve than does a transsternal incision. The pericardium is opened by a vertical incision and the operation continues exactly as it is when using the previously described mediastinal-transpericardial approach to the left main bronchial stump.

MORBIDITY AND MORTALITY

Hemorrhage at the time of operation may occur in a significant number of patients — 17% in the series of 39 operations I and my associates (1987) reported — but it was controlled in all. Recanalization of the bronchus when the excluded stump is not removed may occur. This complication is common if the bronchus is only occluded and not actually divided.

The mortality rate is high — 21% — with this approach, often because of the poor functional status of the patients. In our 1987 series, six patients died of cardiopulmonary insufficiency, two from thrombosis of the remaining sole pulmonary artery and one from recanalization of the bronchus.

PROGNOSIS

When the immediate operative procedure is successful, a 96% cure rate in the surviving patients can be expected. When postoperative deaths are included, however, only an overall 75% success rate is obtained.*

REFERENCES

Abruzzini P: Chirurgische Behandlung der Fisteln des Hauptbronchus. Thoraxchir Vask Chir 10:259, 1963.

Bogush LK, Travin AA, Semenenkov YL: Operatsii na glavnykh bronkhakh cherez polost' perikarda [Operations on the main bronchi via the pericardial cavity.] Moscow: Meditsina, 1972. (In Russian.)

Bruni F, et al: Traitement chirurgical des fistules après pneumonectomie: Intervention modifiée d'Abruzzini. Ann Chir 39:135, 1985.

Padhi R, Lynn R: The management of bronchopleural fistula. J Thorac Surg 39:385, 1960.

Perelman MI, Boguslavskaya TB: Operative approaches to tracheobronchial angles through the sternum and anterior mediastinum to close bronchial fistulas following pneumonectomy. *In* Aktual'nye voprosy tuberkulieza [*In* Current Problems of Tuberculosis.] No. 2. Moscow Central Institute for Advanced Medical Education Publication, 1963, p. 169. (In Russian.)

Perelman MJ, Rymko LP, Ambatiello GP: Bronchopleural fistula: Surgery after pneumonectomy. *In* Grillo HC, Eschapasse H (eds): International Trends in General Thoracic Surgery. Vol. 2. Philadelphia: WB Saunders, 1987, p. 407.

READING REFERENCES

Bogush LK, Trawin AA, Semenenkov YL: Transperikardiale Operationen an den Hauptbronchien und Lungengefässen. Stuttgart: Hippokrates, 1971.

Perelman MI: Transsternal technique for bronchopleural fistula. *In* Grillo HC, et al (eds): Current Therapy in Cardiovascular Surgery. Toronto: BC Decker, 1989, p. 105–106.

Perelman MJ, Ambatiello GP: Transsternaler und kontralateraler Zugang bei Operationen wegen Bronchialfistel nach Pneumonektomie. Thoraxchir Vask Chir 18:45, 1970.

Perelman MJ, Klimansky VA: Operations on the Lungs. *In* Atlas of Thoracic Surgery. Vol. 1. St. Louis: CV Mosby, 1979, pp. 99–225.

Petrowskij BV, Perelman MI: Wiederherstellende und rekonstruktive Operationen am thorakalen Abschnitt von Trached und Bronchien. Langenbecks Arch Klin Chir 332:859, 1968.

---

*Editor's footnote: One should be highly selective in using this procedure. It is perhaps best reserved for right-sided postpneumonectomy bronchial fistulas and is less often indicated for the management of left-sided bronchial fistulas. The author concurs with this statement.

CHAPTER 37

VIDEO-ASSISTED THORACIC SURGERY FOR PULMONARY AND PLEURAL DISEASES

Rodney J. Landreneau, Stephen R. Hazelrigg, Michael J. Mack, Robert J. Keenan, and Peter F. Ferson

Advances in videoscopic instrumentation and endoscopic surgical tools have allowed the rapid expansion in "minimal access," video-assisted operative approaches in nearly every surgical discipline. Thoracic surgery is no exception. Video-assisted thoracic surgery — VATS — has pervaded the practice of general thoracic surgery just as laparoscopic approaches now dominate many aspects of general surgery today.

Video–assisted thoracic surgery has emerged from the well-established pleural diagnostic procedure, "thoracoscopy." It is cogent to provide a brief review of the background of thoracoscopic intervention to place the present use of VATS in proper context. According to Brandt and associates (1985), the first thoracoscopic procedure was performed in 1910 by the Swedish physician, Hans Christian Jacobeus. Braimbridge (1993) noted that Jacobeus used a primitive cystoscope of that day to explore the pleural space and mechanically lyse pleural adhesions to facilitate the "collapse therapy" for pulmonary tuberculosis. Jacobeus presented his expanded series with this technique at the Society of Radiotherapy and Electrocauterization in 1921. Jacobeus used a "two stick" approach to examine the pleural cavity directly and to accomplish electrocoagulative ligation of the offending pleural adhesions that were preventing collapse of the lung. Jacobeus (1922, 1925) subsequently reported his experiences in two articles describing his experiences and those of other investigators with this pleuroscopic technique.

Thoracoscopy was a popular intervention in the management of pulmonary tuberculosis, particularly in Europe, over the next 30 years. Much clinical experience was summarized in many European medical publications of that period, such as those of Fourestier and Duret (1943) and Coulaud and Des Champs (1947), which detailed the technique and results of thoracoscopic intervention. During this same period of enthusiasm with the thoracoscopic approach in Europe,

some vocal and influential thoracic surgeons in the United States did much to forestall the expansion of thoracoscopic intervention in North America. This criticism was led by John Alexander (1937), the first Chief of Thoracic Surgery at the University of Michigan. He was seriously concerned about accounts of several thoracoscopic disasters occurring in the tuberculosis sanitoriums of that day. These institutions were staffed primarily by nonsurgeon physicians who did not have the clinical training, background, or technical support to handle the potentially life-threatening complications that could occur from these "minimally invasive" interventions. He strongly stated his belief that it was wrong to submit the defenseless patient to these procedures, which were being performed by physicians unable to immediately address the life-threatening complications that could rapidly occur.

The development of effective antibiotic therapy for the tubercle bacillus further reduced the use for thoracoscopy by chest physicians and surgeons both in America and in Europe. Thoracoscopic intervention, however, continued to be used in Europe by some pulmonary specialists, including Brandt (1978), Bergquist and Nordenstam (1966), and Swierengor and associates (1974), as a means of diagnosing and managing some pleural and pulmonary parenchymal pathologic conditions.

After a period of near abandonment of this approach over the ensuing 25 years, many thoracic surgeons are re-exploring thoracoscopy, or VATS, as a means of accomplishing many intrathoracic procedures previously done through open thoracotomy. The main goal of these VATS approaches, as postulated by the authors (RJL, 1992a), is to reduce the pain and other post-thoracotomy-related morbidity after thoracic surgical procedures without sacrifice of the therapeutic principles of "open" thoracic surgery. Several diagnostic and therapeutic thoracoscopic applications are being touted as the preferred approach to specific intrathoracic disease processes. Furthermore, several other VATS techniques are being investigated as potential alternatives to traditional open thoracotomy or sternotomy for the management of cardiothoracic pathologic states. The procedures outlined in Table 37–1 summarize the areas of thoracoscopic practice and investigation underway.

Despite this recent enthusiasm with VATS, the authors (RJL, 1993, 1994) question the primary assumption that VATS offers a less morbid means of accomplishing our thoracic surgical diagnostic and therapeutic goals. The equally important issues of VATS — efficacy, cost, and safety — must also be examined closely. Finally, it must be ensured that clinicians are not promoting unnecessary surgery under the auspices that the procedure can be done with little morbidity to patients.

Many articles that attest to the reduced morbidity of VATS are little more than extended case reports providing poorly substantiated subjective commentary of reduced disability following this type of operation. It is now known that many thoracic surgical procedures can be done under video assistance rather than open thoracotomy, but are they truly worthwhile? In general, our strong bias is that the VATS approach is a

benefit for patients when it is used in the proper clinical setting and when it is performed by properly trained surgeons. It is best to approach these VATS applications in the operating room where conversion to open thoracotomy is immediately available if necessary (Table 37–2).

The surgical team preparing to perform VATS interventions must be well trained in the performance of the standard thoracic surgical procedures. Along these lines, we strongly believe that thoracic surgical "standby" help is inappropriate for nonsurgeon physicians. The individuals trained to perform diagnostic and therapeutic transpleural interventions in the Americas and in Europe are, in most circumstances, surgeons skilled in general thoracic surgery. At this time, there is no training precedent or general experience in North America among nonsurgical physicians to perform these intrapleural invasive procedures. It is not ethical, or reasonable, to transfer management of pleural problems to the least technically experienced individuals involved with the care of thoracic surgical patients. It is wise to guard against the potential development of such unwarranted clinical trends, even if the result is a difficult "political" situation. It must be the charge of thoracic surgical educators to instruct future surgeons in the proper use and conduct of these minimally invasive thoracic surgical procedures. Ultimately, hospital administrators and malpractice insurance companies must be made aware of the nature of these VATS interventions so that proper risk management is achieved and patients are protected from unnecessary harm.

Fortunately, objective data regarding the general utility and relative costs — in dollars and in pain — of the VATS approach compared to open thoracotomy are emerging from the studies of the authors and their colleagues (RJL, 1993, 1994; SRH, 1993a, b; and PFF, 1993). Much of this information has been obtained through the efforts of the Video-Assisted Thoracic Study Group and published by one of us (SRH) and colleagues (1993c). This group, working in conjunction with the

Table 37–1. Potential Indications for VATS

Diagnostic
Indeterminate pleural effusion (benign vs. malignant)
Tissue diagnosis
Pleural based masses (metastatic adenocarcinoma versus mesothelioma)
"Closed" wedge resection lung biopsy
Mediastinal lymph node sampling
Biopsy of mediastinal masses
Therapeutic
Pleuropulmonary
Control pleural effusion/empyema
Facilitate pleurodesis (thermal/mechanical/chemical)
Ablate bullous disease
Resect "early stage" lung cancer
Esophageal
Esophagomyotomy
Management of enteric cysts
Resection of esophageal leiomyomata
Antireflux surgery
Video-assisted esophagectomy
Mediastinal
"Limited stage" thymoma resection
Thymectomy for myasthenia gravis
Resect posterior mediastinal masses
Excise bronchogenic/enteric cysts
Pericardiectomy
General/Miscellaneous
Dorsal sympathectomy/splanchnicectomy
Drainage of paravertebral abscess
Orthopedic discectomy
Cardiac
? Mitral valve repair (commissurotomy)
? Video-assisted internal mammary coronary bypass

Table 37–2. Basic Operative Set-up for VATS

General anesthesia
Double-lumen endotracheal tube (or bronchus blocker)
"Open" thoracotomy instrument tray available (open on back table?)
Thoracoscope (10-mm operative scope preferred with a 5-mm operative channel)
High resolution video monitor (× 2; preferably positioned on opposite side of operating table for surgeon and assisting team)
2 to 5 ports of intercostal operative access
Videoscopic instruments (and selected standard surgical instruments)
Endoscopic stapling and clip appliers (*Nd:Yag laser* also useful adjunctive resective tool)
Adequate suction and smoke evacuation system

From Landreneau RJ, et al: Video-assisted thoracic surgery. Basic concepts and intercostal approach strategies. Ann Thorac Surg *102*:800, 1992.

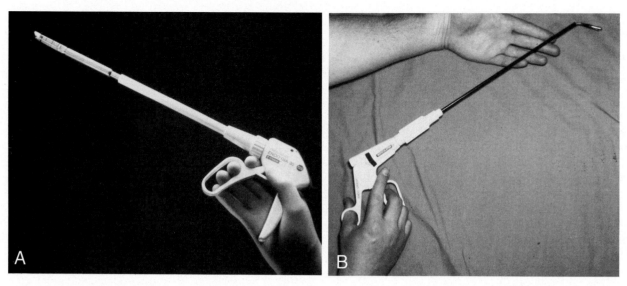

Fig. 37–1. *A*, Endoscopic stapling device (Endo-GIA). *B*, Reticulating hand instrument (United States Surgical Corporation, Norwalk, CT).

Society of Thoracic Surgery and the American Association of Thoracic Surgery, obtained the clinical records of over 1500 patients who underwent VATS over 2 years. Additionally, the aforementioned reports by the authors and their associates objectively compare the perioperative pain differences seen among thoracic surgical patients managed by either VATS or open thoracotomy approaches.

The focus of this chapter is the potential role of VATS in general thoracic surgical practice today, the general operative setup required, and the basic approach strategies important in accomplishing safe and efficacious VATS interventions.

INSTRUMENTATION

The explosion in endoscopic surgical intervention in North America and Europe has fueled industry to invest in both disposable and re-usable hand tools and "accessory" operative instrumentation. Although a vast array of disposable instruments and trocars are available, our strong preference is toward re-usable endoscopic surgical instrumentation. Some disposable endoscopic instruments, such as the endoscopic stapling devices and the multiload endoscopic clip appliers, provide a uniquely important role for many thoracoscopic VATS procedures (Fig. 37–1). The disposable endoscopic scissors are also preferable because of rapid dulling of presently available reusable endoscopic scissors. Certainly, the present medical economic environment dictates judicious use of disposable endoscopic surgical instrumentation by active VATS programs.

An additional problem facing the surgeon attempting VATS intervention relates to the inadequate instrument design of most "pistol grip" endosurgical tools. Although the surgeon can become familiar with these tools, they are awkward to manipulate when detailed dissection is required (Fig. 37–2). Several companies are designing

"coaxial" endosurgical tools that allow for unimpeded access through the intercostal space and also retain the feel of "standard" open surgical tools (Fig. 37–3). As the "user friendliness" of this instrumentation matures, we foresee an even greater use of VATS for more complex thoracic surgical procedures.

We prefer a 10-mm rigid "operating" thoracoscope with a 5-mm biopsy channel, when available (Karl Storz Inc., Olympus Corp., or Wolfe Endoscopic Inc.), to "view only" thoracoscopes/laparoscopes for most VATS procedures (Fig. 37–4). These instruments provide the opportunity for "single stick" diagnostic thoracoscopy and also potentially allow for more complex VATS interventions with one less intercostal access site as noted by us (RJL, 1992, 1993b). When use of the Nd:YAG laser is considered in the VATS procedure, the biopsy channel of the operating thoracoscope allows for

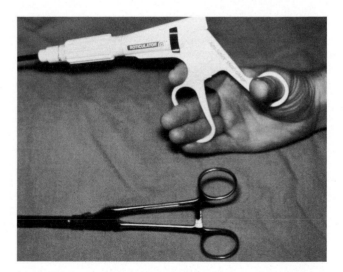

Fig. 37–2. "Pistol grip" handle design used for most manufactured endosurgical instrumentation.

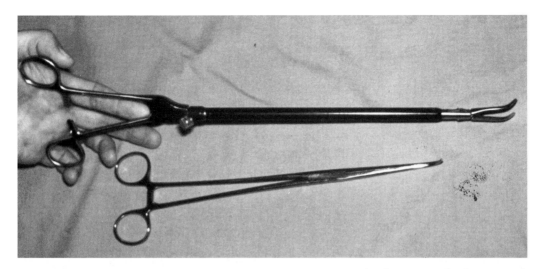

Fig. 37–3. "Coaxial" handle design being developed is tailored to that of standard surgical hand instruments familiar to most thoracic surgeons.

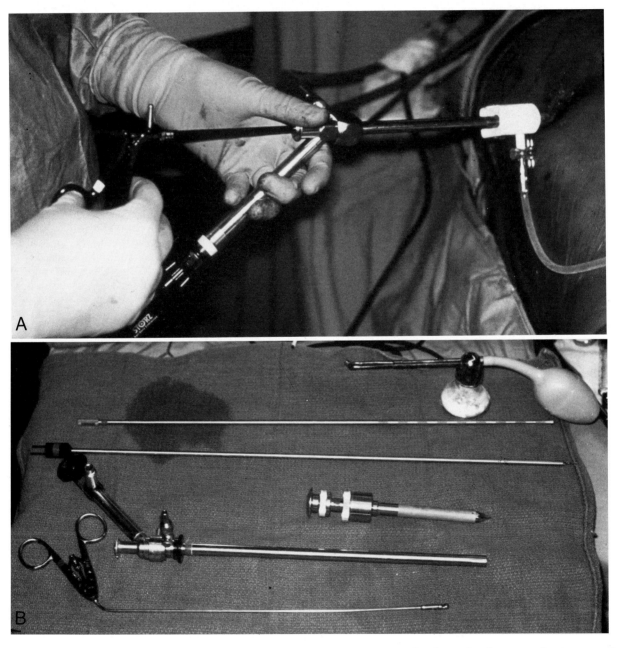

Fig. 37–4. *A*, Ten-millimeter diameter "operating" thoracoscope with biopsy forcep is introduced into the chest cavity for tissue sampling through the 5-mm operative channel. *B*, Operative thoracoscope and basic instrumentation for diagnostic VATS and talc pleurodesis.

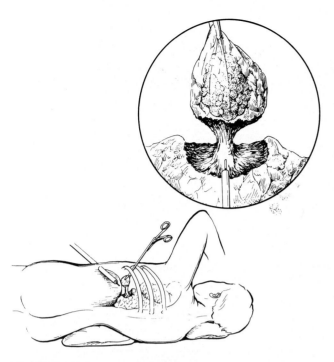

Fig. 37–5. VATS approach for Nd:YAG laser resection of a peripheral lung nodule. *From* Landreneau RJ, et al: Thoracoscopic Nd:YAG laser-assisted pulmonary resection. Ann Thorac Surg 52:1176, 1991.

direct end-on viewing to the laser fiber as the laser beam is applied to the thoracic tissues. Accurate beam application can be a problem when the fiber is introduced through a lateral intercostal access because of the two–dimensional limitations of television.

A brief statement regarding the use of surgical lasers in VATS is justified. Although several laser wavelengths have been applied in general thoracic surgery, the neodymium yttrium aluminum garnet — Nd:YAG — laser wavelength is the most versatile, as reported by LoCicero (1985, 1989) and one of us (RJL, 1991a, b, 1992b) and associates. The Nd:YAG laser can function as a primary — or adjunctive — resective and coag-

ulative tool for many thoracoscopic — VATS — procedures (Fig. 37–5). The aforementioned reports have described the utility of this laser's wavelength in thoracic surgery. We emphasize the importance of developing an appreciation for the Nd:YAG laser wavelength interactions with pulmonary tissues before applying these laser tools clinically. Certainly, the thoracic surgeon should acquire experience with this laser technology in the open thoracotomy setting before applying it to VATS, as pointed out by us (RJL, 1992a). An understanding of basic laser safety practices is also important before using lasers in VATS.

Removal of pathologic tissues from the thoracic cavity can also be a problem encountered with VATS procedures. We usually extract the specimen by placing it into a sterile glove or commercially available plastic sleeved devices that can be introduced into the thoracic cavity through one of the intercostal access sites. Lengthening one of the intercostal access incisions to 3 to 4 cm — without spreading the ribs — can be used to extract larger specimens.

The specific instrumentation used in VATS is characterized in many reports, such as those of Allen (1993) and of Worsey and one of us (RJL) (1993). The thoracic surgeon should review these and similar publications to obtain a basic understanding of the available instrumentation and the specific nuances and limitations regarding their use.

BASIC OPERATIVE STRATEGIES

The availability of this potentially less morbid approach has brought many patients for surgical consultation who would otherwise not be considered operative candidates for "standard" open surgical approaches. Despite the potential advantages of less operative trauma, operative planning for VATS interventions, as with any operative procedure, requires a careful assessment of the patient's physiologic reserve, as stressed by Wernly and DeMeester (1989) and Shields (1993).

Video-assisted thoracic surgery must be respected as a "real" surgical intervention, in which general anes-

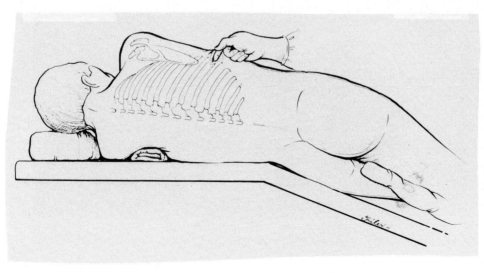

Fig. 37–6. Standard patient positioning for VATS intervention. The patient is severely flexed at the hip to open the width of the intercostal spaces. The index finger is then introduced to ensure that pleural symphysis is not present at the site of introduction of the thoracoscope. *From* Landreneau RJ, et al: Video assisted thoracic surgery: Basic technical concepts and intercostal approach strategies. Ann Thorac Surg *54*:800, 1992.

thesia is usually required, despite the observed potential to reduce incisional trauma for the thoracic surgical patient. Along these lines, a major preoperative concern facing the thoracic surgeon beginning VATS is determining the adequacy of anesthesia team support available. It is imperative that anesthesia personnel be experienced in open thoracic procedures and additionally well versed with the principles of selective one-lung ventilation, as described by Benumof (1983) and in Chapter 21 of this text, during the operative intervention.

A careful preoperative review of the chest radiographs and the computed tomographic scans is vital to formulate the plan for the initial and subsequent intercostal access for the thoracoscopic and surgical instruments, as noted previously by us (RJL, 1993b). The patient is positioned in a full lateral position with the thorax surgically prepared for open thoracotomy should this necessity arise (Fig. 37–6).

We (RJL, 1992a) begin the VATS procedure by choosing an appropriate intercostal site of access for exploratory thoracoscopy. Direct digital exploration of the intercostal access site, rather than blind trocar placement into the chest, is used to identify the presence of local pleural adhesions that can impede the introduction of instruments and potentially result in pulmonary parenchymal injury. Flimsy local adhesions can be separated digitally. More extensive pleural symphysis in the location of the proposed initial access site may require alternative intercostal access. All things being equal, we rely on the sixth or seventh intercostal space in the midaxillary line for "trocar-protected" thoracoscope access to the pleural cavity. Exploratory thoracoscopy is then performed. This initial thoracoscope location usually provides a clear view of the mediastinum, all pleural surfaces, and of the lung. The thoracic surgeon must be prepared to convert to an open thoracotomy if extensive pleural fusion is found.

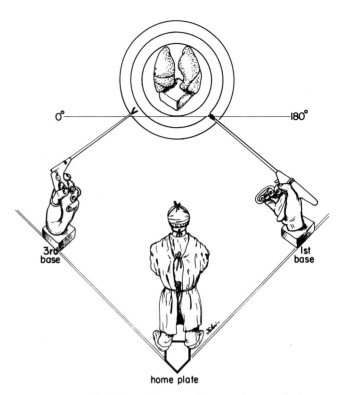

Fig. 37–8. Baseball diamond cartoon depicting the mental schema used to accomplish triangulation of the instruments and thoracoscope for strategic visibility and manipulation of the target pathology. *From* Landreneau RJ, et al: Thoracoscopic resection of 85 pulmonary lesions. Ann Thorac Surg 54:415, 1992.

As we have noted (RJL, 1992a, 1993b), the visibility of the entire thoracic cavity obtained through the VATS approach contrasts favorably with the direct view obtained through a limited axillary, inframammary, or lateral thoracotomy. After the initial thoracoscopic exploration of the pleural cavity is concluded, further intercostal access for VATS instrumentation is achieved under direct thoracoscopic vision (Fig. 37–7).

Carbon dioxide insufflation is rarely needed to conduct VATS. Occasionally, it is used at the beginning of the procedure to facilitate a more complete and expeditious collapse of the lung. If carbon dioxide insufflation is used, the intrapleural pressure is kept below 10 mm Hg to avoid mediastinal tension and hemodynamic compromise.

The primary maneuvers used to accomplish VATS have been described in an earlier review of VATS strategies by our group (RJL, 1992a) (Fig. 37–8). Several basic principles should be applied (Table 37–3). The endoscopic instrumentation and the thoracoscopic camera must be oriented so that they all are being used to face the target pathology from the same direction (Fig. 37–9). Otherwise, difficulties in instrument manipulation occur because of mirror imaging when the instrumentation is directed toward the thoracoscopic camera. Strategic positioning of the thoracoscopic camera and the endoscopic instruments are also vital to the success and efficiency of the procedure.

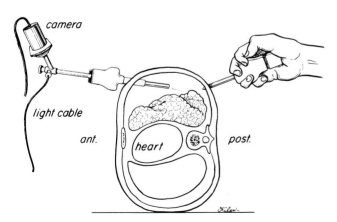

Fig. 37–7. All subsequent instruments/trocars are introduced under direct endoscopic visibility and direction to ensure proper location and to avoid intercostal neurovascular bundle trauma. *From* Landreneau RJ, et al: Video assisted thoracic surgery: Basic technical concepts and intercostal approach strategies. Ann Thorac Surg 54:800, 1992.

Table 37–3. Basic VATS Operative Concepts

Trocar sites and thoracoscope are placed at a distance from lesion to achieve "panoramic" view and room to manipulate the tissue.

Avoid instrument crowding, which may otherwise result in "fencing" during the instrument manipulation.

Avoid *"mirror imaging"* by positioning instruments and thoracoscope within the same 180° arc (approach the lesion in the same general direction with instruments and camera).

Movement/manipulation of instruments (or the camera) should be done serially, rather than randomly or synchronously, to avoid operative chaos. Instruments should only be manipulated when seen directly through the thoracoscope.

From Landreneau RJ, et al: Video-assisted thoracic surgery. Basic concepts and intercostal approach strategies. Ann Thorac Surg 102:800, 1992.

SPECIFIC VATS APPLICATIONS FOR THORACIC SURGICAL PROBLEMS

Management of Pleural Disease

As stated, pleural disease processes were the first to be managed with these minimally invasive surgical approaches. Indeed, diagnostic and therapeutic pleural applications continue to be the most universally accepted use of VATS techniques by us (RJL, 1992a) and others (see Reading References). Truly "video-assisted" techniques are preferable for most VATS procedures.

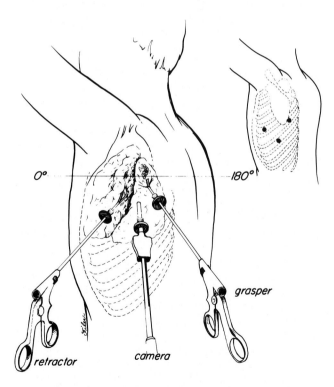

Fig. 37–9. Typical positioning of VATS instruments and the thoracoscopic camera to approach pulmonary parenchymal pathology. Note the triangulation concept in use as a lesion in the superior segment of the lower lobe of the lung is approached. *From* Landreneau RJ, et al: Thoracoscopic resection of 85 pulmonary lesions. Ann Thorac Surg 54:415, 1992.

Television monitors are used to provide an electronically transmitted indirect view of the pleural cavity through an endoscopic camera attached to the eyepiece of the thoracoscope. Such video assistance is not an absolute necessity for some thoracoscopic pleural interventions, as reported by Miller and Hatcher (1978) and Kaiser (1987), as well as Deslauriers (1976) and Lewis (1976) and their associates. The thoracoscope or a standard cervical mediastinoscope can be introduced through a strategically positioned intercostal access site for simple pleural examination and biopsy. The primary drawback of this direct viewing approach is that the procedure is really a one-person manipulation. Others engaged in the procedure are unable to visualize the thoracic pathology and assist directly in the surgical manipulation. In contrast, VATS provides for direct interaction between assistants and surgeon, which allows for the performance of more complex surgical procedures.

Pleural effusive processes often elude diagnosis despite efforts at thoracentesis and closed pleural biopsy techniques. The etiology of fully 40% of pleural effusions remains unidentified despite the use of thoracentesis and closed pleural biopsies. Video–assisted thoracoscopic surgery is a useful means of obtaining a diagnosis in 85 to 90% of persons with these difficult lesions, as reported by us (RJL, 1992a), Kaiser (1987) and Menzies and Charbonneau (1991). This diagnostic utility relates to the superior ability to examine and to perform a biopsy of the pleura nearly throughout its entire area. Treatment of the pleural effusive process can also be done successfully by chemical or mechanical pleurodesis using the VATS approach, as reported by Webb (1992), Boniface (1989), and their colleagues, as well as other investigators (see Reading References).

It is important to comment on the importance of performing a careful bronchoscopic examination during the course of the VATS intervention. An endobronchial lesion may need to be managed independently with laser ablation, radiation therapy, or endobronchial stent to permit expansion of the lung and to facilitate visceral and parietal pleural symphysis. The VATS approach is also useful in managing a number of other pleural processes (Table 37–4). Loculated pleural effusions, early empyemata, pleural based masses, and post-traumatic hemothoraces have all been managed by us (RJK, 1993) with VATS (Fig. 37–10). We must remember that open thoracotomy and decortication of the lung or pleurectomy may be required in some patients. The thoracic surgeon should be prepared for this

Table 37–4. VATS Management of Pleural Disease in 199 Patients

	Benign	Malignant
Effusion	51	72
Empyema	31	—
Biopsy of pleural tumor	—	38
Clotted hemothorax	7	—
Total	89(44.7%)	110(55.2%)

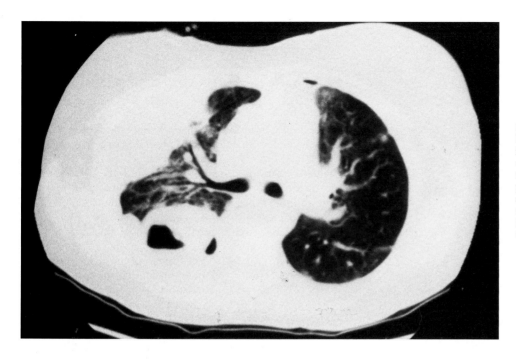

Fig. 37–10. Complex multiloculated pleural effusion well suited for VATS intervention. Multiloculated components are converted to a unilocular process in which pleural symphysis is more readily accomplished. Concomitant pleural biopsies are taken (if needed) to identify the underlying etiology of the effusive process.

possibility when approaching patients with complicated pleural processes, as we (RJK, 1993), as well as Martini (1975), Todd (1980), and their associates have noted.

Spontaneous Pneumothorax and Bullous Emphysema

Although the management of pleural disease processes is the most accepted application for thoracoscopic — or VATS — intervention, the development of minimally invasive approaches to other thoracic surgical problems has been primarily responsible for the recent rush of enthusiasm with VATS techniques by us (RJL, 1992b; MJM, 1992b) and Rogers (1993), Miller (1992), and Lewis (1992) and their colleagues. One of the first thoracic disease processes applicable to VATS intervention to attract the attention of the thoracic surgeon was "primary spontaneous pneumothorax." Earlier reports by Swierenga and co-workers (1974), Steel (1947), and Vanderschueren (1981) described the use of thoracoscopy as a useful approach to accomplish mechanical and chemical pleurodesis for this condition. Many of these reports detail the use of sterile talc as the primary sclerosing agent. Ongoing experience and clinical success with these methods continue to be described by Boutin (1993), Daniel (1990), Viskum (1989), van de Brekel (1993) and their associates. Our primary concern is that inappropriate use of talc sclerosis will be applied for this condition. We are insecure with the idea of attempting management of active bronchopleural fistulae or pneumothoraces associated with "trapped lung" with talc poudrage. Loculated empyemata with persistent bronchopleural fistula are common untoward sequelae with this clinical scenario that often require extensive remedial surgical interventions — decortication — for definitive management.

Torre and Belloni (1989) and Wakabayashi (1993) described the use of the Nd:YAG and carbon diox-

ide — CO_2 — laser to ablate the apical bullae and to thermally effect a mechanical pleurodesis. Nathanson and co-workers (1991) advocated using performed catgut endoscopic ligatures that are thoracoscopically introduced to "loop" beneath the bullae and ligate it at the base of the more normal lung parenchyma. Both the laser and "endoloop" approaches have received mixed reviews by us (RJL, 1992a) given the clinical failures with these techniques. Additionally, these approaches have not been readily translated into the practice of most thoracic surgeons. The endoloop approach has been complicated by loop slippage at the time of expansion of the atelectatic lung at the completion of the procedure, and the laser ablation approach as suggested by Wakabayashi (1994) to apical bullae is not reliably pneumostatic, as one of us (SRH, 1994) has noted.

These reports of laser and "endoloop" management of bullous disease did, however, peak the interest of thoracic surgeons with these VATS approaches to spontaneous pneumothorax. Technologic improvements finally emerged that allowed the surgeon to perform basically the same intervention thoracoscopically as had been accomplished previously through open thoracotomy. Obviously, the primary technologic development allowing for an equivalent VATS management of this condition was the development of an effective endostapling device (Fig. 37–11).

In general, the VATS management of spontaneous pneumothorax we prescribe entails identification of all bullous lesions and performance of a limited stapled wedge resection incorporating a small rim of normal lung tissue beneath the base of the bullae. This procedure is technically identical to that achieved through an open thoracotomy, although instrument use is through small intercostal access sites rather than an open thoracotomy wound, as noted previously (RJL, 1992a; SRH, 1993a).

approaching apical bullae

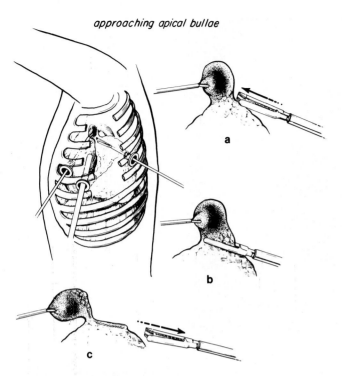

Fig. 37–11. Endostapler application to accomplish VATS resection of discrete apical bullous disease. *From* Hazelrigg SR, et al: Thoracoscopic management of spontaneous pneumothorax. J Thorac Cardiovasc Surg 105:389, 1993.

The basic difference is that our vision during the procedure is "video-optical" rather than direct visualization of the pathologic change.

A report by us (SRH, 1933a) concerned the relative effectiveness and differential morbidity of open thoracic and VATS management of spontaneous pneumothorax. We compared the length of hospital stay, pneumothorax recurrence, narcotic requirements needed to control postoperative pain, and the postoperative morbidity of recent historical control patients managed using limited axillary thoracotomy and a prospective group of patients who underwent VATS management of the spontaneous pneumothorax. All patients in both groups were treated with stapled resection of apical bullous disease and mechanical pleurodesis. Although this study suffers from the usual limitations of retrospective analysis, we found that the patients approached with VATS appeared to have a more favorable outcome with respect to less postoperative narcotic requirement and also had a shorter postoperative hospital stay compared to the historical controls. We also commented on the superior examination of the lung surface that can be achieved with the VATS approach relative to that visible through a limited axillary thoracotomy. In fact, a greater number of bullae were identified in the patients managed with VATS. Conceivably, some bullae may be unnoticed when limited thoracotomy approaches are used. Such unrecognized bullae may have been the source of recurrence among some patients undergoing surgical bullectomy in the past.

Whereas the technical feasibility of the thoracoscopic approach is now without question, we must avoid the urge to recommend surgery for the patient presenting with a first time "primary spontaneous pneumothorax." It is well established, as attested to by the reports of Klassen (1962) and Hagen (1987) and their associates, that the majority of such occurrences can be managed successfully without surgery. Tube thoracostomy evacuation and drainage of the pleural space is successful in 50 to 80% of primary spontaneous pneumothorax patients. Frequently, patients with small — less than 1 inch of pneumothorax — do well without any intervention, other than close observation and followup chest radiographs to document re-expansion of the lung. We continue to follow these clinical decision-making parameters when we are consulted in the care of patients with "primary spontaneous pneumothorax." At present, we limit our thoracoscopic intervention to those patients with recurrent — second episode — pneumothoraces or similar patients with bronchopleural fistulae with or without residual pleural space problems at their first episode of pneumothorax — persistent pneumothorax, air leak, or hemothorax despite proper tube thoracostomy management (Table 37–5).

Nonetheless, our threshold to suggest surgical treatment has changed. Presently, we are inclined to offer surgical intervention earlier in the management of persistent air leaks during the first episode of pneumothorax. We now suggest thoracoscopic management for patients with active air leaks beyond 48 to 72 hours of tube thoracostomy drainage, in contrast to our "historical" management approach of waiting for up to 7 days of chest tube drainage before considering thoracotomy. Mature clinical judgment is necessary in deciding which patients are best suited for this early VATS approach. Although we risk the possibility of doing unnecessary surgery in a few patients who would have ultimately sealed their leak in a day or two, we believe this approach is justified in these select instances because we routinely can have the patient ready for discharge 2 to 3 days after the VATS procedure.

An uncommon but nonetheless important manifestation of primary spontaneous pneumothorax is the development of a second contralateral episode of pneumothorax. In the past, we recommended staged bilateral procedures in this scenario. The thoracic surgical group

Table 37–5. Video-Assisted Thoracic Surgery for Pulmonary Disease in 488 Patients

	Benign	Malignant
Pulmonary nodule	138	227
Metastatic cancer	—	(96)
Wedge resection primary cancer	—	(84)
Wedge resection and open lobectomy	—	(16)
VATS lobectomy	—	(31)
Biopsy diffuse lung disease	61	
Blebs/bullae resection	62	
Total	261 (53%)	227 (47%)

at Stanford University (JBD Mark and W Cannon, personal communication, 1993) described their limited experience with simultaneous bilateral VATS management of such pneumothorax. All of these patients were young college students who recovered remarkably well after this intervention. Although we do not have any experience with this simultaneous VATS treatment approach, we remain intrigued with its potential utility in such selected instances.

It is important to note that "secondary spontaneous pneumothorax" can also be managed with thoracoscopic bullectomy, although the results of VATS intervention in this emphysema population are less satisfactory than that achieved in primary *idiopathic* spontaneous pneumothorax patients. Because these are difficult patients in whom surgical results are poorer — by whatever operative means, we tend to rely on tube thoracostomy management for a longer period before approaching them with either open surgical procedures or VATS. In the patients with secondary pneumothoraces on whom we ultimately choose surgical management, we have achieved success by combining the use of Nd:YAG laser ablation techniques and strategic VATS stapled resection of the offending ruptured bullae to control the pneumothorax.

We have limited experience — 6 patients — with the VATS approach to "giant bullae" of the lung. All of the patients we have approached primarily have all had evidence of dominant bullae crowding and compressing relatively normal parenchyma. A few patients with diffuse emphysema and dominant "giant" bullae have also undergone surgery using the VATS approach in an effort to improve function while they wait for pulmonary transplantation.

The technical aspects of these cases involve initial VATS Nd:YAG laser ablation and shrinkage of the bullae by applying the laser energy in a diffuse non-contact mode — 20 to 30 watts of continuous laser energy — with the laser fiber at a 1- to 2-cm distance from the surface of the bullae. We prefer to introduce the laser fiber through the 5-mm port of the operative thoracoscope, although special laser introducers can be used to apply the beam from an alternate intercostal access. We begin the laser treatment on the edge of the relatively normal parenchymal tissue at the interface with the bullae. The more red parenchyma that is often stained with anthracotic pigment readily absorbs the diffuse laser energy. Parenchymal "shrinkage" can begin at the margin of the bullous area, avoiding inadvertent penetration of the thin bullous membrane. The laser treatment also thickens this more normal parenchymal margin so that a more secure stapler application can eventually be made along the base of the bullae. We try intentionally to avoid entry into the bullae during the course of the procedure and, in most cases, ultimately rely on an endostapler application across the base of the pathologic zone to control the bullous process.

The use of VATS techniques to approach patients with diffuse panacinar emphysema is controversial and at this time is still considered experimental. Future trials will

be necessary before the techniques being explored can be embraced by the thoracic surgical community as legitimate treatment for this end-stage pulmonary condition.

Interstitial/Infiltrative Lung Disease — "Closed" Lung Biopsy

Acute and "chronic" interstitial lung disease encompasses a broad group of clinical conditions that frequently require surgical biopsy to assist in directing appropriate specific therapy. The differential diagnoses potentially accountable for these nonspecific interstitial lung changes is vast. Gaensler and Carrington (1980) as well as Chechani and colleagues (1992), among many others, have stressed that opportunistic bacterial, fungal, or viral infections, lymphangitic spread of malignancy, postchemotherapeutic lung injury, and pulmonary manifestations of connective tissue disease must be included in the differential diagnosis for the patient with progressive pulmonary decline and diffuse pulmonary infiltrates identified by chest radiography. Patients with idiopathic pulmonary fibrosis also frequently require surgical biopsy to confirm the diagnosis. Finally, Magee (1994) has noted that the expanded use of lung transplantation as a treatment of end-stage lung disease also presents a group of patients prone to develop interstitial lung abnormalities and post-transplant pulmonary dysfunction requiring surgical biopsy to determine the etiology of these changes. Specific therapy, rather than an empirical approach to care, is preferable because the appropriate treatment for any one of these conditions can vary significantly, that is, steroids versus antibiotics versus antineoplastics versus specific anti-rejection therapy.

Transbronchial washings and biopsy is a reasonable first approach in the evaluation of these patients, although the results from such bronchoscopic evaluation are relatively nonspecific, as documented by the reports of Wall (1981) and Burt (1981) and their associates. Because of these limitations, surgical biopsy of the lung is often required for diagnosis and to direct appropriate medical therapy for patients with progressive interstitial or infiltrative pulmonary parenchymal disease when simple therapeutic measures fail to reverse the decline in pulmonary function (Fig. 37–12). The classic operative approach of "open" lung biopsy has usually been a limited lateral or transaxillary thoracotomy. Although these open surgical approaches chosen by most surgeons are relatively minor compared to standard posterolateral thoracotomy wounds, they are often physiologically taxing for the patient with limited — and progressively worsening — pulmonary reserve.

It appears that VATS provides a minimally invasive means of surgically obtaining representative pulmonary tissue in these physiologically impaired patients. We now refer to this technique of VATS wedge resection as a "closed" surgical lung biopsy (see Table 37–5). This concept of using thoracoscopic means to obtain pulmonary parenchymal tissue for the diagnosis of interstitial or infiltrative disease is not new. European

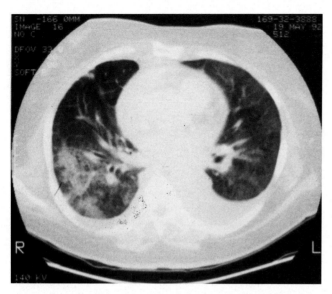

Fig. 37–12. CT scan of the chest from a patient with idiopathic bilateral infiltrative parenchymal lung disease. Careful evaluation of the preoperative CT scan facilitates identification of areas of "averagely" diseased lung that should be chosen for wedge resection biopsy.

investigators, such as Dijkman (1982) and Boutin (1982) and their colleagues, reported the utility of a direct viewing thoracoscopic approach to examine and obtain tissue for endoscopic "cup" biopsies of the lung for this diagnostic evaluation. Most of these reports attest that a histopathologic diagnosis of the disease process was achieved in most patients with acceptable morbidity. The central limitation of this particular thoracoscopic approach relates to the relatively small amount of pulmonary tissue that can be sampled and to postprocedural problems from persistent parenchymal air leak at the biopsy site.

Other surgeons, among whom are Deslauriers (1976) and Daly (1991) and their associates, have suggested the use of very limited intercostal access, or minithoracotomy, to identify the diseased lung and for wedge resection biopsy. After performing a strategically placed minithoracotomy — usually in an anterior parasternal location, these surgeons describe teasing a portion of the lung through this minithoracotomy access and then performing a wedge resection from the exposed tissue outside of the chest wall. This approach has also met with success, although the area that can be sampled is limited and, occasionally, tension on the lung tissue is excessive, which can lead to parenchymal tears along the projected line of wedge resection.

The VATS approach appears to provide another alternative for surgical biopsy of interstitial lung disease that incorporates many of the positive aspects of both the totally endoscopic — thoracoscopic — and the standard open thoracotomy approaches. Video–assisted thoracoscopic surgery overcomes some of the shortcomings of both these other approaches by providing a means of obtaining a truly panoramic inspection of the lung, as well as the ability to perform large, directed wedge resection biopsy of diseased lung with minimal

torque and tension at the biopsy site. Of course, this VATS approach has been primarily facilitated by the development of an effective endoscopic stapling device and improved thoracoscopic video-optics, which were described previously (Fig. 37–13).

The technical concepts for VATS pulmonary wedge resection were detailed in publications by us (RJL, 1993d; PFF, 1993), Dowling (1993), Bensard (1993), and associates. As a summary, wedge resection usually can be accomplished rapidly, for the diagnosis of interstitial or infiltrative disease, with a standard three intercostal access approach. The thoracoscope is introduced through a sixth to eighth interspace access site in the midaxillary line. After thoracoscopic inspection to identify an "averagely" diseased area of the lung, subsequent intercostal accesses are obtained at the fifth to sixth interspace in the anterior and posterior axillary lines to introduce endosurgical — or standard — instruments and the endoscopic stapling device. The position of the stapler and the instruments are aligned to grasp the tissue and accomplish a standard "V" wedge resection of representatively diseased pulmonary tissue (Fig. 37–14). It usually requires two to three applications of the stapler to accomplish the wedge resection. The positions of the stapler and instruments frequently are alternated from their original anterior and posterior fifth intercostal space access to enable a more expeditious wedge resection of the lung. When the operative thoracoscope is used, we frequently can perform the wedge resection using only two intercostal access sites. This approach requires the grasping the lung tissue with forceps through the 5-mm channel of the 10-mm diameter thoracoscope and then introducing the endoscopic stapler from the other intercostal access at approximately 90° to the orientation of the thoracoscope. The stapler is positioned properly across the base of an appropriate thickness of lung tissue that is grasped and the stapler is then fired. A subsequent load of the endoscopic stapler can be introduced through the original intercostal access to complete the wedge resection or, alternatively, the intercostal access position of the thoracoscope and stapler can be reversed to improve the angle of application of the stapler.

As our experience with VATS "closed" wedge resection of interstitial lung disease has matured (Table 37–5), a few key technical points have helped to reduce the time, aggravation, and potential morbidity related to this approach. A right-sided VATS approach is preferable for patients with diffuse interstitial lung disease, primarily because of the increased ability to achieve a wedge resection along a more clearly defined "edge" of lung on the right given the presence of the "extra" horizontal fissure of the middle lobe. Conversely, when asked to perform a lung biopsy in a patient with bilateral discrete nodular disease, we (RJL, 1933b) tend to favor a left-sided VATS approach. In this clinical circumstance, we can identify the target pathology more precisely. The more dependable lung collapse that can be achieved with double-lumen endotracheal tubes or bronchus blocking apparatuses on the left side makes for an easier intraoperative examination of the lung and

3 STICK APPROACH

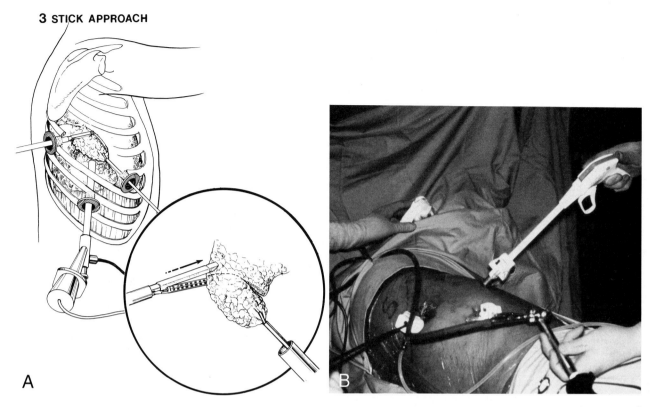

Fig. 37–13. Drawing *(A)* and photograph *(B)* of intercostal access typically used for a "three stick" intercostal access approach for VATS wedge resection of the lung using the endoscopic stapling device. *From* Ferson PF, et al: Thoracoscopic vs. "open" lung biopsy for the diagnosis of infiltrate lung disease. J Thorac Cardiovasc Surg, In press, 1993.

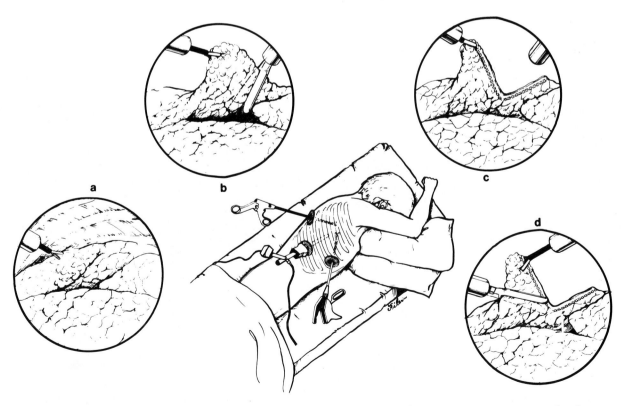

Fig. 37–14. Serial application of the endostapling device to accomplish a standard "V"-wedge resection of the lung. Note that the intercostal access position of the stapling instrument and the grasping tools are reversed to complete the stapled wedge resection expeditiously. *From* Dowling RD, et al: Thoracoscopic wedge resection of the lung. Surg Rounds *16*:341, 1993.

also for more precise application of the endoscopic stapler at specific pathologic areas. Despite our general perception of reduced operative morbidity when the VATS approach is used for surgical lung biopsy, there has been little objective documentation of this benefit. The relative effectiveness and differential morbidity associated with open thoracotomy and VATS techniques for the biopsy of interstitial lung disease were only recently addressed by Bensard and colleagues (1933) as well as by us (PFF, 1993). These authors compared the morbidity of open lung biopsy and of VATS lung biopsy in nonventilator-dependent patients with progressive pulmonary functional decline associated with radiographically defined interstitial lung. Bensard and coworkers reported relatively less postoperative morbidity, a shorter hospital stay, and equivalent diagnostic accuracy when the VATS approach was used to accomplish wedge resection biopsy of interstitial lung disease. Although our biases support the results of these studies, further corroborative work is necessary to define more clearly the benefits of the VATS approach in the diagnosis of interstitial lung disease.

Before leaving this topic, we must clarify the patient subset with diffuse pathologic lung disease we would elect to approach for lung biopsy with these VATS techniques. This approach is most appropriate to assess progressive radiographic interstitial lung changes in patients who are not critically ill and do not require ventilator assistance. The VATS approach is not used for "emergency" lung biopsies in the ventilator-dependent patient with multi-organ failure who is experiencing rapid progression of pulmonary dysfunction in the intensive care unit. The dangers in transfering airway control from a standard endotracheal tube to a double-lumen system in these unstable patients are not warranted. Additionally, most of these unstable patients will not tolerate the necessary single-lung ventilation required for the VATS procedure.

Little benefit is gained by using the VATS approach in these acutely ill, ventilator-dependent patients who are usually dangerously hypoxic, hemodynamically unstable, or both. We recommend performing the usual inframammary thoracotomy or transaxillary thoracotomy expeditiously rather than attempting a VATS approach.

The "Indeterminate" Pulmonary Nodule

The thoracic surgeon frequently is asked to participate in the diagnostic evaluation and the potential therapy for the patient with an indeterminate pulmonary nodule (Fig. 37–15). The primary role for the surgeon usually entails providing tissue for the diagnosis of the newly identified pulmonary lesion. Several characteristics of the clinical history and the patient profile have been established as important in evaluating the patient's cancer risk by Lillington (1992) and Lillington and Caskey (1993). This subject is discussed in detail in Chapter 87.

Because most physicians are not happy to apply a "wait and watch" approach to the newly discovered pulmonary nodule, it becomes imperative to diagnose the indeterminate nodular lesion expediently. Depending on the selection criteria, one third to one half of

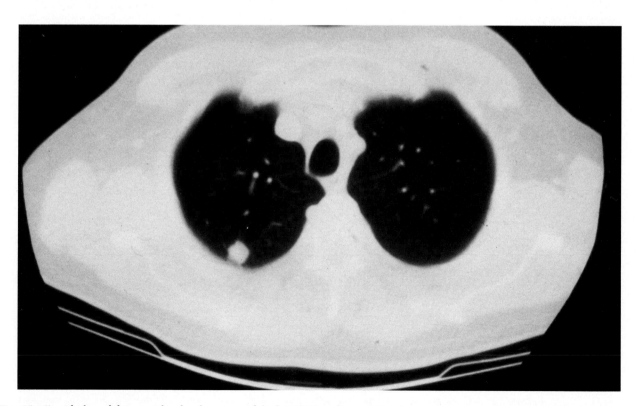

Fig. 37–15. Ideal candidate peripheral pulmonary nodule for VATS wedge resection.

lesions are found to be primary lung cancer, according to Lillington and Caskey (1993), Roth (1992) and Dowling and associates (1992) of our group. The remaining nodules, with a near equal distribution, are either benign processes or sites of metastasis from remote primary tumors.

Spirited discussion regarding the most appropriate diagnostic method for these indeterminant nodules continues. Transbronchial or percutaneous biopsy under fluoroscopic or computed tomographic (CT) guidance is advocated as the first diagnostic maneuver by some physicians. Many reports, including those of Salazar and Westcott (1993) and Midthun and colleagues (1992) emphasize that these are minimally invasive techniques associated with reasonable accuracy in diagnosing malignant nodules. The most troublesome problem with percutaneous biopsy approaches relates to the limited accuracy in determining the benignity of a lesion. Commonly, the information obtained is indeterminate and, as noted by Calhoun and associates (1986), is therefore inadequate to allow surgeons to base future therapeutic decisions on the biopsy findings consistently. Therefore, despite all best efforts to avoid surgical intervention for noncancerous lesions, most patients with peripheral indeterminate pulmonary nodules undergo surgical excision of the lesion.

It is our (RJL, 1993a) opinion that the VATS approach provides an efficient, potentially less morbid surgical means of obtaining excisional biopsy of many indeterminate pulmonary lesions (Table 37–5). We (MJM, 1993) and Allen and colleagues (1994) independently reported the use of the VATS approaches as the "primary" diagnostic method for the indeterminate pulmonary nodule. Both of these reports demonstrated that the VATS approach is a sensitive and specific diagnostic tool for indeterminate peripheral pulmonary nodules. Patients experienced minimal operative morbidity and also appeared to have a shortened hospital stay relative to historical controls approached through lateral thoracotomies. Additionally, we (MJM, 1992a) and Plunkett and associates (1992) emphasized that the use of adjunctive CT-guided needle localization techniques were a helpful adjunct to the identification of small, clinically suspicious lesions that would be difficult to palpate by either open thoracotomy or VATS approaches.

We favor using a primary VATS approach, instead of percutaneous biopsy attempts, for most peripheral pulmonary nodules. This approach is not appropriate management, however, for some peripheral pulmonary lesions. Several anatomic characteristics must be met before suggesting management with VATS wedge excisional biopsy. For some peripheral nodular lesions with radiographic findings highly suggestive of malignancy, it is often unnecessary to obtain a prethoracotomy diagnosis, although we prefer to obtain a preoperative needle biopsy so that the extra step of intraoperative excisional biopsy confirmation of the histology can be avoided and a more expeditious primary resection can be completed. Most importantly, however, if the patient is physiologically unfit for any surgical intervention, a percutaneous biopsy should be considered rather than using the VATS approach to confirm the diagnosis. We, as noted by Shennib and colleagues (1993) of our group, must qualify the latter statement by saying that the VATS approach has allowed us to perform "compromise therapeutic wedge resection" in patients we would not have before considered candidates for any surgical intervention.

Compromise "Primary Wedge Resection" for Bronchogenic Carcinoma

Anatomic lobectomy, performed through an open thoracotomy, according to Ginsberg and associates (1989) and Shields (1993), remains the standard of care for physiologically fit individuals with limited stage lung cancer within the anatomic confines of the pulmonary lobe in question (see Chapter 89). In many reports, however, authors have demonstrated that lesser resections — anatomic segmentectomy or even a wedge resection — may have a survival benefit equivalent to that of lobectomy in the management of small, T1 N0, nonsmall cell carcinomas of the lung (see Reading References for documentation). Miller and Hatcher (1987), however, cautioned against the use of these resectional approaches when the tumor appears to cross segmental boundaries, as the local recurrence rate is significantly higher when this is present.

The potential validity of "compromise resections" for limited stage I — T1 N0 — nonsmall cell carcinoma of the lung was prospectively evaluated by the North American Lung Cancer Study Group and was reported initially by Ginsberg and Rubenstein (1991). They randomized patients with intraoperatively determined peripheral, limited stage I nonsmall cell carcinomas to undergo a lobectomy or either a wedge resection or segmentectomy. Although survival was equivalent, the local recurrence rate after either a wedge or a segmentectomy was significantly higher than when lobectomy was used for the curative resection. These observations were confirmed by the retrospective comparison of these operations by Warren and Faber (1994).

A few studies addressed the validity of the VATS approach for nonanatomic wedge resection of peripheral primary bronchogenic carcinomas. Shennib and colleagues (1993) reported their gratifying experience with the VATS approach to peripheral lung cancers in a few high risk, elderly patients with significant impairment of cardiopulmonary reserve. Adequate resection of the neoplasms were accomplished using the VATS approach in all of these carefully selected patients and no procedure-related morbidities were noted. The authors also believed that adequate intraoperative lymph node sampling could be accomplished as a part of the VATS procedure to stage the malignant process. The experience of Lewis (1993) with VATS resection of small peripheral carcinomas has been similar.

Suffice it to say that wedge resection or segmentectomy by open thoracotomy or the VATS approach may be a legitimate compromise surgical alternative to lobectomy for the patient with significant cardiopulmonary functional impairment (Table 37–5). Careful preoperative and intraoperative staging of the patient is needed to reduce the possibility of missing a more advanced malignancy. Additionally, it is important to ensure that surgical margins are clear of tumor within the extent of the nonanatomic resection performed. The role of adjuvant local radiation therapy — avoiding radiation to the hilum and mediastinum — in reducing the local recurrence rate after VATS resection has yet to be clearly defined. At present, we would reserve thoracoscopic resection for those peripheral, limited stage I primary pulmonary malignancies in patients with severely impaired pulmonary function or those patients with other confounding physiologic problems that seriously increase their risk for standard thoracotomy. The surgeon should be careful to use the same anatomic "criteria for resection" for these peripheral known lung cancers as described for the indeterminate peripheral pulmonary nodule (Table 37–6). Again, the VATS approach is usually not applicable for more deeply seated lesions in close proximity to the pulmonary hilar structures.

We suggest limiting the use of VATS resection in this clinical setting to small — less than 3 cm in diameter — pulmonary lesions located in the outer one third of the pulmonary parenchyma. Stapled wedge resection of a lesion, ensuring a clear margin of normal pulmonary parenchyma, is our standard approach to resection (Fig. 37–16). We also use the Nd:YAG laser alone or in combination with stapled resection techniques to perform excision of the offending lesion when it is located on the flat, thick surface of the lung; stapled resection in this area is impossible alone without risking staple line dehiscence or injuring the underlying lung (Fig. 37–17), as we (RJL, 1992a; 1991a; 1991b, and 1992b), LoCicero (1989) and Keenan (1994) and associates have described.

It is to be emphasized that in all these VATS cases, the thoracic surgeon should be prepared to convert to open thoracotomy if any uncertainty arises regarding the completeness or safety of the VATS resection.

Lobectomy

Although VATS appears to be a "potentially" valid means of accomplishing nonanatomic wedge resection of the lung for the aforementioned selected patients, the general utility and safety of VATS lobectomy remains to be determined (Table 37–5). Certainly, the thoracic surgeon should be familiar with basic VATS strategies and the instrumentation needed for VATS wedge resection of the lung before embarking on the lobectomy.

Table 37–6. Candidate Pulmonary Nodules for VATS Pulmonary Resection

Noncalcified, less than 3 cm in diameter.

Indeterminate etiology after appropriate work-up.

Location in the outer one third of the lung.

Absence of endobronchial extension (with VATS lobectomy?)

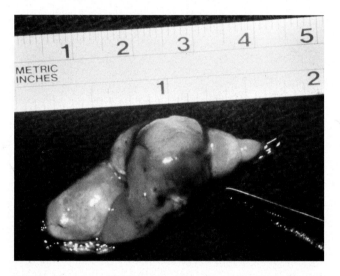

Fig. 37–16. Typical VATS endostapler excisional wedge resection specimen of a peripheral nodule.

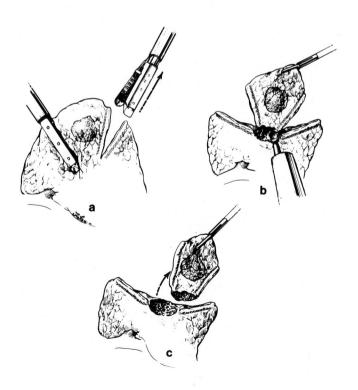

Fig. 37–17. Technique of combined VATS Nd:YAG laser and endostapler resection of a peripheral pulmonary nodule on the flat surface of the lung. *From* Landreneau, RJ et al: Thoracoscopic resection of 85 pulmonary lesions. Ann Thorac Surg 54:415, 1992.

Even more importantly, as pointed out by McKneally (1993), the surgeon must be well experienced with the anatomic and technical nuances of the standard technique for lobectomy before considering these procedures. The different sensory "afferent" input of videoscopic instrument orientation and the limitations of two-dimensional vision can often play tricks on even the most skilled and experienced thoracic surgeon.

To date, Lewis (1992), Roviaro (1992), Kirby (1993), and their associates, as well as McKenna (1994), have described the techniques and early clinical results with VATS lobectomy. A recent prospective, nonrandomized study by Kirby and colleagues (1993) identified a few key points regarding the present use of VATS lobectomy. Lobectomy was accomplished for all lobes of either lung (Fig. 37–18); however, upper lobectomies were technically more challenging than either lower lobe or middle lobe procedures. The authors believed that the patients undergoing VATS lobectomy had relatively little postoperative pain and they experienced an early return to full activity. Compared to historical controls, the overall postoperative hospitalization was slightly shorter. The frequency and nature of postoperative complications were similar, however, to historical control subjects undergoing lobectomy through a standard thoracotomy. Mediastinal nodal sampling to stage the bronchial carcinoma was accomplished in all patients, but radical mediastinal lymphadenectomy was not performed. The primary disadvantages to the VATS approach related to the significantly longer operative time that was necessary to accomplish pulmonary lobectomy and, of course, to the lack of "wide open" access for vascular control of the pulmonary vasculature if an injury should occur.

The videoscopic techniques of VATS lobectomy are nicely described by Kirby and associates (1993) and in the earlier report by Roviaro and colleagues (1992). We summarize by saying that standard segmental pulmonary vascular dissection, control, and ligation were used in all patients. Additionally, independent division and mechanical stapler — EndoGIA — closure of the lobar bronchus was performed according to the principles of standard open lobectomy. Although the present difficulties with VATS lobectomy are likely to be reduced as experience is gained with these approaches, they should be considered investigational at this time, and it is not offered to replace the standard open technique.

The ultimate role of VATS lobectomy in general thoracic surgical practice has yet to be determined. The therapeutic results and safety of these lobectomy techniques will only be defined with the maturation of results from the present clinical studies underway and the broadening of clinical experience with these more advanced VATS procedures by other thoracic surgeons.

CONCLUSIONS

Although a healthy degree of skepticism is important to avoid overzealous use of new technology, thoracic surgeons are the most appropriate group to study the present role of VATS (Table 37–7). In North America, thoracic surgeons presently are asked to evaluate and manage most complicated pleural problems and pulmonary parenchymal mass lesions. Certainly, some of the VATS applications described in this chapter will *not* be found as a reasonable approach to the thoracic pathology toward which they are being directed (Table 37–8). Moreover, the present and potential disadvantages of VATS must be kept in mind (Table 37–9).

The present explosion of interest and emotional discussion in minimally invasive surgical approaches will likely result in thoracic surgeons evolving a spectrum of thoracic surgical procedures and instrumentation aimed at accomplishing less morbid, but equally effective approaches to patients' problems. The concept of using "open" minithoracotomies, with direct viewing of the pulmonary structures in conjunction with periodic

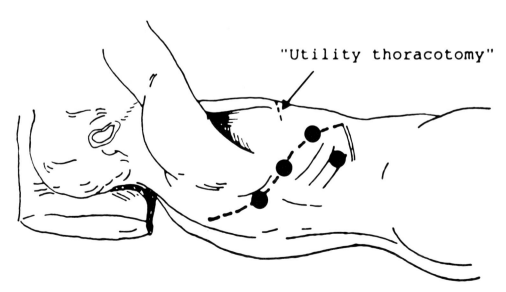

"Utility thoracotomy"

Fig. 37–18. Patient positioning and usual location of the "utility incision" needed to facilitate the performance of VATS lobectomy. *From* Roviaro G, et al: Video-endoscopic pulmonary lobectomy for cancer. Surg Lapar Endo 2:244, 1992.

Table 37–7. Ideal Thoracic Applications for VATS

Diagnosis and management of idiopathic/complex pleural effusions.

Elective "closed" lung biopsy.

Recurrent/complicated "primary" spontaneous pneumothorax.

Alternative to anterior mediastinotomy — "Chamberlain" procedure to evaluate mediastinal adenopathy — adjunct to cervical mediastinoscopy.

Diagnosis and selective management of the indeterminate peripheral pulmonary nodule — less than 3 cm in diameter.

Table 37–8. Limitations of VATS

Hilar pulmonary lesions

Pulmonary parenchymal lesions abutting the upper mediastinum or posterior paravertebral area

"Small" thoracic cavities

Severe emphysema

Ventilator dependency

Noncompliant lung

Small, "deep" parenchymal lesions identified by chest CT scan

Dense pleural symphysis

Table 37–9. Present and Potential Disadvantages of VATS

| Instrumentation |
| Vascular control |
| Pleural seeding |
| Incomplete staging |
| Learning curve |
| Overextension of indications |

video assistance and continuous intrathoracic illumination with the thoracoscope, might become a more prominent approach in the future. Direct videoscopic dissection rather than blind division of pulmonary adhesions in the lateral and posterior costophrenic recesses may also prove useful. Also, we may come to use some of the present endoscopic tools — EndoGIA and endoclip applier — as alternative dissection and resective instruments during open thoracotomy procedures.

In the final analysis, one's conscience must be the guide to what is believed to be the best surgical approach for patients requiring thoracic surgery. These decisions should necessarily be molded on sound clinical data supporting the practice of thoracic surgery.

REFERENCES

Alexander J: The Collapse Therapy of Pulmonary Tuberculosis. Springfield, IL: Charles C Thomas, 1937, pp. 313-316.

Allen MS: Instrumentation for video-assisted thoracic surgery. Ann Thorac Surg, In press, 1993.

Allen MS, et al: Thoracoscopic wedge excision for indeterminate pulmonary nodules. J Thorac Cardiovasc Surg, In press, 1994.

Bensard DD, et al: Comparison of video-assisted lung biopsy to open lung biopsy in the evaluation of interstitial lung disease. Chest 103:765, 1993.

Benumof JL: Physiology of the open chest and one-lung ventilation. In Kaplan JA (ed): Thoracic Anesthesia. New York: Churchill Livingstone, 1983, pp. 287-316.

Bergquist S, Nordenstam H: Thoracoscopy and pleural biopsy in the diagnosis of pleurisy. Scand J Respir Dis 47:64, 1966.

Boutin C: Thoracoscopic management of spontaneous pneumothorax. Am Rev Respir Dis 134:588, 1993.

Boutin C, et al: Thoracoscopic lung biopsy. Experimental and clinical preliminary study. Chest 82:44, 1982.

Boniface E, Guerin JC: Interet du talcage par thoracoscopie dans le traitement symptomatique des pleuresies recidivantes. A propos de 302 cas. Rev Mal Respir 6:133, 1989.

Braimbridge MV: The history of thoracoscopy. Ann Thorac Surg, In press, 1993.

Brandt HJ: Indikation und Technik der Diagnostischen Thorakoskopie. Atemwegs Lungenkrankh 3:150, 1978.

Brandt H, Loddenkemper R, Mai J: Atlas of Diagnostic Thoracoscopy. Indications-Techniques. New York: Thieme, 1985, pp. 1-46.

Burt ME, et al: Prospective evaluation of aspiration needle, cutting needle, transbronchial, and open lung biopsy in patients with pulmonary infiltrates. Ann Thorac Surg 32:146, 1981.

Calhoun P, et al: The clinical outcome of needle aspirations of the lung when cancer is not diagnosed. Ann Thorac Surg 41:592, 1986.

Chechani V, Landreneau RJ, Schaikh S: Diffuse infiltrative lung disease: Where and how many open lung biopsies to perform. Ann Thorac Surg 54:296, 1992.

Coulaud E, DesChamps P: Decouverte pleuroscopique d'une importante perforation pulmonaire Asymptomatique. Guerison Rapide Spontanee. Rev Tuberculose 11:825, 1947.

Daly BDT, et al: Computed tomography-guided minithoracocotomy for the resection of small peripheral pulmonary nodules. Ann Thorac Surg 51:465, 1991.

Daniel TM, Tribble CG, Rodgers BM: Thoracoscopy and talc poudrage for pneumothoraces and effusions. Ann Thorac Surg 50:186, 1990.

Deslauriers J, et al: Mediastinopleuroscopy: A new approach to the diagnosis of intrathoracic diseases. Ann Thorac Surg 22:265, 1976.

Dijkman JH, et al: Transpleural lung biopsy by the thoracoscopic route in patients with diffuse interstitial pulmonary disease. Chest 82:76, 1982.

Dowling RD, Ferson PF, Landreneau RJ: Thoracoscopic resection of pulmonary metastases. Chest 102:1450, 1992.

Dowling RD, et al: Thoracoscopic wedge resection of the lung. Surg Rounds 16:341, 1993.

Ferson PF, et al: Thoracoscopic vs. "open" lung biopsy for the diagnosis of infiltrate lung disease. J Thorac Cardiovasc Surg, In press, 1993.

Fourestier M, Duret M: Necessite de la biopsie pleurale pour le diagnostic de L' endotheliome de la plevre. Presse Med 32:467, 1943.

Gaensler EA, Carrington CB: Open biopsy for chronic diffuse infiltrative lung disease: Clinical, roentgenographic, and physiological correlations in 502 patients. Ann Thorac Surg 30:411, 1980.

Ginsberg RJ, Rubenstein LV: Patients with T1N0 non-small cell lung cancer [abstract 304]. Lung Cancer 7(Suppl):83, 1991.

Ginsberg RJ, Goldberg M, Waters PF: Surgery for non-small cell lung cancer. In Roth JA, Ruckdeschel JC, Weisenburger TH (eds): Thoracic Oncology. Philadelphia: WB Saunders, 1989, pp. 177-205.

Hagen RH, Reed W, Solheim K: Spontaneous pneumothorax. Scand J Thorac Cardiovasc Surg 21:183, 1987.

Hazelrigg SR: Commentary of Wakabayashi A: Thoracoscopic treatment of bullous emphysema using sapphire contact tip neodymium yttrium aluminum garnet laser (contact YAG): Preliminary report. J Thorac Cardiovasc Surg, In press, 1994.

Hazelrigg SR, et al: Thoracoscopic management of spontaneous pneumothorax. J Thorac Cardiothorac Surg 105:389, 1993a.

Hazelrigg SR, et al: Cost analysis for thoracoscopy: Thoracoscopic wedge resection. Ann Thorac Surg, In press, 1993b.

Hazelrigg SR, LoCicero J III, Nunchuck S, and the Video-Assisted Thoracic Surgery Study Group (VATSSG): The Video-Assisted

Thoracic Surgery Study Group Data. Ann Thorac Surg, In press, 1993.

Jacobaeus HC: The practical importance of thoracoscopy in surgery of the chest. Surg Gynecol Obstet 34:289, 1922.

Jacobaeus HC: Die Thorakoskopie und ihre praktische Bedeutung. Ergebn Ges Med 7:112, 1925.

Kaiser LR: Diagnostic and therapeutic use of pleuroscopy (thoracoscopy) in lung cancer. Surg Clin North Am 67:1081, 1987.

Keenan RJ, et al: Video-assisted thoracoscopy for the diagnosis and management of pleural diseases. Am Rev Respir Dis 147:A737, 1993.

Keenan RJ, et al: Video-thoracoscopic resection using the Nd:YAG laser. J Thorac Cardiovasc Surg, In press, 1994.

Kirby TJ, et al: Initial experience with video-assisted thoracoscopic lobectomy. Ann Thorac Surg, In press, 1993.

Klassen KP, Meckstroth CV: Treatment of spontaneous pneumothorax: Prompt expansion with controlled thoracotomy tube suction. JAMA 182:1, 1962.

Landreneau RJ, et al: Nd:YAG laser-assisted pulmonary resections. Ann Thorac Surg 51:973, 1991a.

Landreneau RJ, et al: Thoracoscopic Nd:YAG laser-assisted pulmonary resection. Ann Thorac Surg 52:1176, 1991b.

Landreneau RJ, et al: Video-assisted thoracic surgery: Basic technical concepts and intercostal approach strategies. Ann Thorac Surg 54:800, 1992a.

Landreneau RJ, et al: Thoracoscopic resection of 85 pulmonary lesions. Ann Thorac Surg 54:415, 1992b.

Landreneau RJ, et al: Differences in postoperative pain, shoulder function, and morbidity between video-assisted thoracic surgery and muscle sparing "open" thoracotomies. Ann Thorac Surg, In press, 1993a.

Landreneau RJ, et al: Strategic planning for video-assisted thoracic surgery "VATS". Ann Thorac Surg, In press, 1993b.

Landreneau RJ, et al: Video-assisted thoracic surgical resection of benign pulmonary lesions. Chest Surg Clin North Am 3:283, 1993c.

Landreneau RJ, et al: Prevalence of chronic postoperative pain following pulmonary resection by thoracotomy of video-assisted thoracic surgery. J Thorac Cardiovasc Surg, In press, 1994.

Lewis RJ: The role of video-assisted thoracic surgery (VATS) for primary carcinoma of the lung: Wedge resection to SIS lobectomy. Ann Thorac Surg, In press, 1993.

Lewis RJ, Caccavale RJ, Sisler GE: 100 Consecutive cases of imaged thoracic surgery. Ann Thorac Surg 54:421, 1992.

Lewis RJ, Sisler GE, Caccavale RJ: Imaged thoracic lobectomy: Should it be done? Ann Thorac Surg 54:80, 1992.

Lewis RJ, et al: Direct diagnostic thoracoscopy. Ann Thorac Surg 21:536, 1976.

Lillington GA: Management of solitary pulmonary nodules. Disease-a-Month 37:271, 1992.

Lillington GA, Caskey CI: Evaluation and management of solitary and multiple pulmonary nodules. Clin Chest Med 14:111, 1993.

LoCicero J III, et al: Experimental air leak in lung sealed by low-energy carbon dioxide laser irradiation. Chest 87:820, 1985.

LoCicero J III, et al: Laser-assisted parenchymal sparing pulmonary resection. J Thorac Cardiovasc Surg 97:732, 1989.

Mack MJ, et al: Percutaneous localization of pulmonary nodules for thoracoscopic lung resection. Ann Thorac Surg 53:1123, 1992a.

Mack MJ, et al: Thoracoscopy for the diagnosis of the indeterminate solitary pulmonary nodule. Ann Thorac Surg, In press, 1993.

Magee MJ: Thoracoscopy in the evaluation and treatment of lung transplant recipients. J Heart Lung Transplant, In press, 1994.

McKenna RJ: Thoracoscopic lobectomy for lung cancer. J Thorac Cardiovasc Surg, In press, 1994.

McKneally MF: Video-assisted thoracic surgery: Standards and Guidelines. Chest Surg Clin North Am 3:345, 1993.

Midthun DE, Swenson SJ, Jett JR: Clinical strategies for solitary pulmonary nodules. Annu Rev Med 41:195, 1992.

Miller JI, Hatcher CR: Thoracoscopy: A useful tool in the diagnosis of thoracic disease. Ann Thorac Surg 26:68, 1978.

Miller JI, Hatcher CR: Limited resection of bronchogenic carcinoma in the patient with marked impairment of pulmonary function. Ann Thorac Surg 44:340, 1987.

Nathanson LK, et al: Videothoracoscopic ligation of bulla and pleurectomy for spontaneous pneumothorax. Ann Thorac Surg 52:316, 1991.

Plunkett MB, et al: Peripheral pulmonary nodules: Preoperative percutaneous needle localization with CT guidance. Radiology 185:274, 1992.

Roth JA: Treatment of metastatic cancer to lung. In DeVita VT, Hellman S, Rosenberg SA (eds): Cancer: Principles and Practice of Oncology. Philadelphia: JB Lippincott, 1989, pp. 2261-2275.

Roviaro G, et al: Video-endoscopic pulmonary lobectomy for cancer. Surg Lapar Endo 2:244, 1992.

Salazar AM, Westcott JL: The role of transthoracic needle biopsy for the diagnosis and staging of lung cancer. Clin Chest Med 14:99, 1993.

Shennib H, Landreneau RJ, Mack MJ: Video assisted thoracoscopic wedge resection of T1 lung cancer in high risk patients. Ann Surg, In press, 1993.

Shields TW: Surgical therapy for carcinoma of the lung. Clin Chest Med 14:121, 1993.

Steele JD: Production of pleural adhesions for therapeutic purposes. Am Rev Tub 56:299, 1947.

Swierenga J, Wagenaar JP, Bergstein PG: The value of thoracoscopy in the diagnosis and treatment of diseases affecting the pleura and the lung. Pneumologie 151:11, 1974.

Torre M, Belloni P: Nd:YAG laser pleurodesis through thoracoscopy: New curative therapy in spontaneous pneumothorax. Ann Thorac Surg 47:887, 1989.

van de Brekel JA, Duurkens VAM, Vanderscheuren RGJRA: Pneumothorax: Results of thoracoscopy and pleurodesis with talc poudrage and thoracotomy. Chest 103:345, 1993.

Vanderscheuren RG: Le talcage pleural dans le pneumothorax spontane. Poumon-Coeur 37:273, 1981.

Viskum K, Lange P, Mortensen J: Long term sequelae after talc pleurodesis for spontaneous pneumothorax. Pneumologie 43:105, 1989.

Wakabayashi A: Thoracoscopic treatment of spontaneous pneumothorax. Chest Surg Clin North Am 3:233, 1993.

Wakabayashi A: Thoracoscopic treatment of bullous emphysema using sapphire contact tip neodymium yttrium aluminum garnet laser (contact YAG): Preliminary report. J Thorac Cardiovasc Surg, In press, 1994.

Wall CP, et al: Comparison of transbronchial and open biopsies in chronic infiltrative lung diseases. Am Rev Respir Dis 123:230, 1981.

Warren WH, Faber LP: Segmentectomy vs. lobectomy in patients with stage I pulmonary carcinoma: Five-year survival and patterns of intrathoracic recurrence. J Thorac Cardiovasc Surg, In press, 1994.

Webb WR, et al: Iodized talc pleurodesis for the treatment of pleural effusions. J Thorac Cardiovasc Surg 103:881, 1992.

Wernly JA, DeMeester TR: Preoperative assessment of patients undergoing lung resection for cancer. In Roth JA, Ruckedeschel JC, Weisenburger TH (eds): Thoracic Oncology. Philadelphia: WB Saunders, 1989, pp. 156-176.

Worsey J, Landreneau RJ: Thoracoscopic instruments and ancillary equipment. Endo Surg Allied Tech, In press, 1993.

READING REFERENCES

Boutin C, Viallat JR, Aelony Y: Practical Thoracoscopy. Berlin: Springer, 1991.

Boutin C, et al: Thoracoscopy in malignant mesothelioma. Chest 96:275S, 1989.

Canto A, et al: Points to consider when choosing a biopsy method in cases of pleurisy of unknown origin. Chest 84:176, 1983.

Canto A, et al: Pleural effusion of malignant etiology. Thoracoscopic use of talc as an effective method of pleurodesis. Med Clin 84:806, 1985.

Canto A, et al: Lung cancer and pleural effusion. Clinical significance and study of pleural metastatic locations. Chest 87:649, 1987.

Errett LE, et al: Wedge resection as an alternative procedure for peripheral bronchogenic carcinoma in poor-risk patients. J Thorac Cardiovasc Surg 90:656, 1985.

Ginsberg RJ: Limited resection in the treatment of stage I non-small cell lung cancer: An overview. Chest 96:505, 1989.

Gravelyn TR, et al: Tetracycline pleurodesis for malignant pleural effusions. A 10-year retrospective study. Cancer 59:1973, 1987.

Kessinger A, Wigton RS: Intracavitary bleomycin and tetracycline in the management of malignant pleural effusions: A randomized study. J Surg Oncol 36:81, 1987.

Landreneau RJ: Carcinoma of the lung: Who will benefit from surgery? Postgrad Med 87:117, 1990.

Macchiarini P, et al: Most peripheral, node-negative, non-small cell lung cancers have low proliferative rates and no intratumoral and peritumoral blood and lymphatic invasion. Rationale for treatment with wedge resection alone. J Thorac Cardiovasc Surg 104:892, 1992.

Mack MJ, et al: The present role of thoracoscopy in the diagnosis and treatment of the chest. Ann Thorac Surg 54:405, 1992b.

Martini N, Bains MS, Beattie EJ: Indications for pleurectomy in malignant effusions. Cancer 35:734, 1975.

Menzies R, Charbonneau M: Thoracoscopy for the diagnosis of pleural disease. Ann Intern Med 114:271, 1991.

Miller DL, et al: Video-thoracoscopic wedge resection of the lung. Ann Thorac Surg 54:410, 1992.

Oakes DD, et al: Therapeutic thoracoscopy. J Thorac Cardiovasc Surg 87:269, 1984.

Page RD, Jeffrey RR, Donnelly RJ: Thoracoscopy: A review of 121 consecutive surgical procedures. Ann Thorac Surg 48:66, 1989.

Pastorino U, et al: Limited resection for stage I lung cancer. Eur J Surg Oncol 17:42, 1991.

Read RC, Yoder G, Schaefer RC: Survival after conservative resection for $T_1N_0M_0$ non–small cell lung cancer. Ann Thorac Surg 49:391, 1990.

Ridley PD, Braimbridge MV. Thoracoscopic debridement and pleural irrigation in the management of empyema thoracis. Ann Thorac Surg 51:461, 1991.

Rodgers BM, et al: Thoracoscopy for intrathoracic tumors. Ann Thorac Surg 31:414, 1981.

Rogers DA, Lobe TE, Schropp KP: Video-assisted thoracoscopic surgery in the pediatric patient. Chest Surg Clin North Am 325, 1993.

Thomas P. Thoracoscopy: An Old Procedure Revisited. *In* Kittle CF (ed): Current Controversies in Thoracic Surgery. Philadelphia: WB Saunders, 1986, pp. 101-112.

Todd TRJ, et al: Talc poudrage for malignant pleural effusions. Chest 78:542, 1980.

The Chest Wall

CHAPTER 38

CHEST WALL DEFORMITIES

Robert C. Shamberger

A broad spectrum of congenital chest wall deformities exists. Fortunately, the severe, life-threatening deformities ectopia cordis and asphyxiating thoracic dystrophy are rare in comparison with the more frequent and milder pectus excavatum and carinatum. Congenital anterior thoracic deformities can be considered in five categories: 1) pectus excavatum; 2) pectus carinatum; 3) Poland's syndrome; 4) sternal defects, including ectopia cordis; and 5) miscellaneous conditions, including vertebral and rib anomalies, asphyxiating thoracic dystrophy — Jeune's disease, and rib dysplasia.

PECTUS EXCAVATUM

Pectus excavatum — funnel chest or trichterbrust — is a posterior depression of the sternum and lower costal cartilages. The first and second ribs and the manubrium usually are normal (Fig. 38–1), whereas the lower costal cartilages and the sternum are depressed. In adolescents, the most anterior portion of the osseous ribs may also be curved posteriorly. The extent of sternal and cartilaginous deformity is variable and numerous methods of grading and defining these deformities have been proposed by Hümmer and Willital (1984), Oelsnitz (1981), Welch (1980), Haller (1987), and others, but none has been accepted universally (Fig. 38–2). Asymmetry of the depression is present frequently but may not be appreciated until the time of surgical correction. The right side is often more depressed than the left, and the sternum may be rotated as well. A broad thin chest is present in most children with pectus excavatum as are dorsal lordosis, "hook shoulder" deformity, costal flaring, and poor posture.

Pectus excavatum usually is present at birth or within the first year of life — 86% — as shown in Figure 38–3. The deformity may worsen at adolescence. Waters and associates (1988) identified scoliosis in 26% of 508 patients with pectus excavatum. Hence, all patients seen for pectus deformities should be evaluated clinically for scoliosis. Although initially mild, scoliosis can worsen rapidly at adolescence. Asymmetric pectus ex-

cavatum with a deep right gutter and sternal rotation often is accompanied by more serious right thoracic and left lumbar scoliosis. Correction of the associated pectus excavatum may stabilize the curve in conjunction with exercises or bracing, and avoid spinal fusion.

Congenital heart disease has been identified in 1.5% of our patients undergoing chest wall correction (Table 38–1). The frequency of chest wall deformities among patients with congenital heart disease evaluated at our institution was only 0.17%.

Asthma frequently is identified in patients with pectus excavatum and carinatum. In a recent review of 694 consecutive cases, a subgroup of 35 patients with asthma was identified — 5.2% — which is comparable to the occurrence of asthma in the general pediatric population.

Etiology and Incidence

Ravitch (1977) reported that pectus excavatum may occur as frequently as 1 in 300 to 1 in 400 live births and is rare in blacks. Although the sternal depression appears to be caused by overgrowth of costal cartilages, the mechanism is unexplained. Early investigators such as Lester (1957) attributed its development to an abnormality of the diaphragm, but little evidence supports this theory; the occurrence of pectus excavatum in children born with congenital diaphragmatic hernia was reported by Greig and Azmy (1990). Hecker and associates (1988) described histopathologic changes in the costal cartilages similar to those seen in scoliosis, aseptic osteonecrosis, and inflammatory processes, but the etiology of these findings and their significance is unknown.

An increased familial incidence exists. In a review by the author and Welch (1988b), 37% of 704 patients had a family history of chest wall deformity. Three of four siblings were involved in one family. Scherer (1988) noted that patients with Marfan's syndrome have a high incidence of chest wall deformities that often are severe and usually are accompanied by scoliosis. Currently, no biochemical or genetic markers for this disease are known, so diagnosis must be based on clinical findings.

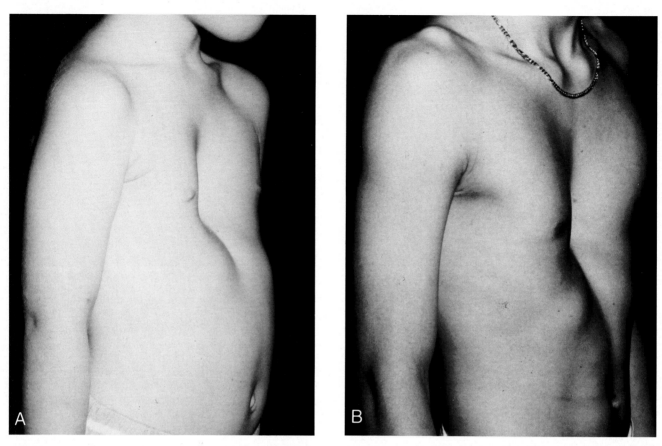

Fig. 38–1. *A,* A 4½-year-old girl with a symmetric pectus excavatum deformity. *B,* A 16-year-old boy with pectus excavatum. Note that the depression extends to the sternal notch.

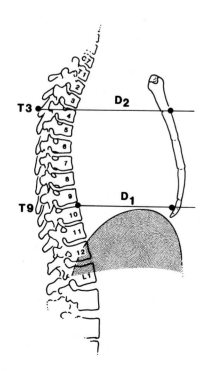

Depression Ratio (DR) $= \dfrac{D_1}{D_2}$

Deformity Grade (DG) $= (1 - DR) \times 10$

Welch Index $= DG + \ldots$

0.5 if Cardiothoracic
Ratio $> 50\%$

Fig. 38–2. Welch Index for grading the severity of pectus excavatum deformities.

Pectus Excavatum

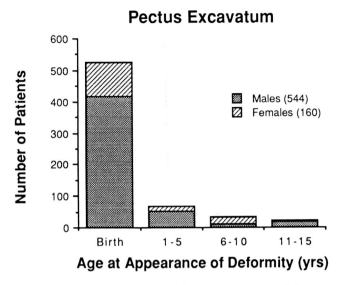

Fig. 38-3. Age at appearance of the pectus excavatum deformity in 704 infants and children.

Patients with abdominal musculature deficiency syndrome — prune belly syndrome — commonly have pectus excavatum, 8 of 43 patients in the experience of Welch and Kearney (1974). Pectus excavatum also occurs with other myopathies and chromosomal defects, such as Turner's syndrome. A summary of the associated musculoskeletal abnormalities is shown in Table 38-2.

Symptoms

Pectus excavatum is well tolerated in infancy and childhood. Chronic upper airway obstruction because of tonsillar and adenoidal hypertrophy may accentuate the depression in an infant with a flexible chest but is not causative. Older children may complain of pain in the area of the deformed cartilages or of precordial pain after sustained exercise. A few patients have palpitations, which presumably are transient atrial arrhythmias.

Table 38-1. Congenital Heart Disease Associated with Pectus Excavatum and Carinatum

Aortic ring	1
Aortic regurgitation	1
ASD primum*	2
ASD secundum	3
Complete atrioventricular canal	3
Dextrocardia	3
Ebstein malformation	1
Idiopathic hypertrophic subaortic stenosis	2
Patent ductus arteriosus	1
Pulmonic stenosis	1
Total anomalous pulmonary venous return	1
Transposition of great arteries	6
Tetrology of Fallot	3
Tricuspid atresia	1
Truncus arteriosus	1
Ventricular septal defect	6

*ASD = atrial septal defect.

Table 38-2. Musculoskeletal Abnormalities in Pectus Excavatum*

Scoliosis	107
Kyphosis	4
Myopathy	3
Marfan's syndrome	2
Pierre Robin syndrome	2
Prune belly syndrome	2
Neurofibromatosis	3
Cerebral palsy	4
Tuberous sclerosis	1
Congenital diaphragmatic hernia	2

*Identified in 130 of 704 cases.

The author and associates (1987) observed that these patients may have mitral valve prolapse and associated atrial arrhythmias.

Pathophysiology

Some authors contend, as does Haller (1970), that no cardiovascular or pulmonary impairment results from pectus excavatum. This contention contrasts, however, with the clinical impression that many patients have increased stamina or level of activity after surgical repair. These findings date back to the surgical repair performed by Sauerbruch in 1913 (1920). The patient was an 18-year-old boy who developed dyspnea and palpitations with limited exercise. Three years following his operation, he could work 12 to 14 hours a day without tiring and without palpitations. Anecdotal reports during the next three decades confirmed this observation. Over the subsequent years, the physiologic abnormality or combination of abnormalities that could explain this symptomatic improvement postoperatively have been sought. Early physiologic measurements of cardiac and pulmonary function were crude and did not yield convincing evidence of a cardiopulmonary deficit. In many early studies, the results fell within the broad range of normal values, if often at the lower limit.

A systolic ejection murmur frequently is identified in patients with pectus excavatum and is magnified by a short interval of exercise. It is attributed to the close proximity between the posterior sternal cortex and the pulmonary artery, which results in transmission of a flow murmur.

Pulmonary Function Studies

As early as 1951, Brown and Cook performed respiratory studies on patients before and after surgical repair. They demonstrated that although vital capacity was normal, the maximum breathing capacity was diminished — 50% or more — in 9 of 11 patients, and that it was increased an average of 31% after surgical repair. Weg and co-workers (1967) evaluated 25 air force recruits with pectus excavatum and compared them with 50 unselected basic trainees. Although the lung compartments of both groups were equal, as were the vital capacities, the maximum voluntary ventilation was significantly lower in those with pectus excavatum than in the control population. Castile and colleagues (1982) evaluated 7 patients with pectus excavatum, 5 of whom were symptomatic with exercise. The mean total lung capacity was 79% of predicted. Flow volume configurations were normal, excluding airway obstruction. Workload tests demonstrated normal response to exercise in the dead space to tidal volume ratio and alveolar-arterial oxygen difference. The measured oxygen uptake, however, increasingly exceeded predicted values as the workloads approached maximum in the four "symptomatic" subjects with pectus excavatum. This pattern of oxygen consumption was different than in normal subjects and the three asymptomatic subjects with pectus excavatum in whom a linear response was seen. The mean oxygen uptake in the symptomatic patients at maximal effort exceeded the predicted values by 25.4%. The three asymptomatic patients on the other hand demonstrated normal linear oxygen uptake during exercise. Increased oxygen uptake suggests increased work of breathing in these symptomatic patients despite the normal or mildly reduced vital capacities. Increases in tidal volume with exercise were uniformly depressed in those with pectus excavatum.

Cahill and co-workers (1984) performed pre- and postoperative studies in children and adolescents with pectus carinatum — 5 patients — and excavatum — 14 patients. No abnormalities were demonstrated in the pectus carinatum group. The low normal vital capacities in excavatum patients were unchanged by operation, but a small improvement in the total lung capacity and a significant improvement in the maximal voluntary ventilation were seen. Exercise tolerance improved in those with pectus excavatum following surgical correction as determined both by total exercise time and the maximal oxygen consumption. In addition, at any given workload, the excavatum patients demonstrated a lower heart rate, stable oxygen consumption, and higher minute ventilation after repair. Mead (1985) studied rib cage mobility by assessing intraabdominal pressure. Normal abdominal pressure tracings in pectus excavatum suggested normal rib cage mobility.

Blickman and colleagues (1985) assessed pulmonary function in 17 children with pectus excavatum by xenon perfusion and ventilation scintigraphy before and after surgery. Ventilation studies were abnormal in 12 children preoperatively and improved in 7 postoperatively. Perfusion scans were abnormal in 10 before repair and improved in 6 after repair. The ventilation-perfusion ratios were abnormal in 10 of the 17 children preoperatively and became normal in 6 after operation.

Electrocardiographic Findings

Electrocardiographic abnormalities are common and are attributed to the abnormal configuration of the chest wall and the displacement and rotation of the heart into the left thoracic cavity. Preoperative findings in 32 patients of Welch (1980) are shown in Table 38–3. Most significant are the cases of conduction blocks or frank arrhythmias. Patients with a history of palpitations should undergo a 24-hour Holter study as well as

Table 38–3. Electrocardiographic Findings in Pectus Excavatum*

Abnormality	Number of Patients
Right axis deviation	15
Depressed ST-T segments (2, 3, AVF)	11
Tall P waves	7
Right bundle branch block	5
Combined block	3
Left ventricular hypertrophy	4
Left atrial hypertrophy	1
Paroxysmal atrial tachycardia	1

*Noted in a group of 32 patients. *From* Welch KJ: Chest wall deformities. *In* Holder TM, Ashcraft KW: Pediatric Surgery. Philadelphia: WB Saunders, 1980.

echocardiography to identify mitral valve prolapse. Resolution of these supraventricular arrhythmias has been anecdotally reported after correction of a pectus excavatum deformity.

Deformity of the chest wall led many authors to attribute the symptomatic improvement in patients postoperatively to initial impairment in pulmonary function. This was difficult to prove, however, with the wide range of cardiopulmonary function that exists from individual to individual and is heavily dependent on physical training and body habitus.

Cardiovascular Studies

Posterior displacement of the sternum can produce a deformity of the heart, particularly anterior indentation of the right ventricle. Early pathologic studies demonstrated this finding (Fig. 38–4). Garusi and D'Ettore (1964), using angiography, showed displacement of the heart to the left side, often with a sternal imprint on the anterior wall of the right ventricle. Howard (1959) demonstrated by angiography its relief by surgical repair. Elevated right atrial and ventricular pressures have been reported by some authors, as have pressure curves similar to those seen in constrictive pericarditis. In 1962, Bevegård evaluated 16 individuals with pectus excavatum by right heart catheterization and workload studies. The physical work capacity in pectus excavatum at a given heart rate was significantly lower in sitting patients than when they were supine. Those with 20% or greater decline in physical work capacity from the supine to the sitting position had shorter sternovertebral distance than those with less decrease in their physical work capacity. The measured stroke volume at rest decreased, with a change from supine to sitting positions, by a mean of 40.3%, similar to normal subjects. In the supine position, the stroke volume increased with exercise 13.2%. In the sitting position, the increase in stroke volume from rest to exercise was 18.5% for the pectus excavatum group, significantly lower — $p < 0.001$ — than the 51% increase seen in normal subjects. Thus, increased cardiac output could be achieved primarily by increased heart rate because of the stroke volume limitations. Intracardiac pressures measured at rest and with ex-

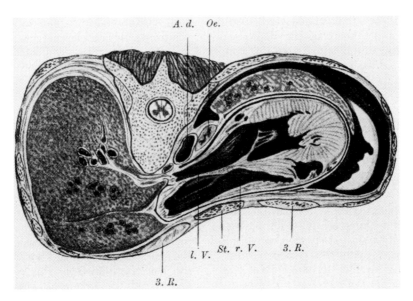

Fig. 38–4. Anatomic drawing from an autopsy of a male with pectus excavatum reported in 1912 demonstrates compression of the heart, particularly the right ventricle by the sternum. *From* Bien G: Zur Anatomie und Actiologie der Trichterbrust. Bertrage Z Pathol Anatomie Allge Pathol 52:567, 1912.

ercise were normal in all subjects despite this apparent limitation of ventricular volume. Gattiker and Bühlmann (1967) confirmed this limitation of the stroke volume in a study of 19 subjects. In upright patients, at a heart rate of 170, the physical work capacity was lower than when they were supine — mean 18% decrease — because of the decrease in stroke volume. Beiser and associates (1972) performed cardiac catheterization in six adolescents and adults with moderate degrees of pectus excavatum. Normal pressures and cardiac index were obtained at rest in the supine position. The cardiac index during moderate exercise was normal, although the response to upright exercise was below that predicted in two, and at the lower limit of normal in three. The cardiac index was 6.8 ± 0.8 L/min/m^2 compared with 8.9 ± 0.3 L/min/m^2 in a group of 16 normal control subjects — $p < 0.01$. The difference in cardiac performance again appeared to be produced primarily by a smaller stroke volume in the group with pectus excavatum in an upright position. Stroke volume was 31% lower and cardiac output was 28% lower during upright as compared with supine exercise. Postoperative studies were performed in three patients; two achieved a higher level of exercise tolerance after repair. The cardiac index was increased an average of 38%. Because heart rate at maximal exercise was not higher after repair, an enhanced stroke-volume response was responsible for this increase.

Radionuclide angiography and workload studies were performed by Peterson and associates (1985) in 13 children with pectus excavatum. Ten of 13 were able to reach the target heart rate before surgical repair, 4 without symptoms. After operation, all but 1 child reached the target heart rate during the exercise protocol and 9 of 13 reached the target without becoming symptomatic. The left and right ventricular end-diastolic volumes were consistently increased after repair at rest and the mean stroke volume was increased 19% after repair. These findings substantiated the ventricular volume changes previously demonstrated by cardiac catheterization, although an increase in the cardiac index was not demonstrated.

Wynn and colleagues (1990) reported data that conflict with earlier studies. They studied eight adolescents before and a mean of 11 months after repair of pectus excavatum and four adolescents with pectus excavatum followed without repair. A statistically significant decrease in total lung capacity was seen in the repaired group. Maximum voluntary ventilation was normal in both groups and did not change significantly with repair. The percentage of predicted work performed increased significantly in the operated group, although the maximum oxygen uptake did not change significantly following repair to explain. Also in conflict with earlier studies was the finding that maximal upright cardiac output, measured by an acetylene-helium rebreathing technique, did not change following repair, and an appropriate increase in stroke volume was noted with exercise both before and after surgical correction. Although it is difficult to rectify the conflicting results in these studies, it is probably correct to place greatest credence on the results of the earlier studies, which most directly measured the critical parameters.

Echocardiographic Studies

Bon Tempo (1975), Salomon (1975), and Schutte (1981) and their associates reported mitral valve prolapse in patients with narrow anterior-posterior chest diameters, anterior chest wall deformities, and scoliosis. Prospective echocardiographic studies in adults with pectus excavatum demonstrated mitral valve prolapse in 6 of 33 subjects — 18% — studied by Udoshi (1979) and in 11 of 17 subjects — 65% — of Saint-Mezard (1986). Anterior compression of the heart by the depressed sternum may deform the mitral annulus or the ventricular chamber and produce mitral valve prolapse in these patients. In 1987, the author and associates reported 23 children with pectus excavatum and mitral valve prolapse confirmed echocardiographically. Postoperative studies failed to demonstrate mitral valve prolapse in 10 — 43%.

Surgical Repair

The first surgical corrections of pectus excavatum were reported by Meyer in 1911 and Sauerbruch in 1920. In 1939, Oschsner and DeBakey summarized early experience with various techniques. In 1949, Ravitch reported a technique that included excision of all deformed costal cartilages with the perichondrium, division of the xiphoid from the sternum, division of the intercostal bundles from the sternum, and a transverse sternal osteotomy securing the sternum anteriorly in an overcorrected position with Kirschner wire fixation in the first two patients and silk suture fixation in later patients. Other surgeons have used internal fixation with Kirschner wires, metallic struts as described by Rehbein and Wernicke (1957), or retrosternal bars reported by Adkins and Blades (1968). No randomized studies have compared the recurrence or complication rates between suture or strut fixation. In large series, Oelsnitz (1981) and Hecker and associates (1981) reported satisfactory repairs in in 90 to 95% of patients with suture fixation.

The "sternal turnover" was first proposed by the Judets (1954) and Jung (1956) in the French literature. Wada and colleagues (1970) reported a large series from Japan in which this technique, which is essentially a free graft of sternum, was used. It is a radical approach and has been associated with major complications if infection occurs. Recent modifications of this technique by Taguchi and co-workers (1975) involved either preservation of the internal mammary vessels by wide dissection or reimplantation of the internal mammary artery. They were developed because of the reported incidence of osteonecrosis and fistula formation in up to 46% of patients over 15 years old. A final method described by Allen and Douglas (1979), which must be mentioned, is that of implantation of silastic molds into the subcutaneous space to fill the deformity. Although the contour of the chest may improve with this approach, extrusion of the molds has occurred, and this method does nothing to increase the volume of the thoracic cavity, improve respiratory mechanics, or relieve pressure on the heart.

In 1958, Welch reported a technique for the correction of pectus excavatum that emphasized total preservation of the perichondrial sheaths and the attachment of the upper sheaths and intercostal bundles to the sternum. Anterior fixation of the sternum was achieved with silk sutures. The technique I use today remains unchanged, except for increased use of strut fixation in older children, those with severe deformities in whom complete correction is difficult to achieve by

suture fixation alone, and all patients with Marfan's syndrome. This technique has the best features of the operations described by Lester (1946), Garnier (1934), and Ravitch (1949).

Surgical Technique

A transverse incision is made below and well within the nipple lines (Fig. 38–5A). In girls, particular attention is taken to place the incision within the projected inframammary crease, thus avoiding the complications of breast deformity and development described by Hougaard and Arendrup (1983). Skin flaps are mobilized by electrocautery to the angle of Louis superiorly and to the xiphoid inferiorly. Pectoral muscle flaps are elevated off the sternum and costal cartilages, preserving the entire pectoralis major and portions of the pectoralis minor and serratus anterior muscles in the flap (Fig. 33–5A). This plane is best defined by identifying the free area just anterior to the costal cartilages at their junction with the sternum. An empty knife handle is used to develop this plane and the muscle flap is then retracted anteriorly with a small right angle retractor (see Fig. 38–5B). Muscle dissection and elevation is extended laterally to the costochondral junctions of the third to fifth ribs. Particular attention is taken to avoid bleeding produced by injury to the intercostal muscles.

Subperichondrial resection of the costal cartilages with specially designed Welch pectus elevators (Codman and Shurtleff, Inc, Randolph, MA), is performed, removing the entire third, fourth, and fifth cartilages to the costochondral junctions (see Fig. 38–5C). The second costal cartilages must be removed if posterior displacement or funneling of the sternum extends to this level, as may be seen in older patients (see Fig. 38–1B). Segments of the sixth and seventh costal cartilages are resected to the point at which they flatten to join the costal arch. Familiarity with the cross-sectional shape of the medial ends of the costal cartilages facilitates their removal. The third cartilage is broad and flat, the fourth and fifth are circular, and the sixth and seventh are narrow and deep.

Two parallel transverse sternal osteotomies extending through the anterior cortex are created using a Hall air drill (Zimmer USA, Inc, Warsaw, IN). These are placed 2 to 4 mm apart (see Fig. 38–5E). The short intervening segment of anterior cortex is then removed and the underlying cancellous bone is rongeured. The attachment of the rectus muscle to the sternum is divided with electrocautery by first elevating the sternum and rectus muscles between towel clips (see Fig. 38–5F). The patient is hand ventilated with small tidal volumes to avoid injury to the pleura as the xiphoid is divided from the sternum with electrocautery, allowing entry into the areolar retrosternal space. The sixth and seventh perichondrial sheaths may be divided at their junction with the sternum if required to adequately displace the sternum forward. I have tried to omit this step if possible to avoid the unsightly depression seen below the tip of the sternum in some patients. The sternal osteotomy

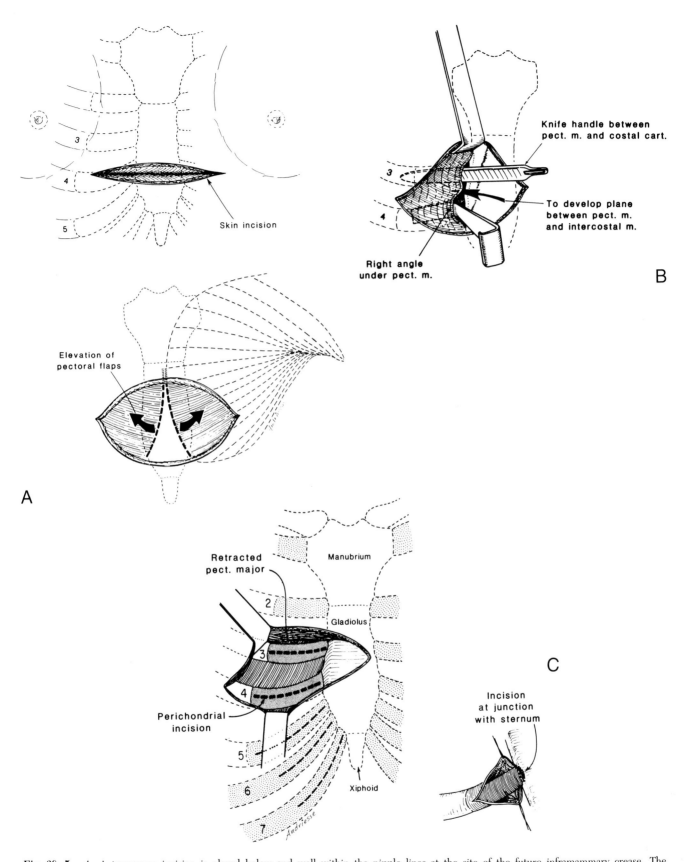

Fig. 38-5. *A*, A transverse incision is placed below and well within the nipple lines at the site of the future inframammary crease. The pectoralis major muscle is elevated from the sternum along with portions of the pectoralis minor and serratus anterior bundles. *B*, The correct plane of dissection of the pectoral muscle flap is defined by passing an empty knife handle directly anterior to a costal cartilage after the medial aspect of the muscle is elevated with electrocautery. The knife handle is then replaced with a right angle retractor, which is pulled anteriorly. The process is then repeated anterior to an adjoining costal cartilage. Anterior distraction of the muscles during the dissection facilitates identification of the avascular areolar plane and avoids entry into the intercostal muscle bundles. *C*, Subperichondrial resection of the costal cartilages is achieved by incising the perichondrium anteriorly. It is then dissected away from the costal cartilages in the bloodless plane between perichondrium and costal cartilage. Cutting back the perichondrium 90° in each direction at its junction with the sternum (inset) facilitates visualization of the back wall of the costal cartilage.

D

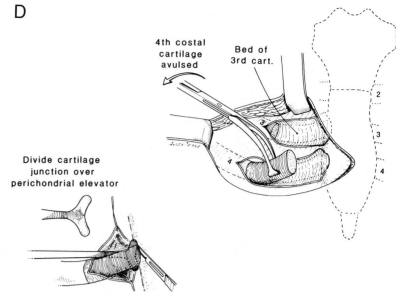

4th costal
cartilage
avulsed

Bed of
3rd cart.

2

3

4

Divide cartilage
junction over
perichondrial elevator

E

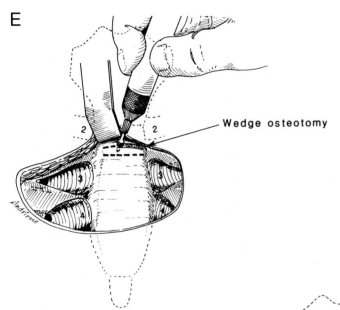

2 2

3 3

4

Wedge osteotomy

Fig. 38–5 (continued).   *D,* The cartilages are divided at the junction of the sternum with a knife with a Welch perichondrial elevator held posteriorly to elevate the cartilage and protect the mediastinum (inset). The divided cartilage can then be held with an Allis clamp, elevated, and avulsed from the costochondral junction. *E,* The sternal osteotomy is created above the level of the last deformed cartilage and the posterior angulation of the sternum, generally the third cartilage but occasionally the second. Two transverse sternal osteotomies are created, 2 to 4 mm apart, through the anterior cortex with a Hall air drill. *F,* The base of the sternum and the rectus muscle flap are elevated with two towel clips and the xiphoid is divided from the sternum with electrocautery. This step allows entry into the retrosternal space and the sixth and seventh perichondrial sheaths can be divided under direct vision, avoiding pleural entry.

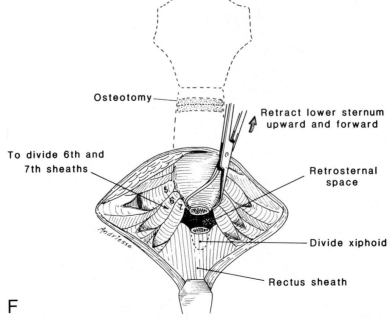

Osteotomy

Retract lower sternum
upward and forward

To divide 6th and
7th sheaths

Retrosternal
space

5
6
7

Divide xiphoid

Rectus sheath

F

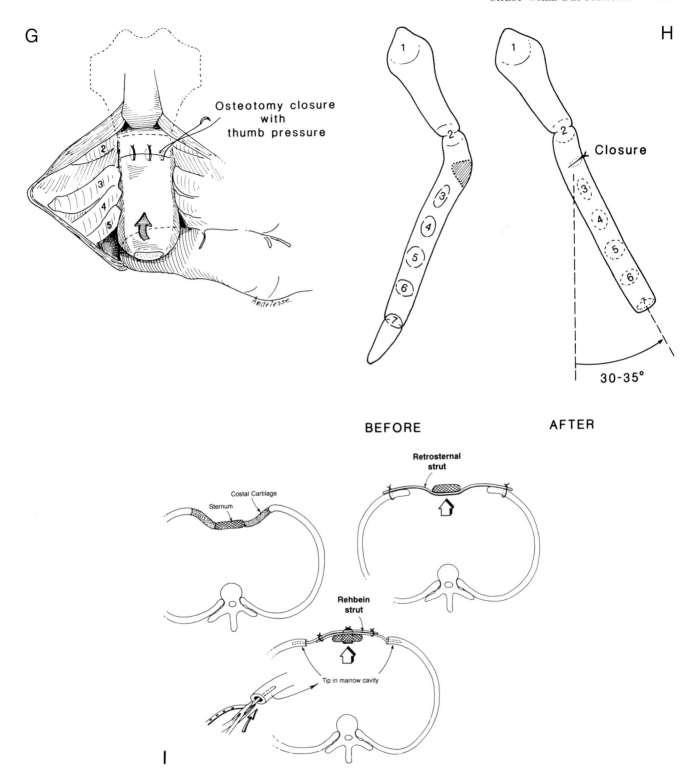

Fig. 38–5 (continued). *G,* The osteotomy is closed with several heavy silk sutures as the sternum is being elevated by the assistant. *H,* Correction of the abnormal position of the sternum is achieved by creation of a wedge-shaped osteotomy, which is then closed, bringing the sternum anteriorly into an overcorrected position. *I,* This figure demonstrates the use of both retrosternal struts and the Rehbein struts. The Rehbein struts are inserted into the marrow cavity (insert) of the third or fourth ribs and are then joined to each other medially to create a metal arch anterior to the sternum. The sternum is sewn to the arch to secure it in its new forward position. The retrosternal strut is placed behind the sternum and is secured to the rib ends laterally to prevent migration.

J

K

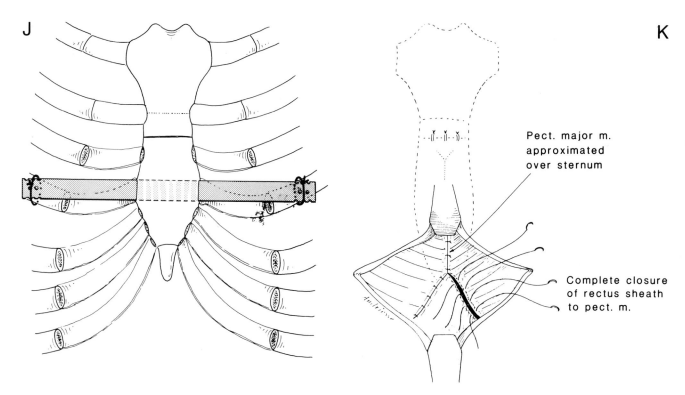

Pect. major m.
approximated
over sternum

Complete closure
of rectus sheath
to pect. m.

Fig. 38–5 (continued). *J*, Anterior depiction of the retrosternal struts. The perichondrial sheath to either the third or fourth rib is divided from its junction with the sternum, and the retrosternal space is bluntly dissected to allow passage of the strut behind the sternum. It is secured with two pericostal sutures laterally to prevent migration. *K*, The pectoral muscle flaps are secured to the midline of the sternum, advancing the flaps to obtain coverage of the entire sternum. The rectus muscle flap is then joined to the pectoral muscle flaps. *From* Shamberger RC, Welch KJ: Surgical repair of pectus excavatum. J Pediatr Surg 23:615, 1988.

is then closed with several heavy — #2 — silk sutures (see Fig. 38–5*G*), intentionally overcorrecting the position of the sternum 30 to 35° (see Fig. 38–5*H*). Alternative methods involve use of the Rehbein struts or retrosternal bars (see Fig. 38–5*I*, *J*).

The wound is then flooded with warm saline and cefazolin solution to remove clots and inspected for a pleural entry. A single limb medium Hemovac drain (Snyder Laboratories, Inc, New Philadelphia, OH) is brought through the inferior skin flap to the left of the sternum and placed in a right parasternal position to the level of the highest resected costal cartilage. The pectoral muscle flaps are then joined to the sternal periosteum in the midline, advancing the flaps inferiorly to cover the previously bare sternum (see Fig. 38–5*K*). The xiphoid is removed from the rectus muscle flap before it is joined to the sternum centrally and to the pectoral muscle flaps laterally to close the mediastinum completely. Perioperative dosage of antibiotics is one dose of cefazolin immediately before and three doses after the operation. The Hemovac drain is removed when the drainage is less than 15 ml for an 8-hour period. All patients are warned to avoid aspirin-containing compounds for 2 weeks before the procedure.

I use either Rehbein struts (Pilling Instruments, Fort Washington, PA) or the retrosternal bars (Baxter Healthcare Co., Deerfield, IL) for internal fixation,

and have not encountered complications with their use. Although correction of pectus excavatum is technically most easily performed in a young child, I have become increasingly concerned about long-term recurrence in these children. Operation is currently delayed until the children are approximately 10 years old. At this age, the chest has less remaining growth and opportunity for recurrence of the pectus excavatum. In contrast, Humphreys and Jaretzki (1980) and Backer and colleagues (1961) found no correlation between the age at repair and frequency of recurrence. Because of the great flexibility of the infant's chest, I believe that correction of pectus excavatum should be performed after 2 years of age. My colleagues and I (1988) currently repair pectus excavatum before cardiac repair in those patients who will require a Fontan procedure or other retrosternal conduit that may be compressed by the sternum. Infants who require other cardiac procedures undergo these operations before correction of their pectus excavatum.

Complications

Complications of pectus excavatum repair that the author and Welch (1988b) reported in 704 patients (Table 38–4) are few and relatively unimportant, except for major recurrence in 17 patients. In 2% of patients, a limited pneumothorax required aspiration or was simply observed. Tube thoracostomy has not been

Table 38–4. Complications of Pectus Excavatum Repair*

Pneumothorax†	11
Wound infection	5
Wound hematoma	3
Wound dehiscence	5
Pneumonia	3
Seroma	1
Hemoptysis	1
Hemopericardium	1
Major recurrence	17
Mild recurrence	23

*Seventy cases in 704 patients.

†Four patients required chest tube placement.

required in the past decade and was needed in only four patients in the entire series. Wound infection is rare with use of perioperative antibiotic coverage.

The most distressing complication following surgical correction of pectus excavatum is major recurrence of the deformity. It is difficult to predict which unfortunate patients will have a major recurrence, but it appears to occur with increased frequency in patients with poor muscular development and an asthenic or "marfanoid habitus." All patients with Marfan's syndrome should be repaired with strut fixation because of the high risk of recurrence reported without struts. Scherer and associates (1988) reported a low recurrence rate — (one of eight cases) — using a retrosternal strut.

Correction of recurrent pectus excavatum is generally a formidable task. Sanger and associates (1968) reported their experience in secondary correction. They resected the regenerated fibrocartilage plate, repeated the osteotomy, and closed the pectoral muscles behind the sternum. Ten patients had an early good result. The author's experience with 12 patients led to a consistent finding. Although recurrences appear symmetric, they are in fact frequently right sided, with a deep right parasternal gutter and sternal obliquity. The third, fourth, and fifth rib ends migrate medially with apparent "foreshortening" of the costal cartilages. Resection of the segments of the third to fifth costal cartilages is necessary to correct the deformity. After clearing the tip of the sternum, resection of the left fibrocartilage plate to the level of the third or second perichondrial sheath allows the sternum to be brought forward and rotated to an acceptable position. Repeat operations were accomplished in 10 of 12 patients without pleural entry. Followup of patients with secondary correction ranged from 10 to 17 years. Of the 12, 8 have acceptable thoracic contour, 2 have a broad shallow depression, and 2 have frank recurrence. I recommend use of strut fixation on all patients with secondary repair, as cartilage regeneration is slower and less adequate than after the primary operation.

Patients are followed to full growth — age 16 years for girls and 19 years for boys (Fig. 38–6). Use of clinical and Moiré photography reported by Shochat and as-

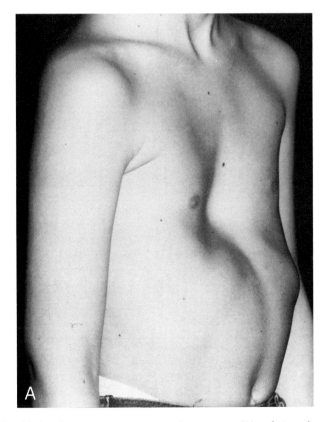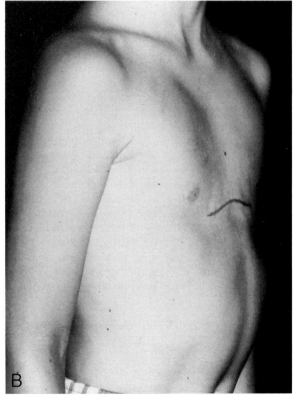

Fig. 38–6. Pectus excavatum repair. Preoperative *(A)* and 6 weeks postoperative *(B)* photographs of a 14-year-old boy.

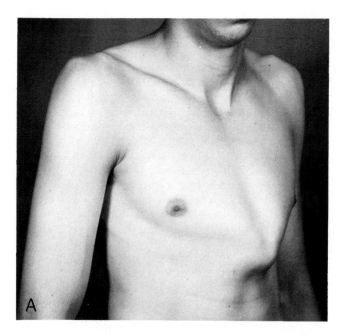

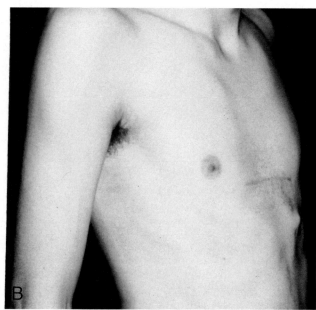

Fig. 38–7. *A*, Symmetric chondrogladiolar pectus carinatum in a 19-year-old male. *B*, Postoperative photograph shows correction of the protruding sternum and costal cartilages.

sociates (1981) for initial evaluation and followup studies leads to improved clinical assessment of results and obviates the need for multiple radiographic examinations.

PECTUS CARINATUM

Pectus carinatum or anterior protrusion of the sternum is less common than pectus excavatum — 16.7% of all chest wall deformities in our group's experience. It consists of a spectrum of abnormal thoracic development often divided into four categories (Table 38–5). The most frequent form, termed chondrogladiolar by Brodkin (1949), consists of anterior protrusion of the body of the sternum with symmetric protrusion of the lower costal cartilages. Howard (1958) described it as appearing as if a giant hand had pinched the chest from the front, forcing the sternum and medial portion of the costal cartilages forward and the lateral costal cartilages and ribs inward (Fig. 38–7). Asymmetric deformities with anterior displacement of the costal cartilages on one side and normal cartilages on the contralateral side are less common (Fig. 38–8). Mixed lesions have a carinate deformity on one side and a depression or excavatum deformity on the contralateral side, often with sternal rotation. These conditions are classified by

some authors as a variant of the excavatum deformities. The most infrequent deformity is the upper chondromanubrial or "pouter pigeon" deformity. It consists of protrusion of the manubrium and second and third costal

Table 38–5. Frequency of Pectus Carinatum Deformities

Chondrogladiolar	
Symmetric	89
Asymmetric	49
Mixed carinatum/excavatum	14
Chondromanubrial	3

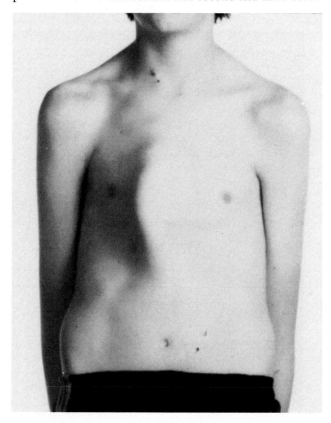

Fig. 38–8. A 12-year-old boy had asymmetric pectus carinatum with protrusion of the costal cartilages only on the right side.

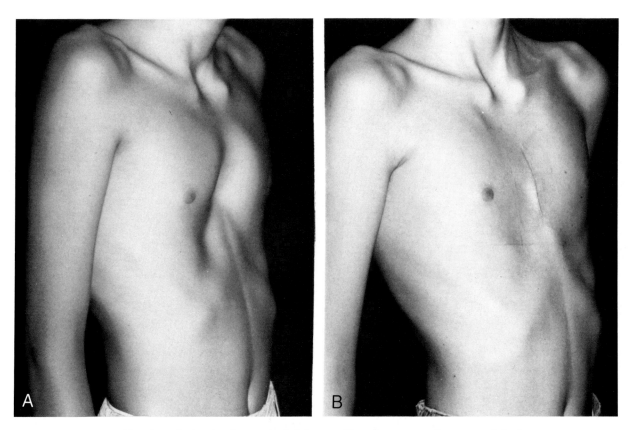

Fig. 38–9. *A,* A 15-year-old male with the chondromanubrial deformity. Note the posterior depression of the lower sternum accentuated by the anterior bowing of the second and third costal cartilages. *B,* After repair, the sternal contour is improved and costal cartilages reform in a more appropriate fashion. *From* Shamberger RC, Welch KJ: Surgical correction of chondromanubrial deformity (Currarino Silverman Syndrome). J Pediatr Surg 23:319, 1988).

cartilages with relative depression of the gladiolus or body of the sternum (Fig. 38–9).

Etiology

The etiology of pectus carinatum is no better understood than that of pectus excavatum. It appears as an overgrowth of the costal cartilages with forward buckling and anterior displacement of the sternum. Again, a clear-cut increased family incidence suggests a genetic basis. In a review of 152 patients by the author and Welch (1987), 26% had a family history of chest wall deformity. A family history of scoliosis was obtained in 12% of the patients. Pectus carinatum occurs more frequently in boys — 119; 78% — than in girls — 33; 22%. Of the associated musculoskeletal anomalies (Table 38–6), scoliosis and other deformities of the spine are most common.

Pectus carinatum usually appears in childhood, and in almost one half of the patients, the deformity was not identified until after the eleventh birthday (Fig. 38–10). The deformity may appear in mild form at birth, and often progresses, particularly during the period of rapid growth at puberty. The chondromanubrial deformity, however, in contrast with the chondrogladiolar form, is often noted at birth and is associated with a short, truncated comma-shaped sternum with absent sternal segmentation or premature obliteration of the sternal sutures (Fig. 38–11). In 1958, Currarino and Silverman described its association with an increased risk of congenital heart disease. In a retrospective review by Lees and Caldicott (1975) of 1915 radiographs, 135 children with sternal fusion anomalies were identified, of which 24 — 18% — had documented congenital heart disease.

Surgical Repair

Correction of carinate deformities has had a colorful history from the first repair by Ravitch (1952) of the upper or chondromanubrial deformity. He resected

Table 38–6. Musculoskeletal Abnormalities in Pectus Carinatum*

Scoliosis	23
Neurofibromatosis	2
Morquio's disease	2
Vertebral anomalies	1
Hyperlordosis	1
Kyphosis	1

*Identified in 30 of 152 cases.

Pectus Carinatum

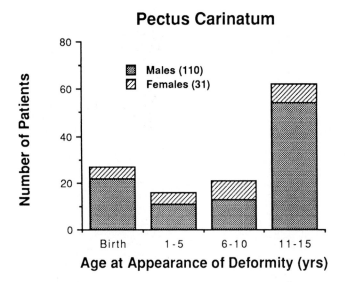

Fig. 38–10. Age at appearance of the pectus carinatum deformity in 141 infants and children. Note the appearance of protrusion in almost one half of the children at puberty.

multiple costal cartilages and performed a double sternal osteotomy. In 1953, Lester reported two methods of repair for chondrogladiolar deformity. The first involving resection of the anterior portion of the sternum was abandoned because of excessive blood loss and unsatisfactory results. The second, a no less radical technique, involved subperiosteal resection of the entire sternum. Chin (1957) and later Brodkin (1958) advanced the transected xiphoid and attached the rectus muscles to

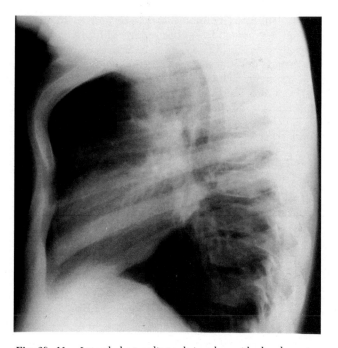

Fig. 38–11. Lateral chest radiograph in a boy with chondromanubrial pectus carinatum. The short, comma-shaped sternum lacking segmentation is apparent.

a higher site on the sternum, the xiphosternopexy. This procedure produced posterior displacement of the sternum in younger patients with a flexible chest wall. Howard (1958) combined this method with subperichondrial costal cartilage resection and a sternal osteotomy. In 1960, Ravitch reported repair of the chondrogladiolar deformity by resection of costal cartilage in a one- or two-stage procedure and "reefing" sutures to shorten and posteriorly displace the perichondrium. A sternal osteotomy was used in one of three cases. In 1963, Robicsek and colleagues reported subperichondrial resection of costal cartilages, transverse sternal osteotomy and displacement, and resection of the protruding lower portion of the sternum. The xiphoid and rectus muscles were reattached to the new lower margin of the sternum, pulling it posteriorly. In 1973, Welch and Vos reported an approach to these deformities that our group continues to use today.

Surgical Technique

The placement of the skin incision, mobilization of the pectoral muscle flaps, and subperichondrial resection of the costal cartilage are identical to the method described for pectus excavatum. Sternal osteotomies through the anterior cortex are created with the Hall drill (Zimmer USA, Inc, Warsaw, IN) to allow posterior displacement of the sternum (Fig. 38–12A). Occasionally, a second osteotomy is required. In patients with the "mixed" deformities, an oblique transverse osteotomy (see Fig. 38–12B) is used to correct both the posterior displacement and rotation of the sternum.

The upper or chondromanubrial deformity must be managed in a special manner, which the author and Welch (1988) have described. In this situation, the costal cartilages must be resected from the second cartilage inferiorly. A generous wedge osteotomy is performed at the point of maximal protrusion of the sternum generally at the level of the second costal cartilage (Fig. 38–13). The superior segment of the sternum can then be displaced posteriorly as the osteotomy is closed, advancing the inferior segment anteriorly. A single limb medium Hemovac drain (Snyder Laboratories, Inc, New Philadelphia, OH) is brought through the inferior skin flap, as with the excavatum patients, with the suction ports in a parasternal position to the level of the highest resected costal cartilage. Closure of the pectoralis muscle flaps and skin flaps and perioperative antibiotic use are as described for repair of pectus excavatum.

Operative Results

Results are overwhelmingly successful in these patients. In a review of 152 cases by the author and Welch (1987), postoperative recovery was generally uneventful. Blood transfusions are rarely required and none has been given in the last 10 years. The complication rate is 3.9% (Table 38–7). Only three patients have required revision, each having additional lower costal cartilages resected for persistent unilateral malformation of the costal arch.

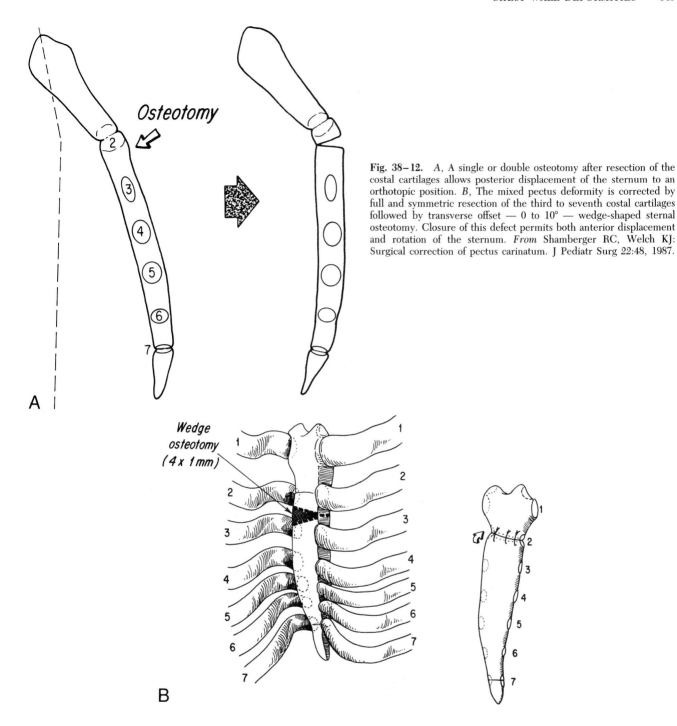

Fig. 38–12. *A,* A single or double osteotomy after resection of the costal cartilages allows posterior displacement of the sternum to an orthotopic position. *B,* The mixed pectus deformity is corrected by full and symmetric resection of the third to seventh costal cartilages followed by transverse offset — 0 to 10° — wedge-shaped sternal osteotomy. Closure of this defect permits both anterior displacement and rotation of the sternum. *From* Shamberger RC, Welch KJ: Surgical correction of pectus carinatum. J Pediatr Surg 22:48, 1987.

POLAND'S SYNDROME

In 1841, Poland described congenital absence of the pectoralis major and minor muscles, associated with syndactyly. Despite prior reports of this entity by Lallemand (1826) and Froriep (1839), it has been labeled Poland's syndrome since 1962, when Clarkson first applied this eponym to a group of these patients. This syndrome often involves the chest wall and breasts. Each of the components of the syndrome may occur with variable severity. The extent of thoracic involvement may range from hypoplasia of the sternal head of the pectoralis major and minor muscles with normal underlying ribs to complete absence of the anterior portions of the second to fifth ribs and cartilages (Fig. 38–14). Breast involvement is frequent, ranging from mild hypoplasia to complete absence of the breast — amastia — and nipple — athelia (see Fig. 38–14). Minimal subcutaneous fat and an absence of axillary hair are often found on the involved side. Hand deformities are frequent, as occurred in the patient described by Poland. They may include hypoplasia — brachydactyly — and fused fingers — syndactyly, primarily of the central three digits. The most severe expression of

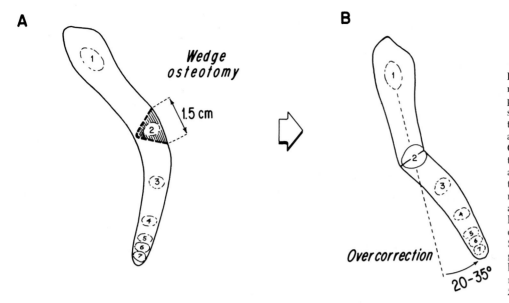

A Wedge osteotomy 1.5 cm

B Overcorrection 20-35°

Fig. 38-13. *A*, The chondromanubrial type of deformity is depicted with a broad wedge-shaped sternal osteotomy placed through the anterior cortex at the obliterated sternomanubrial junction. *B*, Closure of the osteotomy after fracture of the posterior cortex achieves posterior displacement of the superior portion of the sternum, which is secured only by its attachment to the first rib. The lower portion of the sternum is over corrected 20 to 35°. *From Shamberger RC, Welch KJ: Surgical correction of chondromanubrial deformity (Currarino Silverman Syndrome). J Pediatr Surg 23:319, 1988.*

Chondromanubrial (very rare)

the anomaly, mitten or claw deformity — ectromelia, is fortunately rare, as noted by Clarkson (1962) and Walker and associates (1969). Poland's syndrome may also occur in combination with Sprengel's deformity, in which patients have decreased size, elevation, and winging of the scapula.

Poland's syndrome is present from birth and has an estimated incidence, as reported by Freire-Maia and colleagues (1973) and by McGillivray and Lowry (1977), of 1 in 30,000 to 1 in 32,000. Abnormalities in the breast can be defined at birth by absence of the underlying breast bud and the hypoplastic, often superiorly, displaced nipple. The etiology of this syndrome is unknown. Hypoplasia of the ipsilateral subclavian artery has been proposed by Bouvet and associates (1978) as the origin of this malformation, but as suggested by David (1979), decreased blood flow to the extremity may be the consequence rather than the cause of decreased muscle mass of the hypoplastic limb. Whereas some forms of syndactyly have been described as autosomal dominant traits, a similar pattern has not been demonstrated in patients with Poland's syndrome, which generally appears to be sporadic in occurrence. Multiple cases within a family are rare, as described by Sujansky and co-workers (1977), David (1982), and Cobben (1989).

Table 38-7. Complications of Pectus Carinatum Repair*

Pneumothorax†	4
Atelectasis	1
Wound infection	1
Local tissue necrosis	1

*Noted in 7 cases in 152 patients.

†Two patients required chest tube placement.

Poland's syndrome is associated with a second rare syndrome, the Möbius syndrome, involving bilateral or unilateral facial palsy and abducens oculi palsy. Nineteen such cases were identified by Fontaine and Ovlaque (1984), but a unifying etiology is lacking. An unusual association between Poland's syndrome and childhood leukemia has also been reported by Boaz and associates (1971).

In my and my colleagues' (1989) experience with 41 children and adolescents with Poland's syndrome evaluated from 1970 to 1987, 21 were boys. The lesion was right sided in 23, left sided in 17, and bilateral in 1. Hand anomalies were noted in 23 — 56% — and breast anomalies were present in 25 — 61%. In 10 children, the underlying thoracic abnormality required reconstruction, and in three cases, rib or cartilage grafts were needed for complete repair.

Surgical Repair

Assessment of the extent of involvement of the various musculoskeletal components is critical for optimal thoracic reconstruction. If involvement is limited to absence or hypoplasia of the sternal component of the pectoralis major and minor muscles, the functional deficit is minimal and repair is not necessary, except for breast augmentation in females at full growth (Fig. 38-15). If the underlying costal cartilages are depressed or absent, then repair must be considered to minimize the concavity, to eliminate the paradoxic motion of the chest wall if ribs are absent, and, in girls, to provide an optimal base for breast reconstruction. Ravitch (1966) reported correction of posteriorly displaced costal cartilages by unilateral resection of the cartilages, a wedge osteotomy of the sternum allowing rotation of the

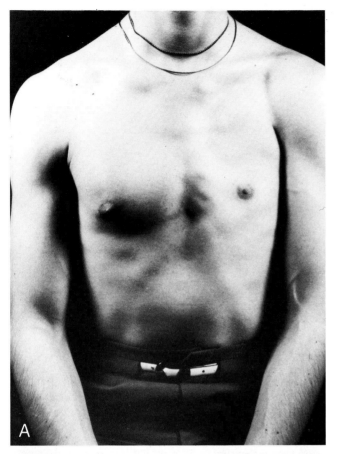

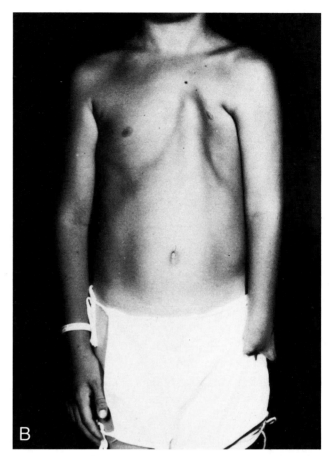

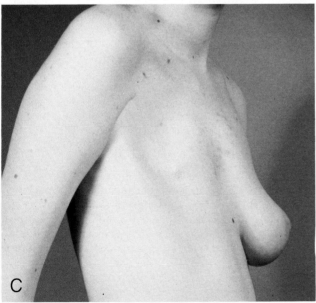

Fig. 38–14. Muscular 15-year-old boy with loss of the left axillary fold, orthotopic sternum, and normal cartilages. He compensates adequately for loss of the pectoralis major and minor muscles. Surgery is not indicated in males with these findings. *B*, Eight-year-old boy with Poland's syndrome. The pectoralis major and minor muscles and the serratus to the level of the fifth rib are absent. The boy has sternal obliquity and the third to fifth ribs are short, ending in points. The corresponding cartilages are absent. The endothoracic fascia lies beneath a thin layer of subcutaneous tissue. Note the hypoplastic nipple and ectromelia of the ipsilateral hand. *C*, Fourteen-year-old girl with Poland's syndrome. Note the high position of the right nipple, amastia, sternal rotation, and depressed right anterior chest. The second to fourth ribs and cartilages were missing, reconstructed with rib grafts. Breast augmentation will be required at full growth.

sternum, and fixation with Rehbein struts and Steinmann pins. Our group has found suitable repair can be achieved in most cases with bilateral costal cartilage resection and an oblique osteotomy, as in the patients with mixed pectus carinatum/excavatum deformity, which allows correction of the rotational deformity (Fig. 38–16). The sternum is then displaced anteriorly, allowing correction of the posteriorly displaced costal cartilages. An unappreciated carinate deformity is often present on the contralateral side that accentuates the ipsilateral concavity (see Fig. 38–15B).

Absence of the medial portion of the ribs can be managed with split rib grafts taken from the contralateral side. These grafts must be secured to the sternum

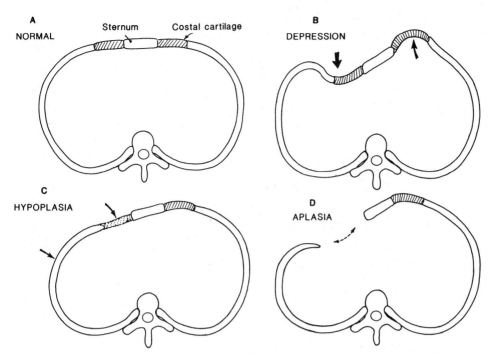

Fig. 38–15. *A,* The spectrum of rib cage abnormality seen in Poland's syndrome is shown. Most frequently, an entirely normal rib cage is seen with only absent pectoral muscles. *B,* Depression of the involved side of the chest wall with rotation and often depression of the sternum. A carinate protrusion of the contralateral side is frequently present. *C,* Hypoplasia of ribs on the involved side but without significant depression may be seen. It usually does not require surgical correction. *D,* Aplasia of one or more ribs is usually associated with depression of adjacent ribs on the involved side and rotation of the sternum.

medially and to the "dagger point" hypoplastic rib ends laterally. The grafts can be covered with a prosthetic mesh if needed for further support. In these cases, it must be remembered that little tissue is present between the endothoracic fascia and the fascial remnants of the pectoral muscles. Coverage of the area can also be augmented with transfer of a latissimus dorsi muscle flap, particularly helpful in girls who will require breast augmentation, as described by Ohmori and Takada (1980) and Haller and associates (1984). It is seldom, if ever, required in boys and has the disadvantage of adding a second posterior thoracic scar and decreasing the strength of the latissimus dorsi muscle.

STERNAL CLEFTS

Sternal defects are rare compared with pectus excavatum and carinatum, yet they have received a great deal of attention in the medical literature because of their dramatic presentation and potentially fatal outcome. Entities involving failure of ventral fusion of the sternum can be divided into three groups: 1) sternal clefts, 2) thoracic ectopia cordis, and 3) thoracoabdominal ectopia cordis.

Cleft Sternum

An infant with cleft sternum has a complete or partial separation of the sternum but a normally positioned intrathoracic heart. This deformity results from failure of fusion of the sternal bars that should occur about the eighth week of gestation. In all such cases, despite the sternal separation, normal skin coverage is present, with an intact pericardium and a normal diaphragm. Omphaloceles do not occur in these patients. The condition causes few functional difficulties. A dramatic increase in the deformity occurs with crying or a Valsalva maneuver. The sternal defects described by the author and Welch (1990) in 109 cases are summarized in Table 38–8. The cleft almost invariably involves the upper sternum, whereas patients with thoracic or thoracoabdominal ectopia cordis have clefts primarily of the lower sternum.

The second distinction between the patients with cleft sternum and those with ectopia cordis is that patients with cleft sternum rarely have intrinsic congenital heart disease. An unexplained association does exist, however, between cleft sternum and cervicofacial hemangiomas, which have been reported in 14 cases since the first description of this association in 1879.

Surgical Repair

Maier and Bortone accomplished the first primary repair in 1949 in a 6-week-old infant. This correction is feasible because the flexibility of the newborn chest allows approximation of the sternum without cardiac compression (Fig. 38–17). A summary of the reported repairs for cleft sternum in 69 cases is shown in Table 38–9.

Reconstruction of cleft sternum using multiple oblique chondrotomies was reported by Sabiston (1958). The chondrotomies increase chest wall dimensions and flexibility. The technique is still useful in older infants and children with a less flexible chest and a widening defect. Meissner (1964) described a variation in which the cartilages are divided laterally and swung medially to cover the defect. Autologous grafts of costal cartilage, split ribs, and segments of the costal arch have been used since Burton (1947) first repaired this defect with

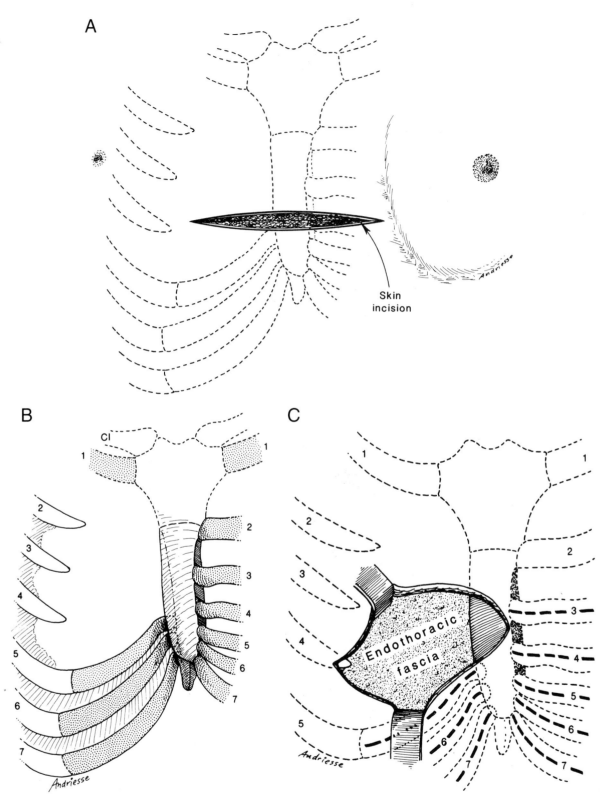

Fig. 38–16. *A*, A transverse incision is placed below the nipple lines and in females in the site of the future inframammary crease. *B*, Schematic depiction of the deformity with rotation of the sternum, depression of the cartilages of the involved side, and carinate protrusion of the contralateral side. *C*, In patients with aplasia of the ribs, the endothoracic fascia is encountered directly below the attentuated subcutaneous tissue and pectoral fascia. The pectoral muscle flap is elevated on the contralateral side and the pectoral fascia, if present on the involved side. Subperichondrial resection of the costal cartilages is then carried out as shown by the dashed line. Rarely, resection must be carried to the level of the second costal cartilage.

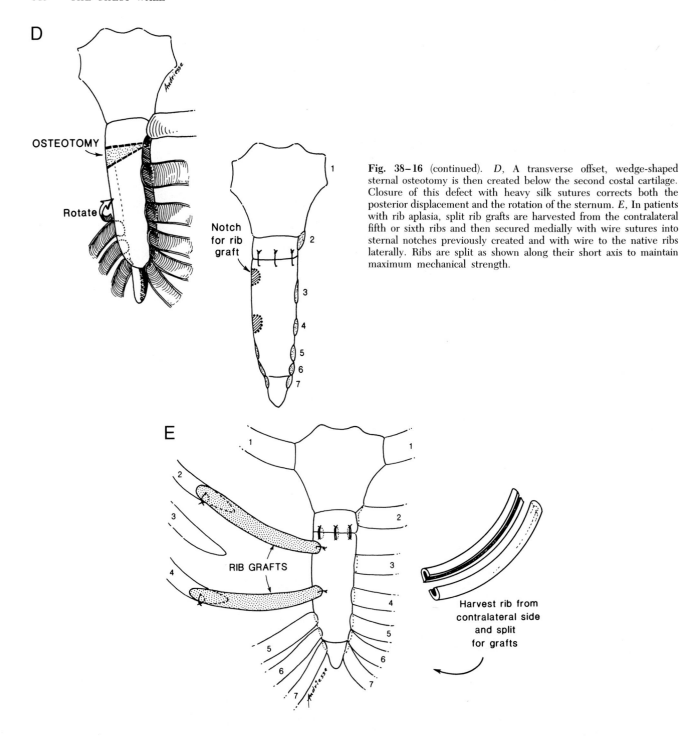

Fig. 38–16 (continued). *D*, A transverse offset, wedge-shaped sternal osteotomy is then created below the second costal cartilage. Closure of this defect with heavy silk sutures corrects both the posterior displacement and the rotation of the sternum. *E*, In patients with rib aplasia, split rib grafts are harvested from the contralateral fifth or sixth ribs and then secured medially with wire sutures into sternal notches previously created and with wire to the native ribs laterally. Ribs are split as shown along their short axis to maintain maximum mechanical strength.

a portion of the costal arch. Repairs with prosthetic material are far less satisfactory because of the risks of infection and inability of these tissues to grow with the patient. Most authors recommend treatment of cleft sternum in the newborn period when simple direct closure is possible without the use of prosthetic materials or grafts.

Ectopia Cordis

Although successful treatment of isolated cleft sternum exists, surgical treatment of ectopia cordis, par-

ticularly thoracic ectopia cordis, has a high mortality rate. The lethal factor in thoracic ectopia cordis, the so-called naked heart, and in thoracoabdominal ectopia cordis, the Cantrell pentalogy, described by Cantrell and associates (1958), is the high incidence of major intrinsic congenital heart disease.

Etiology

The etiology of thoracic ectopia cordis and thoracoabdominal ectopia cordis is much debated. Higginbottom (1975), Opitz (1985), Hersh (1985), Kaplan (1985),

Table 38–8. Sternal Defects Reported in Cleft Sternum

Upper cleft	46
Upper cleft to xiphoid	33
Complete cleft	23
Lower defect with manubrium or middle segment intact	5
Central defect with manubrium and xiphoid intact	2
Skin ulceration noted in only 3 cases	

Table 38–9. Methods of Repair of Cleft Sternum

Primary approximation and repair	25
Primary repair with sliding chondrotomies (Sabiston)	19
Primary repair with rotating chondrotomies (Meissner)	3
Primary repair with other chondrotomy	4
Bone or cartilage graft	8
Prosthetic mesh graft	4
Sternocleidomastoid muscle transposition	3
Transposition of local soft tissues	2
Skin closure with excision of ulcer	1

and their colleagues consider these conditions to result from disruption of the amnion and possibly disruption of the chorionic layer or yolk sac as well. This disruption occurs during the third or fourth week of gestation at a time when cardiac chamber formation is occurring rapidly. This timing may account for the high incidence

of abnormal cardiac development. Von Praagh (personal communication, 1987) has the intriguing notion, based on embryologic studies by Patton (1946) and Bremer (1939), that acute hyperflexion of the craniocervical segment of the embryo pins the heart down in the

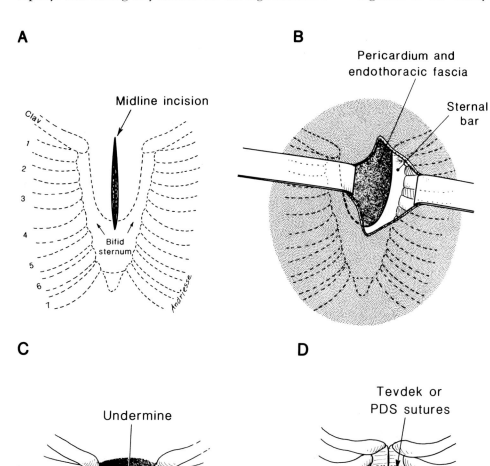

A Midline incision

Clav

1

2

3

4

5

6

7

Bifid sternum

Andriesse

B Pericardium and endothoracic fascia

Sternal bar

C Undermine

± wedge

D Tevdek or PDS sutures

Andriesse

Fig. 38–17. *A,* Repair of bifid sternum is best performed through a longitudinal incision extending the length of the defect. *B,* Directly beneath the subcutaneous tissues, the sternal bars are encountered with pectoral muscles present lateral to the bars. The endothoracic fascia and pericardium are just below these structures. *C,* The endothoracic fascia is mobilized off the sternal bars posteriorly with blunt dissection to allow safe placement of the sutures. Approximation of the sternal bars may be facilitated by excising a wedge of cartilage inferiorly. *D,* Closure of the defect is achieved with a 2-O Tevdek or PDS sutures.

extrathoracic position with the submental cardiac apex. The abnormal fetal configuration produced by oligohydramnios may persist to delivery and oppose traction by the gubernaculum cordis, which normally pulls the cardiac apex into caudal alignment, tying it to the supraumbilical raphe. Chromosomal abnormalities have been reported by Say and Wilsey (1978), King (1980), and Stoll (1986), who also commented on the supraumbilical raphe and gubernaculum cordis.

Thoracic Ectopic Cordis

Thoracic ectopia cordis is one of the most dramatic occurrences in the delivery room (Fig. 38–18). The naked beating heart is external to the thorax. Clearly visible are the atrial appendages, chamber orientation, coronary vasculature, and cephalic orientation of the cardiac apex. The gubernaculum cordis initially extends to the supraumbilical raphe. Thoracic ectopia cordis was first reported by Stenson (1671). This account was later translated by Willius (1948). Stenson identified the four components of the tetralogy of Fallot in this patient with thoracic ectopia cordis, such is the fate of eponyms. Cardiac anomalies are unusually frequent in patients with thoracic ectopia cordis. Table 38–10 is a list of the cardiac anomalies reported to 1990, as reviewed by the author and Welch. Only 4 of 75 patients had no intrinsic cardiac anomalies.

A severe lack of midline somatic tissues is present in these patients, and many attempts at primary closure have failed. Computed tomographic evaluation by Haynor and associates (1984) showed reduced intrathoracic volume in these infants. Regretably, most alleged successes have not been in individuals with true thoracic ectopia cordis but rather in those with thoracoabdominal ectopia cordis. Cutler and Wilens first attempted repair in 1925 by skin flap coverage, but failed because of cessation of cardiac function, presumably from compression of the heart. Only three reported survivors in over 29 attempts have been recorded (Table 38–11).

Table 38–10. Intrinsic Cardiac Lesions Reported in Thoracic Ectopia Cordis

Tetralogy of Fallot	16
Pulmonary artery stenosis	6
Transposition of great arteries and pulmonary artery stenosis or atresia	8
Patent ductus arteriosus (PDA)	2
Tricuspid and pulmonary atresia	3
Ventricular septal defect (VSD), atrial septal defect (ASD)	6
VSD	5
ASD, PDA	4
ASD	1
Truncus arteriosus	3
Coarctation, ASD, PDA	1
Coarctation	1
Aortic hypoplasia	1
Double outlet left ventricle	2
Double outlet right ventricle	2
Aortic stenosis, ASD, PDA	1
Single atrium, single ventricle	3
Double atrium, single ventricle	3
Cor triatriatum	1
Aberrant right subclavian artery	1
Bilateral superior vena cava*	1
Normal	4

*Also present in association with many of the listed anomalies.

The first successful repair of ectopia cordis was achieved by Koop in 1975 and reported by Saxena (1976). An infant with a normal heart had skin flap coverage at 5 hours of age with inferior mobilization of the anterior attachments of the diaphragm. The sternal bands were 2 inches apart and could not be approximated primarily without cardiac compression and compromise. At 7 months of age, an acrylic resin of Dacron and Marlex mesh was inserted to close the sternal cleft, followed by primary skin closure. Necrosis of the skin flaps complicated the postoperative course with infection of the prosthetic material and its subsequent removal. This child survived to age 12 years and is reported to

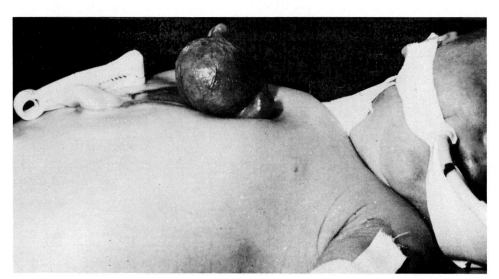

Fig. 38–18. Thoracic ectopia cordis in a high central position. The cardiac apex is cephalad. Any movement of the heart resulted in bradycardia and arrest. The patient had severe aortic overriding and complex tetralogy of Fallot. No significant abdominal wall defect was present.

Table 38–11. Reported Survivors of Thoracic Ectopia Cordis and Their Repair

Authors	Year	Cardiac Lesion	Method of Sternal Closure
Koop and Saxena	1975	None	Skin flap closure at 5 hours. Acrylic resin applied to sternal cleft at 7 months.
Dobell	1986	None	Perinatal skin closure in one stage. Second stage repair with rib grafts.
Amato, Cotroneo, and Gladieri	1988	None	Skin flaps mobilized, diaphragm moved inferiorly, Gortex* membrane used to close defect with skin flaps over it. Child survived but died of aspiration at 11 months of age.

*Gortex, W.L. Gore & Associates Inc., Flagstaff, AZ.

be entirely well. Success in two other patients has been reported. A case of Dobell and associates (1982) is of note in that surgical correction was also performed in two stages. Skin flap coverage was provided as a newborn. At 19 months of age, rib strut grafts were placed over the sternal defect and covered with pectoral muscle flaps. The pericardium was divided from its anterior attachments to the chest wall, allowing the heart to fall back partially into the thoracic cavity. Only in the case reported by Amato and colleagues (1988) was complete coverage achieved in one stage. The unifying theme of successfully managed cases is construction of a partial anterior chest cavity surrounding the heart and avoidance of attempts to return the heart to an orthotopic location. Of note, in the successful cases, intrinsic cardiac lesions and associated abdominal defects were absent. These characteristics do more to distinguish the successful cases from the failures than any differences in surgical techniques. Coverage of the heart with autologous tissues, whether by flap rotation or

bipedical flaps, generally produces excessive compression on the heart, limiting cardiac output either by kinking outflow vessels or impeding cardiac filling. In most instances, attempts are abandoned in the operating room because of severe cardiac impairment. When repair involves the use of autologous tissue grafts — bone or cartilage — or synthetic materials, infection and extrusion of the graft invariably occurs. Ultimate success with this lesion is achieved only by accomplishing tissue coverage of the heart, avoiding posterior displacement into an already limited thoracic space, which requires use of tissues from sites distant from the chest wall. Severe intracardiac defects associated with thoracic ectopia cordis in most cases also limit ultimate survival. Regrettably, as recorded by Kragt (1985) and Mercer (1983) and their associates, the only recent advancement in management of this lesion has been early ultrasonographic diagnosis, including definition of the intracardiac lesions and termination of the pregnancy if acceptable to the parents.

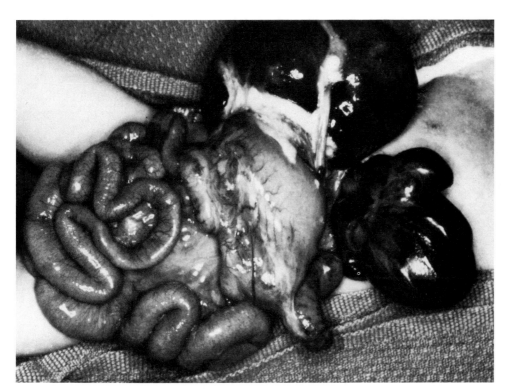

Fig. 38–19. Infant with thoracic ectopia cordis and eventration of the abdominal viscera.

Table 38–12. Abdominal Wall Defects Reported in Thoracic Ectopia Cordis

Omphalocele	36
Diastasis recti (or ventral hernia)*	6
Eventration	4

*Often covered by thin pigmented dermis.

Upper abdominal defects are also frequent in these patients, including an upper abdominal omphalocele or diastasis recti and, rarely, eventration of the abdominal viscera (Fig. 38–19). Associated abdominal defects are summarized in Table 38–12. The presence of abdominal defects should not, however, lead to these lesions being classified as thoracoabdominal ectopia cordis, a designation reserved for those infants in whom the heart is covered at birth.

Thoracoabdominal Ectopia Cordis — Cantrell's Pentalogy

In this group of patients, the heart is covered by a membrane or thin, often pigmented skin with an inferiorly cleft sternum. The heart lacks the severe anterior rotation present in thoracic ectopia cordis. An

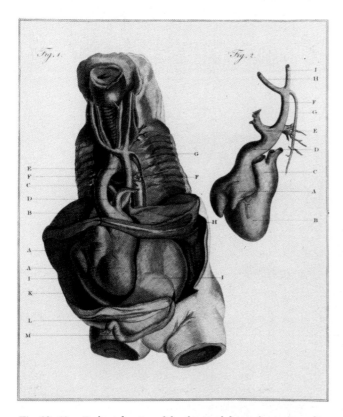

Fig. 38–20. Earliest drawing of the thoracoabdominal ectopia cordis clearly demonstrating the anterior semilunar diaphragmatic and pericardial defects allowing abdominal displacement of the heart. The cardiac defect was a single atrium and single ventricle — cor biloculare with truncus arteriosus. An omphalocele was found as well but is not shown. *From* Wilson J: A description of a very unusual formation of the human heart. Philos Trans R Soc Lond *11*:346, 1798.

Table 38–13. Abdominal Wall Defects Reported in Thoracoabdominal Ectopia Cordis

Omphalocele	64
Diastasis recti (or ventral hernia)	40
Diaphragmatic defect	71
Pericardial defect	46

early report of this lesion by Wilson in 1798 clearly defined the associated somatic defects of the abdominal wall, diaphragm, and pericardium, as shown in Figure 38–20, as well as the intrinsic cardiac anomalies. This group was reviewed by Major (1953) and by Cantrell and co-workers (1958). The five essential features of thoracoabdominal ectopia cordis, now frequently called Cantrell's pentalogy, although described long before their relatively recent review, are a cleft lower sternum; a half-moon anterior diaphragmatic defect resulting from failure of development of the septum transversum; absence of the parietal pericardium; associated adjacent or completely separate omphalocele (Table 38–13); and, in most patients, a major form of congenital heart disease (Table 38–14) (Fig. 38–21). Left ventricular diverticulum occurs with surprising frequency in patients with this anomaly. In many cases, the diverticulum protrudes through the diaphragmatic and pericardial defects, entering the abdominal cavity.

Table 38–14. Intrinsic Cardiac Lesions Reported in Thoracoabdominal Ectopia Cordis

Tetralogy of Fallot	13
Tetralogy of Fallot and diverticulum of left ventricle	1
Diverticulum of left ventricle	16
Diverticulum of left ventricle and ventricular septal defect (VSD)	9
Diverticulum of left ventricle, pulmonary stenosis, VSD	1
Diverticulum of left ventricle, atrial septal defect (ASD)	1
Diverticulum of left ventricle, ASD, VSD	1
Diverticulum of left ventricle, VSD, mitral stenosis	1
Diverticulum left ventricule, hypoplastic left ventricle, VSD	1
VSD	8
VSD, ASD	2
VSD, single atrium	1
ASD	3
ASD, VSD, total anomalous pulmonary venous connection	1
Truncus arteriosus	5
Single atrium, single ventricle	5
Pulmonary atresia, single ventricle	2
Pulmonary atresia, VSD, patient ductus arteriosus	1
Pulmonary stenosis, VSD	3
Tricuspid atresia	4
Double outlet left ventricle	2
Double outlet right ventricle	2
Transposition great arteries, mitral atresia, pulmonary artery hypoplasia	1
Transposition great arteries, pulmonary artery stenosis	2
Transposition great arteries, VSD	1
Aortic stenosis, ASD, VSD	1
Bilateral superior vena cava*	1
Normal	5

*Also present in association with many of the listed anomalies.

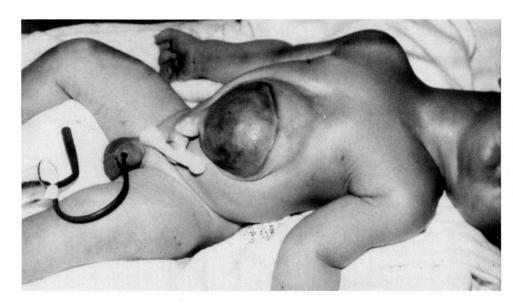

Fig. 38–21. Newborn male with thoracoabdominal ectopia cordis. Note flaring of the lower sternal area merging with a large epigastric omphalocele. The septum transversum and the inferior portion of the pericardium were absent. Tetralogy of Fallot was present.

Successful repair and long-term survival is more frequent in thoracoabdominal ectopia cordis than in thoracic ectopia cordis. Arndt attempted the first repair in 1896, but return of the heart to the thoracic cavity resulted in death. The first successful surgical repair was performed in 1912 by Wieting, who achieved primary closure of the diaphragm and abdominal wall fascia but ignored the ventricular diverticulum. Initial surgical intervention must address the skin defects overlying the heart and abdominal cavity. Primary excision of the omphalocele with skin closure avoids infection and mediastinitis, although several cases have been successfully managed by local application of topical astringents, allowing secondary epithelialization to occur. Several early cases, as in that of Cullerier (1806), document the long-term viability of individuals with thoracoabdominal ectopia cordis with intact skin coverage despite the abnormal location of the heart.

Advances in pediatric cardiac surgery now allow correction of the intrinsic cardiac lesions that were previously fatal. An aggressive approach to these lesions is appropriate. Repair of the abdominal wall defect or diastasis has been achieved by primary closure or prosthetic mesh (Table 38–15). Primary closure may be difficult because of the wide separation of the rectus muscles and their superior attachment to the splayed costal arches. Complete repair of the intracardiac defect is best performed before placement of prosthetic mesh overlying the heart. Complete parietal repair once skin coverage is achieved is important, primarily for mechanical protection of the heart. Early diagnosis by prenatal sonography has not altered the surgical approach or overall mortality of this lesion. Three patients in the series reported by the author and Welch (1990) had severe pulmonary hypoplasia, which was lethal in two. This occurrence has not been reported previously.

Table 38–15. Reported Methods of Repair in Thoracoabdominal Ectopia Cordis

Primary closure of diaphragm and abdominal wall defect	8
Primary closure of skin only and excision of omphalocele	7
Primary closure of diaphragm	4
Primary closure of abdominal wall defect	2
Coverage of abdominal defect with silastic pouch and secondary epithelialization	3
Resection of lower ribs and sternum to increase room in chest with inferior attachment of diaphragm and primary skin coverage	1
Staged repair with initial skin closure with secondary prosthetic mesh closure of the abdominal and thoracic defect	1
Staged repair with initial skin closure with secondary closure of abdominal wall and diaphragm	1

THORACIC DEFORMITIES IN DIFFUSE SKELETAL DISORDERS

Asphyxiating Thoracic Dystrophy — Jeune's Disease

In 1954, Jeune and colleagues described a newborn with a narrow rigid chest and multiple cartilage anomalies. The patient died early in the perinatal period because of respiratory insufficiency. Subsequent authors have further characterized this form of osteochondrodystrophy, which has variable skeletal involvement. It is inherited in an autosomal recessive pattern and is not associated with chromosomal abnormalities. Its most prominent feature is a narrow, "bell-shaped" thorax and protuberant abdomen. The thorax is narrow in both the transverse and sagittal axes and has little respiratory motion because of the horizontal direction of the ribs (Fig. 38–22). The ribs are short and wide and the splayed costochondral junctions barely reach the anterior axillary line. The costal cartilage is abundant and irregular like a rachitic rosary. Microscopic examination

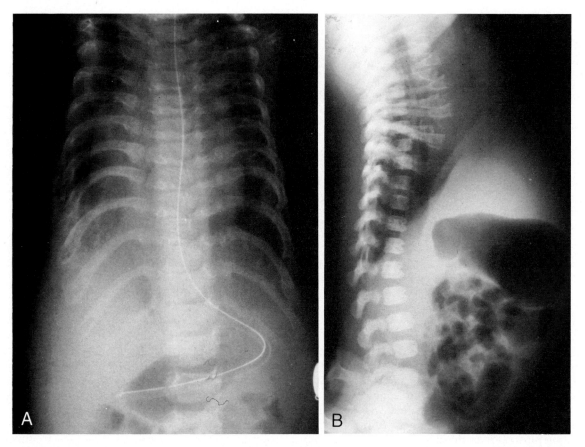

Fig. 38–22. Jeune's disease — asphyxiating thoracic dystrophy. *A*, Anterioposterior radiograph shows the short horizontal ribs and narrow chest. *B*, Lateral radiograph demonstrates the short rib ends at the midaxillary line and abnormal flaring at the costochondral junctions. The patient died of progressive respiratory insufficiency at 1 month of age. No surgical intervention occurred. Postmortem examination revealed alveolar hypoplasia.

of the costochondral junction reveals disordered and poorly progressing endochondral ossification resulting in decreased rib length.

Associated skeletal abnormalities that occur with this syndrome include short stubby extremities with relatively short and wide bones. The clavicles are in a fixed and elevated position and the pelvis is small and hypoplastic with square iliac bones.

The syndrome has variable expression and degree of pulmonary impairment. Although the initial cases reported resulted in neonatal deaths, subsequent reports by Kozlowski and Masel (1976) and others documented a wide range of survival of patients with this syndrome. The pathologic findings in autopsy cases are variable, showing a range of abnormal pulmonary development. In most cases, however, the bronchial development is normal with fewer alveolar divisions, as described by Williams and associates (1984).

Spondylothoracic Dysplasia — Jarcho-Levin Syndrome

Spondylothoracic dysplasia is an autosomal recessive deformity described by Jarcho and Levin in 1938 that is associated with multiple vertebral and rib malfor-

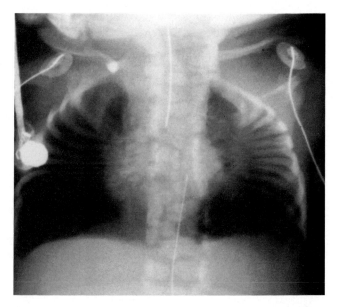

Fig. 38–23. Chest radiograph of an infant with spondylothoracic dysplasia. Severe abnormality of the spine is apparent with multiple alternating hemivertebrae and the "crab-like" ribs.

mations. Death often occurs in early infancy from respiratory failure and pneumonia. Patients have multiple alternating hemivertebrae that affect most if not all of the thoracic and lumbar spine. The vertebral ossification centers rarely cross the midline. Multiple posterior fusions of the ribs as well as remarkable shortening of the thoracic spine result in a "crablike" radiographic appearance of the chest (Fig. 38–23). One third of patients with this syndrome have associated malformations, including congenital heart disease and renal anomalies. Its occurrence has been reported by Heilbronner and Renshaw (1984) primarily in Puerto Rican families — 15 of the 18 reported cases. Bone formation is normal in these patients.

Thoracic deformity is really secondary to the spine anomaly, which results in close posterior approximation of the origin of the ribs. Although most infants with the entity succumb before 15 months of age, as reviewed by Roberts and colleagues (1988), no surgical efforts have been proposed or attempted.

REFERENCES

Pectus Excavatum

Adkins PC, Blades B: A stainless steel strut for correction of pectus excavatum. Surg Gynecol Obstet 113:111, 1968.

Allen RG, Douglas M: Cosmetic improvement of thoracic wall defects using a rapid setting silastic mold: A special technique. J Pediatr Surg 14:745, 1979.

Backer OG, Brünner S, Larsen V: The surgical treatment of funnel chest: Initial and follow-up results. Acta Chir Scand 121:253, 1961.

Beiser GD, et al: Impairment of cardiac function in patients with pectus excavatum, with improvement after operative correction. N Engl J Med 287:267, 1972.

Bevegård S: Postural circulatory changes at rest and during exercise in patients with funnel chest, with special reference to factors affecting the stroke volume. Acta Med Scand 171:695, 1972.

Blickman JG, et al: Pectus excavatum in children: Pulmonary scintigraphy before and after corrective surgery. Radiology 156:781, 1985.

Bon Tempo CP, et al: Radiographic appearance of the thorax in systolic click-late systolic murmur syndrome. Am J Cardiol 236:27, 1975.

Brown AL, Cook O: Cardiorespiratory studies in pre and postoperative funnel chest (pectus excavatum). Dis Chest 20:378, 1951.

Cahill JL, Lees GM, Robertson HT: A summary of preoperative and postoperative cardiorespiratory performance in patients undergoing pectus excavatum and carinatum repair. J Pediatr Surg 19:430, 1984.

Castile RG, Staats BA, Westbrook PR: Symptomatic pectus deformities of the chest. Am Rev Respir Dis 126:564, 1982.

Evans W: The heart in sternal depression. Br Heart J 8:162, 1946.

Garnier C: Traitement chirurgical du thorax en entonnoir. Rev Orthop 21:385, 1934.

Garusi GF, D'Ettorre A: Angiocardiographic patterns in funnel-chest. Cardiologia 45:312, 1964.

Gattiker H, Bühlmann A: Cardiopulmonary function and exercise tolerance in supine and sitting position in patients with pectus excavatum. Helv Med Acta 33:122, 1967.

Grieg JD, Azmy AF: Thoracic cage deformity: A late complication following repair of an agenesis of diaphragm. J Pediatr Surg 25:1234, 1990.

Haller JA, et al: Pectus excavatum: A 20-year surgical experience. J Thorac Cardiovasc Surg 60:375, 1970.

Hecker WC, Procher G, Dietz HG: Results of operative correction of pigeon and funnel chest following a modified procedure of Ravitch and Haller. Z Kinderchir 34:220, 1981.

Hougaard K, Arendrup H: Deformities of the female breasts after surgery for funnel chest. Scand J Thorac Cardiovasc Surg 17:171, 1983.

Howard R: Funnel chest: Its effect on cardiac function. Arch Dis Child 32:5, 1959.

Hümmer HP, Willital GH: Morphologic findings of chest deformities in children corresponding to the Willital-Hümmer classification. J Pediatr Surg 19:562, 1984.

Humphreys II GH, Jaretzki III A: Pectus excavatum: Late results with and without operation. J Thorac Cardiovasc Surg 80:686, 1980.

Judet J, Judet R: Thorax en entonnoir. Un procédé opératoire. Rev Orthop 40:248, 1954.

Jung A: Le traitement du thorax en entonnoir par le "retournement pédiculé" de la cuvette sterno-chondrale. Mém Acad Chir 82:242, 1956.

Lester CW: The surgical treatment of funnel chest. Ann Surg 123:1003, 1946.

Lester CW: The etiology and pathogenesis of funnel chest, pigeon breast, and related deformities of the anterior chest wall. J Thorac Surg 34:1, 1957.

Mead J, et al: Rib cage mobility in pectus excavatum. Am Rev Respir Dis 132:1223, 1985.

Meyer L: Zur chirurgischen behandlung der angeborenen trichterbrust. Verh Berl Med Ges 42:364, 1911.

Ochsner A, DeBakey M: Chone-chondrosternon: Report of a case and review of the literature. J Thorac Surg 8:469, 1939.

Oelsnitz G: Fehlbildungen des brustkorbes. Z Kinderchir 33:229, 1981.

Peterson RJ, et al: Noninvasive assessment of exercise cardiac function before and after pectus excavatum repair. J Thorac Cardiovasc Surg 90:251, 1985.

Ravitch MM: The operative treatment of pectus excavatum. Ann Surg 129:429, 1949.

Ravitch MM: Congenital Deformities of the Chest Wall and Their Operative Correction. Philadelphia: WB Saunders, 1977.

Rehbein F, Wernicke HH: The operative treatment of the funnel chest. Arch Dis Child 32:5, 1957.

Saint-Mezard G, et al: Prolapsus valvulaire mitral et pectus excavatum: Association fortuite ou groupement syndromique? Presse Méd 15:439, 1986.

Salomon J, Shah PM, Heinle RA: Thoracic skeletal abnormalities in idiopathic mitral valve prolapse. Am J Cardiol 36:32, 1975.

Sanger PW, Robicsek F, Daugherty HK: The repair of recurrent pectus excavatum. J Thorac Cardiovasc Surg 56:141, 1968.

Sauerbruch F: Die Chirurgie der Brustorgane. Berlin: Springer, 1920, p. 437.

Schaub VF, Wegmann T: Elektrokardiographische veränderungen bei trichterbrust. Cardiologia 24:39, 1954.

Scherer LR, et al: Surgical management of children and young adults with Marfan syndrome and pectus excavatum. J Pediatr Surg 23:1169, 1988.

Schutte JE, et al: Distinctive anthropometric characteristics of women with mitral valve prolapse. Am J Med 71:533, 1981.

Shamberger RC, Welch KJ: Cardiopulmonary function in pectus excavatum. Surg Gynecol Obstet 166:383, 1988a.

Shamberger RC, Welch KJ: Surgical repair of pectus excavatum. J Pediatr Surg 23:615, 1988b.

Shamberger RC, Welch KJ, Sanders SP: Mitral valve prolapse associated with pectus excavatum. J Pediatr 111:404, 1987.

Shamberger RC, et al: Anterior chest wall deformities and congenital heart disease. J Thorac Cardiovasc Surg 96:427, 1988c.

Shochat SJ, et al: Moiré phototopography in the evaluation of anterior chest wall deformities. J Pediatr Surg 16:353, 1981.

Taguchi K, et al: A new plastic operation for pectus excavatum: Sternal turnover surgical procedure with preserved internal mammary vessels. Chest 67:606, 1975.

Udoshi MB, et al: Incidence of mitral valve prolapse in subjects with thoracic skeletal abnormalities-A prospective study. Am Heart J 97:303, 1979.

Wada J, et al: Results of 271 funnel chest operations. Ann Thorac Surg 10:526, 1970.

Waters PM, et al: Scoliosis in children with pectus excavatum and pectus carinatum. J Pediatr Orthop 9:551, 1989.

Weg JG, Krumholz RA, Harkleroad LE: Pulmonary dysfunction in pectus excavatum. Am Rev Respir Dis 96:936, 1967.

Welch KJ: Satisfactory surgical correction of pectus excavatum deformity in childhood: A limited opportunity. J Thorac Surg 36:697, 1958.

Welch KJ, Kearney GP: Abdominal musculature deficiency syndrome: Prune belly. J Urol 111:693, 1974.

Welch KJ, Chest wall deformities. In Holder TM, Ashcraft KW (eds): Pediatric Surgery. Philadelphia: WB Saunders, 1980.

Wynn SR, et al: Exercise cardiorespiratory function in adolescents with pectus excavatum: observations before and after operation. J Thorac Cardiovasc Surg 99:44, 1990.

Pectus Carinatum

Brodkin HA: Congenital chondrosternal prominence (pigeon breast) a new interpretation. Pediatrics 3:286, 1949.

Brodkin HA: Pigeon breast-Congenital chondrosternal prominence. Arch Surg 77:261, 1958.

Chin EF: Surgery of funnel chest and congenital sternal prominence. Br J Surg 44:360, 1957.

Currarino G, Silverman FN: Premature obliteration of the sternal sutures and pigeon-breast deformity. Radiology 70:532, 1958.

Howard R: Pigeon chest (protrusion deformity of the sternum). Med J Aust 2:664, 1958.

Lees RF, Caldicott WJH: Sternal anomalies and congenital heart disease. AJR Am J Roentgenol 124:423, 1975.

Lester CW: Pigeon breast (pectus carinatum) and other protrusion deformities of the chest of developmental origin. Ann Surg 137:482, 1953.

Ravitch MM: Unusual sternal deformity with cardiac symptoms-operative correction. J Thorac Surg 23:138, 1952.

Ravitch MM: The operative correction of pectus carinatum (pigeon breast). Ann Surg 151:705, 1960.

Robicsek F, et al: The surgical treatment of chondrosternal prominence (pectus carinatum). J Thorac Cardiovasc Surg 45:691, 1963.

Shamberger RC, Welch KJ: Surgical correction of pectus carinatum. J Pediatr Surg 22:48, 1987.

Shamberger RC, Welch KJ: Surgical correction of chondromanubrial deformity (Currarino Silverman syndrome). J Pediatr Surg 23:319, 1988.

Welch KJ, Vos A: Surgical correction of pectus carinatum (pigeon breast). J Pediatr Surg 8:659, 1973.

Poland's Syndrome

Boaz D, Mace JW, Gotlin RW: Poland's syndrome and leukemia. Lancet 1:349, 1971.

Bouvet JP, et al: Vascular origin of Poland syndrome? A comparative rheographic study of the vascularisation of the arms in eight patients. Eur J Pediatr 128:17, 1978.

Clarkson P: Poland's syndactyly. Guy Hosp Rep 111:335, 1962.

Cobben JM, et al: Poland anomaly in mother and daughter. Am J Med Genet 33:519, 1989.

David TJ: Vascular origin of Poland syndrome? Eur J Pediatr 130:299, 1979.

David TJ: Familial Poland anomaly. J Med Genet 19:293, 1982.

Fontaine G, Ovlaque S: Le syndrome de Poland-Möbius. Arch Fr Pediatr 41:351, 1984.

Freire-Maia N, et al: The Poland syndrome — Clinical and genealogical data, dermatoglyphic analysis, and incidence. Hum Hered 23:97, 1973.

Froriep R: Beobachtung eines Falles Von Mangel der Brustdrüse. Notizen aus dem Gebiete der Natur-und Heilkunde 10:9, 1839.

Haller Jr JA, et al: Early reconstruction of Poland's syndrome using autologous rib grafts combined with a latissimus muscle flap. J Pediatr Surg 19:423, 1984.

Lallemand LM: Éphémérides Médicales de Montpellier 1:144, 1826.

McGillivray BC, Lowry RB: Poland syndrome in British Columbia: Incidence and reproductive experience of affected persons. Am J Med Genet 1:65, 1977.

Ohmori K, Takada H: Correction of Poland's pectoralis major muscle

anomaly with latissimus dorsi musculocutaneous flaps. Plast Reconstr Surg 65:400, 1980.

Poland A: Deficiency of the pectoralis muscles. Guy Hosp Rep 6:191, 1841.

Ravitch MM: Atypical deformities of the chest wall- absence and deformities of the ribs and costal cartilages. Surgery 59 :438, 1966.

Shamberger RC, Welch KW, Upton III J: Surgical treatment of thoracic deformity in Poland's syndrome. J Pediatr Surg 24:760, 1989.

Sujansky E, Riccardi VM, Matthew AL: The familial occurrence of Poland syndrome. Birth Defects 13:117, 1977.

Walker JC, Meijer R, Aranda D: Syndactylism with deformity of the pectoralis muscle-Poland's syndrome. J Pediatr Surg 4:569, 1969.

Cleft Sternum

Burton JF: Method of correction of ectopia cordis. Arch Surg 54:79, 1947.

Maier HC, Bortone F: Complete failure of sternal fusion with herniation of pericardium. J Thorac Surg 18:851, 1949.

Meissner F: Fissura sterni congenita. Zentralbl Chir 89:1832, 1964.

Sabiston Jr DC: The surgical management of congenital bifid sternum with partial ectopia cordis. J Thorac Surg 35:118, 1958.

Shamberger RC, Welch KJ: Sternal defects. Pediatr Surg Int 5:156, 1990.

Thoracic Ectopia Cordis

Amato JT, Cotroneo JV, Gladiere R: Repair of complete ectopia cordis (film). Presented at the American College of Surgeons Clinical Congress, Chicago, October 23–28, 1988.

Bremer L: Textbook of Embryology. Philadelphia: WB Saunders, 1939.

Cantrell JR, Haller JA, Ravitch MM: A syndrome of congenital defects involving the abdominal wall, sternum, diaphragm, pericardium, and heart. Surg Gynecol Obstet 107:602, 1958.

Cutler GD, Wilens G: Ectopia cordis: Report of a case. Am J Dis Child 30:76, 1925.

Dobell ARC, Williams HB, Long RW: Staged repair of ectopia cordis. J Pediatr Surg 17:353, 1982.

Haynor DR, et al: Imaging of fetal ectopia cordis: Roles of sonography and computed tomography. J Ultrasound Med 3:25, 1984.

Hersh JH, et al: Sternal malformation/vascular dysplasia association. Am J Med Genet 21:177, 1985.

Higginbottom MC: The amniotic band disruption complex: Timing of amniotic rupture and variable spectra of consequent defects. Pediatrics 95:544, 1979.

Kaplan LC, et al: Ectopia cordis and cleft sternum: Evidence for mechanical teratogenesis following rupture of the chorion or yolk sac. Am J Med Genet 21:187, 1985.

King CR: Ectopia cordis and chromosomal errors. Pediatrics 66:328, 1980.

Kragt H, et al: Case report: Prenatal ultrasonic diagnosis and management of ectopia cordis. Eur J Obstet Gynecol Reprod Biol 20:177, 1985.

Mercer LJ, Petres RE, Smeltzer JS: Ultrasound diagnosis of ectopia cordis. Obstet Gynecol 61:523, 1983.

Opitz JM: Editorial comment following paper by Hersh et al. and Kaplan et al. on sternal cleft. Am J Med Genet 21:201, 1985.

Patten BM: Human Embryology. Toronto: Blakiston, 1946.

Saxena NC: Ectopia cordis child surviving; prosthesis fails. Pediatric News 10:3, 1976.

Say B, Wilsey CE: Chromosome aberration in ectopia cordis (46, xx, 17 qt). Am Heart J 95:274, 1978.

Stensen N: In Acta Medica et Philosophica Hafnienca, Vol. 1, edited by T. Bartholin, 1671-1672, p. 202.

Stoll SC: A supraumbilical midline raphe with sternal cleft in a 47xxx woman. (Letter to the editor.) Genetics, September, 1986.

VonPraagh R, et al: Malpositions of the heart. In Moss AJ, Adams FH, Emmanouilides GC (eds): Heart Disease in Infants, Children, and Adolescents. Baltimore: Williams and Wilkins, 1977, pp. 422-458.

VonPraagh R: Personal communication, 1987.

Willius FA: An unusually early description of the so-called tetralogy of Fallot. Mayo Clin Proc *23*:316, 1948.

Thoracoabdominal Ectopia Cordis, Cantrell's Pentalogy

Arndt C: Nabelschnurbruch mit Herzhernie. Operation durch Laparotomie mit tödlichem Ausgang. Centralbl Gynäkol *20*:632, 1896.

Cantrell JR, Haller JA, Ravitch MM: A syndrome of congenital defects involving the abdominal wall, sternum, diaphragm, pericardium, and heart. Surg Gynecol Obstet *107*:602, 1958.

Cullerier M: Observation sur un déplacement remarquable du coeur; par M. Deschamps, médecin à Laval. J Général Méd. Chir Pharmacie *26*:275, 1806.

Major JW: Thoracoabdominal ectopia cordis. J Thorac Surg *26*:309, 1953.

Wieting: Eine operative behandelte Herzmissbildung. Dtsch Z Chir *114*:293, 1912.

Wilson J: A description of a very unusual formation of the human heart. Philos Trans R Soc Lond [Biol] II:346, 1798.

Miscellaneous Conditions

Heilbronner DM, Renshaw TS: Spondylothoracic dysplasia. J Bone Joint Surg [Am] *66*:302, 1984.

Jarcho S, Levin PM: Hereditary malformation of the vertebral bodies. Bull Johns Hopkins Hosp *62*:216, 1938.

Jeune M, et al: Polychondrodystrophie avec blocage thoracique d'evolution fatale. Pediatrie 9:390, 1954.

Kozlowski K, Masel J: Asphyxiating thoracic dystrophy without respiratory disease: Report of two cases of the latent form. Pediatr Radiol 5:30, 1976.

Roberts AP, et al: Spondylothoracic and spondylocostal dysostosis: Hereditary forms of spinal deformity. J Bone Joint Surg [Br] *70*:123, 1988.

Williams AJ, Vawter G, Reid LM: Lung structure in asphyxiating thoracic dystrophy. Arch Pathol Lab Med *108*:658, 1984.

CHAPTER 39

INFECTIONS OF THE CHEST WALL

Joseph LoCicero, III

Chest wall infections can be either primary problems arising spontaneously or secondary infections caused by previous procedures or pre-existing disease states. The result is the same, with equally devastating potential complications. Management of such infections may be as simple as administering routine antibiotic therapy or may require multiple and prolonged drainage procedures and complex reconstructive operations. Prompt intervention is essential to minimize serious morbidity.

SKIN AND SOFT TISSUE

The thorax accounts for one fifth of the total body surface area and thus can be afflicted with many common nonspecific soft tissue infections. Furuncles and boils common to any hair-bearing surface frequently occur. Superficial infections often develop in minor injuries and burns of the chest as they do elsewhere in the body.

Abscesses

Two potentially serious infections specific to the chest wall and involving large potential spaces are subpectoral and subscapular abscesses. These occasionally present as primary infections, but more often are secondary to a chronically infected thoracotomy incision. They are characterized by local pain, with or without swelling, combined with fever and leukocytosis. Prompt drainage and appropriate antibiotic therapy usually lead to successful resolution. Suction catheters are rarely required because these spaces are obliterated once drained.

Gangrene

Necrotizing soft tissue infections may occur as a complication of empyema or trauma. These infections frequently begin when the pleural material is drained through the soft tissues either by chest tube or thoracotomy. Pingleton and Jeter (1983) reported extensive synergistic gangrene of the chest wall with *Bacteroides*

melaninogenicus and *Streptococcus viridans* following tube thoracostomy for empyema. Delay in recognition led to the patient's demise. The author and Vanecko (1985) reported loss of the pectoralis major and serratus muscles caused by clostridial myonecrosis at the site of a tube thoracostomy in a patient with Boerhaave's syndrome. Radical debridement and daily dressing changes under general anesthesia eventually led to a successful outcome.

Recently, infections of the head and neck and dental manipulation have been identified as sources of necrotizing fasciitis of the chest. Steel (1987) described a case of necrotizing ulceration of the chest wall after dental manipulation successfully treated by surgical debridement and chemotherapy. He noted that the primary suspect organisms were *Str. milleri* and Bacteroides species. Nallathambi and colleagues (1987) reviewed the current literature and discovered 28 chest wall and mediastinal infections related to dental manipulation or phyngeal abscesses. These rapidly progressive, mixed aerobic and anaerobic infections have been associated with a 32% mortality rate. Antibiotic prophylaxis for deep dental manipulations and careful followup for any early signs of sepsis are essential.

Early recognition, radical debridement of all involved necrotic tissue, and treatment with high dose antibiotic therapy — usually penicillin — are all necessary for a good chance for cure. The antibiotic of choice used to be high dose penicillin, but many organisms of the normal flora above the diaphragm have become resistant. Therapy should begin presumptively with a combination including a penicillin, an aminoglycoside, and clindamycin. Once susceptibilities are available, the antibiotic regimen should be tailored accordingly.

Infectious Chest Wall Invasion

With drug resistance and superinfection during antibiotic therapy, virulent organisms occasionally cause a pneumonia that has the capability of direct chest wall invasion. Suchyta and associates (1987) reported a community acquired chronic *Acinetobacter calcoaceti-*

cus pneumonia with direct chest wall involvement discovered only at autopsy. Yuan and associates (1992) successfully treated a patient with pneumonia and extensive chest wall involvement attributed to *Actinobacillus actinomycetemcomitans*. This patient required high dose penicillin therapy for 3 months.

Empyema Necessitatis

Infrequently seen today, this soft tissue infection is caused by an undrained underlying pleural infection. An untreated empyema may eventually burrow through the chest wall and into the subcutaneous tissue of the chest. Suspicion of this entity should be raised by the patient's history and confirmed by physical and radiographic examination of the chest. The soft tissue component may require separate drainage, but often resolves with appropriate drainage of the empyema.

Mondor's Disease

This benign condition is a localized thrombophlebitis occurring in the superficial veins of the breast and anterior chest wall. The true incidence of this entity is unknown. Reports have been infrequent. Because the condition produces few symptoms and signs, most examples are probably not referred to informed examiners for study.

The earliest description was by Fagge (1869). Williams (1931) attributed the disease to thrombophlebitis, and later so did Mondor (1939), for whom the condition is named. Most cases occur in women, and frequently no antecedent cause can be found. Radical mastectomy may predispose to the development of this disease, as Herrman (1966) proposed, whereas benign conditions such as fibrocystic disease have no association with this entity. In a few instances, in which a biopsy was performed, Farrow (1955) described a sclerosing endophlebitis with complete or partial obliteration of the lumen.

Clinically, the disease presents as a cordlike structure in the subcutaneous tissue of the axilla, chest, or abdomen. Its greatest significance may be the possible confusion with inflammatory carcinoma of the breast. It does not tend to recur or lead to thromboembolism. In most subjects, no specific therapy is indicated because it regresses spontaneously.

Miscellaneous

Several other conditions may manifest as infections of the chest wall. Golladay and associates (1985) noted three benign conditions in 24 children who presented with chest wall masses. These included trichinosis, nodular fasciitis, and myositis ossificans, all confirmed by excisional biopsy.

CARTILAGE AND BONY STRUCTURES

Tietze's Syndrome

Painful, nonsuppurative swelling of the costal cartilages without abnormal histologic change is referred to as Tietze's syndrome. This condition, which is not a disease, was described in two patients by Tietze (1921), who attributed the changes to tuberculosis. This has never been confirmed. Since his publication, case reports have been sporadic. Kayser (1956), who reviewed the world literature, could find only 156 cases. The true frequency of this condition is not known, but the symptom complex appears to be common. Peyton (1983) described 76 women in his office practice and 156 men and women visiting an emergency room who complained of this syndrome. Symptoms include chest pain and swelling of the costochondral junction. The junction, usually the second, is usually prominent and is tender to deep palpation. He noted that emotional tension is frequently associated with this symptom complex. Rarely are further tests necessary to confirm this diagnosis, but Edelstein and colleagues (1985) pointed out that computed tomography of the chest is helpful to exclude chest wall masses in these patients.

As might be expected for a condition as vague as this, several invasive treatments have been advocated, from hydrocortisone infiltration to surgical removal of the involved area. The latter hardly seems justified. In most patients, reassurance and symptomatic treatment with compounds containing ibuprofen are sufficient.

Costochondritis

Infections of the costal cartilage cause great debility. They are chronic beyond all expectation and thus demoralizing to the patient and the surgeon alike. When recognized and treated properly, response is rapid, but the required treatment is unseemingly radical for what appears to be such a minor problem. This often leads to delay in appropriate management. Recognizing the basic problem, Moschowitz (1918) pointed out that the chronicity was due less to the type of infecting organism and more to the avascular nature of the cartilage. He urged removal of the cartilage for cure.

Before 1940, most chondritis was spontaneous, usually caused by tuberculosis. Some cases were caused by typhoid or paratyphoid fever. Today most infections are surgical complications. Most follow median sternotomy performed for cardiac procedures; some follow thoracotomy, tube thoracostomy, or chest wall trauma. Occasionally, fungal infections may burrow through the chest wall to cause chondritis.

Because the fifth to the ninth costal cartilages are fused, infections involving any one of these segments dictate a major resection for cure. The xiphoid is partially a cartilaginous structure, and thus may promote bilateral spread of the infection. This avascular hyaline cartilage behaves like a foreign body once infected. When free of perichondrium, it begins to take on a moth-eaten appearance in the depths of a draining wound. The disintegration of the cartilage, however, occurs slowly but the cartilage is never completely reabsorbed. Sequestra characteristic of chronic osteomyelitis do not classically form in chondritis. The cartilage remains exposed and unmoved in the depths of the narrow, granulating wound.

Many organisms have been cultured from costochondritis. The primary infecting organisms include: *Escherichia coli, Streptococcus pneumoniae, Pseudomonas aeruginosa, Mycobacterium tuberculosis*, staphylococci, streptococci, and *Nocardia*. Once the wound is opened and drained, subsequent cultures may grow a variety of organisms, depending on the environment and the antibiotic regimen the patient is receiving.

Usually, the disease manifests as a drainage sinus in the region of the cartilages. Local pain and tenderness are present. As with any other chronic infection, general debility and, perhaps, low grade fever accompany an elevated white cell count. In most patients, the diagnosis is confirmed by tenderness over the cartilages and infection in the vicinity.

The preferred therapy is radical excision, as Murphy (1916) and Moschowitz (1918) advocated. Any involved cartilage should be removed completely (Fig. 39–1). If the lower ribs are involved, all fused segments must be excised. No bare cartilage should remain in the infected wound. The more conservative approach is to pack the wound and reconstruct it later, as Lewis (1967) and Talucci and Webb (1983) advocated. Others, such as Hines and Lee (1983) and Arnold and Pairolero (1984), have shown that the defect may be closed in one stage with a minimal morbidity. Techniques of reconstruction are discussed subsequently.

Osteomyelitis

Although spontaneously appearing osteomyelitis of the sternum or ribs did occur when tuberculosis was prevalent, it is rare today. Even when tuberculosis was more common, osteomyelitis of the sternum was uncommon. In a series of over 1000 patients with bone and joint tuberculosis reported by Wassersug (1941), the sternum was involved in only 1.1%. Today, primary sternal osteomyelitis occurs in heroin addicts. More often, secondary infections, usually following cardiac

surgical procedures, are the etiologic factors; Ochsner and associates (1972) noted a 1.5% infection rate with an overall 10% mortality. The factors implicated in the development of postoperative sternal infections, enumerated by Talamonti and associates (1987), include: diabetes, low cardiac output, use of bilateral internal mammary artery grafts, and most significantly, reoperation for excessive postoperative bleeding. Patients reported by Talamonti and associates (1987) who were explored within 7 hours did not become infected, whereas all patients who were explored after prolonged bleeding — >13 hours or more — became infected.

Manifestations of this condition are similar to those of chondritis. When osteomyelitis involves the sternum, an associated chondritis may occur, which can be mistaken for the principal cause of chronicity. The first sign of postoperative sternal osteomyelitis may be an unstable sternum or serosanguineous discharge.

In chronic sternal osteomyelitis, the most successful results have been achieved by extensive sternal and chondral removal followed by myocutaneous reconstruction. The most commonly used reconstruction is bilateral pectoralis major flap advancement, as described by Johnson and associates (1985). A modified "H" incision is used to mobilize the pectoralis major muscles with the blood supply based on the thoracoacromial artery (Fig. 39–2A) This also allows adequate exposure of the sternum, which is then excised (Fig. 39–2B). If possible, the upper manubrium with the clavicular attachments is left intact. Next, the humeral heads of the pectoralis major muscles are transected and the flaps are advanced over drains to close the defect (Fig. 39–2C). This gives a good cosmetic result with preservation of pulmonary function.

Diagnosis of osteomyelitis of the ribs is usually made because of local inflammatory signs and symptoms or because of a persistently draining sinus. When the infection is secondary to open drainage of an empyema, it can be one cause of a slowly healing wound. Sequestration from ribs affected by osteomyelitis has been reported. The sequestrum may even pass into the lungs, as Roe and Benioff (1955) noted. Confirmation is usually made by chest radiography. Although computed tomography of the chest is usually not necessary for confirmation of the diagnosis, it may help in evaluating possible underlying associated intrathoracic pathology, as suggested by Wechsler and Steiner (1989).

Excision of all diseased bone usually provides adequate treatment for osteomyelitis of the ribs. To prevent the problem following empyema drainage, Churchill (1929) recommended a clean division of the ribs, leaving no rib exposed or unprotected by periosteum. Occasionally, extensive excision may be required. In patients in whom the infection is overwhelming and an extensive excision is required, mechanical ventilation may be necessary until the infection is obliterated and reconstruction can be safely attempted.

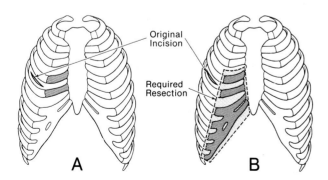

Fig. 39–1. Cartilage resection necessary for proper treatment of costochondritis. *A*, Initial incision and costal involvement. *B*, Delay may lead to secondary costal arch involvement necessitating arch removal.

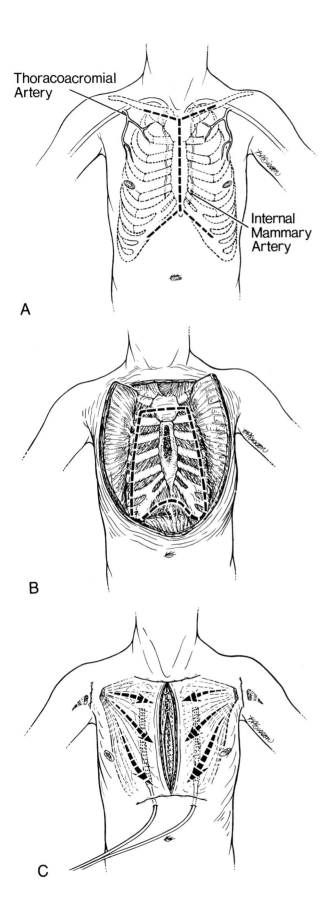

Fig. 39–2. Depiction of one-stage operation for chronic sternal osteomyelitis. *A,* The H-shaped incision used to expose the sternum and costal cartilages. *B,* Bilateral pectoralis major myocutaneous flaps have been raised. The extent of the planned resection is shown. *C,* Humeral detachment of the pectoralis muscles with advancement and closure over suction drains. *From* Johnson P, et al: Management of chronic sternal osteomyelitis. Ann Thorac Surg *40*:69, 1985.

Osteoradionecrosis

One of the most difficult problems encountered by the thoracic surgeon is a large necrotic ulcer of the chest wall following radiation therapy for carcinoma of the breast or other condition. Often, more infection and necrosis exist than are visible externally. Prosthetic materials usually cannot be used in the infected field, and transfer of viable flaps has been difficult. Despite all of precautions taken by radiotherapists, these infections occasionally arise. Treatment requires close cooperation between the thoracic surgeon and the plastic and reconstructive surgeon.

The foremost principle in the treatment of a radionecrotic ulcer is wide surgical excision and primary coverage of the defect, as Arnold and Pairolero (1984, 1989), described. Tissue of the affected area should be sent for pathologic analysis when radiation was performed for a local malignancy to ensure that no residual tumor is present.

Provisions for covering the expected defect with viable tissue must be carefully considered before the surgical procedure. Understanding and use of myocutaneous flaps have advanced. Jurkiewicz and colleagues (1980) described a variety of flaps, including pectoralis major, rectus abdominis and latissimus dorsi flaps (Fig. 39–3). This last flap was first described by Tansini (1906) but was rediscovered by McCraw and colleagues (1978). Hines and Lee (1983) used this flap in five patients and noted that even if the primary blood supply, the thoracodorsal artery, was cut at the time of initial mastectomy, collateral blood supply appeared adequate. They also pointed out that the muscle, albeit smaller and thinner when the thoracodorsal nerve has been resected, remains usable. Other innovative flaps include segmentally split pectoral girdle flaps proposed by Tobin

(1990) and free extended forearm flaps suggested by Schmidt and colleagues (1987).

In most instances, foreign material should be avoided when infection is present. Usually, the resulting paradoxic movement of the chest wall in these patients is minimally debilitating and not worth the risk of secondary infection. Myocutaneous flaps have been beneficial in those situations in which a large portion of the chest wall or sternum must be removed (see Chapter 43).

IMMUNOCOMPROMISED PATIENTS

Patients who are immunocompromised because of malignancy, malnutrition, or human immunodeficiency virus — HIV — infection present special problems. In granulocytopenic patients, findings of severe chest wall infections may be subtle. Aranha and co-workers (1988) recommend antibiotic therapy and surgical debridement with the early findings of erythema, localized tenderness, and temperature elevation. Golladay and Baker (1987) note that in immunocompromised children, invasive aspergillosis is the offending infection one third of the time, with high mortality rates even with early aggressive intervention.

In HIV-infected patients, common organisms often cause serious chest wall infection. Martos and colleagues (1989) reported two cases of tuberculosis of the chest wall. Rodriguez-Barradas and associates (1992) found chest wall infections related to pneumococcal pneumonia. Despite the uniformly fatal nature of the underlying disease, standard surgical principles of aggressive debridement and antibiotic therapy result in gratifyingly good long-term results.

REFERENCES

Arnold PG, Pairolero PC: Intrathoracic muscle flaps: A 10-year experience in the management of life threatening infections. Plast Reconstruct Surg *84*:92, 1989.

Aranha GV, et al: Soft tissue infections in the compromised host. Am Surg *54*:463, 1988.

Churchill E: The technic of rib resection and osteomyelitis of the rib ends. JAMA *92*:644, 1929.

Edelstein G, et al: CT observation of rib abnormalities: Spectrum of findings. J Comput Assist Tomogr *9*:65, 1985.

Fagge CH: Remarks on certain cutaneous affections: With cases. Guy Hosp Rep *15* (3rd series):259, 1869.

Farrow JH: Thrombophlebitis of the superficial veins of the breast and anterior chest wall (Mondor's disease). Surg Gynecol Obstet *101*:63, 1955.

Golladay ES, Baker SB: Invasive aspergillosis in children. J Pediatr Surg *22*:504, 1987.

Golladay ES, et al.: Chest wall masses in children. South Med J *78*:292, 1985.

Herrman JB: Thrombophlebitis of breast and contiguous thoracoabdominal wall (Mondor's disease). NY State J Med *66*:3146, 1966.

Hines GL, Lee G: Osteoradionecrosis of the chest wall: Management of post resection defects using Marlex mesh and a rotated latissimus dorsi: Myocutaneous flap. Am Surg *49*:608, 1983.

Johnson P, et al: Management of chronic sternal osteomyelitis. Ann Thorac Surg *40*:69, 1985.

Kayser HL: Tietze's syndrome: A review of the literature. Am J Med *21*:982, 1956.

Lewis FJ: Chondritis as a postoperative complication. Lancet *87*:247, 1967.

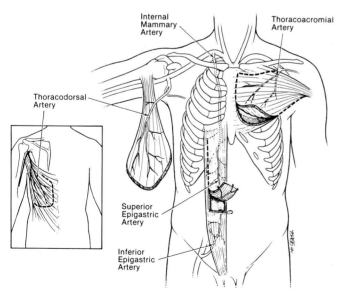

Fig. 39–3. Representation of the most common myocutaneous muscle flaps with their individual blood supply used for chest wall reconstruction.

LoCicero J, Vanecko RM: Clostridial myonecrosis of the chest wall complicating spontaneous esophageal rupture. Ann Thorac Surg 40:396, 1985.

Martos JA, et al: Chondrocostal and chondrosternal tuberculosis in two heroin addicts infected with human immunodeficiency virus. Med Clin (Barc) 93:467, 1989.

McCraw JB, Penix JO, Baker JW: Repair of major defects of chest wall and spine with a latissimus dorsi myocutaneous flap. Plast Reconstr Surg 62:197, 1978.

Mondor MH: Tronculite Sou-cutane Subaigue de la Paroi Thoracique Anteo-Laterale. Mem Acad Chir 65:1271, 1939.

Moschowitz A: The treatment of diseases of the costal cartilages. Ann Surg 68:168, 1918.

Murphy JB: Bone and joint diseases in relation to typhoid fever. Surg Gynecol Obstet 23:119, 1916.

Nallathambi MN, et al: Craniocervical necrotizing fasciitis: Critical factors in management. Can J Surg 30:61, 1987.

Ochsner JL, Mills NL, Woolverton WC: Disruption and infection of the median sternotomy incision. J Cardiovasc Surg 13:394, 1972.

Peyton FW: Unexpected frequency of idiopathic costochondral pain. Obstet Gynecol 62:605, 1983.

Pingleton SK, Jeter J: Necrotizing fasciitis as a complication of tube thoracostomy. Chest 83:925, 1983.

Rodriguez-Barradas MC, et al: Unusual manifestations of pneumococcal infection in human immunodeficiency virus-infected individuals: Past revisited. Clin Infect Dis 14:192, 1992.

Roe BB, Benioff MA: Late hemoptysis from rib sequestrum thirty-four years following empyema drainage. Surgery 38:764, 1955.

Schmidt RG, et al: Chest wall reconstruction with a free extended forearm flap: A case report. J Reconstr Microsurg 3:189, 1987.

Steel A: An unusual case of necrotizing fasciitis. Br J Oral Maxillofac Surg 25:328, 1987.

Suchyta MR, et al: Chronic acinetobacter calcoaceticus var anitratus pneumonia. Am J Med Sci 294:117, 1987.

Talamonti MS, et al: Early re-exploration for excessive postoperative hemorrhage lowers wound complication rates in open heart surgery. Am J Surg 53:102, 1987.

Talucci RC, Webb WR: Costal chondritis of the costal arch Ann Thorac Surg 35:318, 1983.

Tansini I: Sopra il mio nuovo processo di amputazione dell mammella. Riforma Medica (Palermo) 12:757, 1906.

Tietze A: Ueber eine eigenartige Haufung von Fallen mit Dystrophie der Rippenknorpel. Berl Klin Wochenschr 58:829, 1921.

Tobin GR: Segmentally split pectoral girdle muscle flaps for chest wall and intrathoracic reconstruction. Clin Plast Surg 17:683, 1990.

Wassersug JD: Tuberculosis of the sternum. N Engl J Med 225:445, 1941.

Wechsler RJ, Steiner RM: Cross sectional imaging of the chest wall. J Thorac Imaging 4:29, 1989.

Williams GA: Thoraco-epigastric phlebitis producing dyspnea. JAMA 96:2196, 1931.

Yuan A, et al: *Actinobacillus actinomycetemcomitans* pneumonia with chest wall involvement and rib destruction. Chest 101:1450, 1992.

READING REFERENCES

Arnold PG, Pairolero PC: Chest wall reconstruction: Experience with 100 consecutive patients. Ann Surg 199:725, 1984.

Culliford AT, et al: Sternal and costochrondral infections following open heart surgery. J Thorac Cardiovasc Surg 72:714, 1976.

Jurkiewicz MJ, et al: Infected median sternotomy wound: Successful treatment by muscle flaps. Ann Surg 191:738, 1980.

CHAPTER 40

THORACIC OUTLET SYNDROME

Harold C. Urschel, Jr.

Thoracic outlet syndrome refers to compression of the subclavian vessels and brachial plexus at the superior aperture of the thorax. It was designated previously according to presumable etiologies, such as scalenus anticus, costoclavicular, hyperabduction, cervical rib, and first rib syndromes. The various syndromes are similar, and the specific compression mechanism is often difficult to identify; however, the first rib seems to be a common denominator against which most compressive factors operate.

The symptoms are either neurologic, vascular, or mixed, depending on which component is compressed. Occasionally, the pain is atypical in distribution and severity and is experienced predominantly in the chest wall and parascapular area, simulating angina pectoris, as I and my colleagues (1973) noted.

Diagnosis of the nerve compression group, as I and my associates (1971) reported, can be objectively substantiated by determining the ulnar nerve conduction velocity. In the vascular compression group, diagnosis is usually established clinically, rarely requiring the use of angiography.

The ulnar nerve conduction velocity test — UNCV — as described by Jebsen (1967) and Caldwell and associates (1971) has widened the clinical recognition of this syndrome and has improved diagnosis, selection of treatment, and assessment of therapeutic results.

Physiotherapy to improve posture, strengthen shoulder girdle muscles, and stretch neck muscles is used initially in most cases of thoracic outlet syndrome and is often successful in cases of mild compression. Surgical treatment involves extirpation of the first rib, usually through the transaxillary approach, and is reserved, as I and Razzuk (1972) emphasized, for cases of severe compression that have not responded to medical therapy.

ANATOMIC CONSIDERATIONS

The subclavian vessels and brachial plexus traverse the cervicoaxillary canal to reach the upper extremity.

The outer border of the first rib divides this canal into a proximal division composed of the scalene triangle and the space bounded by the clavicle and the first rib — the costoclavicular space. The distal division comprises the axilla. The proximal division is the most critical for neurovascular compression. It is bounded superiorly by the clavicle and the subclavius muscle; inferiorly by the first rib; anteromedially by the border of the sternum, the clavipectoral fascia, and the costocoracoid ligament; and posterolaterally by the scalenus medius muscle and the long thoracic nerve. The scalenus anticus, inserting on the scalene tubercle of the first rib, divides the costoclavicular space into two compartments: an anterior compartment containing the subclavian vein, and a posterior compartment containing the subclavian artery and brachial plexus. The axilla, which is the outer division of the cervicoaxillary canal, with its underlying structures including the pectoralis minor muscle, the coracoid process, and the head of the humerus, is also an area of potential compression.

Compression Factors

A multiplicity of factors may cause compression of the neurovascular bundle at the thoracic outlet. The basic factor, which was pointed out by Rosati and Lord (1961), is deranged anatomy to which congenital, traumatic, and atherosclerotic factors may contribute (Table 40–1).

Bony abnormalities are present in approximately 30% of patients, either as cervical rib, bifid first rib, fusion of first and second ribs, clavicular deformities, or previous thoracoplasty.

Pathologic changes in the configuration of the cervicoaxillary canal alter the normal functional dynamics and serve as the basis of the clinical maneuvers used in the diagnosis of the thoracic outlet syndrome.

Adson or Scalene Test. This maneuver, described by Adson in 1951, tightens the anterior and middle scalene muscles, thus decreasing the interscalene space and magnifying any pre-existing compression of the subclavian artery and brachial plexus. The patient is instructed to: 1) take and hold a deep breath, 2)

Table 40–1. Etiologic Factors in Thoracic Outlet Syndrome

Anatomic
    Potential sites of neurovascular compression
        Interscalene triangle
        Costoclavicular space
        Subcoracoid area

Congenital
    Cervical rib and its fascial remnants
    Rudimentary first thoracic rib
    Scaleni muscles
        Anterior
        Middle
        Minimus
    Adventitious fibrous bands
    Bifid clavicle
    Exostosis of first thoracic rib
    Enlarged transverse process of C7
    Omohyoid muscle
    Anomalous course of transverse cervical artery
    Brachial plexus postfixed
    Flat clavicle

Traumatic
    Fracture of clavicle
    Dislocation of head of humerus
    Crushing injury to upper thorax
    Sudden, unaccustomed muscular efforts involving shoulder girdle
        muscles
    Cervical spondylosis and injuries to cervical spine

Atherosclerosis

---

extend his or her neck fully, and 3) turn his or her face toward the side. Obliteration or diminution in the radial pulse suggests compression.

Costoclavicular Test — Military Position. The shoulders are drawn downward and backward. This maneuver narrows the costoclavicular space by approximating the clavicle to the first rib, thus tending to compress the neurovascular bundle. Changes in the radial pulse with production of symptoms indicate compression.

Hyperabduction Test. When the arm is hyperabducted to 180°, the components of the neurovascular bundle are pulled around the pectoralis minor tendon, the coracoid process, and the head of the humerus. If the radial pulse is decreased, compression should be suspected.

Arm Claudication Test. The shoulders are drawn upward and backward. The arms are raised to the horizontal position with the elbows flexed 90°. With exercises of the hands, numbness or pain is experienced in the hands and forearms if compression is present.

SIGNS AND SYMPTOMS

The symptoms of thoracic outlet syndrome depend on whether the nerves or blood vessels, or both, are compressed at the thoracic outlet.

I and my associates (1971, 1972) observed that symptoms of nerve compression occur most frequently, pain and paresthesia being present in about 95% of patients and motor weakness in approximately 10%. Pain and paresthesia are segmental in 75% of cases, 90% occurring in the ulnar nerve distribution. Pain is usually insidious in onset and commonly involves the neck, shoulder, arm, and hand. In some patients, the pain is atypical, involving the anterior chest wall or the parascapular area, and is termed pseudoangina because it simulates angina pectoris. As I and my associates (1973) reported, these patients have normal coronary arteriograms and decreased ulnar nerve conduction velocities, strongly suggesting the diagnosis of thoracic outlet syndrome. The usual shoulder, arm, and hand symptoms that might have provided the clue for the diagnosis of thoracic outlet syndrome are initially either absent or minimal compared to the severity of the chest pain. Without a high index of suspicion, the diagnosis of thoracic outlet syndrome is frequently overlooked, and many of these patients become "cardiac cripples" without an appropriate diagnosis or develop severe psychologic depression when told that their coronary arteries are normal and that they have no significant cause for their pain.

The two distinct groups of patients with pseudoangina are as follows. Group I patients have symptoms and clinical findings suggesting angina pectoris, but have normal coronary arteriograms and significant depression of ulnar nerve conduction velocity. Group II patients have both significant coronary artery disease, as evidenced by 75% or greater stenosis in one or more of the major coronary arteries on coronary arteriography, and thoracic outlet syndrome, as evidenced by depression of the ulnar nerve conduction velocity. A high index of suspicion of thoracic outlet disease in such individuals must be maintained so that the appropriate methods of diagnosis and management can be exercised. Objective laboratory tests that are important for differentiating these two groups of patients include ECG, exercise stress tests, coronary arteriogram, EMG, UNCV, cine esophagogram and radiographs of the chest.

To understand the symptomatic overlap between coronary artery disease and this atypical manifestation of the thoracic outlet syndrome, that is, pseudoangina, it is necessary to review the neuroanatomy, innervation, and pain pathways of the arm, chest wall, and heart.

At least two types of pain pathways are present in the arm — the commonly acknowledged C5 to T1 cutaneous "more superficial" fibers, and the T2 to T5 afferent spinal fibers, which travel with the sympathetic nerves and transmit "deeper" painful stimuli from the ulnar median and parascapular distribution, as reported by Kuntz (1951). The cell bodies of the two types of afferent neurons are situated in the dorsal root ganglia of the corresponding spinal segments. They synapse in the dorsal gray matter of the spinal cord and the axons of the second order neurons, cross the midline, and ascend in the spinothalamic tract to the brain.

Compression of the "superficial" C8 to T1 cutaneous afferent fibers elicits stimuli that are transmitted to the brain and recognized as integumentary pain or paresthesias in the ulnar nerve distribution. In contrast, compression of the predominantly "deeper" sensory fibers elicits impulses that are interpreted by the brain as deep pain originating in the arm or referred to the chest wall.

The pseudoangina experienced in thoracic outlet compression shares with angina pectoris the same dermatomal distribution in that the heart, arm, and chest wall have afferent fibers convergent on T2 to T5 spinal cord segments and cell bodies that are located in the corresponding dorsal root ganglia. Referred pain to the chest wall is a component in both pseudoangina and angina pectoris. Because somatic pain is more common than visceral pain, the brain interprets activity arriving in a given pathway as a pain stimulus in a particular somatic area.

Two theories attempt to explain the mechanism of referred pain from the heart or arm stimuli to chest wall. The convergence theory holds that somatic and visceral afferents converge on the same spinothalamic neurons; when the same pathway is stimulated by activity in visceral afferents, the signal reaching the brain is the same and the pain is projected to the somatic area. The facilitation effect theory holds that because of subliminal fringe effects, incoming impulses from visceral structures, such as the heart, lower the threshold of spinothalamic neurons receiving afferents from somatic areas, so that minor activity in the pain pathways from the somatic areas — activity that would normally die out in the spinal cord — passes on to the brain and is interpreted as somatic pain rather than pain in the viscera, where the stimulus was initiated.

Symptoms of vascular compression in thoracic outlet syndrome, much less common than those of neurologic compression, include coldness, weakness, easy fatigability of the arm and hand, and pain that is usually more diffuse in distribution. Raynaud's phenomenon is occasionally noted. Venous compression is recognized by edema, venous distention, and discoloration of the arm and hand. Thrombosis of the subclavian vein — "effort thrombosis" or Paget-Schroetter syndrome — is infrequently noted but was described by Lang (1962).

Objective physical findings, in contrast, are more common in patients with primarily vascular rather than neural compression. Loss or diminution of radial pulse and reproduction of symptoms can be elicited with Adson's test, costoclavicular — military position, and hyperabduction maneuvers in most patients with vascular compression. Other possible findings are venous distention and edema, trophic changes, Rayaund's phenomenon, temperature changes, subclavian vein thrombosis, and even arterial occlusion and claudication. In cases of neural compression, the objective neurologic findings, which occur less frequently, consist of hypoesthesia, anesthesia, and occasional muscular weakness or atrophy.

DIAGNOSIS

The basic diagnostic considerations of the thoracic outlet syndrome include the history and physical examination, radiographs of the chest and cervical spine, neurologic consultation, electromyography, and ulnar nerve conduction velocity. On occasion, a cervical myelogram, coronary angiogram, and venograms may be necessary to elicit the diagnosis.

Cardinal for the establishment of the thoracic outlet diagnosis in pseudoangina is the elimination of the possibility of significant coronary artery disease by submaximal exercise stress testing and coronary arteriography when indicated. Subsequently, after excluding pulmonary, esophageal, and chest wall causes, the diagnosis of thoracic outlet syndrome must be entertained and established by the appropriate clinical evaluation and the slowing of the ulnar nerve conduction velocity.

Nerve Conduction Velocity

Motor conduction velocities of the ulnar, median, radial, and musculocutaneous nerves can be reliably measured, as described by Jebsen (1967). Caldwell and associates (1971) improved and adapted to clinical use the technique of measuring UNCV in evaluating patients with thoracic outlet compression. Conduction velocities over proximal and distal segments of the ulnar nerve are determined by recording the action potentials generated in the hypothenar or first dorsal interosseous muscles. The points of stimulation are the supraclavicular fossa, mid-upper arm, area below the elbow, and wrist. The Meditron 201-AD or the TECA B-3 electromyograph, including the coaxial cable with three-needle or surface electrodes, can be used for this examination. The normal average UNCV values are 72 m/sec across the thoracic outlet, 55 m/sec around the elbow, 59 m/sec in the forearm, and 2.5 to 3.5 m/sec at the wrist. In patients with the thoracic outlet syndrome, I and my colleagues (1971) found that the average UNCV value is reduced to 53 m/sec across the outlet, with a range of 32 to 65 m/sec.

Angiography

Simple clinical observations usually suffice to determine the degree of vascular impairment in the upper extremity and, as Lang (1962) noted, peripheral angiography is rarely needed. Bruits in the supra- or infraclavicular spaces suggest stenoses, and absence of pulse denotes total obstruction. In these instances, retrograde or antegrade arteriograms of the subclavian and brachial arterial systems are indicated to demonstrate localized pathologic changes. Using arteriography or phlebography routinely for demonstrating temporary occlusion of the vessels in different arm positions would seem redundant to an adequate clinical examination in most patients, and is associated with some morbidity — unnecessary although minimal. The UNCV is usually depressed in patients with vascular compression

Table 40–2. Differential Diagnosis of Nerve Compression

Cervical spine
  Ruptured intervertebral disc
  Degenerative disease
  Osteoarthritis
  Spinal cord tumors

Brachial plexus
  Superior sulcus tumors
  Trauma — postural palsy

Peripheral nerves
  Entrapment neuropathy
    Carpal tunnel — median nerve
    Ulnar nerve — elbow
    Radial nerve
    Suprascapular nerve

Medical neuropathies

Trauma

Tumor

as well as nerve compression, and serves to satisfy the physician and patient with regard to objective testing; moreover, it is less expensive and safer. In instances of venous stenosis or obstruction, as in the Paget-Schroetter syndrome, phlebography is indicated to discern the extent of thrombosis to determine the status of collateral venous circulation.

Differential Diagnosis

Thoracic outlet syndrome should be differentiated from a variety of neurologic, vascular, pulmonary, and esophageal lesions. It is necessary to differentiate it from lesion of the cervical spine, brachial plexus, and peripheral nerves (Table 40–2).

Several arterial and venous phenomena (Table 40–3) can be confused with thoracic outlet syndrome; however, the differentiation can often be made clinically.

In patients with atypical presentations, such as chest pain, a high index of suspicion of thoracic outlet in addition to angina pectoris must be maintained.

Table 40–3. Differential Diagnosis of Vascular Compression

Arterial
  Arteriosclerosis
    Aneurysm
    Occlusive disease
  Thromboangiitis obliterans
  Embolism
  Functional
    Raynaud's disease
    Reflex vasomotor dystrophy
    Causalgia
    Vasculitis, collagen disease, panniculitis

Venous
  Thrombophlebitis
  Mediastinal venous obstruction
    Malignant
    Benign

THERAPY

Patients with the thoracic outlet syndrome usually should receive physiotherapy before operative intervention. Such therapy must be properly performed because many of these patients receive the same treatment as persons with "cervical syndrome," which often exaggerates the symptoms of thoracic outlet compression. Proper physiotherapy for thoracic outlet compression includes heat massages, active neck exercises, scalenus anticus muscle stretching, strengthening of the upper trapezius muscle, and posture instruction. Because sagging of the shoulder girdle, common among the middle aged, is a major etiologic factor in this syndrome, many of the patients with less severe disease benefit from strengthening the shoulder girdle and improving posture. More than half of the patients seen in consultation required no surgical procedure but improved significantly with conservative management.

Most patients with a UNCV above 60 m/sec improve with conservative management; however, most patients with a UNCV below 60 m/sec require surgical resection of the first rib and correction of other bony abnormalities.

As Roos (1966) and Roos and Owens (1966) suggested, resection of the first rib, with cervical rib when present, is best performed through the transaxillary approach for complete removal, with decompression of the seventh and eighth cervical and first thoracic nerve roots. It can be accomplished without major muscle division, as in the posterior approach advocated by Clagett (1962) or retraction of the brachial plexus, as in the anterior supraclavicular approach suggested by Falconer and Li (1962). The infraclavicular approach does not allow complete removal of the first rib. The transaxillary approach shortens the postoperative disability and provides better cosmetic results when compared with both the anterior and posterior approaches, particularly because 80% of patients are women.

Technique of Transaxillary Resection of First Rib

The patient is placed in the lateral position with the involved extremity abducted to 90° by traction straps wrapped carefully around the forearm and attached to an overhead pulley. An appropriate amount of weight, usually 1 to 2 pounds, depending on the build of the patient, is used to maintain this position without undue traction. Traction can be increased intermittently by the anesthesiologist for exposure. The axilla and forearm are prepared and draped. A transverse incision is made below the hairline between the pectoralis major and the latissimus dorsi muscles and deepened to the external intercostal fascia. Care should be taken to prevent injury to the intercostobrachial cutaneous nerve, which passes from the chest wall to the subcutaneous tissue in the center of the operative field. The dissection is extended cephalad next to the external intercostal fascia up to the first rib. With gentle dissection, the neurovascular bundle is identified and its relation to the first rib and both scalene muscles is clearly outlined to avoid injury to these structures. The insertion of the scalenus anticus muscle on the first rib is dissected and the muscle is divided. The first rib is dissected subperiosteally with a periosteal elevator and carefully separated from the underlying pleura to avoid pneumothorax. The rib is then divided at its middle portion. With use of an alligator forceps, the anterior portion of the rib is pulled away from the vein, the costoclavicular ligament is cut, and the rib is divided at its sternal attachment. The anterior venous compartment is thus decompressed. The posterior segment of the rib is then grasped with alligator forceps and retracted away from its bed to facilitate its dissection and separation from the subclavian artery and brachial plexus posteriorly. The scalenus medius muscle should not be cut from the rib but rather stripped with a periosteal elevator to avoid injuring the long thoracic nerve that lies on its posterior margin. The dissection of this rib segment is carried to its articulation with the transverse process of the vertebra and divided. If the dissection is kept in the subperiosteal plane, no damage occurs to the first thoracic nerve root, which lies immediately under the rib. Complete removal of the neck and head of the first rib is achieved by a long, special double-action pituitary rongeur. The eighth cervical and first thoracic nerve roots can be visualized clearly at this point. If a cervical rib is present, it is removed at this time and the seventh cervical nerve root can be observed. Only the subcutaneous tissues and skin require closure, because no large muscles have been divided. Only occasional, intermittent firm traction is required for exposure, and no evidence of brachial plexus stretching or neuritis has been observed when this technique is used. The patient is encouraged to use the arm normally and can be discharged from the hospital between 2 and 3 days after the surgical procedure.

It is preferable to remove the entire first rib, including its head and neck, to avoid future irritation of the plexus, because a residual portion, particularly if it is long, may cause recurrence of symptoms. The periosteum should be fragmented and destroyed to prevent callus formation and "regeneration" of the rib.

Removal of incompletely resected or "regenerated" rib can best be accomplished through the posterior approach. For lysis of adhesions of the brachial plexus in symptomatic patients with decreased ulnar nerve conduction velocity following previous complete resection of the first rib, the anterior supraclavicular approach is used.

Results

The clinical results of first rib resections in properly selected patients are good in 85%, fair in 10%, and poor in 5%. A good result is indicated by complete relief of symptoms, a fair result by improvement with some residual or recurrent mild symptoms, and a poor result by no change from the preoperative status.

Uniform improvement of symptoms is usually obtained in patients with primarily vascular compression.

In patients with predominantly nerve compression, however, two groups with different rates of improvement are observed. The first group includes patients with the classic manifestations of ulnar neuralgia and elicitation of pulse diminution, in whom an average preoperative UNCV is reduced to 53 m/sec. Ninety-five percent of patients in this group are improved by first rib resection. In the second group are patients with atypical pain distribution who may or may not have shown pulse changes by compression tests, and in whom the average preoperative ulnar nerve conduction velocity was only reduced to 60 m/sec. Surgical intervention is carried out in such patients as a therapeutic trial after prolonged conservative therapy has failed. Although, many patients in the second group are improved, as I and my associates (1971) observed, the fair and poor results all occur in these patients.

The UNCV and clinical status are highly correlated. Patients with good postoperative results have a preoperative average UNCV of 51 m/sec and show return to a normal average of 72 m/sec after operation. In those who have fair results, the preoperative UNCV averages 60 m/sec and increases to an average of only 63 m/sec after operation. In the poor result group, no appreciable change occurs in the postoperative from the preoperative values; in fact, the average conduction time was only 58 m/sec.

No hospital mortality has been directly related to this procedure. Postoperative morbidity after the transaxillary approach includes clinically inconsequential pneumothorax in 15%, hematoma in 1%, and infection in 1%.

PAGET-SCHROETTER SYNDROME

"Effort" thrombosis of the axillary-subclavian vein — Paget-Schroetter syndrome — usually occurs as a result of unusual or excessive use of the arm in addition to the presence of one or more compressive elements in the thoracic outlet, as I and Razzuk (1991) noted.

Historically, Sir James Paget in 1875 in London and von Schroetter in 1884 in Vienna described this syndrome of thrombosis of the axillary-subclavian vein, which bears their names. The word "effort" was added to thrombosis because of the frequent association with exertion producing either direct or indirect compression of the vein. The thrombosis is caused by trauma or unusual occupations requiring repetitive muscular activity as has been observed in professional athletes, linotype operators, painters, and beauticians. Cold and traumatic factors such as carrying skis over the shoulder tend to increase the proclivity for thrombosis. Elements of increased thrombogenicity also increase the incidence of this problem and exacerbate its symptoms on a long-term basis.

For years, patients with "effort" thrombosis were treated with anticoagulants and conservative exercises; if recurrent symptoms developed when they returned to work, they were considered candidates for first-rib resection. Use of thrombolytic agents with early surgical decompression of the neurovascular compression has reduced morbidity, such as postphlebitic syndrome and the necessity for thrombectomy. A review that I and Razzuk (1991) published of 67 patients seen over 25 years showed that 34 were initially treated with heparin sodium and then Coumadin — crystalline warfarin sodium. Recurrent symptoms developed in 21 patients after they returned to work, necessitating transaxillary first-rib resection to relieve symptoms; 8 also underwent thrombectomy. Recently, 33 patients were initially treated with thrombolytic agents and heparin, followed promptly by early first-rib resection. The evaluation and efficacy of this therapy have been established by frequent and repetitive venograms and careful followup of patients. Most of the patients showed improvement with thrombolytic therapy. Remaining stenoses that suggested intravascular thrombosis were usually related to external compression of the vein by the clavicle, costoclavicular ligament, rib, or scalenus anterior muscle. Venous thrombectomy was necessary in only four patients in whom the clot was not controlled by thrombolytic therapy and operative release of compression. No deaths were reported in this series.

Adam and DeWeese (1971) reported long-term results in patients treated conservatively with elevation and Coumadin. They noted a 12% incidence of pulmonary embolism. Development of occasional venous distention occurred in 18%, and late residual arm symptoms of swelling, pain, and superficial thrombophlebitis were noted in 68% of the patients — deep venous thrombosis with postphlebitic syndrome. One patient had phlegmasia cerulea dolens. These findings substantiate our observations (1991) in group 1 that a more aggressive operative approach after thrombolytic therapy is indicated, particularly for younger patients in "precipitating" occupations.

One advantage of urokinase over streptokinase is the direct action of urokinase on the thrombosis distal to the catheter, producing a local thrombolytic effect. Streptokinase produces a systemic effect involving the alteration of serum plasminogen and increasing potential complications. Heparin is given postoperatively until the catheter is removed. A decrease in the need for thrombectomy after use of the thrombolytic agent followed by aggressive surgical intervention is another advantage, as some of the long-term disability is related to morbidity from thrombectomy as well as recurrent thrombosis.

The results in group 2 patients — aggressive thrombolytic therapy with urokinase and surgical resection of the first rib — are in marked contrast to those in group 1 patients. Group 2 patients had no serious complications, and many were able to return to work after 6 weeks.

The natural history of Paget-Schroetter syndrome suggests moderate morbidity with conservative treatment alone. Bypass with vein or other conduits has limited application. Causes other than thoracic outlet syndrome must be treated individually using the basic principles mentioned. Intermittent obstruction of the subclavian vein can lead to thrombosis, and decompression should be used prophylactically.

RECURRENT THORACIC OUTLET SYNDROME

Extirpation of the first rib offers relief of symptoms in patients with thoracic outlet syndrome not improved by physiotherapy. Ten percent of the surgically treated patients develop variable degrees of shoulder, arm, and hand pain and paresthesias that are usually mild and short lasting, and that usually respond well to a brief course of physiotherapy and muscle relaxants. In 1.6% of patients, however, symptoms persist, become progressively more severe, and often involve a wider area of distribution because of entrapment of the intermediate trunk in addition to the lower trunk and C8 and T1 nerve roots. Symptoms may recur from 1 month to 10 years following initial rib resection, but as I and my colleagues (1976) noted, in most instances, recurrence is within the first 3 months. Symptoms consist of aching or burning pain, often associated with paresthesia, involving the neck, shoulder, parascapular area, anterior chest wall, arm, and hand. Vascular lesions are uncommon and consist of causalgia minor and infected false aneurysms.

I (1987) identified two distinct groups of patients requiring reoperation. Pseudorecurrence occurs in patients who never had relief of symptoms after the initial operation. Cases can be separated etiologically as follows: cases in which 1) the second rib was mistakenly resected instead of the first; 2) the first rib was resected, leaving a cervical rib; 3) a cervical rib was resected, leaving an abnormal first rib; or 4) a second rib was resected, leaving a rudimentary first rib. The second group, in whom true recurrence takes place, includes those patients whose symptoms were relieved after the initial operation but who developed recurrence with a significant piece of the first rib remaining, and a second group who had complete resection of the first rib but demonstrated excessive scar formation on the brachial plexus.

Physiotherapy should be instituted in all patients with symptoms of neurovascular compression following first rib resection. If symptoms persist and conduction velocity remains below normal, reoperation is indicated.

Reoperation for recurrent thoracic outlet syndrome is always performed through the posterior thoracoplasty approach to provide better exposure of the nerve roots and brachial plexus, thereby reducing the danger of injury to these structures as well as providing adequate exposure of the subclavian artery and vein. It also provides a wider field for easy resection of any bony abnormalities or fibrous bands and allows extensive neurolysis of the nerve roots and brachial plexus, not always accessible through the limited exposure of the transaxillary approach. The anterior or supraclavicular approach is inadequate for reoperation.

The basic elements of reoperation include: 1) resection of persistent or recurrent bony remnants of either a cervical or the first rib, 2) neurolysis of the brachial plexus and nerve roots, and 3) dorsal sympathectomy. Sympathectomy removes the T1, T2, and T3 thoracic ganglia. The surgeon should avoid damaging the C8 ganglion — upper aspect of the stellate ganglion — which produces Horner's syndrome. This provides relief of major and minor causalgia and alleviates the paresthesias in the supraclavicular and intraclavicular areas. The incidence of the "postsympathetic" syndrome has been negligible in this group of patients. The use of a nerve stimulator to differentiate scar from nerve root is cardinal to avoid damage in reoperation.

The technique of the operation includes a high thoracoplasty incision, extending from 3 cm above the angle of the scapula, halfway between the angle of the scapula and the spinous processes, and caudad 5 cm from the angle of the scapula. The trapezius and rhomboid muscles are divided the length of the incision. The scapula is retracted from the chest wall by incising the latissimus dorsi over the fourth rib. The posterior superior serratus muscle is divided and the sacrospinalis muscle is retracted medially. The first rib remnant and cervical rib remnant, if present, are located and removed subperiosteally. After the rib remnants have been resected, the regenerated periosteum is extirpated. In my experience, most regenerated ribs occur from the end of an unresected segment of rib rather than from periosteum, although the latter is possible. At the initial operation, therefore, it is important to remove the first rib totally to reduce the incidence of bony regeneration in all patients with primarily nerve compression and pain symptoms.

If excessive scar is present after removal of any bony rib remnant, it may be prudent to perform the sympathectomy initially. This involves resection of a 1-inch — 2.5 cm — segment of the second rib posteriorly to locate the sympathetic ganglion. In that way, the first thoracic nerve may be easier to locate beneath rather than through the scar.

Neurolysis of the nerve root and brachial plexus is performed, using a nerve stimulator. Neurolysis is carried down to but not into the nerve sheath. It is extended peripherally over the brachial plexus as far as any scar persists. Excessive neurolysis is not indicated, and opening of the nerve sheath produces more scar than it relieves. To minimize excessive scar, efforts in the initial operation for thoracic outlet should include complete extirpation of the first rib, avoidance of hematomas by adequate drainage either by catheter or by opening the pleura, and avoidance of infection.

The subclavian artery and vein are released if symptoms mediate. The scalenus medius muscle is debrided. The dorsal sympathectomy is completed via extrapleural dissection. Meticulous hemostasis is effected, and a large, round Jackson-Pratt catheter drain is placed in the area of the brachial plexus, although not touching it. This drain is brought out through the subscapular space through a stab wound into the axilla. Methyl-prednisolone acetate — Depo-Medrol — 80 mg is left in the area of the nerve plexus, although the patient is not given systemic steroids unless keloid formation has previously been manifested. The wound is closed in layers with interrupted heavy Vicryl sutures to provide adequate strength, and the arm is kept in a sling to be used gently for the first 3 months. Range-of-motion exercises are prescribed to prevent shoulder limitation; however, overactivity is contraindicated to minimize excessive scar formation.

When the problem is vascular, involving false or mycotic aneurysms, special techniques for reoperation are used. A bypass graft is interposed from the innominate or carotid artery proximally, through a separate tunnel distally, to the brachial artery. Usually, the saphenous vein is used, although other conduits may be selected. The arteries feeding and leaving the infected aneurysm are ligated. At a subsequent stage, the aneurysm is resected through a transaxillary approach with no fear of bleeding or ischemia of the arm.

Special instruments have been devised to provide adequate resection through the transaxillary or posterior route. These include a modified strengthened pituitary rongeur and a modified Leksell double-action rongeur for first rib removal without danger to the nerve root.

The sympathectomy relieves chest wall pain that mimics angina pectoris, esophageal disease, or even a lung tumor by denervating the deep fibers that travel with the arteries and bone.

Results of reoperation have been excellent if an accurate diagnosis was established and the proper procedure was executed. Followup of over 400 patients has ranged from 6 months to 15 years. All patients improved initially after reoperation; in 79%, improvement was maintained for more than 5 years. Symptoms easily managed with physiotherapy developed in 14%; 7% required a second reoperation, in every instance because of rescarring. No deaths occurred, and only one case of significant infection requiring drainage was recorded.

REFERENCES

Adams JT, DeWeese JA: Effort thrombosis of the axillary and subclavian veins. J Trauma 11:923, 1971.

Adson AW: Cervical ribs: Symptoms, differential diagnosis for section of the scalenus anticus muscle. J Int Coll Surg 16:546, 1951.

Caldwell JW, Crane CR, Krusen UL: Nerve conduction studies in the diagnosis of the thoracic outlet syndrome. South Med J 64:210, 1971.

Clagett OT: Presidential address: Research and prosearch. J Thorac Cardiovasc Surg 44:153, 1962.

Falconer MA, Li FWP: Resection of the first rib in costoclavicular compression of the brachial plexus. Lancet 1:59, 1962.

Jebsen RH: Motor conduction velocities in the median and ulnar nerves. Arch Phys Med 48:185, 1967.

Kuntz A: Afferent innervation of peripheral blood vessels through sympathetic trunks. South Med J 44:673, 1951.

Lang EK: Roentgenographic diagnosis of the neurovascular compression syndromes. Radiology 79:58, 1962.

Paget J: Clinical lectures and essays. London: Longmans Green, 1875.

Roos DB: Transaxillary approach for first rib resection to relieve thoracic outlet syndrome. Ann Surg. *163*:354, 1966.

Roos, DB, and Owens, JC: Thoracic outlet syndrome. Arch Surg. *93*:71, 1966.

Rosati, LM, and Lord, JW: Neurovascular Compression Syndromes of the Shoulder Girdle. Modern Surgical Monographs. New York, Grune & Stratton, 1961, p. 168.

Urschel HC Jr: Thoracic outlet syndrome: Reoperation. *In* Grillo HC, Eschapasse, H (eds): International Trends in General Thoracic Surgery: Major Challenges. Vol. 2. Philadelphia: WB Saunders, 1987, p. 374.

Urschel HC Jr, Razzuk, MA: Current concepts: Management of the thoracic outlet syndrome. N Engl J Med *286*:1140, 1972.

Urschel Jr HC, Razzuk M: Improved management of the Paget-Schroetter syndrome secondary to thoracic outlet compression. Ann Thorac Surg *52*:1217, 1991.

Urschel, HC, Jr, et al: Objective diagnosis (ulnar nerve conduction velocity) and current therapy of the thoracic outlet syndrome. Ann. Thorac. Surg. *12*:608, 1971.

Urschel, HC, Jr., et al.: Thoracic outlet syndrome masquerading as coronary artery disease. Ann. Thorac. Surg. *16*:239, 1973.

Urschel, HC, JR., et al.: Reoperation for recurrent thoracic outlet syndrome. Ann. Thorac. Surg. *21*:19, 1976.

Von Schroetter L: Erkrankungen der Gefossl. *In* Nathnogel. Handbuch der Pathologie und Therapie. Wein: Holder, 1884.

READING REFERENCES

Adson AW, Coffey IR: Cervical rig: A method of anterior approach for relief of symptoms by division of the scalenus anticus. Ann Surg 85:839, 1927.

Aziz S, Straehley CJ, Whelan TJ: Effort-related axillosubclavian vein thrombosis. Am J Surg *152*:57, 1986.

Molina JE: Surgery for effort thrombosis of the subclavian vein. J Thorac Cardiovasc Surg *103*:341, 1992.

Rob CG, Standover A: Arterial occlusion complicating thoracic outlet compression syndrome. Br Med J 2:709, 1958.

Roos DB: Experience with first rib resection for thoracic outlet syndrome. Ann Surg *173*:429, 1971.

Telford ED, Mottershead S: Pressure at the cervicobrachial junction. J Bone Joint Surg [Am] *30*:249, 1948.

Urschel Jr HC, Paulson DL, McNamara JJ: Thoracic outlet syndrome. Ann Thorac Surg *61*:1, 1968.

Urschel Jr HC, Razzuk M: The failed operation for thoracic outlet syndrome: The difficulty of diagnosis and management. Ann Thorac Surg *42*:523, 1986.

CHAPTER 41

EXTENDED RESECTION OF BRONCHIAL CARCINOMA IN THE SUPERIOR PULMONARY SULCUS

Kamal A. Mansour

In 1924, Henry K. Pancoast, M.D., then Chairman of Radiology at the University of Pennsylvania, reported four cases of "superior sulcus tumors" and stressed the importance of careful radiographic evaluation of apical chest tumors. It is probable that his 1932 paper is the one that established the syndrome. The tumors occur at a definite location at the thoracic inlet and are characterized clinically "by pain around the shoulder and down the arm, Horner's syndrome and atrophy of the muscles of the hands and present radiographic evidence of a small, homogeneous shadow at the extreme apex, always more or less local rib destruction and often vertebral infiltration."

Much obscurity surrounds the definition of the superior pulmonary sulcus. Teixeira (1983) reported that, as defined by Kubik, the pulmonary sulcus is "nothing but the costovertebral gutter whose superior limit is the first rib arch and whose inferior limit is the insertion of the diaphragm in the thoracic cage." Anatomically defined, Pancoast tumor therefore is a painful apicocostovertebral syndrome and as such should be differentiated from other bronchial carcinomas arising in the upper lobes and invading the chest wall, vena cava, and recurrent laryngeal or phrenic nerves. Paulson (1973) stressed that Pancoast tumors are bronchial carcinomas developing in the extreme periphery of the lung and typically involve, by direct extension, structures in the thoracic inlet including the lower trunk of the brachial plexus, intercostal nerves, the sympathetic trunk and stellate ganglion, subclavian vessels, adjacent ribs, and vertebrae producing severe, steady, and unrelenting pain in the eighth cervical — ulnar surface of forearm and little and ring fingers — and first thoracic nerve root distribution — ulnar aspect of arm to the elbow — and often causing Horner's syndrome (Fig. 41–1).

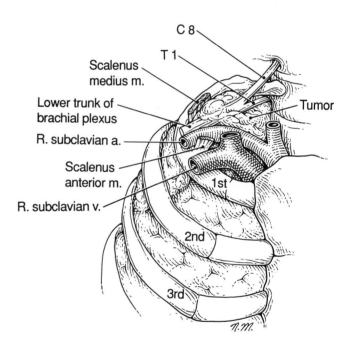

Fig. 41–1. Pancoast tumor located in the superior section of the costovertebral gutter, invading the lower trunk of the brachial plexus, and posterior aspects of the upper ribs.

As is true of bronchial carcinoma in any location, the extent of the tumor and stage of nodal invasion are the dominant factors in prognosis. By definition, carcinomas in the superior pulmonary sulcus are T3 lesions and should be classified as Stage IIIa — T3 N0, T3 N1, T1–3 N2 — and these lesions are usually resectable, or T4 lesions with massive invasion of the vertebral column, and these are classified as Stage IIIb — T4 any N — and these are not truly resectable.

DIAGNOSIS AND
PREOPERATIVE EVALUATION

Tissue diagnosis is necessary to rule out other lesions occurring in the superior pulmonary sulcus such as acute or chronic infections — usually fungal in origin — which may mimic Pancoast syndrome. Stanley and Lusk (1985) reported a case of actinomycosis, and Simpson (1986) and Ziomek (1992) and their associates reported cases that were due to invasive aspergillosis and cryptococcosis, respectively. Gallagher and colleagues (1992) reported a case that was due to a *Staphylococcus aureus* infection.

In the early stages, chest radiography may show a crescentic shadow at the apex of the lung resembling "an apical pleural cap." Regardless of its appearance in the frontal view, an apical lordotic view will show the tumor as a mass with a convex lower border indenting the lung. Destruction of the upper ribs or dorsal vertebrae, together with a unilateral apical lesion is specific for a Pancoast tumor. Bucky films may be required for adequate visualization of the bony structures. Planigraphy and bone scanning are used to delineate the location of the tumor and the extent of involvement of the ribs, paraspinal region, and vertebrae.

Thoracoabdominal computed tomography — CT — scan and magnetic resonance — MR — imaging are used for staging purposes and also to determine the soft tissue extent of the tumor invasion. MR imaging offers the ability to obtain coronal or sagittal planes that give a better delineation of the most superior or inferior extent of the lesion. Both CT and MR imaging can help if there is vascular involvement; however, venous angiography and subclavian arteriography may be resorted to if the MR imaging is not diagnostic. CT and MR imaging are also important in evaluating spinal disease. Noninvasive MR imaging demonstrates tumor replacement of bone marrow and the extent of epidural soft tissue disease. Although CT scans show bone fragments within the canal from pathologic compression fractures, the soft tissue detail is poor. Computed tomographic myelography is invasive but demonstrates both bone detail and cord compression. Enzymann and DeLaPaz (1990) believe it is indicated for patients who are unsuitable for MR — e.g., those with pacemakers, do not have access to emergency MR facilities, or are considered for surgical decompression and stabilization.

Cytohistologic diagnosis has been obtained in a small percentage of cases by sputum examination, bronchoscopic aspirates, brush biopsy, and a transbronchial biopsy. Tissue diagnosis can be obtained by percutaneous needle biopsy. If the tumor is large, it can be biopsied under fluoroscopy using either an anterior or posterior approach. Smaller lesions that are in difficult areas, surrounded by bony or vascular structures, or both, are usually biopsied under CT guidance. Either fluoroscopy or CT-guided biopsies should have a high degree of accuracy with a low incidence of pneumothorax. This is due to the fact that the lung parenchyma is rarely entered.

Transcervical supraclavicular technique described by McGoon (1964) or the supraclavicular thoracotomy described by Dart and colleagues (1977) for removal of specimen from a superior sulcus tumor may be resorted to on rare occasions.

Scalene node biopsy for palpable nodes and mediastinoscopy or limited anterior mediastinotomy, if CT shows mediastinal node enlargement, should be performed as a staging procedure.

PREOPERATIVE IRRADIATION AND
EXTENDED RESECTION

In the 1950s, tumors in the superior pulmonary sulcus were widely believed to be resistant to radiation and inaccessible to complete and curative resection. The average survival time of untreated patients after diagnosis was 10 to 14 months. Radiation therapy alone or following resection left few survivors after 1 year. Since the 1960s, results have been improving. Irradiation used alone has been reported to relieve pain, prolong survival, and in some instances effect a cure. The reports of irradiation combined with incomplete resection have been encouraging, although the results are not always comparable, because less extensive apical chest tumors are frequently confused with typical superior pulmonary sulcus tumors. Preoperative irradiation combined with extended resection, as reported by Shaw and associates (1961), has improved survival dramatically. The reports of many investigators, including Hilaris and colleagues (1974), support this approach (see Chapter 89).

The purpose of preoperative irradiation is to modify the extent of the lesion and sterilize the periphery of the disease at the chest wall level. Using megavoltage equipment, a tumor dose of 3000 rads, given in 10 fractions, is delivered over the tumor in the superior sulcus, the chest wall, and the superior mediastinum beyond the midline.* Two to three weeks after the completion of irradiation, an extended en bloc resection of the carcinoma and chest wall is done, usually including the upper two or three ribs with the intercostal muscles and nerves, the posterior portions of the appropriate thoracic vertebrae, the lower trunk of the brachial plexus, a portion of the stellate ganglion, and the dorsal sympathetic chain. The involved lung is resected by means of either lobectomy or segmental resection depending on the extent of the parenchymal disease.

The pathologic effects of irradiation of the tumor are related to the length of survival after extended resection. Those patients without nodal involvement who had no residual viable carcinoma in the chest wall or margins of resection did well and were long-term

---

*Editor's note: Many radiation therapists believe the initial dose to the tumor should be at least 4000 to 4500 rads.

survivors. Those patients who had viable tumor in the chest wall, the margins of the resection, the perineural lymphatics, or the nerve roots at the intervertebral foramen, however, did poorly and died in less than 2 years, mainly from distant metastases, but also with local recurrence of carcinoma, regardless of postoperative external beam radiation therapy.

Clinical and experimental observations suggest that preoperative irradiation in doses not sufficient to cause gross regression of tumor decreases local recurrence, prevents growth of disseminated tumor cells, and increases survival when compared with irradiation or operation alone.

The theoretical advantages of preoperative over postoperative irradiation depend on the treatment administered before surgical interference and its attendant risks of dissemination, implantation, or inflammation, together with violation of the vascular bed of the tumor, resulting in reduced oxygen tension and consequent diminished radiation sensitivity. Use of additional postoperative radiation in patients who have had preoperative radiation and resection raises the risk of radiation fibrosis and nerve entrapment of the brachial plexus caused by the increased cumulative dose exceeding the tolerance of normal tissues.

CONTRAINDICATIONS FOR SURGICAL RESECTION

Contraindications to surgical intervention follow: extensive involvement of the brachial plexus, the paraspinal region — particularly the intervertebral foramina — and the bodies or laminae of the vertebrae; mediastinal perinodal involvement; soft tissues at the base of the neck; and distant metastases, in addition to the usual cardiopulmonary limitations. Venous obstruction, although not typical of a carcinoma in the superior pulmonary sulcus, is another contraindication to operation. In some instances, patients with ipsilateral involved mediastinal nodes have undergone resection for palliation of pain, but survival has been limited to 2 years. Similarly, resection of an extensively involved subclavian artery may rarely be necessary with grafting, although these patients usually do not survive more than 1 year.

SURGICAL TECHNIQUE

The Classic Posterior Approach — Paulson Operation

The patient is placed on the side with the arm over the head, exposing the axilla and scapular region. A long parascapular incision is made starting just above the level of the spine of the scapula and carried two finger breadths beyond the tip of the scapula and ending in the anterior axillary line (Fig. 41–2). The trapezius and latissimus dorsi muscles are divided, exposing the serratus anterior muscle and rhomboideus major muscle. The serratus anterior muscular attachments to the upper ribs, particularly the second, and the rhomboideus major muscle are divided, thus elevating the scapula and shoulder and exposing the apex of the chest cage. The serratus posterior superior muscle is divided at its insertion on ribs two to five, lateral to their angles and preserved for later use.

The pleural cavity is entered through the space below the planned limit of rib resection. For example, if the third rib is involved, then the incision should be made along the top of the fourth rib, and if the first two ribs are to be removed, then the pleural space should be entered on top of the third rib. The rib spreader is then placed between the undersurface of the scapula and the third or fourth ribs, depending on the situation. Dissection is divided into anterior, superior, and posterior phases.

Anterior dissection should be started first (Fig. 41–3). The third and second ribs and intercostal muscles, nerves, and vessels are divided about 2 inches anterior to the growth and involved lung. The subclavian vein is identified, and dissection is carried medially to divide the first rib anteriorly using a first rib cutter or a Gigli saw.

Superior dissection continues by grasping the first rib using a bone-holding forceps and retracting it downward to expose the attachment of the scalenus anticus to the scalene tubercle of the first rib between the subclavian

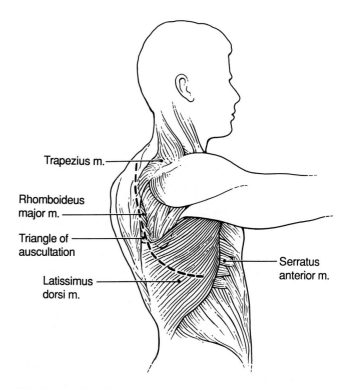

Trapezius m.

Rhomboideus major m.

Triangle of auscultation

Latissimus dorsi m.

Serratus anterior m.

Fig. 41–2. The classic posterolateral thoracotomy incision.

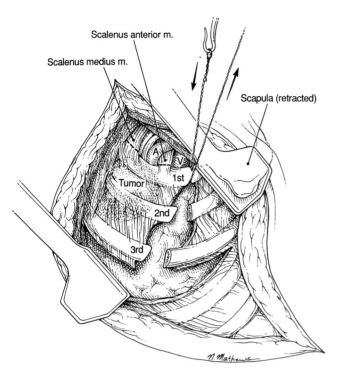

Fig. 41–3. Anterior and superior phases of dissection — division of upper ribs, scalenus anticus and medius muscles, and identification of the subclavian artery and vein by retracting the first rib inferiorly.

vein in front and the subclavian artery behind. The scalenus anticus muscle is then divided, and dissection is carried posteriorly beyond the brachial plexus. At this time the scalenus medius muscle is divided at its attachment into the upper surface of the first rib between the tubercle of the rib and the groove for the subclavian artery.

The posterior phase of the dissection starts by dividing the first rib beyond the extent of the tumor (Fig. 41–4A). With the hand inside the chest, the first rib is cut either at its neck or beyond the attachment of its tubercle to the transverse process of the vertebral body. At this point, the lower trunk of the brachial plexus is identified, as the first rib is retracted downward and divided after the extent of its involvement by the tumor has been determined (Fig. 41–4B). The posterior phase of the dissection continues inferiorly by dividing the second and third ribs. The sacrospinalis muscle is retracted outward, and the transverse processes are divided flush with the tubercles of the ribs or more posteriorly depending on the extent of the tumor. Conversely, the posterior phase of the dissection may start from below upward dividing the third, second, and first ribs in that order. Using chisel and hammer technique, the transverse processes may be divided and a section of the vertebral body may be resected depending on the degree of the tumor invasion. The intercostal nerves and vessels are clipped before division, but if uncontrolled bleeding or spinal fluid leak occurs at the intervertebral foramen, a muscle graft using a small section of an intercostal muscle is sewn over the leak. Bone wax may be used; however, it is not advisable to use oxidized regenerated cellulose (Surgicel; Johnson & Johnson, Summerville, NJ) or absorbable gelatin sponge (Gelfoam; The Upjohn Company, Kalamazoo, MI) because migration or swelling and cord compression are liable to occur with hazardous consequences as has been reported by Tashiro and associates (1987) and Short (1990). It is also not advisable to use the electrocautery in close proximity to the spinal cord because neural injury may result.

The dorsal sympathetic chain is divided posteriorly, and the internal mammary artery is divided as it crosses

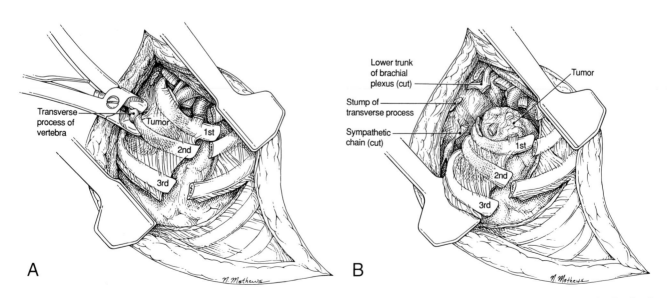

Fig. 41–4. *A,* Posterior approach to resection of the tumor by division of transverse processes of the vertebrae, elevation of the heads of the ribs. *B,* Division of the lower trunk of brachial plexus as the first rib is retracted inferiorly.

the apex of the chest to reach the undersurface of the sternum.

The extended resection of the carcinoma is then completed by the usual technique of upper lobectomy or segmental resection depending on the extent of the disease.

Adequate pleural drainage is established by means of an upper anterior chest tube and a lower posterior tube placed in the ninth interspace so as to lie in the paravertebral gutter. The remaining lung is expanded, and hemostasis is carefully controlled. The chest is closed usually by suturing the serratus posterior superior muscle to the intrinsic dorsal musculature. No synthetic materials are used because the scapula furnishes the posterior support. However, if portions of more than three ribs have been removed, the use of prolene mesh or a soft tissue patch sutured to the margins of the defect under tension is helpful in minimizing paradoxic motion.

Tumor With Mediastinal Node Invasion

The case for mediastinal node resection remains controversial. However, I perform a systematic node dissection for non-small cell carcinoma of the lung even when no perinodal involvement is obvious; this is followed by a course of irradiation therapy to the mediastinum if any nodes prove to be involved by tumor.

Tumor Involvement of the Subclavian Artery

Dissection of the growth away from the subclavian artery may be difficult, but it usually can be accomplished through the adventitial plane. If the artery is invaded, resection of the involved segment with end-to-end anastomosis or interposition graft may be considered. For the latter, a No. 6 or 8 ringed polytetra fluoroethylene — PTFE — graft may be used. Branches of the subclavian artery, including the internal mammary, the thyrocervical, and occasionally the vertebral, may have to be sacrificed.

Tumor Involvement of the Vertebral Bodies

It is usually preferable to elevate the tumor in the plane of its pseudocapsule; however, bony attachments suggestive of tumor involvement are chiselled away carefully. As much as one fourth of the involved vertebral body can be removed without disturbing the spinal support. If CT and preoperative myelography demonstrate destruction of the vertebral body with epidural extensions — Stage IIIb — the disease is usually unresectable. Nevertheless, in selected patients, if the disease is localized to one vertebral body, aggressive treatment is important in delaying or preventing direct compression of the spinal cord. There are some reports of giving preoperative external irradiation of a total dose to the tumor of 4000 rads in 20 fractions. The involved vertebral body is then drilled out with a high-speed drill, and portions of the body above and below are resected. All epidural tumor is resected down to the dura. Nori and associates (1982) suggest that stability of the spine be accomplished by using a bone graft supplemented with methyl methacrylate; after

loading catheters are placed along the resected margins for postoperative irradiation with iridium-192 (^{192}Ir) from the second through the fifth postoperative day.

The Anterior Transcervical Thoracic Approach — Dartevelle's Approach

Recently, Dartevelle and colleagues (1993) described a large L-shaped anterior transcervical thoracic incision, dividing the medial half of the clavicle, for radical resection of upper lobe lesions invading the thoracic inlet (Figs. 41–5 and 41–6). These tumors, however, are located anteriorly and are not typically Pancoast tumors, although the latter may rarely invade the clavicle and subclavian vessels, particularly the subclavian vein (Fig. 41–7). Dartevelle's approach provides

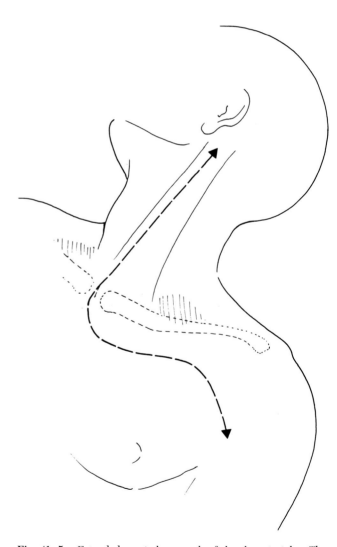

Fig. 41–5. Extended cervical approach of the thoracic inlet. The patient is placed in the supine position. An L-shaped skin incision is made from the angle of the mandible down to the sternal notch, is extended horizontally under the medial half of the clavicle, and eventually prolonged into the deltopectoral groove. *Courtesy of Dartevelle PG.*

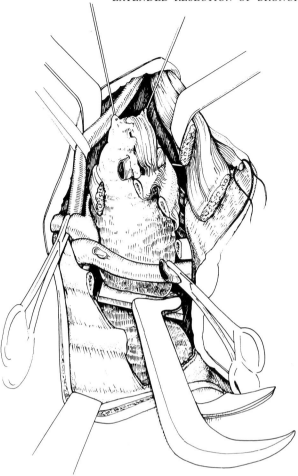

Fig. 41–6. Operative view after en bloc resection of the tumor, chest wall, subclavian artery, and the underlying apex of the upper lobe. *From* Dartevelle PG, et al: Anterior transcervical-thoracic approach for radical resection of lung tumors invading the thoracic inlet. J Thorac Cardiovasc Surg *105*:1025, 1993.

excellent exposure and adequate resection in those patients where only the first and second ribs are involved. In their series of 29 patients, Dartevelle and colleagues (1993) used only the anterior approach in nine patients while the combined approach, i.e., anterior cervical thoracic and classic posterior thoracic, was used in the remaining 20 patients. These authors reported favorable results in patients with invasion of the subclavian vessels.

SURGICAL MORBIDITY AND MORTALITY

In addition to the expected postoperative development of atelectasis caused by pain and interruption of the chest wall, unique complications consist of persistence of spinal fluid leaks and pleural drainage, both of which eventually subside, as do parenchymal air leaks. In the event of a pneumothorax and spinal fluid leak, air may pass into the spinal canal, resulting in meningitis.

Permanent neurologic deficits involving the ulnar nerve, resulting from resection of the lower trunk of the brachial plexus, are not incapacitating. If the extent of the tumor permits preservation of the eighth cervical nerve, the defect secondary to resection of the first and second thoracic nerve roots is not severe. Horner's syndrome, if not present preoperatively, develops postoperatively secondary to resection of the dorsal sympathetic chain and at least a portion of the stellate ganglion. None of these defects are disabling, and all patients surviving over 3 years are relieved of their original pain. There have been no complications of irradiation following the doses recommended.

Operative mortality has been no more than 3%. The stage of nodal involvement, the local extent of the

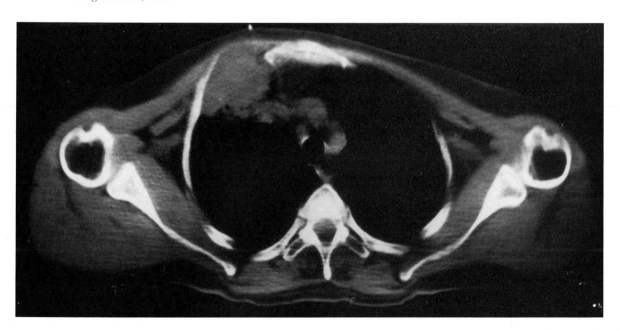

Fig. 41–7. CT scan of the chest showing an anteriorly located apical carcinoma of the right upper lobe invading the thoracic inlet. This is not a Pancoast tumor, and the anterior transcervical thoracic approach would be ideal.

carcinoma, and the pathologic effects of irradiation at the chest wall level are the important factors in prognosis. Paulson (1979) and Miller and associates (1979) of our group report that with the combined preoperative irradiation and extended resection, a 35% survival rate at 5 years is achieved for all patients and 44% for patients without nodal involvement.

REFERENCES

Dart CH, Braitman HE, Lalarb S: Supraclavicular thoracotomy for diagnosis of apical lung and superior mediastinal lesions. Ann Thorac Surg 28:91, 1977.

Dartevelle PG, et al: Anterior transcervical-thoracic approach for radical resection of lung tumors invading the thoracic inlet. J Thorac Cardiovasc Surg 105:1025, 1993.

Enzmann DR, DeLaPaz RL: Tumor. In Enzmann DR, DeLaPaz RL, Rubin JB (eds): Magnetic resonance of the spine. Baltimore: CV Mosby, 1990.

Gallagher KJ, et al: Pancoast syndrome: an unusual complication of pulmonary infection by Staphylococcus aureus. Ann Thorac Surg 53:903, 1992.

Hilaris BS, et al: The value of preoperative radiation therapy in apical cancer of the lung. Surg Clin North Am 54:831, 1974.

McGoon DC: Transcervical technic for removal of specimen from superior sulcus tumor for pathologic study. Ann Surg 159:407, 1964.

Miller JI, Mansour KA, Hatcher CR Jr: Carcinoma of the superior pulmonary sulcus. Ann Thorac Surg 28:44, 1979.

Nori D, Sundaresan N, Bains M, Hilaris BS: Bronchogenic carcinoma with invasion of the spine. JAMA 248:2491, 1982.

Pancoast HK: Importance of careful roentgen ray investigations of apical chest tumors. JAMA 83:1407, 1924.

Pancoast HK: Superior pulmonary sulcus tumor: tumor characterized by pain, Horner's syndrome, destruction of bone and atrophy of hand muscles. JAMA 99:1391, 1932.

Paulson DL: The importance of defining location and staging of superior pulmonary sulcus tumors (editorial). Ann Thorac Surg 15:549, 1973.

Paulson DL: Carcinoma in the superior pulmonary sulcus (editorial). Ann Thorac Surg 28:3, 1979.

Shaw RR, Paulson DL, Kee JL: Treatment of the superior sulcus tumor by irradiation followed by resection. Ann Surg 154:29, 1961.

Short HD: Paraplegia associated with the use of oxidized cellulose in posterolateral thoracotomy incisions. Ann Thorac Surg 50:178, 1990.

Simpson FG, Morgan M, Cooke NJ: Pancoast's syndrome associated with invasive aspergillosis. Thorax 41:156, 1986.

Stanley SL Jr, Lusk RH: Thoracic actinomycosis presenting as a brachial plexus syndrome. Thorax 40:74, 1985.

Tashiro C, et al: Postoperative paraplegia associated with epidural narcotic administration. Can J Anaesth 34:190, 1987.

Teixeira JP: Concerning the Pancoast tumor: what is the superior pulmonary sulcus? Ann Thorac Surg 35:577, 1983.

Ziomek S, et al: Primary pulmonary cryptococcosis presenting as a superior sulcus tumor. Ann Thorac Surg 53:892, 1992.

CHAPTER 42

CHEST WALL TUMORS

Peter C. Pairolero

Chest wall tumors encompass a kaleidoscopic panorama of bone and soft tissue disease. Included among these tumors are primary neoplasms — both benign and malignant — of the bony skeleton, chest wall metastases, neoplasms that invade the chest wall from the lung, pleura, mediastinum, muscle, and breast, and benign non-neoplastic conditions (Table 42–1). Nearly all of these disorders have at one time or another been irradiated either as the treatment of choice or in combination with chest wall resection, and it is common to have patients present with a postradiation necrotic chest wall tumor. The thoracic surgeon is frequently asked to evaluate all of these patients; most to establish a diagnosis, some to treat for cure, and a few to manage necrotic, foul-smelling chest wall ulcers. All are a diagnostic and therapeutic challenge. Surgical extirpation in many of these patients is frequently the only remaining modality of treatment, and this may be compromised by incorrect diagnosis or an inability to reconstruct large chest wall defects. From a practical standpoint, however, treatment for cure is most often limited to resection of primary chest wall tumors.

INCIDENCE

Primary tumors of the chest wall are uncommon, and few series have been reported. Most reports such as

those by Pascuzzi (1957), Groff (1967), and Stelzer (1980) and their associates, excluded patients with soft tissue tumors and included only patients with primary bone tumors. When combined, however, the soft tissues become a major source of chest wall tumors, as Graeber (1982), the author (1985), King (1986), Ryan (1989), Eng (1990), Evans (1990), and Farley (1991) and their associates noted. Indeed, soft tissues are the most common source of primary chest wall malignancy, accounting for nearly 50% of these tumors treated surgically. Altogether, primary tumors of the chest wall, including both bony and soft tissue tumor, account for approximately 2% of all primary tumors found in the body. The reported incidence of malignancy in these tumors varies from approximately 50 to 80%, with the higher malignancy rate found in those series including soft tissue tumors. Malignant fibrous histiocytoma, chondrosarcoma, and rhabdomyosarcoma are the most common primary malignant neoplasms that the thoracic surgeon is asked to manage, and cartilaginous tumors, desmoid, and fibrous dysplasia are the most common primary benign tumors (Table 42–2).

BASIC PRINCIPLES

Signs and Symptoms

Chest wall tumors generally present as slowly enlarging masses. Most are initially asymptomatic, but with continued growth, pain invariably occurs. At first the pain is frequently generalized, and the patient is often treated for a neuritis or musculoskeletal complaint. Nearly all malignant tumors are likely to become painful, as compared to only two thirds of benign tumors. In some instances of rib tumors, a mass may not be apparent on physical examination but instead is detected on radiograph of the chest. On occasion, fever, leukocytosis, and eosinophila accompany some of these tumors.

Diagnosis

The diagnostic evaluation of patients with suspected chest wall tumors should include a careful history and

Table 42–1.   Classification of Chest Wall Tumors

Primary Neoplasms of Chest Wall
   Malignant
   Benign

Metastatic Neoplasms to Chest Wall
   Sarcoma
   Carcinoma

Adjacent Neoplasms With Local Invasion
   Lung
   Breast
   Pleura

Non-neoplastic Disease
   Cyst
   Inflammation

Table 42–2. Primary Chest Wall Tumor

Malignant
  Myeloma
  Malignant Fibrous Histiocytoma
  Chondrosarcoma
  Rhabdomyosarcoma
  Ewing's Sarcoma
  Liposarcoma
  Neurofibrosarcoma
  Osteogenic Sarcoma
  Hemangiosarcoma
  Leiomyosarcoma
  Lymphoma
Benign
  Osteochondroma
  Chondroma
  Desmoid
  Fibrous Dysplasia
  Lipoma
  Fibroma
  Neurilemoma

physical and laboratory examination followed by conventional plain and tomographic chest radiography. Previous radiographs of the chest are important in determining growth rate. In general, magnetic resonance — MR — imaging as pointed out by Fortier and associates (1993), is the preferred method of imaging chest wall tumors. Not only does MR imaging distinguish the tumor from nerves and blood vessels, but it also allows visualization in different planes, such as coronal or sagittal planes. MR imaging, however, does not accurately assess pulmonary nodules or the extent of calcification within the lung. Thus, if the lung parenchyma needs evaluation for metastatic disease, computed tomography — CT — is preferable.

Chest wall tumors that are clinically suspected of being primary neoplasms, either benign or malignant, require tissue diagnosis by histologic examination. Because most malignant primary tumors have a benign counterpart, adequate tissue sampling is mandatory, and an open biopsy provides more thorough sampling than needle aspiration. The biopsy, however, should not interfere with subsequent treatment. An improperly placed biopsy site, extensive soft tissue dissection, and wound infection can all complicate subsequent treatment by delaying definitive resection, radiation, or chemotherapy.

Most pathologists are reluctant to diagnose chest wall tumors on frozen section examination, preferring instead to obtain special stains and multiple tissue sections and to confer with their colleagues. Consequently, definitive diagnosis is frequently not available until several days after the biopsy is obtained.

Small primary neoplasms — 3 to 5 cm — should be diagnosed by excisional biopsy with minimal margins — 1 cm. Chest wall closure for these small lesions is usually straightforward and does not require skeletal reconstruction. If the lesion eventually proves to be benign or is a malignancy better treated with radiation

or chemotherapy, or both, as will be subsequently, discussed no further operative intervention is indicated. However, if malignant and wide radical excision is required, the patient should be returned to the operating room, where the biopsy site is completely excised and a 4-cm margin of chest wall is obtained. Primary chest wall tumors greater than 5 cm should be diagnosed by incisional biopsy. The skin incision should be positioned in such a location that wound healing is not compromised, thereby preventing ulceration and infection. To prevent cancer dissemination, skin flaps should not be elevated and the pleural space should not be entered. Once pathologic examination is complete, treatment can proceed as indicated. Finally, needle aspiration should be reserved only for those patients with a known primary tumor elsewhere and who are clinically suspected of having a metastasis; if nondiagnostic, however, open biopsy is indicated.

Treatment

Wide resection of primary malignant chest wall neoplasm is essential to successful management. The extent of resection should not be compromised because of an inability to close the chest wall defect. Consequently, the mandatory ingredients for successful management of these neoplasms are wide resection and dependable reconstruction, as I and Arnold (1985, 1986) and Arnold and I (1979, 1984) pointed out.

Opinions about what constitutes wide resection do differ. King and associates (1986) analyzed the effect of extent of resection on long-term survival in patients with primary malignant chest wall neoplasm. The percentage of patients with a 4-cm or greater margin of resection remaining free from cancer at 5 years was 56% compared to only 29% for patients with a 2-cm margin (Fig. 42–1). Many surgeons consider a margin of resection free of tumor of several centimeters to be adequate. Although this may be adequate for chest wall metastases, benign tumor, and certain low-grade malignant primary bone

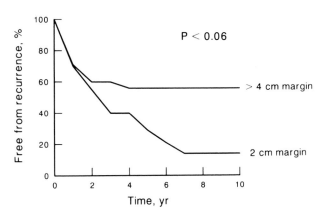

Fig. 42–1. Percentage of patients with malignant chest wall neoplasms remaining free from recurrent cancer by extent of resection margin. Zero time on abscissa represents day of chest wall resection. *From* King RM, et al: Primary chest wall tumors: factors affecting survival. Ann Thorac Surg 41:597, 1986.

neoplasms such as chondrosarcoma, a 2-cm resection margin is inadequate for more malignant neoplasms, such as malignant fibrous histiocytoma and osteogenic sarcoma, that can spread within the marrow cavity or along such tissue planes as the periosteum or parietal pleura. Consequently, all primary malignant neoplasms initially diagnosed by excisional biopsy should have further resection to include at least a 4-cm margin of normal tissue on all sides. High-grade malignancies should also have the entire involved bone resected. For neoplasms of the rib cage, this includes removal of the involved ribs, the corresponding anterior costal arches if the tumor is located anteriorly, and several partial ribs above and below the neoplasm. For tumors of the sternum and manubrium, resection of the entire involved bone and corresponding costal arches bilaterally is indicated. Any attached structures, such as lung, thymus, pericardium, or chest wall muscles, should also be excised.

The role of resection for chest wall metastases and recurrent breast cancer is controversial. Nonetheless, most thoracic surgeons would agree that tumor ulceration is an indication for excision. For these patients, wound hygiene is crucial, and surgical excision is frequently the only treatment option available. The goal in treating patients with necrotic tumor should be a healed wound following local excision. Although the length of survival is not increased after resection, the quality of life is certainly improved.

SPECIFIC TUMORS

Primary Bone Tumors

Primary chest wall tumors historically have included both neoplasms and such non-neoplastic conditions as cysts, infections, and fibromatosis. Although these tumors represent an array of different causes, it is still prudent to combine them because most present similarly, and many have common radiographic features. Primary bone neoplasms constitute the majority of these tumors.

Primary bone neoplasms involving the chest wall are uncommon. In the Mayo Clinic's series of 6034 bone tumors reported by Dahlin and Unni (1986) 355 — 5.9% — occurred in either the ribs — 85% — or the sternum — 15%. Overall, 89% were malignant and only 11% benign. Sternal tumors were slightly more likely to be malignant — 96% versus 88%. The most common benign bone neoplasms were cartilaginous in origin — osteochondroma and chondroma. The most common malignant neoplasms were myeloma, chondrosarcoma, malignant lymphoma, and Ewing's sarcoma.

Benign Rib Tumors

Osteochondroma. This is the most common benign bone neoplasm, constituting nearly 50% of all benign rib tumors. The incidence, however, may actually be higher, because most patients are asymptomatic, and

the tumors are often not removed. Men are affected three times more frequently than women. The neoplasm begins in childhood and continues to grow until skeletal maturity is reached. The onset of pain in a previously asymptomatic tumor may indicate malignant degeneration.

Osteochondromas arise from the metaphyseal region of the rib and present as a stalked bony protuberance with a cartilaginous cap. A rim of calcification may be present at the periphery of the tumor, and there is often stippled calcification within the tumor (Fig. 42–2). Microscopically, bony proliferation occurs to varying degrees, and the thickness of the cartilaginous cap also varies.

All osteochondromas occurring in children after puberty or in adults should be resected. Asymptomatic osteochondromas may occur before puberty, but if pain or increase in size occurs, the tumor should be resected.

Chondroma. Chondromas constitute 15% of all benign neoplasms of the rib cage. Most occur anteriorly at the costochondral junction. Both sexes are affected equally, and the tumor can occur at any age. These neoplasms usually present as a slowly enlarging mass that may be nontender or slightly painful. Radiographically, chondroma is an expansile lesion causing thinning of the cortex. The differentiation between a chondroma and a chondrosarcoma is impossible on clinical and radiographic examination. Grossly, chondroma presents as a lobulated

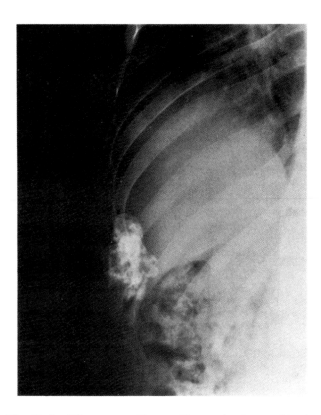

Fig. 42–2. Fifty-two-year-old man with osteochondroma arising in the anterior right ninth rib. Note intact cortex and stippled calcification within the tumor.

mass. Microscopically, the tumor is characterized by lobules of hyaline cartilage. The microscopic differentiation between a chondroma and a low-grade chondrosarcoma can be extremely difficult. All chondromas must be considered malignant and should be treated by wide excision. Although this resection may seem extensive for what may turn out to be a benign tumor, modern reconstructive techniques make the risk negligible, and long-term results are excellent.

Fibrous Dysplasia. This is a cystic non-neoplastic lesion and is probably a developmental abnormality characterized by fibrous replacement of the medullary cavity of the rib. Most cases present as solitary lesions, and when multiple lesions are encountered, Albright's syndrome — multiple bone cysts, skin pigmentation, and precocious sexual maturity in girls — should be suspected.

Fibrous dysplasia is usually manifested by a slowly enlarging, nonpainful mass in the posterolateral rib cage. Both sexes are affected equally. The disease begins in childhood, often in infancy, but is not detected until routine screening chest radiography in young adulthood. Radiographically, there is a characteristic appearance, consisting of expansion and thinning of the bony cortex with a central "ground-glass" appearance (Fig. 42–3). Microscopically, some degree of calcification with bony trabeculation and fibrous formation appears. Treatment should be conservative. Many lesions stop growing at puberty. Local excision is indicated for painful, enlarging lesions.

Histiocytosis X. This is not a neoplasm but is a part of the spectrum of disease involving the reticulo-endothelial system, including eosinophilic granuloma, Letterer-Siwe disease, and Hand-Schüller-Christian disease. Microscopically, all three components are similar and consist of a mixed inflammatory infiltrate of eosinophils and histiocytes.

Eosinophilic granuloma is limited to only bone involvement, whereas Hand-Schüller-Christian disease and Letterer-Siwe disease may have systemic signs and symptoms such as fever, malaise, weight loss, lymphadenopathy, and splenomegaly; leukocytosis, eosinophilia, and anemia are also often present with these two diseases. Most patients with eosinophilic granuloma present with pain limited to the area of skeletal involvement. Histiocytosis X occurs in persons under 50 years of age. Letterer-Siwe disease typically occurs in infants, Hand-Schüller-Christian disease in children, and eosinophilic granuloma in young to middle-aged adults.

Bone lesions occur in all three clinical variants of histiocytosis X. The skull is most commonly involved, but 10 to 20% of patients have rib lesions. The radiographic appearance is similar for all three forms of the disease. The lesion presents as an expansile lesion in the ribs, with periosteal new bone formation and uneven destruction of the cortex producing endosteal scalloping. Confusion with osteomyelitis may occur because of accompanying fever, malaise, and elevated white blood cell count.

Because of the expansile nature of histiocytosis X, excisional biopsy is required to establish the diagnosis. In patients with eosinophilic granuloma, excision alone should result in cure if the lesion is solitary. For patients with multiple lesions of eosinophilic granuloma, low-dose radiation therapy — 300 to 600 rads — to each lesion has been helpful. Characteristically, the other two variants of the disease run a chronic course requiring corticosteroids and chemotherapy.

Malignant Rib Tumors

Myeloma. This is the most common primary malignant rib neoplasm, accounting for one third of all tumors in the Mayo Clinic series reported by Dahlin and Unni (1986). Most myelomas involving the chest wall occur as a manifestation of systemic multiple myeloma, and a patient with a myeloma of the rib cage will almost inevitably develop the manifestations of the systemic disease. Solitary myeloma involving the rib is secondary only to solitary vertebral involvement. Myeloma is most common in the fifth through seventh decades of life and is rare under the age of 30. Two thirds of the patients are men. Pain is the most common symptom and often occurs without a palpable mass. Most patients are anemic, with an increase in the erythrocyte sedimentation rate. Abnormal protein electrophoresis is present in 85% of patients, and up to 50% have hypercalcemia and Bence Jones protein in their urine.

Radiographically, myeloma presents as a punched-out, osteolytic lesion with cortical thinning. Pathologic fracture is common. Grossly, the tumor is typically

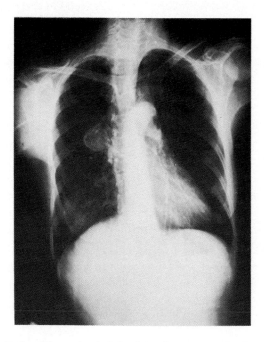

Fig. 42–3. Fibrous dysplasia involving the posterior ribs. Resection necessitated excision of the lateral portion of the adjacent vertebral body.

gray and friable. Microscopically, sheets of closely packed cells with abundant cytoplasm is observed. Mitosis is rare, but hyperchromatism and multinuclear cells are present.

Whether the rib changes are solitary or multiple, local excision is done to confirm the diagnosis, and radiation therapy is the treatment of choice for solitary and both irradiation and chemotherapy for multiple lesions. Five-year survival is approximately 20%.

Chondrosarcoma. Accounting for nearly 30% of all primary malignant bone neoplasms, chondrosarcoma is most frequently a neoplasm of the anterior chest wall, with 75% arising in either the costochrondral arches or the sternum. The tumor most commonly occurs in the third and fourth decades of life and is relatively uncommon in persons under the age of 20. Chondrosarcoma is more frequent in men. Nearly all patients present with a slowly enlarging mass, which has usually been painful for many months. Grossly, chondrosarcoma is a lobulated neoplasm that may grow to massive proportions and consequently may extend internally into the pleural space or outwardly into the muscle and adipose tissue of the chest wall (Fig. 42–4). Microscopically, the findings range from normal cartilage to obvious malignant changes. Lichtenstein and Jaffe (1943) described the characteristic findings of plump, atypical, and multiple nuclei, which may be more apparent in the peripheral areas of a growing tumor (Fig. 42–5). Differentiation from chondroma may be extremely difficult. From a practical standpoint, all tumors arising in the costal cartilages should be considered to be malignant and should be treated by wide resection.

The cause of chondrosarcoma is unknown. Although malignant degeneration of benign cartilaginous tumors — secondary chondrosarcoma — has been reported,

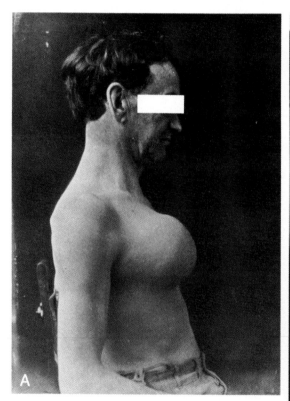
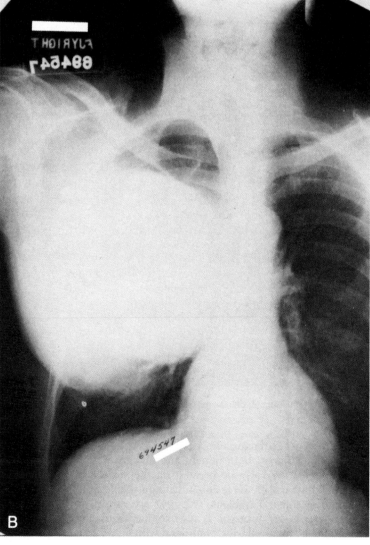

Fig. 42–4. *A*, Fifty-six-year-old man with a huge chondrosarcoma arising from the right anterior third costochrondral arch. *B*, Chest radiograph of the same patient.

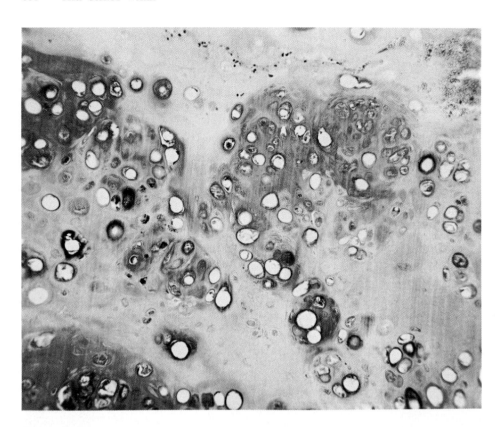

Fig. 42–5. Photomicrograph demonstrating typical cellular changes of chondrosarcoma.

most chondrosarcomas arise de nova. Lichtenstein (1977) was the first to suggest an association between trauma and chondrosarcoma. McAfee and associates (1985) subsequently reported that 12.5% of their patients had sustained severe crushing injury to the ipsilateral chest wall.

Radiographically, chondrosarcoma has a characteristic appearance. The tumor appears as a lobulated mass arising in the medullary portion of the bone (Fig. 42–6). The cortex is often destroyed, and the margins of the tumor are poorly defined (Fig. 42–7). Mineralization of the tumor matrix is common, producing a mottled type of calcification. Pathologic fracture is uncommon. Computed tomography can be helpful in determining the extent of the neoplasms (Fig. 42–8).

Definitive diagnosis of chondrosarcoma can only be made pathologically. Histologic confirmation, however, is sometimes difficult, because most chondrosarcomas are well differentiated. This tendency to be well differentiated may result in misdiagnosis of chondroma and subsequent undertreatment, leading to local recurrences. Generous sampling in the pathology laboratory of different areas within the tumor may facilitate histologic diagnosis. For this reason, excisional biopsy rather than incisional or needle biopsy of all chest wall masses suspected of being chondrosarcoma is indicated.

Chest wall chondrosarcoma typically grows slowly and recurs locally. If it is left untreated, metastases occur late. Prompt, complete control of the primary neoplasm is the main determinant of survival; the

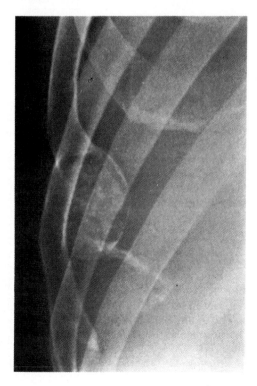

Fig. 42–6. Fifty-three-year-old man with chondrosarcoma of the right anterior sixth rib. Mass had been present 18 months without pain. *From* McAfee MK, et al: Chondrosarcoma of the chest wall: factors affecting survival. Ann Thorac Surg 40:535, 1985.

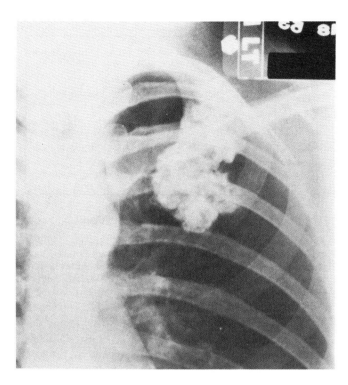

Fig. 42–7. Thirty-two-year-old woman with chondrosarcoma of the left anterior first rib. Both supraclavicular pain and a mass had been present for 2 months. *From* McAfee MK, et al: Chondrosarcoma of the chest wall: factors affecting survival. Ann Thorac Surg *40*:535, 1985.

objective of the first operation should be resection wide enough to prevent local recurrence. This involves resection of a 4-cm margin of normal tissue on all sides. Wide resection results in cure in nearly all patients (Fig. 42–9), with 10-year survival approaching 97%, as McAfee and associates (1985) reported.

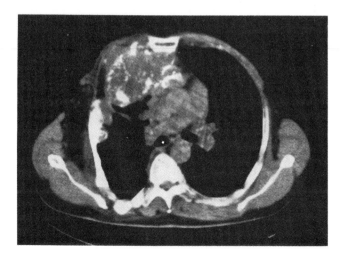

Fig. 42–8. CT scan of a 59-year-old man with chondrosarcoma arising in the right anterior chest wall. Note destruction of cortex and stippling within the neoplasm.

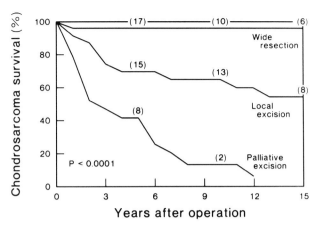

Fig. 42–9. Survival of patients with chest wall chondrosarcoma by extent of operation. Zero time on abscissa represents day of operation. *From* McAfee MK, et al: Chondrosarcoma of the chest wall: factors affecting survival. Ann Thorac Surg *40*:535, 1985.

Ewing's Sarcoma. Ewing's sarcoma involving the rib cage accounts for 12% of all primary malignant neoplasms of the bony thorax. Two thirds of all cases of Ewing's sarcoma occur in persons younger than 20, but young infants rarely develop this tumor. Boys are affected twice as often as girls. Signs and symptoms are common. A painful, enlarging mass is common. Fever, malaise, anemia, leukocytosis, and an increased sedimentation rate may be present. Radiographically, mottled destruction containing both lytic and blastic areas appears. An "onion-skin" appearance of the surface of the bone, caused by elevation of the periosteum and multiple layers of subperiosteal new bone formation, may be seen, but this feature is not pathognomic because it may be found in other bone tumors, both benign and malignant. Radiating spicules may also be present on the surface of the bone, which makes the lesion indistinguishable from osteogenic sarcoma. Pathologic fractures are rare. The radiographic appearance is also similar to that of osteomyelitis. This similarity, combined with fever, leukocytosis, and an increase in sedimentation rate, may lead to the erroneous diagnosis of osteomyelitis.

Ewing's sarcoma tends to be whitish-gray and is soft and not encapsulated. Histologically, the tumor is cellular, and there may be difficulty in distinguishing Ewing's sarcoma from lymphoma. Early spread to the lungs and to other bones is common and occurs in 30 to 75% of patients.

Adequate biopsy is necessary for correct diagnosis. Ewing's sarcoma is radiosensitive, so irradiation is the treatment of choice. Adjuvant chemotherapy is also used. Five-year survival is 40 to 50%.

Osteogenic Sarcoma. Osteosarcoma of the bony thorax is less common than chondrosarcoma and constitutes 6% of all primary malignant bone neoplasms. Unfortunately, it is more malignant and, hence, carries a much less favorable prognosis. Osteogenic sarcoma generally occurs in teenagers and young adults and commonly affects more young men than women. Most patients present with a rapidly enlarging tumor that is often painful. Serum alkaline phosphatase levels are frequently elevated. Radiographically, bone destruction with indistinct borders that gradually merge into adjacent normal bone appears. Calcification characteristically occurs at right angles to the cortex, producing a "sunburst" appearance. Pathologic fractures are rare. Grossly, the tumor is large and lobulated, with extension through cortical bone and into adjacent soft tissue. Microscopically, the predominant component may be bony, cartilaginous, or fibrous.

The treatment of osteogenic sarcoma consists of wide resection of the tumor, including the entire involved bone — rib or sternum — and adjacent soft tissues — lung or muscle. Radiation therapy has not been valuable in managing this neoplasm, and the role of chemotherapy remains controversial. In general, the prognosis is poor; the 5-year survival rate is 20%.

Tumors of the Manubrium, Sternum, Scapula, and Clavicle

Dahlin and Unni (1986) reported that primary neoplasms of the manubrium and sternum constitute 15% of all primary chest wall bone tumors. Nearly all — 96% — are malignant. The majority are chondrosarcomas, myeloma, malignant lymphoma, and osteogenic sarcomas. In addition, the sternum is a frequent site of metastatic neoplasms, such as carcinomas originating in the breast, thyroid gland, or kidney; the last two often present as pulsating tumors. Benign tumors such as chondromas, hemangiomas, and bone cysts have been reported.

The scapula, as Dahlin and Unni (1986) noted, is a common site for primary bone neoplasms, having an incidence of 2.8%, approximately half those of the ribs and sternum combined — 5.9%. Although it is an infrequent site for metastatic tumors, the same kinds of primary bone neoplasms occur in the scapula as in the rib cage. The malignant tumors include myeloma, Ewing's sarcoma, chondrosarcoma, osteogenic sarcoma, and lymphoma.

Primary neoplasms of the clavicle are uncommon, accounting for less than 1% of all primary bone tumors. Ninety percent are malignant. Over two thirds of the malignant tumors are radiosensitive, being either myelomas — 43% — or Ewing's sarcoma — 22%. The clavicle is more likely to be a site of metastatic disease than of primary tumors.

Arnold and I (1978) emphasized that primary malignant neoplasms of the manubrium, sternum, scapula, and clavicle should be treated by wide resection, including all of the involved bone and a 4-cm margin.

Primary Soft Tissue Tumors

Primary soft tissue tumors may arise from any component of the thoracic cage, and a variety have been reported, based on a histologic diagnosis of the predominant cell type. Preoperative differentiation between these neoplasms is difficult. Pain often is present.

Progressive enlargement is usually apparent by both physical and radiographic examination. Wide resection of the tumor and adjacent structures is the treatment of choice.

Benign Soft Tissue Tumors

Various benign tumors involving all chest wall structures has been reported. Predominant among these are fibromas, lipomas, giant cell tumors, neurogenic tumors, vascular tumors, such as hemangiomas with or without arteriovenous fistulas, and less commonly, benign tumors of connective tissue. Malignant degeneration is uncommon, and all should be treated by local excision.

Desmoid. Desmoid tumor deserves special consideration. Forty percent of all desmoids occur in the shoulder and chest wall. Encapsulation of the brachial plexus and the vessels of the arm and neck is common. The tumor often extends into the pleural cavity, markedly displacing mediastinal structures (Fig. 42–10). Initially, the tumor presents as a poorly circumscribed mass with little or no pain. Paresthesias, hyperesthesia, and motor weakness occur later, following neural encasement. Veins or arteries are rarely occluded. Desmoid occurs most commonly between puberty and 40 years of age and is rarely observed in infants or the very old. Men and women are affected equally.

Grossly, the tumor originates in muscle and fascia and frequently extends along tissue planes. Microscopically, a monotonous pattern of elongated spindle-shaped cells infiltrating the surrounding tissue is invariably seen. Most pathologists consider desmoid to be a form of benign fibromatosis, as do Goellner and Soule (1980) and Hayry and associates (1982). Because these tumors invade adjacent structures, however, and because Soule and Scanlon (1962) reported malignant degeneration, some, including Hajdu (1979), consider it to be a low-grade fibrosarcoma. Whatever the cause, the tumor tends to be recurrent if inadequately excised and should be treated with wide resection, like primary malignant chest wall neoplasms. Encapsulation of thoracic outlet structures presents a special problem in management. Enucleation of the tumor

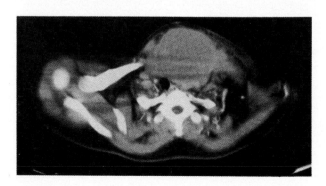

Fig. 42–10. CT scan of a 35-year-old woman with desmoid tumor arising in the left axilla. Note the intrathoracic component displacing the trachea and brachiocephalic vessels to the right.

from these structures followed by radiation therapy is current practice.

Malignant Soft Tissue Tumors

Malignant Fibrous Histiocytoma. As I and Arnold (1985) and King and associates (1986) pointed out, malignant fibrous histiocytoma is the most common primary chest wall neoplasm the thoracic surgeon is asked to evaluate. The tumor characteristically occurs in late adult life, with the majority of cases occurring between the ages of 50 and 70. These neoplasms are rare in childhood, and approximately two thirds occur in men. Malignant fibrous histiocytoma often presents as a painless, slowly enlarging mass. Pregnancy, however, may accelerate the growth rate, resulting in pain. Weiss and Enzinger (1978) reported that fever and leukocytosis with neutropenia or eosinophilia are occasionally present. Excellent circumstantial evidence suggests that some chest wall malignant fibrous histiocytomas are radiation-induced; Weiss and Enzinger (1978) reported the development of this tumor within the irradiated area following therapy for breast cancer, Hodgkins' lymphoma, and myeloma.

Grossly malignant fibrous histiocytoma tends to be lobulated and to spread for considerable distances along fascial planes or between muscle fibers, which accounts for its high recurrence rate following resection. Histologically, the tumor has a highly variable morphologic pattern, ranging from well differentiated, elongated spindle cells to highly anaplastic pleomorphic histiocyte-like cells. The neoplasm is unresponsive to both irradiation and chemotherapy and should be treated by wide resection. Five-year survival is approximately 38% (Fig. 42–11).

Rhabdomyosarcoma. This is the second most common chest wall soft tissue malignant neoplasm and occurs most frequently in children and young adults. These tumors are rare after the age of 45, and men are affected only slightly more often than women. Rhabdomyosarcomas present as a rapidly enlarging

mass that is usually deep-seated and is intimately associated with striated muscle tissue. Generally, the tumor is neither painful nor tender, despite evidence of rapid growth. Both grossly and microscopically, it has few neoplastic characteristics. As with most rapidly growing tumors, the overall appearance reflects the degree of cellularity and the extent of secondary changes such as hemorrhage and necrosis.

Modern therapy has profoundly altered the clinical course of this disease. Wide resection followed by irradiation and multidrug chemotherapy has resulted in 5-year survivals of 70% (Fig. 42–11). Inadequately treated, the tumor rapidly recurs both locally and metastatically.

Liposarcoma. This is primarily a neoplasm of adult life, with the peak incidence between the ages of 40 and 60 years. It rarely occurs in infants and small children. Most patients are men. Malignant degeneration of a pre-existing lipoma is rare. Association with antecedent trauma has been reported.

Grossly, liposarcomas are well encapsulated and lobulated. Microscopically, abundant anaplastic lipoblasts are common. Treatment is with wide excision. Five-year survival is approximately 60%, and recurrence is usually local, reflecting incomplete excision. Radiation therapy and chemotherapy have little to offer.

Neurofibrosarcoma. Chest wall neurofibrosarcoma frequently occurs along the intercostal nerve and is typically a disease of adult life, occurring in persons between 20 and 50 years of age. Three fourths of these neoplasms occur in men, and approximately half are associated with von Recklinghausen's disease. Grossly, the tumor is encapsulated. Microscopically, there is a monotonous pattern of elongated spindle-like cells that spread for considerable distances along the nerve sheath. Treatment is by wide excision.

Leiomyosarcoma. These are primarily neoplasms of adult life but occur less frequently than malignant fibrous histiocytoma and liposarcoma. Approximately two thirds of patients are women. Children rarely develop these tumors. Most neoplasms present as a slowly enlarging mass that may be painful.

Grossly, leiomyosarcomas are whitish-gray and lobulated, with foci of hemorrhage and necrosis. Cyst formation is often present. Microscopically, the tumor appears as swirling, elongated, spindle-like cells. Treatment is with wide excision. Recurrence is both local and metastatic.

CLINICAL EXPERIENCE

During the past 10 years, more than 60 chest wall resections for primary neoplasms were performed at the Mayo Clinic. Nearly two thirds of these neoplasms were malignant. Malignant fibrous histiocytoma and chondrosarcoma were the most common malignant neoplasm, and desmoid tumor was the most common benign tumor. The patients' ages ranged from 12 to 80 years, with a median of 43.5 years. An average of 3.9 ribs were

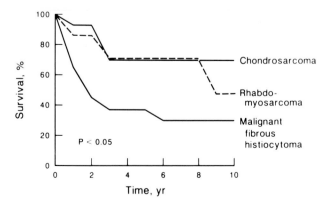

Fig. 42–11. Overall survival of patients with chest wall malignant neoplasms following resection. Zero time on abscissa represents day of chest wall resection. *From* King RM, et al: Primary chest wall tumors: factors affecting survival. Ann Thorac Surg 41:597, 1986.

resected. Total or partial sternectomies were performed in 13 patients. Skeletal defects were closed with prosthetic material in 40 patients and with autogenous ribs in 5. Fifty-four patients underwent 68 muscle transpositions, including 24 pectoralis major, 23 latissimus dorsi, 6 serratus anterior, 3 external oblique, 2 rectus abdominis, 2 trapezius, and 8 other muscles. The omentum was transposed in 8 patients. Patients were generally extubated the evening of the operation or the next day. Two patients required tracheostomy. Most other patients had only minor changes in pulmonary function. Median hospitalization was 9 days. There were no 30-day postoperative deaths.

Long-term survival of patients with malignant primary chest wall tumors depends on cell type and extent of resection. In the Mayo Clinic series, overall 5-year survival was 57%. Wide resection for chondrosarcoma resulted in a 5-year survival of 96% compared to only 70% for patients who had local excision (see Fig. 42–9). Five-year survival for patients with either chondrosarcoma or rhabdomyosarcoma was 70%, in contrast to only 38% for patients with malignant fibrous histiocytoma (see Fig. 42–11). Recurrent neoplasm, however, was an ominous sign; only 17% of patients in whom recurrence developed survived 5 years.

CONCLUSIONS

The key to successful treatment of all chest wall tumors is still early diagnosis with aggressive surgical resection and adequate chest wall reconstruction. This procedure can generally be performed in one operation, with minimal respiratory insufficiency and with low operative mortality. Most importantly, current techniques allow potential long-term survival for all patients with primary chest wall tumor.

REFERENCES

Arnold PG, Pairolero PC: Chondrosarcoma of the manubrium. Resection and reconstruction with pectoralis major muscle. Mayo Clin Proc 53:54, 1978.

Arnold PG, Pairolero PC: Use of pectoralis major muscle flaps to repair defects of anterior chest wall. Plast Reconstr Surg 63:205, 1979.

Arnold PG, Pairolero PC: Chest wall reconstruction: experience with 100 consecutive patients. Ann Surg 199:725, 1984.

Dahlin DC, Unni KK: Bone tumors: general aspects and data on 8,542 cases. Springfield, IL: Charles C. Thomas, 1986.

Eng J, et al: Primary bony chest wall tumours. J R Coll Surg Edinb 35:44, 1990.

Evans KG, et al: Chest wall tumours. Can J Surg 33:229, 1990.

Farley JH Seyfer AE: Chest wall tumors: experience with 58 patients. Mil Med 156:413, 1991.

Fortier M, et al: Chest wall tumors: comparison between MR and CT. Radiology (in press) 1993.

Goellner JR, Soule EH: Desmoid tumors: an ultrastructural study of eight cases. Hum Pathol 11:43, 1980.

Graeber GM, et al: Initial and long-term results in the management of primary chest wall neoplasms. Ann Thorac Surg 34:664, 1982.

Groff DB, Adkins PC: Chest wall tumors. Ann Thorac Surg 4:260, 1967.

Hajdu SI: Pathology of soft tissue tumors. Philadelphia: Lea & Febiger, 1979, p 122.

Hayry P, et al: The desmoid tumor. II. Analysis of factors possibly contributing to the etiology and growth behavior. Am J Clin Pathol 77:674, 1982.

King RM, et al: Primary chest wall tumors: factors affecting survival. Ann Thorac Surg 41:597, 1986.

Lichtenstein L: Bone Tumors. 5th Ed. St. Louis: CV Mosby, 1977, p 186.

Lichtenstein L, Jaffe HL: Chondrosarcoma of bone. Am J Pathol 19:553, 1943.

McAfee MK, et al: Chondrosarcoma of the chest wall: factors affecting survival. Ann Thorac Surg 40:535, 1985.

Pairolero PC, Arnold PG: Chest wall tumors: experience with 100 consecutive patients. J Thorac Cardiovasc Surg 90:367, 1985.

Pairolero PC, Arnold PG: Thoracic wall defects: surgical management of 205 consecutive patients. Mayo Clin Proc 61:557, 1986.

Pascuzzi CA, Dahlin DC, Clagett OT: Primary tumors of the ribs and sternum. Surg Gynecol Obstet 104:390, 1957.

Ryan MB, McMurtrey MJ, Roth JA: Current management of chest-wall tumors. Surg Clin North Am 69:1061, 1989.

Soule EG, Scanlon PW: Fibrosarcoma arising in an extraabdominal desmoid tumor: report of a case. Mayo Clin Proc 37:443, 1962.

Stelzer P, Gay WA Jr: Tumors of the chest wall. Surg Clin North Am 60:779, 1980.

Weiss SW, Enzinger FM: Malignant fibrous histiocytoma: an analysis of 200 cases. Cancer 41:2250, 1978.

CHAPTER 43

CHEST WALL RECONSTRUCTION

Peter C. Pairolero

Reconstruction of chest wall defects has been a constant challenge to the surgeon. Since 1970, numerous authors have made significant contributions to reconstruction of the thorax. Muscle and musculocutaneous flaps of the latissimus dorsi, pectoralis major, serratus anterior, rectus abdominis, and external oblique muscles have been used most frequently. The clarification of the functional anatomy and blood supply of these muscles has resulted in more aggressive resections in the treatment of chest wall tumors and in the surgical amelioration of the ravages of radiation therapy. Reports by McCormack (1981), Larson (1982), Arnold (1986), and their colleagues and by me and Arnold (1985, 1986a,b) confirmed that aggressive resection of the chest wall with immediate, dependable reconstruction is reasonable for managing these problems.

ETIOLOGY

Defects of the chest wall occur almost always as a result of neoplasm, irradiation, or infection (Table 43–1). The chest wall defect produced by resection of most neoplasms involves loss of the skeleton and frequently the overlying soft tissues as well. Infection, radiation necrosis, and trauma produce partial or full-thickness defects, depending on their severity.

Table 43–1.   Etiology of Chest Wall Defects

Neoplasm
    Primary chest wall
    Metastatic chest wall
    Contiguous lung cancer
    Contiguous breast cancer

Infection
    Median sternotomy wound
    Lateral thoracotomy wound
    Osteomyelitis
    Costochondritis

Radiation Necrosis

Trauma

PREOPERATIVE EVALUATION

Chest wall resection and reconstruction is a major undertaking and has the full potential for life-threatening complications. As discussed by Azarow and associates (1989), accurate preoperative assessment is critical because it will allow the detection and treatment of correctable problems. The patient at high risk for developing postoperative complications can often be identified by history and by physical, radiographic, and routine laboratory examinations. The importance of a careful respiratory history cannot be overemphasized. The patient's smoking habits, occupational exposure, and other possible exposure to pulmonary irritants should also be obtained. The presence of dyspnea, cough, sputum, and wheeze should be thoroughly evaluated. The extent of any underlying lung disease should be documented. Routine pulmonary function testing, such as spirometry, should be obtained in all patients. Nonpulmonary risk factors, such as cardiovascular and renal, are equally important. Age itself, however, is relatively unimportant if the patient is otherwise in good health.

CONSIDERATION FOR RECONSTRUCTION

The ability to close large chest wall defects is the main consideration in the surgical treatment of most chest wall afflictions. Excision should not be undertaken if the surgeon does not have the confidence and ability to close the defect. The critical questions of whether or not the reconstructed thorax will support respiration and protect the underlying organs must be answered when considering both the extent of resection and the method of reconstruction. This is true whether the thorax is involved with a neoplasm, an infection, or radiation necrosis. Adequate resection and dependable reconstruction are the mandatory ingredients for successful treatment. These two important items are accomplished most safely, as Arnold and I (1984) noted, by the joint efforts of a thoracic surgeon and a plastic surgeon.

Table 43–2. Considerations for Reconstruction of Chest Wall Defects

Location

Size

Depth
    Partial thickness
    Full thickness

Duration

Condition of Local Tissue
    Irradiation
    Infection
    Residual tumor
    Scarring

General Condition of Patient
    Chemotherapy
    Corticosteroid
    Chronic infection

Life-Style and Type of Work

Prognosis

Reconstruction of chest wall defects involves consideration of many factors (Table 43–2). The location and size are of utmost importance, but the past medical history and local conditions of the wound may drastically alter a reconstructive choice. Primary closure remains the best option available when possible. If the defect is partial thickness and will accept and support a skin graft, reconstruction in this manner is quite reasonable. If a partial thickness defect will not reliably accept a skin graft, a situation that frequently occurs with radiation necrosis, omental transposition with skin grafting is used. If full-thickness reconstruction is required, both the structural stability of the thorax and soft tissue coverage must be considered.

SPECIAL CONSIDERATIONS

Radiation Injury

Radiation therapy has undoubtedly saved many lives and benefited countless other patients. In Arnold's and my experience (1986, 1989), however, the reconstructive surgeon is rarely, if ever, asked to see a recipient of such therapy who has had absolutely no problems. Rather, most patients have impending or actual chest wall ulceration, complicated by the ever-present possibility of recurrent cancer. Certainly, situations arise when resection and reconstruction are reasonable alternatives in spite of the possible presence of metastatic disease. In many of these patients, the quality of life can be vastly improved with such a procedure. It is also important to understand the extent of radiation injury in adjacent tissues. Computed tomography — CT — and magnetic resonance — MR — imaging are helpful because they more accurately delineate the condition of the underlying lung and mediastinum. Such information may, in fact, be more important than the presence or absence of distant metastases. Knowledge of the presence of a mediastinal abscess or destroyed lung is critical for successful chest wall resection and reconstruction. If a history of chest wall bleeding is present, consideration should be given to angiography if there is any suspicion of involvement of the heart or great vessels. Similarly, parasternal ulceration deserves careful evaluation because of potential erosion into the internal mammary vessel, with severe hemorrhage as its sequela.

Infected Median Sternotomy Wounds

Infected median sternotomy wounds are life-threatening complications. Left untreated, these infections can extend to cardiac and aortic suture lines, prosthetic grafts, and intracardiac prostheses. The author and Arnold (1984) and I and my associates (1991) believe that these wounds should be inspected under general anesthesia in the operating room, where the subcutaneous space and sternum are opened and all foreign material is removed. All recesses of the previously dissected mediastinum must be thoroughly explored. However, every effort should be made to avoid entering the pleural spaces if there is no clinical or radiographic evidence of empyema.

After debridement, the sternotomy wound is dressed with gauze moistened with saline solution. The dressing is changed every 4 to 6 hours in the patient's wound. If at any time there is evidence of new or persistent necrotic tissue, the patient is returned to the operating room for further debridement. Secondary closure is performed when the wound is clean.

The author and Arnold (1984) prefer to obliterate the mediastinum with pectoralis major muscle flaps (Fig. 43–1), reserving rectus abdominis muscle transposition as a backup procedure. Most commonly, both pectoralis major muscles are mobilized. The humeral attachments are divided as needed to permit the degree of rotation and advancement required. The overlying skin and subcutaneous tissues are closed either directly or later. Miller and Nahai (1989), however, prefer to leave the medial edge of the pectoralis muscle attached to the chest wall and obliterate the mediastinum by a turnover of the muscle.

SKELETAL RECONSTRUCTION

Reconstruction of the bony thorax is controversial. Differences of opinion exist about who should be reconstructed and what type of reconstruction should be done. In general, all full-thickness skeletal defects that have the potential for paradox should be reconstructed. The decision not to reconstruct the skeleton depends on the size and location of the defect. Defects less than 5 cm in greatest diameter anywhere on the thorax are usually not reconstructed. Posterior defects less than 10 cm likewise do not require reconstruction because the overlying scapula provides support. Larger defects, however, should be reconstructed, and autogenous tissue such as fascia lata or ribs and prosthetic

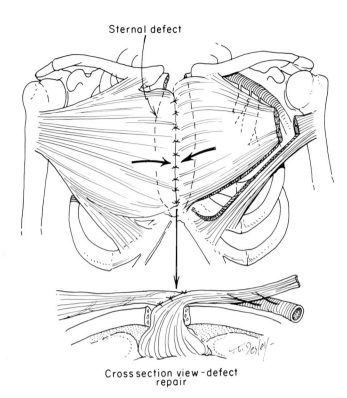

Sternal defect

Cross section view-defect
repair

Fig. 43–1. Use of pectoralis major muscle for infected median sternotomy. The left (nondominant) pectoralis major muscle is separated from its humeral attachment. The lateral aspect of the muscle is left intact to maintain an anterior axillary fold. The left muscle is transposed into the mediastinum to obliterate dead space and is sutured to the right (dominant) pectoralis major muscle, which is advanced to the midline (insert). *From* Pairolero PC, Arnold PG: Management of recalcitrant median sternotomy wounds. J Thorac Cardiovasc Surg 88:357, 1984.

material such as the various meshes, metals, or methyl methacrylate has been used.

Stabilization of the bony thorax is best accomplished with prosthetic material such as Prolene mesh (Ethicon, Inc., Somerville, NJ) or 2-mm polytetrafluoroethylene (Gore-tex) soft tissue patch (W.L. Gore and Associates, Inc., Elkton, MD). Placing either of these materials under tension improves the rigidity of the prosthesis in all directions. The soft tissue patch is superior because it prevents movement of fluid and air across the reconstructed chest wall. Marlex mesh (Daval, Inc., Providence, RI) is used less frequently because when placed under tension, it is rigid in one direction only. Although the author and Arnold (1985, 1986a) believe that reconstruction with rigid materials such as methyl methacrylate-impregnated meshes is not necessary, Mc-Cormack (1989) has been a strong advocate of this procedure.

Full-thickness skeletal defects resulting from excision of tumors of both the sternum and lateral chest wall should be reconstructed if the wound is not contaminated. If the wound is contaminated from previous radiation necrosis or necrotic neoplasm, reconstruction with prosthetic material is not advised, as the prosthesis may subsequently become infected, resulting in oblig-

atory removal. In this situation, reconstruction with a musculocutaneous flap alone is preferred. Similarly, resection of the bony thorax in a patient who has been previously irradiated may not require skeletal reconstruction as the lung frequently adheres to the underlying parietal pleura and paradox does not occur. Covering radiation skin necrosis with soft tissue is frequently adequate.

SOFT TISSUE RECONSTRUCTION

Both muscle and omental transposition can be used to reconstruct soft tissue chest wall defects (Table 43–3). Muscle is the tissue of choice for soft tissue coverage of full-thickness defects for which skeletal reconstruction is not required. Muscle can be transposed as muscle alone or as a musculocutaneous flap. The omentum should be reserved for partial-thickness reconstruction or as a backup procedure for muscle transposition that has failed in full-thickness defects.

Muscle Transposition

Latissimus Dorsi

The latissimus dorsi muscle is the largest flat muscle in the thorax. Its dominant thoracodorsal neurovascular leash has an arc of rotation that allows coverage of the lateral and central back as well as the anterolateral and central front of the thorax, as Campbell (1950) and Bostwick and associates (1979) pointed out. Its dependable musculocutaneous vascular connections also make it a reliable musculocutaneous flap. This muscle flap can cover huge chest wall defects because virtually one half of the back can be elevated on the blood supply of a single latissimus dorsi muscle in the uninjured, nonirradiated patient (Fig. 43–2). The donor site may need skin grafts when large musculocutaneous flaps are elevated, but this represents a small disadvantage when considering that large, robust flaps can be transposed to either the anterior or posterior chest for full-thickness reconstruction. If the dominant blood supply has been compromised from previous trauma or surgery, Fisher and colleagues (1983) showed the muscle can still dependably be transposed on the branch of the adjacent serratus anterior muscle.

Pectoralis Major

The pectoralis major muscle is the second largest flat muscle on the chest wall and in many respects is the

Table 43–3. Autogenous Tissue Available for Chest Wall Reconstruction

Muscle
Latissimus dorsi
Pectoralis major
Rectus abdominis
Serratus anterior
External oblique
Trapezius
Omentum

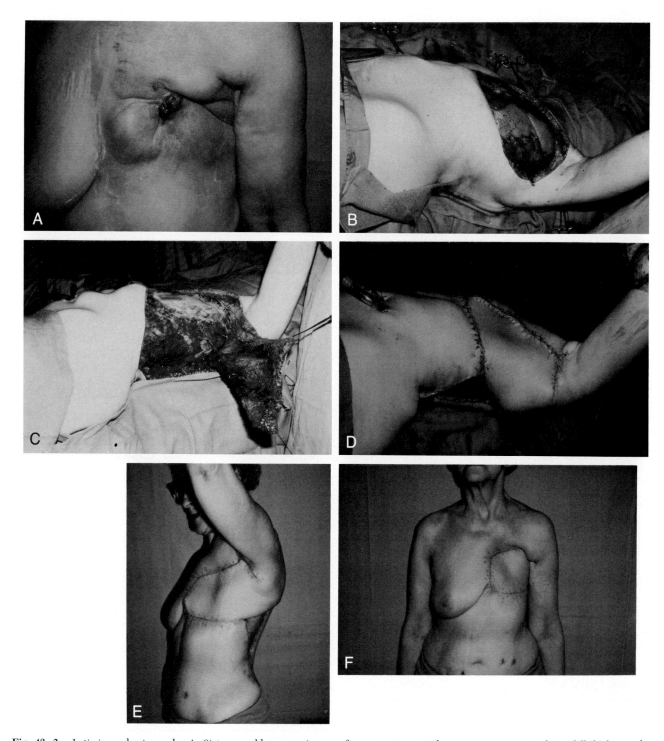

Fig. 43–2. Latissimus dorsi muscle. *A,* Sixty-year-old woman 4 years after mastectomy with recurrent tumor involving full-thickness chest wall. *B,* Intraoperative view at the time of full-thickness chest wall resection. *C,* The thoracic skeleton has been replaced with Prolene mesh and a large left latissimus dorsi musculocutaneous flap elevated. *D,* The musculocutaneous flap has been rotated into place and a portion of the donor site skin grafted. *E* and *F,* Appearance of the chest wall 3 months following resection. *From* Arnold PG, Pairolero PC: Chest wall reconstruction: experience with 100 consecutive patients. Ann Surg *199:*725, 1984.

mirror image of the latissimus dorsi muscle. As Arnold and I (1979) reported, its dominant thoracoacromial neurovascular leash, which enters posteriorly about midclavicle, allows both elevation of the muscle, either as a muscle or musculocutaneous flap, and rotation

centrally for chest wall reconstruction. The pectoralis major muscle is equally as reliable as the latissimus dorsi flap. The author and Arnold (1984, 1986b) showed that it is beneficial in reconstructing anterior chest wall defects such as those resulting from sternal tumor excisions and infected median sternotomy wounds (Fig. 43–3). Generally, only the muscle is transposed, and the skin can be closed primarily, thereby avoiding the distortion created by centralizing the breast. Reconstruction in this manner is more symmetric and aesthetically acceptable. If central skin must be excised, symmetry of the breast can still be maintained, because the transposed muscle readily accepts and supports an overlying skin graft. If necessary, the muscle can also be transposed on its secondary blood supply through the perforators from the internal mammary vessels.

Rectus Abdominis

Use of the rectus abdominis muscle for chest wall reconstruction is based on the internal mammary neurovascular leash. The inferior epigastric vessels must be divided to allow rotation to the chest wall. This muscle can be mobilized and moved either as a muscle or as a musculocutaneous flap (Fig. 43–4) with the skin component oriented either horizontally or vertically or both. The vertical skin flap, however, is more reliable because it is oriented along the long axis of the muscle

and thus maintains more musculocutaneous perforators. The donor site is usually closed primarily.

The author and Arnold (1985) believe the rectus abdominis muscle is most useful in reconstruction of lower sternal wounds. Either muscle can be used, as their arcs of rotation are identical. The muscle that has patent and uninjured internal mammary vessels must be chosen. Angiographic demonstration of vessel patency may help determine which musculocutaneous unit would be most reliable, particularly in previously irradiated patients or in patients with infected sternotomy wounds. Also, in many infected sternotomy wounds, the internal mammary artery may have previously been used for coronary artery bypass.

Serratus Anterior

The serratus anterior muscle is a small flat muscle located in the midaxillary line between the latissimus dorsi and pectoralis major muscles. Its blood supply comes from the serratus branch of the thoracodorsal vessels and from the long thoracic artery and vein. This muscle can be used alone or as an adjunctive muscle

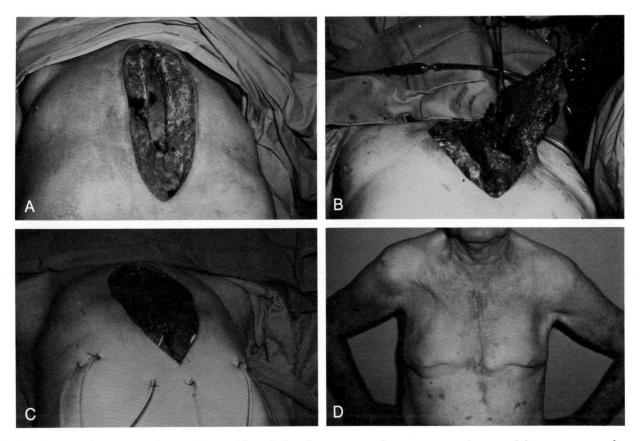

Fig. 43–3. Pectoralis major muscle. A, A 72-year-old man had median sternotomy for coronary artery bypass graft for coronary artery disease. A, Approximately 3 months later, after multiple debridements that removed essentially the central portion of the sternum. B, At the time of closure the left pectoralis major muscle is totally mobilized and separated from the humeral attachment. The right pectoralis major muscle is mobilized over the midaxillary line but not separated from its humeral attachment. C, The two muscles are sutured together in the midline, and a large portion of the left pectoralis major muscle is draped into the defect in the central sternal area. D, Appearance approximately 3 months following closure. *From* Arnold PG, Pairolero PC: Chest wall reconstruction: experience with 100 consecutive patients. Ann Surg 199:725, 1984.

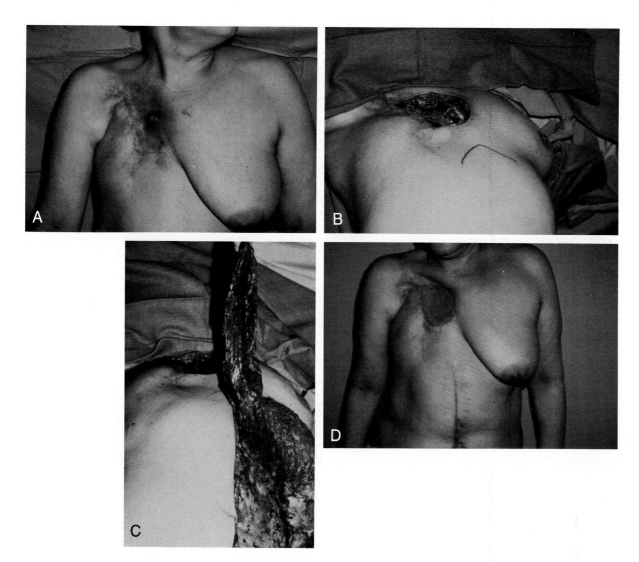

Fig. 43–4. Rectus abdominis muscle. *A,* Forty-nine-year-old woman 5 years following mastectomy and radiation therapy with radionecrotic area on the right chest. *B,* The wound is excised, including a portion of the right sternum and the right anterior chest wall. *C,* Contralateral (left) rectus abdominis muscle is elevated for transposition into the defect. *D,* Four months after closure with split-thickness skin graft over the transposed rectus abdominis muscle. *From* Arnold PG, Pairolero PC: Chest wall reconstruction: experience with 100 consecutive patients. Ann Surg 199:725, 1984.

with the pectoralis major or the latissimus dorsi muscles. As Arnold and colleagues (1984) pointed out, the muscle also augments the skin-carrying ability of either adjacent muscle. The author and colleagues (1983) found that this muscle is particularly useful as an intrathoracic muscle flap.

External Oblique

The external oblique muscle can also be transposed as a muscle or musculocutaneous flap (Fig. 43–5), and it is most useful in closing defects of the upper abdomen and lower thorax. It reaches the inframammary fold without tension but, as Hodgkinson and Arnold (1980) noted, does not readily extend higher. The primary blood supply is from the lower thoracic intercostal vessels, as Lund (1913), Hedblom (1921), Harrington

(1927), Zinninger (1930), Maier (1947), Watson and James (1947), and Bisgard and Swensen (1948) demonstrated. With this muscle, lower chest wall defects can be closed without distorting the breast.

Trapezius Muscle

The trapezius muscle has been useful to close defects at the base of the neck or the thoracic outlet but is not consistently useful for other chest wall reconstructions. Its primary blood supply is the dorsal scapular vessels.

Omental Transposition

Omental transposition, as Jurkiewicz and Arnold (1977) noted, has been most useful in reconstructing partial-thickness chest wall defects, particularly in radiation necrosis that does not involve tumor (Fig. 43–6).

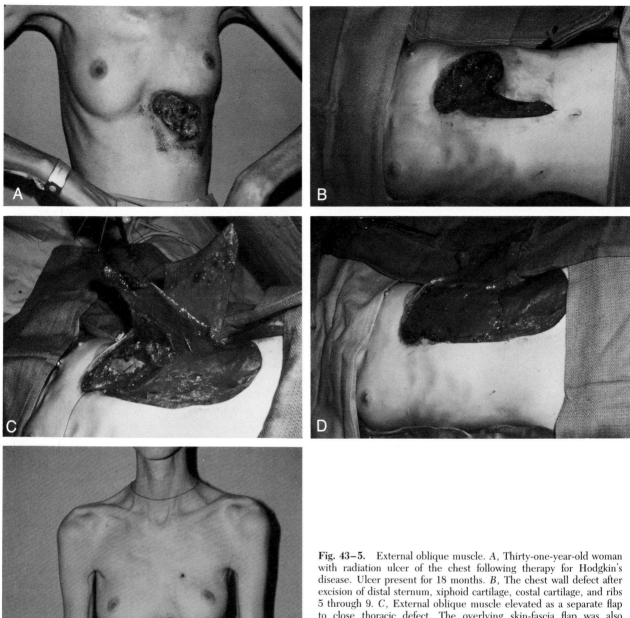

Fig. 43–5. External oblique muscle. *A*, Thirty-one-year-old woman with radiation ulcer of the chest following therapy for Hodgkin's disease. Ulcer present for 18 months. *B*, The chest wall defect after excision of distal sternum, xiphoid cartilage, costal cartilage, and ribs 5 through 9. *C*, External oblique muscle elevated as a separate flap to close thoracic defect. The overlying skin-fascia flap was also advanced to close the cutaneous defect, which was smaller. *D*, Muscle flap sutured into position to close the chest wall defect. *E*, Four months postoperatively. *From* Hodgkinson DJ, Arnold PG: Chest wall reconstruction using the external oblique muscle. Br J Plast Surg 33:216, 1980.

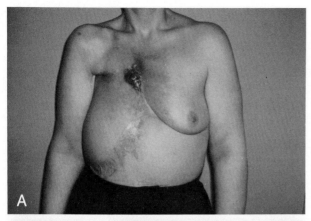

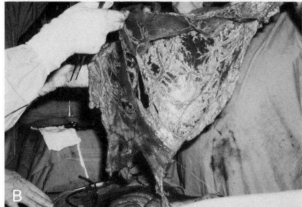

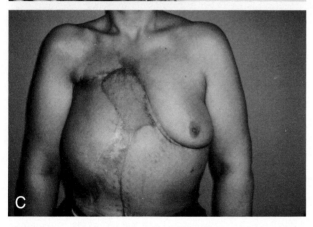

Fig. 43-6. Omentum. A 44-year-old woman had a modified mastectomy with radiation therapy. Radiation necrosis was treated by rotation of a large cutaneous flap based on the right. *A,* Wound breakdown developed, requiring excision of skin and soft tissue only; there was no evidence of recurrent tumor. *B,* Greater omentum was mobilized on right gastroepiploic vessels in preparation for transposition into the defect. *C,* Appearance of chest 6 months after closure, with a stable split-thickness skin graft. *From* Arnold PG, Pairolero PC: Chest wall reconstruction: experience with 100 consecutive patients. Ann Surg *199:*725, 1984.

In this situation, the skin and soft tissue are debrided down to what remains of the thoracic skeleton, which may be either bone or cartilage but frequently is only irradiated ischemic scar. The transposed omentum with its excellent blood supply from the gastroepiploic vessels

adheres to the irradiated wound and readily accepts and supports an overlying skin graft. Because the omentum has no structural stability of its own, it is not particularly useful in full-thickness defects because additional support, such as fascia lata, bone, or prosthetic material, is necessary.

Omental transposition is helpful when planned muscle flaps have failed with partial necrosis. Generally, this results in only a soft tissue defect, and pleural seal with respiratory stability is not required, thus allowing a most threatening situation to be salvaged.

Although infections of the lower sternum are best treated with a rectus abdominis muscle flap, the blood supply, based on the distal aspect of the internal mammary artery, may have been interrupted previously either by use of this artery for coronary revascularization or by ligation with sternal resection. If the internal mammary artery is not intact or if the wound is large, omental transposition is performed, followed by split-thickness skin grafting 48 hours later.

CLINICAL EXPERIENCE

During the past 16 years, Arnold and I have performed 455 chest wall reconstructions at the Mayo Clinic; 195 patients had chest wall tumors, 105 had radiation necrosis, 106 had infected median sternotomy wounds, and 49 had a combination of these. The patients ranged in age from 5 to 85 years, with a mean of 54.2 years. The bony skeleton was resected in 393 patients. An average of 4.9 ribs were resected. Total or partial sternectomies were performed in 155 patients. Skeletal defects were closed with prosthetic material in 150 patients. Three hundred and twenty-four patients underwent 485 muscle transpositions including 301 pectoralis major, 98 latissimus dorsi, 27 serratus anterior, and 18 rectus abdominis. The omentum was transposed in 43 patients.

For each patient, the mean number of operations was 1.8. Most of the multiple operations were debridements in patients with infected wounds. Hospitalization averaged 14.2 days. There were 5 perioperative deaths. Thirteen patients required tracheostomy. Most other patients, as Meadows and associates (1985) reported, had only minor changes in pulmonary function.

Follow-up averaged 56.4 months. No late deaths related to either resection or reconstruction of the chest wall occurred. All patients who were alive 30 days after operation had excellent results at the time of last follow-up or death.

CONCLUSION

Reconstruction of many chest wall defects can be performed in one operation, with minimal respiratory insufficiency, a short hospitalization, and low operative mortality. The key ingredients for successful management are accomplished most safely by the joint efforts of a thoracic and a plastic surgeon.

REFERENCES

Arnold PG, Pairolero PC: Use of pectoralis major muscle flaps to repair defects of the anterior chest wall. Plast Reconstr Surg 63:205, 1979.

Arnold PG, Pairolero PC, Waldorf JC: The serratus anterior muscle: intrathoracic and extrathoracic utilization. Plast Reconstr Surg 73:240, 1984.

Arnold PG, Pairolero PC: Chest wall reconstruction: experience with 100 consecutive patients. Ann Surg 199:725, 1984.

Arnold PG, Pairolero PC: Surgical management of the radiated chest wall. Plast Reconstr Surg 77:605, 1986.

Arnold PG, Pairolero PC: Reconstruction of the radiation-damaged chest wall. Surg Clin North Am 69:1081, 1989.

Azarow KS, Malloy M, Seyfer AE, Graeber GM: Preoperative evaluation and general preparation for chest-wall operations. Surg Clin North Am 69:899, 1989.

Bisgard JD, Swenson SA Jr: Tumors of the sternum: report of a case with special operative technic. Arch Surg 56:570, 1948.

Blades B, Paul JS: Chest wall tumors. Ann Surg 131:976, 1950.

Bostwick J III, et al: Sixty latissimus dorsi flaps. Plast Reconstr Surg 63:31, 1979.

Campbell DA: Reconstruction of the anterior thoracic wall. J Thorac Surg 19:456, 1950.

Fisher J, Bostwick J, Powell RW: Latissimus dorsi blood supply after thoracodorsal vessel division: the serratus collateral. Plast Reconstr Surg 72:502, 1983.

Harrington SW: Surgical treatment of intrathoracic tumors and tumors of the chest wall. Arch Surg 14:406, 1927.

Hedblom CA: Tumors of the bony chest wall. Arch Surg 3:56, 1921.

Hodgkinson DJ, Arnold PG: Chest-wall reconstruction using the external oblique muscle. Br J Plast Surg 33:216, 1980.

Jurkiewicz MJ, Arnold PG: The omentum: an account of its use in the reconstruction of the chest wall. Ann Surg 185:548, 1977.

Larson DL, et al: Major chest wall reconstruction after chest wall irradiation. Cancer 49:1286, 1982.

Lund FB: Sarcoma of the chest wall. Ann Surg 58:206, 1913.

Maier HC: Surgical management of large defects of the thoracic wall. Surgery 22:169, 1947.

McCormack P, et al: New trends in skeletal reconstruction after resection of chest wall tumors. Ann Thorac Surg 31:45, 1981.

McCormack PM: Use of prosthetic materials in chest-wall reconstruction: assets and liabilities. Surg Clin North Am 69:965, 1989.

Meadows JA, III, et al: Effect of resection of the sternum and manubrium in conjunction with muscle transposition on pulmonary function. Mayo Clin Proc 60:604, 1985.

Miller JI, Nahai F: Repair of the dehisced median sternotomy incision. Surg Clin North Am 69:1091, 1989.

Pairolero PC, Arnold PG: Management of recalcitrant median sternotomy wounds. J Thorax Cardiovasc Surg 88:357, 1984.

Pairolero PC, Arnold PG: Chest wall tumors: experience with 100 consecutive patients. J Thorac Cardiovasc Surg 90:367, 1985.

Pairolero PC, Arnold PG: Thoracic wall defects: surgical management of 205 consecutive patients. Mayo Clin Proc 61:557, 1986a.

Pairolero PC, Arnold PG: Primary tumors of the anterior chest wall. Surgical Rounds 9:19, 1986b.

Pairolero PC, Arnold PG, Harris JB: Long-term results of pectoralis major muscle transposition for infected sternotomy wounds. Ann Surg 213:583, 1991.

Pairolero PC, Arnold PG, Piehler JM: Intrathoracic transposition of extrathoracic skeletal muscle. J Thorac Cardiovasc Surg 86:809, 1983.

Watson WL, James AG: Fascia lata grafts for chest wall defects. J Thorac Surg 16:399, 1947.

Zinninger MM: Tumors of the wall of the thorax. Ann Surg 92:1043, 1930.

READING REFERENCES

Blades B, Paul JS: Chest wall tumors. Ann Surg 131:976, 1950.

Boyd AD, et al: Immediate reconstruction of full-thickness chest wall defects. Ann Thorac Surg 32:337, 1981.

Brown RG, Fleming WH, Jurkiewicz MJ: An island flap of the pectoralis major muscle. Br J Plast Surg 30:161, 1977.

Burnard RJ, Martini N, Beattie EJ, Jr: The value of resection in tumors involving the chest wall. J Thorac Cardiovasc Surg 68:530, 1974.

Converse JM, Campbell RM, Watson WL: Repair of large radiation ulcers situated over the heart and the brain. Ann Surg 133:95, 1951.

Fell GE: Forced respiration. JAMA 16:325, 1891.

Graham EA, Singer JJ: Successful removal of an entire lung for carcinoma of the bronchus. JAMA 101:1371, 1933.

Irons GB, et al: Use of the omental free flap for soft-tissue reconstruction. Ann Plast Surg 11:501, 1983.

Jurkiewicz MJ, et al: Infected median sternotomy wound: successful treatment by muscle flaps. Ann Surg 191:738, 1980.

Kiricuta I: L'emploi du grand epiploon dans la chirurgie du sein cancereux. Presse Med 71:15, 1963.

Le Roux BT: Maintenance of chest wall stability. Thorax 19:397, 1964.

Martini N, Starzynski TE, Beattie EJ Jr: Problems in chest wall resection. Surg Clin North Am 49:313, 1969.

McGraw JB, Penix JO, Baker JW: Repair of major defects of the chest wall and spine with the latissimus dorsi myocutaneous flap. Plast Reconstr Surg 62:197, 1978.

Myre TT, Kirklin JW: Resection of tumors of the sternum. Ann Surg 144:1023, 1956.

O'Dwyer J: Fifty cases of croup in private practice treated by intubation of the larynx with a description of the method and of the dangers incident thereto. Med Rec 32:557, 1887.

Parham FW: Thoracic resection for tumors growing from the bony wall of the chest. Trans South Surg Gynecol Assoc 11:223, 1898.

Pickrell KL, Kelley JW, Marzoni FA: The surgical treatment of recurrent carcinoma of the breast and chest wall. Plast Reconstr Surg 3:156, 1948.

Ramming KP, et al: Surgical management and reconstruction of extensive chest wall malignancies. Am J Surg 144:146, 1982.

Rees TD, Converse JM: Surgical reconstruction of defects of the thoracic wall. Surg Gynecol Obstet 121:1066, 1965.

Starzynski TE, Snyderman RK, Beattie EJ Jr: Problems of major chest wall reconstruction. Plast Reconstr Surg 44:525, 1969.

CHAPTER 44

THORACOPLASTY

Thomas W. Shields

The operative removal of the skeletal support of a portion of the chest is called a "thoracoplasty." This procedure is accomplished by the subperiosteal removal of a varying number of rib segments. The removal of the rib segments permits the unsupported portion of the chest wall to sink in toward the mediastinum and, thus, reduces the size of the hemithorax. This results in partial collapse of the underlying lung. Although a great variety of thoracoplasty procedures have been described, the extraperiosteal paravertebral thoracoplasty described by Alexander (1937) is the standard procedure.

At present, this operation is used primarily in the treatment of chronic thoracic empyema when there is either insufficient or no remaining pulmonary tissue to obliterate the pleural space. Even for this purpose, it is used less than it once was, and many surgeons use thoracoplasty only as a procedure of last resort. It is rarely used in patients with pulmonary tuberculosis, except for pleural and occasionally extensive combined pleuropulmonary disease. A limited preresection "tailoring" thoracoplasty and the plombage type of thoracoplasty may be used on rare occasions in a patient with extensive parenchymal disease and markedly reduced pulmonary function.

In the "tailoring" thoracoplasty, a limited number of ribs of the upper portion of the chest are removed a week or so before thoracotomy, when it is expected that the proposed resection would result in an insufficient amount of remaining lung tissue to fill the normal-sized thoracic cage. In a plombage thoracotomy, an inert, foreign substance is placed in a space created beneath the rib cage by extraperiosteal stripping of the ribs of the upper portion of the chest. However, using a foreign substance to obtain collapse in the presence of underlying pleural infection is contraindicated.

When the desired collapse cannot be obtained by a conventional thoracoplasty or the space cannot be obliterated by a muscle flap transposition, and a persistent infected space remains, a Schede thoracoplasty or one of its many modifications may be necessary. A

modification of the standard thoracoplasty, described by Sawamura and reported by Iioka and associates (1985), may even reduce further the need for conventional thoracoplasty or the more deforming Schede procedure in patients with chronic pleural tuberculous or postpneumonic empyema.

OPERATIVE TECHNIQUE

Conventional Thoracoplasty

The standard procedure is that outlined by Alexander (1937). Now that the operation is used to control a chronic thoracic empyema, the procedure is accomplished in one stage. When it was employed to treat pulmonary tuberculosis, it was done in two or more stages to circumvent adverse physiologic changes of paradoxic chest wall motion occurring in the postoperative period. The magnitude of the collapse procedure depends on the size of the empyema cavity. Ordinarily, seven ribs are resected. This allows the scapula and attached extracostal musculature to drop into the space and helps to maintain the collapse. Should fewer ribs be resected, the lower portion of the scapula may have to be excised, so that it does not impinge on the remaining ribs. This would prevent it from falling into the created space to help obtain optimal collapse. Special attention postoperatively must be paid to ensure proper functioning of the ipsilateral shoulder girdle when an extensive thoracoplasty has been done.

With the patient in the lateral decubitus position, a parascapular incision is begun at the level of the spine of the scapula and extended inferiorly and laterally to the midaxillary line. The subjacent extracostal muscles — trapezius, rhomboids, and latissimus dorsi — are incised to expose the rib cage and to allow the scapula to be retracted anteriorly and superiorly (Fig. 44–1). Posteriorly, the attachments of the serratus posterior and erector spinae muscle groups are separated from the ribs of the upper half of the chest. Similarly, the insertions of the serratus anterior muscle are separated from the upper three or four ribs.

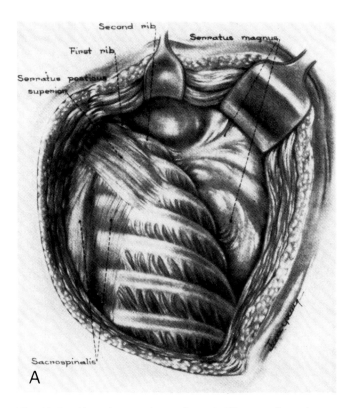

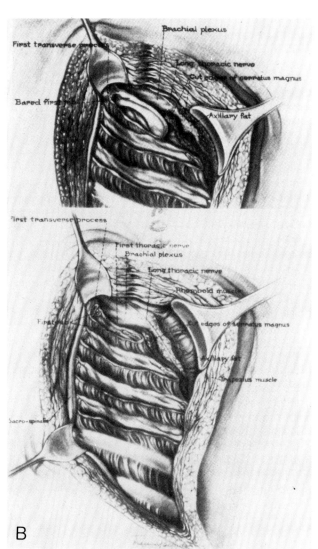

Fig. 44–1. Alexander-type thoracoplasty. *A*, Elevation of scapula to expose chest wall. *B*, Ribs resected as described in text. *From* Alexander J: The Collapse Therapy of Pulmonary Tuberculosis. Springfield, IL: Charles C Thomas, 1937.

After exposure of the rib cage, the posterior half of the third rib is resected after incising and stripping off its periosteal investment. In patients with an empyema, the transverse process of the vertebral body generally need not be excised, but this can be done if necessary to achieve maximal collapse. This excision is facilitated by division of the costotransverse ligaments (Fig. 44–2). The transverse process is best removed by the use of a rongeur after retraction of the sacrospinalis muscles medially. The rib is then resected further posteriorly to the level of the base of the transverse process. Some surgeons also prefer to excise the head of the rib as well, avulsing it from its articulation with the vertebral body. Next, the second rib is resected subperiosteally from the costochondral junction to the vertebral body; the second transverse process may also be removed. It is essential that no residual space remain in the costovertebral sulcus.

The first rib is removed if a limited thoracoplasty is done for obliteration of an apical empyema space that has occurred after a lobectomy. If the procedure is done for the collapse of a chronic postpneumonectomy empyema space, however, the first rib may not have to

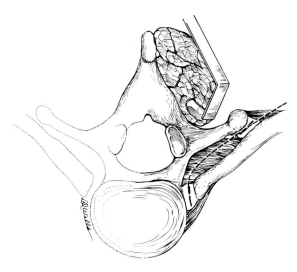

Fig. 44–2. Site of division of the costotransverse ligaments to facilitate removal of the head of the rib and the transverse process.

be removed and, in fact, Deslauriers (personal communication, 1987) believes it should always be left in place to preserve the structural integrity of the neck, shoulder girdle, and upper thorax. If there is any doubt of any apical, residual space remaining, however, the first rib should be removed, as suggested by McMillan (1987). When this is indicated, the first rib is exposed and the periosteum incised on its lower edge. This usually is accomplished by scraping the edge with a periosteal elevator. The flat inferior surface is stripped of its periosteum. Starting far posteriorly, the outer or superior surface is stripped of its periosteum; care must be taken to protect the brachial plexus and subclavian vessels at this time. This is best accomplished by inserting a finger to retract the neurovascular structures away from the rib. Extreme caution is necessary at the scalene tubercle (Fig. 44–3). The rib then is divided at the level of the tip of the transverse process and avulsed from its costochondral junction anteriorly. The head of the first rib and the first transverse process are not resected. A portion of the remaining third rib and segments of the lower ribs are then resected subperiosteally to ensure complete obliteration of the empyema space.

Bjork (1954) and others have suggested the use of an osteoplastic technique of thoracoplasty. Initially, the first rib was divided as well as the second through the fifth ribs; however, now, as described by Conlan (1990), the first rib is left intact, and only a subperiosteal resection of the posterior portions of the second through fifth ribs is carried out. The apex is then freed by extrapleural mobilization and permitted to drop, thus preserving the first rib. The residual lengths of the second to fifth ribs and underlying chest wall are sutured

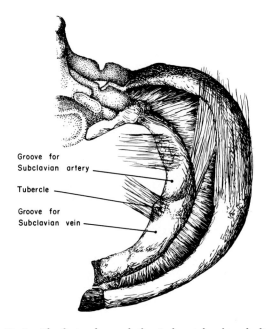

Groove for
Subclavian artery

Tubercle

Groove for
Subclavian vein

Fig. 44–3. The first and second ribs. Scalene tubercle and adjacent important areas are shown.

down to the sixth rib. This gives the chest wall stability, but this step would appear to be unnecessary when the collapse is done to obliterate an empyema cavity.

Thoracomyopleuroplasty

Rather than carry out an Alexander extraperiosteal paravertebral thoracoplasty, Dupon (1990) has suggested the use of thoracomyopleuroplasty — thoracomediastinal plication — originally described by Andrews (1961) (Fig. 44–4). In this technique, only the ribs overlying the empyema space are resected. The remainder of the chest wall, including the apex, is freed as necessary by mobilizing the musculoperiosteal wall from the remaining overlying portions of the rib cage. The empyema space is then entered, and debridement of parietal and visceral surfaces of the space is carried out. The cavity is then obliterated by suturing — mattressing — the pleuromusculoperiosteal wall to the mediastinal or visceral pleura. The thoracotomy incision is then reapproximated down to the space and closed without drainage. The stated advantages are that this procedure is much smaller than the standard thoracoplasty, is a less mutilating procedure, is well tolerated by the poor-risk patient, and obtains similar results.

Grow (1946) and Kergin (1953) reported earlier similar modifications of the thoracoplasty procedure, as that suggested by Andrews (1961). All ribs are resected over the empyema space, but the intercostal bundles are left intact. By incisions through one or more of the exposed periosteal beds, a parietal decortication is accomplished. Superficial curettage of the underlying visceral pleural peel is executed. The intercostal muscle bundles, with their vascular supply intact, are allowed to fall across the visceral surface of the cavity. A bronchopleural fistula, if present, may be excised and closed by suturing a pedicled muscle graft over the opening. The incision is closed loosely over drains lying superficial to the muscle bundles. External pressure dressings are used to ensure apposition of the tissues.

Sawamura Modified Thoracoplasty

A posterolateral thoracotomy incision is made, and all ribs overlying the empyema cavity are exposed. An incision is made through the intercostal bundle overlying the middle of the empyema and carried through the parietal peel into the empyema cavity. All purulent and necrotic tissue is removed. The visceral peel overlying the collapsed lung is removed. Any bronchopleural fistula is closed. The parietal wall is partially decorticated to permit pliability and collapsed to obliterate the space. This is accomplished by stripping the ribs subperiosteally so that the parietal wall consists of parietal pleura, periosteum, and attached intercostal muscles. A percutaneous insertion of a chest tube into the empyema cavity is then carried out. This tube must be isolated from the newly developed extraperiosteal space. The incision in the collapsed parietal wall is closed so that it is airtight. The extraperiosteal space is cleansed and irrigated to prevent subsequent infec-

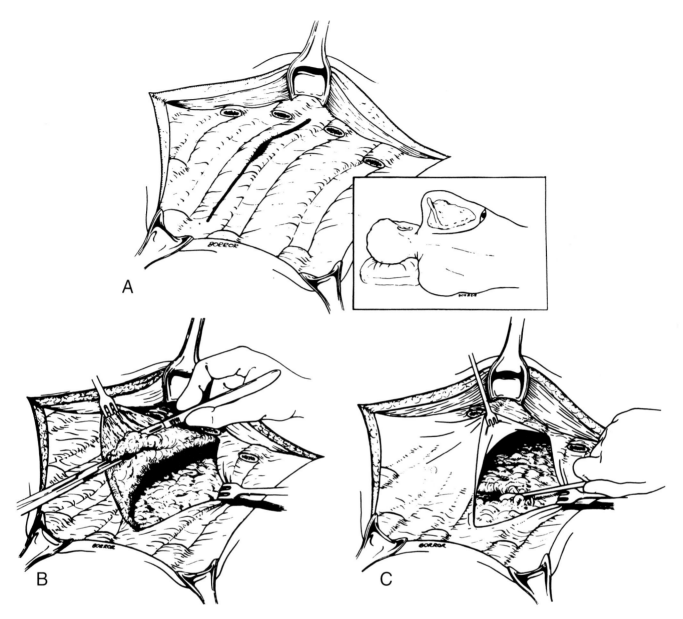

Fig. 44–4. Thoracomyopleuroplasty. *A*, First step is rib resection over the space and incision into empyema space (insert depicts the skin incision). *B*, Second step is currettage and excision of parietal pleura. *C*, Third step is curettage of the visceral or mediastinal pleura.

tion. The muscles and skin of the chest wall are then closed anatomically. After the procedure, the newly created extraperiosteal space fills with exudate, which exerts pressure on the parietal wall to keep it juxtaposed to the underlying lung. With time, this exudate is absorbed, and the lung expands to obliterate the extraperiosteal space (Fig. 44–5).

Tatsumura and associates (1990) have described a somewhat similar technique, except only the parietal wall of the empyema space is decorticated. In reality both of the techniques described by Iioka (1985) — the Sawamura thoracoplasty — and by Tatsumura (1990) and their colleagues are modifications of a pulmonary decortication rather than a thoracoplasty per se.

Plombage Thoracoplasty

This modification of the conventional thoracoplasty was developed to overcome the adverse effects of decostalization of a portion of the chest wall. A foreign substance — paraffin, lucite spheres in a polyethylene bag, or fiberglass — was inserted in a space created between the ribs and the thoracic fascia and freed periosteal and intercostal musculature to maintain optimal collapse. The technique of this procedure was described by Fox and the author (1972) in the first edition of this text. Talamonti and associates (1989) recently have reported the use of an inflatable tissue expander to obtain the degree of collapse desired. The

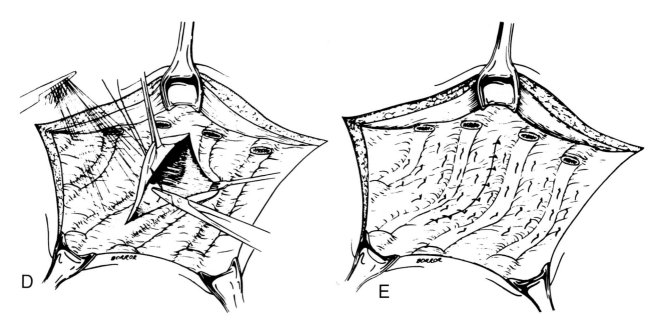

Fig. 44–4 (continued). *D*, Fourth step is the placement of U-type stitch through the pleuromusculoperiosteal layer down to the visceral or mediastinal pleura beginning at the apex and progressing downward and avoiding the intercostal nerves and vessels. *E*, In the last step, all sutures are tied from above downward to oppose the two layers and obliterate the space. *From* Andrews NC: Thoracomediastinal plication: a surgical technique for chronic empyema. J Thorac Surg *41*:809, 1961.

use of a foreign body plomb is contraindicated in the management of a chronic empyema. Consequently, these procedures have been discarded, except in the rare patient with otherwise uncontrollable mycobacterial infection.

Schede Thoracoplasty

The operation described by Schede (1890) for obliteration of a chronic empyema space is rarely, if ever, performed at present, but has been widely modified by many surgeons. The Schede operation consists of radical unroofing of an empyema space by resecting the overlying ribs, intercostal bundles, and subjacent parietal pleural "peel." The extracostal muscles and skin are partially closed over gauze packing. The wound is repacked at intervals. The desired effect is that freshly granulating tissue sets up an obliterative healing process and eventually will close the space.

PHYSIOLOGIC CHANGES AFTER THORACOPLASTY

The immediate physiologic sequelae of a standard extraperiosteal paravertebral thoracoplasty noted previously, when performed to manage parenchymal tuberculosis, were related to the development of an area of paradoxic motion of the chest wall. The effort of breathing increased as the result of the abnormal volume displacement and greater pleural pressure changes necessary to move air in and out of the lungs. If the mediastinum was mobile, mediastinal flutter occurred. *Pendelluft*, that is, air flow from one lung to the other during the ventilatory cycle, may theoretically occur. Maloney and associates (1961), however, reported that,

in the presence of a closed chest, the lung on the side of the paradoxic chest wall motion actually expands on the inspiration. Also, Gaensler (1965) showed, by using a pneumotachographic screen at the carina, that there is no air movement from one lung to the other after a thoracoplasty, as long as the proximal airway is patent.

Retained secretions, however, caused partial airway obstruction. The cough mechanism was reduced in effectiveness as a result of the inability to generate a high positive pressure in the pleural space because of the unsupported portion of the chest wall. The postoperative problems attendant to these changes were directly proportional to the number and length of the segments of rib resected. However, when a thoracoplasty is performed to obliterate a chronic empyema cavity, the rigidity of the underlying visceral and parietal peels prevents paradoxic motion. The early physiologic changes enumerated do not occur, and the procedure can be tolerated by most patients except the very poor-risk patient.

The late physiologic changes after the operation are related not only to the extent of the rib resections and underlying lung collapse but also to the late skeletal deformity that occurs. A greater or lesser degree of rotoscoliosis develops subsequent to the removal of the ribs and the transverse processes. This results in a diminution of function of the contralateral lung. Gaensler and Strieder (1951) found that when a thoracoplasty was done over a nonfunctioning lung, a permanent loss of approximately 27% of the preoperative vital capacity and 21% of maximal voluntary ventilation of the contralateral lung followed.

Iioka and associates (1985) reported improvement in the percent vital capacity and FEV_1 predicted vital

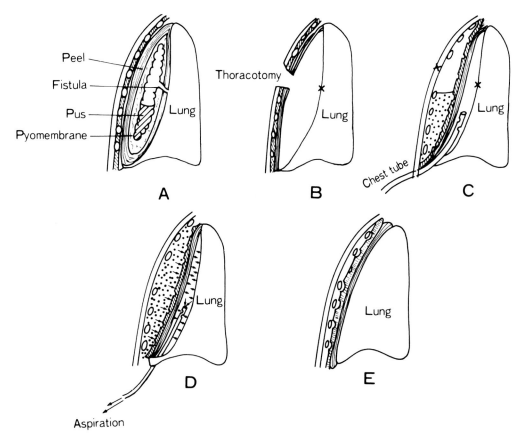

Fig. 44–5. The Sawamura modified thoracoplasty. *A*, The empyema cavity with pulmonary fistulization is encapsulated by pyomembrane and thickened pleura. *B*, The empyema cavity is curetted, and the visceral peel is decorticated. The pulmonary fistula is closed. *C*, The chest tube is inserted into the reducing empyema cavity, and an exudate fills the extraperiosteal space. *D*, The empyema cavity is obliterated by compression of the exudate and by traction of the chest tube aspiration. *E*, The lung consequently expands by absorbing the exudate. *From* Iioka S, et al: Surgical treatment of chronic empyema: a new one-stage operation. J Thorac Cardiovasc Surg 90:179, 1985.

capacity after the Sawamura modified thoracoplasty. This was not as good as they obtained with decortication alone but was superior to the functional results after modified Elosser procedures.

The physiologic changes after a Schede thoracoplasty are related to the unstable chest wall and the degree of paradoxic motion that develops. In addition, sacrifice of the intercostal nerves results in paresis of the ipsilateral abdominal wall.

MORBIDITY

Postoperative morbidity after thoracoplasty is related not only to the type of procedure employed but also to the disease process present. The complications directly related to a conventional thoracoplasty are those caused by injury of the vessels or nerves during removal of the first rib or injury to the thoracic duct with resultant chylous effusion, retention of secretions with atelectasis, and septic complications.

Wound infection is uncommon, but infection of the apical or subscapular space may occur when the operation is performed to treat a chronic empyema. However, even if the empyema space is entered during the procedure, this occurrence is unusual.

MORTALITY

Death after a thoracoplasty is most often related to the underlying chronic disease process rather than to the operation per se. Hopkins and co-workers (1985) reported a 13% mortality rate in their entire series but noted a decline in this figure in the second half of their experience. Young and Ungerleider (1990) reported a mortality rate of 10% and Dupon (1990) a rate of 5.4%. Gregoire and colleagues (1987) reported no deaths in their series of 17 patients. Iioka and associates (1985) reported only one death in 60 patients following a modified Sawamura procedure. Ideally, with modern management, a mortality rate of no more than 5% should occur.

RESULTS

The overall success rate of a thoracoplasty in eliminating intrathoracic space problems has improved over the years. Hopkins and co-workers (1985) reported a failure rate of 33% before 1976 but only 17% since then. Gregoire (1987), from Deslauriers' group, reported an early failure rate of only 12% in 17 patients with chronic postpneumonectomy empyema. In a similar group of patients, Dupon (1990) reported a complete recovery in 84% of cases, and in 2 to 15 years after the procedure, 75% of the patients had returned to normal activity.

REFERENCES

Alexander J: Collapse Therapy of Pulmonary Tuberculosis. Springfield, IL: Charles C Thomas, 1937, p 402.

Andrews NC: Thoraco-mediastinal plication: a surgical technique for chronic empyema. J Thorac Surg *41*:809, 1961.

Bjork VD: Thoracoplasty: a new osteoplastic technique. J Thorac Surg *28*:194, 1954.

Conlan AA: Prophylaxis and management of postlobectomy infected spaces. *In* Deslauriers J, Lacquet LK (eds): Thoracic Surgery: Surgical Management of Pleural Diseases. St Louis: CV Mosby, 1990, p 279.

Dupon H: Andrews technique of thoracomyopleuroplasty. *In* Deslauriers J, Lacquet LK (eds): Thoracic Surgery: Surgical Management of Pleural Diseases. St Louis: CV Mosby, 1990, p 255.

Fox RT, Shields TW: Thoracoplasty. *In* Shields TW (ed): General Thoracic Surgery. 1st Ed. Philadelphia: Lea & Febiger, 1972, p 351.

Gaensler EA: Lung displacement: abdominal enlargement, pleural space disorders, deformities of the thoracic cage. *In* Handbook of Physiology. (Fenn WO, Rahan H, eds). Baltimore: Williams & Wilkins, 1965.

Gaensler EA, Strieder JW: Progressive changes in pulmonary function after pneumonectomy: the influence of thoracoplasty, pneumo-thorax, oleothorax, plastic sponge plombage on the side of pneumonectomy. J Thorac Surg *22*:1, 1951.

Gregoire R, et al: Thoracoplasty: a forgotten role in the management of nontuberculous postpneumonectomy empyema. Can J Surg *30*:343, 1987.

Grow JB: Chronic pleural empyema. Dis Child *12*:26, 1946.

Hopkins RH, et al: The modern use of thoracoplasty. Ann Thorac Surg *40*:181, 1985.

Iioka S, et al: Surgical treatment of chronic empyema: a new one-stage operation. J Thorac Cardiovasc Surg *90*:179, 1985.

Kergin FG: An operation for chronic pleural empyema. J Thorac Surg *26*:430, 1953.

Maloney JV Jr, Schmutzer KJ, Raschke E: Paradoxical respiration and "pendelluft." J Thorac Cardiovasc Surg *41*:291, 1961.

McMillan IKR: Bronchopleural fistula: treatment by space reduction. *In* Grillo HC, Eschapasse H (eds): International Trends in General Thoracic Surgery, Vol II. A Major Challenge. Philadelphia: WB Saunders, 1987, p 440.

Schede M: Die Behandlung der Empyeme. Verh Cong Innere Med Wiesb *9*:41, 1890.

Talamonti MS, et al: A new method of extraperiosteal plombage for atypical pulmonary tuberculosis. Chest *96*:237S, 1989.

Tatsumura T, et al: A new technique for one-stage radical eradication of long-standing chronic thoracic empyema. J Thorac Cardiovasc Surg *99*:410, 1990.

Young WG, Ungerleider RM: Surgical approach to the chronic empyema: thoracoplasty. *In* DesLauriers J, Lacquet LK (eds): Thoracic Surgery: Surgical Management of Pleural Diseases. St Louis: CV Mosby, 1990, p 247.

The Diaphragm

DIAPHRAGMATIC FUNCTION, DIAPHRAGMATIC PARALYSIS, AND EVENTRATION OF THE DIAPHRAGM

Thomas W. Shields

Although the major anatomic function of the diaphragm is the separation of the thoracic and abdominal cavities, its major physiologic function is its role in ventilation. The movement of this musculotendinous structure is responsible for the largest fraction of air moved during inspiration. With quiet breathing, this accounts for approximately 75 to 80% of the total amount of air brought into the lungs. In the supine position it contributes 60% of the minute volume.

Primarily, the diaphragm is a muscle of inspiration, and the downward descent of the central tendon results from a coordinated contraction of all its muscle fibers. The resultant vertical movement is approximately 1 to 2 cm during quiet breathing but may be as great as 6 to 7 cm with deep, forced breathing. It is estimated that each centimeter of vertical movement contributes an intake of approximately 300 to 400 ml of air during normal breathing.

As noted by De Troyer and associates (1982) and Rochester (1985), however, the muscle mass of the diaphragm is considered as comprising two functionally distinct parts — costal and crural. The fiber composition of each is different; the costal muscle thin and the crural portion thicker. Both groups of fibers are innervated by the phrenic nerves, but stimulation by phrenic activity results in two different actions on the chest wall. Contraction of the costal portion causes the diaphragm to flatten and the lower ribs to lift; both activities enlarge the thoracic cavity. The crural portion only causes some downward displacement of the diaphragm and is thus less effective in overall ventilatory activity of the structure.

Some muscular activity of the diaphragm occurs during exhalation. Contraction of the diaphragmatic muscle fibers does not cease abruptly at the onset of expiration but gradually declines during the initial portion of expiration and reaches zero at about the midpoint of expiration. Persistent diaphragmatic activity during the early phase of expiration provides precise regulation of the shift in air flow from inspiration to expiration. During vigorous breathing efforts, activity of the diaphragm also occurs toward the end of maximum expiratory efforts. The muscular activity at this time, as Agostoni and Torri (1962) reported, limits the degree to which the lungs collapse.

PARALYSIS OF THE DIAPHRAGM

Either the right or left hemidiaphragm may be paralyzed without significant respiratory embarrassment in the adult. Although ventilation on the paralyzed side is maintained by transmission of the cyclic pressure changes produced by the functioning hemidiaphragm across the mediastinum, initially a 20 to 30% reduction occurs in the vital capacity and the total lung capacity. Fackler and co-workers (1967) reported the return of these lung volumes to normal after 6 months. Clinically, in the adult, respiratory distress is minimal, although the patient may complain of chest pain and a nonproductive cough. The patient may spontaneously sleep in a semirecumbent position or in the lateral decubitus position with the side of the paralyzed hemidiaphragm down. Bilateral diaphragmatic paralysis may be tolerated by normal adults, but as McCredie and associates (1962) noted, a marked reduction of vital capacity and expiratory flow rates results, particularly while the individual is supine. In the patient with bilateral paralysis, excessive movement of the accessory muscles of respiration may be seen. Rochester (1985) has noted that such individuals are prone to chronic respiratory failure.

In infants and young children, unilateral paralysis may cause severe respiratory embarrassment, and mechanical ventilation is necessary. Bilateral paralysis is even more life threatening and is fatal unless the infant or child receives prompt ventilatory support.

In the infant or child, the lower rib cage, as noted by Hagan and colleagues (1977), may move paradoxically even with quiet respiration. When the infant is in the lateral decubitus position, Robotham (1979) has reported that, with the paralyzed diaphragmatic leaf up, the inward paradoxic motion of the subcostal area of the upper abdomen can be seen readily. In the adult, paradoxic movement of the lower chest wall or abdomen is not evident.

Paralysis of the hemidiaphragm may be suggested by elevation of that leaf of the diaphragm on a standard chest radiograph, and evidence of some basilar atelectasis on the involved side may also be present. Paralysis may be positively identified only by the fluoroscopic observation of paradoxic movement of the paralyzed hemidiaphragm on sudden inspiration. This is best demonstrated by the classic "sniff" test. The sudden inspiratory movement causes the normal hemidiaphragm to descend, whereas the paralyzed hemidiaphragm will move in the opposite direction. In critically ill patients requiring mechanical ventilation, electrophysiologic evaluation of the phrenic nerves has been suggested by Moorthy and associates (1985). This appears to be a reliable and satisfactory method for determining the presence of paralysis of a diaphragmatic leaf under adverse clinical conditions.

Etiology of Diaphragmatic Paralysis

In infants the most common cause of unilateral hemidiaphragmatic paralysis is injury of one of the phrenic nerves during a cardiac procedure. Stone and associates (1987) reported an incidence of only 0.3%, but Watanabe and colleagues (1987) noted one of 1.6%. The incidence was slightly higher for open heart procedures and somewhat lower for closed heart operations — 1.9 versus 1.3%. The Mustard procedure and the Glenn anastomosis had the highest incidences in each respective group. Procedures following previous operations had almost twice the incidence of an initial procedure. Most of the injuries were temporary — 84% — but initially were associated with considerable morbidity and, before modern management, Shoemaker and co-workers (1981) recorded an overall mortality of 20 to 25%; the high rate was due mainly to the underlying cardiac condition. Birth trauma is also an occasional cause of phrenic nerve injury, as is the removal of a mediastinal tumor in an infant or young child.

In adults, posttraumatic injury after a cardiac procedure, particularly with the use of topical hypothermia with ice slush, is the most common cause. Scannell and associates (1963) initially reported two deaths in four patients with cold injury to the phrenic nerves. Subsequently, Dajee and colleagues (1983) reported an incidence of topically hypothermic-induced injury of 9.6% but with no resulting mortality. Usually, the left phrenic nerve is the involved nerve, but right or

bilateral nerve injury does occur. Some degree of paresis probably occurred in even a much higher percentage in the early experience with topical hypothermia. Wheeler and associates (1985) reported the use of a cardiac insulation pad to reduce the incidence of injury. Hypothermic injury, however, is now less of a problem with the avoidance of opening of the pleural space, and, if this does occur, inflation of the lung to protect the nerve from contact with the ice slush has reduced the incidence to below 2% in most centers. When injury does occur, it is generally only temporary but can be permanent in 15 to 25% of patients.

Other traumatic causes of phrenic nerve damage are involvement by tumor: primary carcinoma of the lung, invasive thymoma, malignant germ cell tumors, and non-Hodgkin's lymphoma among others. Surgical injury likewise may occur and has been noted after mediastinotomy, surgical resections both in the thorax and neck, and even after placement of a subclavian or jugular vein catheter or electrode. High cervical spinal cord injuries may also result in diaphragmatic paralysis.

Idiopathic diaphragmatic paralysis is not uncommonly seen in the adult. It frequently is the result of a subclinical viral infection. The paralysis is most often unilateral, but patients with bilateral involvement have been reported by Spitzer (1973), Camfferman (1985), and Celli (1987) and their associates. Piehler and colleagues (1982) reviewed the records of 142 patients with unexplained diaphragmatic paralysis. Less than half were symptomatic. Subsequent improvement was better in those who had pain or cough than in those with dyspnea. The diaphragm returned to a normal position in less than 10%. Only 3.5% had an underlying malignancy and only one patient — 0.7% — had progressive atrophy.

Management of Diaphragmatic Paralysis

In infants and young children, initial therapy is mechanical ventilation, including continuous positive airway pressure. Proper positioning with the involved side down appears helpful. If continued support is required beyond 2 weeks, Watanabe and colleagues (1987) advise operative plication of the involved diaphragmatic leaf, as suggested by Shoemaker and associates (1981) among others. The technique of plication — central pleating, as described by Schwartz and Filler (1978) — which does not require muscle resection and minimizes the possibility of injury to the phrenic nerve branches of the hemidiaphragm, is suggested as the method of choice. The effect of plication of the paralyzed leaf of the diaphragm is the immobilization of the leaf in the flat position to maximally reduce its paradoxic movement with the associated shift of the mobile mediastinum to the contralateral side on inspiration. Ventilatory exchange becomes more efficient, and the infant may be more readily weaned from ventilatory support. The value of early plication has been supported further by the long-term study reported by Stone and colleagues (1987), who showed that plication did not prevent return of diaphragmatic function.

At times, direct repair of a severed nerve may be attempted. Brouillette and associates (1986) reported the successful repair of one transected phrenic nerve but failure of an interposed nerve graft in the other in a patient with bilateral nerve transections during the operative removal of a mediastinal lesion.

In adults and children over 2 years of age, conservative therapy is most often indicated. Surgical intervention and plication of the involved diaphragmatic leaf has been done with good success, however, by Wright and co-workers (1985) in patients with continuing disability. Graham and associates (1990) reported the use of plication in 17 adult patients who had persistent dyspnea and orthopnea that were due to paralysis of a hemidiaphragm with a reduction in the forced vital capacity and lung volume. All showed both subjective and objective improvement. In a 5- to 12-year follow-up in six patients, objective improvement in the lung functions were maintained (Table 45–1). In patients with idiopathic bilateral paralysis, Celli and associates (1987) have reported salutary results by the use of intermittent external negative-positive ventilation.

Therapeutic Use of Phrenic Nerve Paralysis

Therapeutic temporary paralysis of a phrenic nerve has been used in the past for treatment of pulmonary tuberculosis. This procedure can be used to elevate the hemidiaphragm to help obliterate the pleural space after the removal of a portion of the lung when there is insufficient residual lung tissue to fill the pleural space. Temporary paralysis can be obtained postoperatively by percutaneous infiltration about the nerve trunk in the neck with local anesthetic. At times, direct exposure of the nerve in the neck will be required. Additional elevation of the paralyzed diaphragm can be obtained by the induction of a temporary pneumoperitoneum.

EVENTRATION OF THE DIAPHRAGM

Eventration of the diaphragm is a rare anomaly, the cause of which remains to be understood completely. In general, congenital eventration of the diaphragm or the eventration occurring in newborn infants is probably a true congenital defect acquired during the fetal period. Severe cardiorespiratory symptoms in the newborn or neonate with a large unilateral eventration may be present because of secondary hypoplasia of the lung on the involved side. The appropriate resuscitative measures are required to correct acid-base balance, ventilatory insufficiency, and poor systemic perfusions, as in the neonate with a symptomatic congenital posterolateral diaphragmatic hernia (see Chapter 47). Once the condition of the newborn is stabilized, surgical correction of the eventration is indicated.

The repair of the defect is an emergency procedure in newborns or neonates with respiratory distress. It usually is accomplished through a thoracic approach. An incision is made in the circumference of the diaphragm, a few centimeters from the costal margin. The thinned-out diaphragm then is put on a stretch and reattached to the costal margin.

Eventration that occurs in older children and adults is thought to be caused by an acquired complete or incomplete paralysis of the diaphragmatic leaf. More

Table 45–1. Dyspnea Scores and Physiological Measurements Before and After Unilateral Diaphragmatic Plication*

Variable	Before Operation (n = 17)	After Operation (n = 17)	p Value	5- to 10-Year Followup Before (n = 6)	After (n = 6)	p Value
Dyspnea score	7.4 ± 0.8	3.3 ± 0.9	<.001	5.8 ± 0.7	2.4 ± 0.5	<.001
FVC						
Sitting	2.7 ± 0.7	3.2 ± 0.5	<.001	2.9 ± 0.8	3.4 ± 1.0	<.02
Lying	1.9 ± 0.5	2.7 ± 0.6	<.001	2.3 ± 0.6	3.1 ± 1.1	<.05
TLC						
Sitting	4.1 ± 1.6	4.5 ± 1.7	<.002	4.6 ± 1.0	5.4 ± 0.9	<.05
Lying	3.4 ± 0.8	4.2 ± 1.7	<.002	4.2 ± 1.2	5.0 ± 0.9	<.05
FRC	2.5 ± 0.2	2.9 ± 0.2	<.01	2.2 ± 0.9	2.9 ± 0.4	NS
ERV	0.6 ± 0.2	0.9 ± 0.2	<.01	1.1 ± 0.9	1.2 ± 0.3	<.05
RV	1.9 ± 0.2	2.0 ± 0.7	NS	1.7 ± 0.7	1.9 ± 0.2	NS
D_LCO (% predicted)	85 ± 4.5	100 ± 6.9	<.05	87 ± 14.1	98 ± 22.7	<.05
Pa$_{O_2}$	73.1 ± 10.9	85.6 ± 13.2	<.001	75.7 ± 14.3	93.4 ± 10.4	<.01
Pa$_{CO_2}$	39.8 ± 6.7	38.4 ± 6.1	NS	31.4 ± 8.6	38.9 ± 3.6	NS

*Lung values are measured in liters and blood gas estimations in millimeters of mercury.
DLCO = diffusion coefficient; ERV = expiratory reserve volume; FRC = functional residual capacity; FVC = forced vital capacity; NS = not significant; Pa$_{CO_2}$ = arterial carbon dioxide tension; Pa$_{O_2}$ = arterial oxygen tension; RV = residual volume; TLC = total lung capacity.
From Graham DA, et al: Diaphragmatic plication for unilateral diaphragmatic paralysis. A 10-year experience. Ann Thorac Surg 49:248, 1990.

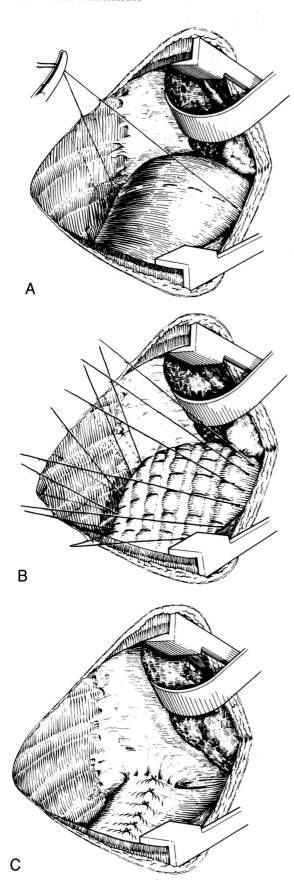

A

B

C

Fig. 45-1. Technique of plication of an eventration of the diaphragm. *A*, Four to six rows of 00 or 000 nonabsorbable sutures are inserted into the hemidiaphragm in an anterolateral to a posterolateral direction. Each row consists of five to six pleats. The branches of the phrenic nerve are avoided when the nerve is still functional. *B*, The sutures are left untied until all rows are in place. *C*, Sutures are tied to plicate and shorten the nonfunctioning leaf. From Spitz L *In* Jackson JW, Cooper DKC (eds): Rob and Smith's Operative Surgery: Thoracic Surgery, 4th Ed. London: Butterworths, 1986, p. 7.

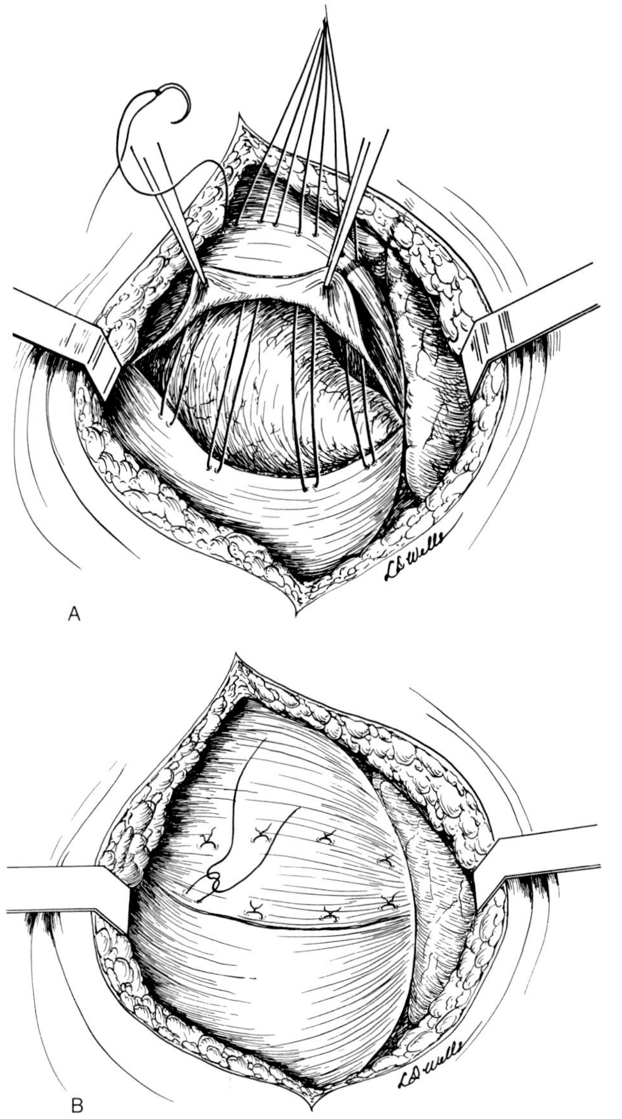

Fig. 45-2. Technique of repair of symptomatic eventration of the diaphragm. *From* Shields TW: The diaphragm. *In* Nora P (ed): Operative Surgery: Principles and Techniques. Philadelphia: Lea & Febiger, 1972.

often than not, localized eventration, which usually occurs on the right, with protrusion of liver through the defect, does not require surgical treatment. With a major hernia or a complete eventration, the patient may have cardiorespiratory or gastrointestinal symptoms, or both, secondary to the elevation of the diaphragmatic leaf. Operative repair is indicated for the older patient who has symptoms. A transthoracic approach is preferred. Entry into the pleural space is made through the bed of the eighth rib or the eighth intercostal space. After any adhesions that may be present are freed, the thinned-out diaphragmatic leaf is repaired by plication (Fig. 45-1). A second method is by incision of the leaf, and the repair then is carried out by imbricating one layer over the other with interrupted sutures of No. 00

or No. 0 silk or other nonabsorbable suture material (Fig. 45-2). Either repair is usually attended with low mortality and morbidity rates; however, plication of the diaphragmatic leaf is the preferred method. Wright (1985) and Graham (1990) and their associates achieved excellent relief of exertional dyspnea and orthopnea following transthoracic diaphragmatic plication of unilateral, nonmalignant diaphragmatic paralysis. There was a significant increase in arterial oxygen tension and all lung volumes except residual volume in the patients (Table 45-1).

Agenesis of the diaphragm and the presence of an accessory diaphragm have been reported by Nazarian (1971) and Geisler (1977) and their colleagues. A syndrome described by Spitz and associates (1975) consists of multiple supraumbilical abdominal wall defects, defects of the lower sternum, deficiency of the anterior diaphragm and diaphragmatic pericardium, and congenital cardiac defects — Cantrell's pentalogy (see Chapter 38).

REFERENCES

Agostoni, E., and Torri, G.: Diaphragm contraction as a limit to maximum expiration. J. Appl. Physiol. *17*:427, 1962.

Brouillette RT, et al: Successful reinnervation of the diaphragm after phrenic nerve transection. J Pediatr Surg *21*:63, 1986.

Camfferman F, et al: Idiopathic bilateral diaphragmatic paralysis. Eur J Respir Dis *66*:65, 1985.

Celli BR, Rassulo J, Corral R: Ventilatory dysfunction in patients with bilateral idiopathic diaphragmatic paralysis: reversal by intermittent external negative pressure ventilation. Am Rev Respir Dis *136*:1276, 1987.

Dajee A, et al: Phrenic nerve palsy after topical cardiac hypothermia. Int Surg *68*:345, 1983.

DeTroyer A, et al: Action of costal and crural parts of the diaphragm on the rib cage in dogs. J Appl Physiol *53*:30, 1982.

Fackler, CD, Perret, GE, and Bedell, GN: Effect of unilateral phrenic nerve section on lung function. J Appl Physiol *23*:923, 1967.

Geisler F, Gottlieb A, Fried D: Agenesis of the right diaphragm repaired with Marlex. J Pediatr Surg *12*:587, 1977.

Graham DR, et al: Diaphragmatic plication for unilateral diaphragmatic paralysis: a 10 year experience. Ann Thorac Surg *49*:248, 1990.

Hagan R, et al: Neonatal chest wall afferents and regulation of respiration. J Appl Physiol *42*:362, 1977.

McCredie M, Lovejoy FW Jr, Kalfrieder NL: Pulmonary function in diaphragmatic paralysis. Thorax *17*:213, 1962.

Moorthy SS, et al: Electrophysiologic evaluation of phrenic nerves in severe respiratory insufficiency requiring mechanical ventilation. Chest *88*:211, 1985.

Nazarian M, et al: Accessory diaphragm: report of a case with complete physiological evaluation and surgical correction. J Thorac Cardiovasc Surg *61*:293, 1971.

Piehler JM, et al: Unexplained diaphragmatic paralysis: a harbinger of malignant disease? J Thorac Cardiovasc Surg *84*:861, 1982.

Robotham JL: A physiologic approach to hemidiaphragm paralysis. Crit Care Med *7*:563, 1979.

Rochester DF: The diaphragm: contractile properties and fatigue. J Clin Invest *75*:1397, 1985.

Scannell SC: Results of open heart operation for acquired aortic valve disease. J Thorac Cardiovasc Surg *45*:47, 1963.

Schwartz MZ, Filler RM: Plication of the diaphragm for symptomatic phrenic nerve paralysis. J Pediatr Surg *13*:259, 1978.

Shoemaker R, et al: Aggressive treatment of required phrenic nerve paralysis in infants and small children. Ann Thorac Surg 32:251, 1981.

Spitz L, et al: Combined anterior abdominal wall, sternal, diaphragmatic, pericardial and intracardiac defects: a report of five cases and their management. J Pediatr Surg 10:491, 1975.

Spitzer SA, Korczym AD, Kalaci J: Transient bilateral diaphragmatic paralysis. Chest 64:355, 1973.

Stone KS, et al: Long-term fate of the diaphragm surgically plicated during infancy and early childhood. Ann Thorac Surg 44:62, 1987.

Watanabe T, et al: Phrenic nerve palsy after topical cardiac hypothermia. Retrospective study of 125 cases. J Thorac Cardiovasc Surg 94:383, 1987.

Wheeler WE, et al: Etiology and prevention of topical cardiac hypothermia-induced phrenic nerve injury and left lower lobe atelectasis during cardiac surgery. Chest 88:680, 1985.

Wright CD, et al: Results of diaphragmatic plication for unilateral diaphragmatic paralysis. J Thorac Cardiovasc Surg 90:195, 1985.

READING REFERENCES

Campbell EJM: The Respiratory Muscles and the Mechanics of Breathing. London: Lloyd-Luke, 1958.

Easton PA, et al: Respiratory function after paralysis of the right hemidiaphragm. Am Rev Respir Dis 127:125, 1983.

Haller JA, et al: Management of diaphragmatic paralysis in infants with special emphasis on selection of patients for operative plication. J Pediatr Surg 14:779, 1979.

Keltz H, Kaplan S, Stone DJ: Effect of quadriplegia and hemidiaphragmatic paralysis on the thoraco-abdominal pressure during respiration. Am J Phys Med 48:109, 1969.

Koontz AR, Levin MB: Agenesis of the right half of the diaphragm. Am Surg 34:657, 1968.

McNamara JJ, et al: Eventration of the diaphragm. Surgery 64:1013, 1968.

Thomas TV: Congenital eventration of the diaphragm. Ann Thorac Surg 10:180, 1970.

CHAPTER 46

PACING OF THE DIAPHRAGM

John A. Elefteriades

The concept of using electrical stimulation of the phrenic nerve to induce contraction of the diaphragm and in this way induce artificial ventilation dates back to a suggestion by Hufeland in his doctoral dissertation entitled "The Use of Electricity in Asphyxia" in 1783. Talonen (1990) has recently reviewed the historical background of diaphragm pacing. In 1818, Ure (1819) demonstrated the feasibility of electrical stimulation of the phrenic nerve in a "freshly hung criminal." "The success of it was truly wonderful. Full . . . breathing instantly commenced. The chest heaved and fell; the belly was protruded and again collapsed, with the relaxing and retiring diaphragm" (Fig. 46–1). In the 1800s, electrical stimulation of the phrenic nerve was popularized by Duchenne de Boulogne (1872) and Beard and Rockwell (1878) as a technique for cardiopulmonary

recuscitation. Said Duchenne, "It is apparent from all my experiments on men and on animals, alive and dead, that stimulation of the phrenic nerve by electrical current can produce contraction of the diaphragm." In 1927, Isreal reported the use of transcutaneous stimulation of the phrenic nerves for ventilation of apneic newborns. In the 1950s, Sarnoff and associates (1950) used electrophrenic respiration extensively to treat victims of the polio epidemic.

Since the early 1970s, the father of modern diaphragm pacing, Glenn, has proven, in a large series of patients cared for at Yale University, that diaphragm pacing is an effective and clinically useful modality. His work has lead to organized programs for diaphragm pacing at a number of centers in the United States and abroad. At the time of Glenn and colleagues' (1988) review of

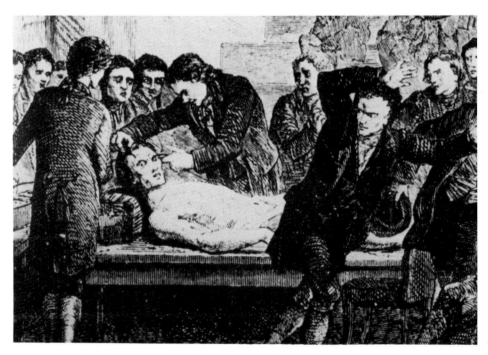

Fig. 46–1. Ure's induction of artificial respiration — Glasgow, 1818 — by galvanic stimulation of the left phrenic nerve in a "freshly hung criminal." *From* Ure A: An account of some experiments made on the body of a criminal immediately after execution, with physiological and practical observations. J Sci Arts (Lond) 6:283, 1819.

worldwide experience, nearly 500 patients had undergone diaphragm pacing.

INDICATIONS

Pacing of the diaphragm has become an accepted form of ventilatory support in two clinical settings: central alveolar ventilation — or, "sleep apnea," in which respiratory drive is deficient — and spinal cord injury — most commonly, quadriplegia, in which, although the drive for respiration exists, injury to the spinal cord itself prevents the transmission of stimuli to the phrenic nerves. These two indications account for the vast majority of clinical cases of diaphragm pacing.

Diaphragm pacing has been used in two additional conditions. Diaphragm pacing was found effective in treating intractable hiccups by Glenn and the author (1991). However, the patients with truly intractable hiccups who require surgical control are few. Diaphragm pacing has also been used, as suggested by Glenn and colleagues (1978) for chronic obstructive pulmonary disease — COPD — specifically, to preserve ventilation despite suppression of the hypoxic drive by oxygen administration. In the case of COPD, however, diaphragm pacing may have a more important role than currently appreciated. Up to the present time, however, central hypoventilation and quadriplegia have accounted for the overwhelming majority of patients undergoing diaphragm pacing.

Diaphragm pacing is *not* indicated in cases in which the phrenic nerve is dysfunctional — traumatic injury, iatrogenic injury, tumor, neuropathy syndromes, in cases in which the muscular apparatus of breathing is dysfunctional — myasthenia gravis, muscular dystrophies, in advanced primary disease of the pulmonary parenchyma, or in obstructive sleep apnea syndromes. Figure 46–2 illustrates schematically the appropriate and inappropriate circumstances for diaphragm pacing.

Central Alveolar Hypoventilation

The various sleep apnea syndromes are still not fully characterized, and miscommunication and confusion persist. Shneerson (1988) has provided a comprehensive review. The most basic distinction is between *obstructive* and *central* sleep apnea. In obstructive sleep apnea, the upper airway closes during inspiration, preventing ventilation; respiratory drive is normal, and respiratory muscle activity is preserved. In obstructive apnea, the brain tells the muscles to breathe, but anatomic closure of the upper airway prevents exchange of air. Obstructive apnea can be caused by tumors of the pharynx, abnormal morphology of the pharynx, obesity, or simply an exaggerated relaxation of the pharyngeal musculature with sleep. In central sleep apnea, there is a failure of respiratory drive; there is no respiratory muscle activity. In central apnea, the brain does not tell the muscles to breathe; the response to hypoxia and hypercapnea is diminished. Central hypoventilation is not usually the sequel of a process affecting the cerebral cortex. It is

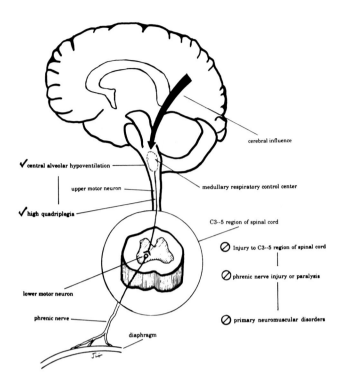

Fig. 46–2. Respiratory control system as regards disorders appropriate or inappropriate for diaphragm pacing. The involuntary medullary respiratory control center is subject to a degree of cerebral voluntary influence. The upper motor neurons of the phrenic system have their cell bodies in the medullary respiratory control center. The axons of the upper motor neurons synapse in the spinal cord with the lower motor neurons, at the level of C3–C5. The phrenic nerve proper is composed of the axons of those lower motor neurons. Check marks indicate appropriate indications for diaphragm pacing. International "*verboten*" symbols identify inappropriate indications.

usually the medullary respiratory control center that is affected, by tumor, infection — encephalitis, stroke, or trauma — including iatrogenic. Some idiopathic cases are thought to represent dysfunction of the medullary chemoreceptors that normally detect hypoxia and hypercarbia.

It has been recognized increasingly that the blunted response to hypoxia and hypercapnia that characterizes central sleep apnea also prevails during the day in many if not most patients — although voluntary contribution to ventilation during the day increases minute volume to a certain extent. For this reason, the term "central hypoventilation" is a better descriptor than "sleep apnea." The term "Ondine's curse" has also been used extensively in the literature to describe this condition. Ondine was an ancient mythological persona, a water spirit, who appears again in modern times in a play by Giraudoux; Ondine's husband was cursed to stop breathing whenever he fell asleep.

The central hypoventilators often, but not always, have a characteristic "Pickwickian" habitus. The chronic hypoxia and hypercapnia — as well as the fragmented sleep pattern itself — lead to daytime somnolence. Over time, chronic hypoxia leads, via hypoxic vasoconstriction, to fixed pulmonary hypertension, at times leading to right heart failure.

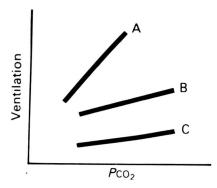

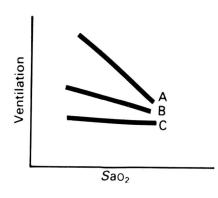

Fig. 46–3. The ventilatory response to hypercapnia and hypoxia. *A*, Normals. *B*, Patients with chest wall disorders. *C*, Central hypoventilators.

The adequacy of respiratory drive can be determined by assessing the ventilatory response to hypercapnia or hypoxia (Fig. 46–3). Ventilation should increase linearly as partial pressure of carbon dioxide — P_{CO_2} — increases. Ventilation should increase linearly as O_2 saturation falls — or exponentially as partial pressure of oxygen — P_{O_2} — falls. Primary weakness of the muscles of respiration can give intermediate responses but is usually easily diagnosed by the standard spirometric tests of pulmonary function. The author and associates' (1993b) policy is to perform a 24-hour respiratory control study, with hourly assessment of asleep/awake status, end-tidal CO_2, and O_2 saturation. A characteristic pattern in central hypoventilation is severe nighttime hypoventilation, with milder daytime hypercarbia as well (Fig. 46–4).

Central alveolar hypoventilation is well treated by diaphragm pacing. The lack of respiratory drive is compensated by the artificially induced ventilation.

Quadriplegia

The lower motor neurons of the phrenic nerve are located in the spinal cord at the level of C3, C4, and C5. Quadriplegia at levels below this range does not disrupt respiration. Quadriplegia involving the C3, C4, and C5 levels may disrupt respiration to a degree dependent on the actual damage to the lower motor neurons of the phrenic nerve. To the extent that the lower motor neurons are damaged, the phrenic nerve becomes dysfunctional; diaphragm pacing per se cannot overcome the damage to the phrenic nerve. Quadriplegia at the C2-3 level or higher does not damage the phrenic nerve motor neurons; quadriplegia at these levels does, however, impair or eliminate spontaneous ventilation — by disrupting the tracts that lead from the medullary respiratory control center to the spinal cord (see Fig. 46–2). The accessory muscles of respiration — intercostals (T1-12), abdominals (T7-L1),

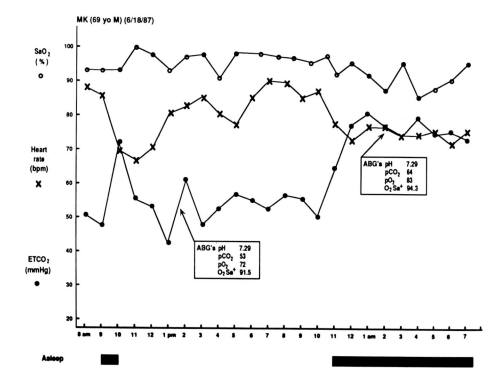

Fig. 46–4. Twenty-four-hour respiratory control study — preoperative — in a central hypoventilator. Note that (1) CO_2 is abnormally high throughout the 24-hour period, (2) CO_2 rises to 69 mmHg during a morning nap, (3) CO_2 is very high throughout the night's sleep — peaking at 78 mmHg at 1 AM, and (4) O_2 saturation falls to 83% at 4 AM, reflecting critically low tidal volume from severe hypoventilation.

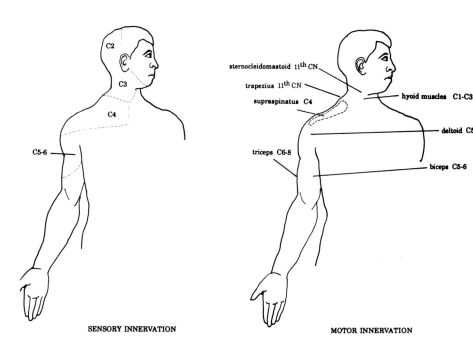

Fig. 46–5. Sensory and motor findings that allow discrimination of "high" quadriplegia. Quadriplegia at C2-3 or higher is well treated by diaphragm pacing.

and pelvic muscles (L1-S2) — are denervated as well by these spinal cord lesions. Only the sternocleidomastoid and trapezius, innervated by the spinal accessory nerve — CN 11, remain functional with quadriplegia at the C2-3 level or higher. The respiratory paralysis from "high quadriplegia" is directly correctable by diaphragm pacing. The neurologic findings that distinguish "high" quadriplegia — C2-3 or higher — are shown in Figure 46–5. In general, in high quadriplegia, sensation is intact only to the clavicles, and motor function disrupted from the deltoid muscle and below.

The publication of Whitehead and colleagues (1985) constitutes one of the best current overall references on high quadriplegia. With increased public awareness of cardiopulmonary resuscitation techniques, improved emergency care delivery systems, widespread availability of positive pressure ventilation, and improved long-term respiratory care, many more patients are surviving the accident that causes quadriplegia and being sustained long term than in earlier eras. The yearly incidence of spinal cord injury in the United States has been estimated at 30 to 35 per million population, or about 6000 to 7000 cases per year. The prevalence of spinal cord injury — patients currently alive — is estimated at 200,000. The majority of injuries are from motor vehicle accidents, with diving accidents, gunshot wounds, falls, and iatrogenic injuries seen as well. Aside from traumatic conditions, developmental abnormalities, vascular abnormalities, infarctions, and transverse myelitis can also produce quadriplegia.

When a patient with high quadriplegia manifests respiratory paralysis and the phrenic nerve is found to be intact by percutaneous testing, diaphragm pacing is indicated if the patient's overall status permits.

PREREQUISITES

Phrenic Nerve Function

Our group regularly receives numerous inquiries about diaphragm pacing for patients with phrenic nerve dysfunction — from tumor, mass, trauma, iatrogenic injury, especially reoperative cardiac surgery, or idiopathic. Unfortunately, current practice cannot offer effective treatment for these patients. *Pacing of the diaphragm requires an intact phrenic nerve.* The intact nerve is stimulated and in turn produces contraction of the diaphragm.

Although experimental studies of direct stimulation of the diaphragm have been performed by Peterson and associates (1986) at Case Western Reserve University, these techniques have not been generally applied clinically. Even these "direct" approaches to diaphragm stimulation probably rely on stimulation of the radicles of the phrenic nerve as it divides in the central portions of the diaphragm. Unlike cardiac muscle, the diaphragm is not an electrical syncytium that propagates an electrical impulse throughout the muscle. Furthermore, even if direct stimulation proves feasible, in cases of phrenic nerve injury, the atrophy of the denervated muscle will likely interfere with any effective diaphragmatic contraction. Thus, no clinical solution for the injured phrenic nerve exists, and an intact phrenic nerve remains essential for diaphragm pacing.

Because an intact phrenic nerve is essential for pacing, testing the status of the nerve assumes paramount importance. Sarnoff (1951) and Shaw (1980) and their colleagues have described the technique for transcutaneous testing of phrenic nerve conduction (Fig. 46–6). The overall technique is similar to that for any electromyelography — EMG — or nerve conduction test. A thimble electrode facilitates the testing of the phrenic

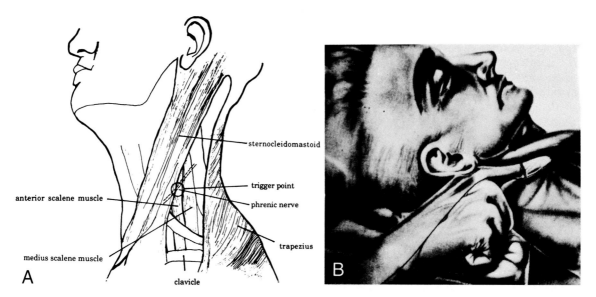

Fig. 46–6. Testing for viability of the phrenic nerve by percutaneous electrical stimulation. *A,* The "trigger point" at the border of the clavicular head of the sternocleidomastoid where the phrenic nerve is accessible to stimulation as it crosses on the scalene muscles. *B,* Application of the "thimble" electrode.

nerve. The "motor point" is located medial to the lateral edge of the clavicular head of the sternocleidomastoid muscle. Stimulation is applied by the thimble electrode, with an emphasis on pushing the sternocleidomastoid medially and directing the current posteriorly. The presence or absence of diaphragm contraction is observed. Intact conduction produces a dramatic and easily recognized contraction of the diaphragm. Measurement of the muscle action potential of the diaphragm and of the phrenic nerve conduction time — the normal for the adult is 7.5 to 10 msec — and even fluoroscopy can be used to confirm diaphragm contraction, but I find simple clinical inspection to be adequate. Failure to elicit a strong diaphragm contraction almost invariably indicates nonviability of the phrenic nerve. In rare cases, the nerve cannot be stimulated percutaneously, and, if pacing is deemed critical, exploration and direct stimulation of the nerve are pursued.

With spinal cord injury, some improvement in phrenic nerve function over time is common, a patient initially respirator-dependent may even become able to breathe spontaneously. Therefore, members of our group wait until at least 3 months after injury before accepting a patient into the pacing program. It usually takes at least this amount of time to establish recovery from injury to other organ systems and to institute effective respiratory, bowel and bladder, skin protective, and physical and psychologic rehabilitation programs, which will be essential in the patient's future.

In some cases of neurologic injury lower than the C3 level, that is, involving the C3-C5 areas where the cell bodies of the phrenic nerve are located, the phrenic nerves may be partially injured but still viable. Pacing may be indicated in *some* of these cases — despite the indications to the contrary in the simplified schematic

representation in Figure 46–2 — although benefit may be limited. The decision to pace under these circumstances must be considered with great care.

Pulmonary Function

It is essential for diaphragm pacing that the ability of the lungs to oxygenate and ventilate be well preserved. Pacing cannot compensate for severe restrictive or obstructive lung disease. In most patients undergoing pacing, measured pulmonary function tests are normal or near normal.

Chest Wall Configuration

For similar reasons, major deformities of the chest wall contraindicate diaphragm pacing by virtue of their interference with ventilatory function.

Diaphragm Function

It is critical that the diaphragm muscle be inherently sound. A diaphragm affected by a primary muscular disorder is not generally appropriate for pacing. In central hypoventilation, I like to demonstrate at least a 5-cm excursion of the diaphragm with spontaneous breathing before embarking on diaphragm pacing. In quadriplegic patients, a brisk downward deflection of the diaphragm with percutaneous stimulation of the phrenic nerve is sought. The atrophy of disuse that affects the diaphragm in quadriplegia can be corrected by gradual conditioning.

Psychosocial Factors

In cases in which injury producing quadriplegia has also resulted in permanent brain injury that impairs cognitive capacity, I have believed that diaphragm pacing is not appropriate. Aside from important issues of health-care allocation, a brain-damaged status prevents appreciation of many of the benefits of diaphragm pacing. For both central hypoventilators and quadriplegics, an attentive and supportive family are essential to success of the pacing program. Considerable involvement of the family in the psychological and physical support of the patient is required.

TECHNIQUES

Pulse Train Stimulation

A cardiac pacemaker delivers a single stimulus, which in turn produces a contraction of the entire heart, by virtue of the electrical syncytium of the ventricular muscle. Skeletal muscles, including the diaphragm, behave differently. A single stimulus produces an ineffective contraction. A train of stimuli is required to produce a summated contraction that is mechanically effective (Fig. 46–7). The pulse train stimulation has a number of critical electrical parameters: rate — the overall number of pulse trains delivered per minute, corresponding, in diaphragm pacing, to the respiratory rate; amplitude — voltage of each stimulus in the train, frequency [Hz] — representing the timing of stimuli with a pulse train, current — milliamperes; pulse width — the length of time that each individual stimulus is maintained; and pulse train duration — the length of time that the pulses continue at the prescribed

frequency, corresponding, in diaphragm pacing to the inspiration duration. The frequency can also be expressed by its inverse, the "pulse interval"; that is: frequency [Hz] = 1000 msec/pulse interval — msec, so that 40 msec corresponds to 25 Hz, 90 msec to 11.1 Hz, 110 msec to 9.1 Hz, and so forth. The muscle contraction lasts only for the duration of the pulse train.

Salmons and Hendriksson (1981), as well as Mannion and Stephenson (1985) have shown that stimulation of the diaphragm or other skeletal muscle by pulse trains over time results in an orderly sequence of histologic, ultrastructural, and biochemical changes. Vascular supply increases, enzyme patterns change, and mitochondrial capacity increases. These changes reflect transformation from a mixture of fast — glycolytic — and slow — oxidative — muscle fibers to exclusively slow fibers. The transition to oxidative fibers allows sustained mechanical work. No nondiaphragmatic skeletal muscle can sustain mechanical work continuously without such conditioning — for example, no one can do push-ups 24 hours a day, day after day. Although the diaphragm does work 24 hours a day in normal respiration, the pattern of recruitment of individual nerve fascicles and motor units — tens to hundreds of muscle fibers per axon — is such that many motor units are dormant during an individual breath, allowing metabolic recovery. With the pulse train stimulation of diaphragm pacing, it is likely that most or all nerve fascicles and all muscle groups are stimulated strongly during each

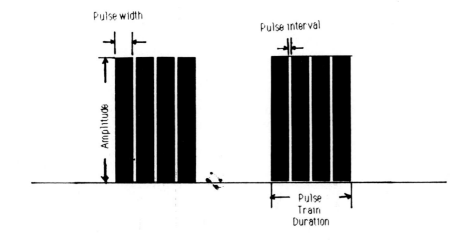

Fig. 46–7. Pulse train stimulation.

Characteristics describing pulse train stimulation.

Rate (bpm): overall number of pulse trains delivered per minute

Amplitude (v): voltage of each stimulus in pulse train

Pulse width (ms): duration of an individual pulse

Pulse interval (ms): duration between pulses in a train

Frequency (Hz): timing of stimuli with a pulse train
(Frequency (Hz) = 1000/pulse interval)

Pulse train duration (ms): overall duration of one train of pulses.

breath, necessitating the adaptive changes described. In addition to the adaptation required for acceptance of pulse train stimulation, in the case of quadriplegia, the diaphragm has often atrophied from disuse during mechanical ventilation and must be restored gradually over time to a functional state.

Apparatus

The generator for diaphragm pacing remains *outside* the body (Fig. 46–8). A table model, about the size of a clock radio, and a portable model, about the size of a personal cassette player are available. The output from the generator is carried via an antenna, the coil of which is taped securely to the patient's skin over the receiver site. The implanted receiver, about the size and shape of a pocket watch, lies subcutaneously over the flat portion of the lower anterolateral ribcage. The

antenna transmits a signal by radiofrequency to the implanted receiver, which generates, via inductive coupling, a stimulating signal. The receiver stimulates the phrenic nerve via an electrode placed underneath the nerve. Despite the external position of the generator and the inductive coupling arrangement for transmission of the signal to the body, the system is reliable and easy to use.

The electrode is a "half-cuff" or 180° model developed at Yale for diaphragm pacing (Fig. 46–9) and subsequently used for skeletal muscle stimulation in other applications. The author prefers not to surround the nerve circumferentially because of the potential for entrapment and injury of the nerve by encircling cicatrix (Fig. 46–10). In a detailed study on the thoracodorsal nerve, Letsou and associates (1992) found no disadvantage in terms of the adequacy of stimulation by a 180° compared to a 360° electrode.

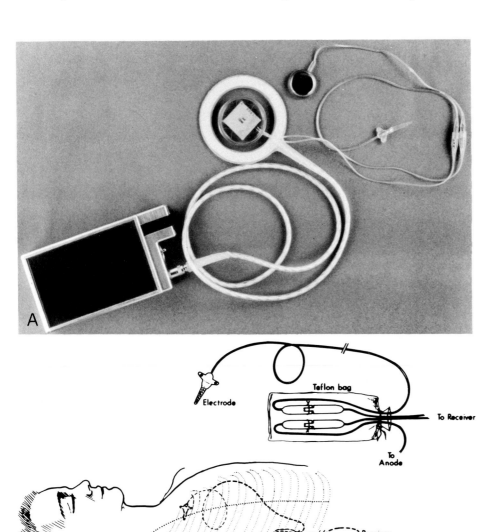

Fig. 46–8. The apparatus for diaphragm pacing. *A,* The hardware. The transmitter, the external antenna, the implantable receiver, and the phrenic nerve electrode are shown. The transmitter remains outside the body, as does the antenna, which is taped securely to the skin over the implanted receiver. *B,* Equipment in place in patient. Note placement of phrenic nerve electrode at the level of the upper thorax. The implanted receiver is situated over a flat portion of the lower chest wall.

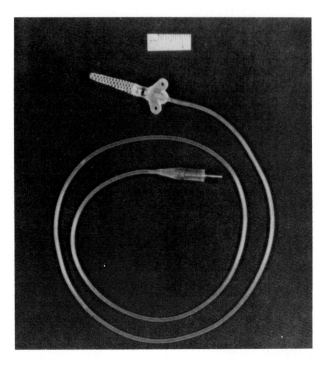

Fig. 46–9. Detail of 180° phrenic nerve electrode.

Commercial Devices

Currently only one commercial manufacturer has diaphragm pacemakers approved for clinical use in this country (Avery Laboratories, Glen Cove, NY). The early model — I107A — is well tested clinically but has exhibited premature receiver failure that is due to deficiencies in hermetic sealing — leading to a need for frequent receiver changes. The later model — I110A — is essentially borrowed from a pain control application, and, while clinically approved for diaphragmatic use, remains unproven for life-sustaining application. Our own laboratory has demonstrated an "uncoupling" of the external antenna from the subcutaneously implanted receiver with only small displacements — 1 to 2 cm — of the magnitude commonly

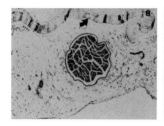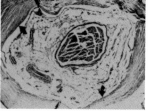

Fig. 46–10. Histologic section of phrenic nerve after long-term stimulation with a 360° electrode *(A)* and a 180° electrode *(B)*. Note circumferential fibrous cicatrice seen with 360° electrode only. 180° electrode elicits only a band of fibrous tissue on the side facing the nerve. Although both nerve fascicles themselves are normal, the potential for damage with the 360° configuration is suggested. Hematoxylin and eosin stain, x 39. From Kim JH, et al: Light and electron microscopic studies of phrenic nerves after long-term electrical stimulation. J Neurosurg 58:85, 1980.

expected in clinical practice. Our group is currently gaining experience with a device manufactured in Finland (Atrotec OY, Tampere, Finland), which is approved for clinical investigation in this country. The early experience has been favorable.

The relatively low volume of implantation of diaphragm pacemakers, with the consequent low profit potential, has limited the development of equipment by commercial manufacturers. The state of development has lagged far behind that of cardiac pacemakers. All units in current clinical use rely on an external transmitter, which generates a radiofrequency signal, which activates a subcutaneously implanted receiver, which generates a signal, which is relayed to an electrode positioned on the phrenic nerve. This is essentially the original system developed at Yale by Glenn and colleagues (1972) and used at Yale since that time. Development of a fully implantable system, as commonly used in cardiac pacing, would represent a major advance. The feasibility of such a system has been demonstrated in the laboratory at Yale by Hogan and colleagues (1976). The requirement for pulse train stimulation complicates design characteristics beyond those for cardiac pacing. The potential for rate-responsive diaphragm pacing — using sensor-based feedback feeding technology, as in modern cardiac pacing — represents an exciting possibility for the future.

Surgical Procedure

Although initially many implants of the electrode were done in the neck, the Yale group has subsequently switched to implantation in the chest. This is because it has been demonstrated that in some cases, accessory radicles — originating below the C3-5 level — join the phrenic nerve late (Fig. 46–11) and would not be stimulated by an electrode situated in the neck as noted by Kelley and associates (1950).

The operation is done through a minithoracotomy anteriorly in the second or third intercostal space (Fig. 46–12). The pectoral muscle is split in the direction of its fibers. The internal mammary artery and vein are divided deliberately to avoid their disruption during spreading of the interspace. A flat spot is identified on the mediastinum above the heart where the phrenic nerve is accessible and where the electrode can "sit" comfortably. Extreme care is taken in the handling of the nerve site — because injury is disastrous. The mediastinal pleura is incised parallel to the nerve and several millimeters away from the nerve and its nutrient vessels; this is done anterior and posterior to the nerve. The electrode is slipped atraumatically behind the mobilized phrenic structures, so that the phrenic bundle rests inside the half-cuff platinum contact of the electrode. Minor oozing from the artery or vein that accompanies the nerve is not treated, because this stops spontaneously and application of cautery could well injure nerve fibers. The Silastic portions of the electrode are secured to the pleura overlying the mediastinum. Perfect lie of the electrode must be obtained, so that no distortion or traction on the nerve results; such

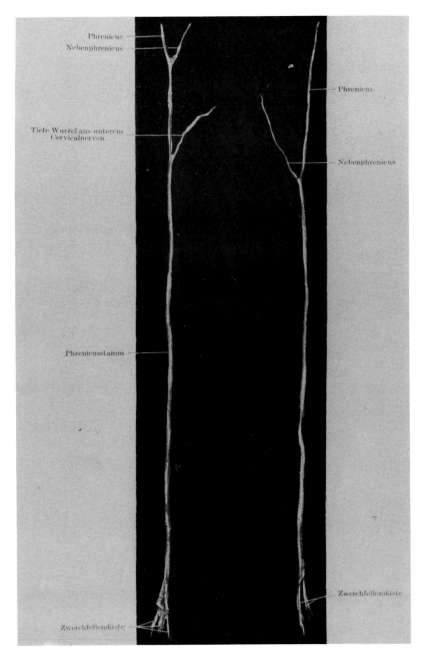

Phrenicus
Nebenphrenicus

Tiefe Wurzel aus unterem Cervicalnerven

Phrenicusstamm

Zwerchfellendäste

Phrenicus

Nebenphrenicus

Zwerchfellendäste

Fig. 46–11. Phrenic nerves removed by the operation of exeresis. This was practiced in the early twentieth century in the treatment of apical tuberculosis. To completely paralyze the diaphragm, surgeons found it necessary to remove all branches of the phrenic nerve, which they accomplished by avulsing the nerves in the neck. The "Nebenphrenicus" is probably the branch of the fifth cervical, the so-called accessory branch, shown here joining the other branches at a high level on the right side and at a low level on the left. On the left side, such a branch would probably not be stimulated by an electrode placed in a cervical location. In the specimen from the right side, note also a branch from the lower cervical cord joining the main trunk. This branch certainly would be missed by stimulation from a cervical location. From Glenn WWL, Sairenji H: Diaphragm pacing in the treatment of chronic ventilatory insufficiency. *In* Roussos C, Macklem PT (eds): The Thorax, Part B. New York: Marcel Dekker, 1985, p. 1434.

distortion or traction could well result over the longterm in injury or dysfunction of the nerve. With careful attention to atraumatic technique, we, as reported by Glenn and associates (1988), have not seen iatrogenic injury or dysfunction of the nerve, although this has been common in centers with limited experience.

The end of the electrode is passed through the chest wall — atraumatically in a chest tube carrier — into a pocket created through a separate incision over a flat portion of the anterolateral lower rib cage. Some redundant wire is looped gently on the surface of the lung within the thorax. Three separate subpockets are made, one for the receiver, one for the indifferent electrode — the "can" is *not* the indifferent electrode, unlike the arrangement with unipolar cardiac pace-

makers, and the junction box — the connection between the receiver and the wires from the nerve electrode and the anode plate. The junction box and excess wire lengths are secured inside a Teflon bag; the wires are very fine — much more so than cardiac pacing wires — and inclusion in the Teflon bag facilitates safe access at the time of receiver change. It is essential that the copper coil on the receiver and the metal plate of the indifferent electrode face outward, away from the body; this optimizes communication between the external antenna and the receiver and avoids unwanted stimulation of chest wall muscles. The subpockets are closed tightly, because the position of the components must be very stable to ensure good communication with the external antenna. As with any

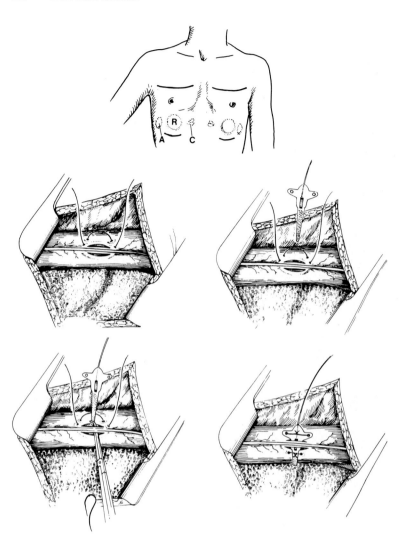

Fig. 46–12. Transthoracic approach to the phrenic nerves for diaphragm pacing. *Top,* Incisions in the second interspace for nerve access. Incisions at the costal margin for implantation of receiver (R), anode plate (A), and connectors (C). *Middle and bottom,* Sequential steps in implantation of 180° electrode behind the phrenic nerve. *Modified from* Glenn WWL: The diaphragm. *In* Glenn WWL (ed): Thoracic and Cardiovascular Surgery. 4th Ed. East Norwalk, CT: Appleton-Century-Crofts, 1983, p. 363.

subcutaneous implantation of foreign bodies, the incision is kept away from the implanted hardware, to prevent pressure on the incision and improper healing or extrusion.

A test of the system is conducted in the operating room to confirm function of the overall system before the patient is undraped. This is performed with a sterile antenna passed to an off-table transmitter. Excellent contraction of the diaphragm with pacing should be confirmed. Threshold should be in the range of 1.0 to 2.0 mamp. Failure to pace or high threshold should lead to re-evaluation for improper connection, injury to the wires, lead dislodgement, or interposition of excess tissue in the cup of the half-cuff electrode.

Extreme care is taken — including the use of prophylactic antibiotics — to prevent infection, which would be disastrous if it led to nerve involvement. We do the right and left implantations at separate sittings, usually about 2 weeks apart.

Electrical and Ventilatory Settings

Inspiration duration — 1.3 sec — and pulse width — 150 sec — are preset at the factory. Inspiration duration can be adjusted to 0.9 sec for children.

Respiratory rate is selected individually for each patient. For bilateral pacing in adults we aim for 6 to 10 breaths per minute. For unilateral pacing, higher rates are required, usually 12 to 14 breaths per minute.

Current is set according to fluoroscopic testing, which is conducted before institution of pacing and at intervals thereafter. A standardized radiographic system is used that can be reproduced from time to time and from patient to patient. A "ruler" with lead numerals "1 through 12" is used, placed behind the patient with the "1" at the dome of the diaphragm. With the tube distance kept constant at 30 cm, reproducible readings result. In the standard fluoroscopic test, maximum voluntary descent of each diaphragm is first determined — for central hypoventilators; quadriplegics usually are not capable of spontaneous diaphragm motion. Movement of 8 to 10 cm is usual for adults. Subsequently, testing of paced ventilation is conducted to determine threshold current — that current that produces a just discernible contraction of the diaphragm — and current for maximal excursion. The maximal descent of the diaphragm by pacing is recorded for future comparison. For clinical conduct of pacing, the current is set just above the current for maximal excursion.

Conduct of Pacing

Pacing can be done unilaterally, bilaterally on alternate sides — usually at 12-hour intervals, or bilaterally simultaneously. Although unilateral pacing may suffice in selected cases — especially in central alveolar hypoventilation, the preference of our group, since the introduction of conditioning to accept low-frequency stimulation, has been for bilateral pacing, usually aiming for 24-hour continuous stimulation.

Pacing is not begun until 2 weeks after the implantations are complete, because it has been found that earlier institution leads to pleural effusions, possibly reflecting bleeding from disruption of immature adhesions by the strong diaphragm contraction elicited by pacing.

With parameters set as described, a program of gradual conditioning is used to allow restoration of diaphragms atrophied by disuse — quadriplegia — and accommodation to pulse train electrical stimulation — quadriplegia and central alveolar hypoventilation. The adaptive processes discussed previously occur over weeks to months. For quadriplegics, pacing is begun at 15 minutes per waking hour. A gradual increase to 30 minutes is carried out. At this point, the pacing period is gradually increased further, with each pacing period followed by an equal period of rest on the ventilator. When the pacing period reaches 12 hours, the rest period is gradually and progressively shortened until full-time pacing is achieved. Changes in pacing period are made about each 7 to 14 days depending on patient tolerance. Along with progressive increases in the pacing period, the frequency of stimuli in the pulse train is decreased progressively — usually to about 7.1 Hz, to minimize diaphragm fatigue and allow longer pacing periods. Concurrently, the number of respirations is decreased progressively to the minimum number that provides adequate ventilation — usually about 7 to 8/min in adults, again to decrease the tendency to fatigue. To maintain adequacy of ventilation, when placed in the sitting position, all quadriplegic patients have a snug abdominal binder applied and the respiratory rate increased by one breath per minute. The entire conditioning phase usually requires 3 to 6 months or longer in quadriplegic patients. Central hypoventilators can be advanced more quickly, because their diaphragms are not atrophied from disuse at the inception of pacing.

Tidal volume, minute volume, end-tidal partial pressure of carbon dioxide — Pco_2, and oxygen saturation are monitored regularly, at least at the beginning and end of each pacing period as well as at regular intervals during pacing. Monitoring is usually done hourly until the patient is well advanced on the pacing protocol. Monitoring is noninvasive by oxygen saturation and CO_2 monitors but is correlated periodically with arterial blood gases obtained by puncture. The author and associates (1993a) have recently described our noninvasive monitoring protocol in detail.

If tidal volume falls or CO_2 rises, this is considered, in the absence of specific correctable pulmonary problems, to be evidence of diaphragm fatigue. The patient is rested temporarily on mechanical ventilation. After at least an overnight rest, pacing is resumed with a shorter pacing period.

In those central hypoventilators who require only part-time — nocturnal — ventilation, the part-time schedule — 8 to 12 hours — can be implemented immediately and fully, as the period off pacing is adequate to prevent diaphragm fatigue. For this part-time pacing, high-frequency pacing — 20 to 25 Hz, (pulse interval) Pi 40 to 50 msec — suffices.

Aftercare

The operation to place the diaphragm pacemaker is straightforward. Unlike the situation with cardiac pacing, however, the device cannot be "turned on" and patient discharged in short order. Careful monitoring during the adaptation phase is required. Even after hospital discharge, the program cannot be effective without concerted and knowledgeable care. Temporary stresses — infection, intercurrent illness, operations related to cutaneous, urologic, or orthopedic complications of quadriplegia — can tax the reserve of diaphragm pacing — which does not automatically adjust to increased respiratory requirements — and lead to institution of positive pressure ventilation. All too often, once positive pressure ventilation is begun, without the involvement of the diaphragm pacing center in patient management, mechanical ventilation — seen as a safer and easier "crutch" — is perpetuated.

Tracheostomy

I believe that the care of all patients with diaphragm pacing is made safer and easier by permanent tracheostomy. It is well-known that pacing can produce upper airway obstruction — extremely vigorous diaphragm contraction combined with lack of coordination with the phasic muscle status of the upper airway. Therefore, all patients are told to leave the stoma open during sleep. Periodic dysfunction of the pacemaker system may occur, and the tracheostomy provides a secure access to the airway for positive pressure ventilation during such times.

Once full-time ventilation is achieved and secure, a Teflon tracheal button can be substituted for the conventional tracheostomy tube (Fig. 46–13). This is a very useful device, which maintains the airway but has the advantages of better cosmetics — hardly visible when in place, normal speech, and reduced tracheal irritation and injury. The inner plug of the button is removed during sleep to ensure an unobstructed airway.

Pacing in Infants and Young Children

Hunt (1978) and Brouillette (1988) and their associates have clarified certain characteristics specific to pacing of infants and young children. Their experience in 32 patients with predominantly central hypoventilation, which can be seen as a congenital condition, demonstrates that pacing is effective; 25 of 32 patients survived

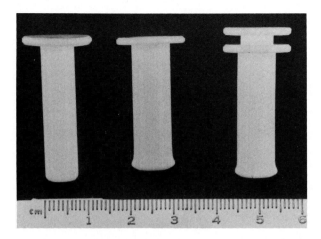

Fig. 46–13. The "tracheal button" used to replace the tracheostomy tube in our patients. The inner plug is shown on the left, the open tube in the middle, and the two components assembled together on the right. The flange of the button sits flush with the skin when the button is in place in the stoma, maintaining patency indefinitely but being minimally apparent cosmetically. *From* Glenn WWL, et al: Long-term ventilatory support by diaphragm pacing in quadriplegia. Ann Surg *183*:566, 1976.

and the vast majority were rehabilitated adequately to allow return to the home. Both Hunt and Brouillette and colleagues have established that pacing of one diaphragm is poorly tolerated — excess mediastinal motion; that a shorter inspiration duration — 0.9 sec — is more efficient; and that full-time bilateral pacing of the infant or young child is not feasible. The difference in tolerance for duration of pacing compared to adults has been attributed by Motoyama (1977) to "immaturity" of the musculoskeletal apparatus for breathing. By age 8 to 10, goals and techniques more closely approximate those for the adult.

RESULTS

The effectiveness of diaphragm pacing as a ventilatory modality has been demonstrated conclusively since 1970, when Glenn and colleagues (1972) first achieved total ventilatory support of a quadriplegic patient with complete respiratory paralysis. The early experience with total ventilatory support involved alternate-side pacing, because bilateral high-frequency ventilation could not be tolerated as a result of diaphragmatic fatigue. Another landmark was achieved in 1980 by Glenn and colleagues (1984) with the introduction of continuous bilateral, low-frequency stimulation of the conditioned diaphragm for complete respiratory support.

The most recent review of the Yale experience by the author and associates (1993a) with bilateral, low-frequency diaphragm pacing in quadriplegia demonstrates a number of very encouraging findings regarding the longterm effectiveness of diaphragm pacing as a means of ventilation. From this experience in 14 patients paced with bilateral low-frequency stimulation for 2 to

10 years — mean 6.5 years, the following specific conclusions are possible: (1) Diaphragm pacing can completely meet ventilatory requirements. Tidal volume meets or exceeds the requirements calculated from the Radford and associates' (1954) nomogram. Arterial blood gases are maintained in normal range. (2) Minute volume is maintained on a long-term basis without decrement (Fig. 46–14). (3) Pacing parameters— threshold and maximum — remain unchanged over time, arguing against theoretical concerns, as expressed by McCreery and Agnew (1990), regarding nerve damage from chronic electrical stimulation. (4) The limited pathologic material available shows no evidence of any significant histologic damage to nerve, diaphragm, or lungs. Thus, the effectiveness of diaphragm pacing as a modality for long-term ventilation has been well documented.

The next question concerns the overall usefulness of diaphragm pacing in clinical practice. Review of the Yale experience and the worldwide experience by Glenn and colleagues (1986, 1988) bear on this point. In the Yale experience, 86 patients have undergone pacing since 1966. More than 93% of the patients have benefitted from diaphragm pacing. In 38 patients — 44% — the ventilatory goal was achieved fully. Partial success, meaning that significant benefit was gained from pacing but another method of ventilatory support was also required, was obtained in another 42 patients — 49%. Pacing-related complications — overpacing, underpacing, phrenic nerve injury, which are avoidable by current techniques — occurred in 8 of 86 patients — 9.3%. With the recognition of the benefits of bilateral, low-frequency stimulation, a number of patients, including some with central alveolar hypoventilation, were converted to this modality after pacing for variable periods on one side at a time.

The review of Glenn and colleagues (1988) of the worldwide experience with diaphragm pacing — there were records of 477 patients who had undergone implantation of a diaphragm pacemaker; detailed analysis was confined to the 165 patients from six major centers for whom complete data were available — allowed the following conclusions. Transcutaneous phrenic nerve stimulation in the neck preoperatively was found to be a reliable predictor of phrenic nerve viability. Pacing was applied during sleep only in 46% of patients, part-time night or day in 15%, and full-time in 27%. Eleven percent of patients did not pace for significant periods of time. Compromised function of the phrenic nerve deemed probably related to the procedure or electrode was seen in 13% of cases. Incidence of nerve dysfunction was lowest with a half-cuff electrode placed in the chest — 3.7%. There has not been an iatrogenic problem of this type in the last 10 years at Yale, where thoracic implantation of a half-cuff electrode is the preferred approach. Infection occurred in 4.5% of surgical procedures. Overall success of diaphragm pacing in meeting ventilatory needs was assessed as follows: complete success 47%, significant ventilatory support 36%, failure or

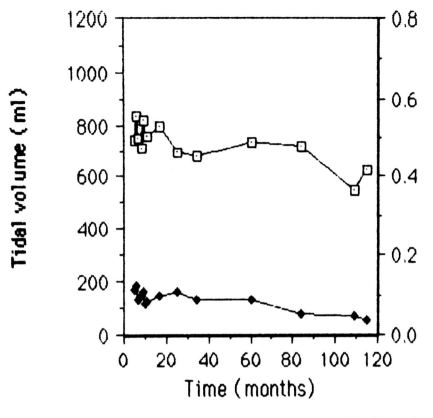

Fig. 46–14. Ten-year assessment of tidal volume and diaphragm acceleration in a quadriplegic patient. (Open squares denote tidal volume, and closed diamonds denote diaphragm acceleration.) Note that tidal volume is well maintained over time. Diaphragm acceleration remains at the desired low levels as well, signifying that the conditioned state of the diaphragm muscle is maintained — with conditioning to oxidative metabolism, fibers become slow twitch.

minimal support 17%. At followup, 59% of the patients were alive.

Another important question is whether diaphragm pacing produces better results than other therapeutic modalities. In particular, it can be asked whether diaphragm pacing improves clinical status or life-expectancy, or both, in central hypoventilation or in high quadriplegia. In the case of central hypoventilation, it is the experience of the group at Yale that without pacing, progressive respiratory deterioration is common. Without treatment, death from hypoventilation may occur. In patients who do survive, common sequellae of prolonged hypoventilation and hypoxia include permanent cerebral dysfunction — from chronic hypoxic injury — and cor pulmonare. No effective medical treatment for patients with true central hypoventilation is known at this time. Positive pressure ventilation, either intermittently or continuously, is the only alternative in cases of life-threatening hypoventilation. Although it is intuitive that treatment of central hypoventilation by positive pressure ventilation impinges on quality of life, direct comparison with diaphragm pacing has not been done. Likewise, although it would seem intuitive that diaphragm pacing could prolong life in these patients and forestall complications, no controlled comparative studies exist.

In the case of quadriplegia, as well, no controlled comparative studies of pacing versus mechanical ventilation have been performed. Such studies would require multi-institutional organization, given the relatively small numbers of patients treated by pacing. In the absence of controlled studies, some inferences can be drawn from accumulated clinical data. Carter and associates (1987a,b), at the Texas Institute for Rehabilitation and Research, compared their experience over 17 years in treating ventilator-dependent spinal cord injury patients with mechanical ventilation — 19 patients — or diaphragm pacing — 18 patients. Overall mortality showed a statistically nonsignificant benefit from pacing — 39% survival with pacing versus 32% with mechanical ventilation. Data on specifics of pacing — especially stimulation frequency — are not given. It is likely that even better results could be attained with our currently favored modality of continuous, bilateral low-frequency stimulation. Data reported by the author and associates (1993a) with continuous, bilateral, low-frequency stimulation in quadriplegia shows an excellent survival — 100% at 9 years, by actuarial methods, among patients completing a pacing protocol. This survival exceeds the 63% 9-year survival expected from Carter and colleagues' (1978a,b) data with mechanical ventilation of respirator-dependent patients.

ADVANTAGES OF DIAPHRAGM PACING

The author and associates (1990, 1993b) have found that diaphragm pacing offers a number of advantages over positive pressure ventilation.

Increased Independence

First and foremost is the increased independence afforded by freedom from the ventilator. The windpipe need no longer be attached to a tubing attached in turn to a ventilator. Central hypoventilators can walk and quadriplegics can travel to school or work, with the portable diaphragm pacemakers functioning. The portable units are about the size and shape of the telemetric transmitters used for ambulatory monitoring of heart rate and rhythm. Recently, one hypoventilator came to Yale on 24-hour positive pressure ventilation from an intensive care setting. Following successful institution of 24-hour bilateral diaphragm pacing, he was discharged fully ambulatory and able to return to work full-time. Many other patients travel regularly for work, school, or pleasure.

Improved Speech

Because positive pressure ventilation requires a tube in the airway, speech is difficult or impossible. With institution of diaphragm pacing, the tracheostomy tube is replaced by the tracheal button. This restores a closed and unobstructed airway. Normal speech is again possible; the movement of air during expiration provides the substrate for this speech. For the patient so incapacitated by high quadriplegia, restoration of speech is tantamount to liberation from isolation.

Avoidance of Tracheal Injury

The problems related to long-term intubation of the trachea — tracheal stenosis, tracheomalacia, tracheo-esophageal fistula, and chronic tracheobronchial infection — are common, serious, and often life-threatening. Surgical correction of these problems is often impossible in the patient dependent on positive pressure ventilation. These problems are eliminated by diaphragm pacing. The tracheal button is noninjurious and nonirritating. Production of irritative secretions ceases. Chronic and progressive injury to the trachea by the tube and its cuff are halted.

Avoidance of Sudden Death
From Ventilator Problems

Physicians experienced in the care of patients dependent on chronic positive pressure ventilation are well aware that sudden death — from tracheostomy occlusion or dislodgement, disconnection of the ventilator tubing, primary malfunction of the ventilator, or power loss — is a common terminal event. The quadriplegic patient, especially, cannot correct such problems by virtue of his immobility; if no attendant is immediately available, death may ensue. Diaphragm pacing eliminates the serious potential for these problems.

Possibility of Improvement in Life Expectancy

Although conclusive data from controlled studies are not available, experience suggests, especially in the case of quadriplegia, for which some historical data are available for comparison, that diaphragm pacing improves survival over that expected with mechanical ventilation.

FUTURE GOALS

Technical Improvement in Stimulating Apparatus

The commercially available systems for diaphragm pacing and their limitations have been described. No fully satisfactory and proven system is currently available. As well, the systems described all involve an external transmitter and an implanted receiver. Development of a fully implantable diaphragm pacing system would constitute a significant advance. Current systems are *asynchronous* with respect to the native respiratory pattern. Development of a *demand*-type unit is certainly feasible. Furthermore, taking a cue from sensor-based cardiac pacemakers currently in widespread clinical use, a physiologically responsive system for diaphragm pacing — which increases rate with increasing respiratory requirement — would clearly be feasible. The relatively small number of diaphragm pacemakers used yearly has limited profit potential and, correspondingly, interest on the part of major manufacturers of cardiac pacing equipment in diaphragm pacing technology. Improved pacing systems applicable to the diaphragm may emerge as a byproduct of the intensive investigation of pacing of skeletal muscle for cardiac support by Higgins and associates (1992) among others.

Comparative Clinical Trials

Direct comparison of diaphragm pacing with other modalities in both central hypoventilation and quadriplegia is necessary. In central hypoventilation, comparison to medical management or mechanical ventilation, or both, could be carried out. In quadriplegia, as no medical management is feasible for apneic patients, comparison with treatment by mechanical ventilation would be necessary. Collaborative studies involving multiple institutions would be required to permit reliable conclusions.

Use of Diaphragm Pacing in COPD

Diaphragm pacing may have a role in the patient with advanced COPD, as suggested by Glenn and co-workers (1978), specifically in sustaining minute volume under treatment with supplemental oxygen in the CO_2-retainer dependent on hypoxic drive. It is possible that such treatment could significantly enhance quality of life by permitting oxygen enrichment in patients for whom this would otherwise be contraindicated.

REFERENCES

Beard GM, Rockwell AD: A Practical Treatise on the Medical and Surgical Uses of Electricity. New York: William Wood, 1878, p 664.

Brouillette RT, et al: Stimulus parameters for phrenic nerve pacing in infants and children. Pediatr Pulmonol 4:33, 1988.

Carter RE: Comparative study of electrophrenic nerve stimulation and mechanical ventilation in traumatic spinal cord injury. Paraplegia 25:86, 1987a.

Carter RE: Respiratory aspects of spinal cord injury management. Paraplegia 25:262, 1987b.

Duchenne GBA: De l'Ectrisation Localisee et de son Application a la Pathologie et a le Therapeutique par Courant Induits et par Courants Galvaniques Interrompus et Continus par le Dr. Duchenne. Paris: Bailliere, 1872.

Elefteriades JA: Discussion of Miller JI, Farmer JA, Stuart W, Apple D. Phrenic nerve pacing in quadriplegia. J Thorac Cardiovasc Surg 99:35, 1990.

Elefteriades JA, Hogan JF, Handler A, Kim Y: Long-term follow-up of bilateral pacing of the conditioned diaphragm in quadriplegia. (Submitted for publication.) 1993a.

Elefteriades JA, Hogan JF, Handler A, Loke JA: Long-term follow-up of bilateral pacing of the diaphragm in quadriplegia. N Engl J Med 326:1433, 1992.

Elefteriades JA, Hogan JF, Loke: The twenty-four hour respiratory control study for diaphragm pacing. (Submitted for publication.) 1993b.

Glenn WWL, Elefteriades JA. The diaphragm: dysfunction and induced pacing. *In* Baue AE, et al (eds): Glenn's Thoracic and Cardiovascular Surgery. (5th Ed.) Norwalk, CT: Appleton-Century-Crofts, 1991.

Glenn WWL, et al: Total ventilatory support in a quadriplegic patient with radiofrequency electrophrenic respiration. N Engl J Med 286:513, 1972.

Glenn WWL, Gee BL, Schachter EN: Diaphragm pacing: application to a patient with chronic obstructive pulmonary disease. J Thorac Cardiovasc Surg 75:273, 1978.

Glenn WWL, et al: Ventilatory support for pacing of the conditioned diaphragm in quadriplegia. N Engl J Med 310:1150, 1984.

Glenn WWL, et al: Twenty years of experience in phrenic nerve stimulation to pace the diaphragm. PACE 9:780, 1986.

Glenn WWL, et al: Fundamental considerations in pacing of the diaphragm for chronic ventilatory insufficiency: a multi-center study. PACE 11:2121, 1988.

Higgins R, et al: Accessory skeletal muscle ventricles for circulatory support: early experience with SMV's in continuity with the circulation. Basic Appl Myol 1:89, 1992.

Hogan JF, Holcomb WG, Glenn WWL: A programmable, totally implantable, battery-powered diaphragm pacemaker: design characteristics. *In* Saha S (ed): Proceedings of the Fourth New England Bioengineering Conference. Elmsford, NY: Pergamon, 1976, p 221.

Hufeland CW: Usum uis electriciae in asphyxia experimentis illustratum. Germany: Göttingen, Dissertatio Inauguralis Medica, 1783.

Hunt CE, et al: Central hypoventilation syndrome: experience with bilateral phrenic nerve pacing in 3 neonates. Am Rev Respir Dis 118:23, 1978.

Isreal F: Uber die Wiederbelebung scheintoter Neugeborener mit Hilfe des elektrischen Stroms. Z Geburtshilfe Gynakol 91:602, 1927.

Kelly WD: Phrenic nerve paralysis: special consideration of the accessory nerve. J Thorac Surg 19:923, 1950.

Letsou GV, et al: Comparison of 180-degree and 360-degree skeletal muscle nerve cuff electrodes. Ann Thorac Surg 54:925, 1992.

Mannion JD, Stephenson LW: Potential uses of skeletal muscle for myocardial assistance. Surg Clin North Am 65:679, 1985.

McCreery DB, Agnew WF. Mechanisms of stimulation-induced neural damage and their relation to guidelines for safe stimulation. *In* Agnew WF, McCreery DB (eds): Neural Prostheses: Fundamental Studies. Englewood Cliffs, NJ: Prentice-Hall, 1990.

Motoyama EK: Pulmonary mechanics during early postnatal years. Pediatr Res 11:220, 1977.

Peterson DK, et al: Intramuscular electrical activation of the phrenic nerve. IEEE Trans Biomed Eng BME 33:342, 1986.

Radford EP, Ferris BG, Kriete BC: Clinical use of a nomogram to estimate proper ventilation during artificial respiration. N Eng J Med 251:877, 1954.

Salmons S, Hendriksson J. The adaptive response of skeletal muscle to increased use. Muscle Nerve 4:94, 1981.

Sarnoff SJ, et al: Electrophrenic respiration in acute bulbar poliomyelitis. AMA 143:1383, 1950.

Sarnoff SJ, et al: Electrophrenic respiration. VII. The motor point of the phrenic nerve in relation to external stimulation. Surg Gynecol Obstet 93:90, 1951.

Shaw RK, et al: Electrophysiological evaluation of phrenic nerve function in candidates for diaphragm pacing. J Neurosurg 53:345, 1980.

Shneerson J: Disorders of Ventilation. Oxford, England: Blackwell Scientific, 1988.

Talonen P: A more natural approach to nerve stimulation in electrophrenic respiration. Doctoral thesis. Tampere University of Technology, Tampere, 1990.

Ure A: An account of some experiments made on the body of a criminal immediately after execution, with physiological and practical observations. J Sci Arts (Lond) 6:283, 1819.

Whiteneck GG, et al: A collaborative study of high quadriplegia. Grant Report, US Department of Education, Rehabilitation Research and Demonstrations — Field Initiated Research. 1985.

CHAPTER 47

CONGENITAL POSTEROLATERAL DIAPHRAGMATIC HERNIAS

Marleta Reynolds

Infants with a congenital diaphragmatic hernia diagnosed at birth have a poor prognosis despite major advances in prenatal diagnosis, neonatal transport systems, and ventilatory support. A better understanding of the pulmonary pathology and pathophysiology associated with the diaphragmatic defect have led to changes in therapy but minimal improvement in survival. Investigations into in-utero correction of the diaphragmatic hernia and the use of inhaled nitric oxide as a potent pulmonary vasodilator are on the forefront of experimental study to reduce the seemingly fixed mortality rates of infants with congenital diaphragmatic hernia.

EMBRYOLOGY

The classic congenital diaphragmatic hernia of Bochdalek is a posterolateral defect in the diaphragm caused by a failure of the pleuroperitoneal canal to close at 8 weeks' gestation (Fig. 47–1). Eighty percent occur on the left side, the remainder on the right, and they occasionally are bilateral. The defect ranges in size from a small circular hole — the characteristic Bochdalek hernia — to total absence of the hemidiaphragm. In moderate-sized defects a small rim of muscle exists posteriorly.

When the intestines return to the abdomen from the yolk sac at 10 weeks' gestation, the intestines and other abdominal viscera may herniate into the chest and alter growth of the ipsilateral lung. If the mediastinum is pushed to the contralateral side of the chest by the abdominal viscera, the contralateral lung may also be affected. Autopsy studies by the author and colleagues (1984) and Nguyen (1983) and Geggel (1985) and their associates of newborns with congenital diaphragmatic hernia demonstrated pulmonary hypoplasia in both lungs. The ipsilateral lung's weight may be 20 to 50% below normal. Geggel and colleagues (1985) reported that the contralateral lung's volume is 12 to 42% below normal. The pulmonary hypoplasia consists of a decrease in the number of bronchioles and arterioles and in the

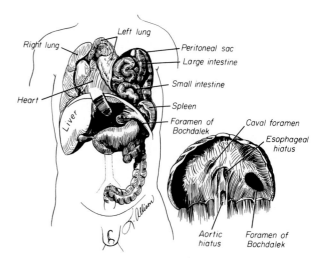

Fig. 47–1. Congenital diaphragmatic hernia of Bochdalek. *From* Shields TW: The diaphragm. *In* Nora P (ed): Operative Surgery: Principles and Techniques. Philadelphia: Lea & Febiger, 1972.

number and size of the alveoli. In addition, the muscularization of the arterioles is abnormal.

Geggel and colleagues (1985) documented a correlation between the extent of arteriolar muscularization and the clinical course of infants with congenital diaphragmatic hernia. Those infants with involvement of only the preacinar arteries exhibited a "honeymoon" period during the postoperative course. Those infants with muscularization extending further out into the interacinar arterioles did not. During the "honeymoon" period, the first 6 to 24 hours, adequate oxygenation is possible. A sudden deterioration coincident with a marked rise in pulmonary vascular resistance and return to fetal circulation follows. Profound hypoxemia, acidosis, and hypercarbia result from the underlying pulmonary hypoplasia. With the return to fetal circulation, blood is shunted right to left across the foramen ovale and patent ductus arteriosus. Further hypoxemia and acidosis result, and a vicious cycle

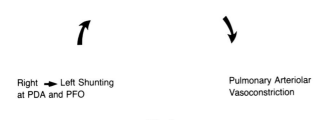

Hypoxemia, Acidosis, Hypercarbia

Right → Left Shunting
at PDA and PFO

Pulmonary Arteriolar
Vasoconstriction

Fig. 47–2. Vicious cycle of persistent fetal circulation.

Table 47–1. Infants With Congenital Diaphragmatic Hernia, 1962–1983

Onset and Severity of Symptoms	Number	Mortality (%)
<6 hours, critical	44	33–83
<6 hours, noncritical	53	6–11
6–24 hours	15	0
>24 hours	32	0
	144	

is established that leads to the infant's death from hypoxia and acidosis (Fig. 47–2).

Nakayama (1985) and the author (1985) and their associates, among others, noted that major associated anomalies exist in at least 22 to 40% of infants treated for congenital diaphragmatic hernia. Puri and Gorman (1984) reported that the incidence increases to 56% if stillborns are included. These anomalies include major chromosomal abnormalities, congenital heart disease, genitourinary anomalies, and other conditions. Anomalies of rotation and fixation of the intestines are always present.

Prenatal diagnosis of congenital diaphragmatic hernia is being made with increasing frequency and accuracy. Berk and Grundy (1982) reported low amniotic fluid lecithin/sphingomyelin ratios in mothers carrying fetuses with congenital diaphragmatic hernia. Ultrasound findings that suggest diaphragmatic hernia include herniated abdominal viscera, abnormal upper abdominal anatomy, and mediastinal shift away from the side of herniation, as Adzick and colleagues (1985b) described. Polyhydraminios was present in 76% of the cases they reported and was a predictor of poor prognosis. Both Adzick (1985b) and Nakayama (1985) and their associates reported that the accuracy in prenatal diagnosis ranges from 50 to 97%, but this may be improved by amniography and single-section computed tomography — CT. Other anomalies can often be identified by ultrasound, as noted by Adzick and colleagues (1985b). Prenatal diagnosis enables the parents to seek genetic and pediatric surgical consultation. Evaluation for in-utero repair may be obtained and plans made for delivery at an institution where neonatologists are in attendance. Unfortunately, as Nakayama and associates (1985) noted, early diagnosis has made little alteration in survival rates.

PRESENTATION

A congenital diaphragmatic hernia may cause life-threatening respiratory distress in the first hours or days of life. The defect can cause respiratory distress or feeding intolerance in later infancy or childhood or may be identified on a radiograph obtained for unrelated reasons in an asymptomatic patient. The morbidity and mortality associated with a congenital diaphragmatic hernia is directly related to the age of the patient at presentation (Table 47–1).

Some babies with congenital diaphragmatic hernia become symptomatic in the delivery room. The diagnosis is suspected if the abdomen is scaphoid and there are heart sounds in the right chest. Radiographs of the baby demonstrate gas-filled loops of intestines in the chest (Fig. 47–3). An oral-gastric tube placed into the stomach to decompress the intestines may appear in the chest, and there is a paucity of gas in the abdomen (Fig. 47–4).

Any baby with respiratory distress at birth who is suspected of having a diaphragmatic hernia should be quickly intubated and ventilated. Mask bagging only

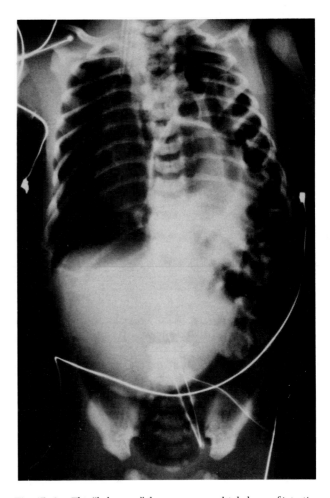

Fig. 47–3. This "babygram" demonstrates multiple loops of intestine in the left side of the chest and a few loops in the abdomen. The mediastinum is shifted to the contralateral side.

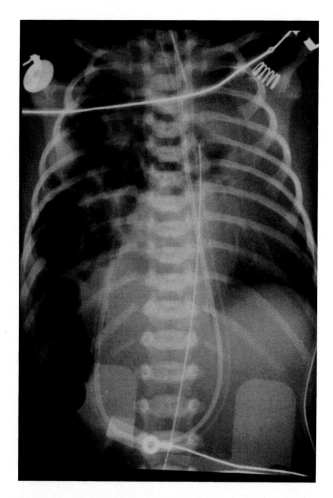

Fig. 47–4. Radiograph demonstrates a right-sided diaphragmatic hernia. The orogastric tube is seen in the right side of the chest, identifying the location of the stomach.

increases the distention of the herniated stomach and intestines and further compromises ventilation.

Mechanical ventilation with 100% FI_{O_2} and low airway pressures — < 25 mmHg with 5 of PEEP — should be used. Vascular access using an umbilical artery catheter is adequate for arterial blood gas sampling and fluid and drug administration. The baby should be rapidly transported to a center with a surgeon, a neonatal intensive care unit equipped to care for such an infant, and extracorporeal membrane oxygenation — ECMO — capabilities. Profound respiratory acidosis is typically found with the first arterial blood gas. Ventilation is individualized to prevent or treat hypercarbia and hypoxemia. Prolonged hypoxemia, acidosis, and hypercarbia produce pulmonary vasoconstriction and persistent fetal circulation. Myocardial dysfunction may necessitate support with dobutamine and renal perfusion with low-dose dopamine. Because dopamine in higher doses may constrict the pulmonary vasculature, it is used only in low doses. Five percent albumin can be used to treat systemic hypotension in boluses of 10 to 15 ml.

A congenital diaphragmatic hernia may be found incidentally in an older infant or child. Newman and

colleagues (1986) found that the older infant or child with a diaphragmatic hernia may also present with respiratory or gastrointestinal symptoms. Diagnosis is made with chest radiograph or barium studies of the gastrointestinal tract. The hernia should be repaired at the time of diagnosis. The lungs of these children are not hypoplastic, and the operative mortality should be 0%.

OPERATIVE CORRECTION

In the past, repair of a congenital diaphragmatic hernia was considered a surgical emergency. Babies were operated on in the delivery room or were taken directly from the transport ambulance to the operating suite. Retrospective analysis of this treatment plan has shown little advantage or improvement in survival. In fact, Sakai and associates (1987) have demonstrated that early surgery causes deterioration in pulmonary mechanics. Nakayama and associates (1991) have shown that preoperative stabilization results in an improvement in pulmonary compliance in a group of babies with delayed repair of the hernia. Glick (1992) and Suen (1993) and their associates have demonstrated that the lungs of fetuses with congenital diaphragmatic hernias are biochemically premature and some babies have been shown to benefit from surfactant replacement therapy during this stabilization period, as reported by Bos and colleagues (1979, 1990). In light of these studies, most centers attempt to stabilize these babies before repair of the diaphragmatic hernia.

Once stable, the neonatal ventilator is moved from the neonatal intensive care unit to the operating room for use during the operation, or the surgery is performed in the intensive care unit. Any sudden deterioration of vital signs during transport, in the operating room, or during the postoperative period usually indicates a pneumothorax on the contralateral side. Gibson and Fonkalsrud (1983) and Srouji and associates (1981) reported that a contralateral pneumothorax or a pneumomediastinum is associated with an increase in mortality and should be prevented with the use of low airway pressures. A tube thoracostomy with a No. 10 French chest tube should be rapidly placed if a pneumothorax is suspected.

The correction of a congenital diaphragmatic hernia is performed through a paramedian incision. The abdominal viscera are returned to the abdomen from the chest, and the hernia sac, if presented, is excised. Extralobar pulmonary sequestrations, often an associated malformation in infants with congenital diaphragmatic hernia, are resected at the time of hernia repair. A small diaphragmatic defect is closed with permanent suture and Teflon pledgets. Larger defects can be closed with polytetrafluoroethylene — PTFE — membrane. When the hemidiaphragm is completely absent, a PTFE membrane can be sutured to the ribs, both anteriorly and posterolaterally. The medial portion of the membrane can be sutured to the contralateral diaphragmatic leaf and the adventitia overlying the aorta and esophagus. A chest tube is placed in the ipsilateral thorax and attached to a three-way stopcock and closed. Topical thrombin and cryoprecipitate are applied to the surgical field to prevent postoperative bleeding if ECMO becomes necessary.

Controversy continues regarding the best method of thoracic drainage. Suggestions have included no chest tube, bilateral prophylactic chest tubes, underwater seal, and tubes exposed to atmospheric pressure. Tyson and associates (1985) recommended "balanced thoracic drainage" to maintain normal intrathoracic pressure. The ipsilateral chest tube attached to a three-way stopcock allows removal of air or fluid, depending on the clinical picture and the finding on radiographs of the chest. I prefer this latter method.

Associated intra-abdominal anomalies should be corrected at the time of hernia repair if the baby's condition is stable. If fascial closure causes compromise of respiratory excursion, a ventral hernia can be created by closing the skin only. Occasionally, even the skin cannot be closed, and a "silo" of silastic sheeting can be used to temporarily contain the abdominal viscera.

POSTOPERATIVE MANAGEMENT

The postoperative management combines all available means to reduce pulmonary vascular resistance, improve oxygenation, and treat persistent fetal circulation. Manual hyperventilation, as Fong and Pemberton (1985) advocated, or ventilator rates of 100 to 150 breaths per minute, as Sawyer (1986) and Vacanti (1984) and their colleagues suggested, produces respiratory alkalosis. Karl and colleagues (1983) reported that high-frequency oscillation with frequencies from 375 to 1800 cycles per minute produced a temporary respiratory alkalosis when other methods failed in four infants with congenital diaphragmatic hernia. They combined hyperventilation with airway pressures not exceeding 25 mmHg. A sodium bicarbonate infusion may be used to treat a metabolic acidosis. Vacanti and colleagues (1984) recommended pancuronium — 0.1 mg/kg/hr — and fentanyl — 1 μg/kg/hr — to control ventilation and reduce pulmonary vascular reactivity. Intravenous fluids are kept to a minimum because the need for multiple drugs quickly exceeds maintenance requirements.

Frequent arterial blood gas determinations coupled with continuous pulse oximetry or transcutaneous partial pressure of oxygen — Po_2 — and of carbon dioxide — Pco_2 — monitoring provide a constant assessment of ventilatory status (Fig. 47–5).

Vasodilators and inotropic drugs may be used for those infants who do not respond. Bloss and colleagues (1980)

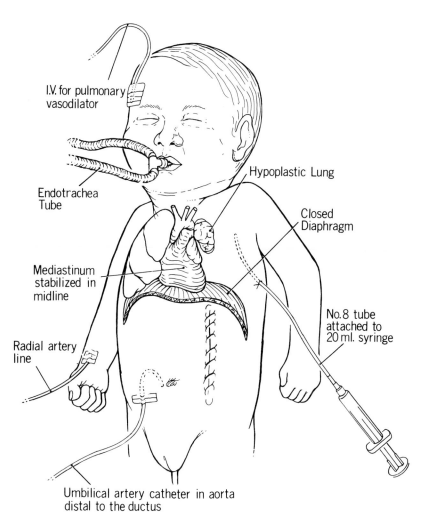

I.V. for pulmonary vasodilator

Endotrachea Tube

Mediastinum stabilized in midline

Radial artery line

Hypoplastic Lung

Closed Diaphragm

No. 8 tube attached to 20 ml. syringe

Umbilical artery catheter in aorta distal to the ductus

Fig. 47–5. Total postoperative management of a poor-risk infant. The mediastinum is stabilized with the pleural catheter, blood gases are monitored above and below the ductus arteriosus, and the intravenous lines are used for the administration of vasodilator drugs. *From* Ramenofsky MD, Luck SR: Diaphragmatic anomalies. *In* Raffensperger JC (ed): Swenson's Pediatric Surgery. 4th Ed. East Norwalk, CT: Appleton-Century-Crofts, 1980, p 675.

reported that tolazoline is useful. I have used sodium nitroprusside and nitroglycerine with some success in a few infants. Drummond and associates (1981) reported that the response to some of these drugs is unpredictable and seldom long-lasting, and I certainly agree. Positive inotropic drugs may be needed to maintain blood pressure when vasodilators are used. Recent reports by Frostell (1991) and Pepke-Zaba (1991) suggest that inhaled nitric oxide is a potent pulmonary vasodilator. Clinical trials are in progress to determine the efficacy and safety in babies with congenital diaphragmatic hernia.

EXTRACORPOREAL MEMBRANE OXYGENATION

Extracorporeal membrane oxygenation — ECMO — has been successfully used in over 60 centers in the United States to treat reversible respiratory failure in newborn infants. Hardesty (1981), Bartlett (1986), Weber (1987), Redmond (1987), and Langham (1987) and their colleagues reported survival rates among infants with congenital diaphragmatic hernia treated with ECMO ranging from 38 to 77%. This wide range in survival rates probably reflects differences in selection criteria and the experience of the particular center. Standard criteria have not been established, but in general include alveolar-arterial oxygen gradient — Aa_{DO_2} — <600 for 12 hours; oxygen index — $O_I \geq 40$; acute deterioration — pH <7.15 or $Pa_{O_2} < 55$ mmHg — for 2 consecutive hours; failure of conventional management; and progressive barotrauma. Contraindication to the use of ECMO, as described by Bartlett and associates (1986), include pre-existing intraventricular hemorrhage, weight less than 2000 g, and congenital or neurologic abnormalities incompatible with normal life.

Several groups have looked retrospectively at survival statistics for infants with congenital diaphragmatic hernia treated with ECMO. Van Meurs (1990), Weber (1987), and Atkinson (1991) and their associates have demonstrated an improved survival using ECMO. O'Rourke and colleagues (1991) did not show an improvement in survival in their group of patients. Trento and associates (1986) noted that once placed on ECMO, infants with congenital diaphragmatic hernia are at greater risk than other infants for bleeding complications. ECMO is reserved for those babies who do not respond to postoperative therapy and for babies who are too unstable to undergo repair. These infants may undergo hernia repair after cessation of ECMO or while they are still receiving ECMO. This group of infants has the worst prognosis (Fig. 47–6).

FACTORS IN SURVIVAL

Several methods have been used to predict survival in infants with congenital diaphragmatic hernia. Biox-Ochoa and colleagues (1977) reported that an arterial blood pH <7.0 with a $Pco_2 > 100$ is an early predictor for a poor outcome. Touloukian and Markowitz (1984) devised a scoring system based on preoperative radiographic findings. The radiographic findings include the side of the diaphragmatic hernia, location of the stomach, presence of pneumothorax, and relative volume of aerated ipsilateral and contralateral lung. A total score can be derived for each patient and identifies the high-risk patient.

Alveolar-arterial oxygen tension differences — Aa_{DO_2} — are used more frequently to predict survival. Harrington (1982) and Manthei (1983) and their associates reported that preoperative and postoperative $Aa_{DO_2} > 500$ mm Hg correlated with little chance of survival. Manthei and colleagues (1983) also noted that initial postoperative improvement, as evidenced by a transient decrease in Aa_{DO_2}, was followed by a sudden rise in Aa_{DO_2}. Expecting this deterioration allows prompt institution of aggressive measures to prevent and treat the decline in oxygenation.

Bohn (1987) used ventilatory parameters to predict survival by plotting Pco_2 versus ventilation index — V_I = ventilation rate × mean airway pressure — in the pre-ECMO era. Wilson and associates (1991) have shown that the best postductal Po_2 — $BPDo_2$ — and the oxygenative/ventilation index — Po_2/mean airway pressure × respiratory rate × 100 — were predictors of mortality. Infants who did not respond to conventional mechanical ventilation — $BPDo_2 < 100$; $BPDPco_2 > 40$ with $V_I > 1000$ — did not benefit from ECMO.

FUTURE PROSPECTS

Because the degree of pulmonary hypoplasia determines survival in infants with congenital diaphragmatic

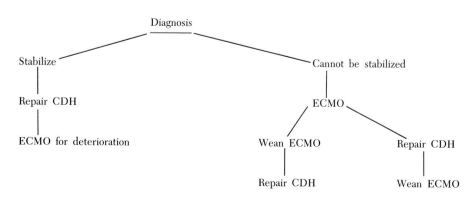

Fig. 47–6. Algorithim for a symptomatic baby with congenital diaphragmatic hernia.

hernia, investigations of in-utero correction began. Harrison (1980a) and Adzick (1985a) and their associates developed a model for congenital diaphragmatic hernia in the fetal lamb and observed that changes identical to those found in humans occurred in the fetal lamb. Harrison and colleagues (1980b) reported that the in-utero correction of the defect in fetal lambs allowed sufficient lung growth for survival. The optimal time predicted for in-utero intervention in humans is between 22 and 28 weeks' gestation. As Harrison and co-workers (1985) pointed out, ultrasound diagnosis of other anomalies and chromosomal analysis are prerequisites for maternal intervention. They have now repaired the diaphragmatic hernia in 14 fetuses and report 4 survivors. Clinical trials continue.

In-utero repair may save those infants who could not otherwise survive because of the severity of the pulmonary hypoplasia and the restructuring of the pulmonary arterioles. Based on the morphometric studies of pathologic specimens and clinical correlation, two types of infants with congenital diaphragmatic hernia become symptomatic at birth. In those infants who do not have a "honeymoon" period and never demonstrate adequate lung function, as evidenced by a Po_2 < 60 mmHg, the muscularization of the arterioles extends into the interacinar arterioles. These infants have the largest diaphragmatic defects and the smallest lungs. Survival in this group is doubtful. Identification of this group of infants in early gestation may allow correction of the defect and improvement in the pulmonary hypoplasia. The other group of infants have a "honeymoon period" and a Po_2 > 60 mmHg in the postoperative period. The pulmonary hypoplasia is not as severe in these infants, and the muscularization of the arterioles extends only into the preacinar arterioles. I believe that ECMO should be available for this group of infants because they can probably survive with this form of aggressive management.

LONG-TERM FOLLOW-UP

The evaluation of lung function in infants surviving repair of congenital diaphragmatic hernia reported by Chatrath (1971), Wurnig (1980), and Freyschuss (1984) and their associates provided some conflicting results. Fifteen-year follow-up in the review by Wurnig and colleagues (1980) identified reduced pulmonary function represented by restrictive or obstructive changes or both. Freyschuss and associates (1984) evaluated 20 patients at 6 to 22 years of age. Most of these patients had required operation at less than 48 hours of age. In these patients, perfusion of the ipsilateral lung was reduced, as was the fractional ventilation. Total lung capacity, FEV_1, and FEV% were normal. Residual volume and FRC were increased. No functional impairment was identified in any patient. This report supports the work of both Wohl and colleagues (1977) and Reid and Hutcherson (1976), who demonstrated decreased blood flow to the ipsilateral lung in similar series of patients. As the number of survivors with congenital diaphragmatic hernia increases, the fate of

the most severely hypoplastic lungs becomes evident (Fig. 47–7). Long-term follow-up should extend to the fourth and fifth decade of life to more accurately predict the eventual outcome.

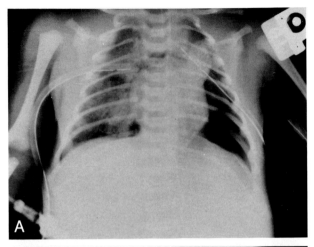

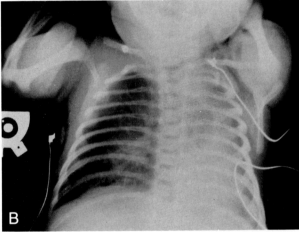

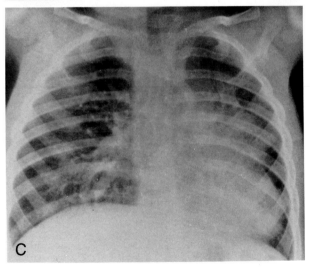

Fig. 47–7. *A*, Early postoperative radiograph shows a small left lung. *B*, One month later. Hyperinflation of the contralateral lung, and the mediastinum has shifted into the ipsilateral chest. *C*, Even 2 years after repair of the diaphragmatic hernia, the contralateral lung and mediastinum are still in the ipsilateral chest. The child was asymptomatic at the time.

REFERENCES

Adzick NS, et al: Correction of congenital diaphragmatic hernia in utero. IV. An early gestation fetal lamb model for pulmonary vascular morphometric analysis. J Pediatr Surg 20:673, 1985a.

Adzick NS, et al: Diaphragmatic hernia in the fetus: prenatal diagnosis and outcome in 94 cases. J Pediatr Surg 20:357, 1985b.

Atkinson JB, et al: The impact of extracorporeal membrane support in the treatment of congenital diaphragmatic hernia. J Pediatr Surg 26:791, 1991.

Bartlett RH, et al: Extracorporeal membrane oxygenation (ECMO) in neonatal respiratory failure. Ann Surg 204:236, 1986.

Berk C, Grundy M: "High risk" lecithin/sphingomyelin ratios associated with neonatal diaphragmatic hernia. Br J Obstet Gynecol 89:250, 1982.

Biox-Ochoa J, et al: The important influence of arterial blood gases on the prognosis of congenital diaphragmatic hernia. World J Surg 1:783, 1977.

Bloss RS, et al: Tolazoline therapy for persistent pulmonary hypertension after congenital diaphragmatic hernia repair. J Pediatr 97:984, 1980.

Bohn DJ, et al: Ventilatory predictors of pulmonary hypoplasia in congenital diaphragmatic hernia confirmed by morphometry. J Pediatr Surg 111:423, 1987.

Bos AP, et al: Surfactant replacement therapy in high-risk congenital diaphragmatic hernia. Lancet 338:1279, 1979.

Bos AP, et al: Congenital diaphragmatic hernia: impact of prostanoids in the perioperative period. Arch Dis Child 65:994, 1990.

Breax CW, et al: Improvement in survival of patients with congenital diaphragmatic hernia utilizing a strategy of delayed repair after medical and/or extracorporeal membrane oxygenation stabilization. J Pediatr Surg 26:333, 1991.

Chatrath RR, El Shafie M, Jones RS: Fate of hypoplastic lungs after repair of congenital diaphragmatic hernia. Arch Dis Child 46:633, 1971.

Drummond WH, et al: The independent effects of hyperventilation tolazoline, and dopamine on infants with persistent pulmonary hypertension. J Pediatr 98:603, 1981.

Fong LV, Pemberton PJ: Congenital diaphragmatic hernia and the management of persistent fetal circulation. Anaesth Intens Care 13:375, 1985.

Freyschuss U, Lannergren K, Frenckner B: Lung function after repair of congenital diaphragmatic hernia. Acta Pediatr Scand 73:589, 1984.

Frostell C et al: Inhaled nitric oxide: a selective pulmonary vasodilator reversing hypoxic pulmonary vasoconstriction. Circulation 83:2038, 1991.

Geggel RL et al: Congenital diaphragmatic hernia: arterial structural changes and persistent pulmonary hypertension after surgical repair. J Pediatr 107:457, 1985.

Gibson C, Fonkalsrud EW: Iatrogenic pneumothorax and mortality in congenital diaphragmatic hernia. J Pediatr Surg 18:555, 1983.

Glick PL, et al: Pathophysiology of congenital diaphragmatic hernia II: The fetal lamb CDH model is surfactant deficient. J Pediatr Surg 27:382, 1992.

Hardesty RL, et al: Extracorporeal membrane oxygenation: successful treatment of persistent fetal circulation following repair of congenital diaphragmatic hernia. J Thorac Cardiovasc Surg 81:556, 1981.

Harrington J, Raphaely RC, Downes JJ: Relationship of alveolar-arterial oxygen tension difference in diaphragmatic hernia of the newborn. Anesthesiology 56:473, 1982.

Harrison MR, Jester JA, Ross NA: Correction of congenital diaphragmatic hernia in utero. I. The model: intrathoracic balloon produces fatal pulmonary hypoplasia. Surgery 88:174, 1980a.

Harrison MR, et al: Correction of congenital diaphragmatic hernia in utero. II. Simulated correction permits fetal lung growth with survival at birth. Surgery 88:260, 1980b.

Harrison MR, et al: Fetal diaphragmatic hernia: fatal but fixable. Semin Perinatol 9:103, 1985.

Harrison MR, et al: Correction of congenital diaphragmatic hernia in utero. VI. Hard-earned lessons. J Pediatr Surg (in press) 1992.

Karl SR, Ballantine TVN, Snider MT: High-frequency ventilation at rates of 375 to 1800 cycles per minute in four neonates with congenital diaphragmatic hernia. J Pediatr Surg 18:822, 1983.

Langham MR Jr, et al: Extracorporeal membrane oxygenation following repair of congenital diaphragmatic hernias. Ann Thorac Surg 44:247, 1987.

Manthei V, Vaucher Y, Crowe CP: Congenital diaphragmatic hernia: immediate preoperative and postoperative oxygen gradients identify patients requiring prolonged respiratory support. Surgery 93:83, 1983.

Nakayama DK, et al: Prenatal diagnosis and natural history of the fetus with a congenital diaphragmatic hernia: initial clinical experience. J Pediatr Surg 20:118, 1985.

Nakayama DK, et al: Effect of preoperative stabilization on respiratory system compliance and outcome in newborn infants with congenital diaphragmatic hernia. J. Pediatr 118:793, 1991.

Newman BM, et al: Presentation of congenital diaphragmatic hernia past the newborn period. Arch Surg 121:813, 1986.

Nguyen L, et al: The mortality of congenital diaphragmatic hernia: is total pulmonary mass inadequate, no matter what? Ann Surg 198:766, 1983.

O'Rourke P, et al: The effect of extracorporeal membrane oxygenation on the survival of neonates with high-risk congenital diaphragmatic hernia: 45 cases from a single institution. J Pediatr Surg 26:147, 1991.

Pepke-Zaba J, et al: Inhaled nitric oxide as a cause of selective pulmonary vasodilation in pulmonary hypertension. Lancet 338:1173, 1991.

Puri P, Gorman F: Lethal nonpulmonary anomalies associated with congenital diaphragmatic hernia: implications for early intrauterine surgery. J Pediatr Surg 19:29, 1984.

Redmond CR, et al: Extracorporeal membrane oxygenation for respiratory and cardiac failure in infants and children. J Thorac Cardiovasc Surg 93:199, 1987.

Reid IS, Hutcherson RJ: Long-term follow-up of patients with congenital diaphragmatic hernia. J Pediatr Surg 11:939, 1976.

Reynolds M, Luck SR, Lappen R: The "critical" neonate with diaphragmatic hernia: a 21-year perspective. J Pediatr Surg 19:364, 1984.

Sakai H, et al: Effect of surgical repair on respiratory mechanics in congenital diaphragmatic hernia. J Pediatr 111:432, 1987.

Sawyer S, et al: Improving survival in the treatment of congenital diaphragmatic hernia. Ann Thorac Surg 41:75, 1986.

Srouji MN, Buck B, Downes JJ: Congenital diaphragmatic hernia: deleterious effects of pulmonary interstitial emphysema and tension extrapulmonary air. J Pediatr Surg 16:45, 1981.

Suen HC, et al: Biochemical immaturity of lungs in congenital diaphragmatic hernia. J Pediatr Surg 28:471, 1993.

Touloukian RJ, Markowitz RI: A preoperative x-ray scoring system for risk assessment of newborns with congenital diaphragmatic hernia. J Pediatr Surg 19:252, 1984.

Trento A, Griffith BP, Hardesty RL: Extracorporeal membrane oxygenation experience at the University of Pittsburgh. Ann Thorac Surg 42:56, 1986.

Tyson KRT, Schwartz MZ, Marr CC: "Balanced" thoracic drainage is the method of choice to control intrathoracic pressure following repair of diaphragmatic hernia. J Pediatr Surg 20:415, 1985.

Vacanti JP, et al: The pulmonary hemodynamic response to perioperative anesthesia in the treatment of high-risk infants with congenital diaphragmatic hernia. J Pediatr Surg 19:672, 1984.

Van Meurs KP, et al: Effect of extracorporeal membrane oxygenation on survival of infants with congenital diaphragmatic hernia. J Pediatr 117:954, 1990.

Weber TR, et al: Neonatal diaphragmatic hernia: an improving outlook with extracorporeal membrane oxygenation. Arch Surg 122:615, 1987.

Wilson JM, et al: Congenital diaphragmatic hernia: predictors of severity in the ECMO era. J Pediatr Surg 26:1028, 1991.

Wohl MEB, et al: Repair of congenital diaphragmatic hernia. J Pediatr 90:405, 1977.

Wurnig P, Balogh A, Hopfgartner L: Fifteen years of surgical therapy for congenital diaphragmatic hernia: results and follow-up. Z Kinderchir 29:134, 1980.

CHAPTER 48

CARDIAL INCOMPETENCE AND ASSOCIATED GASTROESOPHAGEAL REFLUX

Marleta Reynolds

Cardial incompetence is a common abnormality in infants and children. Some degree of "spitting up" is normal in early infancy, but when exaggerated, it may lead to malnutrition, aspiration pneumonia, esophagitis, or sudden death. Boix-Ochoa (1986) demonstrated that children have a lower esophageal sphincter — LES — pressure that is lower than the normal pressure described for adults. Local anatomic defects also play a role as infants with diaphragm and esophageal anomalies have a higher incidence of cardial incompetence. Neurologically impaired children are also prone to have cardial incompetence.

SYMPTOMS

Vomiting is the most common symptom of cardial incompetence and may begin shortly after birth. It usually occurs after feedings and consists of ingested materials. In babies who develop esophagitis, coffee ground emesis may become apparent. Failure to thrive leading to malnutrition develops as formula changes fail to relieve the vomiting.

Chronic aspiration may lead to nocturnal wheezing and chronic cough. Some infants and children are mistakenly treated for asthma. Pneumonia may develop and require hospitalization and parenteral antibiotic therapy. Leape and associates (1977) confirmed an association of respiratory arrest and gastroesophageal reflux in 10 infants less than 6 months of age. Apnea may or may not be related to cardial incompetence.

Strictures of the distal esophagus may develop after prolonged esophagitis but are usually found in older children. I have treated several infants with severe strictures from prolonged reflux. Intolerance to feedings results when the stricture persists untreated (Fig. 48–1).

DIAGNOSIS

A careful history is imperative in differentiating cardial incompetence and associated gastroesophageal reflux from rumination and normal "spit up." A barium esophagram and upper gastrointestinal series with fluoroscopic recording can be diagnostic and should be the initial study of choice to rule out other surgical causes of vomiting. The gastroesophageal scintiscan can accurately diagnose reflux when an esophagram has been normal. Twenty-four hour pH monitoring is the most accurate means to test for gastroesophageal reflux. Esophagoscopy and biopsy of esophageal mucosa confirm the presence of esophagitis.

TREATMENT

Medical Therapy

Conservative therapy can control symptoms in most children with cardial incompetence and gastroesophageal reflux. Dietary manipulations include increasing the frequency and decreasing the volume of feedings, and thickening feedings with rice cereal. The prone upright position is recommended by some authors. Bethanechol and metachlopromide have been recommended by Strickland and Chang (1983) and Orenstein (1992) to improve gastric emptying and esophageal motility. Orenstein (1992) also advocates acid-reducing agents such as the H_2 blockers. The majority of infants grow out of their reflux and do not require surgical treatment.

Surgical Intervention

Approximately 15% of patients with cardial incompetence require surgical intervention to correct persistent gastroesophageal reflux. The incidence of neurologic disorders is high in this subset of patients.

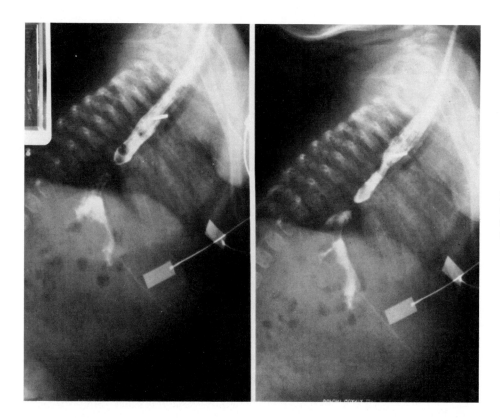

Fig. 48–1. Barium esophagram demonstrates a distal esophageal stricture in a neonate with severe gastroesophageal reflux.

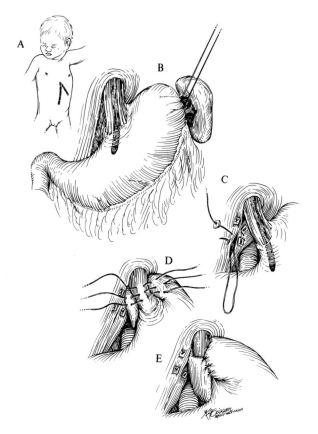

Fig. 48–2. *A,* The operation may be performed through an upper midline or left subcostal incision. *B,* A large catheter is placed in the esophagus and short gastric vessels are ligated and divided. *C,* The diaphragmatic crura are closed with ticron pledgetted suture. *D,* The fundus of the stomach is passed behind the esophagus and sutured to the esophageal wall. *E,* The 360° wrap forms the fundoplication. *From* Raffensperger E (ed): Swenson's Pediatric Surgery. Norwalk CT: Appleton and Lange, 1990.

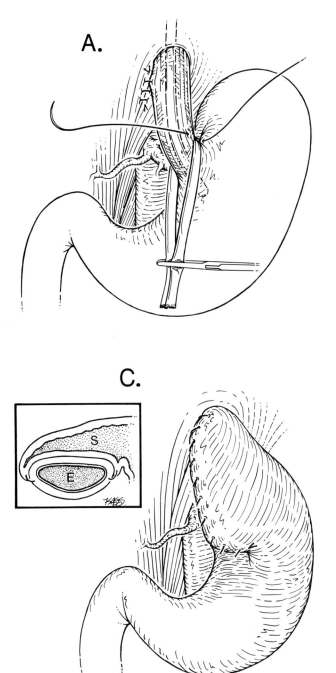

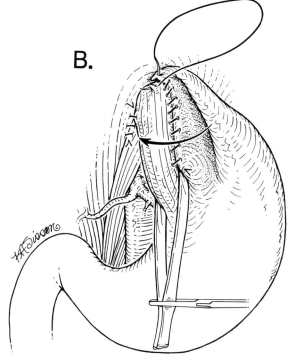

Fig. 48–3. *A,* Exposure of the hiatus is through an upper midline or left subcostal incision. The short gastric vessels are not divided. A suture closes the hiatus and a continuous permanent suture is begun to the left of the esophagus. *B,* The suture is continued up the esophagus, securing the stomach to the esophagus. *C,* The suture continues across and down the right side to achieve a 210° wrap around the anterior wall of the esophagus. *From* Raffensperger E (ed): Swenson's Pediatric Surgery. Norwalk CT: Appleton and Lange, 1990.

Fonkalsrud and colleagues (1985) reported that 32% of the infants and children in their series who required surgical intervention were in this category. For many of those patients who do not respond to medical therapy, a period of nasogastric drip feedings or total parenteral nutrition may be required to improve their nutritional status and make them adequate surgical candidates.

Operations

The Nissen fundoplication and Thal fundoplication are used most frequently to treat cardial incompetence and gastroesophageal reflux in children. Both secure the esophageal hiatus below the diaphragm, create a new angle of His, and provide an artificial valve-like mechanism to recreate a normal LES.

In performing a Nissen fundoplication, I place a mercury bougie into the distal esophagus from the mouth to prevent the wrap from becoming too tight. I approach the hiatus through a left subcostal or midline incision and isolate the distal esophagus. The diaphragmatic crus is sutured with interrupted pledgeted suture and the fundus of the stomach is passed around the gastroesophageal junction after division of several short gastric vessels. The 360° wrap is created with permanent suture, sewing the stomach to itself and the underlying esophagus and diaphragm superiorly (Fig. 48–2).

The Thal fundoplication has been advocated by Ashcraft and colleagues (1984). The 270° wrap is created with a running suture and, at the apex, the diaphragm is incorporated (Fig. 48–3).

Complications of both procedures are not uncommon. Paraesophageal hernias, suture–line dehiscence, bowel obstructions, and recurrent reflux may occur. Good results can be expected, however, in 95% of the patients.

REFERENCES

Ashcraft K, et al: The Thal fundoplication for esophageal reflux. J Pediatr Surg *19*:480, 1984.

Boix-Ochoa J: The physiologic approach to the management of gastric-esophageal reflux. J Pediatr Surg *21*:1032, 1986.

Fonkalsrud EW, Ament ME, Berquist W: Surgical management of the gastroesophageal reflux syndrome in childhood. Surgery *97*:42, 1985.

Grill B, et al: Effectiveness of domperidone therapy on symptoms and upper gastrointestinal motility in infants with gastroesophageal reflux. J Pediatr *106*:311, 1985.

Leape LL, et al: Respiratory arrest in infants secondary to gastroesophageal reflux. Pediatrics *60*:924, 1977.

Orenstein SR: Controversies in pediatric gastroesophageal reflux. J Pediatr Gastroenterol Nutr *14*:338, 1992.

Strickland A, Chang J: Results of treatment of gastroesophageal reflux with bethanechol. J Pediatr *103*:311, 1983.

CHAPTER 49

FORAMEN OF MORGAGNI HERNIA AND UNCOMMON CONGENITAL DIAPHRAGMATIC HERNIAS

Thomas W. Shields and Marleta Reynolds

FORAMEN OF MORGAGNI HERNIA

Anatomy

On each side of the sternum is a potential space, known as the foramen of Morgagni, or the space of Larrey, through which passes the internal mammary artery to become the superior epigastric artery.

This triangular space is between the muscular fibers originating from the xiphisternum and the costal margin that insert on the central tendon of the diaphragm. The left space is less likely to develop a hernia because it is protected by the pericardial sac. The ligamentum teres defines the medial border of the hernia through either space.

Most often, a foramen of Morgagni hernia contains only a piece of omentum that is caught up in the defect and then enlarges as the person grows and produces the mass within the hernia sac. At times, the hernia contains colon and, occasionally, small intestine or other abdominal viscera (Fig. 49–1).

Incidence

Hernias through the foramen of Morgagni are uncommon at any age but are even more rare in the child than in the adult (Fig. 49–2). Berman and associates (1989) reported only 15 infants and children with Morgagni hernias collected over a 20-year period at the Hospital for Sick Children in Toronto. Overall, these hernias represent approximately 3% of all diaphragmatic hernias. They occur more frequently on the right side than on the left and usually contain a sac. Chin and Duchesne (1955) found 30 examples of retrosternal hernias in a mass radiographic survey of the chest. In the past, these hernias probably were frequently unrecognized on routine radiographs of the chest, because the densities they produce in the right

cardiophrenic angle were interpreted as caused by the pericardial fat pad or a pleuropericardial cyst (Fig. 49–3).

Symptoms

A small foramen of Morgagni hernia usually is unrecognized and asymptomatic in young children, although larger ones may produce severe respiratory symptoms in infants. Pokorny and associates (1984) reported only five hernias of this type in infants in a 6-year period at the Texas Children's Hospital. They reviewed 17 additional cases in the literature. Most of these infants were symptomatic, which was due to respiratory distress because of a large hernia.

A foramen of Morgagni hernia is more often symptomatic in older children, adolescents, and adults. Women are affected more commonly than men are, and the obese more often than the thin. Exercise and other athletic activity, as noted by Valases and Sills (1988), may precipitate the occurrence of symptoms. Ellyson and Parks (1986) reported that trauma also could initiate symptomatology.

The patient with a foramen of Morgagni hernia may complain of dull pain in the right subcostal area. Intermittent, partial intestinal obstruction may occur, including gastric volvulus, but complete obstruction is uncommon. Dyspnea is only occasionally observed in patients past early childhood.

Diagnosis

Radiographic studies of the chest reveal a density, either solid or containing air, adjacent to the right or left side of the heart. In small hernias, Lanuza (1971) described the so-called "sign of the cane," which refers to a curvilinear accumulation of fat continuous with the properitoneal fat line of the anterior abdominal wall.

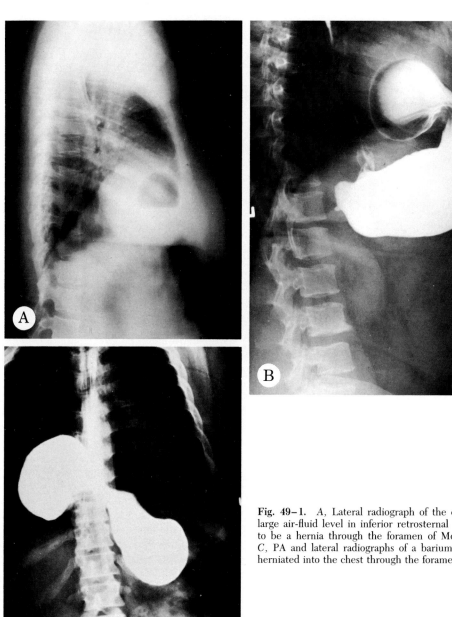

Fig. 49–1. *A,* Lateral radiograph of the chest revealing large air-fluid level in inferior retrosternal area suspected to be a hernia through the foramen of Morgagni. *B* and *C,* PA and lateral radiographs of a barium-filled stomach herniated into the chest through the foramen of Morgagni.

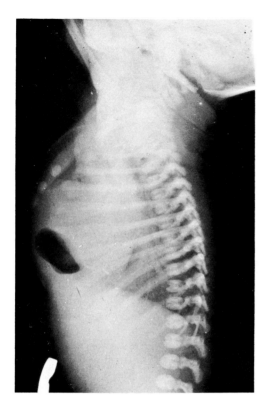

Fig. 49–2. Lateral chest radiograph of the chest in an infant with a congenital foramen of Morgagni hernia that was found to contain most of the stomach at the time of repair.

This sign suggests that a small anterior cardiophrenic mass may be a foramen of Morgagni hernia. A CT examination of an anterior cardiophrenic mass may reveal the presence of bowel (Fig. 49–4), thus confirming the diagnosis. Contrast studies of the large intestine and often of the upper gastrointestinal tract are indicated in the evaluation of some patients. At times, if the diagnosis remains in doubt, a diagnostic pneumoperitoneum may be carried out. If a communication is present between the hernia sac and the peritoneum, air enters the sac and confirms the diagnosis.

Surgical Repair

The abdominal approach for surgical repair of this hernia is chosen if the diagnosis is known preoperatively. A subcostal incision or a right epigastric paramedian incision may be used. With the latter incision, the rectus muscle is retracted laterally to expose the posterior rectus and transversalis fascia. After the abdomen has been opened, the contents of the hernia are reduced into the peritoneal cavity and the margins of the hernial sac are identified. As noted, the ligamentum teres defines the medial border of the hernia. The hernia sac is removed when possible. The repair of the muscular defect is made with interrupted mattress sutures, and usually it is necessary to pull the diaphragm up to the posterior part of the sternum and to the posterior rectus sheath (Fig. 49–5). After repair, the abdomen is closed. In most patients it is not necessary to enter into the chest or to drain the pleural space. Moghissi (1981) reported the repair of an obstructed Morgagni hernia with the combined use of a subcostal and lower median sternotomy, but this approach is not recommended.

Occasionally, a foramen of Morgagni hernia is encountered while the anterior mediastinum is being

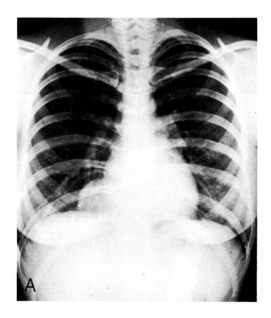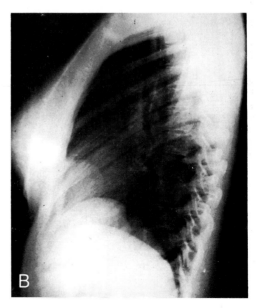

Fig. 49–3. PA (A) and lateral (B) radiographs of the chest of a patient with a foramen of Morgagni hernia that was shown to contain omentum and small bowel.

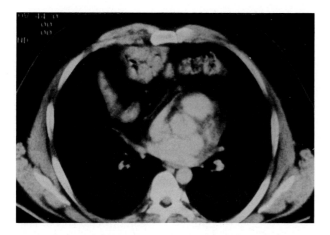

Fig. 49–4. CT of chest revealing the presence of bowel anterior to the heart in a hernia arising from a foramen of Morgagni. Used with permission of Denise Aberle, M.D., University of California at Los Angeles School of Medicine.

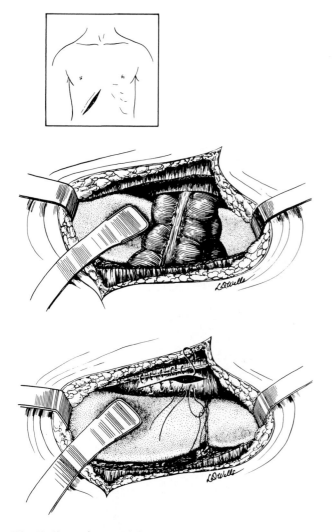

Fig. 49–5. Technique of closure of foramen of Morgagni hernia by the transabdominal approach. *From* Shields TW: The diaphragm. *In* Nora P (ed): Operative Surgery: Principles and Techniques. Philadelphia: Lea & Febiger, 1972.

explored for an undiagnosed mediastinal mass in either the anterior cardiophrenic angle. As soon as the mass has been identified as a foramen of Morgagni hernia, the sac is opened and explored, and the contents are reduced into the peritoneal cavity. The repair is then accomplished in a manner similar to that just described. In this instance it is also best to suture the diaphragm to the posterior part of the sternum and the rectus sheath. Frequently, repair necessitates the passing of the sutures around a rib anteriorly or through a portion of the chest wall. On occasion, because of the size of the defect and a deficiency of available tissue, it is necessary to sew in a small piece of plastic mesh or a soft tissue Gore-Tex patch. A recurrence of a foramen of Morgagni hernia is rare.

MISCELLANEOUS CONGENITAL DIAPHRAGMATIC HERNIAS

Hernias may occur through the central portion of the diaphragm. Partial or localized eventration of the diaphragm with marked thinning of the tissues to form a ring and a hernial sac may also occur. When such a hernia occurs on the right side, a mushroom-like projection of liver that has grown through the opening in the right diaphragmatic leaf may be found. On the radiograph of the chest, this projection is occasionally misinterpreted as a diaphragmatic tumor. Differentiation may be made by instituting a pneumoperitoneum, following which, air appears to surround the liver protrusion. Repair of this type of hernia is unnecessary if clear identification can be made by the pneumoperitoneum. If not, exploration is required to rule out the possibility of a primary tumor of the diaphragm.

If the hernia is on the left side, the stomach is occasionally herniated through the central portion of the diaphragm; it usually is identified as an air-containing cyst on the top of the diaphragm. The hernia may be associated with a partial absence of the pericardium, and the stomach and small intestine may herniate into the pericardial sac and cause cardiac symptoms. In general, when such a defect occurs through the central portion of the left hemidiaphragm or into the pericardial sac, the hernia should be repaired as soon as it is discovered. In infants and children, the repair usually is accomplished through an abdominal approach, similar to that described for the repair of the foramen of Bochdalek hernia. In contrast, in the older child and adult, repair is accomplished through a thoracic approach.

PERITONEAL PERICARDIAL HERNIA

A rare diaphragmatic defect between the peritoneal cavity and pericardial sac has also been reported. Ake and colleagues (1991) reported the prenatal diagnosis of a fetus with such a hernia. The infant was asymptomatic at birth, and the hernia was repaired through the abdomen at 5 days of life. Milne and associates (1990) reported two patients with an identical defect associated with a giant omphalocele. One of us (M.R.) has treated

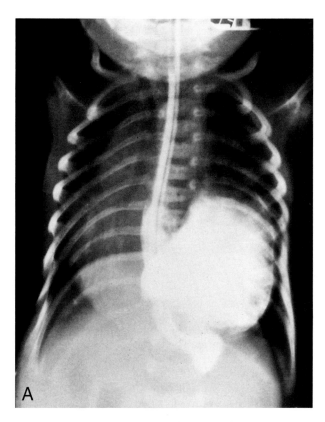 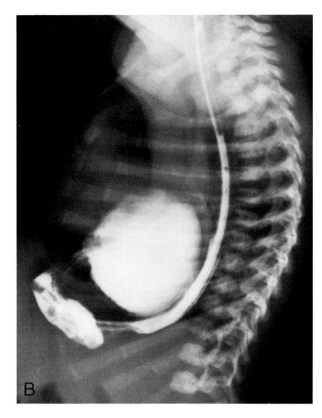

Fig. 49–6. Anteroposterior *(A)* and lateral radiographic *(B)* views of a barium swallow in an infant with a peritoneal pericardial hernia.

an infant with this defect who presented at birth with severe respiratory distress, hypotension, and persistent fetal circulation (Fig. 49–6). Urgent repair was done, and the patient survived. At operation the stomach was found inside the pericardium. Reduction of the stomach immediately improved cardiac function. The defect was closed with interrupted Ticron pledgetted sutures. Milne (1990) suggests that this defect is secondary to failure of fusion of the pars sternalis portion of the septum transversum in the development of the diaphragm. Repair may be performed through the abdomen or chest. The abdominal approach is preferred.

REFERENCES

Ake E, et al.: Short Communication: In utero sonographic diagnosis of diaphragmatic hernia with hepatic protrusion into the pericardium mimicking an intrapericardial tumour. Prenat Diagn 2:719, 1991.

Berman L, et al: The late-presenting pediatric Morgagni hernia. A benign condition. J Pediatr Surg 24:970, 1989.

Chin FF, Duchesne ER: The parasternal defect. Thorax 10:214, 1955.

Ellyson JH, Parks SN: Hernia of Morgagni in trauma patients. J Trauma 26:569, 1986.

Kunar KL, Fosse MA: Herniation through the foramen of Morgagni presenting as cardiomegaly. South Med J 75:694, 1982.

Lanuza A: The sign of the cane: a new radiological sign for the diagnosis of small Morgagni hernias. Radiology 101:293, 1971.

Milne LW, et al: Pars Sternalis diaphragmatic hernia with omphalocele: a report of two cases. J Pediatr Surg 25:726, 1990.

Moghissi K: Operation for repair of obstructed substernocostal (Morgagni) hernia. Thorax 36:392, 1981.

Pokorny WJ, McGill CW, Harberg FJ: Morgagni hernias during infancy. Presentation and associated anomalies. J Pediatr Surg 19:394, 1984.

Valases C, Sills C: Case report: anterior diaphragmatic hernia (hernia of Morgagni). NJ Med 85:603, 1988.

READING REFERENCES

Baran EM, Houston HE, Lynn HB: Foramen of Morgagni hernias in children. Surgery 62:1076, 1967.

Bently G, Lister J: Retrosternal hernia. Surgery 57:567, 1965.

Weber TR, et al: Congenital diaphragmatic hernia beyond infancy. Am J Surg 162:643, 1991.

CHAPTER 50

PARAESOPHAGEAL HIATAL HERNIA

Keith S. Naunheim and Arthur E. Baue

The hiatus for the esophagus is formed by muscle fibers of the right crus to the diaphragm with little or no contribution from the left crus. These fibers overlap inferiorly, where they attach over and along the right side of the median arcuate ligament. This is securely attached to the lateral aspects of the vertebral bodies. The orifice is thus teardrop-shaped, with the point to the right of the aorta and the rounded portion in the midline close to the connecting portion of the central tendon. The crural fibers form a tunnel that encloses the esophagus. The phrenoesophageal ligament is formed by fusion of the endothoracic and endoabdominal fascia at the diaphragmatic hiatus. This ligament holds the distal esophagus in place. The lower esophagus normally resides within the abdomen. Herniation of abdominal contents through the hiatus into the thoracic cavity has been recognized for several centuries.

Bowditch (1853) reported such a case but credited Ambrose Paré with a description of a patient with herniation of the stomach through the esophageal hiatus in 1610. One of the first successful repairs was accomplished by Potempski in 1884 and reported by him in 1889.

CLASSIFICATION

Hiatal hernias are generally classified into four types, the most common of which is the sliding, or type I hiatal hernia.

Type I Hiatal Hernia

In the sliding type of hiatal hernia, the esophagogastric junction moves through the hiatus into the visceral mediastinum so that it occupies an intrathoracic position cephalad to the stomach, which follows it. This occurs because of circumferential weakening of the phrenoesophageal ligament. The factors that may contribute to the development of such a hernia include increased abdominal pressure such as with pregnancy, obesity, vomiting and vigorous esophageal contraction, which may pull the gastroesophageal junction up into the mediastinum. This type of hernia is frequently accompanied by loss of tone and competence of the lower esophageal sphincter, which may result in acid reflux and esophagitis. This may be related to the loss of mechanical advantage at the gastroesophageal junction when it is displaced into the chest. Many sliding hiatus hernias are present without producing symptoms for the patient. There is a peculiar abnormality of incompetence of the gastric cardia or the lower esophageal sphincter without radiologic evidence of a hiatal hernia. This has been called a "patulous cardia" by Hiebert and Belsey (1961). The problems and treatment of reflux esophagitis and a type I hernia is reviewed in Chapter 122.

Type II Hiatal Hernia

The paraesophageal, or type II, hiatal hernia is an uncommon disorder that is distinctly different from sliding hiatal hernia. In a paraesophageal hernia, the phrenoesophageal membrane is not diffusely weakened but focally weakened anteriorly and lateral to the esophagus. The gastric cardia and lower esophagus remain below the diaphragm. The gastric fundus protrudes or rolls through the defect into the mediastinum (Fig. 50–1). Paraesophageal hiatal hernia is by far the less common of these two defects, and Hill (1968) and Ozdemir (1973) and their colleagues and Sanderud (1967) reported it to account for only 3 to 6% of all patients undergoing surgical repair of hiatal hernias. Because most patients with hiatal hernia do not undergo operative correction, probably only 1 to 2% of all hiatal hernias are type II defects. Allen and colleagues (1993) found 147 — 0.32% — paraesophageal hernias with 75% or more of the stomach in the chest in 46,236 patients with hiatal hernia at the Mayo Clinic from 1980 to 1990. In 124 of their patients who had an operation, 51 had a type II hernia — 41%, 52 a type III hernia — 43%, and 17% a type IV hernia.

The term "parahiatal hernia" has been used in the past, but this type of defect seems to be nonexistent. We have never seen a defect in the diaphragm alongside

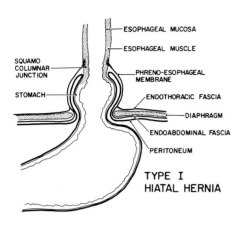

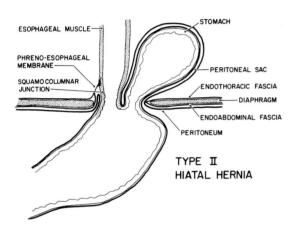

Fig. 50–1. The two types of hiatal hernia. The type I hiatal hernia is not a true hernia in that the endoabdominal fascial lining of the abdomen remains intact. In the type II hernia, a defect in the fascia allows a peritoneal sac to pass through the opening in the hiatus and enter the pleural cavity.

the hiatus with protrusion of stomach into the chest with identifiable crural or diaphragmatic fibers between the hernia orifice and the esophageal hiatus.

Type III Hiatal Hernia

The Type III, or mixed, hiatal hernia is a combination of types I and II, a sliding and rolling hernia. If a type I hiatal hernia enlarges, the attenuated phrenoesophageal membrane may also focally weaken anteriorly, allowing protrusion of the gastric fundus. Rotation of the stomach may result in the body or fundus obtaining a higher position within the chest than the cardia, a situation usually found only in type II hernias. Pearson and colleagues (1983) stated that true type II hernias are rare. They suggested that most are in fact misdiagnosed type III defects with a supradiaphragmatic lower esophageal sphincter. There has been, however, little support in the literature for this controversial viewpoint. How often a type II paraesophageal hernia becomes a type III hernia is not known. Frequently, however, when a patient has a large paraesophageal hernia with rotation of the body and fundus of the stomach into the chest, the esophagogastric junction is

in a location higher than the hiatus of the diaphragm. In such circumstances, however, the esophagogastric junction is in the posterior aspect of the hiatus, and the patient does not usually have symptoms of an attenuated intrinsic sphincter with reflux esophagitis. A type III defect is frequently present when a type II hernia has been present for many years. The mechanism for this seems to be gradual enlargement of the hiatus so that the esophagogastric junction no longer lies within or below the hiatus. Attachments of the esophagogastric junction remain intact posteriorly. Evidence increasingly suggests that a type I, Sliding, hernia is caused by esophageal contraction abnormalities with a pull on the esophagogastric junction; patients with significant or severe esophagitis rarely have a paraesophageal herniation, and patients with a large paraesophageal herniation seldom have significant esophagitis despite a supradiaphragmatic esophagogastric junction.

Type IV Hiatal Hernia

Progressive enlargement of the diaphragmatic opening can eventually lead to herniation of other organs including most commonly the transverse colon and omentum, a type IV hiatal hernia. The spleen and small bowel may also herniate into the chest at times.

ANATOMY AND PATHOPHYSIOLOGY

In a true paraesophageal hiatal hernia, the lower esophagus and cardia remain fixed below the diaphragm in the posterior aspect of the diaphragmatic hiatus. A focal weakening of the phrenoesophageal membrane occurs anterior or lateral to the esophagus, and the combination of negative intrathoracic and positive intraabdominal pressure pushes the abdominal viscera through the defect. The protruding organs are circumferentially covered by a layer of peritoneum that forms a true hernia sac, unlike the type I or sliding hernia, in which the stomach forms the posterior wall of the hernia sac. The intrathoracic migration of stomach evolves by the so-called "organoaxial rotation" (Fig. 50–2). The lesser gastric curve is anchored within the abdomen by the posterior attachments of the lower esophagus, the left gastric artery, and the retroperitoneal fixation of the pylorus and duodenum. These three points define the long axis of the stomach, and they remain relatively fixed in the abdomen in a type II hernia. The greater curvature, however, is relatively mobile and rotates about the "long axis" by moving first anteriorly and then upward, as the hernia evolves. The fundus is the first part of the stomach to protrude upward through the anterior hernia sac. As the hiatal defect enlarges, the body and antrum continue the axial rotation and migrate into the thorax, leaving the cardia and pylorus within the abdomen. The stomach then resides "upside down" within the chest, with the greater curvature pointing cephalad and the cardia remaining below the diaphragm (Fig. 50–3). The stomach may initially occupy a retrocardiac position, but as the hernia enlarges, rotation occurs into the right chest. With huge

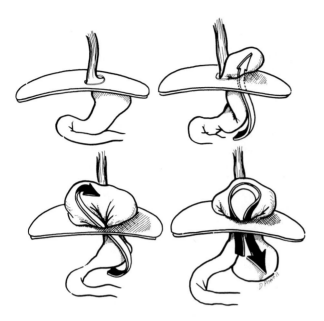

Fig. 50–2. Mechanics of incarceration and strangulation with paraesophageal hernia. Note that the fundus may prolapse back into the abdomen. *From* Postlethwait RW (ed): Surgery of the Esophagus. 2nd Ed. East Norwalk, CT: Appleton-Century-Crofts, 1986.

hernias, most of the stomach lies within the right hemithorax with the greater curvature of the stomach pointing toward the right shoulder. This rotation places an upward tension on the omentum and is why the transverse colon may also herniate into the sac. The organoaxial rotation of the stomach is most commonly

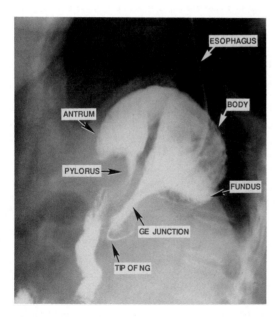

Fig. 50–3. Barium study of the stomach that demonstrates the "up-side down" appearance of the stomach within the thoracic cavity. Note the NG tube extending through the length of the esophagus with the tip at the GE junction below the hiatus. The fundus, body, and antrum are above the diaphragm.

upward into the chest and to the right. This is the path of least resistance because of the aorta to the left and the heart to the left and anteriorly. On occasion however, the stomach may rotate superiorly and not to the right, so that the greater curvature lies transversely behind the heart.

As with any true anatomic hernia, possible complications include bleeding, incarceration, volvulus, obstruction, strangulation, and perforation.

Gastritis and ulceration have been endoscopically visualized in as many as 30% of the patients who have type II hiatal hernias. Wichterman and associates (1979) suggested that these ulcers are the result of poor gastric emptying and torsion of the gastric wall, particularly after repeat incarcerations, which may impair the blood supply and lymphatic drainage. Although brisk bleeding can occur, these ulcers more frequently cause a slow, chronic blood loss with resultant anemia.

The most serious complication of the type II hernia is gastric volvulus associated with incarceration and strangulation. Hill (1968), Ozdemir (1973), and Wichterman (1979) and their colleagues reported that approximately 30% of paraesophageal hernias present with this problem. After a meal, the fundus may prolapse down from the hernia sac and back into the abdomen (see Fig. 50–2). This twists and angulates the stomach in its midportion just proximal to the antrum, resulting in partial or complete obstruction. Distention of the intrathoracic stomach and further rotation of the fundus can result in obstruction at the gastroesophageal junction. Further twisting may lead to pyloric obstruction, which results in an incarcerated gastric segment and closed-loop obstruction. If unchecked, this ultimately leads to strangulation, necrosis, and perforation. Unless this process is recognized and corrected, the resulting mediastinitis and shock are fatal.

Allen and associates (1993) had five patients who required emergency operations for suspected strangulation; three had gastric necrosis and one died. Borchardt's triad (1904) of chest pain, with retching but inability to vomit and inability to pass a nasogastric tube, indicates volvulus of the stomach and was found in three of Allen and associates' patients (1993). Twenty-three of their patients were followed without operation. Four of these patients developed progressive symptoms, and one died of aspiration.

As was mentioned earlier, a type III defect is frequently present when a type II hernia has been present for many years. The mechanism for this seems to be gradual enlargement of the hiatus so that the esophagogastric junction no longer lies within or below the hiatus. The attachment of the esophagogastric junction remains intact posteriorly. Most of these hernias are very large when the diagnosis is made. It may be that the symptoms are so mild or nonspecific when the hernia is small that the patients do not seek medical attention. It may also be that once this type of hernia begins to develop it progresses rapidly to a large size because of negative intrathoracic and positive intraabdominal pressures.

SYMPTOMS

Many type II hernias cause few or no symptoms and remain undiagnosed for years until recognized on a routine radiograph of the chest. Chronic bleeding from gastritis or ulceration of the intrathoracic gastric segment may lead to iron deficiency anemia with resultant fatigue and exertional dyspnea. Most patients, however, present with complaints of postprandial discomfort, caused by an intrathoracic gastric segment that becomes dilated by food and swallowed air. Frequently, these complaints have been present for many years. Patients usually describe sensations of substernal fullness or pressure, and this is often mistaken for angina. Often, this discomfort is accompanied by nausea and is somewhat relieved by belching or regurgitation. Most of the aforementioned authors, as well as Ellis and colleagues (1986), noted that symptoms of gastroesophageal reflux were distinctly uncommon in their patients with type II hiatal hernias. Although Pearson and associates (1983) reported that most of their patients had severe symptoms, it is probably because of the high percentage of combined — type III — hernias in their patient population. True dysphagia is also uncommon. Last, a large type III or IV hernia may occupy a portion of the thoracic cavity and result in postprandial respiratory symptoms of breathlessness with a sense of suffocation. Symptoms may be mild despite a huge hernia. Patients seem to get used to or tolerate these gas-bloat symptoms well.

When gastric volvulus and obstruction occur, patients present in extreme distress. Most such patients give a long history of complaints, such as those outlined previously, but have never sought medical advice. The chief complaints at the time of presentation are severe pain and pressure in the chest or the epigastric region. It is usually accompanied by nausea and may be misdiagnosed as a myocardial infarction. Vomiting may occur, but more frequently the patient complains of retching and an inability to regurgitate. The patient may also complain of the inability to swallow saliva. If the volvulus is allowed to progress, strangulation of the intrathoracic portion of stomach occurs, resulting in a toxic clinical picture including fever, "third spacing" of fluid, and hypovolemic shock. Acute hemorrhagic pancreatitis has also been reported in cases of gastric volvulus and is felt to be caused by distortion of the pancreatic duct with impaired drainage.

DIAGNOSIS

The diagnosis of paraesophageal hiatal hernia is usually first suspected because of an abnormal radiograph of the chest. The most frequent finding is a retrocardiac air bubble with or without an air-fluid level (Fig. 50–4). In a giant paraesophageal hernia, the sac and its contents occasionally protrude into the right thoracic cavity. The differential diagnosis includes mediastinal cyst or abscess and dilated obstructed esophagus as in end-stage achalasia. A barium study of the

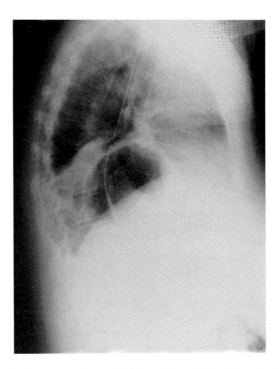

Fig. 50–4. Retrocardiac air bubble and type II hiatal hernia. Note the wedge of atelectatic lung compressed by a large hernia sac.

upper gastrointestinal tract is the diagnostic study of choice. The pathognomonic finding is an "upside down" stomach within the chest (Fig. 50–3). The radiologist must pay careful attention to the position of the cardia; this not only confirms the diagnosis of type II defect but may be important in deciding whether an antireflux procedure should be performed at the same time as an anatomic repair. A barium enema may help determine if any portion of colon is involved.

After the presence of the hernia has been established radiographically, one must determine whether it has a functional effect on the competence of the lower esophageal sphincter. This is best accomplished by endoscopy and esophageal function testing.

Although symptoms of gastroesophageal reflux are rare in patients with a pure type II hiatal hernia, they are occasionally present and may indicate pathologic peptic esophagitis. Preoperative esophageal testing may help confirm or refute this suspicion. Esophageal manometry is useful in determining the location of lower esophageal sphincter — LES — which marks the gastroesophageal junction, an area that can be difficult to locate on barium study. An LES at a supradiaphragmatic level suggests a huge paraesophageal hernia or a type III — "mixed" — paraesophageal and sliding hiatal hernia, which is more likely to have a component of reflux and esophagitis. Ambulatory 24-hour esophageal pH testing can help diagnose gastroesophageal reflux, which is best treated by a fundoplication procedure at the time of surgical correction (Chapter 122).

These test results must, however, be considered in the context of the entire clinical picture. Although

Walther and associates (1984) found pH evidence for pathologic reflux in 9 of 15 patients — 60% — in their paraesophageal hernia series, at endoscopy only 2 patients — 13% — were found to have mild — grade I — esophagitis, which was of questionable clinical significance.

Upper endoscopy can play an important role in the diagnostic workup of these patients. Reports from the literature citing endoscopic results conflict. Pearson and associates (1983) endoscoped all 51 patients with primary incarcerated giant hiatal hernias and found that 30% had grade I esophagitis and an additional 30% had grade II–IV esophagitis, but virtually all these patients had type III or combined hernias. Ellis and colleagues (1986) reported a series that included 39 patients with primary type II defects and found only 5 patients — 13% — with endoscopic evidence of mild to moderate esophagitis, an incidence identical to Walther and associates (1984).

Apparently, pure type II hiatal hernias are infrequently associated with an incompetent lower esophageal sphincter or significant gastroesophageal reflux, which probably occur more frequently in type III defects. Preoperative endoscopy and esophageal motility studies can help establish the location of gastroesophageal junction and LES with relation to the diaphragm. The combination of esophageal pH testing and endoscopy determine whether significant acid reflux exists and whether pathologic esophagitis is present. These tests should be employed before elective operation for any type II hernia patient with symptoms of acid reflux. They should also be routinely used for any patient with known or suspected type III hernia with a supradiaphragmatic LES.

THERAPY

No acceptable medical treatment regimen exists for patients with paraesophageal hiatal hernia. Patients followed expectantly are at great risk, as noted by Skinner and Belsey (1967), who found a 29% mortality in 21 patients treated medically. Because of the serious and life-threatening nature of complications in this disorder, the presence of the defect is, in itself, a surgical indication.

When a patient with a type II hernia presents with gastric volvulus and obstruction, decompression with a nasogastric tube must be promptly performed. In the absence of signs of toxicity, an operation can then be scheduled at the earliest convenience. The inability to decompress a gastric volvulus in this situation constitutes a surgical emergency and mandates immediate operative intervention, whether or not signs of toxicity exist.

Although the necessity for operation is universally recognized, controversy exists regarding what operation should be done and through what approach. The repair can be easily performed through either an abdominal or thoracic approach, and strong proponents for both exist. No matter what the approach, the operative principles for hernia repair apply: reduction of the hernia, resection of the sac, and closure of the defect.

Those who endorse the thoracic approach emphasize the ease of intrathoracic dissection of the hernia contents and sac. In type III defects, the thoracic approach allows the thorough dissection of the esophagus in cases of moderate to severe esophageal shortening; this may allow reduction of a fundoplication beneath the hiatus without the need for a lengthening procedure. The proponents of a transthoracic repair, however, usually neglect to note the increased morbidity and discomfort attendant to the thoracotomy approach. In addition, a transthoracic repair may allow the stomach to rotate organoaxially after it is pushed back into the peritoneal cavity. This then produces a volvulus of the body of the stomach in which the greater curvature adheres to the liver. We are aware of two patients in whom this occurred, and these patients required a laparotomy postoperatively to correct the volvulus; these patients were reported by Wichterman and associates, including one of us (A.E.B.) (1979).

Those who suggest an abdominal approach point out that the procedure is easily performed through the abdomen and that concomitant abdominal procedures can be undertaken simultaneously. In addition, it allows placement of a gastrostomy tube, which obviates the need for a postoperative nasogastric tube and which may also decrease the risk of recurrent volvulus. The only patient in whom this approach might prove difficult is one with a proven type III or "mixed" lesion with known reflux and a foreshortened esophagus. In this case, the thoracic approach could be a better alternative. Familiarity with the dissection of the esophagus as done with a transhiatal esophagectomy, however, allows mobilization of most of the esophagus through an enlarged diaphragmatic hiatus.

The second controversial point deals with the indications for an antireflux operation at the time the anatomic hernia is corrected. Many authors, including Pearson (1983) and Ozdemir (1973) and their associates, have written that they routinely perform an antireflux procedure on all patients regardless of the presence or absence of reflux symptoms. Hill and Tobias (1968) espoused simple anatomic repair alone and had excellent results with no recurrences and no postoperative reflux in 19 patients. Perhaps Ellis and colleagues' (1986) approach is the most enlightened — patients with type II hiatal hernia should undergo preoperative endoscopy, manometry, and pH testing, and only those patients with symptoms or objective evidence of gastroesophageal reflux should be considered for an antireflux repair, usually a Belsey mark IV operation or a loose Nissen wrap. Most patients with a pure paraesophageal hiatal hernia do not have reflux and are well served with a simple hernia reduction and diaphragmatic hiatal repair.

In a recent presentation Williamson and colleagues including Ellis, (1993), reviewed 117 patients with paraesophageal hiatal hernias. The most common presenting symptom was epigastric or substernal pain in 76% of patients. Only seventeen patients underwent antireflux procedures in addition to anatomic repair of the hernia. The antireflux procedures were done for esophagitis determined by symptoms and by esophagoscopy, with a hypotensive lower esophageal sphincter — ≤10 mmHg — or positive 24-hour pH monitoring. Postoperatively, however, 2 of their patients — 1.7% — developed severe reflux symptoms and findings, and 17 others — 14.5% — developed mild and controllable symptoms. They reported the development of a recurrent hernia in 10 of 117 operated patients with good to excellent results in 86% of patients. Allen and associates (1993) in their review reported that 111 — 93.3% — patients had a transthoracic repair with the addition of an uncut Collis-Nissen fundoplication, a Belsey mark IV fundoplication, or a Nissen fundoplication. Eight patients — 6.7% — had an abdominal repair with antireflux procedure. Thus, they routinely performed an antireflux procedure in spite of the fact that only 15% of their patients had esophagitis. The results were similar with all types of repair.

OPERATIVE TECHNIQUE

We prefer and recommend the abdominal approach through an upper midline incision. The left lobe of the liver is mobilized and retracted to the right. The contents of the hernia sac are reduced back into the peritoneal cavity by gentle traction. If resistance is encountered while the hernia contents are being reduced, a small rubber catheter inserted in the hernia sac allows entry of air as downward tension is placed on the contents of the sac. This decreases the suction effect that holds the viscera within the chest. Occasionally in cases of a tight incarceration, the hiatal ring itself may have to be incised to allow return of the organs to the abdominal cavity. This can be done safely on the left side of the crus posteriorly along the side of the aorta.

The hernia sac is dissected free from the thoracic cavity and resected. Once this has been accomplished, the dead space in the mediastinum disappears as the lungs expand. No drainage of this space is necessary. The large diaphragmatic defect is located anterior to the lower esophagus, which usually remains bound to the posterior aspect of the hiatus by fibrous attachments. Care is taken during an ensuing dissection not to damage these posterior attachments, which hold the lower esophagus and its sphincter in an intra-abdominal position. The crural defect is closed beginning anteriorly with a stout 0 interrupted nonabsorbable suture. The closure is continued in a posterior direction until the hiatus just admits the tip of the forefinger beside the esophagus.

If the patient has objective evidence of significant reflux esophagitis preoperatively, an antireflux procedure is now performed. If the posterior attachments of

the lower esophagus are taken down during dissection, then it is likely that the LES has been disturbed and will be incompetent. In these patients we also perform an antireflux procedure at this time, and our procedure of choice is a loose Nissen fundoplication. If there is doubt about whether the esophagogastric junction is below the hiatus, it is best to mobilize the junction and the lower esophagus. Sufficient mobilization allows the junction to be brought 4 to 5 cm below the hiatus. The hiatus can then be narrowed or repaired by approximating the crura, beginning posteriorly over the aorta and behind the esophagus. This displaces the esophagus anteriorly into its normal position as it passes through the hiatus.

The stomach is now fixed within the peritoneal cavity by using two methods. The first is a modified Hill suture plication in which three interrupted nonabsorbable sutures are placed between the lesser curvature of the stomach and the preaortic fascia (Fig. 50–5). These sutures hold the gastroesophageal junction within the abdominal cavity and prevent the development of a type I — sliding — hernia postoperatively. If the esophagus has been mobilized during the repair, then these sutures can be attached to the crural repair posteriorly. The second maneuver is the performance of a Stamm gastrostomy, which serves two functions. First, it removes the need for a nasogastric tube placement. Many patients with incarcerated type II hernias have a prolonged period of postoperative gastric stasis, and a gastrostomy allows continued drainage without the discomfort or complications of an indwelling nasogastric catheter. Second, the gastrostomy fixes the stomach to

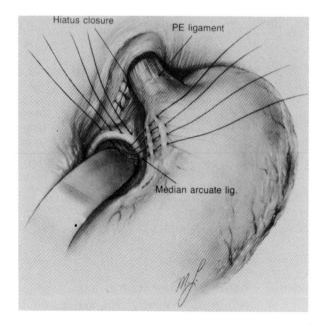

Fig. 50–5. Hill suture plication after reduction of the paraesophageal hernia and repair of the hiatal defect to maintain the position of the gastroesophageal junction within the abdominal cavity. *From* Postlethwait RW (ed): Surgery of the Esophagus. 2nd Ed. East Norwalk, CT: Appleton-Century-Crofts, 1986, p 245.

the anterior wall, thus maintaining its position within the abdominal cavity and preventing an intra-abdominal gastric volvulus, a reported complication of transthoracic repairs. The gastrostomy tube can be removed 8 to 12 days after the operation.

If gangrene or perforation is found at the time of operation, all devascularized tissue must be resected and all infected tissue debrided. Broad-spectrum antibiotics that include anaerobic coverage are strongly advised in this setting because of the possibility of perforation and mediastinal contamination by salivary leakage.

Recently, a few of these paraesophageal hernias have been repaired transabdominally by laparoscopic techniques. Laparoscopic repair of type I hernias has been reported by Cuschieri (1992) from Scotland and is being frequently performed by Dallemagne in Belgium (personal communication). Probably as a result of its relative rarity, laparoscopic paraesophageal hernia repair has been reported only once, by Congreve (1992). This report is anecdotal and includes only information about operative technique and postoperative hospitalization. No data regarding rate of reflux or recurrence are provided. Our own early experience with laparoscopic repair in two patients was frustrating. In one, the repair was not possible, and an open repair was required. The second patient underwent reduction of the hernia and crural closure via laparoscopy combined with placement of a percutaneous endoscopic gastrostomy. Follow-up study after discharge revealed early recurrence with 1 cm of the gastric fundus above the hiatus. The patient fortunately remains free from reflux and from her preoperative symptomatology. As instrumentation improves and experience grows, it is likely to be only a matter of time before repair via the laparoscopic approach becomes routine.

MORBIDITY AND MORTALITY

Elective surgical repair of paraesophageal hernias is safe. A collective review of 300 such patients (Table 50–1) reveals that the operative mortality was less than 1%, a figure similar to that quoted for repair of sliding hiatal hernias. Emergency procedures in cases of gastric volvulus, however, carry a much higher mortality, approximately 14% (Table 50–1). This marked increase in operative risk underscores the need for elective repair at the time of initial diagnosis.

Operative complications are the same as for antireflux procedures, with two additions. In patients with gastric volvulus and obstruction, pulmonary complications apparently increase, probably because of episodes of regurgitation and aspiration. Also, prolonged gastric stasis may persist for a period of 7 to 10 days after operative repair because of lingering inflammation and edema in the released gastric segment.

RESULTS

Long-term results are generally excellent, regardless of whether or not an antireflux procedure is done in

Table 50–1. Operative Mortality for Paraesophageal Hernia Repair

Author	Elective (%)	Emergency (%)
Beardsley & Thompson (1964)	—	3/10 (30)
Sanderud (1967)	0/14 (0)	1/7 (14)
Hill & Tobias (1968)	0/19 (0)	2/10 (20)
Ozdemir et al. (1973)	0/19 (0)	2/12 (16)
Wichterman et al. (1979)	0/16 (0)	1/6 (16)
Carter et al. (1980)	—	1/14 (7)
Pearson et al. (1983)	0/47 (0)	1/4 (25)
Walther et al. (1984)	0/15 (0)	—
Ellis (1986)	1/39 (2)	—
Landreneau et al. (1992)	0/12 (0)	0/5 (0)
Allen et al. (1993)	0/119 (0)	1/5 (20)
Total	1/300 (0.3)	12/83 (14)

Operative mortality reported as number of deaths divided by number of operated patients. Emergency defined as gastric volvulus.

addition to simple repair. Hill and Tobias (1968) performed simple repair and had no recurrence or reflux in 22 patients over a 15-year follow-up. Wichterman and colleagues (1979), who routinely performed concomitant antireflux procedures, noted identical results. Recurrent type I hernias with reflux, however, have been reported by Ozdemir (1973) — 10%, Pearson (1983) — 8%, and their colleagues and Sanderud (1967) — 8% — despite fundoplication at the time of initial repair. Simultaneous fundoplication is therefore apparently ineffective prophylaxis against recurrent herniation with resultant reflux. Fundoplication could be more appropriately used selectively in those patients with documented reflux.

Allen and colleagues (1993) report excellent results in 60% of their patients, good in 33%, fair in 5.2%, and poor in two patients — 1.7%. In Williamson and associates' (1993) report, the results were considered excellent in 53.9%, good in 29.5%, fair in 4.3%, and poor in 12.1%. The poor results in this series were mainly due to symptomatic recurrence of the paraesophageal hernia in 10% and the infrequent development of severe gastroesophageal reflux in 2% of the patients who did not have a concomitant antireflux procedure done at the time of repair.

REFERENCES

Allen MS, Trastek VF, Deschamp C, Pairolero PC: Intrathoracic stomach: presentation and results of operation. Ann Thorac Surg (in press) 1993.

Beardsley JM, Thompson WR: Acutely obstructed hiatal hernia. Ann Surg 159:49, 1964.

Borchardt M: Zur Pathogie und Therapie des Magen Volvulus. Arch Klin Chir 74:243, 1904.

Bowditch HI: Peculiar case of diaphragmatic hernia. Buffalo Med J Month Rev 9:1, 1853.

Carter R, Brewer LA, Hinshaw DB: Acute gastric volvulus: a study of 25 cases. Am J Surg 140:99, 1980.

Congreve DP: Laparoscopic paraesophageal hernia repair. J Laparoendosc Surg 2:45, 1992.

Cuschieri A, Shim S, Nathanson LK: Laparoscopic reduction, crural repair and fundoplication of large hiatal hernia. Am J Surg 163:425, 1992.

Ellis FH, Crozier RE, Shea JA: Paraesophageal hiatus hernia. Arch Surg *121*:416, 1986.

Hiebert CA, Belsey R: Incompetency of the gastric cardia without radiologic evidence of hiatal hernia. J Thorac Cardiovasc Surg *42*:352, 1961.

Hill LD, Tobias JA: Paraesophageal hernia. Arch Surg *96*:735, 1968.

Landreneau RJ, et al: Clinical spectrum of paraesophageal herniation. Dig Dis Sci *37*:537, 1992.

Naunheim KS, Baue AE: Paraesophageal hiatal hernia. *In* Baue AE (ed): Glenns Thoracic and Cardiovascular Surgery. Norwalk, CT: Appleton-Century-Crofts, 1990.

Ozdemir IA, Burke WA, Ikins PM: Paraesophageal hernia: a life-threatening disease. Ann Thorac Surg *16*:547, 1973.

Pearson FG, et al: Massive hiatal hernia with incarceration: a report of 53 cases. Ann Thorac Surg *35*:45, 1983.

Potempski P: Nuovo processo operativo per lar riduzione cruenta della ernie diaframmatiche de trauma e per la sutura delle ferite del diaframma. Bul Reale Accad Med Roma *15*:191, 1889.

Sanderud A: Surgical treatment for the complications of hiatal hernia. Acta Chir Scand *133*:223, 1967.

Skinner DB, Belsey RHR: Surgical management of esophageal reflux and hiatus hernia: long-term results with 1030 patients. J Thorac Cardiovasc Surg *53*:33, 1967.

Walther B, et al: Effect of paraesophageal hernia on sphincter function and its implication on surgical therapy. Am J Surg *147*:111, 1984.

Wichterman K, Geha AS, Cahow CE, Baue AE: Giant paraesophageal hiatal hernia with intra-thoracic stomach and colon: the case for early repair. Surgery *86*:497, 1979.

Williamson WA, Ellis FH Jr, Shahian DM, Streitz JM Jr: Paraesophageal hiatal hernia: is an anti-reflux procedure necessary? Ann Thorac Surg (in press), 1993.

CHAPTER 51

TUMORS OF THE DIAPHRAGM

Thomas W. Shields

INCIDENCE

Primary tumors of the diaphragm are rare. Two major reviews were published by Wiener and Chou (1965) and Olafsson and associates (1971). Most of the tumors are of mesenchymal origin, as one would expect because almost all of the diaphragmatic structure is derived from mesenchymal cells (Table 51–1). Tumors of neural origin do occur, however. McClenathan and Okada (1989), in a review of 13 neural tumors of the diaphragm that had been reported in the literature including one of their own, suggested that these tumors comprise approximately 10% of all primary diaphragmatic tumors. Only 23% of the neural tumors were malignant, whereas when cystic lesions are excluded from the benign tumors, the incidence of malignant mesenchymal tumors is greater than that of the benign mesenchymal tumors.

Table 51–1. Primary Tumors of the Diaphragm

Benign	Malignant
Mesothelial Origin	
Angiofibroma	Chondrosarcoma
	Fibroangioendothelioma
Chondroma	Fibromyosarcoma
	Fibrosarcoma
Fibroma	Hemangioendothelioma
Fibrolymphangioma	Hemangiopericytoma
Fibromyoma	Leiomyosarcoma
Hamartoma	Mesothelioma
Lymphangioma	Myosarcoma
Leiomyoma	Rhabdomyosarcoma
Lipoma	Sarcoma, various cell types
Rhabdomyofibroma	Synovioma
Neurogenic Origin	
Neurilemoma	Neurogenic sarcoma
Neurofibroma	(Neurofibrosarcoma)
Others	
Adenoma	
Cysts	

SYMPTOMATOLOGY

Most diaphragmatic tumors are discovered in adult patients in the fifth to seventh decades of life. No specific sex predilection is noticed. Most benign tumors are asymptomatic, and their presence is suggested only on routine radiographs of the chest. The clinical manifestations of symptomatic diaphragmatic tumors — a few benign and most malignant — are not specific. In general, the patient complains of pain with breathing, although the first evidence of any problem may be a nondescript feeling of fullness in the subcostal area. Cough may also be noted in some patients, as may dyspnea.

Trivedi (1958), Wiener and Chou (1965), as well as McClenathan and Okada (1989) noted that half of the reported neurogenic tumors of the diaphragm were associated with hypertrophic pulmonary osteoarthropathy or clubbing of the fingers, or both. These are rare findings with other diaphragmatic tumors. Wiener and Chou (1965) reported only one patient with clubbing of the fingers in 63 non-neural tumors of the diaphragm.

DIAGNOSIS

The standard radiographic examinations are generally insufficient for positive identification of a diaphragmatic tumor. Computed tomography may be of value in identifying the tumor as originating from the diaphragm. Special studies, such as pneumoperitoneum (Fig. 51–1) and arteriography (Fig. 51–2) have also been used to identify such tumors. Pneumoperitoneum is useful, especially in differentiating diaphragmatic tumors located on the right from tumors of the liver. A liver-spleen scan may also be helpful.

TREATMENT

Surgical removal, when possible, is indicated for all tumors of the diaphragm. In the excision of primary diaphragmatic tumors, the pleural and peritoneal lay-

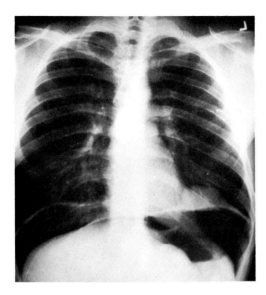

Fig. 51–1. The diagnosis of a diaphragmatic tumor was easily confirmed by a pneumoperitoneum. This tumor was excised and found to be a fibrosarcoma.

ers are excised en bloc along with that portion of the diaphragmatic leaf containing the tumor. Attempts to save the integrity of the peritoneum, as suggested by Butchart (1989) in the resection of a diffuse mesothelioma to avoid spillage of tumor cells into the peritoneum or the placement of a foreign body into a postpneumonectomy space, do not appear to be germane in the

removal of primary tumors. Small defects may be closed primarily. If the tumor is located in the periphery of the diaphragm, the adjacent portion of the diaphragm and part of the chest wall may be removed in continuity. In certain selected instances, enough normal diaphragmatic tissue may be left after the tumor has been removed to permit advancement of the remaining segment up the chest wall for reattachment to the rib cage. In general, with an aggressive approach and with removal of as wide a margin of normal tissue as possible, insufficient tissue for closure will remain. In such cases the defect may be closed with a prosthetic soft tissue patch of Gore-tex or other suitable material — Dacron-Silastic sheeting, preserved dura matter, or Marlex mesh reinforced with woven Dacron. Interrupted sutures are used to secure the prosthetic material to the cut edges of the diaphragm or to the chest wall as necessary. Postoperative radiation therapy may be indicated, depending on the histologic type of the tumor.

The morbidity and mortality rates after excision of diaphragmatic tumors are minimal. Ventilatory loss on the side of the resection is noted, but the magnitude of such losses has not been documented.

PROGNOSIS

The prognosis after resection of benign tumors, as would be expected, is excellent. However, after excision of most, if not all, of the malignant lesions, the prognosis is poor. Recurrence of a malignant lesion is common, and death is the usual result.

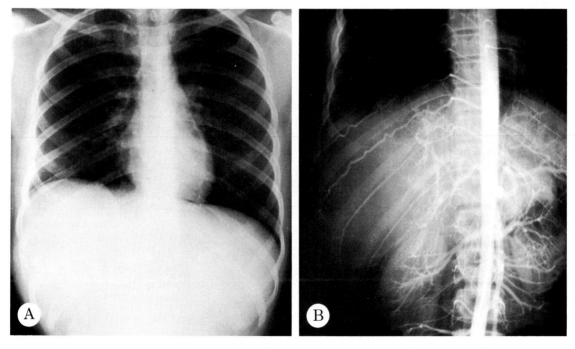

Fig. 51–2. *A,* PA radiograph of the chest revealing an elevated hemidiaphragm. Suggestion of the presence of a mass occupying the lateral three fourths of the right diaphragmatic leaf is noted. *B,* Aortogram of the same patient demonstrates displacement of the normal vascular structures in the liver by a large neurofibroma of the diaphragm. Hypertrophy of the intercostal vessels is visualized clearly on this aortogram.

REFERENCES

Butchart EG: Surgery of mesothelioma of the pleura. *In* Roth JA, Ruckdeschel JC, Weisenburger TH (eds): Thoracic Oncology. Philadelphia: WB Saunders, 1989, p 566.

McClenathan JH, Okada F: Primary neurilemoma of the diaphragm. Ann Thorac Surg *48*:126, 1989.

Olafsson G, Rausing A, Holen O: Primary tumors of the diaphragm. Chest *59*:568, 1971.

Trivedi SA: Neurilemmoma of the diaphragm causing severe hypertrophic pulmonary osteoarthropathy. Br J Tuberc *52*:214, 1958.

Wiener MF, Chou WH: Primary tumors of the diaphragm. Arch Surg *90*:143, 1965.

READING REFERENCES

Clagett OT, Johnson MA III: Tumors of the diaphragm. Am J Surg *78*:526, 1949.

Doyle T: Left basal opacity for diagnosis. Chest *84*:199, 1983.

Sbokes CG, et al: Fibrosarcoma of the diaphragm. Br J Dis Chest *71*:99, 1977.

Sarot IA, Schwimmer D, Schecter DC: Primary neurilemoma of the diaphragm. NY State Med J *69*:837, 1969.

SECTION XI
The Pleura

CHAPTER 52

THE REABSORPTION OF GASES FROM THE PLEURAL SPACE

Yvon Cormier

Under normal circumstances, there are no free gases in the pleural space. A variety of conditions, however, can lead to the accumulation of gases in this cavity. Because the virtual space between the parietal and visceral pleura is under negative pressure, any communication with the surrounding structures — bronchi, alveoli, extrathoracic communication through the chest wall — will immediately cause gases to enter the pleural space, i.e., produce a pneumothorax. The pressure in the pleural space is negative in relation to the atmosphere because of the elastic properties of the lungs, which tend to collapse, and that of the chest wall which, at volumes below 75% of the total lung capacity, tends to expand. In normal individuals, at functional residual capacity when respiratory muscles of the thoracic wall are in the relaxed state, this pressure is about 5 cm/H_2O lower than that of the surrounding atmosphere. This pressure further decreases during inspiration, especially in the presence of airway obstruction. During a Müller maneuver — maximal inspiratory efforts against a closed glottis — pleural pressure can transiently become very negative — lower than 100 cm/H_2O).

When gases enter the pleural space, pressure gradients and the physical laws of gases will favor their eventual reabsorption.

FACTORS DETERMINING GAS REABSORPTION

Gas reabsorption from the pleural space is achieved by a simple diffusion from the pleural space into the venous blood. This diffusion, which can occur in both directions, is possible because the pleura and capillary walls are permeable to gases and because the partial pressures of gases in the pleural space and those in the venous blood can differ. For example, a positive pressure gradient between the gases in the pneumothorax

and those dissolved in the venous blood would favor the passage of those gases from the pneumothorax into the venous blood. There are no active transport mechanisms for gas reabsorption; the only driving forces that determine gas reabsorption are pressure gradients.

The rate of gas reabsorption depends on four variables: 1) diffusion properties of the gases present in the pleural space; 2) the pressure gradients for the gases in the pleural space in relation to the venous blood; 3) the area of contact between the pleural gas and the pleura; and 4) permeability of the pleural surface — e.g., a thickened fibrotic pleura will absorb less than a normal pleura.

Because the solubility and diffusion properties of different gases vary considerably, the speed of reabsorption will depend on the type of gas involved. For example, oxygen — O_2 — will be reabsorbed 62 times faster than nitrogen — N_2. Water vapor — H_2O — and carbon dioxide — CO_2 — will equilibrate almost instantaneously, CO_2 being 23 times more soluble than O_2.

Depending on the clinical situation, a pneumothorax can initially contain room air — i.e., a leak from the outside — or alveolar air — a leak through the lungs. The alveolar air contains different proportions of CO_2, O_2, or N_2 depending on the ventilation of the patient and the presence of supplemental O_2 given to the patient at the time of the leak into the pleural space. If a patient is receiving 100% O_2, the pleural gases will be composed mostly of this gas and contain no N_2, the slowest gas to be reabsorbed. Initial gas compositions in a pneumothorax when the air entry is room air or alveolar air with the patient breathing room air or 100% O_2 are presented in Figure 52–1.

Partial Pressure Of Gases In Venous Blood

Because pressure gradients that will favor gas reabsorption are those between the pneumothorax and

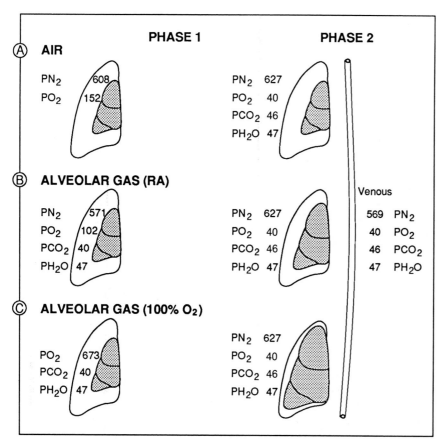

Fig. 52–1. Gas partial pressures initially present in a pneumothorax when air entry was from room air; alveoli, subject breathing room air; and alveoli, subject breathing 100% O_2. After equilibration — phase 1 — the resulting gas partial pressures become identical regardless of the initial gas composition. Note that the volume change of the pneumothorax during phase 1 is least when the pneumothorax was initially constituted with room air; intermediate when with alveolar air, patient breathing room air; and much greater when the patient was breathing 100% O_2.

those in the venous blood, it is also important to consider the venous blood partial gas pressures. Under normal circumstances the total gas pressure in a pneumothorax is within a few millimeters of mercury of that of the atmosphere — 760 mmHg — while that in the venous blood is 702 mmHg, 58 mmHg lower. This positive pressure gradient between the pneumothorax and the venous blood constitutes the driving force responsible for gas reabsorption from a pneumothorax.

Mechanisms Of The Gas Pressure Gradients Between The Pneumothorax And The Venous Blood

A schematic approach will be used here to explain the gas composition in venous blood. Dry room air contains, for all practical purposes, 80% N_2 and 20% O_2. Other gases — CO_2, argon, etc. — are of minute quantities. The normal atmospheric pressure is 760 mmHg — 1031 cm H_2O; therefore the partial pressure of N_2 in dry room air is 608 mmHg, while that of O_2 is 152 mmHg. When room air enters the alveoli, it gains H_2O vapor and CO_2 and loses O_2; the resulting gas composition is now N_2 = 571 mmHg, O_2 = 102 mmHg, H_2O = 47 mmHg, and CO_2 = 40 mmHg. The alveoli being in close communication with the atmosphere, the total gas pressure at this level must equal 760 mmHg. This alveolar gas composition is in contact with the blood at the alveolar capillary level, and gas exchange occurs. The resulting normal arterial gas composition is Pa_{O_2} = 97 mmHg, Pa_{CO_2} = 40

mmHg, and Pa_{N_2} = 569 mmHg, water vapor remains constant at 47 mmHg; the total arterial gas pressure is 753 mmHg. Note that there is a 7-mmHg pressure gradient between the alveolar gas pressure and that of the arterial blood. Our cells consume O_2 and produce CO_2, consuming 300 ml of O_2 for 240 ml of CO_2 produced — a respiratory quotient of 0.8. Despite this small difference between the quantity of O_2 consumed compared to that of CO_2 produced, the metabolic changes will increase the partial pressure of CO_2 by 6 mmHg and decrease that of oxygen by 57 mmHg in its passage through the capillaries from the arterial to the venous system. This large difference in the changes in O_2 and CO_2 partial pressures is due to the difference in the solubility and transport capacity of our blood for these two gases. N_2 is not metabolized and therefore remains unchanged between the arterial and venous blood. Water vapor also remains constant at 47 mmHg. The resulting venous gas pressure is therefore Pv_{O_2} = 40 mmHg, Pv_{CO_2} = 46 mmHg, Pv_{N_2} = 569 mmHg, Pv_{H_2O} = 47 mmHg, for a total gas pressure of 702 mmHg, i.e., 51 mmHg less than that in the arterial blood and 58 mmHg less than that of alveolar or room air total gas pressures. A schematic summary of gas pressures from room air to the venous blood is given in Figure 52–2. A pneumothorax results because of a communication between the pleural cavity and the atmosphere, either via the thoracic wall or the lung. Because of this communica-

Total gas pressure

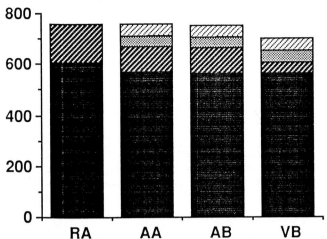

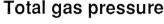

Fig. 52–2. The total and partial gas pressures in room air — RA, alveolar air — AR, arterial blood — AB, and in venous blood — VB. The total pressure for RA and AR is the same, while a small total pressure drop occurs between AR and AB — 7 mmHg — and a further more significant drop is seen between AB and VB — 51 mmHg. The difference between RA and VB therefore equals 58 mmHg.

tion, the initial gas pressure in a pneumothorax will equal that of the atmosphere at 760 mmHg, thus creating a 58-mmHg gradient between the two.

PHASES OF GAS REABSORPTION

There are two phases in the gas reabsorption from the pleural space: phase 1, equilibration of gases partial pressures, and phase 2, constant reabsorption.

Phase 1: Equilibration

The first phase represents the equilibration of gases initially placed into the pleural cavity with that of venous blood. Its duration and the amount of gas reabsorbed during this phase will depend on the composition of the initial gases in the pneumothorax. The second phase is the constant reabsorption rate that follows once the equilibration has occurred.

Regardless of the quality of gases initially in the pneumothorax, the first phase will result in an equilibrating period, after which the composition of the remaining gases in the pneumothorax will all be similar in all situations. It follows, therefore, that gases can enter or leave the pleural cavity as this equilibration takes place. If the initial pneumothorax contained 100% O_2, the N_2 partial pressure will be greater in the venous blood than in the pleural cavity; in this condition the N_2 gradient will favor N_2 to leave the venous blood and enter the pleural space. However, because O_2 is more soluble, more O_2 will leave the pleural cavity than N_2 will enter. Therefore, the total quantity of gases in the pleural cavity will decrease, despite ingoing N_2. If one filled a pleural cavity with 100% N_2, the initial phase of equilibration would produce an increase in the quantity of gases in the pneumothorax because more O_2 and CO_2 would enter the cavity than N_2 would leave. The gas composition at equilibration will be determined by the partial pressures of gases in the venous blood. At this time, the gas composition in the remaining pneumothorax will be the same, regardless of the

composition of the initial gas. The following can be different: the volume reabsorbed during the equilibrating phase (see Fig. 52–1), the greater the quantity of the more soluble gases and the greater the gradient between the pleural space and the venous blood, the faster the reabsorption. The high solubility and reabsorption rate of CO_2 is the reason this gas is infused into the abdominal cavity for laparoscopy.

If a patient receives supplemental O_2 for more than 2 or 3 minutes, the pN_2 in the alveoli and in the blood will decrease proportionally. For example, if a subject received 50% O_2, the partial pressure of N_2 would decrease in the alveolar air, and subsequently in the venous blood, from 569 to about 350 mmHg. Because the Pv_{O_2} does not increase significantly with an increase of inspired O_2, the pressure gradient between a pneumothorax would be greatly increased in such a situation — from 58 mmHg to 277 mmHg in this case.

Phase 2: Constant Reabsorption

If all gases in the pleural space were at equilibrium with the venous gas pressure, the intrapleural total gas pressure would be $O_2 + CO_2 + H_2O + N_2 = 702$ mmHg, or 58 mmHg less than atmosphere. Such a negative pleural pressure — −58 mmHg — is impossible on a long-term basis.

CLINICAL SITUATIONS OF PNEUMOTHORACES

Three potential situations of pneumothoraces will result in different behavior of gas reabsorption from the pleural cavity. The pneumothorax can behave as 1) a closed rigid cavity, 2) a closed collapsible cavity, and 3) an open cavity. Clinical conditions and mechanisms of gas reabsorption under these three conditions will be discussed separately.

Closed Rigid Cavity

In theory, a closed rigid pneumothorax — non-re-expandable lung — could remain air filled. As gases are reabsorbed along each gas partial pressure as previously described, the pressure inside the pleural space would progressively decrease until it stabilizes at a pressure of 58 mmHg lower than the atmosphere. At this negative pressure, no pressure gradient remains to ensure continued reabsorption. Although such a negative pleural pressure is possible on a short-term basis, if this negative pressure is maintained, fluid will eventually seep into the pleural cavity and gradually fill it with liquid, which will subsequently solidify and fibrose. Permanent residual pneumothorax equals a persistent opening as, for example, a bronchopleural fistula.

Closed Collapsible Cavity

This situation is by far the most frequent form of pneumothorax. This condition occurs when gases enter the pleural space, the opening responsible for the pneumothorax becomes occluded, and the lungs are freely re-expandable. As gases are reabsorbed, no new gases enter the pleural space, and the re-expansion of the lungs will compensate for the volume of reabsorbed gases, therefore preventing the appearance of negative intrapleural pressure. All gases will eventually be resorbed, and the lungs will take their normal place, leaving no physical pleural cavity.

As the intrapleural gas pressure tends to decrease as a result of gas reabsorption, the lung will re-expand, and the amount of air in the pleural cavity will progressively decrease until it is all reabsorbed. At the so-called equilibrium, therefore, O_2, CO_2, and H_2O partial pressures are similar in the venous blood and in the pleural cavity. The slower N_2, however, is 58 mmHg higher in the pleural cavity — which is at or very close to atmospheric pressure — than that in the venous blood, which is 58 mmHg subatmospheric. The decreasing volume of the pneumothorax will prevent large intrapleural negative pressures and ensure the persistence of this positive partial pressure gradient between gases in the pleural cavity and the venous blood. The intrapleural pressure will not be allowed to decrease to -58 mmHg as in a closed rigid cavity, where such a gradient would no longer exist and all gas reabsorption would cease. The time required to absorb all gases in a pneumothorax is quite variable and depends on previously described characteristics. It has been estimated that 6% of a pneumothorax is absorbed in 24 hours.

Open Cavity

As long as the communication between the pleural cavity and the lung or through the thoracic wall persists, the lung will not re-expand as all absorbed gases will be replenished from the outside. In this condition, gases in the pleural space will be reabsorbed as for the closed cavity; however, the gases reabsorbed will be determined by what is returned into the pleural cavity. Because the composition of pleural gases will remain constant, what comes in is what will be reabsorbed. For example, if the pleural cavity is opened to the outside,

O_2 and N_2 will be reabsorbed at a proportion of 20:80, corresponding to the gas composition of dry room air.

EFFECTS OF BAROMETRIC PRESSURE ON PLEURAL GASES

People living at different altitudes live in different barometric pressures; for example, the barometric pressure at 11,000 feet above sea level is 500 mmHg compared to 760 mmHg at sea level. However, the gas fractions in the atmosphere always remain the same, regardless of the altitude. For an atmospheric pressure of 500 mmHg, the pN_2 in the atmosphere would be 400 mmHg and the pO_2 100 mmHg — dry air. Changes in these gas pressures from room air to the venous blood would follow the same principle as when the atmospheric pressure is 760 mmHg. At 11,000 feet, the arterial pressure of O_2 would be approximately 60 mmHg and that of venous blood not significantly different from that at sea level — 40 mmHg, giving an arterial to venous oxygen pressure drop of only 20 mmHg compared to 51 mmHg at sea level. Because the O_2 drop between arterial and venous blood is the major cause of the lower total gas pressure in the venous blood and the eventual N_2 gradient between the venous blood and gases in a pneumothorax at equilibrium, this N_2 gradient would therefore be much smaller at this high altitude. Such differences in pressure gradients would decrease the rate of N_2 reabsorption.

Although the proportions of different gases do not change with changing barometric pressures, the volume occupied by a given quantity of gases does. For example, a pneumothorax of 1-liter volume would increase by 33% if the patient was transported in an airplane pressurized at 8000 feet — which is common practice. If a pneumothorax developed in a deep sea diver at 30 feet below the surface, the volume of the pneumothorax would double as the diver resurfaces, and this when no new gases enter the pleural space.

THERAPEUTIC CONSIDERATIONS

The dynamics of gas reabsorption from the pleural space can be used clinically. A potential application is to give 100% O_2 to a patient during a maneuver that is at risk of creating a pneumothorax. A typical example for which this is useful is transthoracic lung biopsy. When 100% O_2 is given during the procedure, any resulting pneumothorax will reabsorb much faster for two reasons: 1) The pneumothorax will be filled with the more soluble O_2; and 2) the pressure gradient between the pneumothorax and the venous blood will be larger, because giving 100% O_2 will wash out N_2 from the alveoli and eventually the venous blood. Giving 100% O_2 to a patient when the pneumothorax is already in place will also increase the rate of gas reabsorption by decreasing Pv_{N_2} and therefore increase the pressure gradient for this gas between the pneumothorax and the venous blood. This beneficial effect, however, will be relatively small and probably not clinically useful.

READING REFERENCES

Cormier Y, Laviolette M, Tardif A: Prevention of pneumothorax in needle lung biopsy by breathing 100% oxygen. Thorax 35:37, 1980.

Dale WA, Rahn H: Rate of gas absorption during atelectasis. Am J Physiol *170*:606, 1952.

Kircher LT, Swartzel RL: Spontaneous pneumothorax and its treatment. JAMA *155*:24, 1954.

Loring SH, Butler JP: Gas exchange in body cavities. *In* Fishman AP, Farhi LE, Tenney MR (eds): Handbook of Physiology, Section 3, The Respiratory System. Washington, DC: American Physiological Society, 1987, p 238.

Piiper J: Physiological equilibria of gas cavities in the body. *In* Fenn NO, Rahn H (eds): Handbook of Physiology. Vol 2, Respiration. Washington, DC: American Physiological Society, 1965, p 1205.

CHAPTER 53

PNEUMOTHORAX

Willard A. Fry and Kerry Paape

Pneumothorax or air in the chest is a phenomenon that has been appreciated since ancient time and has been well discussed by Seremetis (1970), Lindskog and Halas (1957), Killen and Gobbel (1968), Gobbel and associates (1963), and Kittle (1986). Hippocrates and Galen were aware of disease processes involving the pleural space. Adams (1960) notes that Vesalius, in the sixteenth century, was aware of the necessity for positive pressure inflation of the trachea to keep the lungs expanded once the pressure seal of the pleural space had been broken. It was not until the nineteenth century, however, that physicians began to appreciate the various subtleties of disease in the pleural space. The development of the stethoscope by Laennec and the development of radiology by Roentgen brought great advances in the diagnosis of intrathoracic disease, and by 1898, John B. Murphy, in Chicago, stimulated by his European colleagues, wrote about the use of artificial pneumothorax in the treatment of pulmonary tuberculosis. The designation of tuberculosis as the primary etiologic agent for spontaneous pneumothorax was finally put to rest by Kjaergaard in 1932.

The thoracic surgeon is called to treat pneumothorax on a regular basis, and the most common presentations are primary spontaneous and secondary after medical procedures. In some areas, pneumothorax associated with *Pneumocystis carinii* pneumonia is unusually common. Much controversy continues over the best method to treat pneumothorax. In this chapter, we describe the means that we find the most practical and useful and try to list alternatives that we consider appropriate.

ETIOLOGY

The most common cause of primary spontaneous pneumothorax is the rupture of an apical subpleural bleb (Fig. 53–1). The etiology of such blebs is obscure. Some authors have postulated a difference in alveolar pressure in the upright human between the base and the apex

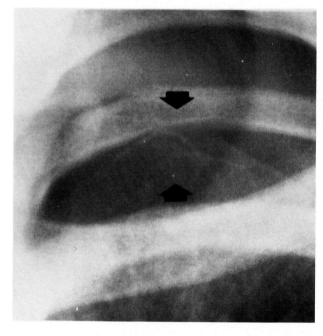

Fig. 53–1. Apical subpleural blebs in a male adolescent with a recurrent spontaneous pneumothorax.

of the lung. In the absence of an associated disorder, spontaneous pneumothorax is rarely seen before puberty. It is more common in men than in women by a factor of six to one, and it is more common in smokers than in nonsmokers, as described by Lindskog (1957) and Bense and associates (1987). The typical patient with a spontaneous pneumothorax is a young, thin man in late adolescence or early adulthood who experiences the sudden onset of chest pain and shortness of breath and who has not been engaging in any unusual or strenuous activity. This clinical picture is in contrast to that of the rarer condition of spontaneous pneumomediastinum, which is invariably associated with strenuous exertion, such as bench-press weight lifting.

The various causes of pneumothorax are listed in Table 53–1. Special mention must be made of secondary spontaneous pneumothorax associated with acquired immune deficiency syndrome — AIDS, because it is prevalent in certain centers, as described by Beers and colleagues (1990), and the question of its precipitation by Pentamidine aerosol has been raised by Sepkowitz (1991), Coker (1993), Shanley (1991), and Renzi (1992), and their associates. The most common sarcomas contributing to pneumothorax are osteosarcoma and synovial sarcomas, as described by Dines and co-workers in 1973. Special mention is made of spontaneous rupture of the esophagus, for if it presents as pneumothorax without gastrointestinal symptoms and the diagnosis is not suspected, an unfavorable outcome is virtually assured. The physician should be alerted by the nature of the accompanying pleural fluid. In the instances of pneumothorax associated with asthma and mucous plugs, the postulated mechanism is obstructive atelectasis of one lobe or segment with hyperinflation of other portions of the lung with resultant parenchymal disruption (Fig. 53–2).

Spontaneous pneumothorax occurring in patients with established chronic obstructive pulmonary disease

Table 53–1. Classification of Pneumothorax

Spontaneous
    Primary
        Subpleural bleb rupture
    Secondary
        Bullous disease — incuding COPD
        Cystic fibrosis
        Spontaneous rupture of the esophagus
        Marfan's syndrome
        Eosinophilic granuloma
        Pneumocystis carinii — especially in AIDS patients
        Metastatic cancer — especially sarcoma
        Pneumonia with lung abscess
        Catamenial
        Asthma — secondary to mucous plugging
        Lung cancer
        Lymphangioleiomyomatosis
    Neonatal

Acquired
    Iatrogenic
        Subclavian — percutaneous — catheterization
            Central lines
            Pacemaker insertion
        Transthoracic needle biopsy
        Transbronchial lung biopsy
        Thoracocentesis
        Chest tube malfunction
        Following laparoscopic surgery
    Barotrauma
    Traumatic
        Blunt trauma
            Motor vehicle accidents
            Falls
        Penetrating trauma
            Gun shot wounds
            Stab wounds

— COPD, especially with bulla formation, is troublesome. These patients tolerate even small degrees of collapse poorly, and they should be treated aggressively rather than by observation, as described by Dines and colleagues in 1970. This group of patients is discussed in detail in Chapter 75. Spontaneous pneumothorax complicating cystic fibrosis is treated differently since the development of effective bipulmonary lung transplantation described by Pasque and associates (1990). Whereas in years past obliteration of the pleural space in cystic fibrosis patients prone to spontaneous pneumothorax was a high priority, less aggressive therapy is now being recommended to facilitate an easier operative field for the lung transplant surgeon.

Catamenial pneumothorax has been described in the reports of Shearin (1974), Maurer (1968), and Lillington (1972), and their colleagues. It is the phenomenon of pneumothorax occurring — and recurring — during the first 3 days of menses. Fleishner and associates (1990) have reviewed the possible causes of this problems. In the classic descriptions, nonovulatory states such as pregnancy and oral contraceptive use were not associated with pneumothorax. We have encountered primary spontaneous pneumothorax complicating pregnancy more often than catamenial pneumothorax. This has also been described by Dhalla and Teskey (1985).

Spontaneous pneumothorax may occur as a rare manifestation of lung cancer. Steinhauslin and Cuttat (1985) described the possible mechanisms. They also noted that lung cancer is estimated to cause only 0.03 to 0.05% of cases of spontaneous pneumothorax. Another rare cause of spontaneous pneumothorax is lymphangioleiomyomatosis, which is seen in young women (see Chapter 99).

Pneumothorax in the neonatal period tends to be treated by the neonatologist and is listed only for completeness. Colombani and Haller (1990) presented a nice review of this subject.

Acquired pneumothorax is most often iatrogenic, except in institutions with a high incidence of civilian trauma. The placement of central lines and pacemakers by percutaneous subclavian vein catheterization, transthoracic needle biopsy, thoracocentesis, and transbronchoscopic lung biopsy are all frequent causes of pneumothorax. Many are directly related to physician experience, but the risk of inducing pneumothorax from such procedures is always present. Breathing high concentrations of oxygen prior to transthoracic needle procedures has been recommended and is discussed in Chapter 52. Farn and associates (1993) described pneumothorax during laparoscopic surgery as a sequela of previous transdiaphragmatic surgical intervention. Another cause of pneumothorax that is often overlooked is chest tube dysfunction attributable to inadequately sophisticated medical personnel. Such situations include failing to refill a water seal bottle with the appropriate amount of water, failing to fill the U-manometer in the Pleur-evac type of chest drainage systems, and not adequately securing a chest tube to the chest drainage

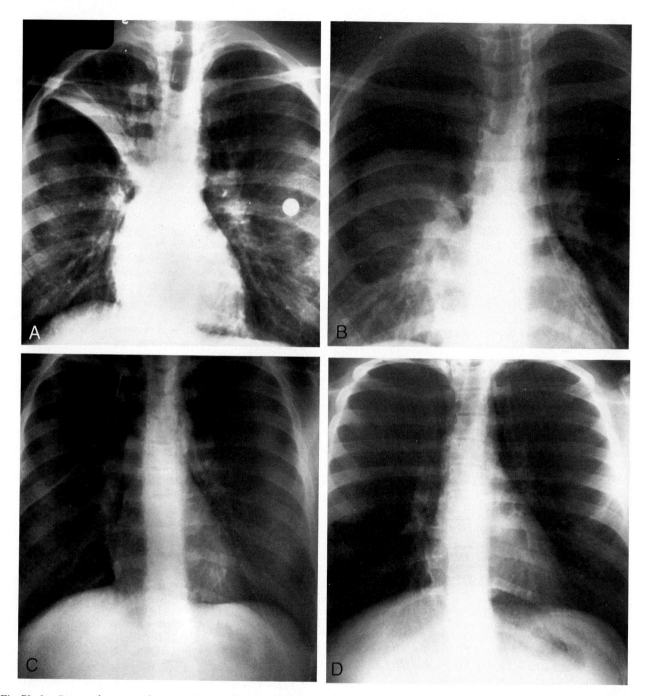

Fig. 53–2. Pneumothorax complicating asthma in a 12-year-old girl. *A*, Right upper lobe atelectasis attributed to mucous plugs. *B*, Pneumothorax attributed to overdistention of nonatelectatic lung. *C*, Re-expansion of the lung by tube thoracostomy with clearing of the atelectasis. *D*, Continued re-expansion of the lung after chest tube removal.

system tubing, permitting the occasional disconnection with resulting potential for an open pneumothorax.

Barotrauma pneumothorax is defined as that occurring in a patient receiving positive pressure ventilation. It is always treated by intervention rather than observation, because patients relying on mechanical ventilation are already in a compromised state, and the positive airway pressure resulting from the mechanical ventilation is a "set-up" for tension pneumothorax. Barotrauma pneumothorax is often attributed to areas of the lung that become overdistended during mechanical ventilation, as other areas are consolidated and poorly ventilated. As a general rule, any barotrauma pneumothorax is an indication for tube thoracostomy, as discussed by Kirby and Ginsberg (1992). This topic is discussed in more detail in Chapter 65.

Traumatic pneumothorax resulting from either blunt or penetrative chest trauma is dealt with in Chapter 64. We, however, urge the placement of a chest tube for traumatic pneumothorax of whatever size whenever there is any other associated injury, because the prompt re-expansion of the collapsed lung immediately eliminates a treatment variable for that patient.

PRESENTATION

The symptoms of spontaneous pneumothorax are the sudden onset of chest pain, shortness of breath, and cough. They can be mild or severe. True tension pneumothorax is relatively uncommon, but it is accompanied by tachycardia, sweating, hypotension, and a pallor that are striking and that result from mediastinal shift, reduced preload, and intense stimulation of the sympathetic nervous system (Fig. 53–3). As previously mentioned, the usual primary spontaneous pneumothorax occurs without warning or precipitating activity. As the lung collapses, the leak is usually obliterated, thereby limiting the amount of collapse and the progression to tension pneumothorax.

The physical findings of a pneumothorax usually vary with the amount of collapse. If the collapse is significant, findings include diminished tactile fremitus, hyperresonance to percussion, and decreased breath sounds on the affected side. In instances of mild collapse, physical findings can be misleadingly normal, so that if the history is suggestive of pneumothorax and yet the physical examination is normal, a chest radiograph should be obtained. In instances of tension pneumothorax, the aforementioned classic physical findings are accentuated and accompanied by a tracheal shift, on palpation of the trachea in the suprasternal notch, to the uninvolved side. A clinical diagnosis of tension pneumothorax made on the basis of appropriate history and physical findings is adequate to allow for the emergency placement of a chest tube without preliminary confirmatory chest radiography, if the clinical situation so demands, and we so instruct our students and house staff.

DIAGNOSIS

The chest radiograph is the standard procedure in making the diagnosis of a pneumothorax. It should be upright and preferable in the posteroanterior —

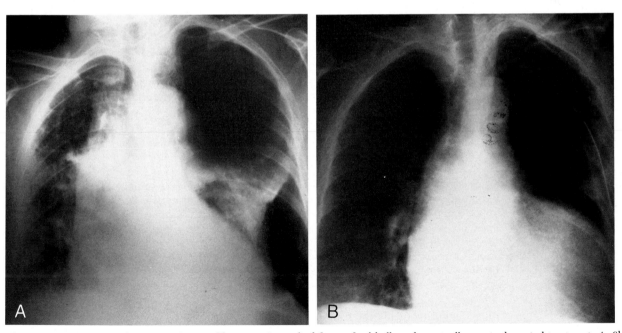

Fig. 53–3. Tension pneumothorax in a 72-year-old woman. It resulted from a focal bulla and eventually required surgical treatment. *A,* Shift of the mediastinum to the right side. A single adhesion kept part of the lung fixed to the chest wall. *B,* Prompt resolution of the pneumothorax with tube thoracostomy. Note return of the mediastinum to its normal position.

PA — projection. It is possible to miss a pneumothorax in a semisupine portable anteroposterior — AP — view. If the patient cannot be upright, a lateral decubitus view with the suspect side positioned up may be helpful. Radiographs obtained in exhalation may accentuate the pneumothorax, but we have not found this technique useful enough in most clinical situations to warrant the double radiographic exposure (see Fig. 53–5). Rhea and colleagues (1982) presented a nomogram for estimating the percent of pneumothorax. In general, the percentage of collapse is underestimated. Skin folds are occasionally misread as pneumothorax. The skin fold artifact, however, has a denser shadow just under the "line," which is the opposite of a pneumothorax, in which the lung is more dense in its central portion. Computed tomography of the lungs gives an excellent evaluation of pneumothorax, as described by Warner (1991) and Lesur (1990) and their associates, but the cost effectiveness of such a procedure must be questioned. Small fluid collections are frequently encountered if the pneumothorax is over 24 hours in duration. The fluid is usually clear, and it is not necessary to analyze it. Large effusions often are bloody and suggest a torn vascular adhesion. Some patients may require immediate operation to control the hemorrhage from a vascular chest wall adhesion that has been torn, because such adhesions have a systemic arterial blood supply.

It is important to exclude a giant bulla in the differential diagnosis, because tube drainage of such bullae is unrewarding.

The physiologic consequences of a pneumothorax range from little, such as 10% spontaneous pneumothorax in a college student, to life threatening, such as a tension pneumothorax in an older patient with already compromised cardiopulmonary function aggravated by mediastinal shift and compression of the contralateral lung. Gustman and co-authors (1983) described a laboratory model of tension pneumothorax resulting in respiratory failure. The consequences of airline travel with the resulting pressure abnormalities are discussed in Chapter 52. In general, patients with a known pneumothorax should not be encouraged to travel by air.

TREATMENT

The various treatment options are listed in Table 53–2. A small spontaneous pneumothorax in an otherwise healthy patient can be observed and followed to its resorption. (Fig. 53–4). Although for some time, as discussed by Carr (1963) and Lippert (1991), and their colleagues, the results of observational therapy have been under question. As discussed in Chapter 52, supplying extra oxygen to such patients theoretically hastens the resolution of the pneumothorax, but the true cost effectiveness of such treatment must be questioned. It is estimated by Kircher and Swartzal (1954) that 1.5% of the air will be reabsorbed over each 24-hour period. Needle or small catheter aspiration of a mild to moderate

Table 53–2. Treatment Options for Pneumothorax

Observation
Needle aspiration
Percutaneous catheter to drainage
Water seal or Pleur-evac type
Heimlich valve
Tube thoracostomy
Water seal or Pleur-evac
Heimlich valve
Tube thoracostomy with instillation of pleural irritant
Video-assisted thoracic surgery (VATS)
Thoracotomy

spontaneous pneumothorax may hasten the resolution, if a persistent leak is absent, as noted by Delius and associates (1989). A plastic needle of the "medicut" or "angiocath" variety is recommended. A tube thoracostomy should be carried out for pneumothoraces over 30% to hasten recovery, or for lesser degrees of collapse in patients with symptoms of associated disorders, such as heart disease or COPD. We prefer to use a 24 to 28F catheter directed toward the apex. If the tube is placed in the anterior to midaxillary line, less muscle tissue has to be traversed. An anterior tube placed through the second interspace does, on the other hand, provide excellent apical air clearance. Anterior tubes are to be avoided in women of almost all ages for cosmetic and esthetic reasons. Foley catheters have been placed in the past, but we no longer recommend its use. A suggestion over the years has been that rubber tubes are more irritating than plastic tubes and that rubber tubes are preferable in patients with primary spontaneous pneumothorax because they promote focal pleural symphysis. We are unaware of any randomized clinical trial that has addressed that issue. Whether the tube is placed by clamp or by trocar is at the discretion of the thoracic surgeon. We tend to prefer the trocar technique for its speed and convenience (Fig. 53–5). Small to medium pneumothoraces can be treated successfully on an outpatient basis, as described by Peters and Kubitschek (1984), as well as by Mercier (1976), Obeid (1954) and Cannon (1981) and their associates, by smaller polyvinyl catheters passed percutaneously; several commercial sets are available. Whether to use a water seal or Pleur-evac drainage system or a Heimlich valve is left to the discretion of the surgeon. We prefer to use a Pleur-evac drainage system and gentle suction of about 20 cm H_2O, only if the lung is not completely re-expanded, to avoid re-expansion pulmonary edema, as described by Matsuura and colleagues (1991), as well as Light (1990) (Fig. 53–6).

Indications for operation are listed in Table 53–3. Surgical treatment of a pneumothorax is recommended for a persistent air leak over 5 to 7 days, for a second recurrence in the usual patient, and for the first episode in a patient with only one lung (Fig. 53–7). Certain occupations suggest that an operation should be performed after the first episode, such as divers and

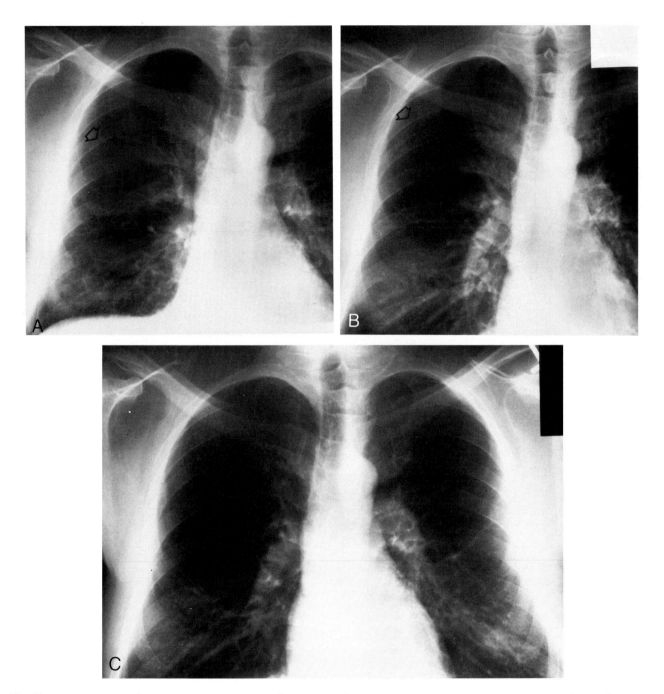

Fig. 53–4. Management of primary spontaneous pneumothorax (arrows) by observation with complete resolution of the collapse. The patient was medically sophisticated, lived near the hospital, and had an occupation that was not physically demanding. *A, B,* and *C* were taken at weekly intervals.

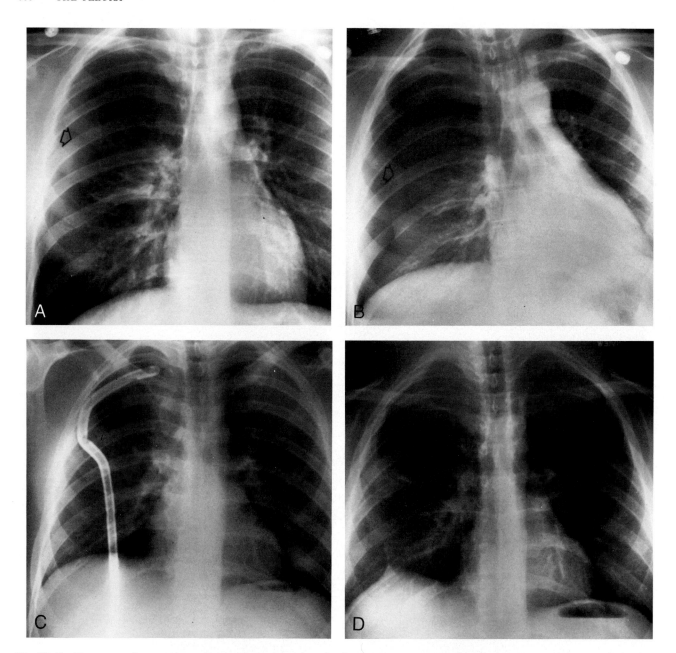

Fig. 53–5. Treatment of primary spontaneous pneumothorax by tube thoracostomy. *A*, On inspiration, significant collapse estimated at 30% in a 22-year-old man. *B*, On exhalation, note accentuation of the pneumothorax, as the pleural air remains constant, whereas the thoracic volume is smaller. Note a slight shift of the mediastinum to the uninvolved side. *C*, Tube thoracostomy with a rubber tube directed to the apex. *D*, Followup chest radiograph demonstrating continued re-expansion of the lung.

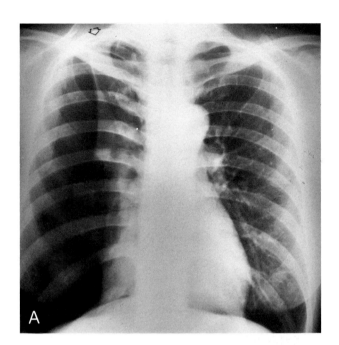

Fig. 53–6. Effect of suction and appearance of re-expansion pulmonary edema in a 52-year-old woman who was a smoker. *A*, Near total collapse from primary spontaneous pneumothorax. An apical adhesion is noted (arrow). *B*, On water seal alone, re-expansion is only minimal.

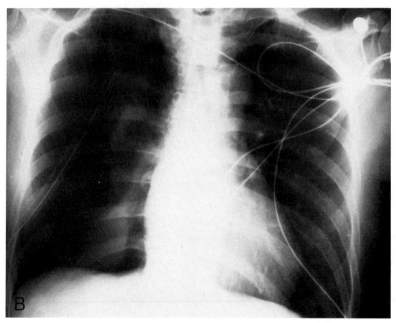

airplane pilots. The chance of recurrence is estimated at 20 to 50% by Seramatis (1970) and Lindskog (1957).

The various surgical options are listed in Table 53–4. The preferred form of surgical treatment is currently the topic of much debate. Various agents have been placed in the pleural space to induce pleural symphysis. The list is long, but includes silver nitrate, talc, hypertonic glucose, urea, oil, nitrogen mustard, and various antibiotics. A clinical trial described by Light in 1990 suggested that intrapleural tetracycline instillation could reduce the incidence of recurrence. We believe, however, that the reduction in recurrence was not overwhelming considering the short followup period. Tetracycline has become difficult to obtain in the United

States, and most tetracycline enthusiasts have switched to doxycycline. Talc has been recommended by Weissberg (1990), van de Brekel (1993) and Almind (1989) and their associates, but talc therapy, whether by tube and slurry or by thoracoscopy with insufflation, should be reserved for malignant effusions, and not benign pneumothorax. Deslauriers (1980), Thomas (1993) and Murray (1993), and their colleagues, as well as Weeden and Smith (1983), reported series of open operations by limited lateral or axillary incision with bleb excision and pleural abrasion or limited apical pleurectomy with excellent results, low recurrence rates, and no mortality. Our experience has been similar. Complete parietal pleurectomy, popularized by Gaensler (1956), should be

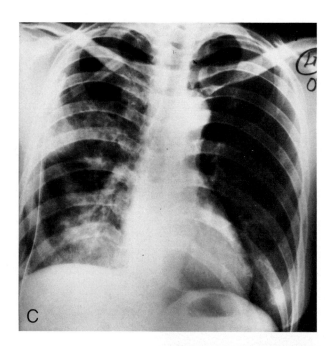

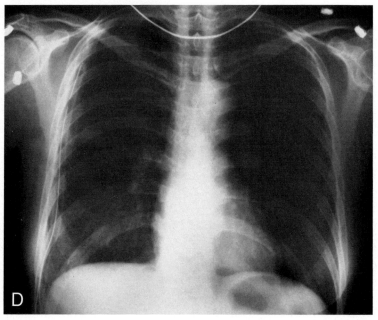

Fig. 53–6. (continued) *C*, After application of suction of −20 cm H₂O, the lung is completely re-expanded. Note the re-expansion pulmonary edema, which was asymptomatic in this case. *D*, 24 hours later, the edema has disappeared.

Table 53–3. **Indications for operative intervention for pneumothorax**

Persistent air leak

Recurrent pneumothorax

First episode in a patient with prior pneumonectomy

First episode with occupational hazard
    Airplane pilot
    Diver

reserved for open treatment failures, for postpneumonectomy patients with a first pneumothorax, and for older patients, usually with COPD, with pneumothorax associated with bullous disease. Mills and Boisch (1963) and Clagett (1968) have raised serious objections to using parietal pleurectomy on a routine basis. Patients with known bilateral pneumothoraces — concurrent or separate — can be considered for bilateral treatment via median sternotomy.

The role of thoracoscopy and video-assisted thoracic surgery — VATS — in the surgical treatment of pneumothorax is evolving, and preliminary reports by Melvin (1992), Nathanson (1993), Inderbitzi (1993), and their associates, as well as by LoCicero (1992), are encour-

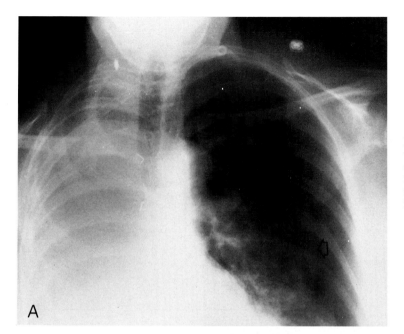

A

Fig. 53–7. Secondary spontaneous pneumothorax in a 50-year-old woman with only one lung. *A*, Significant, symptomatic collapse secondary to metastatic adenocarcinoma of the lung. *B*, Immediate re-expansion by tube thoracostomy. This woman's performance status was good; therefore, she underwent immediate parietal pleurectomy through a small axillary incision.

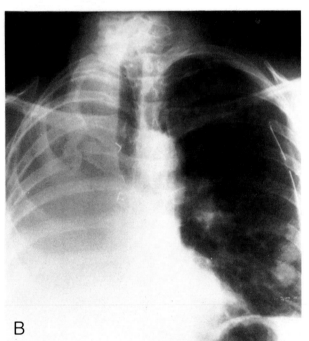

B

Table 53–4. **Surgical Procedures for Pneumothorax***

Pleural abrasion

Parietal pleurectomy
    Apical
    Complete
Talcage
    By slurry
    By insufflation

*All include excision or obliteration of the offending bleb or bulla.

aging. Our results using the VATS approach to the surgical treatment of pneumothorax have been similar. The offending bleb can often be identified and stapled with an endo-GIA through the thoracoscope or with a TA-type stapler through an accessory incision, as described by Lewis and co-workers (1992). Using single-lung anesthesia and a double-lumen endotracheal tube, the anesthesiologist can apply gentle positive pressure to the operated lung to assist in locating the air leak. Pleural abrasion and pleurectomy can also be performed using VATS techniques. At present, our preference is to recommend treatment of the uncomplicated pneumothorax that nonetheless qualifies for surgical treat-

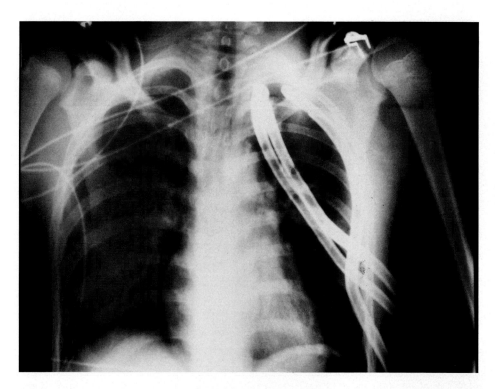

Fig. 53–8. Chest radiograph after VATS bleb excision and pleural abrasion in a 14-year-old boy (same patient as in Fig. 53–1). Three rubber tubes were placed through the three ports. He has had no recurrence.

ment by the VATS approach with stapling of the bleb, if found, or of the ever present apical abnormality and pleural abrasion with dry gauze that has been passed into the chest through the accessory incision. We place rubber chest tubes through the ports — two or three — to encourage pleural irritation, and they usually are removed on the third postoperative day (Fig. 53–8). We prefer a more open surgical approach if we expect to encounter significant bullous disease or unusual adhesion formation, if there has been a previous surgical failure, or if a complete parietal pleurectomy is planned.

The selection of surgical treatment in AIDS patients is more difficult, as described by Gerein (1991), Crawford (1992), and their associates, as well as by Wait and Estrera (1992), because persistent air leak in spite of standard treatment implies a poor prognosis. Hauck and associates (1991) described a thoracoscopic approach using a fibrin glue derivative. Torre and Belloni (1989) described use of a YAG laser thoracoscopically.

Some maneuvers in the treatment of pneumothorax deserve mention. A persistent air leak in a patient with a properly placed chest tube who is a poor operative risk can sometimes be encouraged to close by using pneumoperitoneum, as described by Brooks (1973). Sometimes, high volume suction can "get the lung out" in patients with COPD who are poor operative candidates. The usual Pleur-evac-type drainage systems do not provide this type of suction, but the old-fashioned water seal bottles attached to a high-force suction source such as the Emerson apparatus will accomplish the task.

Finally, we plea for patience on behalf of the thoracic surgeon. Sometimes waiting a few more days allows an air leak to seal. On the other hand, if surgical treatment is going to be necessary, the sooner it is performed, the sooner that patient can resume a routine lifestyle.

REFERENCES

Adams WE: Pulmonary reserve and its influence on the development of lung surgery. J Thorac Cardiovasc Surg 40:141, 1960.

Almind M, Lange P, Viskum, K: Spontaneous pneumothorax: Comparison of simple drainage, talc pleurodesis, and tetracycline pleurodesis. Thorax 44:627, 1989.

Beers MF, Sohn M, Swartz M: Recurrent pneumothorax in AIDS patients with pneumocystis pneumonia. Chest 98:266, 1990.

Bense L, Eklund G, Wiman LG: Smoking and the increased risk of contracting spontaneous pneumothorax. Chest 92:1009, 1987.

Brooks JW: Open thoracotomy in the management of spontaneous pneumothorax. Ann Surg 177:798, 1973.

Cannon WB, Mark JBD, Jamplis RW: Pneumothorax: A therapeutic update. Am J Surg 142:26, 1981.

Carr DT, Silver AW, Ellis Jr FH: Management of spontaneous pneumothorax: With special reference to prognosis after various kinds of therapy. Mayo Clin Proc 38:103, 1963.

Clagett OT: The management of spontaneous pneumothorax. J Thorac Cardiovasc Surg 55:761, 1968.

Coker RJ, et al: Pneumothorax in patients with AIDS. Respir Med 87:43, 1993.

Colombani PM, Haller JA: Neonatal pneumothorax. In Deslauriers J, Lacquet LK (eds): Thoracic Surgery: Surgical Management of Pleural Diseases. St. Louis: CV Mosby, 1990, p 149.

Crawford BK, et al: Treatment of AIDS-related bronchopleural fistula by pleurectomy. Ann Thorac Surg 34:212, 1992.

Delius RE, et al: Catheter aspiration for simple pneumothorax. Arch Surg 124:833, 1989.

Deslauriers J, et al: Transaxillary pleurectomy for treatment of spontaneous pneumothorax. Ann Thorac Surg 30:569, 1980.

Dhalla S, Teskey JM: Surgical management of recurrent spontaneous pneumothorax during pregnancy. Chest 88:301, 1985.

Dines DE, Clagett OT, Payne WS: Spontaneous pneumothorax in emphysema. Mayo Clin Proc 45:481, 1970.

Dines DE, et al: Malignant pulmonary neoplasms predisposing to spontaneous pneumothorax. Mayo Clin Proc *48*:541, 1973.

Farn J, Hammerman AM, Brunt LM: Intraoperative pneumothorax during laparoscopic cholecystectomy: A complication of prior transdiaphragmatic surgery. Surg Lap Endosc *3*:219, 1993.

Fleisher AG, Clement PB, Nelems B: Catamenial pneumothorax: Patholophysiology and management. *In* Deslauriers J, Lacquet LK (eds): Thoracic Surgery: Surgical Management of Pleural Diseases. St. Louis: CV Mosby, 1990, p. 132.

Gaensler EA: Parietal pleurectomy for recurrent spontaneous pneumothorax. Surg Gynecol Obstet *102*:293, 1956.

Gerein AN, et al: Surgical management of pneumothorax in patients with acquired immunodeficiency syndrome. Arch Surg *126*:1272, 1991.

Gobbel Jr WG, et al: Spontaneous pneumothorax. J Thorac Cardiovasc Surg *46*:331, 1963.

Gustman P, Yerger L, Wanner A: Immediate cardiovascular effects of tension pneumothorax. Am Rev Respir Dis *127*:171, 1983.

Hauck H, Bull PG, Pridun N: Complicated pneumothorax: Short- and long-term results of endoscopic fibrin pleurodesis. World J Surg *15*:146, 1991.

Inderbitzi RG, et al: Thoracoscopic pleurectomy for treatment of complicated spontaneous pneumothorax. J Thorac Cardiovasc Surg *105*:84, 1993.

Killen DA, Gobbell Jr WG: Spontaneous Pneumothorax. Boston: Little, Brown, 1968, pp. 1–35.

Kirby TJ, Ginsberg RJ: Management of the pneumothorax and barotrauma. Clin Chest Med *13*:97, 1992.

Kircher Jr LT, Swartzel RL: Spontaneous pneumothorax and its treatment. JAMA *155*:24, 1954.

Kittle CF: The Surgical Management of Recurrent or Persistent Pneumothorax. *In* Current Controversies In Thoracic Surgery. Philadelphia: WB Saunders, 1986, pp. 41–42.

Kjaergaard H: Spontaneous pneumothorax in the apparently healthy. Acta Med Scand (Suppl)*43*:159, 1932.

Lesur O, et al: Computed tomography in the etiologic assessment of idiopathic spontaneous pneumothorax. Chest *98*:341, 1990.

Lewis RJ, et al: One hundred consecutive patients undergoing video-assisted thoracic operations. Ann Thorac Surg *54*:421, 1992.

Light RW: Reexpansion Pulmonary Edema in Pleural Diseases. 2nd Ed. Philadelphia: Lea & Febiger, 1990, pp. 256–257.

Light RW, et al: Intrapleural tetracycline for the prevention of recurrent spontaneous pneumothorax. JAMA *264*:2224, 1990.

Lillington GA, Mitchell SP, Wood GA: Catamenial pneumothorax. JAMA *219*:1328, 1972.

Lindskog GE, Halasz NA: Spontaneous pneumothorax. Arch Surg *75*:693, 1957.

Lippert HL, et al: Independent risk factors for cumulative recurrence rate after first spontaneous pneumothorax. Eur Respir J *4*:324, 1991.

LoCicero J: Minimally invasive thoracic surgery, video-assisted thoracic surgery and thoracoscopy. Chest *102*:330, 1992.

Matsuura Y, et al: Clinical analysis of reexpansion pulmonary edema. Chest *100*:1562, 1991.

Maurer ER, Schaal JA, Mendez Jr FL: Chronic recurrence of spontaneous pneumothorax due to endometriosis of the diaphragm. JAMA *168*:2013, 1968.

Mercier C, et al: Outpatient management of intercostal tube drainage in spontaneous pneumothorax. Ann Thorac Surg *22*:163, 1976.

Melvin WS, Krasna MJ, McLaughlin JS: Thoracoscopic management of spontaneous pneumothorax. Chest *102*:1877, 1992.

Mills M, Baisch BF: Spontaneous pneumothorax. Ann Thorac Surg *1*:286, 1965.

Murphy JB: Surgery of the lung. JAMA *31*:151, 208, 281, 341, 1898.

Murray KD, et al: A limited axillary thoracotomy as primary treatment for recurrent spontaneous pneumothorax. Chest *103*:137, 1993.

Nathanson LK, et al: Videothoracoscopic ligation of bulla and pleurectomy for spontaneous pneumothorax. Ann Thorac Surg *52*:316, 1991.

Obeid FN, et al: Catheter aspiration for simple pneumothorax (CASP) in the outpatient management of simple traumatic pneumothorax. J Trauma *25*:882, 1985.

Pasque MK, et al: Improved technique for bilateral lung transplantation: Rationale and initial clinical experience. Ann Thorac Surg *49*:785, 1990.

Peters J, Kubitschek KR: Clinical evaluation of a percutaneous pneumothorax catheter. Chest *86*:714, 1984.

Renzi PM, et al: Bilateral pneumothoraces hasten mortality in AIDS patients receiving secondary prophylaxis with aerosolized pentamidine. Chest *102*:491, 1992.

Rhea JT, DeLuca SA, Greene RE: Determining the size of pneumothorax in the upright patient. Radiology *144*:733, 1982.

Sepkowitz KA, et al: Pneumothorax in AIDS. Ann Intern Med *114*:455, 1991.

Seremetis MG: The management of spontaneous pneumothorax. Chest *57*:65, 1970.

Shanley DJ, et al: Spontaneous pneumothorax in AIDS patients with recurrent *Pneumocystis carinii* pneumonia despite aerosolized pentamidine prophylaxis. Chest *99*:502, 1991.

Shearin RPN, Hepper NGG, Payne WS: Recurrent spontaneous pneumothorax concurrent with menses. Mayo Clin Proc *49*:98, 1974.

Steinhauslin CA, Cuttat JF: Spontaneous pneumothorax a complication of lung cancer? Chest *88*:709, 1985.

Thomas P, et al: Résultats du traitement chirurgical des pneumothorax persistants ou récidivants. Ann Chir *47*:136, 1993.

Torre M, Belloni P: Nd:YAG laser pleurodesis through thoracoscopy: New curative therapy in spontaneous pneumothorax. Ann Thorac Surg *47*:887, 1989.

van de Brekel JA, Duurkens VAM, Vanderschueren RGJRA: Pneumothorax: Results of thoracoscopy and pleurodesis with talc poudrage and thoracotomy. Chest *103*:345, 1993.

Wait MA, Estrera A: Changing clinical spectrum of spontaneous pneumothorax. Am J Surg *164*:528, 1992.

Warner BW, Bailey WW, Shipley RT: Value of computed tomography of the lung in the management of primary spontaneous pneumothorax. Am J Surg *162*:39, 1991.

Weeden D, Smith GH: Surgical experience in the management of spontaneous pneumothorax, 1972–82. Thorax *38*:737, 1983.

Weissberg D: Role of chemical methods to induce adhesive pleuritis. *In* Deslauriers J, Lacquet LK (eds): Thoracic Surgery: Surgical Management of Pleural Diseases. St. Louis: CV Mosby, 1990, p. 130.

CHAPTER 54

THE PHYSIOLOGY OF PLEURAL FLUID PRODUCTION AND BENIGN PLEURAL EFFUSION

Richard W. Light

The author (1990) has estimated that more than 1 million cases of pleural effusions occur annually in the United States. The possibility of a pleural effusion should be considered whenever a patient with an abnormal chest radiograph is evaluated. Increased densities on the chest radiograph are frequently attributed to parenchymal infiltrates when they actually represent pleural fluid. Free pleural fluid is best demonstrated with lateral decubitus chest radiographs. If, on the lateral decubitus chest radiograph, the distance between the inside of the chest wall and the outside of the lung is greater than 10 mm, a diagnostic thoracentesis is usually indicated. If this distance is less than 10 mm, the pleural effusion is probably not clinically significant and a thoracentesis is not indicated. The presence of loculated pleural fluid is best demonstrated with ultrasonography.

FORMATION AND REABSORPTION OF PLEURAL FLUID

Pleural fluid has several possible origins. It can originate in the capillaries in the parietal or visceral pleura. It can come from the interstitial spaces of the lung, or it can come from the peritoneal cavity through small holes in the diaphragm. Wiener-Kronish and co-workers (1984) have reported that the rate of entry of fluid into the pleural space is about 0.01 ml/kg/hr.

Capillary Origin

The movement of fluid across the pleural membranes is believed to be governed by Starling's law of transcapillary exchange. When this law is applied to the pleura

$$Q_f = L_p \cdot A[(P_{cap} - P_{pl}) - \sigma_d(\pi_{cap} - \pi_{pl})]$$

where Q_f is the liquid movement; L_p is the filtration coefficient per unit area or the hydraulic water con-

ductivity of the membrane; A is the surface area of the membrane; P and π are the hydrostatic and oncotic pressures, respectively, of the capillary — cap — and pleural — pl — space; and σ_d is the solute reflection coefficient for protein, a measure of the membrane's ability to restrict the passage of large molecules. Kinasewitz and colleagues (1984) have estimated that σ_d is approximately 0.80 in humans.

Estimates for the magnitude of the pressures affecting fluid movement in and out of the pleural space are shown in Figure 54–1. When the parietal pleura is considered, a gradient for fluid filtration is normally present. The hydrostatic pressure in the parietal pleura is approximately 30 cm H_2O, whereas the pleural pressure is about −5 cm H_2O. The net hydrostatic pressure gradient is therefore 30 − (−5) = 35 cm H_2O and favors the movement of fluid from the capillaries in the parietal pleura to the pleural space. Opposing this hydrostatic pressure gradient is the oncotic pressure gradient. The oncotic pressure in the plasma is ap-

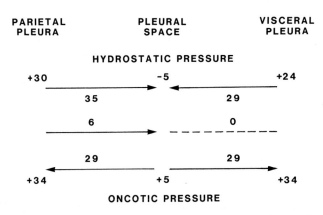

Fig. 54–1. Diagram of the various pressures that influence the movement of fluid in and out of the pleural space in humans. *From* Light RW: Pleural Diseases. Philadelphia: Lea & Febiger, 1990, p 14.

proximately 34 cm H_2O. Because the oncotic pressure of the small amount of pleural fluid is about 5 cm H_2O, the net oncotic gradient is $35 - 5 = 29$ cm H_2O. Thus the net gradient is $35 - 29 = 6$ cm H_2O, favoring the movement of fluid from the capillaries in the parietal pleura to the pleural space.

Albertine and co-workers (1982) have shown that the blood supply to the visceral pleura in humans is from the bronchial artery rather than the pulmonary artery. The net gradient for fluid movement across the visceral pleura in humans is probably close to zero. The pressure in the visceral pleural capillaries is approximately 6 cm H_2O less than that in the parietal pleural capillaries because the former drain into the pulmonary veins. Because this is the only pressure that differs from those affecting fluid movement across the parietal pleura and because the net gradient for the parietal pleura is 6 cm H_2O, it follows that the net gradient for fluid movement across the visceral pleura is approximately zero. It is also quite likely that the filtration coefficient — L_p — for the visceral pleura is substantially less than that for the parietal pleura because Albertine and co-workers (1982) have shown that the capillaries in the visceral pleura are much farther from the pleural space than are those in the parietal pleura.

Interstitial Origin

In recent years, convincing evidence has been presented that the origin of a substantial percentage of pleural fluid is the interstitial spaces of the lung. Broaddus and co-workers (1990) have demonstrated that when sheep — a species with pleurae very similar to that in humans — were volume overloaded by administration of 20% of their body weight as Ringer's lactate, transudative liquid flowed across the visceral pleura of the isolated, in situ lungs. The pleural fluid contained the same protein concentration as did the lung lymph and the interstitial edema liquid in the lung. The volume of pleural fluid constituted about 25% of all edema formed in the lung. In other experiments Allen and colleagues (1989) have shown that with high-pressure pulmonary edema in sheep, pleural fluid accumulates only after pulmonary edema develops. In the clinical situation Wiener-Kronish and co-workers (1985) have shown that in patients with congestive heart failure, the presence of pleural effusions on ultrasound correlates more closely with the pulmonary venous pressure than with the systemic venous pressure and that the likelihood of pleural effusions increases as the severity of the pulmonary edema on chest radiographs increases.

Exudates found in association with increased permeability pulmonary edema probably also originate from the lung interstitium. When Wiener-Kronish and associates (1988) induced increased permeability edema in sheep by the infusion of oleic acid, pleural fluid accumulated only after pulmonary edema developed. In this report there was no detectable injury to the visceral pleura by morphologic studies. They found that approximately 20% of the excess lung liquid that formed

after oleic acid-induced lung injury was cleared from the lung through the pleural space. Other researchers have come to similar conclusions. Amouzadeh and colleagues (1991) concluded that the high-protein pleural effusion that developed in rats after the administration of xylazine had its origin in the parenchymal interstitial spaces of the lung. Bernaudin and associates (1986) made similar conclusions about the exudative pleural effusions induced by hypoxia in rats.

Peritoneal Origin

Fluid that is free in the peritoneal cavity can move directly into the pleural space if there are holes in the diaphragm. This mechanism is responsible for the pleural effusions that occur in conjunction with cirrhosis and ascites, pancreatic ascites, Meigs' syndrome and peritoneal dialysis.

Lymphatic Clearance

Figure 54–1 might lead one to conclude that pleural fluid should continuously accumulate because the Starling equation favors fluid formation through the parietal pleura and there is no gradient for fluid absorption through the visceral pleura. Fluid clearance via the pleural lymphatics is thought to explain the lack of fluid accumulation normally. Wang (1975) demonstrated that, at least in rabbits, the pleural space is in communication with the lymphatic vessels by means of stomas located within the *parietal* pleura. No such stomas are present in the *visceral* pleura. Gaudio and co-workers (1988) were unable to demonstrate these stomas in parietal pleura from humans. Stewart (1965) demonstrated that proteins, cells, and all other particulate matter are removed from the pleural space by these lymphatics in the parietal pleura.

Most fluid that enters the pleural space is removed via the lymphatics. Broaddus and co-workers (1988) produced artificial hydrothoraces in awake sheep by injecting an autologous protein solution at a volume of 10 ml/kg with a protein level of 1.0 g/dl. They found that the hydrothorax was removed almost completely by the lymphatics in a linear fashion at a rate of 0.28 ml/kg/hr. This linearity suggests that the lymphatics operate at maximum capacity once the pleural liquid exceeds a certain threshold volume. Note that the capacity for lymphatic clearance is 28 times as high as the normal rate of pleural fluid formation.

In the experiments of Broaddus and colleagues (1988) previously referred to, the fluid that was introduced into the pleural space had an oncotic pressure of about 5 cm H_2O. From Figure 54–1 one might speculate that if fluids with oncotic pressures other than 5 had been introduced, the equilibrium would have been altered such that fluid would enter the pleural space from visceral pleura in animals with high pleural fluid oncotic pressures and would leave the pleura space through the visceral pleura in animals with very low pleural fluid oncotic pressures. This does not appear to be the case. Aiba and co-workers (1984) produced artificial pleural effusions in dogs with protein levels ranging from 0.1

to 9.0 g/dl. Even when the induced pleural effusion had an oncotic pressure of 0.1 g/dl, there was no increase in the concentration of protein with time, indicating that the very low oncotic pressure did not induce a rapid efflux of fluid out of the pleural space. When the protein concentration of the induced effusions was greater than 4 g/dl, the concentration of protein in the pleural fluid did decrease with time, indicating a net transfer of protein free fluid into the pleural space. However, the net amount of fluid entering the pleural space, even with a protein level of 9.0 g/dl, was only 0.22 ml/kg/hr. This degree of fluid flux is similar to the lymphatic clearance of 0.22 ml/kg/hr reported in the same studies. These observations explain why protein levels and hematocrits remain relatively stable in individuals with hemothoraces.

The amount of fluid that can be cleared through these lymphatics is substantial. Stewart (1963) found that the mean lymphatic flow from one pleural space in seven patients was 0.40 ml/kg/hr, whereas Leckie and Tothill (1965) found that the mean lymphatic flow was 0.22 ml/kg/hr in seven patients with congestive heart failure. In both these studies, marked variability was noted from one patient to another. If these results from patients with congestive heart failure can be extrapolated to the normal person, a 60-kg individual should have the capacity to absorb approximately 20 ml/hr or 500 ml/day from each pleural space through the lymphatics.

In summary if the experimental results in sheep can be extrapolated to humans, it appears that a small amount — 0.01 ml/kg/hr — of fluid constantly enters the pleural space from the capillaries in the parietal pleura. Almost all of this fluid is removed by the lymphatics in the parietal pleura, which can remove approximately 0.20 ml/kg/hr. Very little net fluid movement occurs across the visceral pleura. A pleural effusion will develop when the amount of pleural fluid that enters the pleural space exceeds the amount that can be removed via the lymphatics. Accordingly, pleural effusions can develop and are due to increased pleural fluid formation, decreased lymphatic clearance from the pleural space, or a combination of these two factors. The three primary origins of pleural fluid are the pleural capillaries, the pulmonary interstitial spaces, and the peritoneal cavity.

DIFFERENTIAL DIAGNOSIS

Pleural effusions can occur as complications of many different diseases (Table 54–1). The initial step in evaluation of the patient is the differentiation between exudative and transudative effusions.

SEPARATION OF EXUDATES FROM TRANSUDATES

When it is found that a patient has a pleural effusion that measures more than 10 mm on the decubitus radiograph, a diagnostic thoracentesis should usually be performed. If the patient has obvious congestive heart

Table 54–1. Differential Diagnoses of Pleural Effusions

I. Transudative pleural effusions
  A. Congestive heart failure
  B. Pericardial disease
  C. Cirrhosis
  D. Nephrotic syndrome
  E. Peritoneal dialysis
  F. Superior vena cava obstruction
  G. Myxedema
  H. Pulmonary emboli
  I. Sarcoidosis
  J. Urinothorax
II. Exudative pleural effusions
  A. Neoplastic diseases
    1. Metastatic disease
    2. Mesothelioma
  B. Infectious diseases
    1. Bacterial infections
    2. Tuberculosis
    3. Fungal infections
    4. Viral infections
    5. Parasitic infections
  C. Pulmonary embolization
  D. Gastrointestinal disease
    1. Esophageal perforation
    2. Pancreatic disease
    3. Intra-abdominal abscesses
    4. Diaphragmatic hernia
    5. Postabdominal surgery
    6. Endoscopic variceal sclerotherapy
  E. Collagen vascular diseases
    1. Rheumatoid pleuritis
    2. Systemic lupus erythematosus
    3. Drug-induced lupus
    4. Immunoblastic lymphadenopathy
    5. Sjögren's syndrome
    6. Wegener's granulomatosis
    7. Churg-Strauss syndrome
  F. Postcardiac injury syndrome
  G. Asbestos exposure
  H. Sarcoidosis
  I. Uremia
  J. Meigs' syndrome
  K. Yellow nail syndrome
  L. Drug-induced pleural disease
    1. Nitrofurantoin
    2. Dantrolene
    3. Methysergide
    4. Bromocriptine
    5. Procarbazine
    6. Amiodarone
  M. Trapped lung
  N. Radiation therapy
  O. Electrical burns
  P. Urinary tract obstruction
  Q. Iatrogenic injury
  R. Ovarian hyperstimulation syndrome
  S. Chylothorax
  T. Hemothorax

failure, consideration can be given to postponing the thoracentesis until the heart failure is treated. If such a patient, however, is febrile or has pleuritic chest pain or if the effusions are not of comparable size on both sides, a thoracentesis should be performed without delay. Shinto and I (1990) have shown that the characteristics of pleural fluid associated with heart failure change very little with diuresis over several days.

The first question to be answered with a diagnostic thoracentesis is whether the patient has a transudative or an exudative pleural effusion. Broaddus and I (1992) have modified the classic definitions of the transudates and exudates to take into account the newer theories concerning the formation and reabsorption of pleural fluid. By this new definition, transudative effusions arise from increased hydrostatic pressures or decreased oncotic pressure, while exudative effusions result from increased permeability. This differentiation can be made by simultaneous analysis of the protein and lactic acid dehydrogenase — LDH — levels in the pleural fluid and in the serum. Exudative pleural effusions meet at least one of the following criteria, whereas transudative pleural effusions meet none, according to the classic definitions of the author and colleagues (1972): 1) pleural fluid protein/serum protein > 0.5, 2) pleural fluid LDH/serum LDH > 0.6, and 3) pleural fluid LDH > ⅔ upper normal limit for serum. If none of these criteria are met, the patient has a transudative pleural effusion and the pleural surfaces and the lung can be ignored while the congestive heart failure, cirrhosis, or nephrosis is treated. Remember, however, that a transudative pleural effusion can result from pulmonary embolization. The most cost-effective use of the laboratory for a patient with a pleural effusion is to initially measure only the pleural fluid protein and LDH levels and store the remaining pleural fluid. Then, if it is ascertained that an exudative pleural effusion is present, other diagnostic tests such as cytology, amylase, glucose, cell count, and differential and cultures can be obtained.

DIFFERENTIATING EXUDATIVE PLEURAL EFFUSIONS

Once it has been determined that a patient has an exudative pleural effusion, one should attempt to determine which of the diseases listed in Table 54–1 is responsible, remembering that pneumonia, malignancy, and pulmonary embolization account for the great majority of all exudative pleural effusions. It is recommended that the following tests be obtained on the pleural fluid from a patient with an undiagnosed exudative pleural effusion: glucose level, amylase level, LDH level, differential cell count, microbiologic studies, and cytology. In selected patients, other tests on the pleural fluid, such as the pH, antinuclear antibody level, adenosine deaminase level, rheumatoid factor level, and lipid analysis may be of value.

Appearance of Pleural Fluid

The gross appearance of the pleural fluid should always be described and its odor noted. If the pleural fluid smells putrid, the patient has a bacterial infection — probably anaerobic — of the pleural space. If the pleural fluid is bloody, a pleural fluid hematocrit should be obtained, and if this is greater than 50% that of the peripheral blood, the patient has a hemothorax, and one should consider inserting chest tubes. If the pleural fluid is turbid, milky, or bloody, the supernatant should be examined after centrifugation. If the supernatant is clear, then the turbidity was due to cells or debris in the pleural fluid. If the turbidity persists, then the patient probably has a chylothorax or a pseudochylothorax.

Pleural Fluid Glucose

The presence of a reduced pleural fluid glucose level — < 60 mg/dl — narrows the diagnostic possibilities to six: parapneumonic effusion, malignant effusion, tuberculous effusion, rheumatoid effusion, hemothorax, or a pleural effusion that is due to paragonimiasis. If a patient with a parapneumonic effusion has a pleural fluid glucose level < 40 mg/dl, tube thoracostomy should be performed. Most patients with rheumatoid pleural effusions will have a pleural fluid glucose level below 30 mg/dl.

Pleural Fluid Amylase

An elevated — above the upper normal limit of serum — pleural fluid amylase indicates that the patient has esophageal perforation, pancreatic disease, or malignant disease. The best screening test for a ruptured esophagus is probably the pleural fluid amylase. The origin of the amylase in this instance is the salivary glands. It is very important to establish this diagnosis expeditiously, because the mortality rate exceeds 50% if the mediastinum is not explored within 24 hours of the perforation. Approximately 10% of patients with acute pancreatitis have an accompanying pleural effusion, and in an occasional patient, the chest symptoms will dominate the clinical picture and the elevated pleural fluid amylase will be the first clue that the primary problem is pancreatic rather than pulmonary. Patients with chronic pancreatic disease may develop a sinus tract between the pancreas and the pleural space, which leads to a chronic illness dominated by a large pleural effusion. Unless the pleural fluid amylase level is measured, one may wrongly ascribe the chronic illness and the large pleural effusion to malignancy. The pleural fluid amylase level is elevated in approximately 10% of malignant pleural effusions.

Pleural Fluid Lactic Acid Dehydrogenase

The pleural fluid LDH level is not useful in the differential diagnosis of exudative pleural effusion. Nevertheless, it is recommended that a pleural fluid LDH level be measured every time a diagnostic thoracentesis is performed because the level of LDH in the pleural fluid is a good indicator of the degree of inflammation in the pleural space. If the pleural fluid LDH level increases with serial thoracentesis, the degree of inflammation is worsening, and one should be more aggressive in pursuing the diagnosis.

Pleural Fluid White Cell Count and Differential

The absolute pleural fluid white blood cell count is of limited utility. Counts >10,000/µl are most common with parapneumonic effusions but are also seen with pancreatitis, pulmonary embolism, collagen vascular disease, malignancy, and tuberculosis. The differential cell count on the pleural fluid is of more utility than is the absolute cell count. If the pleural fluid contains predominantly polymorphonuclear leukocytes, then it is due to an acute disease process such as pneumonia, pulmonary embolization, pancreatitis, intra-abdominal abscess, or early tuberculosis. If the pleural fluid contains predominantly mononuclear cells, then malignancy, tuberculosis, or a resolving acute process is probably responsible for the effusion. The majority of patients with pleural fluid eosinophilia have had either blood or air in their pleural space. If neither air nor blood is present in the pleural space, several unusual diagnoses should be considered. Benign asbestos pleural effusions are frequently eosinophilic. Patients with pleural effusions secondary to drug reactions — nitrofurantoin or dantrolene — typically have pleural fluid eosinophilia. The pleural fluid of patients with pleural paragonimiasis is typically eosinophilic with a low glucose, low pH, and a very high LDH level. No diagnosis is ever determined for approximately 20% of exudative pleural effusions, and interestingly, pleural fluid eosinophilia is found in approximately 40% of these effusions. The demonstration that more than 50% of the white blood cells in an exudative pleural effusion are small lymphocytes indicates that the patient probably has a malignant or a tuberculous pleural effusion and thus serves as a strong indication for needle biopsy of the pleura if the cytology of the pleural fluid is negative.

Pleural Fluid Cytology

Pleural fluid cytology is quite useful in establishing the diagnosis of malignant pleural effusion because the diagnosis can be established in 40 to 90%, depending on the tumor type, the amount of fluid submitted, and the skill of the cytologist. Wirth and co-workers (1991), among others, have shown that the use of immunohistochemical tests using monoclonal antibodies facilitates the differentiation of adenocarcinoma cells, benign mesothelial cells, and malignant mesothelial cells. Rijken and associates (1991) reported that the demonstration of aneuploidy in cells from pleural fluid is strongly suggestive of the diagnosis of malignant pleural effusion but that approximately one third of patients with malignant pleural disease do not have aneuploidy of their pleural fluid cells.

Culture and Bacteriologic Stains

Pleural fluid from patients with undiagnosed exudative pleural effusions should be cultured for bacteria — both aerobically and anaerobically, mycobacteria, and fungi. A Gram stain of the fluid should also be obtained. Countercurrent immunoelectrophoresis — CIE — is used to identify bacterial antigens in pleural fluid and to thus establish a presumptive bacteriologic diagnosis in patients with parapneumonic effusions. CIE has proved to be quite valuable in children with parapneumonic effusions. It is less useful in the adult population because anaerobic organisms are responsible for many parapneumonic effusions in this population and no antigens from these organisms are available for routine use.

Pleural Fluid pH and P_{CO_2}

The pleural fluid pH is most useful in determining whether chest tubes should be inserted in patients with parapneumonic effusions. If the pleural fluid pH is < 7.00, the patient invariably has a complicated parapneumonic effusion, and tube thoracostomy should be instituted. If the pleural fluid pH is > 7.20, the patient will probably not require tube thoracostomy. The pleural fluid pH can be reduced to < 7.20 with seven other conditions: 1) systemic acidosis, 2) esophageal rupture, 3) rheumatoid pleuritis, 4) tuberculous pleuritis, 5) malignant pleural disease, 6) hemothorax, or 7) paragonimiasis. When the pleural fluid pH is used as a diagnostic test, it must be measured with the same care as arterial pH. The fluid should be collected anaerobically in a heparinized syringe and placed in ice for transfer to the laboratory to avoid spontaneous acid generation by the fluid.

Immunologic Studies

About 50% of patients with systemic lupus erythematosus — SLE — and 5% of patients with rheumatoid arthritis will have a pleural effusion during the course of their disease. The best screening test for lupus pleuritis is measurement of the pleural fluid antinuclear antibody titer. Patients with lupus pleuritis will have a titer equal to or greater than 1:160 or a pleural fluid titer equal to or greater than the serum titer. Only patients with rheumatoid pleuritis have a pleural fluid rheumatoid factor titer equal to or greater than 1:320 or equal to or greater than the serum titer.

Other Diagnostic Tests on Pleural Fluid

It appears that the demonstration of an elevated — >70 U/L — pleural fluid adenosine deaminase — ADA — level is virtually diagnostic of tuberculous pleuritis while levels < 40 U/L virtually rule out this diagnosis. If the supernatant of the pleural fluid is cloudy, levels of cholesterol and triglycerides in the pleural fluid should be obtained to differentiate chylothorax from pseudochylothorax. With chylothorax the pleural fluid triglyceride levels are usually elevated > 110 mg/dl. With pseudochylothorax, the pleural fluid cholesterol level is elevated. Various reports have advocated measuring other enzymes and proteins in the pleural fluid including carcinoembryonic antigen, hyaluronic acid, lysozyme, and alkaline and acid phosphatase. However, none have proven to be useful in the differential diagnosis or management of patients with pleural effusions.

INVASIVE TESTS FOR UNDIAGNOSED EXUDATIVE PLEURAL EFFUSIONS

In the majority of patients, the cause of the pleural effusion will be apparent after the initial clinical assessment and a diagnostic thoracentesis. If the diagnosis is not apparent, the following invasive tests might be considered: needle biopsy of the pleura, pleuroscopy, bronchoscopy, and open biopsy of the pleura. It is important to remember that no diagnosis is established for approximately 20% of exudative pleural effusions that resolve spontaneously leaving no residua. Three factors should influence the vigor with which one pursues the diagnosis in patients with undiagnosed exudative effusions: 1) The symptoms and clinical course of the patient: if the symptoms are minimal or if they are improving, a less aggressive approach is indicated; 2) the trend of the pleural fluid LDH level: if the pleural fluid LDH tends to increase with serial thoracenteses, a more aggressive approach is indicated because the process is getting worse; 3) the attitude of the patient: if the patient is desperate to know why he has developed a pleural effusion, an aggressive approach should be taken.

Needle Biopsy of the Pleura

With special needles, small specimens of the parietal pleura can be obtained relatively noninvasively. Because this procedure is useful mainly to establish the diagnosis of malignant or tuberculous pleural effusion, it is indicated when one of these two diagnoses is suspected but not yet proved. In patients with tuberculous pleuritis, the initial biopsy is positive for granulomas in 50 to 80%. The demonstration of granulomas on the pleural biopsy is virtually diagnostic of tuberculous pleuritis. When tuberculous pleuritis is suspected, a portion of the pleural biopsy specimen should be cultured for mycobacteria because this will increase the overall diagnostic yield. The needle biopsy of the pleura will be positive in about 40% of patients with malignant pleural disease, and overall the yield from pleural fluid cytology is higher. A prudent approach to the patient with a suspected malignant pleural effusion is to perform a pleural biopsy and repeat pleural fluid cytology only if the cytology obtained at the time of the initial diagnostic thoracentesis is nondiagnostic.

If no diagnosis is obtained after routine laboratory tests including cytology and one-needle biopsy of the pleura, what can be said concerning the patient? Poe and co-workers (1984) reported on 143 such patients, whom they followed 12 to 72 months after the appearance of the pleural effusion. During the observation period, 29 patients were diagnosed with malignant pleural disease and 1 with tuberculous pleuritis. In all 29 patients with malignancy, the diagnosis was strongly suggested by clinical criteria such as weight loss, constitutional symptoms, or a history of a previous cancer. Poe and associates (1984) concluded that most patients with undiagnosed exudative pleural effusions in this situation in whom the clinical picture does not suggest malignancy are best managed by observation.

Thoracoscopy

With this procedure — discussed in more detail in Chapter 17, the pleural surfaces can be directly visualized through a scope introduced through a small incision in the chest wall after a pneumothorax is induced on the side of the pleural effusion. In the past few years, the equipment for thoracoscopy has improved dramatically. The same equipment can be used for thoracoscopy as is used for endoscopic cholecystectomy. It is anticipated that with the better equipment, more and more thoracic procedures will be done through the thoracoscope and accordingly this procedure will be used more and more to diagnose and treat diseases of the pleura.

Thoracoscopy is excellent at establishing the diagnosis of malignancy. When the series of Menzies and Charbonneau (1991) and the series of Hucker and associates (1991) — each with 102 cases — are combined, the diagnosis of malignancy was established in 99 of 117 patients — 85% — with malignancy including 51 of 56 — 91% — of those with mesothelioma. When one does a diagnostic thoracoscopy, one should be prepared to insufflate talc at the time of the procedure because this is the most effective way to prevent recurrence of the pleural effusion.

Bronchoscopy

Bronchoscopy is at times useful in the evaluation of patients with an undiagnosed exudative pleural effusion. Not all patients with an undiagnosed pleural effusion should undergo bronchoscopy. Chang and Perng (1989) demonstrated that bronchoscopy was useful only if the patient had a parenchymal abnormality or hemoptysis. Patients with an undiagnosed pleural effusion should undergo computed tomography — CT — of the chest. Then bronchoscopy is performed only if the CT scan demonstrates parenchymal abnormalities or if the patient has hemoptysis. At the time of bronchoscopy, special attention is paid to those portions of the lung in which the parenchymal abnormalities were demonstrated.

Open Biopsy of the Pleura

Thoracotomy with direct biopsy of the pleura provides the best visualization of the pleura and the best biopsy specimens. The main indication for open pleural biopsy is progressive undiagnosed pleural disease. Open pleural biopsy does not always provide a diagnosis in patients with pleural effusions. Ryan and co-workers (1981) reported that between 1962 and 1972, 51 patients with pleural effusion at the Mayo Clinic had no diagnosis after an open pleural biopsy. In 31 of these patients, there was no recurrence of the pleural effusion and no cause ever became apparent. However, 13 of the patients were eventually proven to have malignant disease.

BENIGN CONDITIONS CAUSING PLEURAL EFFUSION

The remainder of this chapter deals with specific conditions that cause pleural effusion. The reader is referred to the following chapters for a discussion of other diseases of the pleura: Chapter 55 for parapneumonic effusion, Chapter 57 for tuberculous pleural effusion, Chapter 59 for chylothorax, Chapter 61 for mesothelioma and Chapter 63 for malignant pleural effusions.

TRANSUDATIVE PLEURAL EFFUSIONS

Transudative pleural effusions occur because of increased hydrostatic or decreased oncotic pressures.

Congestive Heart Failure

Congestive heart failure is responsible for more pleural effusions than any other disease process. The pleural effusions that occur with congestive heart failure tend to be bilateral and of approximately the same size on each side. Almost all patients with pleural effusions secondary to congestive heart failure have left ventricular or biventricular failure. Patients with congestive heart failure and pleural effusion should undergo diagnostic thoracentesis if the effusions are not bilateral and comparable in size, if the patients are febrile, or if they have pleuritic chest pain to verify that the fluid is transudative. Otherwise, the effusion can be observed while the heart failure is treated and it will usually resolve.

A rare patient with congestive heart failure will have a persistent pleural effusion despite intensive therapy. If such patients are dyspneic and if their dyspnea is relieved by a therapeutic thoracentesis, consideration can be given to attempting a pleurodesis with a sclerosing agent such as a minocycline.

Hepatic Hydrothorax

Pleural effusions occur in approximately 5% of patients with cirrhosis and ascites. The predominant mechanism responsible for the pleural effusion is the direct movement of peritoneal fluid through small holes in the diaphragm into the pleural space. The effusions are usually right sided and frequently are large enough to produce severe dyspnea. If medical management of the cirrhosis and ascites does not control the pleural effusion, there are several alternatives, but all are far from ideal. Pleurodesis with an agent such as minocycline following tube thoracostomy may be attempted. Runyon and co-workers (1986) believe that this procedure is contraindicated in these patients because of the danger of hypovolemia and even death.

An alternative treatment is the insertion of a peritoneojugular shunt. As reported by Ikard and Sawyers (1980), however, these shunts frequently do not control the effusion because fluid will preferentially move to the pleural space, which is due to its negative pressure, rather than to the central veins. The most aggressive approach for these patients is to perform a thoracotomy, repair the diaphragmatic defects, and abrade the pleural surface in an attempt to effect a pleurodesis. This major

surgical procedure obviously carries significant risk for these patients with their severe underlying medical problems.

Nephrotic Syndrome

Pleural effusions that are due to decreased plasma oncotic pressure occur in about 20% of patients with the nephrotic syndrome. The possibility of pulmonary emboli should always be considered in patients with this syndrome, and a lung scan or a pulmonary arteriogram, or both, should be obtained to exclude this diagnosis. Optimally, treatment of the nephrotic syndrome will result in an increased level of protein in the serum and resolution of the pleural effusion.

Peritoneal Dialysis

Large pleural effusions occasionally complicate peritoneal dialysis. The mechanism appears to be a diaphragmatic defect as it is for the hydrothorax seen with cirrhosis and ascites. Frequently one wants to continue the dialysis in these patients. Such cases are best managed, as recommended by Chow and associates (1988), by chemical pleurodesis induced by a tetracycline derivative combined with a short period of small-volume, intermittent peritoneal dialysis.

EXUDATIVE PLEURAL EFFUSIONS

Pleural Effusions That Are Due to Pulmonary Embolization

The diagnosis most commonly overlooked in the differential diagnosis of a patient with an undiagnosed pleural effusion is pulmonary embolization. The symptoms of patients with pleural effusions accompanying pulmonary embolization are no different from those in patients with emboli but without pleural effusion. Dyspnea is reported by more than 80% of the patients and is usually greater than one would expect from a similar-sized effusion with a different etiology.

There is nothing characteristic about the pleural fluid associated with pulmonary embolization. It may be a transudate or an exudate; may be bloody or clear; and may contain mostly neutrophils, lymphocytes, or other mononuclear cells. Any patient with an undiagnosed pleural effusion should undergo perfusion lung scanning. Ideally, the pleural fluid should be removed before the lung scan because its presence complicates interpretation of the scan. If the perfusion scan is abnormal, a ventilation lung scan should be obtained. If doubt persists, pulmonary arteriography should be performed. The treatment of the patient with a pleural effusion secondary to pulmonary embolism is the same as for any patient with pulmonary emboli. If the pleural effusion increases in size with treatment, the patient probably has recurrent emboli or another complication such as a hemothorax or a pleural infection.

Pleural Effusions Secondary to Diseases of the Gastrointestinal Tract

Esophageal Perforation

The possibility of esophageal rupture should be considered in acutely ill patients with pleural effusion, because the mortality from this condition approaches 100% if it is not appropriately diagnosed and treated within 48 hours. Esophageal rupture occurs spontaneously in patients who have vomited or iatrogenically after endoscopy or insertion of a Blakemore tube. Patients with esophageal rupture are acutely ill with chest pain and dyspnea owing to chemical pleuritis. Subcutaneous emphysema in the suprasternal notch is very suggestive of the diagnosis. The best screening test for esophageal rupture appears to be the level of amylase in the pleural fluid. The pleural fluid amylase level is elevated because of saliva with its high amylase content entering the pleural space. The diagnosis is confirmed with the demonstration of esophageal disruption via contrast studies. Ginai (1986) has demonstrated that Hexabrix — meglumine and sodium ioxaglate — is the contrast agent of choice because it minimizes the inflammatory reaction and bronchospasm.

The treatment of choice for esophageal perforation is exploration of the mediastinum with primary repair of the esophageal tear and drainage of the pleural space and mediastinum. Large doses of parenteral antibiotics should be given to treat the mediastinitis and the pleural infection. If exploration of the mediastinum is delayed more than 48 hours after rupture, primary repair is usually not possible because of the damaged tissue. Such patients may be managed with T-tube intubation of the esophageal defect, as suggested by Naylor and associates (1990) (see Chapter 117 for a detailed discussion of this problem).

Acute Pancreatitis

Approximately 10% of patients with acute pancreatitis will have an exudative pleural effusion that arises from diaphragmatic inflammation and the transdiaphragmatic transfer of the exudative fluid arising from acute pancreatic inflammation. At times respiratory symptoms consisting of pleuritic chest pain and dyspnea may dominate the clinical picture. If the pleural effusion does not resolve within 2 weeks of starting appropriate therapy for the pancreatitis, the possibility of a pancreatic abscess or a pancreatic pseudocyst should be considered.

Chronic Pancreatic Disease

Patients with chronic pancreatic disease on occasion develop a sinus tract from their pancreas through the diaphragm into the mediastinum and then into the pleural space. The clinical picture of patients with chronic pancreatic disease and pleural effusion is usually dominated by chest symptoms such as dyspnea, cough, and chest pain. Rockey and Cello (1990) found that most patients do not have abdominal symptoms,

because the pancreaticopleural fistula decompresses the pseudocyst. The pleural effusion is usually massive and recurs rapidly after thoracentesis. The effusion is most commonly left sided but may be right sided or bilateral.

The diagnosis is suggested by a high pleural fluid amylase level and is confirmed by abdominal CT scan or ultrasound. Endoscopic retrograde cholangiopancreatography — ERCP — usually documents the fistulous tract or other pathology in the pancreas.

Patients with chronic pancreatic pleural effusions should be given a trial of conservative therapy for 2 to 3 weeks. Rockey and Cello (1990) recommended that this therapy consist of nasogastric suction, no oral intake, suppression of pancreatic secretion with atropine, and repeated therapeutic thoracenteses. Pederzoli and associates (1986) reported that the administration of a continuous infusion of somatostatin may decrease the secretions through the fistula and facilitate closure. If conservative treatment fails, which Parekh and Segal (1992) reported is much more common when the patient has severe pancreatitis, a laparotomy should be performed. The anatomy of the pancreatic ductal system should be assessed preoperatively with ERCP or at the time of operation with an operative pancreatogram. If a sinus tract is found, it should be ligated or excised. The pancreas should be partially resected, drained with a Roux-en-Y loop, or both. Faling and colleagues (1984) suggested an alternate approach whereby the pancreatic pseudocyst was drained by percutaneous catheter drainage. Decortication of the pleura may be necessary for some patients.

Intra-abdominal Abscess

Pleural effusions frequently accompany intra-abdominal abscesses including subphrenic — 80%, pancreatic — 40%, intrasplenic — 35%, and intrahepatic — 20%. The pleural fluid is a sterile exudate with predominantly neutrophils. The possibility of an intra-abdominal abscess should be seriously considered in a patient with a persistent neutrophilic pleural effusion and no parenchymal infiltrates. The diagnosis is best established by abdominal CT scan, and treatment consists of antibiotics plus drainage.

Pleural Effusions After Surgical Procedures

After Fontan Procedure

With this procedure the right ventricle is bypassed by an anastomosis between the superior vena cava, the right atrium, or the inferior vena cava and the pulmonary artery. This surgery is usually performed for tricuspid atresia or univentricular heart. As reported by Laks and co-workers (1984), a transudative pleural effusion occurs postoperatively in nearly every patient and is a significant problem postoperatively in many patients. The treatment of choice for this condition is probably the insertion of a pleuroperitoneal shunt, as suggested by Sade and Wiles (1990).

After Abdominal Surgery

The author and George (1976) reported that the incidence of pleural effusion in the 2 to 3 days following abdominal surgery is approximately 50%. The incidence of postoperative pleural effusion is greater in patients undergoing upper abdominal surgery, in patients with postoperative atelectasis, and in those patients with free abdominal fluid at surgery. The pleural effusion in the postoperative period is probably due either to diaphragmatic irritation or the transdiaphragmatic movement of intra-abdominal fluid. If a patient develops a significant amount of fluid postoperatively, a diagnostic thoracentesis should be performed to rule out pleural infection as a cause of the effusion. The possibility of pulmonary embolization should also be considered. If the effusion develops more than 72 hours postoperatively, it is probably not related to the surgical procedure itself, and alternate explanations must be found such as pulmonary embolization, intra-abdominal abscess, or hypervolemia.

After Coronary Artery Bypass Surgery

Peng and co-workers (1992) and Hurlbut and associates (1990) have reported that the incidence of pleural effusion following coronary artery bypass surgery exceeds 40%. The incidence is comparable whether saphenous vein graphs or internal mammary artery grafts are used. The pathogenesis of the effusions is unknown, but Peng and co-workers (1992) have speculated that they are due to pericardial inflammation. The effusions are predominantly small and on the left side. In almost all cases, the effusions resolve spontaneously without treatment over several weeks.

After Endoscopic Variceal Sclerotherapy

In recent years endoscopic variceal sclerotherapy — EVS — has become one of the principal forms of therapy for patients who have bled from ruptured esophageal varices. Edling and Bacon (1991) have reported that small pleural effusions complicate this procedure approximately 50% of the time. The pleural effusion is thought to result from the extravasation of the sclerosant into the esophageal mucosa, which results in an intense inflammatory reaction in the mediastinum and pleura. The effusions can be right sided, left sided, or bilateral, and the fluid is exudative. If the effusion persists for more than 24 to 48 hours and is accompanied by fever or if the effusion occupies more than 25% of the hemithorax, a thoracentesis should be done to rule out an infection or an esophagopleural fistula. The latter diagnosis is suggested by a high pleural fluid amylase level.

Pleural Effusions That Are Due to Miscellaneous Diseases

AIDS and Pleural Effusion

Pleural effusions are relatively uncommon in patients with AIDS. As reported by Strazzella and Safirstein (1991) parapneumonic effusions are the most common cause of pleural effusion in patients with AIDS, and these parapneumonic effusions are more likely to be complicated in patients with AIDS than in immunocompetent patients. Other common causes of pleural effusions in patients with AIDS include Kaposi's sarcoma, tuberculosis, cryptococcosis, lymphoma and rarely *Pneumocystis carinii* infection.

Rheumatoid Pleuritis

Approximately 5% of patients with rheumatoid arthritis have a pleural effusion sometime during their life. Most effusions occur in the older man with subcutaneous nodules. The pleural fluid with rheumatoid pleuritis is very distinctive, being characterized by a glucose level < 30 mg/dl, a high LDH level — >700 IU/L, a low pH — <7.20, and a high rheumatoid factor titer — ≥1:320. The pleural effusion usually resolves spontaneously within 3 months. No controlled study has documented the efficacy of any treatment.

Lupus Erythematosus

Approximately 40% of patients with SLE or drug-induced SLE will develop a pleural effusion during the course of their disease. The pleuritis may be the first manifestation of the underlying disease. Most patients with lupus pleuritis have pleuritic chest pain and are febrile. The pleural fluid antinuclear antibody — ANA — titer is at least 1:160 and the pleural fluid/serum ANA ratio is at least 1 in most patients with lupus pleuritis. Patients with lupus pleuritis should be treated with prednisone 80 mg every other day with rapid tapering once the symptoms are controlled.

After Cardiac Injury Syndrome

The postcardiac injury syndrome, also called "the postpericardiectomy" or "the postmyocardial infarction" — Dressler's — syndrome, is characterized by pericarditis, pleuritis, or pneumonitis, or a combination of these, that occurs after injury to the myocardium or pericardium. The syndrome typically develops about 3 weeks after the injury but can occur anytime between 3 days and 1 year. The pleural fluid is an exudate that is frequently serosanguineous or bloody. The treatment of choice is the use of anti-inflammatory agents such as aspirin or indomethacin. Patients with this syndrome following coronary artery bypass procedures should be treated with corticosteroids because the pericarditis may cause graft occlusion.

Asbestos Exposure

Pleural effusions develop in approximately 3% of individuals who have had moderate to heavy asbestos exposure. The resulting exudative pleural effusion usually develops between 5 and 20 years of the initial exposure. Patients with pleural effusion are usually asymptomatic. The diagnosis of benign asbestos effusion is one of exclusion and requires the following: asbestos exposure, exclusion of other causes — infection, pulmonary embolism, malignancy, and a follow-up of at least 2 years to verify that it is benign.

Drug Reactions

The administration of nitrofurantoin, dantrolene, methysergide, and bromocriptine at times is associated with a syndrome characterized by fever, dyspnea, chest pain, and peripheral blood and pleural eosinophilia, which develop weeks to months after initiation of therapy. Discontinuation of the offending medication will result in resolution of the syndrome.

Uremia

Uremia may be complicated by a fibrinous pleuritis and pleural effusion. Approximately 3% of uremics will have an exudative pleural effusion, and there is no close relationship between the degree of uremia and the occurrence of a pleural effusion. After dialysis is initiated, the effusion gradually disappears within 4 to 6 weeks in the majority of patients.

REFERENCES

Aiba M, Inatomi K, Homma H: Lymphatic system or hydro-oncotic forces. Which is more significant in drainage of pleural fluid? Jpn J Med 23:27, 1984.

Albertine KH, et al: Structure, blood supply, and lymphatic vessels of the sheep's visceral pleura. Am J Anat 165:277, 1982.

Albertine KH, Wiener-Kronish JP, Staub NC: The structure of the parietal pleura and its relationship to pleural liquid dynamics in sheep. Anat Rec 208:401, 1984.

Allen S, Gabel J, Drake R: Left atrial hypertension causes pleural effusion formation in unanesthetized sheep. Am J Physiol 257 (2 Pt 2):H690, 1989.

Amouzadeh HR, et al: Xylazine-induced pulmonary edema in rats. Tox Appl Pharmacol 108:417, 1991.

Bernaudin JF, et al: Protein transfer in hyperoxic induced pleural effusion in the rat. Exper Lung Res 210:23, 1986.

Broaddus VC, et al: Removal of pleural liquid and protein by lymphatics in awake sheep. J Appl Physiol 64:384, 1988.

Broaddus VC, Light RW: What is the origin of pleural transudates and exudates? (Editorial.) Chest 102:658, 1992.

Broaddus VC, Wiener-Kronish JP, Staub ND: Clearance of lung edema into the pleural space of volume-loaded anesthetized sheep. J Appl Physiol 68:2623, 1990.

Chang S-C, Perng RP: The role of fiberoptic bronchoscopy in evaluating the causes of pleural effusions. Arch Intern Med 149:855, 1989.

Chow CC, et al: Massive hydrothorax in continuous ambulatory peritoneal dialysis: diagnosis, management and review of the literature. NZ Med J 27:475, 1988.

Edling JE, Bacon BR: Pleuropulmonary complications of endoscopic variceal sclerotherapy. Chest 99:1252, 1991.

Faling LJ, et al: Treatment of chronic pancreatic pleural effusion by percutaneous catheter drainage of abdominal pseudocyst. Am J Med 76:329, 1984.

Gaudio E, et al: Surface morphology of the human pleura. A scanning electron microscopic study. Chest 92:149, 1988.

Ginai AZ: Experimental evaluation of various available contrast agents for use in the gastrointestinal tract in case of suspected leakage. Effects on pleura. Br J Radiol 59:887, 1986.

Hucker J, et al: Thoracoscopy in the diagnosis and management of recurrent pleural effusions. Ann Thorac Surg 52:1145, 1991.

Hurlbut D, et al: Pleuropulmonary morbidity: internal thoracic artery versus saphenous vein graft. Ann Thorac Surg 50:959, 1990.

Ikard RW, Sawyers JL: Persistent hepatic hydrothorax after peritoneojugular shunt. Arch Surg 115:1125, 1980.

Kinasewitz GT, et al: Role of pulmonary lymphatics and interstitium in visceral pleural fluid exchange. J Appl Physiol 56:355, 1984.

Laks H, et al: Experience with the Fontan procedure. J Thorac Cardiovasc Surg 88:939, 1984.

Leckie WJH, Tothill P: Albumin turnover in pleural effusions. Clin Sci 29:339, 1965.

Light RW: Pleural Diseases. Philadelphia: Lea & Febiger, 1990.

Light RW, et al: Pleural effusions: the diagnostic separation of transudates and exudates. Ann Intern Med 77:507, 1972.

Light RW, George RB: Incidence and significance of pleural effusion after abdominal surgery. Chest 69:621, 1976.

Menzies R, Charbonneau M: Thoracoscopy in the diagnosis and management of recurrent pleural effusions. Ann Thorac Surg 52:1145, 1991.

Naylor AR, et al: T tube intubation in the management of seriously ill patients with oesophagopleural fistulae. Br J Surg 77:40, 1990.

Parekh D, Segal I: Pancreatic ascites and effusion. Risk factors for failure of conservative therapy and the role of octreotide. Arch Surg 127:707, 1992.

Pederzoli P, et al: Conservative treatment of external pancreatic fistulas with parenteral nutrition alone or in combination with continuous intravenous infusion of somatostatin, glucagon or calcitonin. Surg Gynecol Obstet 163:428, 1986.

Peng M-J, et al: Postoperative pleural changes after coronary revascularization. Comparison between saphenous vein and internal mammary artery grafting. Chest 101:327, 1992.

Poe RH, et al: Sensitivity, specificity, and predictive values of closed pleural biopsy. Arch Intern Med 144:325, 1984.

Rijken A, et al: Diagnostic value of DNA analysis in effusions by flow cytometry and image analysis. Am J Clin Pathol 95:6, 1991.

Rockey DC, Cello JP: Pancreaticopleural fistula. Report of 7 cases and review of the literature. Medicine 69:332, 1990.

Runyon BA, Greenblatt M, Ming RHC: Hepatic hydrothorax is a relative contraindication to chest tube insertion. Am J Gastroenterol 81:566, 1986.

Ryan CJ, et al: The outcome of patients with pleural effusion of indeterminate cause at thoracotomy. Mayo Clin Proc 56:145, 1981.

Sade RM, Wiles HB: Pleuroperitoneal shunt for persistent pleural drainage after Fontan procedure. J Thorac Cardiovasc Surg 100:621, 1990.

Shinto RA, Light RW: The effects of diuresis upon the characteristics of pleural fluid in patients with congestive heart failure. Am J Med 88:230, 1990.

Stewart PB: The rate of formation and lymphatic removal of fluid in pleural effusions. J Clin Invest 42:258, 1963.

Strazzella WD, Safirstein BH: Pleural effusions in AIDS. NJ Med 88:39, 1991.

Wang NS: The preformed stomas connecting the pleural cavity and the lymphatics in the parietal pleura. Am Rev Respir Dis 111:12, 1975.

Wiener-Kronish JP, et al: Protein egress and entry rates in pleural fluid and plasma in sheep. J Appl Physiol 56:459, 1984.

Wiener-Kronish JP, et al: Relationship of pleural effusions to pulmonary hemodynamics in patients with congestive heart failure. Am Rev Respir Dis 132:1253, 1985.

Wiener-Kronish JP, et al: Relationship of pleural effusions to increased permeability pulmonary edema in anesthetized sheep. J Clin Invest 82:1422, 1988.

Wirth PR, Legier J, Wright GI Jr: Immunohistochemical evaluation of seven monoclonal antibodies for differentiation of pleural mesothelioma from lung adenocarcinoma. Cancer 67:655, 1991.

CHAPTER 55

PARAPNEUMONIC EMPYEMA

Thomas W. Shields

Pleural exudates commonly occur in patients with pneumonia. Light and associates (1980) estimate that a pleural effusion occurs in approximately 40% of patients with bacterial pneumonia. Many of these effusions are sterile and resolve with appropriate antibiotic therapy of the underlying pneumonia, but in a variable percentage of patients — depending on the virulence of the infecting organism, the status of the defense mechanisms of the host, and the timing and appropriateness of therapy, the effusion will progress into a complicated parapneumonic effusion or into a frank empyema thoracis. These empyemas represent 50% or greater of all empyemas seen in clinical practice (Table 55–1).

Light (1983, 1991) defines a complicated parapneumonic effusion as one in which the fluid is not grossly purulent and the Gram stain of the pleural effusion is negative but nonetheless a closed tube thoracostomy is required for its resolution, or as a similar effusion in which the bacteriologic culture becomes positive. When the parapneumonic effusion is yellow and clear, and the specific gravity is greater than 1.018, a white blood count is greater than 500 cells/mm^3, and a protein level is

greater than 2.5 g/dl, a complicated parapneumonic effusion is most likely present. Light (1990) suggested that if the pH is below 7.2 or the lactic dehydrogenase — LDH — level is above 1000 IU/L, these findings support this assumption.

A parapneumonic empyema is defined as the presence of a grossly purulent effusion or one in which the Gram stain is positive. The white blood cell count is greater than 15,000 cells/mm^3, the protein level is greater than 3 g/dl, the pH is less than 7.0, the pleural fluid glucose level is below 50 mg/dl, and the LDH is greater than 1000 IU/L.

Either of these effusions may be present in association with an acute lung abscess or bronchiectasis. Similarly, although not truly a parapneumonic process, an empyema may occur as a result of an iatrogenic infection of an originally sterile pleural transudate, a sterile exudative effusion associated with an underlying malignant process, or an effusion or hemothorax following thoracic trauma. When this occurs, the management — with modifications as required — is the same as that of either a true parapneumonic complicated effusion or a frank empyema thoracis.

PATHOPHYSIOLOGY

Andrews and colleagues (1962), reporting for the American Thoracic Society, classified thoracic empyema into three stages: 1) exudative or the acute phase, 2) fibrinopurulent or the transitional phase, and 3) organizing or the chorionic phase. The three phases cannot be sharply defined and in actuality represent a continuous evolving process that may progress at varying speeds and may be modified or arrested by therapeutic interventions.

The exudative phase is represented by accumulation of a small to moderate amount of pleural fluid as a result of increased permeability of the visceral pleura contiguous to an underlying parenchymal infection. The exudative fluid is sterile but contains a small number of polymorphonuclear leukocytes. The pleural fluid

Table 55–1. Incidence of the Various Causes of Empyema

Cause	Percent
Pyogenic pneumonia	50
Lung abscess rupture	1–3
Secondary to generalized sepsis	1–3
Pulmonary tuberculosis	1
Pulmonary mycotic infection	1
Post-traumatic	3–5
Postsurgical (esophagus, lungs, mediastinum)	25
Extension from subphrenic abscess	8–11
Secondary to bronchopleural fistula of spontaneous pneumothorax	<1
Secondary to parasitic infestation	<1
Retained foreign bodies in bronchial tree	<1
Miscellaneous	1

From Miller JI Jr: Pleural diseases. *In* Shields TW (ed): General Thoracic Surgery. 3rd Ed. Philadelphia: Lea & Febiger, 1989, p. 634.

glucose level and pH are normal and the LDH level is below 1000 IU/L. Without appropriate treatment of the underlying pulmonary infection, the effusion will evolve into the second or fibropurulent stage with infection of the fluid and the accumulation of greater amounts of fluid. This collection will contain large numbers of white blood cells and cellular debris, and bacteria may or may not be identified by Gram stain. Fibrin is deposited in layers on both pleural surfaces of the involved area, and loculation of the fluid collection may occur relatively early in this phase. As the process evolves, the pleural fluid pH and glucose level fall and the LDH level increases progressively higher. The final or the organization phase is represented by ingrowth of fibroblasts and capillaries into the deposited fibrin layers to produce a firm, inelastic membrane termed the pleural peel. The pleural fluid is thick and viscous and contains at least 75% sediment on standing in a jar after its removal from the chest. The pH of the fluid is generally below 7.0 and the glucose level is less than 40 mg/dl. The organizing phase may begin as early as 7 to 10 days after the onset of the parapneumonic effusion and be complete in 4 to 6 weeks.

BACTERIOLOGY

Before the development of effective antibiotics, the most common causative organisms of empyema were *Streptococcus pneumoniae* and hemolytic streptococci. In the late 1950s and early 1960s, *Staphylococcus aureus* was the most common causative organism. In the 1970s and onward, anaerobic organisms assumed the majority role in culture-positive parapneumonic empyemas. Bartlett and co-workers (1974) reported that in 83 untreated adult patients with parapneumonic effusion, only anaerobic organisms were isolated in 35%, both anaerobic and aerobic organisms in 41%, and aerobic organisms alone in 24%. Most patients — 72% — had more than one organism cultured from the effusion. An exception to these findings is in children under the age of 2 years in whom the *Staphylococcus* bacterium remains the most common causative organism. The more commonly isolated organisms are listed in Table 55–2.

CLINICAL FEATURES

The clinical symptomatology of a parapneumonic empyema is frequently difficult to distinguish from those of the underlying disease process in the lung. The range of presentation may be wide, from the absence of symptoms related to involvement of the pleura to a severe febrile illness with toxemia. Empyemas from aerobic organisms tend to manifest acutely, with chest pain, fever, cough, tightness in the chest, and occasionally shortness of breath. In patients with anaerobic infections, the course tends to be more insidious and chronic, but severe toxemia may develop. In cases of long duration, weight loss and anemia may be common. In many patients, the presence of the empyema is manifested by failure of response or even a worsening

Table 55–2. Frequency of Causative Organisms of Parapneumonic Empyemas

Organism	n(%)
Peptostreptococcus	5(12)
Staphylococcus epidermidis	5
Streptococcus viridans	4(10)
Peptococcus	3(7)
Diphtheroids	3
Staphylococcus aureus	3
Streptococcus pyogenes	2(5)
Haemophilus influenzae	2
Fusobacterium nucleatum	2
Acinetobacter	2
Bacteroides	2
Enterobacter aerogenes	1(2)
Klebsiella pneumoniae	1
Pseudomonas	1
Microaerophilic streptococci	1
Micrococcus species	1
Steptococcus pneumoniae	1
Clostridium species	1
Anaerobic gram-positive cocci	1
Anaerobic gram-positive bacilli	1
Total	42

From Ali I, Unruh H: Management of empyema thoracis. Ann Thorac Surg 50:335, 1990.

of the patient's clinical condition despite what has been presumed to be adequate antibiotic therapy based on results of sputum or blood cultures. A sudden expectoration of a large amount of purulent sputum may occur because of the development of a bronchopleural fistula.

Physical findings consist of decreased breath sounds, restricted respiratory excursions, and dull percussion note over the involved area. With passage of time, the affected hemithorax is contracted and its movement is limited. Clubbing of the fingers may occur. A chest wall abscess may develop as a result of erosion of the empyema through the chest wall — an empyema necessitans.

Late in the course of the disease, pericarditis, mediastinal abscess, disseminated infection, and multiorgan failure may occur.

DIAGNOSIS

The diagnosis of a parapneumonic empyema is suggested by the patient's history and clinical course. The presence of a parapneumonic effusion is confirmed by radiographic, computed tomographic — CT, and ultrasonographic studies as necessary.

Radiographic Features

Standard posteroanterior and lateral radiographs are essential for identification and localization of the presence of the effusion. The fluid appears as a homogeneous opacity that is in a dependent position. Small amounts of fluid are best seen on the lateral upright radiograph, which reveals blunting of the posterior costophrenic sulcus. Lateral decubitus radiographs demonstrate

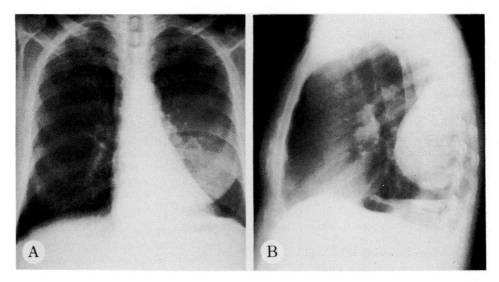

Fig. 55–1. *A*, Posteroanterior radiograph of patient with encapsulated pleural effusion. *B*, Lateral radiograph showing D-shaped configuration of the encapsulated fluid.

whether or not the fluid is free within the pleural space. Light and colleagues (1980) report that the amount of the fluid can be semiquantitated by measuring the distance between the inside of the chest wall and the outside of the lung when the patient has the involved side in the inferior position. When the involved side is superior, one can assess how much the radiodensity is the fluid and how much is the consolidated lung. If no free flow of fluid is observed in the decubitus views, the effusion can be assumed to be encapsulated. LeRoux and Dodds (1964) pointed out that a localized effusion may be suggested by a posteriorly located D-shaped opacity with the convex border toward the hilus (Fig. 55–1). Large pleural effusions are accompanied by a shift of the trachea and mediastinal structures toward the unaffected side and the effusion may occupy most of the affected side (Fig. 55–2); however, aerated lung may be seen anteriorly on the lateral radiograph. Loculation of the effusion is difficult to assess on the standard views unless a bronchopleural fistula is present and multiple air fluid levels are present. In a patient in whom the parapneumonic effusion is associated with a lung abscess, the differentiation between a pyopneu-mothorax because of a bronchopleural fistula and the abscess itself may be difficult. It is essential, in such a situation, that the radiographs are taken with the patient in a true upright position. The contrasting feature of a pyopneumothorax, as emphasized by Swenson and associates (1991), is that the fluid level in a typical abscess has equal air-filled widths on both the posteroanterior and lateral chest radiographs, whereas this rarely is the case with an air-fluid level in the pleural space.

Computed tomography is of great value in the overall evaluation of the parapneumonic effusion. It may define the extent of the involvement of the pleural space precisely, as well as the presence and location of loculated fluid collections (Fig. 55–3), and is helpful in differentiating between a pleural fluid collection containing air from a bronchopleural fistula and a pulmonary abscess. Stark and associates (1983) reported that empyemas conform to the shape of the chest wall and most have thin smooth walls, especially their inner margins. In contrast, lung abscesses are spherical and, at least initially, have thick irregular walls.

The most important value of the CT scan is the demonstration of loculated pockets, the presence of which influences therapeutic management, as will be noted. Light (1990) recommends the use of sonography for the determination of the presence of loculation. The choice of one diagnostic technique over the other depends on the expertise at any given institution.

Ancillary radiographic studies with the use of contrast material placed into the pleural space and bronchog-

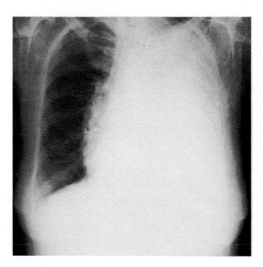

Fig. 55–2. Massive effusion opacifying the left hemithorax and displacing the mediastinum to the right with compression of the contralateral lung.

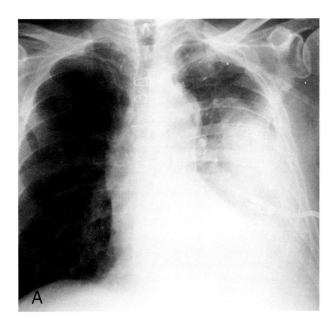

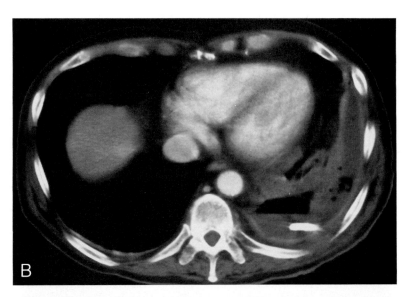

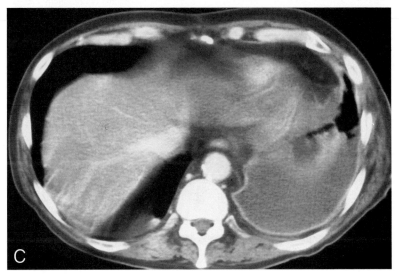

Fig. 55–3. *A,* Posteroanterior chest radiograph showing unresolved empyema with a small drainage catheter in place. *B* and *C,* CT scans at different levels revealing multiple loculated fluid collections with several small air fluid levels.

raphy may be necessary in various clinical situations when major invasive surgical procedures are thought indicated.

Thoracentesis

The diagnosis of a parapneumonic empyema is established by a thoracentesis. The appropriate site is selected by examination of the radiographs and CT scans. A large 18- or 19-gauge needle is used to carry out the thoracentesis. Approximately 20 to 50 ml of fluid is removed into a heparinized syringe, its odor is noted, and aliquots are sent to the laboratory for determination of the specific gravity, the pH, and the glucose, LDH, and protein levels. A white cell count and differential is obtained. A Gram stain is done immediately and aerobic and anaerobic cultures are plated.

The gross appearance of pus, a malodorous, fetid smell, or a positive Gram stain for bacteria immediately establishes the diagnosis. When the pleural fluid is clear and yellow, the diagnosis must await the positive laboratory findings described previously. When antibiotics have been administered prior to the thoracentesis, Miller (1989) noted that approximately 50% of the patients have negative cultures. Nonetheless, antibiotic sensitivity studies should be done on all specimens.

MANAGEMENT

The principles of treatment of a complicated parapneumonic effusion or a parapneumonic empyema is evacuation of the fluid, obliteration of the pleural space, and augmentation of the host's natural defenses with the use of the appropriate antibiotic(s), nutritional support,

and any other supportive measures as required to control the underlying disease process and to restore the normal mobility of the lung.

Choice of Antibiotics

Until positive cultures and sensitivity results are obtained, the selection of the antibiotic is guided by the findings on the Gram stain of the exudate, the odor of the fluid — malodorous fluid is associated with anaerobic infection — and a Gram stain of the sputum. Early on, the antibiotic levels in the pleural fluid, as noted by Taryle and associates (1981), are comparable to those in the serum so that normal dosage schedules may be used. Light (1990) suggested that if an anaerobic infection is suspected, clindamycin — 600 mg every 6 hours — should be included as one of the antibiotics. Once a dominant organism(s) is identified, Bergeron (1990) suggests the use of the antibiotic(s), as listed in Table 55–3.

Aspiration

In an early stage of a parapneumonic fluid collection in an adult, when the fluid is thin and there are no loculations, a single therapeutic thoracentesis combined with the use of appropriate antibiotic therapy may be sufficient to control the disease. As noted, however, if it is a complicated parapneumonic effusion or a frank empyema, closed tube thoracostomy drainage will be required. In children, Bergeron (1990) as well as others reported that intermittent aspirations with pleural lavage every 2 to 3 days may be effective in controlling the process.

Table 55–3. Choice of Antibiotics Against Pathogens in Empyema

Pathogen	First Choice	Alternative
Gram-positive bacteria		
Streptococcus pneumoniae	Penicillin	Erythromycin, clindamycin
Staphylococcus aureus (BL−)*	Penicillin	Cefazolin-clindamycin
Staphylococcus aureus (BL+)	Oxacillin	Cefazolin, clindamycin
Staphylococcus aureus (methicillin resistant)	Vancomycin	Teicoplanin,† daptomycin,† ciprofloxacin fusidic acid, coumermycin,† rifampin, and aminoglycosides
Staphylococcus epidermidis (BL−)	Penicillin	Cefazolin, clindamycin
Staphylococcus epidermidis (BL+)	Oxacillin	Cefazolin, clindamycin
Staphylococcus epidermidis (methicillin resistant)	Vancomycin	Teicoplanin,† daptomycin, ciprofloxacin, coumermycin,† rifampin, and aminoglycosides
Streptococcus faecalis	Ampicillin-gentamicin	Vancomycin
Gram-negative bacteria		
Pseudomonas aeruginosa	Ceftazidime	Imipenem, aztreonam, aminoglycosides, ticarcillin, and ciprofloxacin
Escherichia coli, Proteus mirabilis	Cefazolin	Cefamandole, cefoxitin, ampicillin (if sensitive)
Haemophilus influenzae	Cefamandole	Cefuroxime, ampicillin (if sensitive), trimethroprim-sulfamethazole
B. fragilis	Clindamycin or metronidazole	Cefoxitin

*BL(+ or −) beta-lactamase producer or nonproducer.
†Under investigation.
From Bergeron MG: The changing bacterial spectrum and antibiotic choices. *In* Deslauriers J, Lacquet LK (eds): Surgical Management of Pleural Diseases. St. Louis: CV Mosby, 1990, p. 197.

Chest Tube Drainage

Closed chest tube drainage is the recommended initial step in the management of either a complicated parapneumonic effusion or an empyema. It should be carried out early to prevent increased morbidity from the progression of the process. Light (1990, 1991) suggested that the criteria for its use are as follows: 1) presence of gross pus in the pleural space, 2) bacterial organisms visible on Gram stain of the pleural fluid, 3) a pleural fluid glucose level less than 50 mg/dl, and 4) a pleural fluid level pH below 7.00 and 0.15 units lower than the arterial pH. Chest tube drainage should also be considered if the pH is below 7.20 or if the pleural fluid LDH level is above 1000 IU/L.

When the fluid is grossly purulent, no attempt should be made to remove all of the pus by the thoracentesis. Removal requires immediate placement of a chest tube in the most dependent area of the empyema cavity. Although a small pig-tailed catheter is frequently used by the interventional radiologist, particularly when the fluid is thin, it is more appropriate to use a large-bore No. 28 to 32 F chest tube in patients who require drainage. The chest tube is connected to an underwater seal suction system to establish closed drainage. A moderate level of suction is generally applied.

When this approach is successful, the purulent fluid is evacuated and the lung expands to obliterate the pleural space. The clinical signs of infection subside and the overall condition of the patient improves. Repeat chest radiographs in 48 to 72 hours confirms a decrease in the amount of fluid and beginning re-expansion of the lung. The chest tube may be removed when the drainage is clear and is less than 50 ml in amount for a 24-hour period, and when the chest radiograph shows complete expansion of the lung; this may occur in 4 to 10 days after initiation of therapy. When a small residual pocket remains, its actual size should be evaluated by a sinogram with contrast medium administered through the chest tube. When the pocket is larger than the tube and enough time has elapsed for adhesions to have developed to seal off the pocket from the remainder of the pleural space, the chest tube is cut and converted to open drainage. The chest tube should be secured in place to prevent it from being dislodged either out of or into the residual cavity. This is best done by placing a safety pin through the tube and securing the pin by tape to the skin of the chest wall. In a number of days to a few weeks, the cavity is completely obliterated and the tube can be removed.

If the situation fails to improve within 48 hours after the initial placement of the chest tube, either inappropriate antibiotic therapy has been used or loculation of the empyema has occurred within the pleural space resulting in inadequate drainage. The antibiotics are changed as necessary and a CT scan or a sonogram of the chest should be obtained. When loculation of the empyema is demonstrated, the surgeon has a number of choices as to the next step in the management of the patient. Fibrinolytic therapy, thoracoscopy or video-assisted thoracoscopy to break up the loculations, or early open surgical debridement of the empyema cavity are the three major options.

Therapy of Loculated Empyemas

Fibrinolytic Enzymes

The use of fibrinolytic enzymes in the management of thoracic empyemas was suggested by Tillett and Sherry in 1949. These authors reported that the instillation of streptokinase and streptodornase aided in the evacuation of thick pus and fibrin from the empyema cavity by breaking up any loculations that were present. Creech (1953) and Bergh (1977) and their associates confirmed the value of the use of these enzymes. The use of this combination of agents, however, was usually associated with pyogenic and adverse systemic reactions — some of these toxic effects could be alleviated by the oral use of salicylate before instillation of the enzymes — and the results of the use of the enzymes were less satisfactory in most institutions than those reported in the literature. Consequently, the use of these agents fell into disfavor. With the development of a more purified streptokinase enzyme, however, and experience with the use of urokinase as a fibrinolytic agent, the role of these two enzymes as adjunctive measures in the management of loculated empyemas has been reported with greater frequency in the late 1980s and early 1990s. Mitchell (1989), Willsie-Ediger (1990), Aye (1991), and Rosen (1993) and their associates reported success rates of up to 80% with the use of streptokinase in patients with loculated empyemas, despite the fact that in most series, only small chest catheters were used for chest drainage. Similar salutatory results — success rates of 90% — were reported with the use of urokinase by Moulton (1989) and Lee (1991) and their colleagues.

The instillation of the fibrinolytic agent into the empyema space is accomplished by placing the patient in the lateral decubitus position with the affected side up; the chest tube is clamped, and the agent is instilled into the tube using a syringe and a 21-gauge needle. The tube remains clamped for 6 to 8 or more hours. The tube is then unclamped and the system is returned to suction drainage. The instillation is done daily for 5 to 7 days as a rule depending on the patient's response (Fig. 55–4). The recommended dose of streptokinase is 250,000 units in 100 ml of 0.9% saline; for urokinase, the dose is 100,000 units in 100 ml of 0.9% saline. The use of streptokinase may still be associated with postinstillation fever and chest pain and occasionally other toxic systemic symptoms. Specific IgG antistreptokinase antibodies may occur with intrapleural instillation, which may be of some significance to the patient at a later date. On the other hand, urokinase is both nonantigenic and nonpyrogenic. Because of these aforementioned factors, the use of urokinase, despite the limited number of treated cases reported, may be the

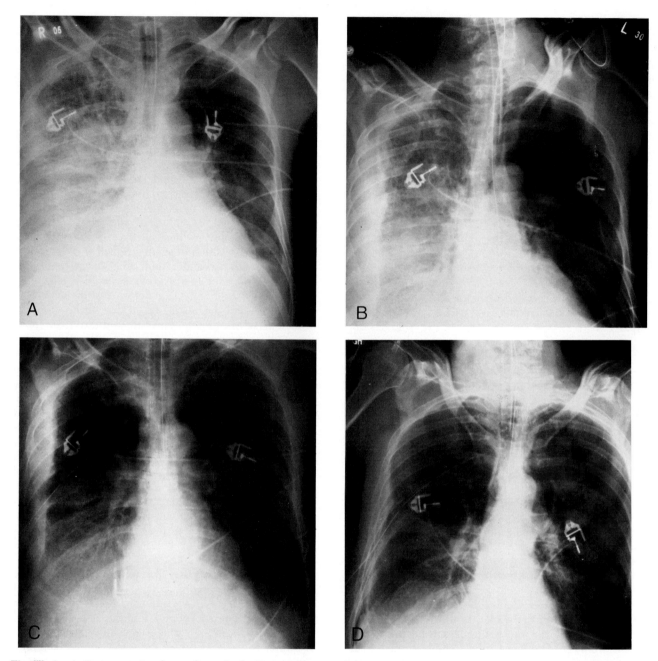

Fig. 55–4. *A,* Posteroanterior chest radiograph of a 50-year-old man with *H. Influenzae* pneumonia reveals diffuse parapneumonic effusion. *B,* Patient's condition became worse despite cefamandole therapy. Chest radiograph reveals the persistence of the pleural fluid with possible loculated collection laterally. Thoracentesis revealed the presence of a "complicated" effusion. *C,* Chest tube thoracostomy was carried out with some clearing of the effusion, but loculated collection persisted laterally. *D,* Chest radiograph reveals almost complete clearing of pleural involvement 5 days after instillation of streptokinase into the pleural space.

enzymatic agent of choice for the patient with a loculated, non- or poorly draining empyema.

The response to therapy and subsequent management of the chest tube is that as described previously. It is to be emphasized that the use of the fibrinolytic enzymes is an adjunctive measure to improve the drainage of the empyema cavity and does not change the underlying principle of the use of a closed tube thoracostomy in the management of an empyema.

Thoracoscopic and Video-Assisted Thoracoscopy

Hutter and associates (1985) and Ridley and Braim-bridge (1991) recommended the use of thoracoscope-aided debridement and irrigation for the management of loculated empyemas, although it was successful in only 60% of patients. At present, a video-assisted thoracoscopic surgical — VATS — approach has come into favor in place of thoracoscopy alone in managing complicated empyemas. Mack and colleagues (1992) recommended early — within 3 weeks of onset — debridement and decortication by the VATS approach. This method has been used successfully several times at Northwestern University, although occasionally it has been technically difficult to completely free all areas. Apparently VATS debridement should be reserved for those patients in whom enzymatic therapy has failed.

Thoracotomy

When loculations are initially apparent, some surgeons have resorted to early limited thoracotomy for removal of the fibrinous debris and the purulent exudate as well as for the placement of the chest tube for subsequent drainage. This approach has been used successfully in adults by Mayo and McElvein (1966), as well as by Hoover (1986) and Van Way (1988) and their associates, and in children by Raffensperger and colleagues (1982). The aggressive approach would seem best suited for children who tolerate the long-term effects of pleural disease poorly. Rosen and associates (1993), however, reported excellent results with the use of intrapleural streptokinase in pediatric patients.

Management of Incomplete Lung Re-expansion

Unfortunately at times, either because of delay in treatment, or failure thereof, or the late recognition of the empyema, the inflammatory process has progressed to the organization stage. The occurrence of a complicating bronchopleural fistula also usually results in progression to this organization — chronic — stage.

The incidence of the progression to this stage is variable, but it is less than 5% in well-managed patients. Because of the thick inelastic peel on the visceral pleura, the underlying compressed, atelectatic lung is unable to re-expand. As a consequence, a persistent cavity of greater or lesser size remains and the empyema remains unresolved. A major surgical procedure is then required. The procedures are empyemectomy, standard surgical decortication or one of its modifications, and rarely, in the case of a parapneumonic empyema, a muscle flap transposition or a thoracoplasty. Initially, open drainage of the persistent pleural pocket is carried out, unless an empyemectomy of a suitable, small, residual empyema is to be attempted.

Open Drainage

One of two methods can be used to obtain satisfactory open drainage. The first involves simple rib resection, in which segments of one to three ribs overlying the lowest part of the empyema cavity are resected and a large-bore chest tube is inserted into the empyema cavity; this tube is often initially connected to the appropriate underwater seal drainage apparatus and later converted to open drainage. When this technique is used, the pocket to be drained must be located accurately radiographically. The tube should be placed dependently and back no further than the posterior

axillary line. If the tube is not dependent, a successful outcome is rarely seen.

The second method is the open flap procedure, as Elosser originally described in 1935 and also reported in 1969, which provides better drainage in that it creates a skin-lined fistula that provides drainage without tubes. This procedure is usually elected after closed tube thoracostomy drainage or simple rib resection when long-term open drainage is necessary. It is also useful when open tube drainage would be uncomfortable, such as when the tube would be located high in the axilla or in the paravertebral area. Symbas and colleagues (1971) modified the Elosser procedure, and made a significant advance in converting the original U-shaped flap to an inverted U-shaped flap.

In performing the open flap drainage procedure, the incision must be planned carefully to be effective. The inverted U-shaped flap of skin is 6 to 7 cm long with a base 6 to 8 cm wide. The base of the flap is parallel to the most dependent portion of the empyema cavity. The top of the inverted U-shaped flap is placed two to three intercostal spaces or ribs above the base of the cavity. The inverted U is performed by incising down through skin, subcutaneous tissue, and all muscles and fascia to the rib cage. Three inches of two to three ribs, including the periosteum, are resected. The tongue of the flap is completely debrided of all tissue, except underlying subcutaneous tissue. The underlying tongue is tacked down to the bottom of the empyema space, using #0 polydioxane suture. The margins of the flap are approximated with interrupted polydioxane suture to close the skin over the exposed rib ends.

Open flap drainage is easier to care for, and generally cleaner, than open tube drainage. The cavity is packed daily, depending on the rate of soilage. Pseudomonas infection frequently develops, and the use of packing soaked in 1% acetic acid provides good control of this organism.

Empyectomy

A small residual cavity can be excised completely without opening into the cavity. The technique as described by Morin and Petsikas (1990) is straightforward. The removal of the parietal peel is done mainly with blunt dissection in the plane of the endothoracic fascia. Posteriorly, at the junction of the chest wall and the mediastinum, care must be taken to avoid injuring the posterior mediastinal structures such as the aorta, the esophagus, the azygos vein, and, superiorly, the vagus and phrenic nerves. The visceral peel can be removed with meticulous dissection using a combination of blunt and sharp dissection to achieve complete resection of the peel with minimal lung trauma. As this step is completed, the lung expands and regains its full volume. The thoracic incision is closed in the standard manner and closed tube drainage of the pleural space is carried out as with other thoracic procedures.

Decortication

The success of pulmonary decortication depends primarily on three factors: 1) the pleural irritation or inflammation results in a fibroelastic "peel" that traps the lung; 2) the visceral pleura remains relatively normal; and 3) the lung must be expansile so that the space can be obliterated by pulmonary re-expansion when decortication is complete. The technique of decortication is described in Chapter 58. On entering the chest, the decision is made whether both the parietal and visceral pleural peels need to be removed, or whether decortication can be limited to the visceral pleura. In general, only the visceral peel must be removed in the early phases of chronic empyema. If a rigid, thickened parietal pleura restricts the mobility of the thoracic cage, it should be removed as well. Generally, an extrapleural dissection is then required. If both the parietal pleura and the visceral peel are to be removed, the practical approach is to open the empyema cavity, evacuate the contents, define its limits, and then decorticate the lung.

When a chronic pathologic process is present or the underlying lung disease prevents lung re-expansion, complete obliteration of the pleural space by decortication cannot be accomplished. Successful obliteration of the persistent space may be accomplished by combining the decortication with a small modified thoracoplasty or a muscle flap transposition. In this situation, a small modified two- or three-rib extraperiosteal thoracoplasty can be performed. To close the remaining pleural space, however, a muscle flap transposition of serratus anterior or latissimus dorsi can be done with excellent results. The technique is discussed in Chapter 56. Several modifications of standard decortication to permit eradication of a longstanding chronic empyema with a collapsed lung that will not readily expand were suggested by Iioka (1985) and Tatsumura (1990) and their colleagues. The Sawamura operation described by Iioka and associates (1985) (see Chapter 44) and the modified decortication described by Tatsumura and colleagues (1990) are similar, except in the former only the curetted, cleaned-out empyema space is drained postoperatively, whereas in the latter, both the empyema space and the newly created space between the chest wall and the parietal peel are drained. Fortunately, the aforementioned procedures are rarely needed in the management of a chronic parapneumonic empyema.

Thoracoplasty

Thoracoplasty in the treatment of parapneumonic empyema is rare. The technique is described in Chapter 44. A thoracoplasty should not be performed unless it is absolutely necessary, because space obliteration by muscle flap transposition is thought to produce less late morbidity for the patient. Previously, patients with empyematous spaces unresponsive to decortication underwent a standard thoracoplasty, either the standard extrapleural type or one of the Schede type. In the latter procedure, all underlying ribs and intercostal structures and the parietal pleura and peel are removed to allow the space to fill in with granulation tissue.

MORBIDITY AND MORTALITY

The morbidity of a promptly recognized and adequately treated parapneumonic empyema is low. Blasco and associates (1990) reported satisfactory resolution in 93% of patients treated with antibiotics and drainage; only 5% of their patients required a major surgical procedure. In patients who develop loculated empyemas, however, the morbidity is increased, as noted by Light (1990) and others. The presence of alcoholism, debility, drug addiction, immunosuppression, and other serious co-morbid conditions, as well as delayed recognition of the empyema, increases the chance of failure of initial therapy.

The mortality rate is affected similarly by the aforementioned conditions. Uncontrolled sepsis is a frequent cause of death. In the series of Blasco and associates (1990), the mortality rate was 2%. This rate is lower than that reported by Leblanc and Tucker (1984) and Jess and colleagues (1984): 15 and 33%, respectively. In these two reports, however, not all the empyemas were parapneumonic nor were all the deaths related to the effects of the empyema. In the series reported by Leblanc and Tucker, only 4% of the deaths were attributed to sepsis.

REFERENCES

Ali I, Unruh H: Management of empyema thoracis. Ann Thorac Surg 50:355, 1990.

Andrews NC, et al: Management of nontuberculous empyema: A statement of the subcommittee on surgery. Am Rev Respir Dis 85:935, 1962.

Aye RW, Forese DP, Hill LD: Use of purified streptokinase in empyema and hemothorax. Am J Surg 161:560, 1991.

Bartlett JG, et al: Bacteriology of empyema. Lancet 1:338, 1974.

Bergeron MG: The infected pleural space: The changing spectrum and antibiotic choices. In Deslauriers J, Lacquet LK (eds): Thoracic Surgery: Surgical Management of Pleural Diseases. St Louis: CV Mosby, 1990, p 197.

Bergh NP, et al: Intrapleural streptokinase in the treatment of haemothorax and empyema. Scan J Thorac Cardiovasc Surg 11:265, 1977.

Blasco E, Paris F, Padilla J: Acute postpneumonic empyema treated by intercostal tube drainage with suction and pleural washing but without rib resection. In Deslauriers J, Lacquet LK (eds): Thoracic Surgery: Surgical Management of Pleural Diseases. St Louis: CV Mosby, 1990, p 220.

Creech O, et al: The intrathoracic use of streptokinase-streptodornase. Am Surg 19:128, 1953.

Elosser L: An operation for tuberculous empyema. Surg Gynecol Obstet 60:1096, 1935.

Elosser L: An operation for tuberculous empyema. Ann Thorac Surg 5:355, 1969.

Hoover EL, et al: Reappraisal of empyema thoracis. Chest 90:511, 1986.

Hutter JA, Harari D, Braimbridge MV: The management of empyema thoracis by thoracoscopy and irrigation. Ann Thorac Surg 39:517, 1985.

Iioka S, et al: Surgical treatment of chronic empyema: A new one-stage operation. J Thorac Cardiovasc Surg 90:179, 1985.

Jess P, Bryntz S, Moller AF: Mortality in thoracic empyema. Scand J Thorac Cardiovasc Surg *18*:85, 1984.

Leblanc KA, Tucker WY: Empyema of the thorax. Surg Gynecol Obstet *158*:66, 1984.

Lee KS, et al: Treatment of thoracic multiloculated empyemas with intracavitary urokinase: A prospective study. Radiology *179*:771, 1991.

LeRoux BT, Dodds TC: A Portfolio of Chest Radiographs. Edinburgh: E and S Livingston, 1964.

Light RW: Pleural Diseases. Philadelphia: Lea & Febiger, 1983.

Light RW: Definitions, pathology and significance of parapneumonic effusions. *In* Deslauriers J, Lacquet LK (eds): Thoracic Surgery: Surgical Management of Pleural Diseases. St. Louis, CV Mosby, 1990, p 173.

Light RW: Management of parapneumonic effusions. Chest *100*:892-893, 1991.

Light RW, et al: Parapneumonic effusions. Am J Med *69*:507, 1980.

Mack MJ, et al: Present role of thoracoscopy in the diagnosis and treatment of diseases of the chest. Ann Thorac Surg *54*:403, 1992.

Mayo P, McElvein RB: Early thoracotomy for pyogenic empyema. Ann Thorac Surg *2*:649, 1966.

Miller JI Jr: Infections of the pleura. *In* Shields TW (ed): General Thoracic Surgery. 3rd Ed. Philadelphia: Lea & Febiger, 1989, p. 633.

Mitchell ME, et al: Intrapleural streptokinase in management of parapneumonic effusions: Report of series and review of literature. J Fla Med Assoc *76*:1019, 1989.

Morin JE, Petsikas D: Surgical technique: Empyemectomy. *In* Deslauriers J, Lacquet LK (eds): Thoracic Surgery: Surgical Management of Pleural Diseases. St. Louis: CV Mosby, 1990, p 277.

Moulton JS, Moore PT, Mencini RA: Treatment of loculated pleural effusions with transcatheter intracavitary urokinase. AJR Am J Roentgenol *153*:941, 1989.

Raffensperger JG, et al: Mini-thoracotomy and chest tube insertion for children with empyema. J Thorac Cardiovasc Surg *84*:477, 1982.

Read CA, Sporn TA, Yeager H: Parapneumonic empyema: A pitfall in diagnosis. Chest *101*:1712, 1992.

Ridley PD, Braimbridge MV: Thoracoscopic debridement and pleural irrigation in the management of empyema thoracis. Ann Thorac Surg *51*:461, 1991.

Rosen H, et al: Intrapleural streptokinase as adjunctive treatment for persistent empyema in pediatric patients. Chest *103*:1190, 1993.

Stark DD, et al: Differentiating lung abscess and empyema: Radiography and computed tomography. AJR Am J Roentgenol *141*:163, 1983.

Swenson SJ, et al: Radiology in the intensive-care unit. Mayo Clin Proc *66*:396, 1991.

Symbas PN, et al: Nontuberculous pleural empyema in adults. Ann Thorac Surg *12*:69, 1971.

Taryle DA, et al: Antibiotic concentrations in human parapneumonic effusions. J Antimicrob Chemother *7*:171, 1981.

Tatsumura T, et al: A new technique for one-stage radical eradication of longstanding chronic thoracic empyema. J Thorac Cardiovasc Surg *99*:410, 1990.

Tillett WS, Sherry S: The effect in patients of streptococcal fibrinolysin (streptokinase) and streptococcal desoxyribonuclease on fibrinous, purulent and sanguinous pleural effusions. J Clin Invest *28*:173, 1949.

Van Way C, Narrod J, Hopeman A: The role of early limited thoracotomy in the treatment of empyemas. J Thorac Cardiovasc Surg *96*:436, 1988.

Willsie-Ediger SK, et al: Use of intrapleural streptokinase in the treatment of thoracic empyema. Am J Med Sci *30*:296, 1990.

CHAPTER 56

POSTSURGICAL EMPYEMAS

Joseph I. Miller, Jr.

The second most frequent cause of empyema is the postsurgical development of infection in the pleural space following surgery of the esophagus, lungs, or mediastinum (Table 56–1). This accounts for 20% of all cases of empyema. It most frequently follows pneumonectomy, occurring in 2 to 12% of patients. It may occur in 1 to 3% of patients following lobectomy. LeRoux and associates (1986) reports that, in 8 to 11% of patients, the preceding lesion causing an empyema thoracis is an unrecognized subphrenic abscess in the patient who has undergone an abdominal, urologic, or pelvic operation. Empyema may occur secondary to a spontaneous pneumothorax with a persistent bronchopleural fistula; it may occur following parasitic infection or secondary to retained foreign bodies in the bronchial tree, or it may have a number of miscellaneous causes. The etiology of empyema in 215 patients is given in Table 56–2.

Factors that may promote the development of a postsurgical empyema are listed in Table 56–3.

Table 56–1. Etiology of Surgical Empyema

I. Postresectional
   A. Post open lung biopsy or wedge resection
   B. Postsegmentectomy
   C. Postlobectomy
   D. Postpneumonectomy
II. Infection Secondary to General or Thoracic Surgical Procedures or Intra-abdominal complications
   A. Gastric or pancreatic
   B. Esophageal
   C. Cardiac
   D. Pulmonary
   E. Others
      1. Perforated intra-abdominal viscus
         a. Duodenal ulcer
         b. Diverticulum of the colon
         c. Appendiceal abscess
      2. Other causes of peritonitis

Table 56–2. Etiology of Empyema in 215 Patients

Event or State	Number	Percent
Pulmonary infection	122	57
Following surgical procedures	42	20
Following trauma	13	6
Spontaneous pneumothorax	7	3
Esophageal perforation	5	2
Following thoracentesis	4	2
Subdiaphragmatic infection	4	2
Undetermined	18	8
	215	100

Compiled from Snider GL, Saleb SS: Empyema of thorax in adults: review of 105 cases. Chest 54:12, 1968, and Hall DP, Elkin RG: Empyema thoracis: a review of 110 cases. Am Rev Respir Dis 88:785, 1963.

Table 56–3. Factors That Promote Development of Postsurgical Empyema

Delay in diagnosis
Improper choice of antibiotics
Loculation or encapsulation by a dense inflammatory reaction
Presence of a bronchopleural fistula
Foreign body in the pleural space
Chronic infection
Entrapment of lung by thick visceral peel
Inadequate previous drainage or premature removal of a tube.

POSTSURGICAL EMPYEMA — NONRESECTIONAL

The development of nonresectional thoracic surgical empyema is related to the predisposing cause. It may follow esophageal surgery with resultant leak into the pleural space; it may develop subsequent to subdiaphragmatic surgery on the stomach, pancreas, or spleen with the accumulation of fluid in the subdiaphragmatic space. It may occur subsequent to rupture of an infected pleural bleb or secondary to lung abscess.

Infection in the pleural space unrelated to a pulmonary resection can generally be treated in the same manner as a nonsurgical empyema with correction of the underlying cause, appropriate antibiotics, and drainage with closed chest tube thoracostomy.

EMPYEMA AFTER RESECTION

Empyema that complicates pulmonary resection must be considered separately from empyema that occurs spontaneously or after trauma. When empyema complicates a pulmonary resection that is less than a pneumonectomy, the ability of the remaining lung to fill the pleural space after management of the empyema by drainage or decortication, and thereby to obliterate the pleural space, depends on the state of the remaining lung and its location, apical or basal. Empyema after upper lobectomy nearly always requires more than simple drainage, which nearly always suffices after lower lobectomy. After pneumonectomy, the empyema space is inevitably large and nearly always permanent. In these circumstances, alternative methods of treatment include sterilization, permanent drainage, thoracoplasty, and obliteration of the space by muscle flap transposition.

The incidence of empyema after pulmonary resection varies with the indications for the resection — inflammatory or neoplastic disease, with or without preoperative radiation. With resection for pulmonary tuberculosis, sputum conversion having been achieved, the incidence of bronchopleural fistula with empyema in the series Lynn (1958) reported was 6.7% after lobectomy. When sputum was still positive for acid-fast organisms, Teixera (1968) reported it was 10%.

With pneumonectomy, as opposed to lesser resections, LeRoux and associates (1986) reported that the incidence of empyema varies between 2 and 13%. When pneumonectomy is completed through an empyema, the incidence of continued pleural infection is 45%.

Although empyema may occur at any time postoperatively, even years later, most empyemas develop in the early postoperative period. The pleural space may be contaminated at the time of pulmonary resection, with the development of a bronchopleural or esophagopleural fistula, or from blood-borne sources. After pulmonary resection, less than a pneumonectomy, empyema occurs more often when the pleural space is incompletely filled by expansion of the remaining lung, mediastinal shift, and elevation of the diaphragm. Symptoms and signs vary, and if resection was performed for neoplastic disease, they may be difficult to distinguish from those caused by dissemination of tumor. The possibility of empyema must be considered in any patient with clinical features of infection after pulmonary resection. Expectoration of serosanguineous liquid and purulent discharge from the wound or the drain sites is almost diagnostic. On the radiograph of the chest, there is usually a pleural opacity, with or without a fluid level, when resection has been less than a pneumonectomy. After pneumonectomy, a fall in the fluid level early postoperatively, or the appearance of a new fluid level when the pneumonectomy site was uniformly opaque, strongly suggests an infected pleural space with bronchopleural fistula. The timing of surgical intervention and the type of operative procedure undertaken are tailored to the individual patient. An algorithm for the management of postresectional empyema is given in Figure 56–1.

General Principles of Treatment

When the diagnosis of postresectional empyema, with or without a bronchopleural fistula, is made, surgical drainage by closed chest tube thoracostomy and institution of appropriate antibiotic therapy is crucial. Once adequate drainage has been established and the patient stabilized — usually in 10 to 14 days, the course of management can be determined. If a bronchopleural fistula is present, the fistula should be closed by a

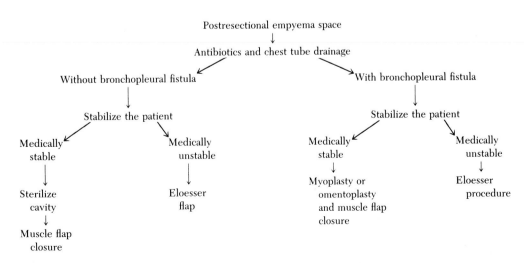

Fig. 56–1. Management of postresectional empyema.

myoplasty or omentoplasty, followed by single-stage muscle flap closure of the remaining space. If the patient is medically unstable, the closed chest tube thoracostomy can be converted to open drainage by an Eloesser procedure.

If the patient has only an empyema space without a bronchopleural fistula, the cavity is sterilized by irrigation with the appropriate antibiotic solution, as determined by the antibiotic sensitivities of the chest tube drainage, and a single-stage muscle flap closure of the remaining cavity is performed. A complete discussion of muscle flap closure is given later in this chapter. If the patient is medically unstable, closed chest tube thoracostomy can be converted to an open Eloesser flap.

Postpneumonectomy Empyema

Postpneumonectomy empyema remains a problem. It is associated with a bronchopleural fistula in approximately 40% of patients, and in only 20% of patients does the bronchopleural fistula close spontaneously. One of the most important advances in the treatment of this complication was the report by Clagett and Geraci (1963) in which they described rib resection with antibiotic irrigation and closure of the space in 6 to 8 weeks. Stafford and Clagett (1972) reported a success rate of 75 to 88% in using this method in sterilization of the empyema and permanent closure. My own experience with this method has not achieved that success rate. When the offending organism is *Staphylococcus aureus*, there is a fair chance of success, but when multiple bacterial organisms are present, the rate of success is only about 20%.

Figure 56–2 presents an algorithm for treatment of the postpneumonectomy empyema space. Once the diagnosis of postpneumonectomy empyema, with or without bronchopleural fistula, has been established,

prompt pleural drainage by closed chest tube thoracostomy is mandatory. Chest tube thoracostomy is continued until the mediastinum becomes stabilized, generally requiring approximately 2 weeks. Thereafter, open drainage or another modality of therapy for the empyema space can be undertaken safely without shift of the mediastinum. Once the patient is medically stable and has entered into the chronic phase at 3 to 4 weeks, if no bronchopleural fistula is present, a modified Clagett procedure is performed. A second small chest tube is inserted into the second intercostal space, and a continuous inflow-outflow irrigation system is established through the pleural cavity. The irrigant is based on antibiotic sensitivities to the pleural drainage. This is generally 2 g of cephalosporin in 500 cc of D_5W, running at a rate of 50 cc an hour through the inflow catheter, with continuous drainage through the outflow catheter. Occasionally, if gram-negative organisms are present, I use 0.25% neomycin as the irrigant. This method achieves sterilization of the space in approximately 50% of patients. If the method is successful and the return irrigant is negative on 3 consecutive days after 2 weeks of irrigation, the chest tubes can be removed, and pleural fluid is allowed to reaccumulate to fill the remaining space. If the modified Clagett technique fails, a complete muscle flap closure of the pneumonectomy space can be performed.

If a patient with a postpneumonectomy empyema has a bronchopleural fistula, it is likewise treated during the acute phase with closed chest tube thoracostomy, with conversion to open drainage at the appropriate time when mediastinal stabilization has occurred. If the fistula closes, one can attempt the aforementioned modified Clagett sterilization of the cavity. In the patient in whom the bronchopleural fistula persists, the fistula and space are then managed by transposition of muscle flaps into

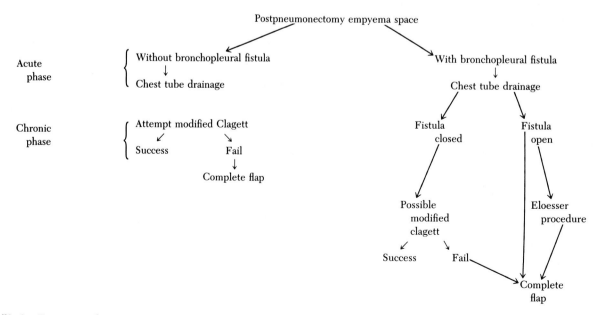

Fig. 56–2. Treatment of postpneumonectomy empyema space.

the empyema space, as I and my associates (1984) reported.

Muscle Flap Closure of the Postpneumonectomy Empyema Space

I believe that the best way to treat a postpneumonectomy space is single-stage muscle flap closure, completely obliterating the pneumonectomy space by the transposition of the thoracic skeletal muscles.

Abrashanoff (1911) reported extrathoracic muscle transposition for closure of a bronchopleural fistula. Since then, muscle flaps have been used to obliterate spaces, close a bronchopleural fistula, and reinforce tracheobronchial and esophageal anastomosis. In the late 1970s, our group used extrathoracic muscle flaps to close bronchopleural fistula and postlobectomy empyema cavities, but not until 1980 did we attempt to fill an entire pneumonectomy space with muscle flaps.

Because of their excellent blood supply and ability by pedicle flap to reach almost any location in the pleural space, muscle flaps are ideal tissue to fill a contaminated space. The extrathoracic muscle flaps used in various combinations in our (1984) patients in order of frequency are the latissimus dorsi, the serratus anterior, the pectoralis major, the omentum, and the rectus abdominis. The percentage of flap coverage of normal pneumonectomy space in the adult by each flap is latissimus dorsi — 30 to 40%; serratus anterior — 10 to 15%; pectoralis major — 20 to 30%; pectoralis minor — 0 to 2%; omentum — 5 to 15%; and the rectus abdominis — 5 to 15%. These figures are based on clinical estimation of coverage at the time of operation and cadaver studies.

Extrathoracic muscle flaps require a route of entry when transposed into the thoracic cavity. Segments of rib, determined by the blood supply of the muscles (Fig. 56–3), are resected, to prevent kinking and constriction and consequent swelling and ischemia of the muscle when the muscle is transposed into the pleural space.

Specific Muscle Flaps and Omentum

Omentum. The omentum can be brought into the pleural space as a flap or a free graft. It is the flap of choice to cover an open bronchial stump because of the excellent vascular supply. Neovascularization is evident in the stump within 48 hours after placement of an omental flap around a closed stump. The omental flap is usually brought up through a separate anterior opening in the diaphragm and is laid over the bronchial stump; tacking sutures are placed around the flap (Fig. 56–4). Normally, I do not use this flap unless an open bronchial stump is present or there is not enough muscle available to fill the space.

Pectoralis Major. The pectoralis major flap is one of the two most commonly used extrathoracic muscle flaps. It has a dual blood supply from the predominant thoracoacromial artery to the major pedicle, and from the internal mammary to the major pedicle and secondary pedicles. It can be used as a reverse turnover flap or placed directly into the wound. It

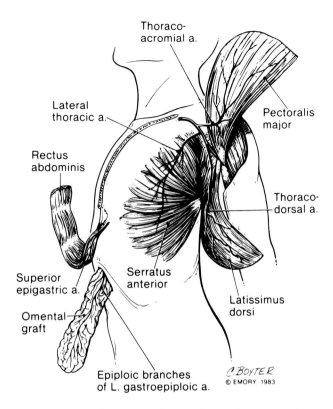

Fig. 56–3. Extrathoracic muscle flaps that can be used in closure of a postpneumonectomy empyema cavity. a = artery. *From Miller JI, et al: Single-stage complete muscle flap closure of the postpneumonectomy empyema space: a new method and possible solution to a disturbing complication. Ann Thorac Surg 38:227, 1984.*

requires a 5-cm rib resection for entry into the chest. It is the flap of choice for sternal infections and ranks after the latissimus dorsi and serratus anterior for the pleural space.

Latissimus Dorsi. The latissimus dorsi flap is the most commonly used flap for thoracic defects. Its predominant blood supply is from the thoracodorsal artery. It can be used as a turnover flap or placed directly into the wound. It may be brought through the incision or through a separate small rib resection.

Serratus Anterior. This is my second choice of flap for filling a pneumonectomy space and is particularly good for filling a small space. The entrance into the chest is through the primary chest incision.

Rectus Abdominis. In general, the rectus abdominis is used for closure of the lowest third of sternal defects. It is held in reserve for problems involving the pleural space in case a residual space remains. It is generally the last flap applied.

Surgical Technique of Single-Stage Complete Muscle Flap Closure

Single-stage muscle flap closure is performed for a persistent postpneumonectomy empyema space at approximately 3 months for benign disease and 6 months to 1 year for malignant disease. The six basic steps for complete flap closure are 1) appropriate antibiotics are

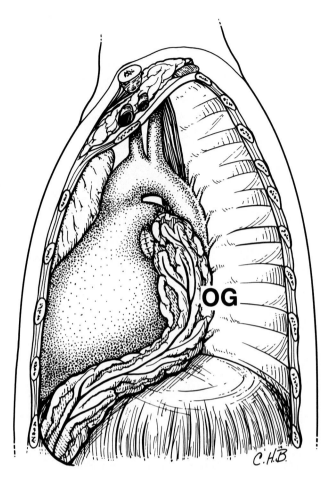

Fig. 56–4. The omental flap is brought through an anterior opening in the diaphragm and placed over the bronchial stump. OG = omental graft. *From* Miller JI, et al: Single-stage complete muscle flap closure of the postpneumonectomy empyema space: a new method and possible solution to a disturbing complication. Ann Thorac Surg 38:227, 1984.

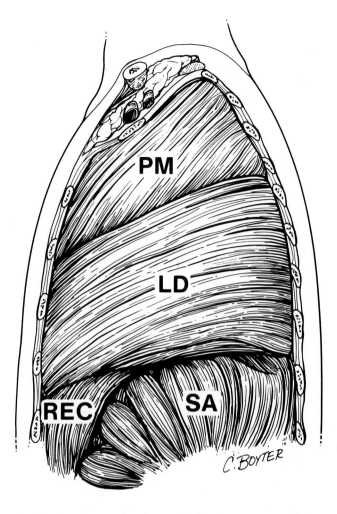

Fig. 56–5. An entire pleural space filled with muscle flaps and their usual anatomic location. PM = pectoralis major; LD = latissimus dorsi; REC = rectus abdominis; SA = serratus anterior. *From* Miller JI, et al: Single-stage complete muscle flap closure of the post-pneumonectomy empyema space: a new method and possible solution to a disturbing complication. Ann Thorac Surg 38:227, 1984.

given, based on the sensitivities of the pleural drainage; 2) the original incision is re-opened; 3) the cavity is debrided widely so that good granulation tissue is present; 4) a bronchopleural fistula is identified, and if present, the edges are freshened, and the fistula is closed, if technically possible. An omental flap is brought up through the anterior diaphragmatic incision (see Fig. 56–4) and tacked around the fistula with 3-0 Prolene sutures; 5) appropriate muscle flaps are then swung to fill the pleural space; and 6) the procedure is begun with a latissimus dorsi flap and followed with any necessary flaps to fill the entire space, depending on the anatomic location and size of the space. The filling of the entire pleural space is shown in Figure 56–5. Mathes and Nahai (1982) discussed in detail the technique of flap mobilization in their excellent work on muscle and musculocutaneous flaps.

All extrathoracic muscle flaps require a route of entry into the chest. The location of the opening is usually determined by the blood supply of the muscle and should be placed so that the blood supply is under no

tension after transposition. Generally, 4 to 5 cm of the appropriate rib is all that must be resected to allow for flap entry. Figure 56–6 shows the typical site of entry for the pectoralis major and latissimus dorsi flaps. The sine qua non for success with single-stage complete muscle flap closure is that the entire space must be filled. If a space is left, it is usually just beneath the fifth or sixth rib in the midaxillary line and can be closed by a short resection of the ribs over it without cosmetic deformity. Following transposition of the muscle flaps, the wound is closed primarily, and chest tubes are connected to Pleuro Vac suction for 7 to 10 days. Appropriate antibiotics are given.

The two predominant points in this surgical technique are that no residual space can be left and that a sufficient number of flaps must be available so that any intrathoracic space can be filled. To date, I have used this technique in over 35 patients, with only 6 — 17.2% — failures.

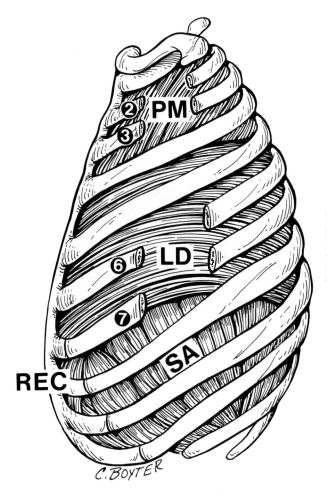

Fig. 56–6. Usual sites of rib resection for entrance of the pectoralis major (PM) and latissimus dorsi (LD) flaps into the pleural spaces. REC = rectus abdominis; SA = serratus anterior. *From* Miller JI, et al: Single-stage complete muscle flap closure of the postpneumonectomy empyema space: a new method and possible solution to a disturbing complication. Ann Thorac Surg 38:227, 1984.

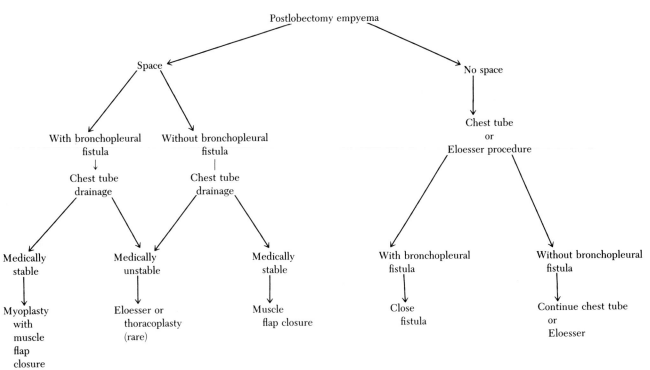

Fig. 56–7. Treatment of postlobectomy empyema.

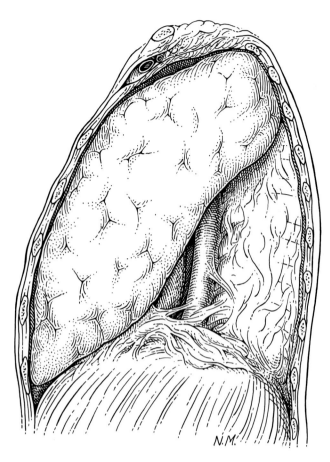

Fig. 56–8. A residual empyema cavity after a lower lobectomy.

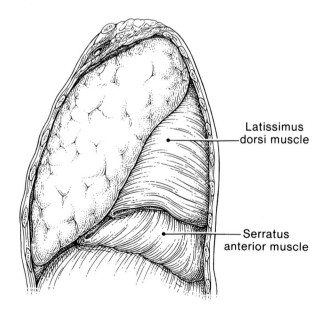

Latissimus dorsi muscle

Serratus anterior muscle

Fig. 56–9. Flap closure of a lower lobectomy empyema cavity with the latissimus dorsi and serratus anterior muscles.

Postresectional Lobectomy Empyema

Our group's algorithm for the treatment of the postresectional empyema space following lobectomy is given in Figure 56–7. The basic principles that apply to the pneumonectomy space apply to the management of the empyema space following resectional lobectomy. In general, a persistent lower lobectomy space (Fig. 56–8) can be easily closed and filled by application of the serratus anterior and latissimus dorsi flap. This is illustrated in Figure 56–9. If a bronchopleural fistula is present, this is closed by myoplasty, using a pedicled intercostal muscle flap, followed by obliteration of the space with the latissimus dorsi and serratus anterior muscles. If an upper lobe space persists following lobectomy, with or without bronchopleural fistula, the fistula is closed with a pedicle intercostal muscle flap, followed by a reverse pectoralis major turnover flap into the superior space through the second intercostal space.

REFERENCES

Abrashanoff: Plastische Methode der Schliessung von Fistelgangen, welche von inneren Organen kommen. Zentralbl Cir 38:186, 1911.

Clagett OT, Geraci JE: A procedure for the management of postpneumonectomy empyema. J Thorac Cardiovasc Surg 45:141, 1963.

LeRoux BT, et al: Suppurative diseases of the lung and pleural space. Part 1. Empyema thoracis and lung abscess. Curr Probl Surg 23:6, 1986.

Lynn RB: The bronchial stump. J Thorac Surg 36:70, 1958.

Mathes SJ, Nahai F: Clinical applications for Muscle and Musculocutaneous Flaps. St Louis: CV Mosby, 1982.

Miller JI, et al: Single-stage complete muscle flap closure of the postpneumonectomy empyema space: a new method and possible solution to a disturbing complication. Ann Thorac Surg 38:227, 1984.

Stafford EG, Clagett OT: Postpneumonectomy empyema: neomycin instillation and definitive closure. J Thorac Cardiovasc Surg 63:771, 1972.

Teixera J: The present status of thoracic surgery in tuberculosis. Dis Chest 53:19, 1968.

READING REFERENCES

Beck C: Thoracoplasty in America and visceral pleurectomy with report of a case. JAMA 28:58, 1897.

Bowditch HI: Paracentesis thoracis: an analysis of 25 cases of pleuritic effusion. Am Med Monthly p. 3, 1853.

Eggers C: Radical operation for chronic empyema. Ann Surg 77:327, 1923.

Fowler GR: A case of thoracoplasty for the removal of a large cicatricial fibrous growth from the interior of the chest, the result of an old empyema. Med Record 44:938, 1893.

Graham EA, Bell RD: Open pneumothorax: its relation to the treatment of acute empyema. Am J Med Sci 156:939, 1918.

Hewitt C: Drainage for empyema. Br Med J 1:317, 1876.

Hippocrates: In Major Classic Descriptions of Disease. Springfield, IL: Charles C Thomas, 1965.

Hood RM: History of empyema management. In Hood RM (ed): Surgical Diseases of the Pleura and Chest. Philadelphia: WB Saunders, 1986.

Lawrence GH: Empyema. In Lawrence GH (ed): Problems of the Pleural Space. Philadelphia: WB Saunders, 1983.

Trousseau A: Lectures on clinical medicine delivered at the Hotel-Dieu, Paris. McCormick JR (trans). London: The New Sydenham Society 3:198, 1870.

CHAPTER 57

TUBERCULOUS AND FUNGAL INFECTIONS OF THE PLEURA

Walter L. Barker and Thomas W. Shields

TUBERCULOSIS OF THE PLEURA

Tuberculous effusions, according to Hood (1965), are rare and account for only 1 to 3% of exudative pleural effusions. They are a sequel to a primary parenchymal infection in which a subpleural foci of disease ruptures into and thus involves the pleural space or, as De Meester (1983) suggested, from shedding of the bacilli into the pleural space from an involved hilar node or nodes. Delayed hypersensitivity appears to play an important role in the pathogenesis.

Myobacterial infection of the pleural surfaces and pleural space, on the other hand, occurs to a greater or lesser extent in most patients with postprimary pulmonary tuberculosis. Variable amounts of fine to dense adhesions occur between the two pleural surfaces over the area of parenchymal involvement. When the disease is uncontrolled, extension of the infection through the pleura and into the pleural space may result in granulomatous involvement of the pleural surface. Deposition of fibrous tissue between the two pleural layers may occur, which entraps the underlying lung. Calcification of parts of or of the entire rim of the fibrous peel may occur (Fig. 57–1). Lastly, and more devastating to the patient, is the secondary contamination of the involved pleural space by one or more pyogenic organisms resulting in a mixed tuberculous/pyogenic empyema. The pyogenic contamination occurs most often because of the development of a bronchopleural fistula, but occasionally, it develops as the result of inappropriate and unnecessary repeated attempts to drain a tuberculous pleural effusion. A thick fibrous peel containing many areas of necrotic grumous material is present and loculated fluid-containing spaces within the peel or residual pleural space may be observed. A loculated pyopneumothorax is occasionally observed. Almost all of the patients who develop this advanced pleural disease have extensive tuberculous as well as pyogenic infection of the under-

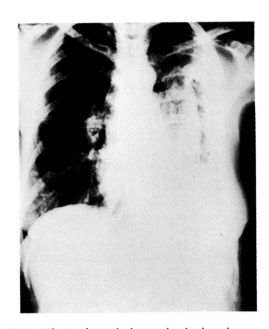

Fig. 57–1. Chest radiograph showing basal tuberculous empyema with a bronchopleural fistula. Extensive calcification in the wall is visible. *From* Langston HT, Barker WL, Graham AH: Pleural tuberculosis. J Thorac Cardiovasc Surg 54:511, 1967.

lying lung; the presence of a destroyed lobe or entire lung is a common feature.

Pleural involvement by tuberculosis has often been referred to as a tuberculous empyema. Because of the disparity in the presentations of pleural involvement, however, the definition of tuberculous empyema is difficult at best. In a strict sense, a tuberculous empyema must be a purulent effusion caused by the tubercle bacillus; it is questioned whether or not this actually ever occurs. Pleural involvement by tuberculosis, as noted, presents so many and varied aspects that the term tuberculous empyema should be discarded, and the infection should be simply referred to as pleural tuberculosis.

"Tuberculosis of the pleura" more often than not invokes the picture of a pleural effusion; however, tuberculosis may extend across the pleura without causing the formation of fluid or producing the classic appearance of pleural disease in the chest radiograph. It is thus difficult to segregate for study the various types of pleural tuberculosis in the classic sense. Because it is generally conceded that pleural tuberculosis is the result of extension of tuberculosis to the pleura from a subadjacent pulmonary lesion, the physician is concerned really with the impact that such extension — however manifested — has on the course and management of the underlying pulmonary tuberculosis. The addition of a pyogenic infection, as noted, often complicates the picture, and the superimposition of communication between pleura and bronchus compounds the patient's misery, as well as poses a further challenge to the patient's physician. Thus, if in addition to the pleural problems, one considers that the underlying lung is affected to a varying extent, a complex combination of possibilities immediately is apparent.

Clinical Presentations

Generally, four manifestations of pleural tuberculosis occur: 1) pure pleural tuberculosis, 2) pure pleural disease with mixed tuberculous/pyogenic infection, 3) pleuroparenchymal tuberculosis, and 4) mixed tuberculous/pyogenic pleural disease with parenchymal infection.

Pure Pleural Tuberculosis

In many parts of the world, tuberculosis remains the most common cause of pleural effusions. In the United States, the incidence is lower and more urban in distribution. In a series reported by Light and colleagues (1972), 13% of exudative pleural effusions in a hospital setting were related to tuberculosis.

The patients with a tuberculous effusion are usually young with recent skin tuberculin — PPD — test conversion and radiographic evidence of variable amounts of pleural fluid accumulation. The effusion is most often unilateral, and as many as one third of patients have an identifiable pulmonary infiltrate. This effusion may be obscured on the radiograph by the fluid accumulation, but it can be identified by computed tomography — CT, although the latter cannot usually identify tiny peripheral subpleural granulomas. The patient may be acutely or chronically ill. The former state is characterized by cough and chest pain; the latter by low grade fever, weakness, and weight loss. The effusion is exudative. Thoracentesis usually yields thin, opalescent, exudative fluid with a differential white cell count in excess of 50% lymphocytes and less than 10% eosinophils; mesothelial cells are uncommon — less than 5%. The pH and glucose studies are not of diagnostic significance, although both levels may be low. Elevated levels of adenosine deaminase — ADA — > 70 U/L or gamma-interferon and

are suggestive of the diagnosis. Smears for tubercle bacilli are most often negative and culture recovery of organisms is reported in only 20 to 30% of patients. A major diagnostic step is pleural needle biopsy. The demonstration of granulomata, caseating or not, is generally accepted as indicative of tuberculosis. Light (1983) reported that granulomata are present in 60 to 80% of patients. When parenchymal disease is present, cultures of the sputum or from gastric aspirates should be done. In the absence of demonstrable acid-fast organisms, these effusions are still considered tuberculous in origin. Tuberculous pleural effusions should be medically treated for at least 6 months to avoid the development of active parenchymal tuberculosis, to alleviate symptoms, and to prevent fibrothorax.

In 20 to 40% of patients with a tuberculous pleural effusion, the initial intermediate PPD skin test may be negative. In the absence of anergy or an immunocompromised host, however, the skin test becomes positive in 2 or at most 3 months. When the skin test is initially negative but the clinical course and characteristics of the pleural exudate suggest tuberculosis as the cause, despite the absence of confirmatory evidence of organisms or granulomata, the effusion is often termed "idiopathic." About 25% of the idiopathic exudates prove to be tuberculous. Initially, all "idiopathic" exudative effusions that meet the aforementioned criteria in young patients should be treated empirically. If a repeat skin test is negative at 2 or 3 months, antituberculous chemotherapy may be discontinued.

Only about 5 to 10% of patients with pure pleural tuberculosis develop active parenchymal disease if adequate antituberculosis therapy is initiated promptly. If untreated, although the effusion may resolve, most patients subsequently develop postprimary pulmonary tuberculosis.

Pure Pleural Disease with Mixed Tuberculous/Pyogenic Bacterial Flora

This category is unusual, because most instances of mixed infection are associated with underlying parenchymal disease. When it occurs in the absence of parenchymal disease, the mixed infection usually represents contamination from repeated thoracenteses or placement of ill-advised chest tubes.

Pleuroparenchymal Tuberculosis

Many patients present with combined parenchymal infiltrates, consolidation, and cavitation in association with extensive pleural fibrosis or fluid, or both (Fig. 57–2). These patients usually are ill. Ordinarily, the sputum and pleural aspirates are positive. The radiographs reveal parenchymal disease with pleural extension and even free fluid. The course of the disease and the goals of therapy are primarily directed to the management of the parenchymal processes.

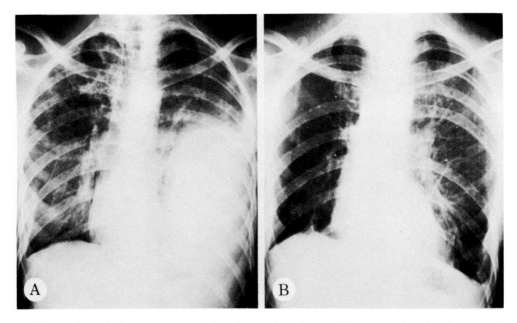

Fig. 57-2. *A,* Initial chest radiograph showing cavernous tuberculosis in the right apex, diffuse parenchymal infiltration, and a bilateral pleural process more extensive on the left than on the right. *B,* Radiograph appearance of the same patient after staged bilateral decortication and right upper lobectomy. *From* Cherniak NS, Barker WL: *In* Gordon BL (ed): Clinical Cardiopulmonary Physiology. 3rd Ed. New York: Grune & Stratton, 1969.

Mixed Tuberculous/Pyogenic Empyema with or without Parenchymal Disease and with or without Bronchopleural Fistula

These patients are symptomatic and may be extremely ill and toxic; occasionally, the patient is moribund. The mixed infection may result from contamination from repeated thoracenteses or ill-advised chest tube insertions, as stated previously, or, most often, from frank perforations of peripheral tuberculous cavities. The empyema is basically a pyogenic pleural process in a patient with pulmonary tuberculosis. The pulmonary tuberculosis often is far advanced and is associated with superimposed pyogenic or fungal infection. A destroyed lobe or entire lung is often present (Fig. 57-3).

Treatment

Medical Therapy

The basis of all tuberculosis therapy is proper medical management with antituberculosis chemotherapy. The drugs must be effective, used in proper combination and dosage, and maintained for sufficient time (see Chapter 78). Barring mycobacterial resistance, combinations of rifampin, ethambutol, and isoniazid — INH — are the mainstays of medical treatment. Resistant organisms may require as many as five drugs, including streptomycin, cycloserine, and pyrizinamide — PZA — to bring about bacteriologic control. In general, therapy should be continued for a minimum of 3 to 6 months or longer before considering any major surgical intervention.

Surgical Therapy

Because of the distortions that are incident to the presence of a space-occupying pleural lesion, as well as to its obscuring effects, some of the usual diagnostic studies are less reliable than those made in patients who do not have pleural disease. The following significant points in this regard need to be emphasized.

First, in determining the necessity for surgical intervention insofar as pleural residuals are concerned, the standard radiograph in the lateral projection is of utmost value. If obscuration by pleural disease is seen on the posteroanterior projection but is not recognized on the lateral projection, it can be surmised that the process is diffuse around the entire pleural sac and thus the thickness of the pleural peel is not great. If progressive clearing of the pleural process is seen on serial radiographs, and motion, as determined clinically, is returning to the chest wall, complete resolution of this process is likely, the benefits of decortication of the lung are doubtful, and surgical intervention is unnecessary.

If, on the other hand, the pleural shadow is seen as a localized lesion, particularly in the posteroinferior gutter where effusions are expected to be thickest by virtue of dependent accumulation, decortication is likely to be required even if some clearing has taken place. Such encapsulated pleural processes are not likely to resolve completely unless small at the outset.

Second, laminagrams in both the anteroposterior and lateral projections cannot be interpreted with the same accuracy as those made in patients whose disease is strictly pulmonary. This lack occurs because distortion

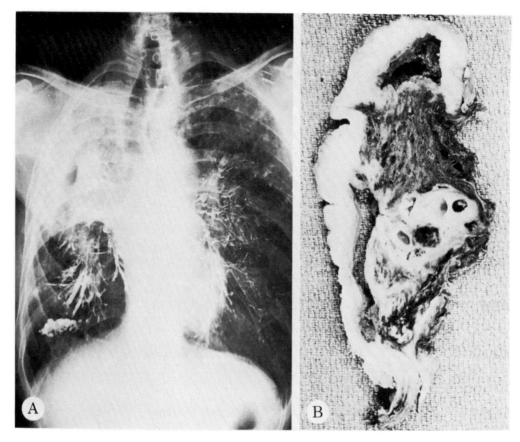

Fig. 57–3. *A,* Far-advanced pulmonary tuberculosis with severe right-sided pleural disease including empyema with bronchopleural fistula. The classic appearance of pleural effusion is not present. *B,* Cross section of pleuropneumonectomy specimen that has been removed. *From* Langston HT, Barker WL, Graham AH: Pleural tuberculosis. J Thorac Cardiovasc Surg 54:511, 1967.

and loss of volume in the lobes or segments results in shifting of boundaries, and also because of the obscuration by the pleural shadows themselves. Therefore, these studies are not indicated.

Third, bronchograms also are often of poor quality because of incomplete filling. The areas of collapsed and enfolded lung are prone to ventilate poorly and, thus, the contrast material has difficulty in entering the depths of the bronchial tree in such areas because of the poor ventilatory exchange. Blunting, "beading," and crowding of the branches of the bronchial tree are seen. Any bronchial diseases compatible with bronchiectasis should not be diagnosed in these patients unless the bronchographic findings are characteristic, and unmistakable.

Fourth, the CT scan, as reported by Pugatch and colleagues (1978), is the most appropriate examination in differentiating pleural and parenchymal lesions. Moreover, the status of the underlying lung — cavitary lesions, bronchiectasis, carnification, destroyed lung — can be evaluated readily by CT. Computed tomography is the most significant radiographic diagnostic procedure (Fig. 57–4).

Pure Pleural Tuberculosis

In most cases of pure pleural tuberculosis, treatment with careful thoracenteses and avoidance of tube tho-

racostomy in association with nutritional support and proper antituberculous chemotherapy resolves or significantly ameliorates most pleural residuals in about 3 months.

Decortication is considered when clinical toxicity is controlled and thoracentesis fails to yield fluid or to alter the radiographic picture. The lateral chest radiograph and, more recently, the CT scan of the chest is particularly informative in identifying significant "pockets," especially in the posterior basal gutter. Ill-defined and rapidly fading pleural shadows or "peels" usually clear spontaneously and do not justify surgery. We think that after 3 to 6 months of pharmacologic control, and with a pleural residual occupying one fourth to one third of the hemithorax, decortication should be carried out to avoid undue delays in resolution. Ignoring the localized residual pleural pocket subjects the patient to constant threat of local exacerbation consisting of thoracic aching or pain and systemic reaction with fever and clinical illness at varying intervals, not to mention perforation of the pleural exudate into the bronchus with spread of parenchymal disease occurring months or even years later. The dictum of our late colleague H.T. Langston was, "Do not put off simple decortication, today, for complicated pleuropneumonectomy, tomorrow." The technique of decortication is described in Chapter 58. In addition to obvious clinical and radiologic

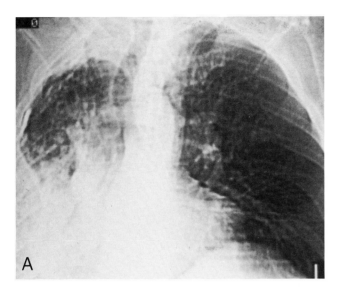
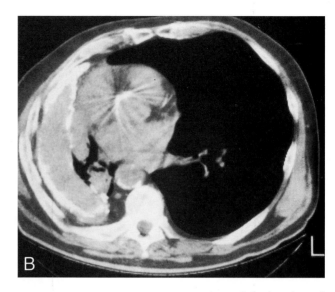

Fig. 57–4. *A*, Posteroanterior chest radiograph showing extensive pleuroparenchymal tuberculosis. *B*, CT scan shows shift of mediastinal structures to the right, empyema space with thickened calcified peel, and complete collapse of the adjacent lung.

benefits, functional improvement after a decortication can be significant.

Pure Pleural Disease with Mixed Tuberculous/Pyogenic Flora

Admittedly, this situation is unusual. The management is basically the same as with pure pleural tuberculosis but with the addition of proper antibiotic therapy. Clinical toxicity may mandate early closed tube thoracostomy or open drainage, especially if the drainage procedure can be considered definitive or if the pleural disease can be expected to heal before any operation that ultimately might be required. Indications for decortication are similar to those described for pure pleural tuberculosis (Fig. 57–5).

Pleuroparenchymal Tuberculosis

The presence of pleural and parenchymal residuals after appropriate antituberculous medication requires more complicated surgical programs. Medical therapy is extended to 6 to 12 months or more and is directed primarily toward the underlying parenchymal disease — cavities, infiltrates, carnification. Should the parenchymal disease clear, pleural residuals can be approached independently. When control of the parenchymal disease permits anatomic delineation of indicated surgical targets, surgery, including resection, resection/decortication, and even pleuropneumonectomy, is carried out, depending on the anatomic extent of disease. Surgical success is predicated on exchanging an actively infected pleural space for one that is fresh and merely contaminated. Antituberculosis drugs, antibiotics, local tissue and host immunity, and particularly complete excision of infected tissue contribute to ultimate success. When the pleural disease is of such extent as to require extrapleural pneumonectomy, however, we have recorded mortality rates of over 20% and an empyema rate of over 15% among the survivors.

At times, although no active underlying parenchymal disease is present, the lung is not re-expandable and resection is not indicated. In this situation, the use of various modifications of a decortication procedure have been suggested. Dupon (1990) reported the use of the Andrew's thoracomyopleuroplasty (1961) (see Chapter 44) in 56 patients with chronic tuberculous disease of the pleura with a low mortality and a satisfactory recovery rate. Iioka (1985) and Tatsumura (1990) and their colleagues suggested the use of a one-stage radical eradication of a longstanding chronic empyema in which the chest wall is left itact for patients with this clinical problem.

Mixed Tuberculous/Pyogenic Empyema with Parenchymal Disease With or Without a Bronchopleural Fistula

Mixed infections of the pleura — primarily a pyogenic infection — in association with significant parenchymal tuberculous disease are most often associated with bronchopleural fistulas, cavitary and bronchiectatic disease, carnification, and destroyed lobes or entire lung. These patients are the most severely ill and have the worst prognosis. Basic therapy still consists of antituberculosis drugs and appropriate antimicrobial therapy to address the pyogenic component. We believe, however, that even though antibiotic therapy can produce clinical remissions, it does not provide long-term control of such compounded pathologic states.

Similarly, we tend to avoid pleural drainage. If the patient is toxic with symptoms of associated large bronchial fistulas, or if drainage can be considered definitive and provide pleural healing before an operation for parenchymal residuals might be required, tube thoracostomy or even rib resection-dependent drainage can be carried out.

Patients with mixed tuberculous and pyogenic disease, however, usually present with chronicity char-

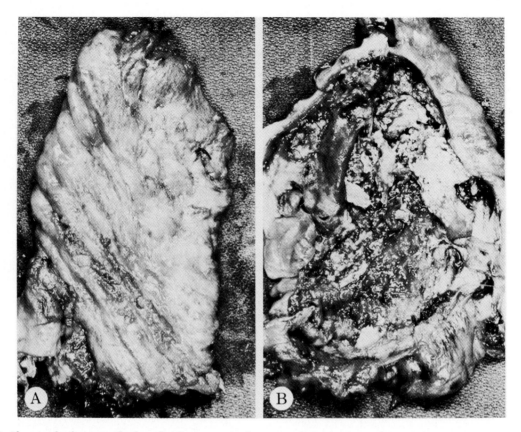

Fig. 57–5. *A,* Photograph of an excised tuberculous empyema sac that occupied the entire hemithorax. *B,* View of the interior of tuberculous empyema showing calcific wall and content. *From* Langston HT, Barker WL, Graham AH: Pleural tuberculosis. J Thorac Cardiovasc Surg 54:511, 1969.

acterized by a contracted chest wall, thickened and calcified pleura, and carnified and entrapped lung. Simple decompression of the pleural space has little prospect of promoting pulmonary expansion. Therefore, surgical intervention requires major resection as well as decortication of the pleural space. We avoid drainage even in the face of chronic bronchial fistulas. Although antimicrobial therapy may not be definitive, toxicity and constitutional symptoms can be controlled with its use. Furthermore, in our experience, complications after pleuropneumonectomy seem particularly more likely to occur in those patients who have had preliminary drainage and who still have a sinus tract at the time of operation.

Rather than performing a pleuropneumonectomy in a patient with a mixed empyema and a destroyed lung, Odell and Henderson (1985) recommended doing the pneumonectomy through the empyema space. In Odell's report (1990) of this approach, 34% of the patients having a pneumonectomy in relation to an empyema developed — or continued to have — a postpneumonectomy empyema. Approximately one third of these empyemas were eventually sterilized using maneuvers similar to the Clagett procedure, one third required a thoracoplasty, and the remaining one third were managed by permanent open drainage. Rarely, a Schede type of thoracoplasty was used.

Finally, collapse therapy — a standard thoracoplasty — in the absence of appropriate drainage has little chance of success in controlling the parenchymal processes let alone the compounded pleural infection, and it is not recommended. Thus, we prefer to avoid both prior drainage or collapse therapy and proceed to resection/decortication up to and including extrapleural pneumonectomy. Surgical intervention is carried out only after prolonged medical preparation and provided the patient is physiologically acceptable for the procedure.

A summary of our approach in the management of the four combinations of pleural tuberculosis with or without parenchymal involvement is provided in Table 57–1.

Results

When surgery is required for pleural disease alone, mortality is low and serious postoperative complications such as empyemas or bronchopleural fistulas are minimal. With the presence of associated parenchymal disease, the mortality and morbidity rates rise in proportion to the extent of the disease and the complexity of the surgical procedure required. These rates can be as high as 20 to 40%, respectively. Postresection empyemas and bronchopleural fistulas occur most often after pleuropneumonectomy, especially for those re-

Table 57–1. **Treatment of Pleural Tuberculosis**

Type		Status of Underlying Lung	Basic Treatment	Effect of Basic Treatment			Surgical Procedure Indicated
Pleural tuberculosis	Pure tuberculous	No lesion demonstrable	Anti-TB regimen and thoracentesis	No lesion remains			None
				Pleural residual			Decorticate
		Tuberculous lesion present	Anti-TB regimen and thoracentesis	Pleura clear	Lung clear		None
					Lung diseased		Individualize according to extent of involvement
				Pleura diseased	Lung clear		Decorticate
					Lung diseased		Individualize decortication and resection to pleuropneumonectomy
	Mixed tuberculous and pyogenic	No lesion demonstrable	Thoracentesis, anti-TB regimen, anti-pyogenic regimen, ?enzymes?	No lesion remains			None
				Pleural residual			Drain and/or decorticate
		Tuberculous lesion present	Thoracentesis, anti-TB regimen, anti-pyogenic regimen, ?enzymes?	Pleura clear	Lung clear		None
					Lung diseased		Individualize
				Pleura diseased	Lung clear		Drain and/or decorticate
					Lung diseased		Pleuropneumonectomy drain and/or resection plus decortication

From Langston HT, Correll NO: *In* Steele JD (ed): Surgical Treatment of Pulmonary Tuberculosis. 2nd Ed. Springfield IL: Charles C Thomas, 1957.

quiring preoperative drainage, those with a persisting sinus tract at the time of the operation, or those in which drug-resistant tuberculous organisms are present.

Postresectional surgical complications are usually from bacterial infection. Occasionally, fungal disease, especially aspergillosis, occurs. Should a tuberculous complication occur, by either contamination of the pleural space with tubercle bacilli or contralateral tuberculous spread, chemotherapeutic control should be regained before considering further operations that may require opening fresh tissue planes. Management of residual space problems, empyema — pyogenic or fungal, or a postoperative bronchopleural fistula may require collapse procedures or muscle transfers, as described by Pairolero (1983) and Miller (1984) and their associates. Long-term open drainage should be avoided, but may be the fate of some unfortunate patients.

In conclusion, Odell (1990) succinctly summarized this subject as follows: "Pulmonary tuberculosis involved the pleura in more than a quarter of all thoracic surgical patients with pulmonary tuberculosis. The disease is predominantly treated medically with antituberculous therapy, and with patience, the majority improve. In those not improving, there is almost always an underlying reason, either a destroyed lung or lobe or an inadequately drained pleural space; these conditions should be actively looked for and treated. Only when the patient is fit and in an optimal condition should more major surgical procedures be considered. *The procedures are demanding and require considerable skill. Other procedures that, in the Western world, would be considered obsolete, are necessary; these procedures still have a role in the patient with pulmonary tuberculosis.*"

FUNGAL INFECTIONS OF THE PLEURA

Light and associates (1972) reported that fungal disease accounts for approximately 1% of all pleural effusions. The effusion or, more often, contiguous involvement of the visceral and parietal pleural layers is the result of direct extension of underlying parenchymal fungal disease. Most often, it is unilateral, but in immunocompromised patients, especially in AIDS patients, bilateral disease can occur. Diagnostic studies are standard and include skin and serologic tests, as well as pleural fluid cultures for fungal diseases.

Aspergillosis

Pleural involvement is seen occasionally in aspergillosis patients as the result of rupture of a cavity containing the fungus into the pleural space or as either an early complication of lung resection for an aspergilloma or pulmonary tuberculosis with secondary contamination with the organism or a late complication of a lung resection, a thoracoplasty, or, as in the series reported by Bisson (1990), a very late — up to 40 years — sequela of a therapeutic pneumothorax. Although in a literature review by Herring and Pecora (1976) found only 24 cases of pleural aspergillosis recorded between 1958 and 1970, Bisson (1990) recorded 48 patients and Massard and colleagues (1992, 1993) recorded 19 patients with pleural aspergillosis. Both of these large series were reported from France. The patients in the series by Massard and colleagues were treated at their unit in Strasburg, France over a 15-year period. In this series, approximately one third of the patients presented with an early aspergillosis empyema following a lung resection, and two thirds of the cases followed as a complication of a remote pulmonary resection or of a previous thoracoplasty. Thirteen patients underwent curettage and thoracoplasty, 2 had a decortication, 1 had a pleuropneumonectomy, and 3 did not have any operative intervention. Bleeding was a significant problem in 62.5% of the operations. Space problems were common after the thoracoplasties and the decortications were unsuccessful. Two patients died in the postoperative period. Multiple procedures were required to control the residual space problems and the occasional bronchopleural fistula; the same was true in Bisson's (1990) series. Ultimately, success was obtained in 14 of Massard's 16 patients who had undergone an operation. Surgical therapy, although successful, carries a high morbidity rate and a significant — 10 to 12.5% — mortality rate in this disease. In the United States, Utley (1993) reported the use of a one-stage completion pneumonectomy with an extensive 8 rib thoracoplasty to obliterate the pleural space in 2 patients with a bronchopleural fistula, an aspergillous empyema, and fungal cavities in the remaining ipsilateral lobe following previous resection for carcinoma. Both procedures were successful.

Coccidioidomycosis

Miller (1989) noted that approximately 20% of patients with parenchymal coccidioidomycosis have evidence of pleural involvement — blunting of the costopleural angle — on routine radiography. Pleural effusions, generally small and unilateral, occasionally are observed. An empyema may occur as a result of rupture of a cavity with a resultant bronchopleural fistula or may occur after surgical resection of the disease. Amphotericin B or ketoconazole may be used to cover any indicated procedure, which in most instances would be resection of the offending parenchymal disease and obliteration of the pleural space. Utley (1993) reported the successful use of a combined completion pneumonectomy and thoracoplasty in one such patient who had had a left lower lobectomy for coccidioidomycosis 10 years previously. Secondary pyogenic contamination of the pleural space is to be avoided.

Cryptococcosis

Young and associates (1980) noted only 30 cytococcal pleural effusions in a review of the literature. When it occurs, the effusion is generally unilateral but may involve 50% of the affected hemithorax.

Other Fungi

Pleural involvement by histoplasmosis, Nocardia, or Candida organisms is rare. O'Neill and associates (1992) reported 20 patients with positive cultures for Candida in over 1250 patients with pleural fluid cultures in a 5-year period. Of these, the authors thought in only 9 patients was the positive culture indicative of a Candida empyema as a complication of esophageal rupture or mediastinitis or as an infection in patients with immunosuppression. The treatment of choice was appropriate surgical drainage and amphotericin B. In the aforementioned series, when two or more other body sites were involved with Candida infection, the patient died of multisystem organ failure, whereas all those with no or only one other body site involved survived.

Although likewise rare, Nelson and Light (1977) reported that as many as 26% of patients with pulmonary blastomycosis showed pleural changes on chest radiographs. Cutaneous sinus formation associated with pleural disease may occur in patients with blastomycosis.

Cutaneous sinus formation with exudation of "sulfur" granules is characteristic of actinomycotic involvement of the pleural space. Therapy with penicillin is the initial approach. Surgical intervention should be avoided when possible.

General Therapeutic Principles

Initial therapy in fungal involvement of the pleura is with the appropriate antifungal agent directed primarily to control the primary pulmonary parenchymal disease (see Chapter 79). Open drainage is to be avoided unless the patient is toxic, because of the possibility of a complicating mixed fungal-pyogenic empyema. If, however, the patient tolerates the pleuroparenchymal fungal disease and the drug regimen without systemic toxicity, open drainage is not indicated. The objectives are to avoid secondary pyogenic contamination and to obviate the high morbidity and mortality associated with surgical resection, which require extrapleural resections, excision of sinus tracts, and subsequent chest wall reconstruction when the disease is not under medical control.

REFERENCES

Andrews NC: Toraco-mediastinal plication (a surgical technique for chronic empyema). J Thorac Surg *41*:809, 1961.

Bisson A: Pleural aspergillosis. *In* Deslauriers J, Lacquet LK (eds): Thoracic Surgery: Surgical Management of Pleural Disease. St. Louis: CV Mosby, 1990, p. 448.

DeMeester TR: The pleura. *In* Sabiston D (ed): Textbook of Thoracic Surgery. Philadelphia: WB Saunders, 1983.

Dupon H: Andrews technique of thoracomyopleuroplasty. *In* Deslauriers J, Lacquet LK (eds): Thoracic Surgery: Surgical Management of Pleural Disease. St. Louis: CV Mosby, 1990, p. 255.

Herring M, Pecora D: Pleural aspergillosis: A case report. Ann Surg *42*:300, 1976.

Hood RM: Tuberculosis of the pleura. *In* Surgical Diseases of the Pleura and Chest Wall. Springfield IL: Charles C Thomas, 1965.

Iioka S, et al: Surgical treatment of chronic epyema: A new one-stage operation. J Thorac Cardiovasc Surg *90*:179, 1985.

Light RW, et al: Pleural effusions: The diagnostic separation of transudates and exudates. Ann Intern Med *77*:507, 1972.

Light RW: Tuberculous pleural effusions. *In* Light RW (ed): Pleural Diseases. Philadelphia: Lea & Febiger, 1983.

Massard G, et al: Pleuropulmonary aspergilloma: Clinical spectrum and results of surgical treatment. Ann Thorac Surg *54*:1159, 1992.

Massard G, et al: Operative management of pleural aspergilloma. Presented at the 29th Annual Meeting of the Society of Thoracic Surgeons. San Antonio, TX, January 26, 1993.

Miller JI, Jr: Infections of the pleura. In Shields TW (ed): General Thoracic Surgery. 3rd Ed. Philadelphia: Lea & Febiger, 1989, p. 633.

Miller JI, et al: Single-stage complete muscle flap closure of the postpneumonectomy empyema space: A new method and possible solution to disturbing complication. Ann Thorac Surg *38*:227, 1984.

Nelson O, Light RW: Granulomatous pleuritis secondary to blastomycosis. Chest *71*:433, 1977.

Odell JA, Henderson BJ: Pneumonectomy through an empyema. J Thorac Cardiovasc Surg *89*:423, 1985.

Odell JA, Pleural tuberculosis. In Deslauriers J, Lacquet LK (eds): Thoracic Surgery: Surgical Management of Pleural Disease. St. Louis: CV Mosby, 1990, p. 459.

O'Neill BV, Wiedemann HP, Basheda SG: Candida empyema: An unrecognized entity (abst). Presented at 58th Annual Scientific Assembly of the American College of Chest Physicians, Chicago, October 26, 1992, p. 108S.

Pairolero PC, Arnold PG, Piehler JM: Intrathoracic transposition of extrathoracic muscle. J Thorac Cardiovasc Surg *86*:809, 1983.

Pugatch RD, et al: Differentiation of pleural and pulmonary lesions using computed tomography. J Comput Assist Tomogr *2*:601, 1978.

Tatsumura T, et al: A new technique for one-stage radical eradication of long standing chronic thoracic empyema. J Thorac Cardiovasc Surg *99*:410, 1990.

Utley JR: Completion pneumonectomy and thoracoplasty for bronchopleural fistula and fungal empyema. Ann Thorac Surg *55*:672, 1993.

Young EJ, et al: Pleural effusions due to *Cryptococcus neoformans*; a preview of the literature and report of two cases with cryptococcal antigen determinations. Am Rev Respir Dis *121*:743, 1980.

READING REFERENCES

Barker WL, Neuhaus H, Langston HT: Ventilatory improvement following decortication in pulmonary tuberculosis. Ann Thorac Surg *1*:532, 1965.

Deschamps C, et al: Surgical approach to chronic empyema: Decortication and muscle transposition. *In* Deslauriers J, Lacquet LK (eds): Thoracic Surgery: Surgical Management of Pleural Diseases. St. Louis: CV Mosby, 1990.

Langston HT: Empyema Thoracis. Ann Thorac Surg *2*:766, 1965.

Langston HT, Correll NO: The surgical treatment of pleural tuberculosis. *In* Steele JD (ed): Surgical Management of Pulmonary Tuberculosis. Alexander Monograph Series # 1. Springfield IL: Charles C Thomas, 1957.

Langston HT, Barker WL: Pleuro-pulmonary tuberculosis. *In* Effler DB (ed): Surgical Diseases of the Chest. 4th Ed. St. Louis: CV Mosby, 1978.

Langston HT, Barker WL, Graham AA: Pleural tuberculosis. J Thorac Cardiovasc Surg *54*:511, 1967.

Langston HT, Barker WL, Pyle MM: Surgery for pulmonary tuberculosis. *In* Lewis Practice of Surgery. Vol. V. Hagerstown: Prior, 1968, p. 56.

Langston HT, Barker WL, Pyle M: Surgery in pulmonary tuberculosis — 11 year review of indications and results. Ann Surg *164*:567, 1966.

Lord FT: Section 3, Diseases of the Pleura. *In* Diseases of the Bronchi, Lungs and Pleura. Philadelphia: Lea & Febiger, 1925, p. 642.

CHAPTER 58

DECORTICATION OF THE LUNG

Thomas W. Shields

Decortication of the lung consists of the removal of a restrictive, fibrous membrane or layer of tissue from the pleural surface of the lung. The layer also may be removed from the chest wall and diaphragm. The procedure is used in the treatment of fibrothorax resulting from either organized hemothorax or empyema. The empyema may be the result of an infected post-traumatic hemothorax or may be postoperative or parapneumonic in origin. The empyema may be associated with a specific granulomatous disease process, such as tuberculosis.

The purpose of the procedure is to free the encased — "trapped" — lung and, as a result of the re-expansion of the lung, to obliterate the pleural space. If the operation is performed because of an organizing hemothorax, its objective is the preservation of pulmonary function and prevention of delayed suppurative complications. If done for empyema, the major goal is to free the lung for expansion, thereby obliterating the pleural space, eliminate much of the by-products of suppuration, expediting recovery, and preserving lung function.

TECHNIQUE

Pulmonary decortication is best carried out through a standard posterolateral thoracotomy at the midchest level. The operation can be performed with or without rib resection. Rib resection provides the best visualization at the pleural level because the intercostal space is often narrowed by the pleural process.

If the entire pleural sac is to be excised, the extrapleural plane can be sought immediately and the parietal wall of the sac separated from it. Ultimately, the edge of the visceral peel is reached, and care is to be exercised in turning these margins and beginning the separation of the visceral surface. Particular care should be taken in separating the pleural sac along the gutters of the mediastinum, along the pericardium, and, especially, at the diaphragmatic area where cleavage planes are often difficult to follow and avulsion of the

diaphragm can occur with entry into the retroperitoneal area.

Although somewhat less than ideal from a theoretic standpoint, a practical approach to the management of decortication is to incise through the parietal peel to gain entry into the space within the organized pleural mass. The content of this space is then evacuated, and appropriate cultures or samples are taken as required.

After the visceral coat is mechanically cleaned, an area over one of the lobes is selected for incision, avoiding a fissure if possible. With the use of a small scalpel, the peel is incised carefully down to the loose plane that lies immediately beneath the cicatricial coat and just above the visceral pleura (Fig. 58–1). The visceral pleura must be left intact, and care must be taken to avoid separation of the visceral pleura from the underlying pulmonary parenchyma. If an artificial plane is established, numerous air leaks and bleeding — both difficult to control — will occur. Once this loose areolar plane is entered, the opening is enlarged, and decortication is carried out mainly by blunt dissection, although sharp dissection is used at any point where intimate adherence exists between the visceral pleura and the peel. At the limits of the visceral investment, where it is met by the parietal portion of the pleural mass, the peel thins out and becomes merely a fibrous pleural symphysis obliterating the anatomic pleural space.

When the visceral pleura has been decorticated, attention is directed to separation of the parietal peel and underlying parietal pleura in the loose connective tissue plane between the latter and the endothoracic fascia of the chest wall, ultimately cutting the thinned-out pleural obliteration in the gutters. Separating the peel from over the diaphragm is usually less satisfactory because the cleavage plane is often much more difficult to follow.

The necessity of removing the parietal peel has been debated. It is true that, in uninfected hemothoraces and other sterile pleural processes, the complete re-expansion of the lung, so as to obliterate the pleural space,

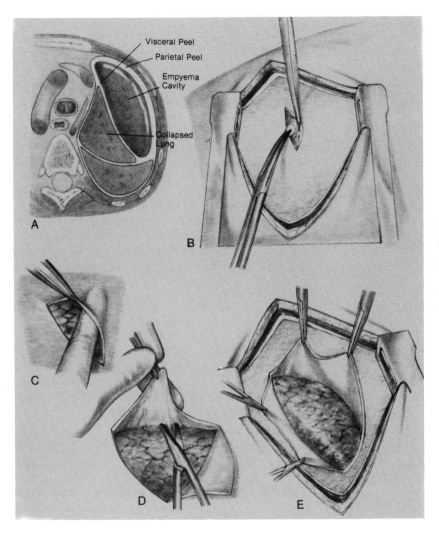

Visceral Peel
Parietal Peel
Empyema Cavity
Collapsed Lung

A

B

C

D

E

Fig. 58-1. Decortication of the pleura. A, Cross-sectional diagram of empyema cavity and relationship of chest wall and underlying lung. B, Incision of visceral peel with beginning dissection of peel. C, Finger dissection of peel. D, Sharp dissection as necessary. E, Progressive decortication with expansion of underlying lung. From Hood RM: Techniques in General Thoracic Surgery. Philadelphia: WB Saunders, 1985.

sets the stage for the resorption of even dense pleural coats. When dealing with an infection, a complete operation does indeed have a strong logical appeal.

During decortication, the anesthetist should expand the lung progressively, so that it is possible to recognize any areas of binding adhesions that still may be enfolding and distorting the lung and that would militate against the lung's assumption of increased or relatively normal volume. Such unfolding of the lung by severance or stripping of deforming symphyses has been termed "secondary decortication."

Injury to lung parenchyma must be repaired but should be minimal unless rather severe parenchymal disease or dense adhesions have been present between it and visceral peel. Adequate closed-tube drainage and the addition of suction to the closed drainage system promote prompt expansion of the lung in spite of leaks.

Objections may be voiced against making a direct opening into the pleural pocket, because this would offer the danger of contamination of the operative field by the content of the pleural mass. This hazard is probably not as great as might be presumed, because the operative area can be fairly well cleansed at the conclusion of the procedure by copious irrigation. Local tissue immunity, no doubt, plays a protecting role, and the expanded lung, which obliterates the pleural space, provides further protection. Appropriate antibiotics also are indicated in an attempt to avoid the development of postoperative suppuration.

TIMING OF THE SURGICAL INTERVENTION

The decision as to the timing of the decortication depends on the nature of the underlying process producing the fibrinous peel, the age of the patient, and the status of underlying lung — diseased or not involved in the pathologic process. This latter is best determined by bronchoscopy and computed tomographic examination, as reported by Gustafson and associates (1990). Young children tolerate continued tube drainage poorly, and the development of scoliosis is noted with prolonged pleural infection in the pediatric age group. This has led Sensenig (1963), Kosloske (1980), Mayo (1982) and their colleagues, as well as Foglia and Randolph (1987), to advocate early thoracotomy and decortication in a poorly responding empyema in children. A posttraumatic infected hemothorax is likewise an indication for decortication. An uninfected traumatic hemothorax may be observed for 4 to 6 weeks before surgical intervention, as initially suggested by Samson and Burford (1947), although many, such as Milfeld and associates (1978) and Webb and Jones (1983), question the advisability of waiting this long. (See Chapter 64 for management of acute hemithorax.) The timing of surgical intervention to control a parapneumonic or postoperative empyema varies greatly with the clinical situation and is discussed in detail in Chapters 55 and 56.

ADDITIVE PROCEDURES

Necessary parenchymal resection for the removal of any underlying lung disease may be carried out following removal of the visceral peel. At times, if inadequate lung tissue remains to fill the pleural space, a concomitant thoracoplasty may be advisable. However, it would appear more prudent to transpose a pedicled muscle flap from the chest wall, as summarized by Deschamps and associates (1990) and presented in Chapter 56. Parenchymal resection or thoracoplasty definitely increase the risk of postoperative complications.

PHYSIOLOGIC RESULTS

In the presence of a significant fibrothorax, pulmonary function is markedly deranged. There is interference both in the mechanics of ventilation and in perfusion of the "captive" lung. Actually, perfusion is reduced to a greater extent than is ventilation.

The physiologic improvement obtained with successful decortication varies. The extent of disease of the underlying lung at the time of the development of the fibrothorax is the most important factor in determining the eventual outcome. The functional improvement may be good after decortication of a traumatic hemothorax but may be only fair to poor after the procedure in patients with nontuberculous or tuberculous empyema. Iioka and associates (1985) reported significant improvement in both percent VC and the FEV_1/predicted VC in 20 patients who underwent successful decortication of a chronic empyema. The duration of the presence of the fibrothorax appears not to be important, although it has been suggested that the shorter the duration of the pleural disease, the better is the eventual return of function.

In patients in whom the decortication proves successful, pulmonary function studies reveal an increase in the lung volumes and improved ventilatory capacity. An improved perfusion and oxygen uptake on the side operated on has been recorded by Swoboda and colleagues (1990). These investigators found that before operation the perfusion of the affected side in nine patients was reduced to a mean of 23% — range, 10 to 40% — and that after decortication the mean perfusion was increased to 37.8% — range, 26 to 48%. Functional improvement may continue for many months

after the operation. Postoperative breathing exercises appear to be especially beneficial in these patients.

MORBIDITY AND MORTALITY

The incidence of nonfatal complications is approximately 10%. The major problems are related to sepsis, persistent air leak, and bleeding. Injury to lung or to vessels in the chest wall resulting in important hemorrhage postoperatively is rare but can defeat the purpose of the operation by recreating a second pleural clot, which may organize and again delay obliteration of the pleural space. Wound infection and empyema with or without a bronchopleural fistula are the most common septic complications. Persistent air leaks for 10 to 14 days, caused by injury of the underlying lung during the operation, are not uncommon, but with adequate drainage of the pleural space and re-expansion of the lung to obliterate the pleural space, serious septic complications do not occur.

The mortality rate after decortication should approach zero but has been reported to be as high as 8% by Benfield (1981). When death occurs, it is usually related to hemorrhage or to septic complications. Both hemorrhage and sepsis are more likely to occur when the procedure has been technically difficult or if a supplementary procedure has been carried out at the same time.

RESULTS

It is difficult to state categorically the results to be expected after a decortication for the management of a chronic empyema. Yeh and associates (1963) reported 25 successful results and no deaths after 27 decortications and Benfield (1981) reported 42 cures in 46 patients. Iioka and colleagues (1985) reported a 100% success rate in a highly selected population of 20 patients. Therefore, a successful outcome of over 90% should be expected after decortication of a chronic empyema in selected patients. In patients with a clotted hemothorax, good results should exceed 95%.

REFERENCES

Benfield GFA: Recent trends in empyema thoracis. Br J Dis Chest 75:358, 1981.
Deschamps C, et al: Surgical approach to chronic empyema: decortication and muscle transposition. In Deslauriers J, Lacquet LK (eds): Thoracic Surgery: Surgical Management of Pleural Diseases. St Louis: CV Mosby, 1990.
Foglia RP, Randolph J: Current indications for decortication in treatment of empyema in children. J Pediatr Surg 22:28, 1987.
Gustafson RA, et al: Role of lung decortication in symptomatic empyemas in children. Ann Thorac Surg 49:940, 1990.
Iioka S, et al: Surgical treatment of chronic empyema. A new one-stage operation. J Thorac Cardiovasc Surg 90:179, 1985.
Kosloske AM, Cushing AH, Shuck JM: Early decortication for anaerobic empyema in children. J Pediatr Surg 15:422, 1980.
Mayo P, Saha SP, McElvein RB: Acute empyemas in children treated by open thoracotomy and decortication. Ann Thorac Surg 34:401, 1982.

Milfeld DJ, Mattox KL, Beall AC: Early evacuation of clotted hemothorax. Am J Surg *136*:686, 1978.

Samson PC, Burford TH: Total pulmonary decortication. J Thorac Surg *16*:127, 1947.

Sensenig DM, Rossi NP, Ehrenhaft JL: Decortication for chronic nontuberculous empyema. Surg Gynecol Obstet *117*:443, 1963.

Swoboda L, et al: Decortication in chronic pleural empyema. Investigation of lung function based on perfusion scintigraphy. Thorac Cardiovasc Surg *38*:359, 1990.

Webb WR, Jones JW: Thoracic trauma. In Glenn WWL, et al (eds): Thoracic and Cardiovascular Surgery. 4th Ed. Norwalk, CT: Appleton-Century-Crofts, 1983.

Yeh TJ, Hall D, Ellison RG: Empyema thoracis: a review of 110 cases. Am Rev Respir Dis *88*:785, 1963.

READING REFERENCES

Barker WL, Neuhaus H, Langston HT: Ventilatory improvement following decortication in pulmonary tuberculosis. Ann Thorac Surg *1*:532, 1965.

Burford TH: Hemothorax and hemothoracic empyema. *In* Surgery World War II, Thoracic Surgery, Vol. 2. Washington, DC, Office of the Surgeon General, Department of the Army, 1965, p 237.

Burford TH, Parker EF, Samson PC: Early pulmonary decortication in the treatment of post-traumatic empyema. Ann Surg *112*:163, 1945.

Carroll D, et al: Pulmonary function following decortication of lung. Am Rev Tuberc *63*:231, 1951.

Cherniak NS, Barker WL: Cardiopulmonary function in tuberculosis.

In Gordon BL (ed): Clinical Cardiopulmonary Physiology. New York: Grune & Stratton, 1969, p. 600.

Delorme E: Noveau traitment des empyemes chronique. Gaz d' Hosp *67*:94, 1894.

Fowler GR: A case of thoracoplasty for the removal of a large cicatricial fibrous growth from the interior of the chest, the result of an old empyema. Med Rec *44*:838, 1893.

Gordon J, Welles ES: Decortication in pulmonary tuberculosis including studies of respiratory physiology. J Thorac Surg *18*:337, 1949.

Hood RM: Pleural decortication. *In* Surgical Diseases of the Pleura and Chest Wall. Hood RM (ed): Philadelphia: WB Saunders, 1986.

Morton JR, Boushy SF, Guinn GA: Physiological evaluation of results of pulmonary decortication. Ann Thorac Surg *9*:321, 1970.

Patton WE, Watson TR Jr, Gaensler EA: Pulmonary function before and at intervals after surgical decortication of the lung. Surg Gynecol Obstet *95*:477, 1952.

Samson PC: Pleural complications of thoracic trauma. *In* Hood RM (ed): Management of Thoracic Injuries. Springfield, IL: Charles C Thomas, 1969, p 34.

Samson PC, et al: Technical consideration in decortication for the pleural complications of pulmonary tuberculosis. J Thorac Surg *36*:431, 1958.

Rudstrom P, Thoren L: Decortication of lung. Acta Chir Scand *100*:437, 1955.

Savage T, Fleming HA: Decortication of lung in tuberculous disease. Thorax *10*:293, 1955.

Siebens AA, et al: The physiologic effects of fibrothorax and the functional results of surgical treatment. J Thorac Surg *32*:53, 1956.

CHAPTER 59

CHYLOTHORAX

Joseph I. Miller, Jr.

Chylothorax is the presence of lymphatic fluid in the pleural space resulting from a leak of the thoracic duct or one of its major divisions. This condition is being recognized more frequently, after both cardiac and general thoracic surgery. Increased understanding of the physiology, pathogenesis, diagnosis, and management of chylothorax have decreased the initial 50% mortality to a mortality of 10% in major medical centers.

COMPOSITION OF CHYLE

The term "chyle" comes from the Latin "chylus," meaning "juice." It is the lymph that originates in the intestine. The fat contained in the intestinal lymph gives chyle its characteristic appearance. Thoracic duct lymph is not pure chyle, but a mixture of lymphatic fluid originating in the intestine, liver, abdominal wall, and lower extremities. Ninety-five percent of the volume of the thoracic duct lymph originates in the liver and the intestinal tract. Under normal circumstances, the amount of lymph originating in the extremities is negligible.

The primary function of the thoracic duct is the transport of digestive fat to the venous system. Munk and Rosenstein (1891) observed a thoracic duct fistula and recognized that the thoracic duct lymph was clear during fasting but became milky following a fatty meal. About 60 to 70% of the ingested fat is absorbed by the intestinal lymphatic system and conveyed to the blood stream by the thoracic duct. The composition of chyle is listed in Table 59–1. The main component of chyle is fat.

Thoracic duct lymph contains from 0.4 to 5 g of fat per 100 ml and 50 to 70% of absorbed fat is conveyed to the blood stream by way of the thoracic duct. This is made up of neutral fat, free fatty acids, sphingomyelin, phospholipids, cholesterol, and cholesterol esters. The total amount of cholesterol ranges from 65 to 220 mg/100 ml.

Those fatty acids with less than 10 carbon atoms in the chain are absorbed directly by the portal venous

Table 59–1. **Composition of Chyle**

Component	Amount (per 100 ml)
Total fat	0.4–5 g
Total cholesterol	65–220 mg
Total protein	2.21–5.9 g
Albumin	1.2–4.1 g
Globulin	1.1–3.6 g
Fibrinogen	16–24 g
Sugar	48–200 g
Electrolytes	Similar to plasma
	Amount
Cellular elements	
Lymphocytes	400–6800/mm^3
Erythrocytes	50–600/mm^3
Antithrombin globulin	>25% plasma concentrate
Prothrombin	>25% plasma concentrate
Fibrinogen	>25% plasma concentrate

system. This particular fact forms the basis for the use of medium-chain triglycerides as an oral diet in the conservative management of chylothorax. Neutral fat, as Ross (1961) noted, is found in the lymph in the form of minute globules that are less than 0.5 mm in diameter. Ingested fat passes from the intestine to the systemic circulation in about 1.5 hours, with a peak absorption at 6 hours after ingestion.

Ross (1961) and Roy and associates (1967) reported that the total protein content of thoracic duct lymph ranges from 2.2 to 5.9 g/100 ml, approximately half of that found in the plasma. Thoracic duct lymph contains as much as 4% protein, consisting of albumin, globulin, fibrinogen, and prothrombin, with an albumin ratio of 3 to 1. Sugar concentration in thoracic duct lymph ranges from 40 to 200 g/100 ml. The electrolyte composition is similar to that found in plasma, with sodium, potassium, chloride, calcium, and inorganic phosphorus being the predominant electrolyte components.

Antithrombin globulin, prothrombin, and fibrinogen are all present in human thoracic duct lymph in

714

concentrations greater than 25% of plasma levels. Stutt-man and associates (1965) reported that factors V and VIII are present in concentrations of approximately 8.9% and 4.5%, respectively, in thoracic lymph.

The main cellular elements of thoracic duct lymph are lymphocytes. They range from 400 to 6800 cells/mm^3. As Hyde and colleagues (1974) noted, most of these lymphocytes are T-lymphocytes. Thoracic duct lymphocytes differ qualitatively and quantitatively from peripheral blood lymphocytes in their reactivity to antigenic stimulation.

In clear lymph, there are approximately 50 red cells/mm^3, whereas in the postabsorptive states, as Shafiroff and Kau (1959) reported, the number may increase to 600 red cells/mm^3 of thoracic duct lymph. In addition, fat-soluble vitamins, antibodies, en-zymes — including pancreatic lipase, alkaline phos-phatase, SGOT, and SGPT — and urea nitrogen are also present in thoracic duct lymph. Because of the numerous constituents of thoracic duct lymph, it is readily apparent why the persistent loss of this fluid can interfere with nutrition and immunity.

PHYSIOLOGY OF THE THORACIC DUCT

The function of the thoracic duct is the transport of ingested fat to the venous system. Volume and weight of flow of lymph have been estimated to be 1.38 ml/kg of body weight/hour. Crandall and associates (1943) found that the rate of flow increases following ingestion of food and water, and also during abdominal massage, with a maximum flow of 3.9 ml/min and a minimum flow of 0.38 ml/min. Hepatic lymph increases by 150% following meals, whereas intestinal lymph increases to up to 10 times the basal flow following fatty meals. Starvation and complete rest decrease the flow of thoracic duct lymph.

The forward flow of chyle from the cisterna chyli to the entrance into the left subclavian-internal jugular vein junction is influenced by several factors: 1) The inflow of chyle into the lacteal system creates a vis a tergo, which is in turn produced by the intake of food and liquid into the intestine and is augmented by intestinal movement. 2) Negative intrathoracic pressure on inspiration and the resultant gradient between this negative pressure and positive intra-abdominal pressure helps the upward flow of chyle. 3) Muscular contrac-tions of the thoracic duct wall are probably the most important factor. Contractions of the duct wall occur every 10 to 15 seconds independent of respiratory movements. The intraductal pressure ranges from 10 to 25 cm H$_2$O, and with obstruction, as Shafiroff and Kau (1959) observed, it may rise to 50 cm H$_2$O. These rhythmic contractions cause the duct to empty into the subclavian vein. The thoracic duct valves, located throughout its course but which are mostly in the upper portion, permit only upward unidirectional flow.

The flow of chyle varies greatly with the content of the meal and is particularly increased when the fat content of the food is high. Volumes up to 2500 ml of chyle in 24 hours have been collected from the can-nulated human thoracic duct. Most of the body's lymphocytes are transported through the thoracic duct system back to the venous system.

The lymph circulation performs the vital function of collecting and transporting excess tissue fluid, extrav-asated plasma protein, absorbed lipids, and other large molecules from the interstitial spaces back to the blood stream.

ETIOLOGY OF CHYLOTHORAX

There have been numerous classifications of chylo-thorax. Most have been based on information obtained at postmortem examination. In 1971, Bessone and colleagues suggested classifying chylothorax into 1) congenital chylothorax; 2) postoperative traumatic chy-lothorax; 3) nonsurgical traumatic chylothorax; and 4) nontraumatic chylothorax. DeMeester (1983), however, has published a more thorough classification (Table 59–2).

Congenital Chylothorax

Chylothorax in the neonate, although rare, is the leading cause of pleural effusion in this age group. In most cases, the exact cause cannot be ascertained. Birth trauma or congenital defects in the duct wall or both may be precipitating factors. Increased venous pressure in birth trauma, causing thoracic duct rupture, has been suggested as a possible cause. In rare incidences, malformations of the lymphatic system, particularly in the thoracic duct itself, have been shown to be the cause

Table 59–2. Etiology of Chylothorax

Congenital
    Atresia of thoracic duct
    Thoracic duct-pleural fistula space
    Birth trauma
Traumatic
    Blunt
    Penetrating
    Surgical
        Cervical
            Excision of lymph nodes
            Radical neck dissection
        Thoracic
            Ligation of patent ductus arteriosus
            Excision of coarctation
            Esophagectomy
            Resection of thoracic aortic aneurysm
            Resection of mediastinal tumor
            Left pneumonectomy
        Abdominal
            Sympathectomy
            Radical lymph node dissection
Diagnostic procedures
    Lumbar arteriography
    Subclavian vein catheterization
Neoplasms
Miscellaneous

of congenital chylothorax. The thoracic duct may be absent or atretic, and in occasional instances, multiple dilated lymphatic channels with abnormal communications have been noted, as well as multiple fistulae between the thoracic duct and pleural space.

Traumatic Chylothorax

The second major cause of chylothorax is traumatic chylothorax, which may occur with either blunt or penetrating trauma or after a surgical procedure. The most common form of nonpenetrating injury to the thoracic duct is produced by a sudden hyperextension of the spine with rupture of the duct just above the diaphragm. Sudden stretching over the vertebral bodies may be enough in itself to tear the duct, but usually the duct has been fixed as a result of prior disease or malignancy. This may be secondary to a blast or blunt trauma. Episodes of vomiting or a violent bout of coughing can also result in tearing of the thoracic duct. Biet and Connolly (1951) believe this is generally caused by a shearing of the thoracic duct by the right crus of the diaphragm. These are the most commonly mentioned causes of chylothorax resulting from nonpenetrating injuries to the chest. Penetrating injury from a gunshot or a stab wound to the thoracic duct is unusual and is apt to be overshadowed by damage to other structures of more immediate importance.

Operative Injuries

Injury at operation is fairly common. Chylothorax has been reported following almost every known thoracic surgical procedure, including operations on the aorta, esophagus, heart, lungs, and sympathetic nervous system. Injury has also been reported following surgery in the neck, after such operations as radical neck resection and scalene node biopsy. It has also been reported following abdominal operations of sympathectomy and radical lymph node dissection. In addition, it has been reported with translumbar aortography and subclavian venous catheterization. An occasional instance has been reported after an attempt to introduce a cannula into the left internal jugular vein.

Often a latent interval of 2 to 10 days passes between the time of injury and the development of a chylothorax that becomes clinically evident. This is because of the accumulation of lymph in the posterior mediastinum until the mediastinal pleura ruptures, usually on the right side at the base of the pulmonary ligament. Once established, the thoracic duct pleural fistula does not tend to close, in contrast to the dictum that in the absence of obstruction a fistula will close. Spontaneous sealing of a fistula after a closed injury may be expected in only approximately 50% of patients, and death generally ensues in the remaining patients unless the fistula is surgically closed.

Intraoperatively, the duct is most vulnerable to damage in the upper part of the left chest, particularly, as Higgins and Molder (1971) noted, with procedures involving mobilization of the aortic arch, the left subclavian artery, or the esophagus. The classically described course of the duct explains why damage to it below the level of the fifth or sixth thoracic vertebra usually results in a right-sided chylous effusion, and why damage above this level usually results in effusion on the left side.

Neoplastic Chylothorax

Ross (1961) stated that the thoracic duct can be involved in both benign and malignant disease by direct lymphatic permeation in continuity with the primary growth, by direct invasion of the duct by the primary growth, or by tumor embolus in the main duct. The chylothorax may be either unilateral or bilateral. De-Meester (1983) reported that the predominant mechanism of the leak is by rupture of distended tributaries because of back pressure from the neoplastic obstruction or actual erosion of the duct itself. It has been most frequently reported following lymphosarcoma, retroperitoneal lymphoma, or primary carcinoma of the lung. Rarely, malignant chylous leaks may fill the pericardial sac with chyle and produce signs and symptoms of cardiac tamponade.

Miscellaneous Causes

Infections, filariasis, pancreatic pseudocysts, thrombosis of the jugular and subclavian veins, cirrhosis of the liver, and tuberculosis can all cause chylothorax.

Benign lymphangiomas arising in the thoracic duct may also produce single or multiple cyst-like spaces filled with chyle.

Pulmonary lymphangiomatosis, reported by Cunn (1973) and Silverstein (1974) and their associates, is a rare cause of chylothorax. This condition is seen in women of reproductive age who have shortness of breath as the major complaint. Pneumothorax and hemoptysis can be seen in addition to chylothorax, and these women usually die of pulmonary insufficiency within 10 years of presentation.

PATHOLOGIC PHYSIOLOGY

Chylothorax can cause cardiopulmonary abnormalities, as well as serious metabolic and immunologic deficiencies. The accumulation of chyle in the chest can result in compression of the underlying lung, with a reduction of vital capacity and mediastinal shift, resulting in shortness of breath, and occasionally, symptoms of marked respiratory distress. In general, the development is insidious, and symptoms occur gradually. In contrast, with rapid accumulation, shock, tachypnea, tachycardia, and hypotension can occur. Chyle is thought to be bacteriostatic because of its lecithin and fatty acid content, and therefore is usually sterile. Because it is nonirritating, chyle does not tend to form a peel that can result in a trapped lung.

The loss of protein, fat-soluble vitamins, and fat contained in chyle can lead to serious metabolic defects and death in patients with chylothorax. Shafiroff and Kau (1959) emphasized that the loss of lymphocytes and antibodies can also interfere with the immunologic status of a patient with chylothorax.

DIAGNOSIS

The diagnosis of a chylothorax is suggested by the presence of a nonclotting milky fluid, which is obtained from the pleural space at thoracentesis or chest tube insertion. The diagnosis is confirmed by the finding of free microscopic fat and fat content of the fluid higher than that of the plasma. In traumatic chylothorax, the chyle may initially appear blood-stained, and this may be misleading. On microscopic examination, the presence of fat globules that clear with alkali and ether, or stain with Sudan-3, is diagnostic. Lymphocytes are the predominant cells found in chyle, while in traumatic chylus effusion, red blood cells are at least initially present. Chylous effusions must be distinguished from pseudochyle and cholesterol pleural effusions. Boyd (1986) noted that pseudochyle occurs with malignant tumors or infection and is milky in appearance because of the presence of lecithin-globulin complex. Pseudochyle contains only a trace of fat, and fat globules cannot be seen with Sudan-3 stain smears. Milky pleural effusions also can be seen secondary to tuberculosis, and Bower (1968) reported it to occur in rheumatoid arthritis. Cholesterol pleural effusions that are seen in these two disease entities acquire their milky appearance from a high concentration of cholesterol crystals. If it is still difficult to distinguish chyle from pseudochyle or cholesterol pleural fluid, a test consisting of feeding a patient a fat stained with green No. 6 dye, which will stain the chylous effusion approximately 1 hour after ingestion of the dye, is a helpful diagnostic test. Obtaining cholesterol and triglyceride levels of the fluid can help because most chylous effusions have a cholesterol/triglyceride ratio of less than 1, whereas nonchylous effusions have a ratio greater than 1. In addition, if the fluid has a triglyceride level of more than 110 mg/100 ml, there is a 99% chance that the fluid is chyle. If the triglyceride level is less than 50 mg/100 ml, Staats and colleagues (1980) noted that there is only a 5% chance that the fluid is chyle.

Another helpful index in determining if a leak is related to a chylous leak is the rate of fluid accumulation in the chest. The rate of accumulation in the chest from a chylous fistula exceeds 400 to 500 ml/day and is an average of approximately 700 to 1200 ml/day in a 70-kg adult. The flow rate is obviously proportionately less in infants and children, depending on the body surface area. A detailed analysis of the effusion should produce values similar to those listed in Table 59–1 if the effusion is indeed a chylous effusion. Once a chylothorax is diagnosed, a complete history and physical examination should be performed to discern the etiology. Chylothorax in a postoperative period generally develops 7 to 14 days postoperatively. Surgery in the region of the aorta, esophagus, or posterior mediastinum should suggest the presence or the possibility of a chylothorax.

Blunt trauma 2 to 6 weeks earlier should also suggest the presence of a potential chylothorax.

In nontraumatic chylothorax, an extensive search for the cause of the pleural effusion must be undertaken. Computed tomography and lymphangiography are diagnostic techniques that are helpful in the study of chylothorax. Occasionally, lymphangiography details the exact site of leakage and also the anatomic abnormalities of the thoracic duct. A CT examination of the chest is a good way to demonstrate the presence of mediastinal disease that could cause a chylothorax. A mediastinal mass or enlarged mediastinal nodes, as well as primary lung cancer, could easily be demonstrated by this technique.

MANAGEMENT

The ideal management of the patient with chylothorax is unknown. The disease occurs in various situations, and opinion about which types of chylothorax should be treated operatively is diverse: the postsurgical or posttraumatic types only, or the nontraumatic types as well. Whether young children should undergo surgery is also controversial. The development of a lymphatic leak in the thorax certainly necessitates decisive management if considerable morbidity and mortality are to be avoided. Well-standardized guidelines have emerged that have enhanced the understanding and treatment of this difficult clinical problem.

Table 59–3 lists the various modalities used in the treatment of chylothorax. They can be divided into conservative therapy, operative therapy, and radiation therapy.

Current treatment of chylothorax is thoracic duct ligation, introduced by Lampson and associates (1948). They showed that the mortality rate from chylothorax decreased from 50 to 15%. Before this report of successful control of traumatic chylothorax by direct ligation of the thoracic duct, the mortality rate for this condition was 45%; nontraumatic chylothorax had a mortality rate of 100%. Treatment of the condition before 1948 consisted of thoracentesis or closed chest

Table 59–3. Modalities Used in Treatment of Chylothorax

Conservative
    Nothing by mouth
    Medium-chain triglycerides
    Central hyperalimentation
    Drainage of pleural space
        Thoracentesis
        Closed chest tube thoracostomy
    Complete expansion of lung
Operative
    Direct ligation of thoracic duct
    Mass ligation of thoracic duct tissue
    Pleuroperitoneal shunting
    Pleurectomy
    Fibrin glue
Radiation therapy

tube thoracostomy and a low-fat diet. Today the crucial decision in the management of these patients is when to advocate surgical intervention. There is no unanimous opinion on whether to operate or, if surgery is not undertaken initially, on how long conservative management should be used before resorting to surgical intervention.

Conservative therapy consists of maintaining effective thoracostomy tube drainage with good expansion of the lung. The most important aspect is to maintain adequate nutrition, as loss of chylous fluid causes electrolyte imbalance and increases nutritional needs. Central hyperalimentation is routinely used while keeping the patient NPO. Any oral feedings increase output through the fistula. There is no standard of how long conservative therapy should be tried before considering operative intervention. Williams and Burford (1964) as well as Selle and associates (1971) recommended that 14 days is a maximum limit for conservative therapy before surgical intervention. In approximately 50% of patients, the thoracic duct leak closes spontaneously, and the other 50% require surgical intervention. When chest tube drainage is consistently greater than 500 ml per day for two weeks, surgical intervention is definitely indicated, except for those patients for whom thoracotomy is contraindicated, such as those with vertebral fractures or with nonresectable tumors. If a lung is entrapped and pleural synthesis cannot be achieved with re-expansion by closed chest tube thoracostomy, then early surgical intervention is indicated. If chylous drainage is still present after a period of carefully supervised nonoperative conservative therapy, patients with congenital, traumatic, or postoperative chylothorax should undergo surgical treatment.

OPERATIVE THERAPY OF A CHYLOUS FISTULA

Several techniques may be used to control a chylous fistula, singly or in a combination: direct ligation of the thoracic duct, mass ligation of the thoracic duct, pleuroperitoneal shunting, and pleurectomy. Occasionally, decortication may be required when the lung is entrapped. Stenzel and colleagues (1983) suggested that fibrin glue be applied in some instances.

In unilateral chylothorax, the chest should be opened on the side of the effusion. When the effusion is bilateral, it is more prudent to explore the right side first, with ligation of the duct low in the right chest. Exploration of the left side is done later, if necessary. Ross (1961) stated that the easiest way to find the duct and the leakage point is to give the patient 100 to 200 ml of olive oil through a nasogastric tube 2 to 3 hours before the operation — what remains in the stomach at the time of anesthetic induction can be removed by the same nasogastric tube. This causes filling of the duct with milky chyle, which is readily recognized throughout the course of the operation. An alternative method is to inject a 1% aqueous solution of Evans blue dye into the leg. This causes staining of the thoracic duct

within 5 minutes that lasts up to 12 minutes. The disadvantage of the dye is that the adjacent tissues are also stained when there is free escape of chyle.

Ligation of the thoracic duct just above the diaphragm throughout the right chest is currently favored by most authors, including Selle (1971), Patterson (1981), and Milson (1985) and their associates, regardless of the site of the chylous leak. As noted, the thoracic duct is a single structure from T12 to T8 in over 75% of all patients.

The three techniques used to control the leak of chyle are direct closure of the fistula, suture of the leaking mediastinal pleura, and supradiaphragmatic ligation of the duct. The best method is to find the actual point of leakage and to close it with nonabsorbable sutures with the use of Teflon pledgets, compressing the leakage point in the adjacent tissue between the two pledgets, and, if possible, allowing the main portion of the duct to remain patent. Either of the first two techniques, and particularly the second, should be combined with supradiaphragmatic ligation of the duct. This alone is entirely effective in instances in which no attempt has been made to directly close the fistula. The most favorable site for elective ligation is low in the right chest just above the right crus of the diaphragm where the duct lies on the vertebral column between the aorta and the azygos vein (Fig. 59–1).

If a definite source of leak cannot be identified when the right chest is explored, despite use of the previously described ingestion of fat — milk or cream — or olive oil before surgery, then supradiaphragmatic ligation of

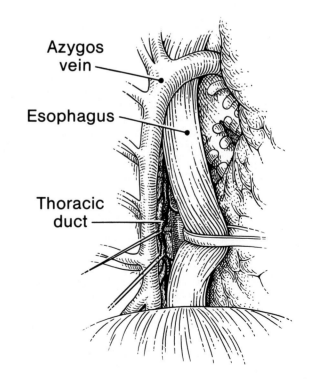

Fig. 59–1. Surgical anatomy of the thoracic duct in the right suprahepatic location.

the duct should be performed. This method was originally described by Murphy and Piper (1977) and subsequently championed by Patterson and colleagues (1981).

Supradiaphragmatic Ligation of the Thoracic Duct

A standard posterolateral thoracotomy incision is made, going through the bed of the resected right sixth rib. Generally, the pleura has a shaggy appearance because of fibrin deposits. After these deposits are cleaned off, the pulmonary ligament is divided between clamps and the pulmonary ligament swept upward to the level of the inferior pulmonary vein. The retropleural area is often thickened up to 1 to 2 cm and should be biopsied, if this is the case. It is best to ligate the duct en masse by going around the duct, taking a generous bite of tissue around the duct, and going close to the vertebral bodies, but avoiding the esophagus, aorta, and azygos vein. This suture should be tied with large pledgeted sutures on either end, as shown in Figure 59–2. This effects a mass ligature in the area between the azygos vein and the aorta just above the diaphragm. One must take care not to enter the wall of the esophagus. In effect, all tissue between the azygos vein and the aorta is ligated in the mass ligature.

A parietal pleurectomy is performed to achieve pleural synthesis. At the same time, if the underlying lung is trapped, it is decorticated. Two chest tube catheters are placed into the thoracic cavity and the chest closed in the usual fashion. In general, the chest tubes can be removed in 5 to 7 days, and recovery is rapid.

Other Techniques to Control Chylothorax

Milson and associates (1985) and Weese and Schouten (1984) reported the successful use of pleuroperitoneal

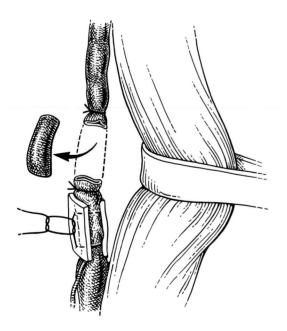

Fig. 59–2. Mass ligation of the thoracic duct using Teflon pledgets with nonabsorbable suture.

shunting with the double-valve Denver peritoneal shunt in the treatment of chylothorax. I have used this method with success.

Stenzel and colleagues (1983) reported the successful use of fibrin glue in one case of postsurgical chylothorax after an extrapleural ligation of the patent ductus arteriosus.

In nontraumatic chylothorax, the cause must be determined, and if neoplasm or infection is the cause, it must be treated specifically with radiation therapy, chemotherapy, or antibiotic therapy. If chylous drainage persists in these situations, pleural synthesis by catheter drainage of the pleura with instillation of nitrogen mustard or other irritants can be tried. In some cases, even though not desirable, thoracic duct ligation or pleurectomy may be needed to control the chylothorax. Radiation therapy has been successful in managing chylothorax in patients with mediastinal lymphoma and carcinoma. Irradiation of the pleural lymphatics to 2000 rads causes closure of the thoracic duct leak in most cases. I have observed four patients with nontraumatic chylothorax in whom no malignancy could be found who received radiation therapy to the pleural lymphatics to 2000 rads with success in all cases.

GUIDELINES FOR MANAGEMENT

In an excellent review of the indications for surgery, Selle and colleagues (1971) established the following guidelines: 1) Idiopathic cases in the neonate usually respond well to thoracentesis. 2) Nontraumatic chylothorax, exclusive of the neonatal group, usually suggests a widespread fatal illness, and operative intervention is usually ineffective and should, therefore, be avoided. 3) In cases resulting from trauma, an initial trial of nonoperative therapy is indicated. Transthoracic ligation of the duct is indicated when the average daily chyle loss has exceeded 1500 ml a day in adults for more than 5 days. 4) If the chyle flow has not diminished within 14 days or if nutritional complications appear imminent, surgery is indicated. Figure 59–3 lists my approach in the management of chylothorax. Thoracentesis is performed to confirm the diagnosis. Once the diagnosis of chylothorax has been established, a chest tube is inserted by closed thoracostomy. The patient is kept NPO, and nutritional replacement is begun, using central hyperalimentation. Rarely is the patient allowed to drink, and if so, a medium-chain triglyceride diet is used. This method is continued for 2 weeks. If drainage greater than 500 ml/day persists, and the underlying cause is nonmalignant, the patient is taken to the operating room for surgical control of the leak in the aforementioned manner. A success rate of greater than 90% may be expected with surgical intervention. Moreover, the mortality rate should be zero.

If the drainage is less than 250 ml/day, and appears to be decreasing, I may continue to try conservative therapy for 1 more week. If the leakage stops, the chest tube is removed. If this is to be done, one should give a trial of a high-fat diet before removing the chest tube.

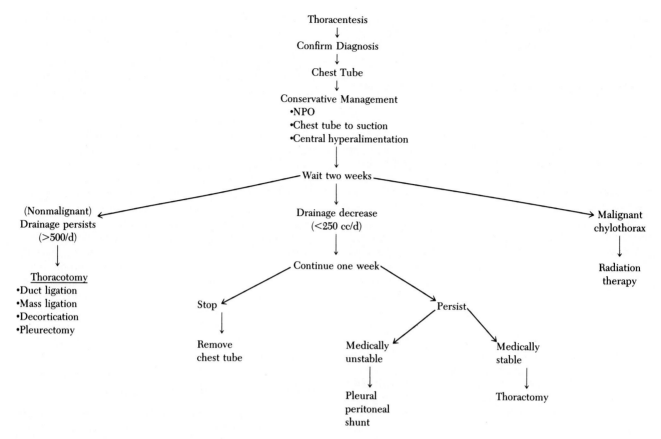

Fig. 59–3. Management of chylothorax.

If leakage persists at this time, pleuroperitoneal shunting could be performed if the patient is a medically compromised candidate, or thoracotomy and the previously mentioned procedures can be performed. If conservative therapy fails to control the chylothorax after 2 weeks and the underlying condition is a malignancy, then irradiation is administered. Generally, radiation therapy to the amount of 2000 rads controls most cases of this variety of chylothoraces.

REFERENCES

Bessone LN, Ferguson TB, Burford TH: Chylothorax: a collective review. Ann Thorac Surg *12*:527, 1971.

Biet AB, Connolly NK: Traumatic chylothorax: a report of a case and a survey of the literature. Br J Surg *39*:564, 1951.

Bower BC: Chyliform pleural effusion in rheumatoid arthritis. Am Rev Respir Dis *47*:4515, 1968.

Boyd A: Chylothorax. *In* R.M. Hood, et al (eds): Surgical Disease of the Pleura and Chest Wall. Philadelphia: WB Saunders, 1986.

Crandall L Jr, Barker SB, Graham DC: A study of the lymph from a patient with thoracic duct fistula. Gastroenterology *1*:1040, 1943.

Cunn B, Liebow AA, Friedman PJ: Pulmonary lymphangiomatosis: a review. Am J Pathol *79*:398, 1973.

DeMeester TR: The pleura. *In* Sabiston DC, Spencer EC (eds): Surgery of the Chest. 4th Ed. Philadelphia: WB Saunders, 1983.

Higgins CB, Molder DG: Chylothorax after surgery for congenital heart disease. J Thorac Cardiovasc Surg *61*:411, 1971.

Hyde PV, Jerky J, Gishen P: Traumatic chylothorax. S Afr J Surg *12*:57, 1974.

Lampson RS, et al: Traumatic chylothorax: a review of the literature and report of a case treated by mediastinal ligation of the thoracic duct. J Thorac Surg *17*:778, 1948.

Milson JW, et al: Chylothorax: an assessment of current surgical management. J Thorac Cardiovasc Surg *89*:221, 1985.

Munk I, Rosenstein A: Zur Lehre von der Resorption in Darm nach Untersuchungen an einer Lymph (chylus) fistel beim Menschen. Virchuis Arch Pathol Anat *123*:484, 1891.

Murphy TO, Piper CA: Surgical management of chylothorax. Ann Surg *43*:719, 1977.

Patterson GA, et al: Supradiaphragmatic ligation of the thoracic duct in intractable chylous fistula. Ann Thorac Surg *32*:44, 1981.

Ross JK: A review of surgery of the thoracic duct. Thorax *16*:12, 1961.

Roy PH, Carr DT, Payne WS: The problem of chylothorax. Mayo Clin Proc *42*:457, 1967.

Selle JG, Synder WA, Schreiber JT: Chylothorax. Ann Surg *177*:245, 1971.

Shafiroff GP, Kau QY: Cannulation of the human thoracic lymph duct. Surgery *45*:814, 1959.

Silverstein EF, et al: Pulmonary lymphangiomyomatosis. Am J Roentgenol Radium Ther Nucl Med *120*:832, 1974.

Staats RA, et al: The lipoprotein profile of chylous and unchylous pleural effusion. Mayo Clin Proc *55*:700, 1980.

Stenzel W, et al: Treatment of post surgical chylothorax with fibrin glue. J Thorac Cardiovasc Surg *31*:35, 1983.

Stuttman LJ, Dumont AE, Shinowara G: Coagulation factors in human lymph and plasma. Am J Med Sci *250*:292, 1965.

Weese JL, Schouten JT: Internal drainage of intractable malignant pleural effusions. Wis Med J *83*:21, 1984.

Williams KR, Burford TH: The management of chylothorax. Ann Surg *160*:131, 1964.

READING REFERENCES

Blalock A, Cunningham RS, Robinson CS: Experimental production of chylothorax by occlusions of the superior vena cava. Ann Surg *104*:359, 1936.

Donini I, Batteggati M: The Lymphatic System. London: Piccin Medical Books, 1972, p II–26.

Goorwitch J: Traumatic chylothorax and thoracic duct ligation. J Thoracic Surg *29*:467, 1955.

Klepser RG, Berny JF: The diagnosis and surgical management of chylothorax with the aid of lipophilic dyes. Dis Chest *25*:409, 1954.

CHAPTER 60

LOCALIZED FIBROUS TUMORS OF THE PLEURA

Thomas W. Shields

Localized fibrous tumors of the pleura have previously been most often classified as localized mesotheliomas of the pleura, either benign or malignant. The malignant variety also has been classified by some investigators, including Martini and associates (1987), as fibrosarcomas. Scharifker and Kaneko (1979), among others, have suggested that the cell origin of these tumors is a noncommitted mesenchymal cell present in the areolar tissue subadjacent to the mesothelial lining of the pleura and is not from the mesothelial cells of the pleura, as the earlier name implies. The most appropriate term for the malignant variety is "a localized malignant fibrous tumor of the pleura."

The studies of Dalton (1979), Said (1984), Dervan (1986), Keating (1987), and England (1989) and their associates, as well as the studies of Witkin and Rosai (1989), El-Naggar (1989), and Steinetz (1990) and their colleagues, have supported this concept of the mesenchymal origin of both the benign and malignant localized fibrous tumors of the pleura. Additional, but oblique, support of this concept is the observation that a history of asbestos exposure is lacking in the patients with these tumors, which is in marked contrast to those patients with diffuse malignant mesothelioma, in whom asbestos exposure is recorded in over 60%.

BENIGN LOCALIZED FIBROUS TUMORS OF THE PLEURA

Pathologic Characteristics

Gross Features

Most benign localized fibrous tumors arise from the visceral pleura on a stalk and project into the pleural space in a pedunculated manner. Sessile attachment to the pleura occurs, and inward growth into the lung parenchyma may infrequently be seen. Yousen and Flynn (1988) reported three intraparenchymal localized fibrous tumors, only one of which was attached to the visceral pleura. They theorized that the other two may

have arisen from mesenchymal cells in the interlobular septa or even de nova in the lung tissue. Localized fibrous tumors may also occasionally develop within a fissure. The benign tumors also may arise from the mediastinal, diaphragmatic, or costal portions of the parietal pleura. Tumors in these locations, however, including those arising within a fissure or growing into the lung, often prove to be malignant. Grossly, the benign tumors may have vascular adhesion between it and the adjacent visceral or parietal pleura. They are almost always solitary and are ovoid or round. The external surface may be smooth or bosselated. According to England and associates (1989), a thin, membranous capsule is present in about one half the cases. The size may vary greatly from a small nodule to a huge mass that may completely fill the hemithorax. On cut section, the mass is composed of dense, whorled fibrous tissue that may contain cyst-like structures filled a clear viscid fluid in 10 to 15% of cases. Calcifications may be present within the tumor.

Histologic Features

Microscopically, one or more histologic patterns can be seen. The most common pattern seen is the "patternless pattern" described by Stout (1971). Fibroblast-like cells and connective tissue are observed in varying proportions and are arranged in a disorderly or random pattern (Fig. 60–1). The tumor cells are spindle or plump ovoid cells with round-to-oval nuclei and small nucleoli. Collagen and elastin bundles are readily identified. Pleomorphism and mitosis are very infrequently seen. The second most common pattern is described as hemangiopericytoma-like and is often combined with the "patternless pattern." In this variety, closely packed tumor cells are arranged around open or collapsed, irregular branching capillaries. Other uncommon patterns, always mixed with one of the aforementioned patterns, are described as storiform, herringbone, leiomyoma-like, or neurofibroma-like.

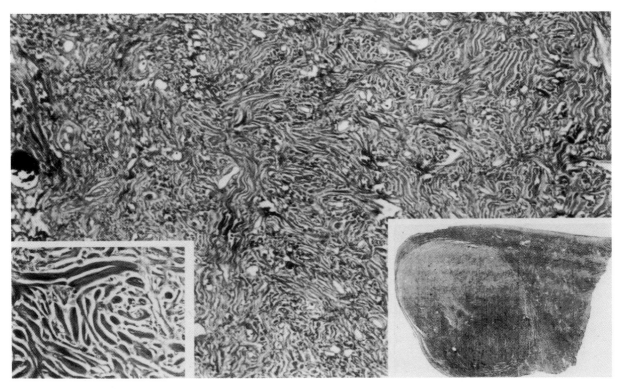

Fig. 60–1. Localized benign fibrous tumor of pleura with dense, wirelike strands of collagen sprinkled with plump fibroblast-like cells (insert bottom left) forming a "patternless pattern." Scanning lens view shows varying cellularity of tumor (insert, bottom right). *From* England DM, Hochholzer L, McCarthy MJ: Localized benign and malignant fibrous tumors of the pleura: a clinicopathologic review of 223 cases. Am J Surg Pathol 13:640, 1989.

Ultrastructural Features

Ultrastructurally, single to clusters of fusiform-to-round cells are found interspaced between focal or abundant collagen. The cells, according to Said and colleagues (1984), most closely resemble mesenchymal cells of fibroblastic type. Keating and co-workers (1987) noted that no basal lamina, intracellular junctions, or microvilli are seen. The observations of El-Naggar (1989) and Steinetz (1990) and their associates support the fibroblastic nature of these cells.

Immunohistologic Features

Immunohistochemically, the localized fibrous tumors are positive for vimentin and weakly to variably positive for muscle-specific actin. The cells have negative reactions to cytokeratin, epithelial membrane antigen carcinoembryonic antigen — CEA — factor VIII related antigen, neurofilament, and S-100 protein. The immunohistochemical differences between these tumors and the diffuse malignant mesotheliomas are shown in Table 60–1. The lack of reactivity to factor VIII related antigen and to neurofilament and S-100 protein differentiate the tumor from a true hemangiopericytoma or a neurogenic tumor, respectively.

Flow-Cytometric DNA Studies

El-Naggar and colleagues (1989) described a diploid DNA pattern in all 12 nonrecurrent benign fibrous

Table 60–1. Differentiation of Localized Fibrous Tumor and Diffuse Mesothelioma of the Pleura: Immunoreactivity

	Localized Fibrous Tumor	Mesothelioma
Vimentin	+	+ +
EMA	−	(+)*
Actin	(+)*	
Cytokeratin	−	+ +
CEA	−	−

*(+) Variably or weakly positive.

CEA = carcinoembryonic antigen; EMA = epithelial membrane antigen.

tumors in their study. The S-phase was low in all 12 as well.

Clinical Features

Benign localized fibrous tumors of the pleura occur with equal frequency in both sexes, although Milano (1990) reported a greater incidence in women. The tumor may occur in any age group but is more common in the fifth to eighth decades of life. More than one half of the tumors are asymptomatic. Previously, Briselli and associates (1981), in a review of 368 patients with these tumors recorded in the literature, including 8 of their own cases, noted that 64% were reported to have had symptomatic lesions. However, this included many patients diagnosed late, and in addition, 12% of these patients had malignant lesions. Okike (1978) and England (1989) and their colleagues reported that chronic cough, chest pain, and dyspnea were the more common complaints (Table 60–2). Chest pain is most often manifested when the lesion arises from the parietal pleura. Occasionally, in a patient with a large tumor, symptoms of bronchial compression and atelectasis may occur. Okike and colleagues (1978) recorded the occurrence of hypertrophic pulmonary osteoarthropathy in 20% of their patients. Briselli and associates (1981), in their collective review, reported an incidence of 22%. Frequently, the tumor is of large size — greater than 7 cm — when this is observed.

Hypertrophic Pulmonary Osteoarthropathy

This symptom complex occurs in association with many intrathoracic disease processes. Clagett and colleagues (1952) at the Mayo Clinic reported that hypertrophic pulmonary osteoarthropathy occurred in 66% of cases of localized fibrous tumor of the pleura, although their latter data presented by Okike and associates (1978) noted this association in only 20% of instances. Nonetheless, this pattern contrasts markedly with the overall 5% incidence of hypertrophic pulmonary osteoarthropathy in bronchial carcinoma, as reported in one of the lead articles in Lancet ("Lead Article," 1959). I have observed the incidence to be only 2 to 3% in this latter disease.

Osteoarthropathy describes a "rheumatoid-like" disease of the bones and joints. It is frequently associated with clubbing of the fingers, but it may be present without clubbing. Gynecomastia is similarly seen with hypertrophic pulmonary osteoarthropathy yet also occurs as a solitary extrathoracic manifestation of an intrathoracic neoplasm.

The classic findings in hypertrophic pulmonary osteoarthropathy include stiffness of the joints, edema over the ankles and occasionally of the hands, arthralgia, and pain along the surfaces of the long bones — especially the tibia. At times, the joint and bone pain is severe.

Table 60–2. Symptoms of Benign Localized Fibrous Tumors of the Pleura

Symptom	Okike et al (1978) (52 Patients)	England et al (1989) (138 Patients)
Asymptomatic	28	92
Chronic cough	17	16
Chest pain	12	26
Dyspnea	10	15
Fever	9	1
Hypertrophic pulmonary osteoarthropathy ± clubbing	10	—
Pleurisy	3	—
Weight loss	3	3
Hemoptysis	1	0
Pneumonitis	1	—

The joint and bone involvement is usually bilateral. The distal ends of the ulna and radius are most frequently involved, and radiographic evidence of the periosteal thickening is most commonly seen here. The bones of the hands, ankles, knees, elbows, and shoulders are involved in that approximate order. Finger pressure on the anterior surface of the distal tibia often elicits pain in advance of any radiologic changes.

Clinical symptoms vary from minimally detectable stiffness of the wrists to systemic toxicity. Some of the systemic manifestations seem to be related to one or more endocrine, collagen, or immunologic mechanisms of the body that are not directly related to the osteoarthropathy. Chills and spiking temperature, markedly elevated sedimentation rate, and malaise with obvious systemic toxicity may be present.

Hypertrophic pulmonary osteoarthropathy may be associated with clubbing of the fingers and toes, although many investigators believe the latter is not actually part of the syndrome. Martinez-Lavin (1987), as well as Shneerson (1981), however, have suggested that the two processes are related and arise from the same underlying cause, most likely the overproduction or lack of metabolism by the lung of a growth-like hormone.

Clubbing

Clubbing is the enlargement of the distal phalanges, usually of both the hands and feet. Diner (1962) described periosteal new growth with lymphocytic and plasma cell infiltration of connective tissue around the nail beds, resulting in increased fibrous tissue between the nail bed and phalanx. Van Hazel (1940) reported the digital arteries to be enlarged and elongated 10 to 15 times normal. Also, Cudkowicz and Armstrong (1953) noted the presence of arteriovenous anastomosis in the distal finger segments near the junction of the dermis and the subcutaneous tissue.

Clinically, the distal phalanx is enlarged — especially widened — with a loss of the obtuse angle that the nail bed normally forms with the plane of the proximal skin surface. A spongy sensation on depression of the proximal nail bed is characteristic.

According to Martinez-Lavin (1987), a common denominator appears to be present in the various processes associated with clubbing. These processes can be broadly classified into pulmonary, cardiac, and extrathoracic. Only the first category will be discussed.

Neoplastic lesions of the lung causing clubbing are generally associated with hypertrophic pulmonary osteoarthropathy, whereas the congenital structural and inflammatory pulmonary lesions associated with clubbing rarely show signs of arthropathy. Non-neoplastic pulmonary disorders seen with clubbing include pulmonary arteriovenous fistula, lung abscess, bronchiectasis, empyema, pulmonary infarction, emphysema, chronic bronchitis, chronic inflammation of the lung, sarcoidosis, idiopathic pulmonary fibrosis, diffuse interstitial fibrosis, primary pulmonary hypertension, pneumoconioses, and atelectasis.

Etiology

The etiology of hypertrophic pulmonary osteoarthropathy and clubbing remains an enigma. A single cause for these two frequently associated yet distinct phenomena seems unlikely. Flavell (1956) reported relief from the pain of hypertrophic osteoarthropathy following division of the vagus nerve at the hilus of the lung in patients with inoperable pulmonary neoplasms. Diner (1962) described dramatic relief of symptoms following cervical or thoracic vagotomy. Ginsburg (1958) found that blood flows in the hand and foot were similar in a control group and in patients with hypertrophic pulmonary osteoarthropathy. Lovell (1950), however, demonstrated increased blood flow in patients with clubbing secondary to congenital cyanotic heart disease. These patients had dilated venous plexuses in the skin of the nail-bed area, accompanied by increased caliber in the digital arteries and abnormal arteriovenous communications.

Although the cause of these conditions remains unknown, several observations may be made. First, clubbing of the fingers has some connection with arteriovenous shunting. Whether these abnormal arteriovenous communications permit a substance that is normally altered or detoxified in the lung to appear in the systemic circulation or whether small emboli that are usually filtered out by the lung are allowed to appear there is unanswered, but certainly the latter is highly debatable. Cudkowicz and Armstrong (1953) demonstrated precapillary bronchopulmonary anastomosis in patients with clubbing. Desaturation of the blood per se seems an unlikely explanation because the incidence of clubbing in severely emphysematous patients is so low. Second, there is circumstantial evidence in the relationship of hypertrophic pulmonary osteoarthropathy and involvement of the pleura. This aspect is borne out by the occurrence of the syndrome in some patients with localized fibrous tumors of the pleura, as well as in patients with peripheral bronchial carcinomas. A neoplastic process involving the pleura, the embryologic origin of which is pluripotential, may elaborate a substance that elicits osseous articular responses. This same neoplastic process might also create an arteriovenous fistula, producing clubbing. It has been suggested by Steiner (1968) and Gosney (1990) and their colleagues that ectopic production of a growth hormone-like substance by a tumor may result in the development of clubbing, as well as in pulmonary osteoarthropy.

The clinical significance of hypertrophic pulmonary osteoarthropathy is greater in its diagnostic than its therapeutic implications. Removal of the pulmonary lesion for the most part gives dramatic remission of the arthralgia and peripheral edema. In the series reported by Okike and associates (1978), 8 of 10 patients with localized fibrous tumors experienced complete relief of the symptom complex after operative removal of the tumor. Osseous radiographic changes regress much more slowly. Recurrence of a localized fibrous tumor is usually heralded by a return of the symptoms present with the original osteoarthropathy.

Hypoglycemia

A large benign localized fibrous tumor of the pleura may be associated with a severe *hypoglycemia*. An incidence of 3 to 4% has been stated. In addition, a number of diverse mesenchymal tumors also have been reported to have an infrequent association with this condition. In 1968 Devroede and Tirol reported that 58 examples of hypoglycemia secondary to a mesenchymal tumor had been recorded in the literature up to that time. According to Silverstein and associates (1964), most of those were fibrosarcomas, although examples of neurofibroma, rhabdomyosarcoma, liposarcoma, leiomyosarcoma, hemangiopericytoma, and mesothelioma were also noted.

As in the instances of hypoglycemia from other causes, the patient can present with varying symptoms of central nervous system deprivation of glucose. Convulsions, syncope, and even coma may occur. Death may result if the severe hypoglycemia is not corrected promptly.

Nelson and co-workers (1975) reviewed the numerous theories to explain the mechanism of hypoglycemia. Among these are increased glucose consumption by the tumor, a defect in glucose regulators, that is, adrenocorticotropic hormone, growth hormone, or glucagon; ectopic secretion of insulin by the tumor, the presence of a stimulator of insulin release, or a potentiator of circulating insulin; the inhibition of glycogenolysis; the inhibition of lipolysis and hepatic gluconeogenesis; and the presence of nonsuppressible insulin-like activity/insulin growth factors I and II.

Most of these theories have been disproved, and Nelson and co-workers (1975) suggested that increased glucose use by the tumor was probably a partial explanation. Bunn and Ridgway (1989), however, report that tumor use of glucose to a degree that causes hypoglycemia has not yet been substantiated. Currently, these latter authors believe the most likely, although far from established, mechanism is tumor production of nonsuppressible insulin-like active substances — called somatomedins — and insulin-like growth factors. Somatomedins are reported by Van Wyk and associates (1974) to be a family of peptide hormones produced by the liver under growth hormone regulation. Zaph (1981), Gordon (1981), and Li (1983) and their colleagues have reported these substances in various examples of extrapancreatic tumor hypoglycemia. Recently, Cole (1990) and Strøm (1991) and their associates have demonstrated insulin-like growth factors in one patient each who had associated hypoglycemia with a benign fibrous pleural tumor. The hypoglycemia was relieved in each with removal of the tumor. The relief of the hypoglycemia associated with a benign fibrous tumor is typical after complete removal of the tumor.

Galactorrhea

This is a rare finding in patients with fibrous tumors of the pleura. It has been reported, however, by Brisilli (1981) and McCaughey (1980) and their associates.

Radiographic Features

The appearance of a localized fibrous tumor of the pleura is for the most part indistinguishable from that of other nodules of the lung (Fig. 60–2). A circumscribed mass of varying size usually is located in the lung periphery or in the projection of an interlobar fissure. The larger neoplasms may have irregular shapes, although the margins are usually sharply defined. These tumors arise, more often from a pedicle from the visceral pleura. Occasionally, movement of the mass may be demonstrated with changes in position when the tumor is on a stalk. Zirinsky and Hsu (1982) demonstrated this change in location by computed tomography — CT — examination. However, CT examination *per se* has little to add to the standard radiographic examination of these lesions. Mendelson and colleagues (1991) have reviewed the CT findings relative to this tumor. Infrequently, a pleural effusion may be present. In the collective review of England and associates (1989), 8% of 138 patients had a pleural effusion and was the initial clinical finding.

Diagnosis

The nature of the solitary lesion is established most often at the time of thoracotomy and subsequent histologic examination. It is doubtful that tissue obtained by percutaneous transthoracic needle biopsy would be sufficient for precise diagnosis, although, Milano (1990) has suggested that it may occasionally be diagnostic. I do not recommend the procedure.

Treatment

Localized fibrous tumors of the pleura are usually amenable to surgical resection (Fig. 60–3). Tumors that are considered benign on the basis of being localized may, however, be malignant both histologically and clinically, so adequate removal of the original lesion must be ensured. Nothing in my experience suggests that lobectomy is preferable to local resection of a pedunculated lesion arising from the visceral pleura. If the lesion is within the lung parenchyma, however, resection of the lobe is advisable. A segmentectomy is occasionally sufficient, but even a bilobectomy may be necessary when the lesion is located within a fissure. Localized fibrous tumors of the mediastinal, diaphragmatic, and parietal pleura should be excised as widely as can be accomplished satisfactorily because these locations are more often associated with a malignant lesion.

Prognosis

Almost all patients, with benign localized fibrous tumors of the pleura are cured by adequate excision of the lesion. England and associates (1989) noted only two recurrences in 98 patients — 2% — and in both patients a second curative resection was possible. Any recurrences, however, must be viewed with suspicion.

MALIGNANT LOCALIZED FIBROUS TUMORS OF THE PLEURA

Incidence

The relative incidence of malignant localized fibrous tumors as compared to that of the benign lesions is unknown. Thirty-six percent of the fibrous pleural tumors reviewed by England and associates (1989) were malignant, but all of the 223 cases had been referred

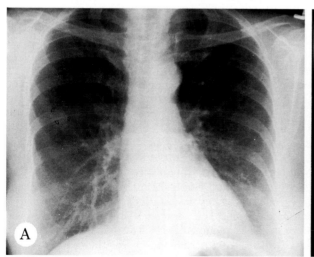
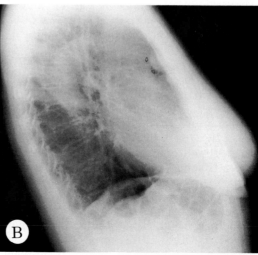

Fig. 60–2. PA and lateral radiographs of the chest of a 68-year-old woman revealing a small peripheral mass in the anterior aspect of right upper lobe. At thoracotomy the mass was found to be a pedunculated fibrous tumor attached to the visceral pleura of the right upper lobe.

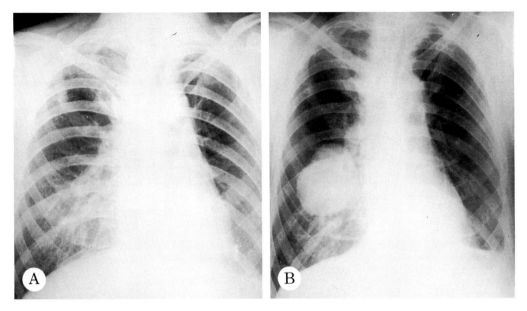

Fig. 60–3. *A*, Radiograph of chest revealing 3-cm solitary nodule at the level of the fifth interspace anteriorly in the right lung. *B*, Radiograph of the same patient 10 years later, revealing marked enlargement of the mass. At thoracotomy a benign fibrous tumor was readily removed.

to the Armed Forces Institute of Pathology for study and represent a biased data base. In the review of 360 cases by Briselli and colleagues (1981) the incidence of malignant tumors was 12%. In the report from the Mayo Clinic by Okike and co-workers (1978), the incidence was 13%; these latter figures may represent a more appropriate incidence of malignancy.

Pathologic Characteristics

Gross Features. The malignant variety as compared to the benign tumors tend to be large in size, to be more often located atypically — from the parietal pleura, intralobar in location, or to exhibit inverted growth into the pulmonary parenchyma — and to show areas of necrosis and hemorrhage (Table 60–3).

Microscopic Features. The malignant fibrous tumors of the pleura in contrast to the benign tumor show an increased cellularity, cellular pleomorphism, and an increased number of mitotic figures (Table 60–3). El-Naggar and associates (1989) observed higher mitotic counts than in the benign tumors. Extensive areas of myxomatous change, hemorrhage, and necrosis are also commonly seen.

Other Features. The malignant tumors are often positive for vimentin. Staining for cytokeratins is negative. The ultrastructural findings are not truly distinguishable from those tumors of the benign variety. Flow-cytometric DNA studies showed an elevated S-phase in contrast to a low S-phase in benign lesions according to the study of El-Naggar and associates (1989).

Clinical Features

Most of these patients — approximately three-quarters — in contrast to those with localized benign me-

Table 60–3. Pathologic Features that Distinguish Benign and Malignant Localized Fibrous Tumor of Pleura

Feature	Benign (n = 141) n	Benign (n = 141) (%)	Malignant* (n = 82) n	Malignant* (n = 82) (%)
Gross				
Pedunculated	73	(52)	21	(26)
Atypical location†	67	(48)	55	(67)
Size (>10 cm)	34	(24)	45	(55)
Necrosis and hemorrhage	21	(15)	53	(65)
Microscopic				
Increased cellularity	18	(13)	62	(76)
Pleomorphism‡	14	(10)	69	(84)
Mitosis (>4 mf/10 hpf)	2	(1)	63	(77)

*For all features, the differences between benign and malignant tumors are statistically significant by the chi-square test (p <.05).

†Tumor attached to parietal pleura, fissure, or mediastinum, or inverted into peripheral lung.

‡Pleomorphism expressed as increased nuclear grades.

From England DM, Hochholzer L, McCarthy MJ: Localized benign and malignant fibrous tumors of the pleura. A clinicopathologic review of 223 cases. Am J Surg Pathol 13:640, 1989.

sotheliomas, have symptoms. Chest pain, cough, dyspnea, and fever are the most common symptoms. Osteoarthropathy rarely, if ever, occurs with the localized malignant lesion. Hypoglycemia, however, is more commonly seen in patients with the malignant than the benign fibrous tumors of the pleura. An incidence of 11% as compared to 3%, respectively, is found according to the data of England and associates (1989).

Radiographic Features

The radiographic findings in patients with the malignant fibrous tumors of the pleura are similar to those seen in patients with the benign variety, except the lesions tend to be larger and pleural effusion is seen more often. An incidence of associated pleural effusion of 32% was recorded by England and associates (1989). Occasionally, rib erosion may occur as the result of invasion of the chest wall.

Diagnosis

In most instances, the diagnosis is not apparent until histologic examination of the resected specimen. Invasion of the chest wall or other adjacent structures within the chest grossly establishes the malignant nature of the lesion. Recurrence of lesion originally thought to be benign must be regarded as suggesting the true malignant nature of the lesion (Fig. 60–4).

Treatment

Wide local excision, including pulmonary and pleural resections, is carried out as indicated. Resection of a lesion arising from the parietal pleura should include the adjacent chest wall. When complete resection is possible, postoperative adjuvant therapy — irradiation or chemotherapy — is not indicated. When the resection is incomplete, Martini and associates (1987) suggest that radiation therapy both internal — brachy-

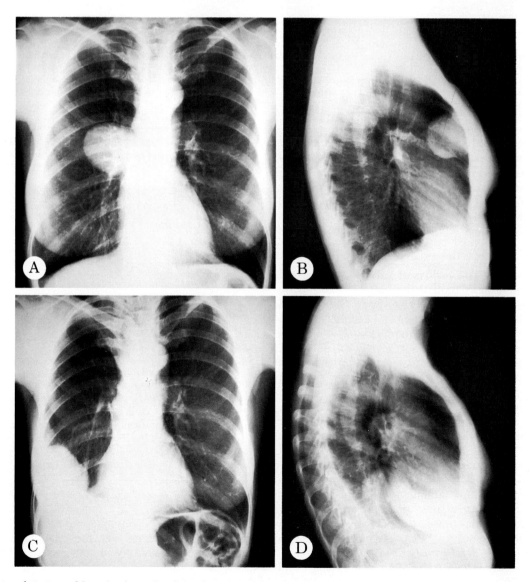

Fig. 60–4. *A* and *B,* PA and lateral radiographs of the chest revealing a large solitary mass, which was diagnosed as a benign fibrous tumor on its removal by a right upper lobectomy. *C* and *D,* PA and lateral radiographs of the chest 6 months after removal of the tumor, revealing rapid recurrence of the tumor, which required a pneumonectomy for its complete removal. The mass was frankly malignant on histologic examination. The patient succumbed from recurrent malignant fibrous tumor of the pleura.

therapy — and external should be used. Localized recurrence of a solitary malignant fibrous tumor should be evaluated for possible resection.

Prognosis

Okike and colleagues (1978) reported only a 12% long-term survival in patients with localized malignant tumors. England and associates (1989), however, reported a survival of 45% among 71 patients they considered to have had malignant lesions; most of the survivors had either pedunculated or well-circumscribed tumors. Chest wall or pericardial invasion does not preclude long-term survival if a complete excision can be carried out. Pleural effusion is a poor prognostic feature in the patients with a malignant fibrous tumor of the pleura.

Martini and colleagues (1987) reported 10 patients with long-term survival following complete resection of the tumor. England and associates (1989) concur that the most important indicator of clinical outcome is whether the tumor can be initially totally excised. Patients with incomplete excision all die of their disease.

Recurrences of even completely excised lesions do occur. Initially, these are almost always local at the site of excision. However, spread to other sites within the thorax or into the abdomen occurs. Lymph node metastases are seen as are blood-borne metastases in patients with persistent or recurrent disease. The sites of metastases recorded, in order of decreasing frequency, are the liver, central nervous system, spleen, peritoneum, adrenal gland, gastrointestinal tract, kidney, intra-abdominal lymph nodes, and bone. Most patients with recurrent disease survive less than 5 years.

REFERENCES

Arkless D, Goranow I, Krastinow G: Hypoglycemia in an intrathoracic fibroma. Med Bull Vet Admin 19:225, 1942.

Arrigoni MC, et al: Benign tumors of the lung: A ten-year surgical experience. J Thorac Cardiovasc Surg 60:589, 1970.

Barclay N, Ogbeide M, Grillo A: Gross hypertrophic pulmonary osteoarthropathy in a 7-year-old child. Thorax 25:484, 1970.

Barrett NR: The pleura. Thorax 25:515, 1970.

Berne AS, Heitzman ER: The roentgenologic signs of pedunculated pleural tumors. AJR Am J Roentgenol 87:892, 1962.

Briselli M, Mark EJ, Dickersin R: Solitary fibrous tumors of the pleura: eight new cases and review of 360 cases in the literature. Cancer 47:2678, 1981.

Brown WJ, Johnson LC: Post inflammatory "tumors" of the pleura: three cases of pleural fibroma of the interlobar fissure. Milit Surg 109:415, 1951.

Bunn PA Jr, Ridgway EC: Paraneoplastic syndromes. In DeVita VT Jr, Hellman S, Rosenberg SA (eds): Cancer: Principles and Practice of Oncology. 3rd Ed. Philadelphia: JB Lippincott, 1989, p 1896.

Clagett OT, McDonald JR, Schmidt HW: Localized fibrous mesothelioma of the pleura. J Thorac Surg 24:213, 1952.

Cole FH, et al: Benign fibrous pleural tumor with elevation of insulin-like growth factor and hypoglycemia. South Med J 83:690, 1990.

Cudkowicz L, Armstrong JB: Finger clubbing and changes in the bronchial circulation. Br J Tuberc Dis Chest 47:277, 1953.

Cudkowicz L, Wraith DC: A method of study of the pulmonary circulation in finger clubbing. Thorax 12:313, 1957.

Dalton WR, et al: Localized primary tumors of the pleura: An analysis of 40 cases. Cancer 44:1465, 1979.

Dervan PA, Tobin B, O'Connor M: Solitary localized fibrous mesothelioma: evidence against mesothelial cell origin. Histopathology 10:867, 1986.

Devroede J, Tirol AF: Grant pleural mesothelioma associated with hypoglycemia and hyperthyroidism. Am J Surg 116:130, 1968.

Diner WC: Hypertrophic osteoarthropathy. JAMA 181:555, 1962.

El-Naggar AK, et al: Localized fibrous tumor of the serosal cavities: immunohistochemical, electron-microscopic and flow-cytometric DNA study. Am J Clin Pathol 92:561, 1989.

England DM, Hochholzer L, McCarthy MJ: Localized benign and malignant fibrous tumors of the pleura: a clinicopathologic review of 223 cases. Am J Surg Pathol 13:640, 1989.

Flavell G: Reversal of pulmonary hypertrophic osteoarthropathy by vagotomy. Lancet 1:260, 1956.

Ginsburg J: Observations on the peripheral circulation in hypertrophic pulmonary osteoarthropathy. Q J Med 27:335, 1958.

Gordon P, et al: Hypoglycemia associated with non-Iet cell tumors and insulin like growth factors. N Engl J Med 305:1452, 1981.

Gosney MA, Gosney JR, Lye M: Plasma growth hormone and digital clubbing in carcinoma of the bronchus. Thorax 45:545, 1990.

Hernandez FJ, Fernandez BB: Localized fibrous tumors of pleura: a light and electron microscopic study. Cancer 34:1667, 1974.

Keating S, et al: Solitary fibrous tumor of the pleura: an ultrastructural and immunohistochemical study. Thorax 42:976, 1987.

Lead article: Lancet 2:389, 1959.

Lewis MI, et al: The case of the moving intrathoracic mass. Chest 88:897, 1985.

Li TCM, et al: Surgical cure of hypoglycemia associated with cystosarcoma phylloides and elevated NSILP. Am J Med 74:1080, 1983.

Lovell RRH: Observations on the structure of clubbed fingers. Clin Sci 9:299, 1950.

Maier HC, Barr D: Intrathoracic tumors associated with hypoglycemia. J Thoracic Cardiovasc Surg 44:321, 1962.

Marie P: De l'ostéoarthropathie hypertrophiante pneumonique. Rev Med Paris 10:1, 1890.

Martinez-Lavin M: Digital clubbing and hypertrophic osteoarthropathy: a unifying hypthesis. J Rheumatol 14:6, 1987.

Martini N, et al: Pleural mesothelioma: current review. Ann Thorac Surg 43:113, 1987.

McCaughey WET, Kannerstein M, Chrug J: Tumors of submesothelial origin. In Tumors and Pseudotumors of the Serous Membranes. Bethesda MD: Armed Forces Institute of Pathology, 1980, p 81.

Mendelson DS, et al: Localized fibrous pleural mesothelioma: CT findings. Clin Imaging 15:105, 1991.

Milano MJ: Benign mesothelioma. In Deslauriers J, Lacquet LK (eds): Thoracic Surgery: Surgical Management of Pleural Disease. St Louis: CV Mosby, 1990.

Nelson R, et al: Hypoglycemic coma associated with benign pleural mesothelioma. J Thorac Cardiovasc Surg 69:306, 1975.

Okike N, Bernatz PE, Woolner LB: Localized mesothelioma of the pleura. Benign and malignant variants. J Thorac Cardiovasc Surg 75:363, 1978.

Said JW, et al: Localized fibrous mesothelioma: an immunohistochemical and electron microscopic study. Hum Pathol 15:440, 1984.

Scharifker D, Kaneko M: Localized fibrous "mesothelioma" of pleura (submesothelial) fibroma: a clinicopathologic study of 18 cases. Cancer 43:627, 1979.

Shneerson JM: Digital clubbing and hypertrophic osteoarthropathy: the underlying mechanisms. Br J Dis Chest 75:113, 1981.

Silverstein MN, Wakin KE, Bahn RC: Hypoglycemia associated with neoplasia. Am J Med 36:415, 1964.

Spry CI; Williamson DH, James ML: Pleuromesothelioma and hypoglycemia. Proc R Soc Med 61:1105, 1968.

Steiner H, Dahlback O, Waldenstrom J: Ectopic growth hormone production and osteoarthropathy in carcinoma of the bronchus. Lancet 1:783, 1968.

Steinetz C, et al: Localized fibrous tumors of the pleura: correlation of histopathological, immunohistochemical and ultrastructural features. Pathol Res Pract *186*:344, 1990.

Sternon I, Paramentier G, Rutsaert J: Comas hypoglycemiques et mesotheliome pleural benin. Acta Clin Belg *26*:44, 1971.

Stout AP: Tumors of the pleura. Harlem Hosp Bull *5*:54, 1971.

Strøm EH, et al: Solitary fibrous tumor of the pleura. An immunohistochemical, electron-microscopic and tissue culture of a tumor producing insulin-like growth factor I in a patient with hypoglycemia. Pathol Res Pract *187*:109, 1991.

Van Hazel W: Joint manifestations associated with intrathoracic tumors. J Thorac Surg *9*:495, 1940.

Van Wyk JJ, et al: The somatomedians: a family of insulin-like hormones under growth hormone control. Recent Prog Horm Res *30*:259, 1974.

Von Bamberger E: Ueber Knochenveranderungen bei chronischen Lungen- und Herzkrankheiten. Z Klin Med *18*:193, 1890.

Wierman H, Clagett OT, McDonald JR: Articular manifestations in pulmonary diseases. JAMA *155*:1459, 1954.

Witkin FB, Rosai J: Solitary fibrous tumor of the mediastinum, a report of 14 cases. Am J Surg Pathol *13*:547, 1989.

Yousen SA, Flynn DS: Intrapulmonary localized fibrous tumor: intraparenchymal so-called localized fibrous mesothelioma. Am J Clin Pathol *89*:365, 1988.

Zaph J, Walter H, Froesch ER: Radioimmunological determination of insulin-like growth factors I and II in normal subjects and in patients with growth disorders and extrapancreatic tumor hypoglycemia. J Clin Invest *68*:1321, 1981.

Zirinsky K, Hsu JT: Flopping mass in an asymptomatic woman. Chest *81*:733, 1982.

CHAPTER 61

DIFFUSE MALIGNANT MESOTHELIOMA

Valerie W. Rusch

Diffuse mesothelioma is an uncommon and usually lethal cancer for which there is currently no standard treatment. The first report of a primary pleural tumor, presumably a mesothelioma, is attributed to Lieutaud in 1767, but there was no accurate pathologic description until Klemperer and Rabin (1937) classified mesotheliomas as either localized or diffuse. Cell culture experiments by Stout and Murray (1942) demonstrated the mesothelial origin of these tumors. However, mesothelioma was largely regarded as a medical curiosity until 1960, when Wagner and co-workers reported 33 cases of diffuse malignant pleural mesothelioma in asbestos mine workers from the North Western Cape Province of South Africa. Subsequent studies, especially work by Selikoff and associates (1965) and Whitwell and Rawcliffe (1971) in the United States, confirmed that asbestos exposure was the major risk factor for malignant mesothelioma. The epidemiology of diffuse mesothelioma is now well understood, but its biologic behavior remains an enigma, and the treatment of this cancer is still controversial. Although mesothelioma is uncommon, its incidence is increasing because of the large number of individuals who were exposed to asbestos during the 1930s to 1960s in asbestos mines and asbestos-related industries, before the causal relationship between asbestos and mesothelioma was recognized. There are now an estimated 2000 to 3000 cases per year in the United States. It is important for thoracic surgeons to be knowledgeable about mesothelioma because they are often called on to make the diagnosis and to recommend treatment.

EPIDEMIOLOGY AND INCIDENCE

The relationship between asbestos exposure and interstitial lung disease was first recognized in 1906, when deaths among asbestos textile workers from pneumoconiosis were reported in England and France by Murray (1907) and Auribault (1906). Scattered case reports by Wedler (1943a,b), Cartier (1952), and Van der Schoot (1958) during the 1940s and 1950s suggested a possible link between asbestos exposure and diffuse malignant mesothelioma, but this was not clearly established until Wagner and associates' reports (1960, 1986). Wagner had been appointed Asbestosis Research Fellow at the South Africa Pneumoconiosis Research Unit in 1954 and had been charged with determining if all types of asbestos caused the same diseases. An increasing incidence of a rapidly fatal pleural tumor in patients hospitalized at the Tuberculosis Hospital in the asbestos mining region of South Africa led Wagner and associates to study pleural biopsies on these patients. The surprise finding of mesothelioma in these biopsies prompted a careful epidemiologic investigation. Asbestos exposure was the single factor common to all of these cases. Subsequently, Wagner went to Great Britain to study this problem further, and he again demonstrated an epidemiologic relationship between asbestos exposure and mesothelioma among asbestos workers and insulators.

The second and equally dramatic demonstration of the relationship between asbestos exposure and mesothelioma, as described by Layman (1992) and Musk and colleagues (1989) occurred in Western Australia where, during a 23-year period, from 1943 to 1966, approximately 7000 individuals who worked at the Wittenoom asbestos mines experienced unprotected exposure to asbestos. The first case of mesothelioma was recognized in 1960. By the end of 1986, 94 cases of mesothelioma, 141 cases of lung cancer, and 356 successful compensation claims for asbestosis had been recorded among the former asbestos miners and millers. An additional 692 cases of mesothelioma have been predicted to occur in this cohort between 1987 and 2020. The Wittenoom asbestos industry is regarded as the worst industrial disaster in Australian history.

As reported by de Klerk and Armstrong (1992), the type of asbestos fiber plays a critical role in the risk of developing mesothelioma. Asbestos is part of the family of silicate fibers and includes two mineralogic groups: amphibole and serpentine fibers. Chrysotile asbestos is the only member of the serpentine group,

Table 61–1. Nonasbestos Causes of Mesothelioma

Agent	Species Tumor Observed in or Induced In*
Naturally occurring mineral fibers Zeolites (eronite)	Man, rat
Minerals	
Nickel	Rat
Silica powder	Rat
Beryllium	Rat, ?man
Radiation	Man, rat
Organic chemicals	
Polyurethane, polysilicone	Rat
Sterigmatocystin (aflatoxin B_1-related compound)	Rat
Ethylene oxide	Rat
N-methyl-N-nitrosourea	Guinea pig
N-methyl-N-nitrosourethane	Mouse
3-Methylcholanthrene	Mouse
Methyl nitrosamine	Rat
1-Nitroso-5, 6-dihydrouracil	Rat
Diethylstilbesterol	Monkey
Stilbesterol	Dog
3, 4, 5-Trimetholxycinnamaldehyde	Rat
Mineral oil	Man
Liquid paraffin	Man
Viruses	
MC 29 avian leukosis virus	Chicken
SV 40	Hamster
Chronic inflammation	
Recurrent lung infections	Man
Tuberculous pleuritis	Man
Recurrent diverticulitis	Man
Familial Mediterranean fever	Man
Nonspecific industrial exposure	
Shoe industry workers	Man
Petrochemical-oil industry workers	Man
Stone cutters	Man
Leather factory or textile workers	Man
Occupations involving exposure to copper, nickel, fiberglass, rubber or glass dust	Man
Co-carcinogens	
3-Methylcholantrene-asbestos	Rat
Radiation-asbestos	Rat
N-methyl-N-nitrosourea-asbestos	Rat
Hereditary predisposition	Man

*Note: In some instances, the tumors induced in animals by various agents may represent sarcomas and not mesotheliomas.
From Hammar SP, Bolen JW: Pleural neoplasms. *In* Dail DH, Hammar SP (eds): Pulmonary Pathology. New York: Springer Verlag, 1988, p 979.

while crocidolite, amosite, tremolite, anthophyllite, and actinolite asbestos belong to the amphibole group. Pooley (1987) reports that these minerals differ considerably in their structure and composition. Serpentine fibers are large, curly shaped fibers that do not travel beyond the major airways, while amphibole fibers are narrow and straight fibers that migrate through the lymphatics of the pulmonary parenchyma and accumulate in the interstitial spaces and the subpleural region. It is the amphibole fibers, especially crocidolite asbestos — "blue asbestos," that have been most clearly associated with malignant mesothelioma. Chrysotile appears to be a far greater risk factor for the development of lung cancer, perhaps because of its physical characteristics.

Crocidolite asbestos is found only in South Africa and Western Australia but has been exported to other countries all over the world for various industrial uses. Chrysotile — "white asbestos" — accounts for 97% of worldwide asbestos production and is mined principally in the Ural mountains in Russia, Quebec Province in Canada, Zimbabwe and Swaziland in South Africa, the Italian Alps, and Cyprus. Churg and DePaoli (1988) and McDonald and co-workers (1989) report that chrysotile itself is not thought to cause mesothelioma but is often contaminated with amphibole fibers such as tremolite or amosite — "brown asbestos".

There are many different situations in which individuals can be exposed to asbestos because it has over a thousand uses, as reported by Huncharek (1992). However, as discussed by Andersson (1985), Malker (1985), and McDonald (1980) and their associates, the areas of the world that have a high incidence of mesothelioma are those with asbestos mines, and countries that have shipyards, insulation, construction, and automobile industries that use large amounts of asbestos. In North America, the highest incidence areas include the provinces of Quebec and British Columbia in Canada, which have asbestos mines, and Seattle, Hawaii, San Francisco-Oakland, New York-New Jersey, and New Orleans in the United States, which have either large shipyards or asbestos industries. It is difficult to document a relationship between the duration or intensity of asbestos exposure and the risk of developing mesothelioma, but Levine (1981) has reported that patients with peritoneal mesothelioma often have a history of heavier exposure than do patients with pleural disease.

Mesothelioma is also caused by other naturally occurring and man-made silicate fibers that share the physical properties of amphibole asbestos fibers; that is, a diameter of less than 0.25 μm and a length greater than 5.0 μm. The most notable example of this is erionite, a zeolite fiber that is found in volcanic deposits of central Turkey and is the major building material of homes in that area. Baris (1987) found that in Karain, Turkey, a village with a population of 604, malignant mesothelioma was the single most common cause of death, with 62 cases recorded over the 11-year period from 1970 to 1981.

There are other less common causes of malignant mesothelioma. Lerman and colleagues (1991) record that radiation exposure at periods ranging from 10 to 31 years before the development of mesothelioma is the most clearly documented of these causes, but extravasation of radioactive thorium dioxide — Thoratrast — during radiologic procedures, and exposure to isoniazid in utero have also been anecdotally reported by Antman (1983, 1984) and Anderson (1985) and their co-workers. A variety of other substances, some of which are summarized by Peterson and associates (1984) and Hammar and Bolen (1988) in Table 61-1, are thought to be possible risk factors for malignant mesothelioma, based on epidemiologic or experimental animal studies. Of great importance, however, is that smoking does not appear to be a risk factor for malignant mesothelioma. This is in distinct contrast to lung cancer, in which asbestos and smoking act as synergistic carcinogens.

The peak incidence for the majority of individuals who develop mesothelioma is in the sixth decade of life. Because most patients develop mesothelioma as a result of occupational exposure to asbestos, the increased incidence of this disease has occurred in men. In the United States, the incidence in women remains at the baseline level of 3 cases per million, while in men it has risen to 15 cases per million inhabitants per year. Malignant mesothelioma is predominantly a disease of adults because of the long latency period — at least 20 years — between exposure to causative agents and the development of cancer, but Fraire and colleagues (1988) report that it can occur in childhood. In that setting, it seems to be idiopathic. Malignant mesothelioma sometimes develops in young adults because of exposure to risk factors during childhood, as reported by Kane and colleagues (1990).

PATHOLOGY AND MOLECULAR BIOLOGY

Mesotheliomas arise from multipotential mesothelial or subserosal cells that can develop into either an

Table 61-2. Histologic Classification of Mesothelioma

Epithelial
Tubulopapillary
Epithelioid
Glandular
Large cell—giant cell
Small cell
Adenoid-cystic
Signet ring
Sarcomatoid
(Fibrous, sarcomatous, mesenchymal)
Mixed epithelial-sarcomatoid (biphasic)
Transitional
Desmoplastic
Localized fibrous mesothelioma

From Hammar SP, Bolen JW: Pleural neoplasms. *In* Dail DH, Hammar SP (eds): Pulmonary Pathology. New York: Springer-Verlag, 1988, p 979.

epithelial or a sarcomatoid neoplasm. In contrast to localized fibrous tumors of the pleura (see Chapter 60), diffuse mesotheliomas almost always have an epithelial component. However, they exhibit a wide array of histologic patterns (Table 61–2) and often have a mixture of epithelial and sarcomatoid features (Figs. 61–1 and 61–2). In a review of 819 cases, Hillerdal (1983) reported that 50% were of epithelial type, 34% were of mixed type, and 16% were of the sarcomatoid type. The histologic appearance of mesotheliomas is easily confused with that of other neoplasms, and there is often disagreement among pathologists when light microscopy is used as the sole method of diagnosis: the reclassification rate of tumors originally diagnosed as mesotheliomas ranges from 30 to 84% when these specimens are reviewed by panels of reference pathologists. The usual challenge for the pathologist is to distinguish epithelial mesotheliomas from metastatic adenocarcinoma. However, as Cantin and associates (1982) report, very early mesotheliomas can be difficult to distinguish from benign mesothelial hyperplasia, and the rare desmoplastic form of mesothelioma often resembles benign fibrosis because of its predominantly fibroblastic cell type and sparsely cellular appearance. Several standard histochemical stains help to distinguish malignant mesothelioma from other tumors. Pulmonary adenocarcinomas usually stain positively with mucicarmine, whereas mesothelioma does not. About 20% of epithelial mesotheliomas produce an acidic mucosub-

stance, hyaluronic acid, which can be seen either within or between cells with an alcian blue or colloidal iron stain.

Immunohistochemistry and electron microscopy, however, have become the standard approach to diagnosis. Wirth (1991), Battifora (1985), and Mezger (1990) and their colleagues report that useful immunohistochemical stains include antibodies to high and low molecular weight cytokeratins, to vimentin, human milk fat globule, to carcinoembryonic antigen — CEA, and to Leu-M1. Mesotheliomas stain positively for low molecular weight cytokeratins, a feature that distinguishes them from sarcomas. They always fail to stain for CEA, a feature that distinguishes them from adenocarcinomas. If immunohistochemical stains yield equivocal results, electron microscopy will usually lead to a definitive diagnosis. Burns and associates (1985) have emphasized that the most prominent feature of mesotheliomas is that they have numerous, long, sinuous microvilli, whereas adenocarcinomas have short, straight microvilli that are covered by a fuzzy glycocalyx.

Relatively little is understood about the biology of diffuse malignant mesothelioma. Burmer and co-workers (1989) reported that approximately 65% of malignant mesotheliomas were diploid on flow cytometry and had surprisingly low proliferative rates. One study by Tammilehto (1992), however, has shown low S-phase fraction to be an independent prognostic

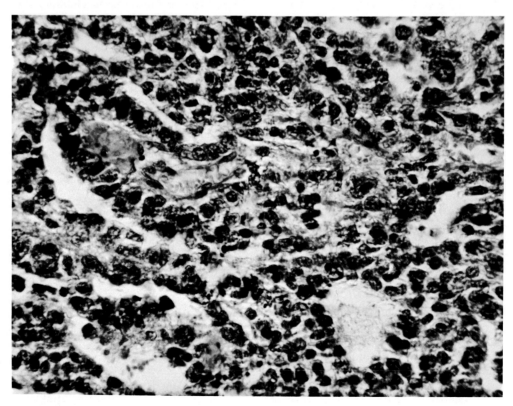

Fig. 61–1. Photomicrograph of epithelial type of malignant mesothelioma.

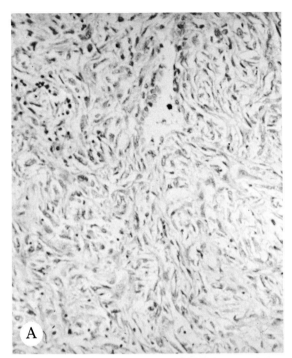

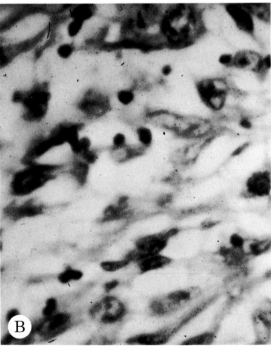

Fig. 61–2. Photomicrograph of a malignant mesothelioma of the sarcomatous variety. *A*, Low-power magnification. *B*, High-power magnification.

factor. Molecular biologic information has been derived mostly from mesothelioma cell lines, although chromosomal abnormalities have also been studied in primary tumor specimens. These abnormalities include alterations — usually deletions — on chromosomes 1, 3, 4, 9, 11, 14, and 22, as reported by Popescu

(1988) and Hagemeijer (1990) and their co-workers. Additional copies of the short arm of chromosome 7 have also been seen by Tiainen and colleagues (1989) and may be an indicator of poor prognosis. Overexpression of the platelet-derived growth factors — PDGF, and of their receptors, has been a consistent finding by Gerwin and associates (1987) in human mesothelioma cell lines compared to normal cell lines. Abnormalities of the tumor suppressor gene, p53, have also been reported by Cote and co-investigators (1991). Transfection experiments conducted by Reddel and colleagues (1989) using the activated c-Ha-*ras* — HRAS1 — oncogene EJ-*ras* in a human mesothelial cell line suggest that activation of this oncogene may play a critical role in the malignant transformation of mesothelial cells. How these preliminary pieces of information will fit together in the overall sequence of carcinogenesis in mesothelioma remains to be seen.

CLINICAL AND RADIOLOGIC PRESENTATION

The clinical presentation of diffuse malignant mesothelioma is insidious and nonspecific. Mesothelioma has traditionally been portrayed as a diffuse, massive tumor that causes excruciating chest pain. In fact, these signs and symptoms are seen only when mesothelioma becomes advanced. In the early stages of disease, dyspnea is the predominant symptom and is related to the presence of an effusion. When the effusion is drained, patients are asymptomatic. As the tumor grows, patients develop ill-defined, mild but continuous chest discomfort, which they are unable to localize or clearly describe. Dyspnea may actually improve during this phase of the disease because, with tumor growth, the pleural surfaces fuse, and the effusion resolves. Only when the tumor becomes locally advanced does the patient develop severe chest pain, which is related to infiltration of the chest wall and intercostal nerves. This is accompanied by a sense of chest tightness, of being unable to take a deep breath, probably caused by encasement of the lung and the development of restrictive lung disease. Dyspnea returns and worsens at this point. In the final stages of disease, both dyspnea and chest pain become severe and unremitting. These symptoms are related to encasement of the chest wall, lung, and mediastinum, with compression of the uninvolved lung. Direct extension of the tumor though the pericardium with associated pericardial effusion or myocardial metastases may aggravate the dyspnea. The symptoms of locally advanced pleural disease can also be compounded by the development of ascites from direct extension of the tumor through the diaphragm or a contralateral pleural effusion from metastatic disease. Elmes and Simpson (1976) and Ruffie and associates (1989) report a variety of other symptoms, such as bone pain, which can occur in terminal patients who develop extrathoracic metastases.

Thus, dyspnea and chest pain are the most common presenting symptoms, occurring in 90% of patients. Weight loss occurs in about 30% of patients but is seen only in the advanced stages of the disease. Uncommon symptoms include cough, weakness, anorexia, fever, hemoptysis, hoarseness, dysphagia, and Horner's syndrome. A few cases presenting with a spontaneous pneumothorax have been reported by Sheard and colleagues (1991).

In the early stages of disease, the findings on physical examination are nonspecific. Dullness to percussion and decreased breath sounds may be noted because of the presence of a pleural effusion, but the chest examination is otherwise normal. In the late stages of disease when tumor encases the hemithorax, the excursion of the chest with respiration diminishes, and the chest wall is noticeably contracted. Diffuse dullness to percussion and decreased breath sounds are present over the entire hemithorax. There is a subtle fullness of the intercostal spaces. Palpable soft tissue masses may be found in the chest wall if the tumor has grown through the intercostal spaces or has implanted in the site of a previous thoracentesis or thoracotomy incision. Palpable supraclavicular nodes and obvious ascites may be present if the tumor has metastasized to these areas, as described by Law and colleagues (1982).

Paraneoplastic syndromes are uncommon, but autoimmune hemolytic anemia, hypercalcemia, hypoglyce-

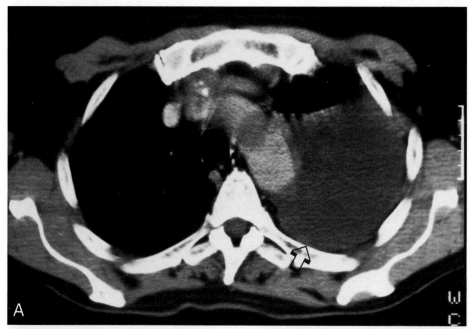

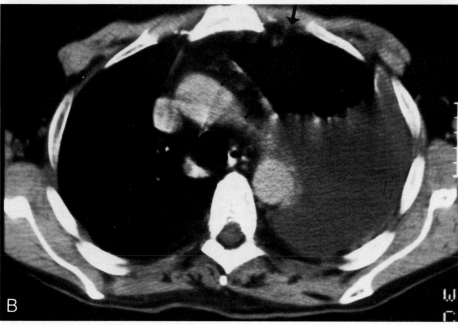

Fig. 61–3. CT scans of an early-stage diffuse mesothelioma. *A,* The CT scan at the level of the aortic arch shows a large left pleural effusion (arrow) with no evidence of pleural disease. *B,* The second CT scan at the level of the aortopulmonary window shows mild pleural thickening and irregularity (arrows) in addition to the effusion. At thoracotomy, there was diffuse studding of the pleura with tumor nodules that were 1 to 2 mm in size.

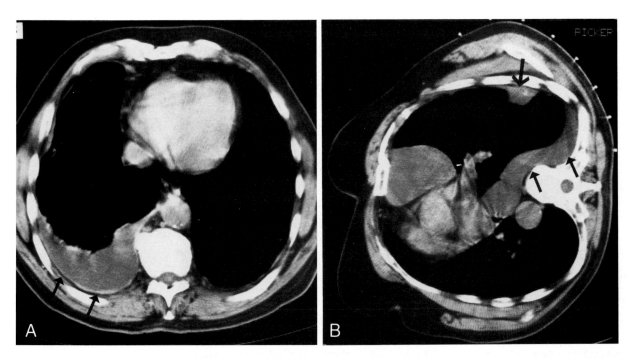

Fig. 61–4. CT scans of another early-stage mesothelioma. *A*, There is a large pleural effusion with diffuse mild pleural thickening and irregularity (arrows). *B*, A CT scan obtained with the patient in the lateral position shows a dominant chest wall mass (large arrow) and a freely flowing effusion (small arrow).

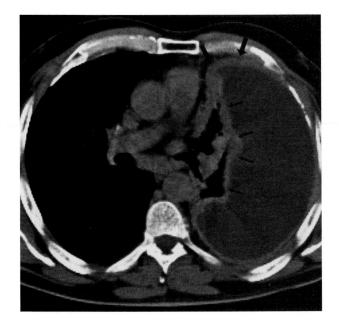

Fig. 61–5. CT scan of a more locally advanced mesothelioma. There is a thick confluent pleural peel along the chest wall (large arrows), encasing the collapsed lung and extending into the fissure (small arrows).

mia, inappropriate secretion of antidiuretic hormone — SIADH, and hypercoagulability not related to thrombocytosis, have been reported by Ruffie and associates (1989). Olesen and Thorshauge (1988) found that thrombocytosis, defined as a platelet count ≥400,000 /μl occurs in about 30 to 40% of patients, is sometimes associated with a leukemoid reaction, but does not seem to increase the risk of thromboembolic episodes.

Mesothelioma patients often have abnormal electrocardiographic — ECG — and echocardiographic findings. In a review of 64 patients, Wadler and co-workers (1986) found that 55 patients — 89% — had an abnormal ECG. Sinus tachycardia was seen in 42%, non-life-threatening ventricular or atrial arrhythmias occurred in 17% of patients, while over a third of patients had some form of bundle branch block. Although pericardial invasion or myocardial involvement was a common finding at autopsy in these patients, most ECG abnormalities occurred more than 6 months before death, suggesting that they are not solely related to the presence of advanced disease. Echocardiography was somewhat insensitive but highly specific for involvement of the pericardium or myocardium by tumor: Three patients who had pericardial effusions by echocardiogram had pericardial and myocardial involvement at autopsy, whereas five patients who had pericardial tumor at autopsy had a normal echocardiogram premortem.

No tumor markers are routinely used for malignant mesothelioma. Serum hyaluronan may be elevated in some patients, a not surprising finding given the positive

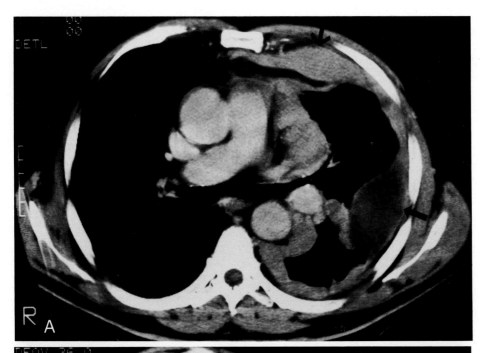

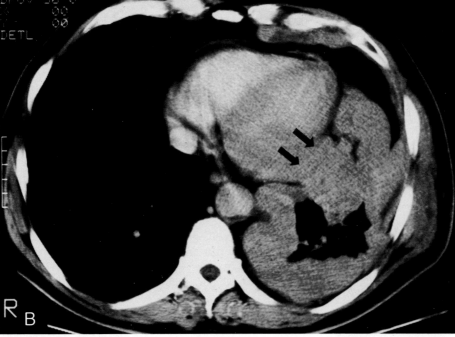

Fig. 61–6. CT scan of another locally advanced mesothelioma. *A*, The CT scan at the level of the pulmonary artery shows a thick irregular confluent pleural peel (large arrow) with a loculated pleural effusion (small arrow). *B*, The CT scan at the level of the mid-heart shows massive tumor encasing and collapsing the lung and suggests invasion of the pericardium (arrows).

staining for hyaluronic acid seen in many epithelial mesotheliomas. In one study of 37 patients, Dahl and colleagues (1989) found that a rise in serum hyaluronan had a sensitivity of 65% and a specificity of 85% as a predictor of progressive disease. Hyaluronan can be measured using a commercial kit, but the kit is not readily available in most hospitals. CA-125 has been anecdotally reported by Blackstein (personal communication, 1992) to be a serum marker in malignant mesothelioma, but the utility of this has not been investigated in large numbers of patients.

The radiographic appearance of malignant mesothelioma is variable and nonspecific. In early-stage mesothelioma, a large pleural effusion is often the only sign of disease (Fig. 61–3). Subtle pleural thickening or small discrete pleural-based masses may be seen on CT (Fig. 61–4). Subsequently, larger pleural-based masses become evident and are often intermixed with multiloculated effusions. Gotfried and colleagues (1983) note that rarely, a dominant pleural-based mass may be the initial presentation, but ultimately the involvement of the pleura is always diffuse. Eventually, a thick irregular pleural rind develops, with encasement of the lung and obliteration of the pleural space (Fig. 61–5). Mediastinal adenopathy, direct extension of the tumor into the mediastinum, involvement of the pericardium with pericardial effusion, and extension into the chest wall or through the diaphragm are seen in very locally advanced tumor (Fig. 61–6). Rabinowitz (1982), Mirvis (1983), Law (1982), and Alexander (1981) and their colleagues reported that CT permits a far better appreciation of the extent of the disease, than does standard radiography, which cannot demonstrate many of these abnormalities. CT is currently the most accurate noninvasive way to stage patients, to assess response to treatment, and to detect recurrent disease postoperatively, but, as reported by the author and associates (1988), is often inaccurate in diagnosing chest wall involvement or extension through the diaphragm. It is hoped that magnetic resonance imaging — MR scan — will prove more accurate in this regard.

DIAGNOSIS

A thoracentesis is usually the initial diagnostic procedure because most patients present with a pleural effusion. Pleural fluid cytology is positive for malignancy in only 30 to 50% of patients. Percutaneous pleural biopsy yields a diagnosis of malignancy in up to a third of cases, but, as emphasized by Wirth (1991), Battifora (1985), and Mezger (1990) and their colleagues, usually does not provide the pathologist a large enough specimen on which to perform the immunohistochemical or electron microscopic studies that are so critical to a definitive diagnosis. As described by Boutin and associates (1991b, 1993) thoracoscopy is the optimal diagnostic procedure because it yields a diagnosis in at least 80% of patients but does not commit the patient to a major surgical procedure. The appearance of the pleural space is variable and depends on the extent of disease and the cell type. In the earliest stages of mesothelioma, involvement of the pleura is microscopic, and the only visible finding is a large pleural effusion. As the disease progresses, the thoracoscopic appearance evolves from pleural studding with a free pleural space and a large pleural effusion, to larger but still discrete masses with multiloculated pleural effusions, to a confluent irregular sheet of tumor with obliteration of the pleural space. The tumor ranges in appearance from being soft, friable, and hypervascular, to being densely fibrotic, depending on the mixture of cell types. No clinical findings are pathognomonic of malignant mesothelioma.

Thoracoscopy is not technically feasible in the patient whose pleural space is obliterated by locally advanced tumor. The small incision that is usually made for thoracoscopy is then simply used for open pleural biopsy, which may be facilitated by resection of short segment of the overlying rib. Because mesothelioma has a notorious propensity to implant in the chest wall, this incision should be placed in line with a possible subsequent thoracotomy incision, so that it can be excised at the time of the definitive operation. Placing the thoracoscopy incision in a random manner complicates the local management of this disease by placing the patient at risk for chest wall recurrence. Exploratory thoracotomy is rarely necessary and is ideally avoided, because it exposes some patients who have metastatic adenocarcinoma to the unnecessary morbidity of a major operation. Most importantly, the surgeon must submit pleural biopsies fresh to the pathologist so that they can be placed in the appropriate fixatives for immunohistochemistry and electron microscopy.

No additional studies or procedures beyond thoracoscopy and CT scans of the chest and abdomen are routinely necessary to diagnose and stage patients with malignant mesothelioma. Bronchoscopy is done only to

Table 61–3. Staging Proposed by Butchart and Colleagues

Stage I	Tumor confined within the "capsule" of the parietal pleura, i.e., involving only ipsilateral pleura, lung, pericardium, and diaphragm
Stage II	Tumor invading chest wall or involving mediastinal structures, e.g., esophagus, heart, opposite pleura Lymph node involvement within the chest
Stage III	Tumor penetrating diaphragm to involve peritoneum; involvement of opposite pleura Lymph node involvement outside the chest.
Stage IV	Distant blood-borne metastases.

From Butchart EG, et al: Pleuropneumonectomy in the management of diffuse malignant mesothelioma of the pleura: experience with 29 patients. Thorax *31*:15, 1976.

Table 61–4. Staging Proposed by Chahinian

Stage I	$T_1 N_0 M_0$
Stage II	$T_{1-2} N_1 M_0$ $T_2 N_0 M_0$
Stage III	T_3 any N, M_0
Stage IV	T_4, any N, M_0, any M_1

T = primary tumor;
T_1 = limited to ipsilateral pleura only (parietal pleura, visceral pleura);
T_2 = superficial local invasion (diaphragm, endothoracic fascia, ipsilateral lung, fissures);
T_3 = deep local invasion (chest wall beyond endothoracic fascia);
T_4 = extensive direct invasion (opposite pleura, peritoneum, retroperitoneum);
N = lymph nodes;
N_0 = no positive lymph node;
N_1 = positive ipsilateral hilar nodes;
N_2 = positive mediastinal nodes;
N_3 = positive contralateral hilar nodes;
M = metastases;
M_0 = no metastases;
M_1 = metastases, blood-borne or lymphatic.

From Chahinian AP: Therapeutic modalities in malignant pleural mesothelioma. *In* Chretien J, Hirsch A (eds): Diseases of the Pleura. New York: Masson, 1983.

Table 61–5. Staging System Proposed by UICC (Union Internationale Contre le Cancer)

T — primary tumor and extent

T_x	Primary tumor cannot be assessed
T_0	No evidence of primary tumor
T_1	Primary tumor limited to ipsilateral parietal and/or visceral pleura
T_2	Tumor invades any of the following: ipsilateral lung, endothoracic fascia, diaphragm, pericardium
T_3	Tumor invades any of the following: ipsilateral chest wall muscle, ribs, mediastinal organs or tissues
T_4	Tumor extends to any of the following: contralateral pleura or lung by direct extension, peritoneum or intra-abdominal organs by direct extension, cervical tissues

N — lymph nodes

N_x	Regional lymph nodes cannot be assessed
N_0	No regional lymph node metastases
N_1	Metastases in ipsilateral bronchopulmonary or hilar lymph nodes
N_2	Metastases in ipsilateral mediastinal lymph nodes
N_3	Metastases in contralateral mediastinal, internal mammary, supraclavicular or scalene lymph nodes

M — metastases

M_x	Presence of distant metastases cannot be assessed
M_0	No (known) distant metastasis
M_1	Distant metastasis present

Mesothelioma staging system*

Stage I
  T_1, N_0, M_0
  T_2, N_0, M_0

Stage II
  T_1, N_1, M_0
  T_2, N_1, M_0

Stage III
  T_3, N_0, M_0
  T_3, N_1, M_0
  T_1, N_2, M_0
  T_2, N_2, M_0
  T_3, N_2, M_0

Stage IV
  Any T, N_3, M_0
  T_4, any N, M_0
  Any T, any N, M_1

*Staging solely on clinical measures is designated cTNM. Staging that can be done on clinical pathologic information is designated as pTNM. Clinical and pathologic groups are identical.

From Rusch VW, Ginsberg RJ: New concepts in the staging of mesotheliomas. *In:* Deslaurier J, Lacquet LK (eds): Thoracic Surgery: Surgical Management of Pleural Diseases. St Louis: CV Mosby, 1990, p 340.

exclude the possibility of a primary lung cancer with endobronchial tumor. It is uniformly normal in patients with mesothelioma, as noted by Lewis and co-workers (1981). Mediastinoscopy may demonstrate involved mediastinal nodes but will not be routinely indicated until nodal involvement is confirmed to have a negative impact on survival and therefore is important in selecting patients for treatment. Additional imaging studies such as bone scans are indicated only to evaluate specific symptoms; that is, localized bone pain or laboratory abnormalities such as an elevated alkaline phosphatase. As a general rule, distant metastases are seen only in patients who have very locally advanced intrathoracic tumor.

NATURAL HISTORY AND STAGING

An understanding of the natural history is critical to the evaluation and development of therapy for any cancer. Our understanding of the natural history and prognostic factors in malignant mesothelioma is poor, because it is an uncommon tumor and, in part, because there is no accurate, universally accepted staging system. The staging system used most often is the one proposed by Butchart and colleagues in 1976 (Table 61–3). Unfortunately, the descriptors for the primary tumor and for the involvement of lymph nodes are imprecise. A stage I tumor, for instance, could include patients who have minimal pleural studding, a free pleural space, and a pleural effusion, as well as patients who have a thick, confluent sheet of tumor with obliteration of the pleural space but without invasion of the mediastinum or opposite pleura. Yet clinical experience suggests that the latter represents a much more locally advanced tumor. In addition, the exact incidence and prognostic implications of lymph node involvement have not been clearly established in malignant mesothelioma. The inclusion of "lymph node involvement within the chest" in stage II, and "lymph node involvement outside the chest" in stage III is empiric. A recent report of 44 patients, by Sugarbaker and associates (1992), all of whom had Butchart's stage I disease and underwent extrapleural pneumonectomy, adjuvant chemotherapy, and radiation, showed a significantly poorer survival among the 10 patients who had positive mediastinal nodes. These data need to be confirmed in larger numbers of patients subjected to systematic lymph node dissection.

Dimitrov and McMahon (1987) describe several other proposed staging systems, including a TNM-based system by Chahinian (1983) (Table 61–4). This system is more precise than the Butchart system but does not fully reflect the usual findings at thoracotomy. For instance, it is uncommon to find patients who have a "T1" tumor, as defined by Chahinian, with involvement of the parietal and visceral pleural surfaces but with sparing of the diaphragm, because mesothelioma is a diffuse disease and because the area of greatest tumor burden is usually in the lower half of the hemithorax and on the diaphragm.

In an effort to improve and unify the staging system for malignant mesothelioma, the UICC has proposed another TNM-based system (Table 61–5). The T-status descriptors are more detailed than in previous systems, and the descriptors for nodal involvement in this system are borrowed directly from the current international staging system for non-small cell lung cancer. Even this system is not definitive, however, and needs to be confirmed or modified by careful clinicopathologic correlation.

Another confounding issue is that most published reports do not stage patients by CT scan and assess them only by symptoms, physical examination, and chest radiographs. The inaccuracy of such a clinical assessment leads to a heterogeneous patient population. Finally, many series record outcome in small numbers of patients, seen over long periods of time, and treated in a highly individualized manner. Little wonder that reported survival rates vary widely. Law and co-workers (1984) reported a median survival of 18 months for 64 patients treated with supportive care, with no differences in survival according to cell types. Twelve of the 64 patients survived longer than 5 years, but the diagnosis of mesothelioma in this study was based on histology alone, and less than a third of all patients were staged by CT scan. Hulks and colleagues (1989) reported a median survival of 30 weeks for 68 patients treated with supportive care. They based their pathologic diagnosis on immunohistochemistry as well as histology. No CT scanning was performed, and patients were classified principally according to their symptoms. Patients who presented with dyspnea lived significantly longer than did patients who presented with pain — median survival of 44 versus 22 weeks, probably reflecting the extent of disease at diagnosis. Cell type did not appear to influence survival.

Other authors, notably Tammilehto (1992), Ruffie (1989), Adams (1986), and Antman (1988) and their

colleagues, have tried to identify prognostic factors in malignant mesothelioma but have done this mainly in the setting of retrospective reviews of patients with different stages of disease, treated with widely varying regimens. Contrary to the data reported by Law (1982) and Hulks (1989) and their associates, epithelial histology has generally been a favorable prognostic factor. Absence of chest pain and good performance status are also thought to be favorable prognostic factors but probably just reflect an early stage of the disease. Other factors, including female gender and age less than 50 years, have incidentally been cited as favorable prognostic factors. In several series, a platelet count greater than 400,000 appears to have a negative impact on survival.

Malignant mesothelioma was long thought to be a tumor that remained localized to the chest, as described by Nauta and colleagues (1982). Several autopsy series have now disproven this. Ruffie and co-investigators (1989) found that 45 of 92 — 49% — patients had distant metastases at autopsy. The liver was the most common site, and the contralateral lung the second most common site of distant disease, but metastases in sites as widely disseminated as the prostate, brain, and thyroid were also found. Elmes and Simpson (1976) found distant metastases in 48 of 148 — 33% — patients at autopsy. The metastases were widely disseminated, but the liver and the contralateral lung were once again the most common sites of disease. Similar findings have been reported by Roberts (1976) and by Whitwell and Rawcliffe (1971). The uncommon but definite occurrence of brain and spine metastases has been emphasized in several reports, notably Walters and Martinez (1975), Kaye (1986), and Ruffie (1989) and their associates. Virtually all patients have advanced local or regional disease at death. As pointed out by Nauta and colleagues (1982), however, the symptoms related to locoregional tumor are usually the most difficult to palliate, and therefore the most obvious clinically. Patients with malignant mesothelioma face a dual problem: control of the locoregional tumor throughout the course of their disease and prevention of distant metastases as a late manifestation of their cancer.

TREATMENT

As for any other cancer, the treatment options for malignant mesothelioma include surgery, radiation, chemotherapy, immunotherapy, supportive care, or some combination of these modalities. However, the choice of treatment is influenced by factors that do not apply to some other malignancies: the location and extent of the tumor, and the general medical condition of these patients who are usually older and often have serious underlying diseases. The assessment of treatment regimens for malignant mesothelioma is hampered by a lack of large prospective clinical trials. Most patients have been treated in a highly individualized manner. Reported series are usually small and retrospective.

Radiation Therapy

It is difficult to evaluate the success of radiation therapy as the only treatment because it has usually been given in conjunction with surgical resection or chemotherapy. Radiation therapy as the sole treatment is generally used to palliate an area of symptomatic tumor in the chest wall or mediastinum.

According to Brady (1981), Ball and Cruickshank (1990), and Gordon and co-workers (1981), the use of radiation therapy is limited by the volume of the primary tumor that involves the entire hemithorax, and by proximity of the tumor to many vital structures that are intolerant of high doses of radiation. For the most part, radiation doses to the affected hemithorax have been kept at 4500 cGy or less to prevent toxicity to the heart, esophagus, lung, and spinal cord. Maasilta (1990) has documented the severe pulmonary toxicity caused by higher dose hemithoracic irradiation. The radiographic changes, and the deterioration in pulmonary function and oxygenation that develop over the year following radiation therapy, are compatible with a total loss of lung function on the irradiated side. Sinoff and associates (1982) have shown that the toxicity of irradiation may also be potentiated by the administration of chemotherapy, including drugs such as doxorubicin.

One way to circumvent these problems is to administer radiation therapy as adjuvant treatment after surgical resection of gross tumor. A variety of techniques can be used to minimize the radiation dose to the lung. The largest and most consistent experience with this approach has been reported by Hilaris (1983) and Kutcher (1987) and their colleagues at the Memorial Sloan-Kettering Cancer Center. Following subtotal resection of gross tumor by pleurectomy/decortication, any residual tumor was implanted intraoperatively with ^{125}I or ^{192}Ir implants. Patients then received external beam irradiation to the entire hemithorax using a mixed photon-electron beam technique to a total dose of 4500 cGy, attempting to spare the underlying lung. In a report by Mychalczak and co-workers (1989), 105 patients treated in this manner from 1976 to 1988 experienced a median survival of 12.6 months with 1- and 2-year actuarial survivals of 52 and 23%, respectively. However, the 27 patients who had pure epithelial histology and minimal gross residual disease requiring only external beam irradiation without brachytherapy had a median survival of 15 months, and 1- and 2-year survivals of 68 and 35%, respectively. There were 19 complications including 12 cases of radiation pneumonitis and 8 patients with pericarditis and tamponade. Unfortunately, the most common site of relapse was local. Ipsilateral recurrent pleural tumor was seen in 64 of the 105 patients — 63%. Both this experience and some experimental work by Soubra and associates (1990) indicate that a low-dose mixed photon-electron beam may be theoretically attractive but often does not succeed in sparing the pulmonary parenchyma and fails to provide long-term local control for most patients.

Table 61-6. Single-Agent Response Rates (>50% Regression) in Malignant Mesothelioma

Agent	Number Responding/Evaluable
Anthracyclines	
Doxorubicin	29/164
Detorubicine	9/21
Alkylating agents	
Cyclophosphamide	4/14
Mechlorethamine	2/6
Thiotepa	1/7
Melphalan	2/3
Procarbazine	2/6
Mitomycin C	2/12
Decarbazine (DTIC)	1/4
Cisplatin	5/49
Dibromodulcitol	0/5
Nitrosoureas	
BCNU	0/2
Methyl CCNU	0/3
ACNU	0/2
Streptozotocin	0/1
Vincas and related compounds	
Etoposide (VP16)	
Vindesine	0/8
	1/37
Antimetabolites	
5-Fluoracil	4/28
Methotrexate, high dose	4/9
Methotrexate, standard	0/1
Bakers antifol	0/3
Dichloromethotrexate	0/1
5 Azacytadine	0/7
Bleomycin	1/6
Actinomycin D	0/3
Ara C, high dose	1/1
Miscellaneous	
Maytansine	0/5
Methyl-G	1/2
Glucosamine	0/2
Hydroxyurea	0/1
DDMP	0/2
Bruceantin	0/1
MAMSA	1/19
Cycloencine	2/7
AZQ	0/20

From Antman KH et al.: Mesothelioma. Updates 3:9, 1989.

External beam radiation therapy can also be safely administered to higher total doses when the lung is resected along with the pleural tumor by extrapleural pneumonectomy. At the Dana Farber Cancer Institute, Sugarbaker and colleagues (1991) reported that 31 patients have received 5500 cGy of radiation to sites of residual disease or to the ipsilateral hemithorax, following extrapleural pneumonectomy without experiencing significant toxicity. These patients had 1- and 2-year survivals of 70 and 48%, respectively, but also received postoperative adjuvant chemotherapy, making it hard to assess the specific contribution of radiation therapy. The sites of relapse were not listed in this report.

The successful use of fast neutron therapy to control local bulky disease has been described in a case report by Blake and co-workers (1985), but this has not yet been confirmed in larger series. Small-series studies have been reported on the intrapleural use of radioactive colloidal compounds including radioactive gold — [198]Au — and chromic phosphate — [32]P, but as described by Brady (1981), these seem ineffective in treating any substantial tumor bulk within the pleural cavity.

Overall, the contribution of radiation therapy to the local control of malignant mesothelioma has been disappointing. It is generally agreed that hemithoracic radiation is not a feasible form of *primary treatment* for malignant mesothelioma, because the doses of irradiation that might be effective in controlling the tumor cannot be safely tolerated by the underlying lung or surrounding mediastinal structures. Radiation therapy may play a role in adjuvant treatment, particularly after extrapleural pneumonectomy, when it becomes possible to deliver higher dose irradiation to the hemithorax. It may also be helpful as a form of palliation in patients who have very locally advanced tumor with painful involvement of the chest wall.

Chemotherapy

Numerous phase II studies of chemotherapeutic agents have been performed in malignant mesothelioma. These have been well summarized by Antman and associates (1989) (Table 61–6) and more recently reviewed in detail by Krarup-Hansen and Hansen (1991). Response rates as high as 30 to 40% have been reported in small single-institution studies, but in pooled data from multiple studies, response rates are generally in the 20% range. The results of these studies are influenced by the inclusion of patients with varying stages of disease and different mesothelioma cell types, and by the lack of use of CT scanning to assess response. Dimitrov (1982), Chahinian (1978), Dabouis (1981), Raghavan (1990), and Umsawasdi (1991) and their associates have shown that active agents include doxorubicin, detorubicin, ifosfamide, cisplatin, carboplatin, mitomycin, methotrexate, 5-azacytidine, and 5-fluorouracil. Combination treatment has not proven clearly superior to a single agent. Chahinian and colleagues (1987) reported the initial results of a randomized phase III trial that found a 13% response rate for the combination of cisplatin and doxorubicin compared to a 28% response rate for cisplatin and mitomycin. The long-term results of this trial have not yet been published. Overall, the response rates for currently available chemotherapy drugs in malignant mesothelioma remain disappointing.

Immunotherapy

Interferons are known to have a direct antiproliferative effect on mesothelioma cell lines. Studies by Sklarin and co-workers (1988) on mesothelioma xenografts in nude mice have shown the efficacy of recombinant human alfa-2a-interferon combined with mitomycin C. These experimental data have prompted the development of clinical trials using interferon, either alone or in combination with chemotherapy. Two phase II trials designed to evaluate the value of systemically administered alfa-interferon in conjunction with chemotherapy in patients with advanced disease are currently in progress. The first trial, being performed at Memorial Sloan-Kettering Cancer Center combines alfa-interferon with cisplatin. The second trial, being performed at the National Cancer Institute, combines alfa-interferon with cisplatin and tamoxifen.

The use of gamma-interferon as an intrapleural treatment in patients with early stage disease has recently been reported by Boutin and associates (1991a). Twenty-two patients were treated with a solution of gamma-interferon — 40 × 106 U — infused into the pleural space twice weekly for 2 months. Response was assessed by serial CT scans and by repeat thoracoscopy. A 56% overall response rate was observed. These promising initial results will undoubtedly stimulate additional clinical trials in the next few years. Intrapleural immunotherapy, however, requires a free pleural space to be effective and therefore can be administered only to patients with early stage disease who have a free-flowing effusion and minimal tumor involving the pleural surfaces.

Surgery

Because of the limitations of radiation and chemotherapy, surgical resection is still the mainstay of treatment for malignant mesothelioma. Three operations have been performed: extrapleural pneumonectomy — also termed "pleuropneumonectomy," pleurectomy/decortication, and a palliative limited pleurectomy.

Extrapleural pneumonectomy is an en-bloc resection of the pleura, lung, ipsilateral hemidiaphragm, and pericardium. As described by the author and co-investigators (1991), pleurectomy/decortication is an attempt to remove all gross pleural disease without removing the underlying lung. The hemidiaphragm and pericardium are also removed and reconstructed if necessary. A palliative pleurectomy involves limited resection of the parietal pleura to control a pleural effusion by creating a durable pleurodesis. The details of the surgical technique for these operations are described in Chapter 62 and will not be reviewed here.

One operation performed for strictly palliative purposes is thoracoscopy and talc poudrage. As reported by Ruffie (1989) and Boutin (1991b) and their colleagues, this is highly effective in controlling effusions and provides excellent palliation for patients whose general medical condition precludes more aggressive treatment.

The Role of Surgical Resection

Complete resection of all gross tumor seems to convey a modest but definite improvement in survival in several large series. However, the value of extrapleural pneumonectomy as compared to pleurectomy/decortication remains controversial. Extrapleural pneumonectomy has the aesthetic appeal of removing the tumor en bloc, but either operation, if performed well in properly selected patients, allows the removal of all gross tumor. On the other hand, resection of the tumor with microscopically negative margins, as can be achieved with a lung, breast, or colon cancer, is simply not feasible in malignant mesothelioma, because the margins of resection are vital structures such as the aorta, cavae, and esophagus.

In an initial report by Butchart and associates (1976), extrapleural pneumonectomy carried an operative mortality of 30%. More recent data show a substantial reduction in this mortality, probably reflecting better patient selection and improved perioperative care. Preoperative CT scanning, careful pulmonary function testing, ventilation/perfusion lung scanning, and improved methods of evaluating cardiac function noninvasively now allow us to select patients who have completely resectable tumors and have the cardiopulmonary reserve to tolerate the operation safely. Intraoperative monitoring and anesthetic management are much better than they were 20 years ago. In a recent prospective multi-institutional study reported by the author and co-investigators (1991), the mortality rate was 15%. However, as reported by Sugarbaker (1991), DeValle (1986), and DeLaria (1978) and their colleagues, as well as by Butchart (personal communication, 1991), mortality rates as low as 6% have been achieved in single-institution retrospective studies in which patients have been carefully selected and operated on by surgeons specialized in this area. The operative mortality and overall survival after extrapleural pneumonectomy as reported in several series are shown in Table 61–7.

In contrast, in the experience reported by McCormack and associates (1982) at Memorial Sloan-Kettering, pleurectomy/decortication is associated with a mortality of 1.8%. These data parallel those reported for pulmonary resections for lung cancer, which have shown that operative mortality is directly related to the extent of resection and is 5 to 10% for a standard pneumonectomy. Both operations, and particularly extrapleural pneumonectomy, are complex and are not performed frequently by most surgeons. Therefore, patients may benefit by referral to centers dedicated to the treatment of malignant mesothelioma.

The focus of the controversy with regard to surgical treatment is the relative value of an extrapleural pneumonectomy compared to a pleurectomy/decortication: Is the higher operative mortality of extrapleural pneumonectomy justified by a better overall survival? One problem is that extrapleural pneumonectomy is applicable to relatively few patients — probably about 20 to 25% of all mesothelioma patients who have resectable tumors, according to the author and co-investigators (1991) and Butchart (personal communication, 1991). Underlying cardiopulmonary disease and other medical problems often preclude pneumonectomy in patients who can tolerate pleurectomy/decortication. Pneumonectomy, however, can facilitate some types of adjuvant treatment, especially postoperative irradiation, which can be administered in a much higher total dose after pneumonectomy than after pleurectomy/decortication.

On the other hand, some patients do not have a tumor that is technically resectable by pleurectomy/decortication. A confluent sheet of tumor encasing the lung with obliteration of the pleural space is resectable only by extrapleural pneumonectomy. This situation can often be recognized by the preoperative CT scan (Figs. 61–3 and 61–4) and by a preoperative ventilation/perfusion lung scan showing minimal function on the affected side. Whether a patient who has early stage disease that is technically completely resectable by either extrapleural pneumonectomy or by pleurectomy/decortication is better served by one operation versus the other is simply unknown. This question remains unresolved, but ultimately, the long-term outcome of such a patient after complete resection of all gross tumor may be determined not by the operation but by the type and effectiveness of the adjuvant treatment.

Combined Modality Treatment

Extrapleural pneumonectomy and pleurectomy/decortication are by definition cytoreductive operations. The author and co-investigators (1991) have shown that patients treated with surgical resection alone relapse rapidly. Therefore, most treatment regimens have focused on multimodality treatment. Unfortunately, it is difficult to evaluate the results of combined modality treatment, because most series, including Achatzy (1989), Chahinian (1982), and Alberts (1988) and their associates, report small numbers of patients treated in a highly individualized manner over long periods of time. In addition to the Memorial Sloan-Kettering experience with pleurectomy/decortication and radiation therapy described previously, another large and rela-

Table 61–7. Results of Extrapleural Pneumonectomy

Reference	N	Patient Mortality (%)	Two-Year Survival (%)	Median Survival
Wörn (1974)	62	Not stated	37	Not stated
Butchart et al (1976)	29	31	10	4 months*
DeValle (1986)	33	9	24	13.5 months
Vogt Moykopf (1987)	55	5.5	16	10 months
			(at 3 years)	
LCSG (1991)	20	15	33	10 months
Sugarbaker et al (1991)	31	6	48	Not stated

*For Butchart: overall median, 4 months; median of survivors of surgery, 8 months.

tively uniform experience with combined modality treatment has been reported by the Dana Farber Cancer Center. From 1980 to 1990, Sugarbaker and colleagues (1991) performed extrapleural pneumonectomy in 31 patients, followed by chemotherapy with cisplatin, doxorubicin, and cyclophosphamide and subsequent hemithoracic radiation. The survival rates were 70% at 1 year and 48% at 2 years. The Dana Farber group continues to use this approach and have now seen similar results in a total of 44 patients. As reported by Sugarbaker and colleagues (1992), epithelial histology and lack of involvement of hilar and mediastinal nodes define the patient population with the best prognosis. The results obtained with this trimodality treatment in a highly selected group of patients are the best reported to date in patients with malignant mesothelioma.

There are finally efforts to perform prospective clinical trials of multimodality treatment in malignant mesothelioma. Several novel treatment strategies have recently been under investigation. At the National Cancer Institute, Pass (1993) has recently completed a phase I trial evaluating the use of photodynamic therapy immediately after completion of either pleurectomy/decortication or extrapleural pneumonectomy. Photodynamic therapy seeks to improve local control by eliminating microscopic residual disease immediately after surgical resection. This approach is based on experimental data with mesothelioma cell lines, reported by Keller and co-workers (1990). A previous small clinical trial reported by Ris and colleagues (1991) has already suggested the feasibility of this approach.

Another novel approach is a phase II trial recently performed at Memorial Sloan-Kettering Cancer Center. Patients received a single dose of intrapleural cisplatin — 75 mg/m^2 — and mitomycin — 8 mg/m^2 — after complete resection of all gross tumor by pleurectomy/decortication. Additional chemotherapy was then administered systemically starting 1 month postoperatively using two cycles of cisplatin 50 mg/m^2/week × 4 and mitomycin 8 mg/m^2 × 1. This approach of surgical resection and brief, but very intensive, chemotherapy sought to address the dual problem of local control and eventual distant metastases experienced by most mesothelioma patients. It was based on the established use of intraperitoneal chemotherapy in ovarian cancer and on a smaller but successful experience with intracavitary chemotherapy in both pleural and peritoneal mesothelioma, reported by Lederman (1987), Markman (1986), and Mintzer (1985) and their associates. The author and co-investigators (1992) found that the first 23 patients treated during this trial tolerated the treatment well but that only 12 patients were alive and free of disease with a median follow-up of 11.2 months. Sites of relapse were primarily local.

SUMMARY

Diffuse malignant mesothelioma is an uncommon cancer that is increasing in incidence because of the occupational exposure to asbestos of many individuals from the 1930s through the 1960s. It is important for thoracic surgeons to be familiar with mesothelioma because they are often involved in making the diagnosis and recommending treatment. In the early stages of disease, the clinical presentation is nonspecific. The tissue diagnosis is best established by thoracoscopy and pleural biopsy. CT scanning of the chest and abdomen is the most accurate noninvasive way to evaluate the extent of disease.

The treatment of diffuse mesothelioma remains controversial, in part because the natural history and prognostic factors are poorly understood. Current staging systems are inadequate and do not stratify patients well. Chemotherapy and radiation therapy are relatively ineffective as primary treatment and, by default, surgical resection remains the mainstay of therapy for patients fit enough to tolerate it. Extrapleural pneumonectomy or pleurectomy/decortication allow the complete resection of all gross tumor in properly selected patients but will need to be coupled with effective adjuvant treatment to achieve long-term control of disease. Prospective clinical trials evaluating novel therapeutic strategies are needed to improve the currently dismal survival rates of patients with malignant mesothelioma.

REFERENCES

Achatzy R, et al: The diagnosis, therapy and prognosis of diffuse malignant mesothelioma. Eur J Cardiothorac Surg 3:445, 1989.

Adams VI, et al: Diffuse malignant mesothelioma of pleura. Cancer 58:1540, 1986.

Alberts AS, et al: Malignant pleural mesothelioma: a disease unaffected by current therapeutic maneuvers. J Clin Oncol 6:527, 1988.

Alexander E, et al: CT of malignant pleural mesothelioma. AJR Am J Roentgenol 137:287, 1981.

Anderson EA, et al: Malignant pleural mesothelioma following radiotherapy in a 16-year-old boy. Cancer 56:273, 1985.

Andersson M, Olsen JH: Trend and distribution of mesothelioma in Denmark. Br J Cancer 51:699, 1985.

Antman KH, et al: Multimodality therapy for malignant mesothelioma based on a study of natural history. Am J Med 68:356, 1980.

Antman KH, et al: Mesothelioma. Updates 3:9, 1989.

Antman KH, et al: Malignant mesothelioma following radiation exposure. J Clin Oncol 1(11):695, 1983.

Antman KH, et al: Mesothelioma following Wilms' tumor in childhood. Cancer 54:367, 1984.

Antman K, et al: Malignant mesothelioma: prognostic variables in a registry of 180 patients, the Dana-Farber Cancer Institute and Brigham and Women's Hospital experience over two decades, 1965–1985. J Clin Oncol 6:147, 1988.

Auribault M: Bulletin de l'Inspection du Travail, 1906, p. 126.

Ball DL, Cruickshank DG: The treatment of malignant mesothelioma of the pleura: review of a 5-year experience, with special reference to radiotherapy. Am J Clin Oncol 13:4, 1990.

Baris YI: Asbestos and Erionite Related Chest Diseases. Ankara, Turkey: Semik Ofset Matbaacilik, 1987.

Battifora H, Kopinski MI: Distinction of mesothelioma from adenocarcinoma. Cancer 55:1679, 1985.

Blake PR, Catterall M, Emerson PA: Pleural mesothelioma treated by fast neutron therapy. Thorax 40:72, 1985.

Boutin C, et al: Activity of intrapleural recombinant gamma-interferon in malignant mesothelioma. Cancer 67:2033, 1991a.

Boutin C, et al: Thoracoscopic diagnosis and staging of pleural malignant mesothelioma: a prospective study of 188 consecutive patients. Cancer (in press) 1993.

Boutin C, Viallat JR, Aeolony Y (eds): Practical thoracoscopy. Heidelberg: Springer-Verlag, 1991b.

Brady, LW: Mesothelioma — the role for radiation therapy. Semin Oncol 8:329, 1981.

Burmer GC, et al: Flow cytometric analysis of malignant pleural mesotheliomas. Hum Pathol 20:777, 1989.

Burns TR, et al: Ultrastructural diagnosis of epithelial malignant mesothelioma. Cancer 56:2036, 1985.

Butchart EG, et al: Pleuropneumonectomy in the management of diffuse malignant mesothelioma of the pleura. Thorax 31:15, 1976.

Cantin R, Al-Jabi M, McCaughey WTE: Desmoplastic diffuse mesothelioma. Am J Surg Pathol 6:215, 1982.

Cartier P: *In:* Smith WE: Survey of some current British and European studies of occupational tumor problems. Arch Indust Hygiene Occup Med 5:242, 1952.

Chahinian AP: Therapeutic modalities in malignant pleural mesothelioma. *In* Chretien J, Hirsch A (eds): Diseases of the Pleura. New York: Masson, 1983.

Chahinian AP, et al: Diffuse pulmonary malignant mesothelioma: response to doxorubicin and 5-azacytidine. Cancer 42:1687, 1978.

Chahinian AP, et al: Diffuse malignant mesothelioma: Prospective evaluation of 69 patients. Ann Intern Med 96:746, 1982.

Chahinian AP, et al: Cisplatin with adriamycin or mitomycin for malignant mesothelioma: A randomized phase II trial. Proc ASCO 6:183, 1987.

Christ F, Weinbrenner J, Reiser M: The radiological image of pleural lipomas with special reference to computed tomography. ROFO 155:58, 1991.

Churg A, DePaoli L: Environmental pleural plaques in residents of a Quebec chrysotile mining town. Chest 94:58, 1988.

Cote RJ, et al: Genetic alterations of the P53 gene are a feature of malignant mesotheliomas. Cancer Res 51:5410, 1991.

Dabouis G, LeMevel B, Corroller J: Treatment of diffuse pleural malignant mesothelioma by Cis Dichloro Diammine Platinum (CDDP) in nine patients. Cancer Chemother Pharmacol 5:209, 1981.

Dahl IMS, et al: A longitudinal study of the hyaluronan level in the serum of patients with malignant mesothelioma under treatment. Cancer 64:68, 1989.

de Klerk NH, Armstrong BK: The epidemiology of asbestos and mesothelioma. *In* Henderson DW et al (eds): Malignant Mesothelioma. New York: Hemisphere, 1992.

DeLaria GA, et al: Surgical management of malignant mesothelioma. Ann Thorac Surg 26:375, 1978.

DeValle MJ, et al: Extrapleural pneumonectomy for diffuse, malignant mesothelioma. Ann Thorac Surg 42:612, 1986.

Dimitrov NV, et al: High-dose methotrexate with citrovorum factor and vincristine in the treatment of malignant mesothelioma. Cancer 50:1245, 1982.

Dimitrov NV, McMahon S: Presentation, diagnostic methods, staging, and natural history of malignant mesothelioma. *In* Antman K, Aisner J (eds): Asbestos-Related Malignancy. Orlando, FL: Grune & Stratton, 1987.

Elmes PC, Simpson MJC: The clinical aspects of mesothelioma. Q J Med 45:427, 1976.

Fraire AE, et al: Mesothelioma of childhood. Cancer 62:838, 1988.

Gerwin BI, et al: Comparison of production of transforming growth factor-β and platelet-derived growth factor by normal human mesothelial cells and mesothelioma cell lines. Cancer Res 47:6180, 1987.

Gordon W, et al: Radiation therapy in the management of patients with mesothelioma. Int J Radiat Oncol Biol Phys 8:19, 1981.

Gotfried MH, Quan SF, Sobonya RE: Diffuse epithelial pleural mesothelioma presenting as a solitary lung mass. Chest 84:99, 1983.

Hagemeijer A, et al: Cytogenetic analysis of malignant mesothelioma. Cancer Genet Cytogenet 47:1, 1990.

Hammar SP, Bolen JW: Pleural neoplasms. *In* Dail DH, Hammar SP (eds): Pulmonary Pathology. New York: Springer-Verlag, 1988.

Hilaris BS, et al: Pleurectomy and intraoperative brachytherapy and postoperative radiation in the treatment of malignant pleural mesothelioma. Int J Radiat Oncol Biol Phys 10:324, 1983.

Hillerdal G: Malignant mesothelioma 1982: review of 4710 published cases. Br J Dis Chest 77:321, 1983.

Hulks G, Thomas JSJ, Waclawski E: Malignant pleural mesothelioma in western Glasgow 1980–6. Thorax 44:496, 1989.

Huncharek M: Changing risk groups for malignant mesothelioma. Cancer 69:2704, 1992.

Kane MJ, Chahinian AP, Holland JF: Malignant mesothelioma in young adults. Cancer 65:1449, 1990.

Kaye JA, et al: Malignant mesothelioma with brain metastases. Am J Med 80:95, 1986.

Keller SM, Taylor DD, Weese JL: *In vitro* killing of human malignant mesothelioma by photodynamic therapy. J Surg Res 48:337, 1990.

Klemperer P, Rabin CB: Primary neoplasms of the pleura. A report of five cases. Arch Pathol 11:385, 1937.

Krarup-Hansen A, Hansen HH: Chemotherapy in malignant mesothelioma: a review. Cancer Chemother Pharmacol 28:319, 1991.

Kutcher GJ, et al: Technique for external beam treatment for mesothelioma. Int J Radiat Oncol Biol Phys 13:1747, 1987.

Law MR, et al: Computed tomography in the assessment of malignant mesothelioma of the pleura. Clin Radiol 33:67, 1982.

Law MR, et al: Malignant mesothelioma of the pleura: a study of 52 treated and 64 untreated patients. Thorax 39:255, 1984.

Law MR, Hodson ME, Heard BE: Malignant mesothelioma of the pleura: relation between histological type and clinical behavior. Thorax 37:810, 1982.

Layman L: The blue asbestos industry at Wittenoom in Western Australia: A short history. *In* Henderson DW et al (eds): Malignant mesothelioma. New York: Hemisphere, 1992.

Lederman GS, et al: Long-term survival in peritoneal mesothelioma: the role of radiotherapy and combined modality treatment. Cancer 59:1882, 1987.

Lerman Y, et al: Radiation associated malignant pleural mesothelioma. Thorax 46:463, 1991.

Le Roux BT: Pleural tumors. Thorax 17:111, 1962.

Levine RL (ed): Asbestos: An Information Resource (NIH Publication No. 81-1681). Bethesda, MD: National Institutes of Health, 1981.

Lewis RJ, Sisler GE, Mackenzie JW: Diffuse, mixed malignant pleural mesothelioma. Ann Thorac Surg 31:53, 1981.

Maasilta P: Deterioration in lung function following hemithorax irradiation for pleural mesothelioma. Int J Radiat Oncol Biol Phys 20:433, 1990.

Malker HSR, et al: Occupational risks for pleural mesothelioma in Sweden, 1961–79. J Natl Cancer Inst 75:61, 1985.

Markman M, et al: Cisplatin administered by the intracavitary route as treatment for malignant mesothelioma. Cancer 58:18, 1986.

McCormack PM, et al: Surgical treatment of pleural mesothelioma. J Thorac Cardiovasc Surg 84:834, 1982.

McDonald JC, et al: Mesothelioma and asbestos fiber type. Cancer 63:1544, 1989.

McDonald AD, McDonald JC: Malignant mesothelioma in North America. Cancer 46:1650, 1980.

Mezger J, Lamerz R, Permanetter W: Diagnostic significance of carcinoembryonic antigen in the differential diagnosis of malignant mesothelioma. J Thorac Cardiovasc Surg 100:860, 1990.

Mintzer DM, et al: Phase II trial of high-dose cisplatin in patients with malignant mesothelioma. Cancer Treat Rep 69:711, 1985.

Mirvis S, et al: CT of malignant pleural mesothelioma. AJR Am J Roentgenol 140:665, 1983.

Murray M: *In* Report of the Departmental Committee on Compensation for Industrial Diseases. London: HMSO, 1907, p 127.

Musk AW, et al: The incidence of malignant mesothelioma in Australia, 1947–1987. Med J Aust 150:242, 1989.

Mychalczak BR, et al: Results of treatment of malignant pleural mesothelioma with surgery, brachytherapy, and external beam irradiation. Proceedings of 12th winter mid-meeting of the American Endocurietherapy Society, Hilton Head, SC, December 6–9, 1989.

Nauta RJ, et al: Clinical staging and the tendency of malignant pleural mesotheliomas to remain localized. Ann Thorac Surg 34:66, 1982.

Olesen LL, Thorshauge H: Thrombocytosis in patients with malignant pleural mesothelioma. Cancer 62:1194, 1988.

Pass H: Intrapleural photodynamic therapy results of a Phase I trial. J Surg Oncol (in press) 1993.

Peterson JT, Greenberg SD, Buffler PA: Non-asbestos related malignant mesothelioma. Cancer 54:951, 1984.

Pooley FD: Asbestos mineralogy. *In* Antman K, Aisner J (eds): Asbestos-Related Malignancy. Orlando, FL: Grune & Stratton, 1987.

Popescu NC, Chahinian AP, DiPaolo JA: Nonrandom chromosome alterations in human malignant mesothelioma. Cancer Res *48*:142, 1988.

Rabinowitz JG, et al: A comparative study of mesothelioma and asbestosis using computed tomography and conventional chest radiography. Radiology *144*:453, 1982.

Raghavan K, et al: Phase II trial of carboplatin in the management of malignant mesothelioma. J Clin Oncol *8*:151, 1990.

Reddel RR, et al: Tumorigenicity of human mesothelial cell line transfected with EJ-ras oncogene. J Natl Cancer Inst *81*:945, 1989.

Ris H-B, et al: Photodynamic therapy with chlorins for diffuse malignant mesothelioma: initial clinical results. Br J Cancer *64*:1116, 1991.

Roberts GH: Distant visceral metastases in pleural mesothelioma. Br J Dis Chest *70*:246, 1976.

Ruffie P, et al: Diffuse malignant mesothelioma of the pleura in Ontario and Quebec: a retrospective study of 332 patients. J Clin Oncol *7*:1157, 1989.

Rusch VW, Piantadosi S, Holmes EC: The role of extrapleural pneumonectomy in malignant pleural mesothelioma: a Lung Cancer Study Group trial. J Thorac Cardiovasc Surg *102*:1, 1991.

Rusch VW, Godwin JD, Shuman WP: The role of computed tomography scanning in the initial assessment and the follow-up of malignant pleural mesothelioma. J Thorac Cardiovasc Surg *96*:171, 1988.

Rusch V: Pleurectomy/decortication for malignant mesothelioma. Paper presented at Cine clinics, meeting of the American College of Surgeons, October 1991.

Rusch V, et al: A phase II trial of intrapleural and systemic chemotherapy after pleurectomy/decortication for malignant pleural mesothelioma. J Clin Oncol *11*:352, 1992.

Rusch V, Piantadosi S, Holmes EC: The role of extrapleural pneumonectomy in malignant pleural mesothelioma. J Thorac Cardiovasc Surg *102*:1, 1991.

Scharifker D, Kaneko M: Localized fibrous "mesothelioma" of pleura (submesothelial fibroma). Cancer *43*:627, 1979.

Selikoff IJ, Churg J, Hammond EC: Relation between exposure to asbestos and mesothelioma. N Engl J Med *272*:560, 1965.

Sheard JDH, Taylor W, Pearson MG: Pneumothorax and malignant mesothelioma in patients over the age of 40. Thorax *46*:584, 1991.

Sinoff C, et al: Combined doxorubicin and radiation therapy in malignant pleural mesothelioma. Cancer Treat Rep *66*:1605, 1982.

Sklarin NT, et al: Augmentation of activity of *cis*-Diamminedichloroplatinum(II) and mitomycin C by interferon in human malignant mesothelioma xenografts in nude mice. Cancer Res *48*:64, 1988.

Soubra M, et al: Physical aspects of external beam radiotherapy for the treatment of malignant pleural mesothelioma. Int J Radiat Oncol Biol Phys *18*:1521, 1990.

Stout AP, Murray MR: Localized pleural mesothelioma. Arch Pathol *34*:951, 1942.

Sugarbaker DJ, et al: Extrapleural pneumonectomy, chemotherapy, and radiotherapy in the treatment of diffuse malignant pleural mesothelioma. J Thorac Cardiovasc Surg *102*:10, 1991.

Sugarbaker D, et al: Trimodality therapy of malignant pleural mesothelioma. J Clin Oncol *11*:295, 1992.

Tammilehto L: Malignant mesothelioma: Prognostic factors in a prospective study of 98 patients. Lung Cancer *8*:175, 1992.

Tiainen M, et al: Chromosomal abnormalities and their correlations with asbestos exposure and survival in patients with mesothelioma. Br J Cancer *60*:618, 1989.

Umsawasdi T, et al: A case report of malignant pleural mesothelioma with long-term disease control after chemotherapy. Cancer *67*:48, 1991.

Van der Schoot HC: Asbestosis en pleuragezwellen. Ned Tijdschr Geneeskd *102*:1125, 1958.

Vogt-Moykopf I, Etspüler W, Bülzebruck H: Des diffuse maligne Pleuramesotheliom: Diagnostik, Therapie und Prognose. Z Herz Thorax Gefässchir *1*:67, 1987.

Wadler S, et al: Cardiac abnormalities in patients with diffuse malignant pleural mesothelioma. Cancer *58*:2744, 1986.

Wedler HW: Asbestose und Lungenkrebs. Dtsch Med Wochenschr *69*:575, 1943a.

Wedler HW: Uber den Lungenkrebs bei Asbestose. Dtsch Arch Klin Med *191*:189, 1943b.

Wagner JC: Mesothelioma and mineral fibers. Cancer *57*:1905, 1986.

Wagner JC, Slaggs CA, Marchand P: Diffuse pleural mesothelioma and asbestos exposure in North Western Cape Province. Br J Indust Med *17*:260, 1960.

Walters KL, Martinez AJ: Malignant fibrous mesothelioma. Acta Neuropathol *33*:173, 1975.

Whitwell F, Rawcliffe RM: Diffuse malignant pleural mesothelioma and asbestos exposure. Thorax *26*:6, 1971.

Wirth PR, Legier J, Wright GL: Immunohistochemical evaluation of seven monoclonal antibodies for differentiation of pleural mesothelioma from lung adenocarcinoma. Cancer *67*:655, 1991.

Wörn H: Möglichkeiten und Ergebnisse der chirugischen Behandlung des malignen Pleuramesothelioms. Thoraxchirurgie 1974; 22:391, 1974.

CHAPTER 62

TECHNIQUE OF PLEURAL PNEUMONECTOMY IN DIFFUSE MESOTHELIOMA

David J. Sugarbaker and Simon C. Body

Historically, the technique of extrapleural pneumonectomy has been described for over 40 years, initially by Sarot (1949) for the treatment of tuberculous empyema and in the last two decades for other noninfectious pleural diseases such as malignant pleural mesothelioma — diffuse mesothelioma. Worn (1974), Bamler and Maassen (1974), Butchart (1976), DeLaria (1978), Faber (1986), DaValle (1986), and others have described both the surgical approach and the pathophysiologic and histologic consequences of extrapleural pneumonectomy for malignant pleural mesothelioma. All authors, however, have reported a high perioperative mortality and morbidity when compared with that of nonextrapleural pneumonectomy (Table 62–1). There has been considerable discussion by Falkson (1988), Harvey (1990), and Sugarbaker (1991) and their colleagues on the histologic indications and treatment rationale for combination protocols using extrapleural pneumonectomy, chemotherapy, and radiotherapy. Essential to all discussions of the surgical approach to patients with malignant mesothelioma has been the evidence of a need to debulk the tumor mass and an inability to demonstrate that clear surgical margins are necessary for a curative procedure. In addition, the last 20 years have been notable for improvements in preoperative preparation, intraoperative management, and postoperative care of patients with this extremely complex disease. These improvements have been reflected in decreases in perioperative mortality, morbidity, and length of hospital stay.

The patient selection, technique, and clinical results in our experience with malignant pleural mesothelioma are as follows: The surgical technique for right-sided extrapleural pneumonectomy will be described in detail and is supplemented by the variations that are required in a left-sided approach.

PATIENT SELECTION AND PREPARATION

Surgical resection is only appropriate in Butchart (1976) stage I patients (Fig. 62–1). Extension of the disease into the mediastinum or through the diaphragm — stages II, III — prohibits resection. Survival in these groups beyond 1 year is extremely low. Surgical resection combined with postoperative cyclophosphamide, doxorubicin, and cisplatin — CAP — chemotherapy and radiation therapy has been shown to improve survival, as noted by one of us (D.J.S.) and colleagues (1991, 1993). Protocols involving a trimodality treatment plan demonstrate better short- and long-term survival than surgery alone.

Table 62–1. Reported Mortality With Extrapleural Pneumonectomy

	Series					
	Butchart (1976)	Worn (1974)	Bamler & Maassen (1974)	DeLaria et al (1978)	DaValle et al (1986)	Sugarbaker et al (1991, 1992, 1993)
Number of patients	29	62	17	11	33	52
Epithelial histopathology	11	—	—	9	20	32
2-Year survival	3(10.3%)	23(37%)	6(35%)	2(18%)	8(24%)	9(17.3%)
5-Year survival	1(3.5%)	6(10%)	—	—	2(6%)	2(3.8%)
Operative mortality	31%	—	23%	0%	9.1%	5.8%

I	Within the "capsule" of the parietal pleura: ipsilateral pleura, lung, pericardium, diaphragm.
II	Invading chest wall or mediastinum: esophagus, heart, opposite pleura. + Lymph nodes within the chest.
III	Through diaphragm to peritoneum. Opposite pleura. + Lymph nodes outside the chest.
IV	Distant blood-borne metastases.

Fig. 62–1. Butchart staging system for malignant pleural mesothelioma. *From* Butchart EG, et al: Pleuropneumonectomy in the management of diffuse malignant mesothelioma of the pleura. Experience with 29 patients. Thorax 31:15, 1976.

Cell type and node status have only recently been shown by one of us (D.J.S.) and associates (1993) to be of prognostic value. Patients with epithelial cell pleural mesothelioma enjoyed a survival advantage over patients with mixed or pure sarcomatous cell type treated with surgery, chemotherapy, and radiation therapy. Furthermore, regardless of cell type, the presence of nodal involvement at the time of surgical resection is a predictor of poorer survival. This survival stratification has led the authors to propose a new staging system that takes into account these new prognostic factors (Fig. 62–2). This revised staging system is derived from a traditional treatment strategy that achieves local control in this series by using pleuropneumonectomy followed by radiation therapy and control of systemic disease with chemotherapy — CAP.

Patients with malignant pleural mesothelioma who are to be selected for extrapleural pneumonectomy require accurate preoperative assessment. As a result of the obliterative nature of the pleural disease, pulmonary function tests, notably FEV_1 and FVC, may not fully reflect postoperative pulmonary function. These patients may have complete functional pneumonectomy before their surgery. For patients in whom lung function is borderline — predicted postoperative FEV_1 <1 liter,

the use of quantitative ventilation/perfusion scanning, when combined with knowledge of FEV_1 and FVC, results in a reliable prediction of the postoperative lung function remaining. Doxorubicin chemotherapy induces a dose-dependent, irreversible decrease in biventricular function in some patients. It is appropriate in this group to measure left and right ventricular function by standard echocardiography to both assess pre-existing alterations in ventricular function and provide a baseline for monitoring cardiac toxicity during postoperative chemotherapy.

Preoperative chest magnetic resonance — MR — imaging and computed tomography — CT — are essential to determine the extent of intrathoracic and extrathoracic disease preoperatively. Determining the presence of transdiaphragmatic extension or mediastinal invasion, especially of the vena cavae, trachea, esophagus, or aorta, as well as invasion of the paravertebral sulcus, is required to determine operability in these patients. The presence of mediastinal invasion or abdominal disease precludes surgical resection because no long-term survivors have been reported in this setting. Chest MR imaging has been shown by Patz and associates (1992) to be of value, in addition to CT scanning, in making these determinations. Careful pre-

STAGE I	Disease confined to within "capsule" of the parietal pleura: ipsilateral pleura, lung, pericardium, diaphragm* or chest wall disease limited to previous biopsy sites.
STAGE II	All of Stage I with positive intrathoracic (N1 or N2) lymph nodes.
STAGE III	Local extension of disease into: chest wall or mediastinum; heart, or through diaphragm, peritoneum; with or without extrathoracic or contralateral (N3) lymph node involvement.
STAGE IV	Distant metastatic disease.

Fig. 62–2. A proposed staging system for mesothelioma patients based on survival of 52 patients. Butchart stage II and III (Butchart, 1976) are combined into stage III. Stage I represents resectable patients with negative nodes. Stage II patients are resectable but have positive nodal status. *From* Sugarbaker DJ, et al: Node status has prognostic significance in the multimodality therapy of diffuse, malignant mesothelioma. J Clin Oncol (in press) 1993. *From Antman, K, Pass HI, Recht A: Benign and malignant mesothelioma. *In* DeVita VT Jr, Hellman S, Rosenberg SA (eds): Cancer: Principles and Practice of Oncology. 3rd Ed. Philadelphia, JB Lippincott, 1989.

operative selection is required if the appropriate patients are to be selected for these aggressive treatment regimens.

TECHNIQUE OF RIGHT PLEUROPNEUMONECTOMY

After induction of anesthesia and placement of a left-sided Robertshaw double-lumen tube, the patient is positioned in a left lateral decubitus position in preparation for an extended right posterolateral thoracotomy. A nasogastric tube should be placed to facilitate palpation of the esophagus during the dissection.

These patients are monitored with arterial lines, continuous oximetry, and a central venous line. Thoracic epidural catheters are placed preoperatively and may be used for intraoperative management as well as postoperative pain control.

Before making the thoracotomy incision, a limited subcostal incision is made to explore for possible transdiaphragmatic involvement if this possibility has been suggested by the preoperative MR imaging. Laparoscopic exploration may be preferred by surgeons with experience in this technique. Should peritoneal involvement be discovered, the procedure should be terminated and no attempt at thoracic resection made. The diaphragm may be distended with the tumor, but frank invasion into the peritoneal space should be documented with biopsy before abandoning the procedure.

An incision is made along the bed of the sixth rib (Fig. 62–3). The incision is taken from 2 cm lateral to the costovertebral junction along the bed of the sixth rib to the costochondral junction. After periosteal stripping, the sixth rib is excised in its entirety to provide adequate exposure. The periosteum is then incised, and a widely based extrapleural dissection is advanced superiorly toward the apex of the thorax using both sharp and blunt dissection. The anterior component of the dissection is completed first, both superiorly and inferiorly toward the diaphragm. The posterior dissection is delayed until adequate exposure has been obtained anteriorly. This is to avoid an uncontrolled approach to the mediastinal structures in the posterior portion of the visceral compartment. After adequate initial exposure has been obtained, two chest retractors are placed anteriorly and posteriorly within the chest. Combined sharp and blunt dissection continues toward the apex of the hemithorax. The brachial triangle is exposed carefully to avoid the subclavian artery and vein, and the plane of dissection is maintained carefully.

On the anterior border, the internal mammary artery and vein are protected from injury because they easily can be avulsed from the superior vena cava and the subclavian artery. Posterosuperiorly, the dissection is carried from the apex of the hemithorax down to the azygos vein. The dissection is extrapleural until the right main stem bronchus and upper lobe are identified (Fig. 62–4). The extrapleural tissues are then dissected from

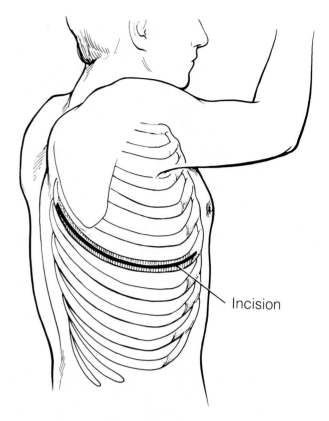

Fig. 62–3. The extended right thoracotomy incision. *From* Sugarbaker DJ, Mentzer SJ, Strauss G: Extrapleural pneumonectomy in the treatment of malignant pleural mesothelioma. Ann Thorac Surg 54:941, 1992.

the superior vena cava and azygos vein. The anterior dissection at the base of the lung is completed when the circumferential diaphragmatic margin is dissected. The diaphragm is incised at its lateral margin in a circumferential fashion as far as the anterior border of the pericardium. Care should be taken to maintain continuity of the pleural envelope, and, in some situations, this requires dissection of the pleural envelope off the diaphragm before the division of the diaphragm (Fig. 62–5). The diaphragm is dissected off the peritoneum with a sponge stick (Fig. 62–6). When the diaphragm has been incised anteriorly to the pericardium, it is then divided along the caval-esophageal hiatuses. Frequently, this requires entering the pericardium to delineate the inferior vena cava. Then, just lateral to the inferior vena cava and the esophagus, the diaphragm and pleural envelope are divided (Fig. 62–7). At this point the diaphragmatic incision has been completed.

If the pericardium has not already been opened, it is then incised and entered anteromedially to the phrenic nerve and hilar vessels (Fig. 62–8). The main pulmonary artery is then dissected free from the superior vena cava and superior pulmonary vein (Fig. 62–9). The right pulmonary artery is then divided intrapericardially between two lines of vascular staples (Fig. 62–9) as one of us (D.J.S.) and colleagues (1992)

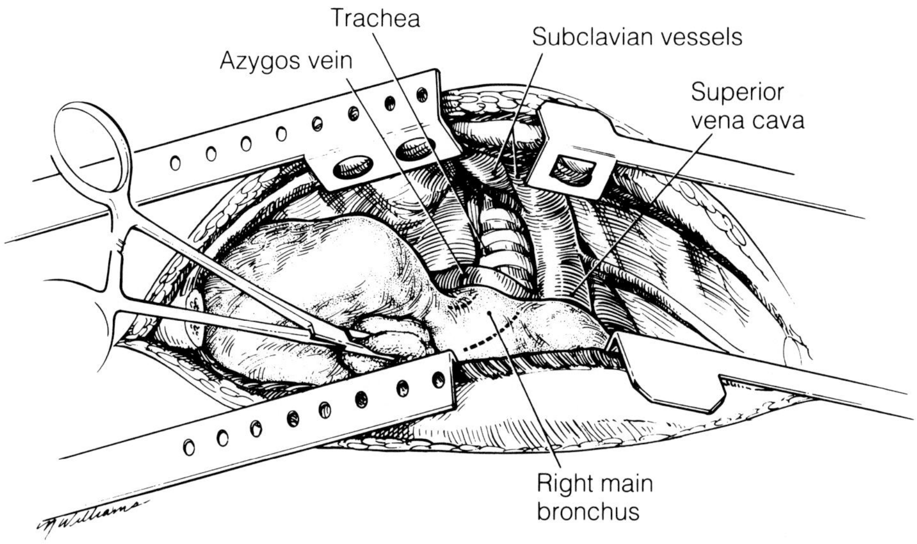

Trachea

Azygos vein

Subclavian vessels

Superior
vena cava

Right main
bronchus

Fig. 62–4. The right main stem bronchus identified. *From* Sugarbaker DJ, Mentzer SJ, Strauss G: Extrapleural pneumonectomy in the treatment of malignant pleural mesothelioma. Ann Thorac Surg *54*:941, 1992.

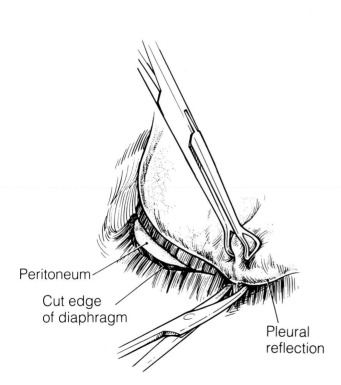

Peritoneum

Cut edge
of diaphragm

Pleural
reflection

Fig. 62–5. Dissection of the pleural envelope off the diaphragm. *From* Sugarbaker DJ, Mentzer SJ, Strauss G: Extrapleural pneumonectomy in the treatment of malignant pleural mesothelioma. Ann Thorac Surg *54*:941, 1992.

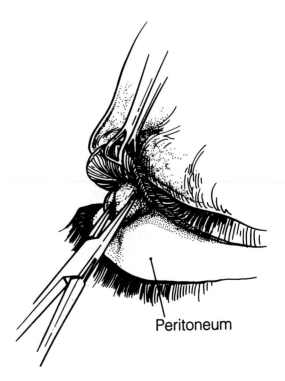

Peritoneum

Fig. 62–6. The peritoneum wiped off the diaphragm with a sponge. *From* Sugarbaker DJ, Mentzer SJ, Strauss G: Extrapleural pneumonectomy in the treatment of malignant pleural mesothelioma. Ann Thorac Surg *54*:941, 1992.

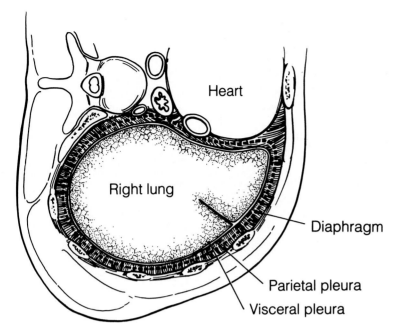

Fig. 62–7. Diaphragm and pleural envelope divided lateral to inferior cava and esophagus. *From* Sugarbaker DJ, Mentzer SJ, Strauss G: Extrapleural pneumonectomy in the treatment of malignant pleural mesothelioma. Ann Thorac Surg *54*:941, 1992.

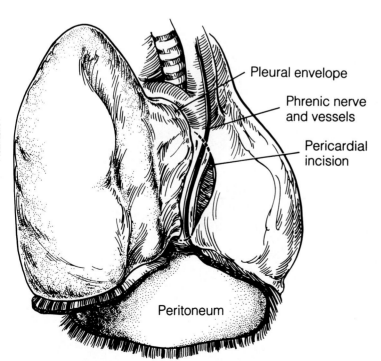

Fig. 62–8. The pericardium is opened anteromedially to the phrenic nerve and hilar vessels. *From* Sugarbaker DJ, Mentzer SJ, Strauss G: Extrapleural pneumonectomy in the treatment of malignant pleural mesothelioma. Ann Thorac Surg *54*:941, 1992.

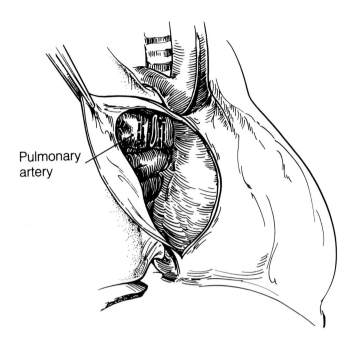

Fig. 62–9. The intrapericardial right pulmonary artery is divided by two staple lines. *From* Sugarbaker DJ, Mentzer SJ, Strauss G: Extrapleural pneumonectomy in the treatment of malignant pleural mesothelioma. Ann Thorac Surg *54*:941, 1992.

have described. Next, the superior and inferior pulmonary veins are each stapled between two lines of vascular staples. The pericardium is divided posterior to the hilum; this completes the pericardial resection. The surgical specimen is then brought forward anteriorly. Now dissection is continued posteriorly to the

pericardium and lateral to the esophagus. At this point, we perform a subcarinal node dissection. The right main bronchus is then dissected as far as the carina and stapled (Fig. 62–10), and subsequently the specimen is removed. The surgical specimen is examined by the pathologist for the status of the resection margins in several areas.

A pericardial fat pad is raised from the anterior superior aspect of the pericardium (Fig. 62–11) and is placed over the bronchial stump. The pericardium on the right side is always reconstructed with a fenestrated patch to prevent cardiac herniation; this is done with a prosthetic patch and running 0 monofilament suture (Fig. 62–11). If the abdominal peritoneum remains intact, then sutures of 0 vicryl are used in a reefing fashion (Fig. 62–12) to strengthen the underlying peritoneum. Following this reinforcement, the sutures are anchored to the chest wall (Fig. 62–12), and no further reconstruction is necessary. If the peritoneum was incised during the dissection, a prosthetic impermeable patch is placed and sewn with a running monofilament 0 suture (Fig. 62–13). Use of permeable patches in this situation can result in peritoneal fluid filling the right pneumonectomy space, which may result in a severe mediastinal shift or cardiac tamponade.

If an area of gross disease cannot be resected following pneumonectomy, it is outlined with radio-opaque clips for subsequent irradiation. The chest is then closed in the usual fashion to ensure an airtight closure, and a red rubber catheter is placed in the residual pleural space until the skin is closed. In the immediate postoperative period before extubation, the pneumonectomy space is reduced in size by removal of 750 cc of air in

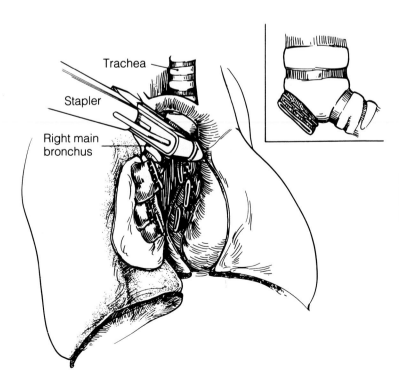

Fig. 62–10. The main bronchus is dissected to the carina and stapled. *From* Sugarbaker DJ, Mentzer SJ, Strauss G: Extrapleural pneumonectomy in the treatment of malignant pleural mesothelioma. Ann Thorac Surg *54*:941, 1992.

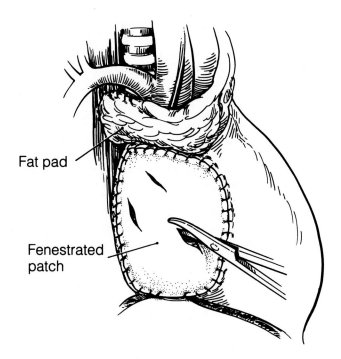

Fat pad

Fenestrated
patch

Fig. 62–11. A pericardial fat pad has been sewn to cover the bronchial stump; the pericardium is closed with a patch, and fenestrations are made in the patch. *From* Sugarbaker DJ, Mentzer SJ, Strauss G: Extrapleural pneumonectomy in the treatment of malignant pleural mesothelioma. Ann Thorac Surg *54*:941, 1992.

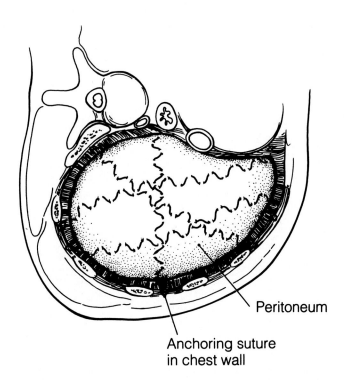

Peritoneum

Anchoring suture
in chest wall

Fig. 62–12. Reconstruction of the diaphragm using multiple sutures of 0 vicryl in reefing fashion is carried out; the sutures are anchored to the chest wall. *From* Sugarbaker DJ, Mentzer SJ, Strauss G: Extrapleural pneumonectomy in the treatment of malignant pleural mesothelioma. Ann Thorac Surg *54*:941, 1992.

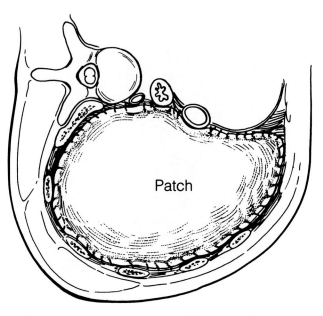

Patch

Fig. 62–13. A prosthetic impermeable patch is sewn in place where the peritoneum has been removed. *From* Sugarbaker DJ, Mentzer SJ, Strauss G: Extrapleural pneumonectomy in the treatment of malignant pleural mesothelioma. Ann Thorac Surg *54*:941, 1992.

women and 1000 cc in men with the use of a 50 cc syringe attached to the red rubber catheter with a three-way stopcock. In the recovery room, the chest radiograph is obtained to check for midline position of the heart and mediastinal structures. If these are not midline on the radiograph, then air can be instilled or removed to balance the mediastinum; subsequently the catheter can be removed. If a hemothorax is present, then a standard chest tube is placed and is water sealed to monitor drainage overnight; it is usually removed the next day.

LEFT PLEUROPNEUMONECTOMY

It is appropriate in this situation to place an endobronchial blocker for lung isolation because the placement of a right double-lumen tube can be difficult. The dissection for a diffuse mesothelioma of the left hemithorax is similar to that on the right, but there are some subtle differences. Technically, the dissection is easier, which is due to the position of the caval and esophageal hiatuses. During dissection of the posteromedial aspect of the specimen, it is important to enter the correct plane in the pre-aortic region to avoid avulsion of the intercostal vessels. It is also important to assess tumor involvement of the aorta at this time because aortic involvement may preclude resection. It is important to clearly define the aorta at the diaphragmatic hiatus during the dissection; otherwise, serious bleeding can result from injury to the aorta or intercostal vessels.

The left main pulmonary artery is dissected and divided extrapericardially (Fig. 62–14), using two vascular staple lines. The pulmonary veins are dissected,

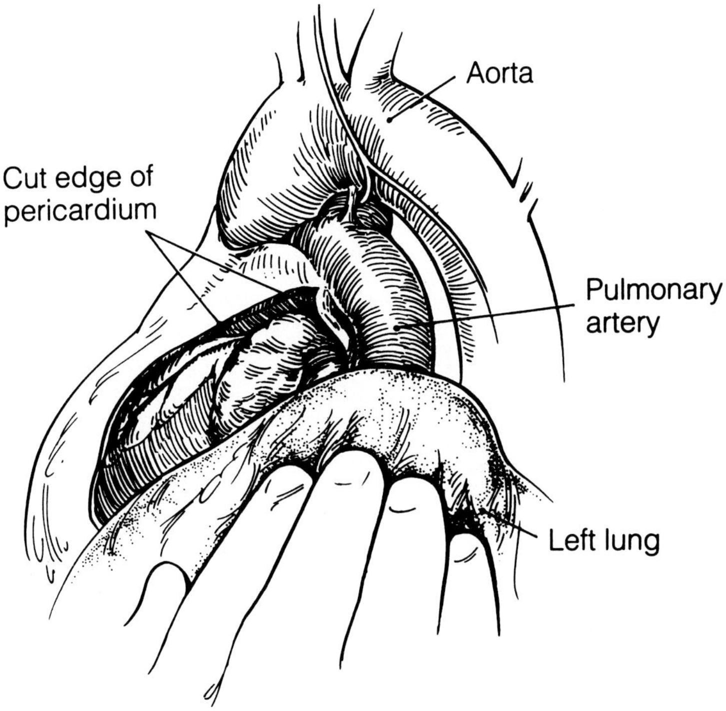

Fig. 62–14. The left main pulmonary artery extrapericardial and extrapleural ready to be dissected and divided. *From* Sugarbaker DJ, Mentzer SJ, Strauss G: Extrapleural pneumonectomy in the treatment of malignant pleural mesothelioma. Ann Thorac Surg 54:941, 1992.

however, intrapericardially, and the pericardial resection is then completed posteriorly. The left main stem bronchus must be dissected up to the carina to ensure a short bronchial stump. The pericardium, however, is not routinely reconstructed on the left side, because the risk of cardiac herniation is low on the left, which is due to the native cardiac position in the left hemithorax.

Because of the reduced size of the left hemothorax, less air is removed at the end of the procedure — 500 cc in women; 750 cc in men.

HEMOSTASIS

Routine blood loss during this procedure is 750 cc for a right pneumonectomy and 500 cc for a left pneumonectomy. Surgical hemostasis is best achieved by rapid packing of areas that have been dissected. Once the specimen is out, Surgicel (Johnson & Johnson, Arlington, TX) can be placed over the raw, bleeding chest wall surface and packed. Liberal use of the electrocautery is needed to coagulate the numerous small vessels in the extrapleural plane.

POSTOPERATIVE MANAGEMENT

The goals of postoperative management are not dissimilar from those with patients undergoing other standard pneumonectomy procedures. These are to control pain and minimize intravascular volume changes. We routinely use thoracic epidural catheters for the first 3 to 5 days postoperatively. Pain control is vital to minimize postoperative atelectasis and its resulting pulmonary dysfunction. Patients are monitored

in a thoracic stepdown unit with arterial lines, central venous lines, continuous oximetry, and respiratory rate monitors (Marquett Electronics, Milwaukee, WI). Nursing is on a one-to-two basis with regular chest physiotherapy. Patients are placed with the operated side down for 2 days postoperatively. Deep vein thrombosis prophylaxis is carried out by the use of pneumatic stockings (Kendall Healthcare Products Co., Mansfield, MA).

Patients are routinely placed on a 1-liter, 24-hour fluid restriction for 3 to 5 days postoperatively. This is due to the tendency of these patients to retain fluid and to have mild episodes of capillary leak in the remaining lung, which can lead to desaturation. Desaturation of oxygen levels is usually treated with diuresis or chest physiotherapy and occasionally bronchoscopy. Daily chest radiographs are closely evaluated for mediastinal shift that might lead to tamponade or in-flow obstruction. Contralateral infiltrates are treated aggressively in this patient population. The nasogastric tube is removed on day 1 based on clinical findings. Aspiration can be a fatal complication in this group of patients, given their limited pulmonary reserve.

CLINICAL RESULTS AND DISCUSSION

We have reported our series of pleuropneumonectomy with a consistent postoperative mortality rate comparable to standard pneumonectomy as reported by Ginsberg and associates (1983) (Table 62–1). Clearly, patient selection is an important factor in this lowered mortality, as are advances in anesthesia and surgical techniques. As noted, one of us (D.J.S.) and colleagues (1993) have recently reported the prognostic importance of cell type and node status in these patients. These data have led us to propose a modified staging system for this disease (Fig. 62–2). This staging system would define patients that are stage I or II as potentially resectable. This patient population, while technically resectable, could theoretically be further distinguished by preresectional lymph node biopsy via mediastinoscopy or thoracoscopy. The aggressive treatment of both node-negative and node-positive patients regardless of cell type will be enhanced by the development of more active adjuvant chemotherapeutic agents.

REFERENCES

Antman K, Pass HI, Recht A: Benign and malignant mesothelioma. *In* DeVita VT Jr, Hellman S, Rosenberg SA (eds): Cancer: Principles and Practice of Oncology. 3rd Ed. Philadelphia: JB Lippincott, 1989.

Bamler KJ, Maassen W: The percentage of benign and malign pleura-tumors among the patients of a clinic of lung surgery with special consideration of the malign pleuramesothelioma and its radical treatment, including results of a diaphragma substitution of preserved dura mater [Ger]. Thoraxchir Vask Chir 22:386, 1974.

Butchart EG, et al: Pleuropneumonectomy in the management of diffuse malignant mesothelioma of the pleura. Experience with 29 patients. Thorax 31:15, 1976.

DaValle MJ, et al: Extrapleural pneumonectomy for diffuse, malignant mesothelioma. Ann Thorac Surg 42:612, 1986.

DeLaria GA, et al: Surgical management of malignant mesothelioma. Ann Thorac Surg 26:375, 1978.

Faber LP: Malignant pleural mesothelioma: operative treatment by extrapleural pneumonectomy. *In* Kittle CF (ed): Current Controversies in Thoracic Surgery. Philadelphia: WB Saunders, 1986.

Falkson G, Alberts AS, Falkson HC: Malignant pleural mesothelioma treatment: the current state of the art. Cancer Treat Rev 15:231, 1988.

Ginsberg RJ, et al: Modern thirty-day operative mortality for surgical resections in lung cancer. J Thorac Cardiovasc Surg 86:654, 1983.

Harvey JC, et al: Malignant pleural mesothelioma: a survival study. J Surg Oncol 45:40, 1990.

Patz EF Jr, et al: Malignant pleural mesothelioma: value of CT and MR imaging in predicting resectability. AJR Am J Roentgenol 159:961, 1992.

Sarot IA: Extrapleural pneumonectomy and pleurectomy in pulmonary tuberculosis. Thorax 4:173, 1949.

Sugarbaker DJ, et al: Extrapleural pneumonectomy, chemotherapy, and radiotherapy in the treatment of diffuse malignant pleural mesothelioma. J Thorac Cardiovasc Surg 102:10, 1991.

Sugarbaker DJ, et al: Node status has prognostic significance in the multimodality therapy of diffuse, malignant mesothelioma. J Clin Oncol (in press) 1993.

Sugarbaker DJ, Mentzer SJ, Strauss G: Extrapleural pneumonectomy in the treatment of malignant pleural mesothelioma. Ann Thorac Surg 54:941, 1992.

Worn H: Möglichkeiten und Ergebnisse der chirurgischen Behandlung des malignen Pleuramesotheliomas. Thoraxchir Vask Chir 22:391, 1974.

CHAPTER 63

MALIGNANT PLEURAL EFFUSIONS

Steven A. Sahn

DEFINITION AND INCIDENCE

Malignant pleural effusions are diagnosed by finding malignant cells in the pleural fluid or pleural tissue by closed needle biopsy, by biopsy through thoracoscopy or thoracotomy, or at autopsy. In some cases of documented malignancy with pleural effusion, malignant cells cannot be demonstrated in either pleural fluid or pleural tissue and probably are not present at the time of the diagnostic procedure. The author (1987a) believes these effusions are best termed "paramalignant" because they are associated with and caused by the malignancy but do not result from pleural invasion. Paramalignant effusions can be caused by a direct local effect of the tumor, by systemic manifestations of the malignancy, or by therapy (Table 63–1). Impaired pleural space lymphatic drainage is the most important mechanism responsible for both paramalignant and malignant pleural effusions.

As the author (1988) noted, lymphomas account for approximately 10% of all malignant pleural effusions and are the most common cause of chylothorax. Both Hodgkin's disease and non-Hodgkin's lymphoma have been associated with pleural effusions with variable incidences and usually through different mechanisms. Pleural effusions result more commonly from impaired lymphatic drainage of the pleural space in Hodgkin's disease, whereas direct pleural involvement tends to be more common in non-Hodgkin's lymphoma. These observations were recorded by Weick (1973), Jenkins (1981), and Xaubet (1985) and their associates.

Diffuse malignant mesothelioma arises from mesothelial cells or possibly from a precursor cell that is situated in the submesothelial connective tissue. The association

Table 63–1. Causes of Paramalignant Pleural Effusions

Cause	Comment
Local Effect of Tumor	
Lymphatic obstruction	Predominant mechanisms of pleural fluid accumulation
Bronchial obstruction with pneumonia	Parapneumonic effusion; does not rule out operability in lung cancer
Bronchial obstruction with atelectasis	Transudate; does not rule out operability in lung cancer
Chylothorax	Disruption of thoracic duct; chyle in pleural space; lymphoma most common cause
Superior vena cava obstruction	Transudate; due to increased systemic venous pressure
Systemic Effect of Tumor	
Pulmonary embolism	Hypercoagulable state
Low plasma oncotic pressure	Serum albumin <1.5 g/dl; associated with anasarca
Results of Therapy	
Radiation therapy	6 weeks to 6 months — radiation pleuritis
	Late — mediastinal fibrosis, SVC obstruction, constrictive pericarditis
Drug reactions	
Methotrexate	Pleuritis, pleural thickening or effusion occurs with low or high dose therapy
Procarbazine	Blood eosinophilia; hypersensitivity reaction
Cyclophosphamide	Pleuropericarditis
Mitomycin	Aggregates of lymphocytes and eosinophils in pleura; prompt relief of symptoms with drug withdrawal
Bleomycin	Resolves in weeks to months

From Sahn SA: Malignant pleural effusions. Semin Respir Med 9:43, 1987.

of asbestos exposure and malignant mesothelioma was established in 1960 by the report of Wagner and colleagues. McDonald and co-workers (1970) recorded that the incidence of malignant mesothelioma is approximately one per million per year in the general population that is not exposed to asbestos. Emont and associates (1970) reported that the incidence can rise 20-fold in certain populations and is even higher in shipyard communities.

Virtually all cancers metastasize to the pleura. Lung cancer is the most common to involve the pleura because of its proximity to the pleural surface and, as Meyer (1966) suggested, its propensity to invade the pulmonary arteries and embolize to the visceral pleura. Breast cancer also frequently metastasizes to the pleura, causing approximately 25% of malignant pleural effusions. Ovarian carcinoma and gastric cancer are next in frequency, and each represents <5% of malignant pleural effusions. As the author (1988) has pointed out, approximately 7% of patients with malignant pleural effusions, however, have an unknown primary site at the time of the initial diagnosis of the malignant effusion.

PATHOGENESIS

Impaired lymphatic drainage of the pleural space is the most important mechanism responsible for accumulation of large amounts of pleural fluid in malignancy. The lymphatic system can be blocked at any point from the stoma of the parietal pleura to the mediastinal and parasternal — internal mammary — lymph nodes. The autopsy studies by Meyer (1966) and Chernow and the author (1977) clearly demonstrated the association of mediastinal lymph node involvement and the presence of substantial pleural fluid. Conversely, these studies showed evidence of pleural involvement with tumor in the absence of pleural effusions, lending support to this mechanism. Furthermore, as Meyer (1966) noted, pleural effusions usually do not occur when the pleura is involved by sarcoma because of the absence of lymphatic metastasis. Weick and associates (1973) noted that Hodgkin's disease tends to cause pleural effusions by lymphatic obstruction, and Xaubet and associates (1985) noted that non-Hodgkin's lymphoma tends to produce effusions by both lymphatic obstruction and direct pleural invasion.

The inflammatory response to pleural tumor invasion results in increased microvascular permeability and produces small volumes of pleural effusion. Chretien and Jaubert (1985) suggested that oxygen radicals, arachidonic acid metabolites, proteases, lymphocytes, and immune complexes are probably causative.

Pleural effusion is an early manifestation of a malignant mesothelioma and probably results from a combination of increased capillary permeability from direct pleural invasion and impaired lymphatic drainage of the pleural space. As the tumor progresses and the visceral and parietal pleura fuse, the fluid diminishes or disappears.

Autopsy series have shown that in patients with carcinoma of the lung, pleural metastasis is almost always found on both the visceral and parietal pleural surfaces. Meyer (1966) noted that rarely is only the visceral pleural surface involved, and isolated parietal pleural metastases were never identified. Visceral pleural metastasis in lung cancer appears to be either through contiguous spread or through pulmonary arterial invasion and embolization. Once seeded with tumor, these malignant cells migrate from the visceral to parietal pleural surface by either preformed or tumor-induced pleural adhesions. Alternatively, free tumor cells shed from the visceral pleural surface can adhere to the parietal pleura and multiply. Chernow and the author (1977) reported that adenocarcinoma of the lung is the most common cell type to involve the pleura, because of its peripheral location. When bilateral pleural metastases occur in lung cancer, hepatic spread and parenchymal invasion in the contralateral lung also usually occur. Once contralateral lung metastasis occurs, pulmonary artery invasion and embolization follow, as in the ipsilateral lesion. The data concerning the laterality of the pleural effusion in relation to the primary lesion support this mechanism. Chernow and the author (1977) pointed out that in lung cancer, pleural effusions occur either ipsilaterally or bilaterally and virtually never occur solely in the contralateral pleural space. With other cancers, pleural involvement is usually from tertiary spread from established liver metastases with no predilection for side. Fentiman and associates (1981) summarized the conflicting data in breast carcinoma, with some studies showing a high incidence of ipsilateral pleural effusion and others no predilection for side. Probably two mechanisms are operative: chest wall lymphatic invasion resulting in ipsilateral effusion, and hepatic spread with bilateral or contralateral hematogenous spread.

CLINICAL PRESENTATION

The most common presenting symptom of patients with carcinoma or lymphoma of the pleura and a large pleural effusion is dyspnea on exertion. In diffuse pleural mesothelioma, patients generally present with the insidious onset of either dyspnea or chest pain. Taryle and colleagues (1976) noted that almost all patients with a malignant mesothelioma present with some symptoms whereas Chernow and the author (1977) and Weick and associates (1973) reported that up to 25% of patients with carcinoma or lymphoma of the pleura, respectively, may be relatively asymptomatic when the pleural effusion is discovered on a routine chest radiograph.

Because malignant involvement of the pleura signals advanced disease, these patients frequently have weight loss and appear chronically ill. Chernow and the author (1977) found that pleural effusion provided the initial diagnosis of cancer in almost 50% of these patients.

Patients with carcinoma of the pleura may have chest pain caused by involvement of the parietal pleura, ribs, or chest wall. Elmes and Simpson (1976) emphasized, however, that the chest pain associated with malignant mesothelioma is more common and impressive but is nonpleuritic and frequently referred to the upper abdomen or shoulder.

Physical examination may show cachexia and lymphadenopathy in cancer and lymphoma but may be unremarkable in malignant mesothelioma, except for the findings of a moderate to large pleural effusion.

RADIOGRAPHS OF THE CHEST

The pleural effusion associated with lung cancer is ipsilateral to the primary lesion. This may be because of direct pleural involvement, mediastinal lymph node infiltration, or an endobronchial lesion with pneumonia or atelectasis. With other primary sites, with the possible exception of breast cancer, there appears to be no ipsilateral predilection and bilateral effusions are common, and as Chernow and the author (1977) pointed out, are usually the result of mediastinal lymph node metastasis.

Patients with carcinomatous pleurisy usually present with a moderate to large effusion — 500 to 2000 ml; 10% have effusions <500 ml and a similar number have massive pleural effusion — complete opacification of the hemithorax. Malignancy is the most common cause of a massive pleural effusion; in a series by Maher and Berger (1972), 67% of 46 massive pleural effusions were caused by malignancy. The radiographic finding of bilateral effusions with a normal heart size suggests malignancy, most commonly carcinoma, which Rabin and Blackman (1957) noted. Benign effusions associated with this radiographic finding include lupus pleuritis, esophageal rupture, cirrhosis with ascites, nephrotic syndrome, and constrictive pericarditis.

When an apparently large pleural effusion is present — 1500 ml — with an absence of contralateral mediastinal shift, malignancy is almost always the cause and the patient has a poor prognosis. The following diagnoses should be considered in this context: (1) carcinoma of the ipsilateral main stem bronchus causing atelectasis; (2) a fixed mediastinum caused by malignant lymph nodes; (3) malignant mesothelioma — the density represents mostly tumor with a small effusion; and (4) extensive tumor infiltration of the ipsilateral lung radiographically mimicking a large effusion.

As Whitcomb and associates (1972) and MacDonald (1977) described, in Hodgkin's disease, patients with pleural effusions usually have associated lymphadenopathy and parenchymal infiltrates. In contrast, Jenkins and colleagues (1981) reported that in non-Hodgkin's lymphoma, intrathoracic lymphadenopathy occurs in few of the cases associated with either pulmonary disease or pleural effusions.

Heller and colleagues (1970) noted that in malignant mesothelioma the initial chest radiograph usually shows a moderate to large unilateral pleural effusion. Following therapeutic thoracentesis, the pleura may show thickening or nodularity. Evidence of asbestos exposure, such as interstitial lung disease or pleural plaques, may be identified in the contralateral lung and pleura. Radiographic clues suggesting that the large effusion may be caused by mesothelioma rather than carcinoma are pleural nodularity; absence of contralateral mediastinal shift with an apparent large effusion; and a tendency for loculation.

PLEURAL FLUID CHARACTERISTICS

Malignant pleural effusions may be serous, serosanguineous, or grossly bloody. A grossly bloody effusion suggests direct pleural involvement, whereas a serous effusion results from either lymphatic obstruction or an endobronchial lesion with atelectasis. Light and coworkers (1973b) suggested that when the red blood cell count in the pleural fluid is >100,000/µl in the absence of trauma, malignancy is the most likely diagnosis. Most of the nucleated cells — 2500 to 4000/µl — in pleural fluid, as Yam (1967) noted, are lymphocytes, macrophages, and mesothelial cells; more than 50% of the cellular population are lymphocytes in about one half of the cases. The percentage of PMNs is usually <25% of the cell population, but on rare occasions, when there is intense pleural inflammation, the PMN may predominate. Deresinski (1978) reported that pleural fluid eosinophilia is inexplicably rare — approximately 5% — in bloody, malignant pleural effusions.

Carcinomatous pleural effusions usually are exudates, with a protein concentration of about 4 g/dl; Chernow and the author (1977) and Light and associates (1972), however, reported protein concentrations from 1.5 to 8 g/dl. Approximately 5 to 10% of malignant pleural effusions are transudates. These transudative malignant effusions are caused by early stages of lymphatic obstruction, atelectasis from bronchial obstruction, or concomitant congestive heart failure. When an effusion meets exudative criteria by LDH but not protein, Light and associates (1972) emphasized that malignancy should be suspected. Good and colleagues (1980) stated that approximately one third of patients with malignant pleural effusions have a low pleural fluid pH — <7.30, range of 6.95 to 7.29 — and a low glucose concentration — <60 mg/dl or pleural-fluid-to-serum ratio of <0.5 — at presentation. These effusions usually have been present for several months and are associated with a large tumor burden and fibrosis of the pleural surface. Good and colleagues (1985) suggested that the abnormal pleural membrane reduces glucose entry into the pleural space and impairs glucose end product efflux, resulting in a local acidosis. Furthermore, the author and Good (1988) noted that low pH-low glucose malignant effusions are associated with short survival, ease of diagnosis by cytology and pleural biopsy, and a poor response to intrapleural sclerosing agents.

Pleural effusions caused by lymphoma have characteristics similar to those of carcinoma of the pleura. These effusions, however, tend to be less hemorrhagic and less likely to result in pleural fluid acidosis and low glucose concentrations. The author and Good (1988) pointed out that a pleural effusion in malignant mesothelioma is more likely to have a low pH and low glucose content and greater protein and LDH concentrations than effusions from carcinoma of the pleura. Because of an overlap of values in an individual patient, however, these data are not helpful in separating carcinoma from mesothelioma.

DIAGNOSIS

From the author's (1988) compilation of several large series totaling over 500 cases of malignancy, pleural fluid cytology had a diagnostic yield of 66% and percutaneous pleural biopsy 46%. When both procedures were performed, a positive diagnosis was obtained in 73%. Several observations can be made from these data: 1) pleural fluid cytology is more sensitive than pleural biopsy; 2) the tests are complementary, but pleural biopsy adds little to cytologic examination; 3) the lower yield from pleural biopsy results from sampling error and possibly operator technique; and 4) the wide range of incidence of positive results with both tests probably relates to imprecise handling of specimens, expertise of the cytopathologist, and the possibility that the pleural effusion was paramalignant at the time of the procedure. Repeat cytologic examination and pleural biopsy may be diagnostic, and Salyer (1975) and Boutin (1981) and their colleagues urged that a second procedure be done if suspicion for malignancy is high. Repeat thoracentesis for cytology a few days following the first procedure provides freshly shed cells and less degenerative mesothelial cells. Repeat pleural biopsy provides a greater sampling area. From the thoracoscopy data of Canto (1983), the yield of pleural biopsy probably could be increased by performing the procedure as close to the diaphragm and midline as possible because pleural metastases tend to originate near the diaphragm and spread cephalad toward the costal pleura.

Some patients with exudative pleural effusions remain without a diagnosis following repeat cytologic examination and pleural biopsy. Options at this time include observation, thoracoscopy, or open pleural biopsy. Recommending an invasive procedure is easier psychologically for the physician but creates morbidity for the patient. Thoracoscopy, as Boutin and associates (1985) reported, has a high yield — 80 to 97% — in malignant pleural disease when multiple biopsies are taken, frozen sections of each biopsy are examined, and the visceral pleura is also biopsied. Open pleural biopsy requires a thoracotomy with associated morbidity, a low incidence of mortality, and economic burden. Treatable causes of exudative effusions such as tuberculous pleurisy and pulmonary embolism must be excluded before invasive procedures are performed. Patients with a positive tuberculin skin test and a lymphocyte-predominant exudate should be treated with antituberculous drugs, because approximately 5 to 10% of patients with tuberculous pleurisy are not diagnosed bacteriologically following pleural fluid and tissue culture and pleural histologic examination. Furthermore, if tuber-

culous pleurisy is untreated, 65% of patients will develop active tuberculosis within 5 years. Bronchoscopy should be done before thoracoscopy or open pleural biopsy if there is absence of contralateral shift with a large effusion, evidence of ipsilateral volume loss, or a pulmonary lesion in addition to the pleural effusion. According to Feinsilver and associates (1986), the value of bronchoscopy in an undiagnosed pleural effusion without the aforementioned factors is limited.

An alternate approach is observation with repeat cytology and pleural biopsy at a later time if the effusion has not regressed. Malignant pleural effusions almost never resolve spontaneously; an increase in the size of the pleural effusion heightens the suspicion of malignancy. Furthermore, if the clinician "misses" a malignant pleural effusion for several weeks, in almost no situation has a disservice been done to the patient who has widespread, incurable disease. The diagnosis of a malignancy that characteristically is responsive to therapy, such as breast, prostate, thyroid, small cell, and germ cell cancer and lymphoma, however, must be considered carefully. Screening tests such as mammography, prostatic-specific antigen, and thyroid scan should be done as appropriate.

Measurements of carcinoembryonic antigen, hyaluronic acid, and LDH isoenzymes have no diagnostic value. Chromosomal analysis of pleural fluid is expensive and not available in all laboratories but may be helpful in the diagnosis of lymphoma, leukemia, and mesothelioma.

The antemortem diagnosis of malignant mesothelioma requires both clinical and histologic observations. Diagnosis from exfoliative cytology is difficult, and Whitaker (1978) questions its value. Even when malignancy is diagnosed, it may be impossible to differentiate metastatic adenocarcinoma from a malignant mesothelioma. Percutaneous needle biopsy does not consistently yield a definitive diagnosis and frequently prompts a misleading diagnosis of adenocarcinoma. High levels of hyaluronic acid are reported to establish the diagnosis of mesothelioma; however, Rasmussen and Faber (1967) observed that most patients with mesothelioma have intermediate levels, frequently seen in metastatic carcinoma and other inflammatory diseases. Thoracoscopy has been recommended, but the pathologist may be unable to reach a diagnosis; usually thoracotomy is required to obtain adequate tissue for examination. Mesotheliomas, as Edge and Choudhury (1978) noted, tend to invade surgical sites. Prophylactic irradiation should be given postoperatively. On occasion, even after adequate tissue has been examined from the thoracotomy, diagnosis remains uncertain. The subsequent course or biopsy from a tumor implant at the surgical site often provides the diagnosis.

Most pathologists can confidently diagnose a sarcomatous or mixed histologic variant but have difficulty in differentiating the epithelial form of mesothelioma from the more common metastatic adenocarcinoma. Special tissue stains, newer immunologic techniques, and electron microscopy aid in the antemortem diagnosis of patients with the epithelial variety of mesothelioma (see Chapter 61).

PROGNOSIS

Establishing the diagnosis of a malignant pleural effusion portends a poor prognosis. Patients with carcinoma of the lung, stomach, and ovary generally survive only a few months from the time of diagnosis of the malignant effusion, whereas patients with breast cancer may survive several months to years, depending on the response to chemotherapy. Patients with lymphomatous pleural effusions tend to have a survival intermediate between breast cancer and other carcinomas.

The author and Good (1988) observed that patients with low pH-low glucose malignant effusions survive only a few months, whereas those with a normal pH and glucose survive for about 1 year. Thus, the biochemical findings in the pleural fluid provide the clinician with information that is helpful in deciding on a rational plan of palliative treatment.

Even though a pleural effusion is an ominous sign in lung cancer, usually ruling out operability, Decker and colleagues (1978) reported that approximately 5% of these patients have a paramalignant effusion or effusion from another cause and may be operative candidates. The burden falls to the clinician to diagnose the cause of the pleural effusion before making a decision about possible curative surgery. Circumstances suggesting that the pleural effusion in lung cancer is paramalignant and that the patient may still be cured by resection are squamous cell type, radiographic volume loss, serous effusion, transudate, and parapneumonic effusion. If the cause of the effusion cannot be established clinically, thoracoscopy should be done to investigate the etiology.

TREATMENT

When the pleural effusion has been documented to be malignant or paramalignant and the patient is not a surgical candidate, the clinician must make a decision concerning palliative therapy. Factors that must be considered in this decision are the patient's general condition, symptoms, and expected survival. Management options range from observation in the asymptomatic patient to thoracotomy with pleurectomy and pleural abrasion. Some asymptomatic patients develop progressive pleural effusions, producing dyspnea that requires therapy, but others reach a new steady state of pleural fluid formation and absorption and do not progress to a symptomatic stage requiring therapy. In the debilitated patient with a short expected survival, based on the extent of disease, general status, and the biochemical characteristics of the fluid, it is more prudent to perform a therapeutic thoracentesis periodically on an outpatient basis than to recommend hospitalization and tube thoracostomy or thoracoscopy

with instillation of a sclerosing agent, with their associated morbidity and cost.

Pleurectomy and pleural abrasion are virtually completely effective in obliterating the pleural space and controlling recurrence of the effusion. Pleural abrasion should be carried out in most patients who undergo thoracotomy for an undiagnosed pleural effusion and are found to have malignancy, because this prevents the subsequent development of a symptomatic pleural effusion. Pleurectomy, however, even when indicated, as Martini and colleagues (1975) discussed, is a major surgical procedure associated with substantial morbidity and some mortality. Thus, this procedure should be reserved for patients with an expected survival of several months, who are in relatively good condition, who have a trapped lung, or who have failed a sclerosing-agent procedure.

Technique of Pleurectomy*

Beattie (1963) described pleurectomy well. The thorax is entered by a posterolateral incision, with entrance into the pleural space preferably by an intercostal incision in the fifth or sixth interspace. The extrapleural dissection is begun in the plane between the parietal pleura and the extrathoracic fascia at the margins of the intercostal incision before the rib spreader is inserted. The parietal pleura is then stripped circumferentially to the mediastinum; more tumor tends to be present at the diaphragmatic costopleural junction than at the apical pleura, and it is recommended that the upper half of the pleural dissection be completed first. Care must be taken in continuing the pleural dissection over the mediastinal surface to avoid injury to the phrenic, recurrent laryngeal, or sympathetic nerves or stellate ganglion. Damage to the vascular structures of the mediastinum likewise must be avoided. Dissection is continued down from the apex to the pulmonary hilus, which completes the initial phase of the procedure. The inferior portion of the parietal pleura is then dissected free. Care must be taken at the costophrenic sulcus not to remove the diaphragmatic attachment to the chest wall. It is unnecessary, as well as often impossible, to remove the diaphragmatic pleura, but the reflection of the pleura posteriorly on the lower mediastinal surface in association with the pulmonary ligament should be freed to the inferior border of the hilus. Dissection of the mediastinal pleura from pericardium is difficult and should not even be attempted in the region of the phrenic nerve. If the lung is free and ventilates well, no visceral pleural dissection is indicated. If, on the other hand, the lung is bound down with fibrin, a standard decortication is necessary. After hemostasis is obtained satisfactorily, pleural drainage and closure are completed in the standard manner.

The procedure is applicable only to a highly selected group of patients in good general condition whose

---

*Addendum by the Editor, T.W. Shields

malignant pleural effusion has failed to respond to other local therapy. Best results are obtained when the primary lesion is a carcinoma of the breast or, occasionally, a melanoma. Results vary but are more often poor in patients with carcinoma of the lung. Complications are frequent, as high as 23%, and mortality rates are significant, 10 to 18%. When decortication of the lung is necessary in conjunction with the pleurectomy, the mortality rate is significantly increased.

Chemotherapy or Irradiation

In general, systemic chemotherapy is disappointing for the control of malignant pleural effusions. Nonetheless, patients with lymphoma, according to Weick (1973) and Xaubet (1985) and their associates; breast cancer, from the reports of Fentiman (1981) and Jones (1975) and their colleagues; or small cell carcinoma of the lung, as Livingston and co-workers (1982) noted, may respond well to chemotherapy. Information about steroid receptors obtained from malignant pleural fluid in patients with breast cancer can provide a source for determining potential response to hormonal manipulation. In general, radiation therapy is of limited value in controlling carcinomatous malignant pleural effusions. Roy and associates (1967) suggested, however, that when there is predominantly mediastinal node involvement, irradiation may be valuable for patients with lymphoma or small cell carcinoma of the lung or when the effusion is a chylothorax.

Pleurodesis

For most patients, the most effective and least morbid method, short of pleurectomy or pleural abrasion, for controlling a symptomatic, malignant pleural effusion is chest tube drainage with instillation of a sclerosing agent. Tetracycline hydrochloride was most commonly used, but in 1991 Lederle Laboratories, the only manufacturer of intravenous and intramuscular tetracycline hydrochloride, ceased production of this drug as a result of the unavailability of the sterile tetracycline salt, which was now required by the FDA. Walker and associates (1993) reported that other tetracyclines, minocycline 300 mg and doxycycline 500 mg, have produced complete response rates of 86% — 6 of 7 — and 72% — 43 of 60 — respectively. Most patients treated with intrapleural doxycycline have required more than one instillation compared to only a single dose of minocycline. The most common adverse effects of the tetracycline drugs have been chest pain and fever. The chest pain can be ameliorated or abolished with narcotics and midazolam. The effectiveness of the tetracyclines depends primarily on their fibrogenicity rather than antineoplastic activity. Dryzer and colleagues (1993b) have shown in the rabbit model that both tetracycline and minocycline produce a marked inflammatory response and extensive pleural fibrosis and symphysis in a dose-dependent manner as the author and Good (1981) have previously pointed out.

If the clinician has documented that therapeutic thoracentesis results in relief of dyspnea and the rate of recurrence and the return of symptoms is rapid, instillation of minocycline or doxycycline should be considered. If the expected survival is several months, the patient is not debilitated, and the pleural fluid pH is >7.30, the patient is a good candidate for pleurodesis. Attempting pleurodesis is useless if the lungs cannot be expanded fully; this would occur in main stem bronchial obstruction with atelectasis or a trapped lung. The author and Good (1988) have reported that the documentation of a low pleural fluid pH — <7.30 — not only suggests a limited survival but a poor response to the pleurodesis agent. The large tumor bulk and fibrosis involving the pleural surfaces in the low-pH effusions diminishes the effectiveness in producing pleural symphysis, which is at least partially due to the inability of fibroblasts to migrate into the pleural space.

The technique for instillation of a sclerosing agent is critical for a successful result in the properly selected patient (Table 63–2). The pleural surfaces must be in close contact at the time inflammation is induced and remain in close contact over the ensuing 48 to 72 hours; this is best accomplished with chest tube drainage of the pleural space. If the effusion is large, the fluid should be drained slowly over the first several hours with intermittent clamping of the tube to decrease the risk of unilateral pulmonary edema. Pulmonary edema is most likely to occur when there is an endobronchial obstruction or trapped lung that does not allow the lung to expand to the chest wall with removal of fluid, resulting in a precipitous drop in intrapleural pressure. Furthermore, pleurodesis should not be attempted in the aforementioned situations because it is unlikely to be successful. Minocycline 300 mg or doxycycline 500 mg should be instilled into the pleural space when the pleural effusion is absent or minimal and the lung is expanded fully. Lorch and colleagues (1988), working in the author's laboratory, have radiolabeled tetracycline and demonstrated that following intrapleural instillation, the tetracycline is distributed completely throughout the pleural space within seconds and that the distribution is not enhanced by rotation of the patient. This study suggested that the patient need not be rotated through various positions following tetracycline instillation to ensure

Table 63–2. Procedure for Pleurodesis

1. Place chest tube in midaxillary line directed toward diaphragm.
2. Remove fluid in controlled manner under water seal.
3. Assess tube position on radiograph to position patient for optimal drainage.
4. Connect chest tube to suction (−20 cm H_2O).
5. Demonstrate minimal tube drainage at bedside and lung expansion and small or absent effusion on radiograph.
6. Give IV narcotic and midazolam.

With patient supine:
7. Instill Minocycline 300 mg in 50 ml of saline through chest tube and clamp for 1 hour.
8. Connect chest tube to suction (−20 cm H_2O).
9. Remove chest tube when drainage <100 ml/day.

adequate distribution of the pleurodesis agent. In a follow-up clinical study from our group, Dryzer and colleagues (1993a) showed no difference in success rate with both tetracycline and minocycline in those patients not rotated compared to those who were rotated through various positions following drug instillation. Thus, the author's recommendation is that patients receiving chemical pleurodesis need not be rotated through various positions following instillation, thus avoiding discomfort for the patient and additional personnel time. No studies have evaluated the optimum dwell time; a 1-hour dwell time for the pleurodesis agent should be adequate. The chest tube should be removed when pleural space drainage is <100 ml of fluid per day. With appropriate patient selection and the use of proper technique, the malignant effusion should be controlled in over 80% of patients. Success should not be defined as the production of total pleural symphysis but as diminishing the reaccumulation of pleural fluid so that dyspnea is relieved. Wooten and associates (1988) noted that both tetracycline and lidocaine, the latter used by some clinicians in an attempt to ameliorate chest pain, are absorbed systemically and reach therapeutic levels by 30 to 60 minutes; a history of allergic reactions to either drug is a contraindication to its use. The dose of lidocaine should not exceed 150 mg or 3 mg/kg, whichever is less. Strange and associates (1993), in the author's laboratory, recently have found similar rapid absorption of minocycline from the rabbit pleural space.

Walker and colleagues (1993) have reported that the insufflation of talc through the thoracoscope has resulted in a complete response in 91% of 131 patients with malignant pleural effusions. Talc is thought to cause pleural symphysis as a result of a reactive pleuritis. Only asbestos-free USP talc should be used for intrapleural administration. In most patients, talc has been administered under general anesthesia, but it can be given under local. The most common adverse effects have been fever and chest pain. Rinaldo and co-workers (1983), however, reported adult respiratory distress syndrome following the instillation of saline suspensions of large quantities of talc through a chest tube. Granulomatous pneumonitis has been noted by Factor (1975) following talc instillation. Reflux pulmonary edema and brain microembolization have also been reported. Other disadvantages of talc include the need for and the expense of thoracoscopy, the cost of operating room use, the expense and risk of general anesthesia, and the potential hazards from induced pneumothorax.

The average wholesale price of talc is less than one dollar. Minocycline 300 mg and doxycycline 500 mg cost about $80.00 each. In contrast, the usual one unit/kg dose of bleomycin costs $1100.00. Thus, cost consideration must be kept in mind in the management of the malignant effusion.

The management of malignant mesothelioma is discussed in Chapter 61. Judgment in the management of these patients is the keynote of appropriate care.

REFERENCES

Bartlett JG, Finegold SM: Anaerobic infections of the lung and pleural space. Am Rev Respir Dis *110*:56, 1974.

Beattie EJ, Jr: The treatment of malignant pleural effusions by partial pleurectomy. Surg Clin North Am *43*:99, 1963.

Black LF: The pleural space and pleural fluid. Mayo Clin Proc *47*:493, 1972.

Boutin C, Cargnino P, Viallat JR: Thoracoscopy in malignant effusion. Am Rev Respir Dis *124*:588, 1981.

Boutin C, et al: Thoracoscopy. *In* Chretien J, Bignon J, Hirsch A (eds): The Pleura in Health and Disease. New York: Marcel Dekker, 1985, p 587.

Brandstetter RD, Cohen RP: Hypoxemia after thoracentesis: a predictable and treatable condition. JAMA *242*:1060, 1979.

Broaddus C, Staub NC: Pleural liquid and protein turnover in health and disease. Semin Respir Med *9*:7, 1987.

Bynum LJ, Wilson JE, III: Characteristics of pleural effusions associated with pulmonary embolism. Arch Intern Med *136*:159, 1976.

Campbell GD, Webb WR: Eosinophilic pleural effusion. Am Rev Respir Dis *90*:194, 1964.

Canto A, et al: Points to consider when choosing a biopsy method in cases of pleurisy of unknown origin. Chest *84*:176, 1983.

Chernow B, Sahn SA: Carcinomatous involvement of the pleura: an analysis of 96 patients. Am J Med *63*:695, 1977.

Chretien J, Jaubert F: Pleural responses in malignant metastatic tumors. *In* Chretien J, Bignon J, Hirsch A (eds): The Pleura in Health and Disease. New York: Marcel Dekker, 1985, p 489.

Chusid EL, Siltzbach LE: Sarcoidosis of the pleura. Ann Intern Med *81*:190, 1974.

Clarkson B: Relationship between cell type, glucose concentration, and response to treatment in neoplastic effusions. Cancer *17*:914, 1964.

Collins TR, Sahn SA: Thoracentesis: complications, patient experience, and diagnostic value. Chest *91*:817, 1987.

Daniels AC, Childress ME: Pleuropulmonary amebiasis. Calif Med *85*:369, 1956.

Decker DA, et al: The significance of a cytologically negative pleural effusion in bronchogenic carcinoma. Chest *74*:640, 1978.

Deresinski SC: Eosinophils, pleural effusions, and malignancy. Ann Intern Med *89*:424, 1978.

Dryzer SR, et al: Rotational maneuvers do not improve success in chemical pleurodesis. Am Rev Respir Dis (in press) 1993a.

Dryzer SR, et al: A comparison of the inflammatory response between tetracycline and three doses of minocycline on the rabbit pleura. Am Rev Respir Dis (in press) 1993b.

Edge JR, Choudhury SL: Malignant mesothelioma of the pleura in Barrow-in-Furness. Thorax *33*:26, 1978.

Elmes PC, Simpson MJC: The clinical aspects of mesothelioma. Q J Med *45*:427, 1976.

Emont et al: Epidemiology of primary malignant mesothelial tumors in Canada. Cancer *26*:914, 1970.

Estenne M, Yernault J-C, Detryer A: Mechanism of relief of dyspnea after thoracocentesis in patients with larger pleural effusions. Am J Med *74*:813, 1983.

Factor SM: Granulomatous pneumonitis. A result of intrapleural instillation of quinacrine and talcum powder. Arch Pathol *99*:499, 1975.

Feinsilver SH, Barrows AA, Braman SB: Fiberoptic bronchoscopy and pleural effusion of unknown origin. Chest *90*:516, 1986.

Fentiman IS, et al: Pleural effusion in breast cancer: a review of 105 cases. Cancer *47*:2087, 1981.

Good JT Jr, et al: The diagnostic value of pleural fluid pH. Chest *78*:55, 1980.

Good JT Jr, Taryle DA, Sahn SA: The pathogenesis of low glucose, low pH malignant effusions. Am Rev Respir Dis *131*:737, 1985.

Heller RM, Janower ML, Weber AL: The radiological manifestations of malignant pleural mesothelioma. Am J Roentgenol *108*:53, 1970.

Jenkins PF, et al: Non-Hodgkin's lymphoma, chronic lymphatic leukemia, and the lung. Br J Dis Chest *75*:22, 1981.

Jones SE, Durie BGM, Salmon SE: Combination chemotherapy with adriamycin and cyclophosphamide for advanced breast cancer. Cancer 36:90, 1975.

Kaye MD: Pleuropulmonary complications of pancreatitis. Thorax 23:297, 1968.

Light RW, Ball WC, Jr: Glucose and amylase in pleural effusions. JAMA 225:257, 1973a.

Light RW, Erozan YS, Ball WC: Cells in pleural fluid: their value in differential diagnosis. Arch Intern Med 132:854, 1973b.

Light RW, et al: Parapneumonic effusions. Am J Med 69:507, 1980.

Light RW, et al: Pleural effusions: the diagnostic separation of transudates and exudates. Ann Intern Med 77:507, 1972.

Livingston RB, et al: Isolated pleural effusion in small cell lung carcinoma: favorable prognosis. Chest 81:208, 1982.

Lorch DG, Sahn SA: Pleural effusions due to diseases below the diaphragm. Semin Respir Med 9:227, 1987.

Lorch DG, et al: The effect of patient positioning on the distribution of tetracycline in the pleural space during pleurodesis. Chest 93:527, 1988.

McDonald JB: Lung involvement in Hodgkin's disease. Thorax 32:664, 1977.

McDonald JB, et al: Epidemiology of primary malignant mesothelial tumors in Canada. Cancer 26:914, 1970.

Magnussen H, et al: Transpleural diffusion of inert gases in excised lung lobes of the dog. Respir Physiol 20:1, 1974.

Maher GG, Berger HW: Massive pleural effusions: malignant and non-malignant causes in 46 patients. Am Rev Respir Dis 105:458, 1972.

Martini N, Bains MS, Beattie EJ, Jr: Indications for pleurectomy in malignant effusion. Cancer 35:734, 1975.

Maulitz RM, et al: The pleuropulmonary consequences of esophageal rupture: an experimental model. Am Rev Respir Dis 120:363, 1979.

Metzger JB, Garagusi VF, Kermin DM: Pulmonary oxalosis caused by *Aspergillus niger*. Am Rev Respir Dis 129:501, 1984.

Meyer PC: Metastatic carcinoma of the pleura. Thorax 21:437, 1966.

Miller KS, Tomlinson JR, Sahn SA: Pleuropulmonary complications of enternal tube feedings: two reports, review of the literature, and recommendations. Chest 88:230, 1985.

Potts DE, Levin DC, Sahn SA: Pleural fluid pH in parapneumonic effusions. Chest 70:328, 1976.

Potts DE, et al: The acidosis of low glucose effusions. Am Rev Respir Dis 117:665, 1978.

Rabin CB, Blackman NS: Bilateral pleural effusion. Its significance in association with a heart of normal size. J Mt Sinai Hosp 24:45, 1957.

Rasmussen KN, Faber V: Hyaluronic acid in 247 pleural fluids. Scand J Respir Dis 48:366, 1967.

Rinaldo JE, Owens GR, Rogers RM: Adult respiratory distress syndrome following intrapleural instillation of talc. J Thorac Cardiovasc Surg 85:523, 1983.

Reda MG, Baigelman W: Pleural effusion in systemic lupus erythematosus. Acta Cytol 24:553, 1980.

Roy PH, Carr DT, Payne WS: The problem of chylothorax. Mayo Clin Proc 42:457, 1967.

Sahn SA: Malignant pleural effusions. Clin Chest Med 6:113, 1985a.

Sahn SA: Pathogenesis and clinical features of diseases associated with a low pleural fluid glucose. *In* Chretien J, Bignon J, Hirsch A (eds): The Pleura in Health and Disease. New York, Marcel Dekker, 1985b, p 267.

Sahn SA: Pleural fluid pH in the normal state and in diseases affecting the pleural space. *In* Chretien J, Bignon J, Hirsch A (eds): The Pleura in Health and Disease. New York, Marcel Dekker, 1985c, p 253.

Sahn SA: Malignant pleural effusions. Semin Respir Med 9:43, 1987a.

Sahn SA: Pleural fluid analysis: narrowing the differential diagnosis. Semin Respir Med 9:22, 1987b.

Sahn SA: Malignant pleural effusions. *In* Fishman AP (ed): Pulmonary Diseases and Disorders, 2nd Ed. New York: McGraw-Hill, 1988.

Sahn SA, Good JT, Jr: The effect of common sclerosing agents on the rabbit pleural space. Am Rev Respir Dis 124:65, 1981.

Sahn SA, Good JT Jr: Pleural fluid pH in malignant effusion: diagnostic, prognostic and therapeutic implications. Ann Intern Med 108:345, 1988.

Salyer WR, Eggleston JC, Erozan YS: Efficacy of pleural needle biopsy and pleural fluid cytopathology in the diagnosis of malignant neoplasm involving the pleura. Chest 67:536, 1975.

Spriggs AI, Boddington MM: Absence of mesothelial cells from tuberculous pleural effusions. Thorax 15:169, 1968.

Stark DD, et al: Biochemical features of urinothorax. Arch Intern Med 142:1509, 1982.

Stelzner TJ, et al: The pleuropulmonary manifestations of the postcardiac injury syndrome. Chest 84:383, 1983.

Strange C, et al: Minocycline and tetracycline are rapidly absorbed through the rabbit pleural space. Am Rev Respir Dis (in press) 1993.

Taryle DA, Lakshminarayan S, Sahn SA: Pleural mesotheliomas. An analysis of 18 cases and review of the literature. Medicine (Baltimore) 55:153, 1976.

Wagner JC, Sleggs CA, Marchand P: Diffuse pleural mesothelioma and asbestos exposure in the North Western Cape Province. Br J Ind Med 17:260, 1960.

Walker PB, Vaughan LM, Sahn SA: Chemical pleurodesis for the treatment of malignant pleural effusions: Review of the world's literature. (Submitted) Ann Intern Med 1993.

Weick JK, et al: Pleural effusion in lymphoma. Cancer 31:848, 1973.

Whitaker D: The cytology of malignant mesothelioma in Western Australia. Acta Cytol 22:67, 1978.

Whitcomb ME, et al: Hodgkin's disease of the lung. Am Rev Respir Dis 106:79, 1972.

Wooten SA, et al: Systemic absorption of tetracycline and lidocaine following intrapleural instillation. Chest 94:960, 1988.

Xaubet A, et al: Characteristics and prognostic value of pleural effusions in non-Hodgkin's lymphomas. Eur J Respir Dis 66:135, 1985.

Yam LT: Diagnostic significance of lymphocytes in pleural effusions. Ann Intern Med 66:972, 1967.

Yamada S: Über die serose Flüssigkeit in der Pleurahöhle der gesunder Menschen. Z Gesamte Exp Med 90:342, 1933.

READING REFERENCES

Antman KH: Multimodality treatment for malignant mesothelioma based on a study of natural history. Am J Med 68:356, 1980.

Hillerdal G: Malignant mesothelioma 1982: review of 4710 published cases. Br J Dis Chest 77:321, 1983.

Schienger M, et al: Mesotheliomes pleuraux malins. Bull Cancer (Paris) 56:265, 1969.

Thoracic Trauma

CHAPTER 64

BLUNT AND PENETRATING INJURIES OF THE CHEST WALL, PLEURA, AND LUNGS

Felix Battistella and John R. Benfield

Thoracic trauma has challenged physicians since earliest recorded medical history. The Edwin Smith Papyrus, of approximately 3000 BC, described three cases involving chest injuries. Hippocrates and Galen proposed treatments for blunt and penetrating thoracic injuries that persisted for centuries. For example, Galen's recommendation of open packing of penetrating chest injuries with a poultice was followed until the thirteenth century, when Theodoric advised debriding and closing chest wounds. In the sixteenth century, Ambroise Paré advocated delayed closure of chest wounds when there had been significant bleeding. During the seventeenth century, numerous irrigating cannulas were developed and used for the treatment of empyema. Johannes Scultetus (1674) described these in *The Surgeon's Storehouse*. During this time, physicians employed professional "wound suckers" to drain intrathoracic collections. It was not until 1707 that Anel adapted a syringe to the instruments used in sucking wounds, thus eliminating the need for human wound suckers.

A major step forward in the nineteenth century occurred when closed drainage of the chest was developed. The use of cannulas eventually lead to the development of the chest tubes. Although the underwater-seal method was first described by Playfair in 1875, the use of closed chest drainage systems did not become popular until World War II.

Perhaps the most famous chest wound was reported by William Beaumont in 1825. His patient, after treatment of a close-range gunshot wound to the lower chest, developed a chronic gastric fistula that subsequently allowed Beaumont's classic observations regarding gastric physiology.

The discovery of x-rays by Roentgen in 1895 ushered in a new era in the diagnosis of thoracic pathology. The twentieth century brought the development of endotracheal intubation and the introduction of mechanical ventilators in the 1950s. Control of thoracic pain was achieved with the introduction of intercostal nerve blocks by Latteri, and recently, the use of epidural analgesia has become widespread.

Overall mortality from chest wounds has decreased from 62% during the Civil War to 4 to 7% in recent civilian experience. Among other developments, this improved survival was associated with the description of "wet lungs" by Burford and Burbank in 1945. The term "traumatic respiratory insufficiency" was subsequently used to describe the entity that is currently referred to as "adult respiratory distress syndrome — ARDS." To this day, ARDS and multisystem organ failure are the major barriers in the quest for improved survival of multiple-trauma victims.

EPIDEMIOLOGY

Although trauma is known to be the leading cause of death in the first four decades of life, statistics regarding the true incidence of chest trauma are scant. It has been estimated by LoCicero and Mattox (1989) that 20 to 25% of trauma deaths, and approximately 16,000 deaths per year, are attributable to thoracic injuries. In recent years, according to Shorr and associates (1987), blunt trauma from motor vehicle accidents has accounted for 70 to 80% of thoracic injuries. Besson and Saegesser (1983) have noted that up to one third of patients hospitalized following automobile accidents have evidence of significant chest trauma.

When considering blunt thoracic trauma, the victims' age is a critical variable. Children's elastic and flexible chest walls simultaneously protect them from rib and sternal fractures and enhance their exposure to force on the thoracic viscera. Thus, Nakayama and colleagues (1989) stress that children are at high risk for significant intrathoracic injuries. Elderly patients have brittle chest walls that are subject to significant injury secondary to low-energy trauma while affording poor protection for the underlying viscera. Hence, as noted by Shackford (1986), old people suffer a significant mortality rate, even from minor chest wall injuries.

Penetrating thoracic injuries are rare in children and in old people but are increasingly common in young adults. Most civilian gunshot wounds are from low-velocity handguns. These do not transfer significant energy to the surrounding tissues. In military situations, and occasionally in civilian settings, high-velocity gunshot wounds and close-range shotgun wounds dissipate large amounts of lateral shock wave energy that result in considerable amounts of devitalized tissues that require debridement.

Although most chest trauma can be managed without thoracotomy, Shackford (1986), as well as Kish and co-workers (1976) emphasize that thoracic injuries require prompt evaluation and treatment to avoid preventable mortality. This chapter will address only injuries of the chest wall, pleura, tracheobronchial tree, and lungs. Diaphragmatic and esophageal injuries are discussed in Chapters 68 and 117, respectively.

EVALUATION AND MANAGEMENT

General Considerations

The priority for evaluation and management of any trauma victim is to assess the airway and to establish adequate ventilation. Arterial blood gas determinations are useful when circumstances allow; however, decisions as to airway management should be based on rather simple clinical observations. A respiratory rate greater than 30/min or labored respirations should trigger evaluation for easily correctable causes of respiratory distress. Immediate intubation and mechanical ventilation are required for patients with a respiratory rate greater than 35/min or for patients with labored respirations, profound shock, or severe head injuries. Circulation should be assessed and supported with the necessary resuscitative measures almost simultaneous to airway management. In hemodynamically unstable patients, evaluation of the thorax for reversible causes of shock is critical (Table 64–1).

The circumstances surrounding the accident should be ascertained, because they may assist in giving clues toward arriving at a correct diagnosis. For example, patients requiring extrication from behind steering wheels, or crushed by automobiles, are likely to have life-threatening intrathoracic injuries. Rapid deceleration accidents increase the index of suspicion for shearing injuries of the thoracic aorta or main stem bronchi. In hemodynamically unstable patients, evaluation of the chest begins with examination of the neck veins. Distention of these veins differentiates compressive shock that is due to tension pneumothorax or cardiac tamponade from hypovolemic shock, which is usually associated with collapsed veins. Inspection of the chest wall during spontaneous respirations may reveal paradoxic motion associated with a flail chest. Palpation may reveal less conspicuous instability of the chest wall, or it may demonstrate crepitus that is due to subcutaneous emphysema associated with pneumothorax. Point tenderness can be elicited over rib, sternal, or clavicular fractures.

Isolated thoracic injury following blunt thoracic trauma is uncommon (Table 64–2). Associated extrathoracic injuries have been reported by Shorr and colleagues (1987), Besson and Saegesser (1983), and Glinz (1991), among others, in more than 75% of thoracic trauma patients. Glinz (1991) recorded that among 200 patients, with systolic blood pressures less than 100, over half had significant intra-abdominal injuries fully or in part responsible for the hemodynamic instability.

The location of penetrating wounds should be noted, but they should not be probed. If the wound is located below the fifth rib, evaluation of the abdomen is necessary because the possibility of diaphragmatic penetration and intra-abdominal injury must be excluded. Visualization of the diaphragm to exclude injury can be accomplished by a variety of means including video-assisted thoracotomy — thoracoscopy, laparoscopy, laparotomy, or thoracotomy. In patients with multiple injuries that involve the chest and abdomen who have been hemodynamically unstable, we recommend laparotomy as the first avenue of intervention. This approach allows control of abdominal bleeding, which is often easily corrected, before proceeding with further evaluation and perhaps operative intervention for complex intrathoracic injuries.

All critically injured patients, except those who require resuscitative thoracotomy in the emergency department, or patients with clinical evidence of a tension pneumothorax, should have an immediate radiograph of the chest. In addition to looking for the common post-traumatic abnormalities, particular attention is paid to possible findings that may be easily

Table 64–1.   Etiology of Shock After Thoracic Trauma

Tension pneumothorax
Hemothorax
Cardiac tamponade
Myocardial dysfunction that is due to contusion
Air emboli
Injury to the great vessels
Large pulmonary contusion
Ruptured diaphragm

Table 64–2.   Injuries Associated With Blunt Thoracic Trauma (Compilation of Several Series)*

Type of Injury	Percentage
Cranial injury	44
Abdominal injury	21
Extremity fractures	54
Pelvic fractures	12
Spinal fractures	6

*Galan, et al. (1992), Kulshrestha, et al. (1988), and Glinz (1986).

Table 64–3. Frequently Overlooked Chest Radiograph Findings in the Polytrauma Victim

Soft tissue injuries
Skeletal injuries
Ruptured diaphragm
Widened mediastinum
Foreign bodies
Mediastinal air

overlooked (Table 64–3). Up to 35% of patients with ruptured diaphragms may initially have normal or minimally abnormal chest radiographs. Penetrating wounds should be identified with radiopaque markers before radiographs are obtained. The initial location of bullets is noteworthy because they may embolize (Fig. 64–1).

Stab wounds and low-velocity gunshot wounds lead to minimal chest wall trauma unless associated with injury to an intercostal or internal mammary artery. These injuries are typically managed expectantly unless there is continued bleeding. Persistent hemorrhage from the aforementioned arteries is an indication for thoracotomy with ligation of the offending vessel. High-velocity gunshot wounds or close-range shotgun wounds, on the other hand, lead to devastating chest wall injuries as well as significant injuries to the underlying structures. Management of such injuries almost always requires operation, as will be discussed in greater detail.

Trauma to the lower chest wall raises concern about possible intra-abdominal injuries. Penetrating injuries below the fifth rib may be associated with diaphragmatic hernias as well as injuries to intra-abdominal organs. In hemodynamically stable patients, thoracoscopy can be used to assess the integrity of the diaphragm; if it has been violated, laparotomy should be performed to inspect the abdominal contents. Hemodynamically unstable patients with penetrating lower chest wall injury should undergo urgent laparotomy. Blunt trauma to the lower thorax is also associated with a significant number of injuries to the underlying abdominal organs.

Chest wall injuries are most commonly the result of a motor vehicle accident and are often associated with injuries to the underlying structures, as pointed out by Campbell (1992), as well as injuries to other areas of the body (Table 64–2). In the series reported by Glinz (1991), more than three fourths of patients hospitalized with thoracic trauma had other associated injuries. These associated injuries take precedence over chest wall injuries. On completion of the initial evaluation and treatment of life-threatening injuries, attention should be directed to pain control and pulmonary physiotherapy. Inadequate pain management and poor pulmonary hygiene lead to the various complications associated with chest wall injuries resulting from ventilatory compromise.

Mediastinal and Subcutaneous Emphysema

Injuries to the tracheobronchial tree, esophagus, and lungs can all lead to mediastinal emphysema. Although rupture of the lung substance following a penetrating injury typically leads to a pneumothorax, blunt rupture

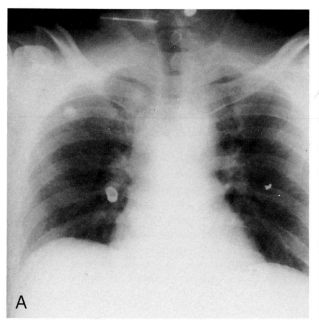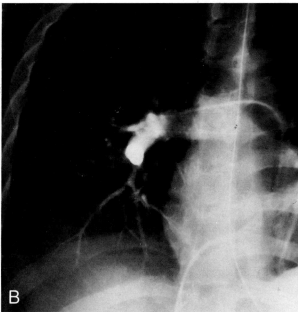

Fig. 64–1. Foreign body embolization. *A*, This chest radiograph depicts two foreign bodies lodged in the pulmonary arteries following a gunshot wound to the abdomen, where the iliac vein was injured. *B*, Pulmonary angiogram confirms the foreign body's location within the pulmonary artery.

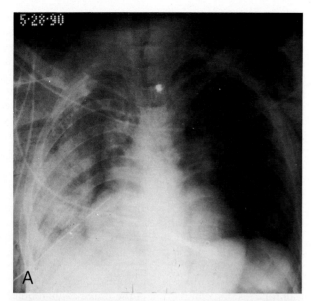

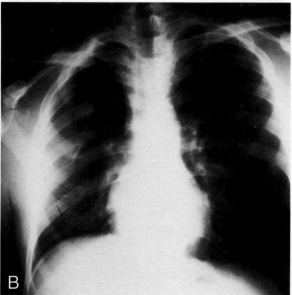

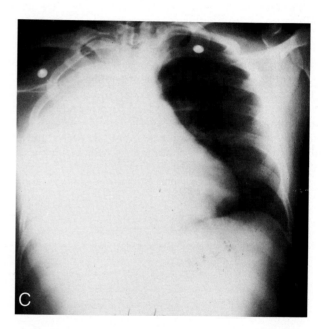

Fig. 64–2. Delayed recognition of bronchial rupture. Chest radiographs. *A,* Significant amount of subcutaneous emphysema and mediastinal air following a crushing injury of the chest. *B,* Partial aeration following the chest tube removal approximately 2 weeks later; the patient was discharged from the hospital doing well. *C,* Total collapse of the right lung 3 days later, when a stenotic obstruction of the right main stem bronchus from a torn bronchus was recognized.

can involve part of the lung facing the hilar vessels or the bronchi. Air will then dissect back along the bronchi and vessels to the mediastinum. If the leak is large, air will migrate into the subcutaneous space of the neck, from where it can extend to the face and torso down to the inguinal ligament, and occasionally to the external genitalia. Tracheobronchial injury should be suspected when there is a large amount of mediastinal air, especially if it seems to increase with mechanical ventilation (Fig. 64–2). Both the tracheobronchial tree and the esophagus should be assessed in the victim of penetrating injury to the mediastinum. Treatment and management should address the etiology of the mediastinal or subcutaneous emphysema. Decompression incisions in the skin are rarely, if ever, indicated.

INJURIES OF THE CHEST WALL, PLEURA, AND LUNGS

Rib Fractures

Rib fractures have been reported by Kemmerer (1961) and Conn (1963) and their associates in 35 to 40% of thoracic trauma victims, thus making them the most common significant thoracic injury. The diagnosis is based primarily on clinical findings. Posttraumatic pleuritic chest pain is usually diagnostic of rib fractures; these can be localized by palpation. We consider the added expense of films made for the purpose of showing rib detail unnecessary. It is nonetheless important to quantitate the severity of rib fracture(s) for prognosis and to assist in making a judgment as to possible types of associated injuries. Chest radiographs are used largely to identify associated intrathoracic injuries.

Fractures of the first and second ribs indicate the possible existence of additional significant intrathoracic injury. Although routine aortography was advocated for patients with upper rib fractures, we agree with Poole (1989) that it is not needed unless there are other signs of injury to the thoracic aorta or great vessels. However, as noted by Richardson and colleagues (1975) fractures of the upper ribs and scapula are hallmarks of severe trauma that have been associated with a mortality rate up to 36%. According to the aforementioned authors concomitant injuries to the head — 53%, abdomen — 33%, and thorax — 64% — are found in a significant number of these patients.

Management of upper rib fractures is directed at identifying associated injuries and at controlling the associated pain that leads to splinting of the chest wall and hypoventilation. Decreased excursions of the chest wall and poor pulmonary hygiene may lead to atelectasis, pneumonia, and respiratory failure. Our experience, as that of Wisner (1990), has shown that the prompt use of epidural analgesia results in a lower morbidity and mortality than parenteral narcotics, particularly in elderly patients. Early mobilization, deep inspiratory efforts, and frequent coughing should be encouraged. Pulmonary physiotherapy, nasotracheal suctioning, and prompt bronchoscopy should be instituted in patients unable to clear secretions. Although young patients with single rib fractures might be managed with oral narcotics, more significant injuries may require parenteral narcotics. In general, young patients with multiple rib fractures, or the older patient with fewer than three fractured ribs, will obtain adequate relief of discomfort with patient-controlled intravenous analgesia using the narcotic of choice. Old patients with three or more rib fractures, or patients with pre-existing compromised pulmonary status are best managed with epidural analgesia. In the experience of Mackersie and co-workers (1987), Worthley (1985), and Wisner (1990), continuous administration of epidural analgesia is universally useful in patients with severe chest wall injuries such as multiple bilateral rib fractures, flail chests, or a combined thoracoabdominal injury.

Alternative methods for controlling pain following thoracic trauma include intercostal nerve blocks, intrapleural catheter analgesia, or transcutaneous electric nerve stimulation. Each of these modalities has disadvantages. Intercostal nerve blocks require repeated administration, and each injection exposes patients to the risk of pneumothorax. Intrapleural regional analgesia with a catheter in the pleural cavity achieves adequate pain control without sedation or respiratory depression. However, catheter placement carries the risk of pneumothorax. Transcutaneous electric nerve stimulation is of no benefit immediately after trauma, and so this method should be limited to controlling pain in the chronic setting.

Wilson (1977) and Garcia (1990) and their colleagues have documented that the outcome of treatment, and therefore the prognosis for rib fractures is related to the number of ribs injured, the patient's age, and the underlying pulmonary status. Conn and associates (1963) and Worthley (1985) have noted that the mortality rate from isolated rib fractures in the elderly has been as high as 10 to 20%. Rib fractures in children, as recorded by Nakayama and co-workers (1989), have been associated with a mortality rate of 5%. Thus, the full significance of rib fractures has too often been inadequately recognized. Morbidity and mortality from rib fractures can be minimized if associated injuries are identified and treated promptly and adequate pain control is achieved. These principles are especially important in the care of elderly patients.

Flail Chest

Instability of the chest wall from unilateral or bilateral multiple rib fractures, or from disruptions of the costochondral junctions, results in an estimated 5% of patients with thoracic trauma according to the data of LoCicero and Mattox (1989). The force needed to create a flail chest depends on the compliance of the ribs; old people may suffer an unstable chest wall after low-energy impacts, whereas, as noted by Nakayama and associates (1989), flail chest occurs in less than 1% of children following severe thoracic trauma.

Paradoxic chest wall motion leads to a reduction in vital capacity and to ineffective ventilation that, along with associated pulmonary contusion, can lead to ARDS. Early documentation of respiratory compromise with frequent monitoring of respiratory rate, oxygen saturation, and arterial blood gasses is crucial. *The "clinical appearance" of patients with flail chest may be misleading.* Objective information obtained from arterial blood gas determinations should be the supervening guide to therapy. Unless there is evidence of rapid improvement after brief observation with aggressive pain management, we recommend endotracheal intubation and ventilator assistance for patients whose respiratory rate is greater than 30, whose Pa_{O_2} is less than 60 torr, or whose Pa_{CO_2} is more than 45 torr.

Treatment of the unstable chest wall remains somewhat controversial. Previous attempts at external stabilization of the involved segment including the use of sand bags and towel clips are now considered anachronistic. Internal stabilization using positive pressure ventilation was introduced by Avery and associates in 1956, and this method became the routine until the current recommendations. We now use the same therapeutic guidelines for flail chest as for simple rib fractures, that is, aggressive pain control and selective endotracheal intubation with mechanical ventilation. The reports of other surgeons, including those of Trinkle (1975), Shackford (1976), Freedland (1990), and Clark (1988) and their associates, and our experience, have taught us that *prophylaxis and early intervention must be the guiding principles.* Endotracheal intubation and mechanical ventilation are instituted early, based primarily on physiologic evidence of ventilatory insufficiency, respiratory fatigue, or deterioration. Mechanical ventilation is instituted for treatment of respiratory insufficiency rather than for its ability to splint chest wall instability, and it is maintained until pain control permits vigorous pulmonary hygiene and early mobilization of the patient. Patients are given aggressive pulmonary physiotherapy with incentive spirometry, deep coughing, suctioning, humidification of air, and chest percussion with postural drainage. Bronchoscopy is used liberally to remove retained secretions promptly and to expand areas of collapse.

Operative fixation of flail segments has not gained widespread acceptance, although several techniques have been developed by Haasler (1990) as well as by Paris (1991) and Landreneau (1991) and their colleagues. We use operative fixation of flail chest wall segments when thoracotomy is being done for other indications. In addition, we employ internal fixation for patients with isolated extensive flail segment associated with poorly controlled pain.

Survival after flail chest injuries has improved with selective ventilatory support and improvements in pain management. The mortality rate of about 30 to 40% reported by Shackford (1976) and Thomas (1978) and their associates in the mid-1970s fell to 11 to 16% in the late 1980s, as recorded by Freedland (1990) and Clark (1988) and their colleagues. Associated injuries, such as underlying pulmonary contusion, as pointed out by Clark and associates (1988), continue to contribute significantly to the persistently high mortality rate, perhaps causing it to be twice as high in patients with associated injuries as compared to individuals with isolated chest wall trauma. Other commonly associated injuries, such as central nervous system injuries and intra-abdominal trauma, contribute to mortality and increase the likelihood that mechanical ventilation will be needed.

Landercasper and co-workers (1984) noted that flail chest injuries may have long-term consequences. Impaired pulmonary function has been documented in long-term survivors. Subjective abnormalities included 63% of patients reporting dyspnea and 49% reporting persistent pain. Objective evidence of chronic disability included 57% of patients having abnormal spirometry and 70% of individuals with abnormal treadmill testing. The etiology of these abnormalities is unclear, and it is unknown whether internal stabilization of the chest wall would reduce their incidence.

Traumatic Asphyxia

Traumatic asphyxia results from a severe crush injury of the thorax. It manifests itself with facial and upper chest petechiae, subconjunctival hemorrhages, cervical cyanosis, and occasionally with neurologic symptoms. Temporary impairment or loss of vision, presumed to be due to retinal edema, may be present rarely. Factors implicated in the development of these striking physical characteristics include thoracoabdominal compression,

following deep inspiration, against a closed glottis. This results in venous hypertension in the valveless cervicofacial venous system. Williams (1968) and M.C. Lee (1991) and their associates recommend that treatment be primarily supportive; however, associated injuries should be excluded.

Sternal Fractures

Sternal fractures, according to Otremski and colleagues (1990) occur in approximately 4% of patients involved in motor vehicle accidents. Older patients and front-seat vehicle occupants involved in frontal collisions are at greatest risk. The fracture is typically transverse and is located in the upper and middle portions of the body of the sternum. Diagnosis can be made on physical examination with the identification of localized tenderness, swelling, and deformity. Radiographic confirmation of these fractures requires a lateral view because they are rarely apparent on the anteroposterior chest film (Fig. 64–3).

These fractures, like other chest wall injuries, as noted by Buckman and co-workers (1987), are frequently associated with other significant intra- and extra-thoracic injuries. Injury to the underlying myocardium has been variably reported depending on the diagnostic test used to identify its presence. Although the clinical significance of abnormal test results in hemodynamically stable patients has been challenged by the studies of Wisner and associates (1990), myocardial injury should be considered in the hemodynamically unstable patient with evidence of anterior chest wall injury.

Treatment of sternal fractures is similar to that for rib fractures, and it consists primarily of pain control and pulmonary hygiene. If the fracture is severely displaced, open reduction through a midline incision with internal fixation using cross wires is indicated. In the rare patient with a flail sternum that is due to disruption of the costochondral junctions, internal fixation or external fixation, as recommended by Shackford (1976) and Henley (1991) and their colleagues respectively, have been advocated to minimize the need for positive pressure ventilation.

Scapular and Clavicular Fractures

Fractures of the scapula are uncommon, and they are due to a significant force of impact. This results in an 80 to 90% incidence of associated injures according to MaGahan (1980) and Thompson (1985) and their associates; Armstrong and Van der Spuy (1983) report a 10% mortality rate. Because of the high incidence of concurrent brachial plexus injuries, a careful neurovascular exam should be documented. Treatment consists of shoulder immobilization with subsequent early range of motion exercises. Guttentag and Rechtine (1988) have pointed out that surgical repair may be indicated when glenohumeral joint function is impaired.

Clavicular fractures, on the other hand, are common and often isolated. Isolated fractures rarely, if ever, compromise ventilation, and treatment by stabilization with a figure-of-eight dressing splint plus analgesia is

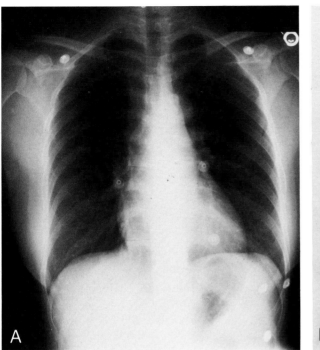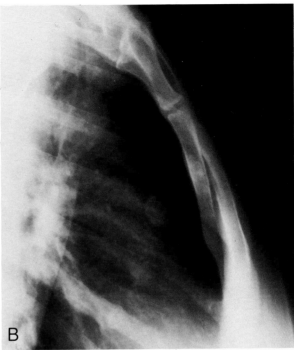

Fig. 64–3. Sternal fracture. *A*, PA chest radiograph fails to reveal the fracture sustained by this patient following a head-on motor vehicle accident. *B*, lateral projection shows the fracture with the two overriding fragments.

effective and usually without complications. Only rarely is operative repair necessary for severely displaced fractures. Damage to the underlying subclavian vessels or the brachial plexus is rare; but this possibility needs to be considered.

Penetrating Chest Wall Wounds

Wounds from stabbings or low-velocity gunshot wounds are quite different from the large chest wall defects associated with penetration from high-velocity missiles or shotgun wounds. Sucking chest wounds present life-threatening emergencies, and they are often associated with devastating intra-thoracic injuries. The equilibration of intra-thoracic pressure with atmospheric pressure associated with an open pneumothorax leads to decreased alveolar ventilation. A patient's inability to ventilate can be corrected in part temporarily by covering the defect. In the field, this can be accomplished by covering the wound using a plastic sheet that is taped on three sides, leaving one side free to act as a one-way valve. In the emergency department, the wound can be covered with an impermeable dressing, and a chest tube can be placed to re-expand the lung. Management of large open wounds requires operative debridement with removal of devitalized tissue, foreign bodies — such as shotgun wadding materials, and bone fragments, followed by chest wall closure. Often, this can be accomplished by mobilizing the surrounding tissues; however, large soft tissue defects will require rotational or free myocutaneous flaps. The pectoralis muscle, latissimus dorsi, or rectus abdominis flaps can

be used in this setting (Fig. 64–4). The use of synthetic materials such as Marlex, Gortex, or methyl-methacrylate may be appropriate for elective chest wall reconstruction, but we do not recommend their use after acute trauma because of the risk of infection from the contamination associated with the injury.

Most low-velocity handgun and stab wounds can be managed nonoperatively, usually requiring only tube thoracostomy. Although the appearance of gunshot wounds should be described in detail, it is best to avoid describing wounds as "entrance" or "exit" wounds because appearance can be deceiving. We prefer to leave this determination to the discretion of the forensic pathologist, because often it is of great medical-legal importance.

High-velocity missiles from military weapons or rifles are associated with surprisingly large lateral shock waves that cause extensive tissue injury and temporary cavities that often are not externally apparent. Therefore, these injuries require enhanced suspicion of significant internal viscus injury, debridement of surface wounds, and liberal use of exploratory thoracotomies when the indications for operation are marginal. We have experienced instances of delays in proceeding with thoracotomy after high-velocity bullet wounds with subsequent adverse consequences. However, we cannot recall a single instance of regret for having proceeded with early operation in this setting.

Asymptomatic penetrating chest wall wounds, of the type usually seen in civilian practice, without evidence of intrathoracic injury can be observed in the emergency

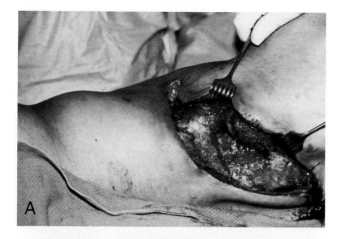

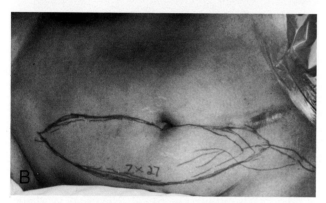

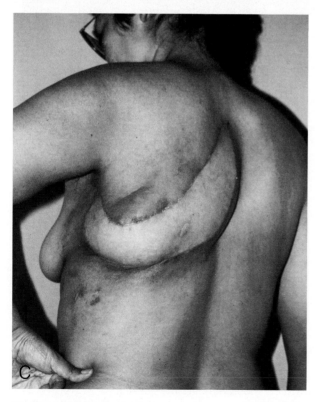

Fig. 64–4. Myocutaneous flap. *A,* Post-traumatic chest wall defect. *B,* rectus abdominis myocutaneous flap. *C,* postoperative result.

department with a repeat chest radiograph obtained 6 hours after the initial chest film. If re-evaluation shows no evidence of deterioration, patients may not need to be admitted to the hospital, and appropriate follow-up can be accomplished with outpatient visits, as documented by the data of Ordog (1983), Karanfilian (1981), Weigelt (1982), and Ammons (1986) and their colleagues. Delayed evidence of hemothorax or pneumothorax under such circumstances can be expected in about 7 to 9% of patients.

Pneumothorax

Simple Pneumothorax

Posttraumatic pneumothoraces may not always come to attention in critically injured victims in the noisy resuscitation room. The chest radiograph should be inspected carefully for the presence of lung markings extending to the periphery. We recommend chest tube drainage of posttraumatic pneumothoraces, even for small collections of air, especially in patients who will require positive pressure ventilation. When a large air leak is present or re-expansion of the lung is difficult, a tracheobronchial injury should be suspected and bronchoscopy should be performed.

Tension Pneumothorax

Physical examination in patients with a tension pneumothorax will usually reveal severe respiratory distress, distended neck veins, a deviated trachea, and absent breath sounds on the affected side. In such cases placement of a thoracostomy tube before obtaining a chest radiograph will help to restore the patient's blood pressure because decompression with a chest tube is an immediately effective treatment. Tension pneumothorax should be suspected in any patient with chest wall trauma receiving general anesthesia when there is a sudden cardiopulmonary deterioration that is associated with a marked increase in ventilatory pressures. Some surgeons routinely insert thoracotomy tubes in patients with rib fractures, even though there is no evidence of underlying pulmonary injury or the presence of a pneumothorax to prevent the possible occurrence of a tension pneumothorax, if the injured patient is to undergo a general anesthetic.

Hemothorax

Massive intrathoracic hemorrhage that is recognized during emergency department resuscitative thoracotomy requires rapid assessment of the bleeding source. Temporary placement of a large vascular clamp on the hilum of the lung may prove lifesaving while the patient is transported to the operating room.

More commonly, recognition of a hemothorax relies on the chest radiographic findings. Because initial radiographs are obtained with the patient in the supine position, it may be difficult to detect a small hemothorax. In patients with moderate-sized collections, the chest film may reveal a slight opacification of the affected hemithorax. Treatment is directed at correcting the hypovolemia and at evacuating the blood from the pleural cavity. Initial drainage of the pleural space should be established with a chest tube. If the chest cavity is adequately drained with a No.-36 French chest tube, and bleeding has stopped, this should be ample treatment. However, thoracotomy is indicated if the initial chest tube output is greater than 1500 ml or if the hourly output continues without abatement at greater than 200 ml/hour for 2 to 4 hours. If progressive opacification of the chest radiograph develops, this indicates an inadequately drained hemothorax, and thoracotomy should be undertaken to prevent the formation of a fibrous peel and to reduce the risk of empyema. It is best to lean in the direction of proceeding with operation in doubtful cases.

Sources for intrathoracic bleeding include intercostal vessels, pulmonary parenchymal injuries, major pulmonary vessels, and injury to the heart or great vessels. Most pulmonary parenchymal injuries can be managed simply by evacuating the hemothorax and allowing the lung to re-expand. The pulmonary distention, associated with re-expansion of the lung, tamponades parenchymal bleeding following most injuries. If a thoracotomy is needed because of injury to the intercostal vessels or the internal mammary artery, management requires adequate exposure. Often, the exposure can be enhanced by cutting a rib or two posteriorly. In patients who are exsanguinating, this can be done using a large rib shear without skeletonizing the ribs. In patients with large chest wall injuries whose bleeding is diffuse and difficult to localize, ligation of the intercostal vessels near their origins may be a lifesaving maneuver. If bleeding from intercostal vessels occurs at the level of the intervertebral foramen, control may require laminectomy; packing of the foramen should be avoided because it may place patients at risk for spinal cord injury and subsequent paraplegia.

If inflation of the lung fails to control pulmonary parenchyma bleeding, the patient may require pulmonary resection. In the patient with large pulmonary lacerations, contusion, and significant bleeding, hemorrhage can be controlled with standard anatomic lobar or segmental resection. Thompson (1988) and Bowling (1985) and their associates report that pneumonectomy in the trauma victim carries a mortality rate approaching 100% and should be considered a last resort. Gunshot wounds in the periphery of the lung may be amenable to wedge resections. Central penetrating injuries with massive pulmonary hemorrhage may require intrapericardial control of the pulmonary artery and the pulmonary veins. Occasionally, in moribund patients, rapid control of pulmonary bleeding can be achieved by using stapling devices.

If a major air leak is present, the source should be identified. Small air leaks from the lung periphery will usually resolve without need for repair. Lacerations of the trachea or major bronchi, as will be discussed, require repair with 4-0 or 3-0 absorbable sutures. It is

usually best to begin by gaining control of the pulmonary vasculature so that the airway can be exposed with relative leisure, and under the best possible conditions.

Air Embolism

Thomas and Roe (1973) and Yee (1983) reported that air embolism often follows penetrating and blunt chest injury. In the experience of Swanson and Trunkey (1989), it occurred in 4% of all major thoracic trauma cases. Sixty-five percent of cases resulted from penetrating injuries to the chest, and 35% of cases from blunt chest trauma, almost invariably because of lacerations of the lung secondary to rib fractures.

The key to diagnosis is to have a high index of suspicion. The pathophysiology is a fistula between a bronchus and a pulmonary vein. In those patients who are breathing spontaneously, the pressure differential is from the pulmonary vein to the bronchus so that air is not aspirated into the vascular system; hemoptysis may occur in approximately one fourth of such patients. When the patient is intubated with positive pressure, however, the pressure differential is from the bronchus to the pulmonary vein, resulting in air being carried to the left side of the heart and being ejected into the aorta, causing systemic air embolism. These patients present in one of three ways: 1) focal or lateralizing neurologic signs; 2) sudden cardiovascular collapse, and 3) froth when the initial arterial blood specimen is obtained. Any patient who has a chest injury but does not have a head injury, and yet has focal or lateralizing neurologic findings, should be assumed to have air embolism. Confirmation may be obtained by fundoscopic examination showing air in the retinal vessels. When a patient comes into the emergency room in extremis and an emergency thoracotomy is carried out, air should always be looked for in the coronary vessels. If this is found, the hilum of the offending lung should be immediately clamped to stop the ingress of air into the left side of the heart.

The treatment of air embolism is immediate thoracotomy, preferably in the operating room, although many of these patients have emergency-room thoracotomies. The hilum of the affected lacerated lung is cross clamped, and the left ventricle is vented to remove any residual contained air. Other resuscitative measures in patients who have had cardiac arrest from air embolism include internal cardiac massage to re-establish perfusion and to clear the coronary vessels of any contained air. One milliliter of 1:1000 epinephrine can be injected intravenously or down the endotracheal tube to provide an alpha-adrenergic effect, driving air out of the systemic microcirculation. Definitive treatment is to oversew the lacerations of the lung, and in some instances a lobectomy and rarely a pneumonectomy may be required. Using aggressive diagnosis and treatment, Swanson and Trunkey (1989) report a 55% salvage can be achieved in patients with air embolism secondary to penetrating trauma and 20%

salvage in patients with air embolism from blunt trauma.

Pulmonary Contusion

Pulmonary contusion, which usually results from blunt trauma, consists of hemorrhage into the alveolar and interstitial spaces. Contusions can result from penetrating injury, especially high-velocity missile wounds (Fig. 64–5). Although Nakayama and co-workers (1989) have reported that pulmonary contusions can occur as isolated injuries in children, in adults they are typically associated with other injuries and with an overall mortality rate of 22 to 30%, as has been recorded by Besson and Saegesser (1983), as well as by Stellin (1991). Many contusions are small and contribute little to patients' morbidity, but large contusions lead to hypoxia and the need for mechanical ventilation. The increased use of computed tomography — CT — scanning in the evaluation of acute chest trauma, as described by Wagner and Jamieson (1989), has improved sensitivity in making the diagnosis over plain radiographs.

Pulmonary contusion should be suspected in any patient with significant chest wall injury, and it can be confirmed by radiologic evaluation. Most clinically significant contusions will appear on the initial chest radiographs and may be difficult to differentiate from aspirations. Several characteristics will aid in distinguishing between the two entities. Pulmonary contusions are usually present on the initial film. The first post-trauma chest radiograph of patients suffering from aspiration may be normal, with the development of an infiltrate occurring over the next several hours. Infiltrates that are due to aspiration may be confined by anatomic pulmonary segments, while those associated with pulmonary contusions outline the area of impact, which may or may not correspond to the lobar or segmental anatomy of the lung. Among the most helpful features that permit distinction between contusion and aspiration pneumonia is the nature of the tracheobronchial secretions: Aspiration is associated with copious secretions that usually contain particulate matter, whereas contusions may be associated with bloody secretions. Initial care for both conditions is supportive and is based on serial physiologic measurements and sequential radiographs. Patients with aspiration, however, will often benefit from early bronchoscopy.

Pulmonary hematoma is another condition that may be difficult to differentiate from pulmonary contusion because of the surrounding intraparenchymal hemorrhage. However, over 24 to 48 hours ensuing the injury, hematomas typically develop into a discrete mass with distinct margins. Computed tomographic scans can be helpful in distinguishing between contusion and hematoma. In most cases, the hematoma itself will not interfere with gas exchange and with time will resorb spontaneously. Rarely, these hematomas can become secondarily infected and present as an abscess requiring drainage.

Computed tomographic evaluation of the chest following blunt trauma has been advocated by Toombs (1981) and Wagner (1988) and their colleagues as a more sensitive and accurate means of diagnosing pulmonary contusions. Additionally, CT has led to the finding that pulmonary lacerations are frequently associated with pulmonary contusions. A classification system has been

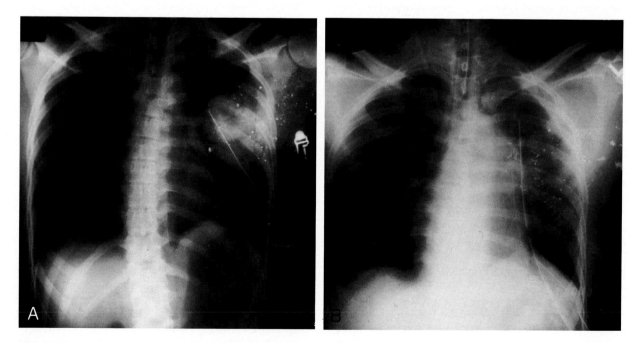

Fig. 64–5. High-velocity missile wounds. *A*, Chest radiograph shows a significant injury from a high-power rifle wound sustained through a bulletproof vest. *B*, Postoperative chest radiograph. The contusion and pulmonary parenchymal bleeding was confined to the upper lobe that was resected.

proposed to quantitate injury and thus allow comparison of various treatment modalities. However, present treatment recommendations for pulmonary contusion do not depend on CT findings. Thus, neither the risk involved in transport, for patients who are unstable or who require intensive support, nor the expense of CT studies is warranted.

Our current recommendations for treatment include ventilatory support, as needed, based on clinical and laboratory findings. Associated injuries to the chest wall, pleura, and lungs should be identified and treated. Fluid administration should be adequate to resuscitate shock; oxygen delivery and consumption should be made optimal. Because of increases in capillary endothelial permeability associated with pulmonary contusion, some authors have encouraged fluid restriction. Judicious administration of fluids with cardiovascular monitoring is appropriate, particularly in elderly patients; however, fluid restriction and the administration of diuretics in the treatment of pulmonary contusion is appropriate only in patients with evidence of fluid overload. Filling pressures should be returned to normal, using either blood products or crystalloid or colloid solutions, to maintain adequate oxygen delivery. Massive pulmonary contusions associated with large shunt fractions and hypoxemia with differential lung compliances between the affected and unaffected lungs can be managed with dual lung ventilation, or rarely, even with resection of the affected lung.

Occasionally, pulmonary injuries will require lung resections to control massive intrathoracic hemorrhage. This is particularly true for high-velocity missile injuries as documented by war-time experiences recorded by Fisher and associates (1974). Contusions surrounding low-velocity gunshot wounds seen in the civilian experience can usually be managed without the need for operation. In all cases, the extent of resection should be as conservative as possible, and according to anatomic boundaries, if feasible.

TRACHEOBRONCHIAL TRAUMA

Mechanisms

The self-healing potential of the large airways was first described by Winslow in 1874 when he reported evidence of a remote bronchial injury that had healed in a canvasback duck that subsequently had been killed by a hunter. Since that time, progress has been made in the recognition and treatment of airway injuries, and an increased incidence of this injury has been reported, which is in part due to improvements in prehospital care. In spite of improved recognition, bronchial injury remains rare, with less than a 1% incidence in major trauma victims. Injuries to the tracheobronchial tree occur following both blunt and penetrating injuries, with the latter predominating. Cervical tracheal injuries are more common from both mechanisms than is the intrathoracic portion of the tracheobronchial tree.

Injuries to the large airways following penetrating trauma are usually associated with other major injuries, especially vascular, which require early operative intervention. This often leads to the diagnosis of the tracheobronchial injury at the time of exploration. Partial tears of the airway following blunt trauma are often missed on initial evaluation; these can present months to years later with a stenosis of the airway and collapse or infection, or both, of the distal portion of the lung.

Blunt injuries to the intrathoracic airway usually occur within 2 cm of the carina. Penetrating injuries can occur along any portion of the airway. Although direct trauma to the airway is responsible for penetrating as well as blunt injuries to the cervical trachea, several mechanisms are postulated in the genesis of blunt intrathoracic injuries. These include the following: 1) linear rupture of the membranous portion of the trachea following an abrupt increase in large airway pressures that is due to thoracic compression in a patient with a closed glottis; 2) disruption of the trachea at points of fixation — the carina and the cricoid — that is due to the shearing forces seen with rapid deceleration, or 3) laceration or transection of the trachea near the carina that is due to lateral traction on the lungs with crushing chest injuries that acutely decrease the anterior-posterior diameter of the thoracic cavity.

Diagnosis

The degree of challenge in diagnosing tracheobronchial trauma depends on the location of the injury. Injuries to the cervical trachea can readily be made on the basis of history and physical findings. Symptoms associated with injury to the cervical trachea can include subcutaneous emphysema, dyspnea, dysphonia, and hemoptysis. Once an adequate airway is established, penetrating injuries with these findings should be explored. Blunt injuries to the cervical trachea can be evaluated with bronchoscopy and CT of the neck.

Timely diagnosis of injuries to the intrathoracic tracheobronchial tree requires a high index of suspicion. At times, the injury to the intrathoracic tracheobronchial tree may manifest with massive air leaks following tube thoracostomy. The findings may, however, be much more subtle, and therefore partial tears of a main stem bronchus are often missed at the time of initial presentation. For example, subcutaneous emphysema, pneumomediastinum, air outlining a bronchus, deviation of an endotracheal tube, or the "fallen lung sign" — collapse of the lung toward the lateral chest wall, as described by Unger and colleagues (1989), can all be clues to the presence of a tracheobronchial injury. Inability to re-expand the lung following tube thoracostomy or a persistent air-leak in the postinjury period may also be indicative of a tracheobronchial injury. Patients with tracheobronchial tears that are not recognized progress to develop either a suppurative lung infection or a complete collapse of the affected lung. Management of delayed presentations of bronchial injuries is discussed in the section on complications following thoracic trauma.

Patients with suspected tracheobronchial injuries should undergo immediate bronchoscopy to evaluate the airways. Either rigid or flexible bronchoscopy can be used, and the examination is best performed in the operating room by an experienced endoscopist. Any blood or clots found in the airway should be cleared because this can interfere with detection of an injury and can impede ventilation. Not only is bronchoscopy a sensitive diagnostic tool for the detection of tracheobronchial injuries, but it can often aid in establishing a secure airway. Bronchoscopy is nearly always diagnostic for major trauma to the tracheobronchial tree, as noted by Hara and Prakash (1989), as well as by Velly and associates (1991).

Treatment

Although surgical intervention is indicated in most patients with documented injuries to the large airways, small tracheobronchial tears involving less than one third of the circumference can be managed nonoperatively if the lung is fully re-expanded following tube thoracostomy and if the patient does not require high-pressure mechanical ventilation. These patents should be watched closely for signs of respiratory insufficiency and for evidence of infection, especially mediastinitis.

Injuries to the cervical trachea can usually be managed through a collar incision. The development of skin flaps below the platysma will allow exposure of the entire cervical trachea, and with some dissection, the proximal retrosternal trachea can be mobilized into the field for repair. Injuries should be debrided and repairs should be made with fine interrupted absorbable suture. Conversion of a major tracheal injury with tissue loss into a tracheostomy may be required. Injuries near the thyroid cartilage should be examined for possible laryngeal injury and should be managed with a tracheostomy. When performed, the tracheostomy should be brought out through a separate incision, if possible, to avoid contaminating the entire wound. Injuries to the cervical trachea, away from the larynx, can be repaired primarily with interrupted absorbable suture. The repair can be stinted for short periods of time with an endotracheal tube.

Combined injuries to the trachea and esophagus should have viable tissue such as a strip of sternocleidomastoid muscle interposed between the repairs. Should the injury extend down into the mediastinum, further exposure can be obtained by performing a median sternotomy or a partial sternotomy with a trap door to expose the proximal intrathoracic trachea. The entire chest therefore should be prepared for possible inclusion in the operative field.

Exposure of the mediastinal trachea, the carina, and the right main stem bronchus is best achieved through a right posterior-lateral thoracotomy through the fourth intercostal space. The proximal left main stem bronchus can be dealt with through a right thoracot-

omy; however, complete transection of the left main stem bronchus is best exposed through a standard left thoracotomy.

The first priority on identifying the injury should be to establish an adequate airway so that the repair can be accomplished safely. This is best achieved by selectively cannulating and ventilating the uninjured lung. If the area of injury involves the carina or the trachea, the repair can be performed over the endotracheal tube. Although some authors have advocated the use of cardiopulmonary bypass for the repair of tracheobronchial injuries, we disagree with this recommendation. The systemic anticoagulation required for cardiopulmonary bypass is best avoided, if possible, in polytrauma victims. Adequate ventilation and oxygenation can be achieved with either single or double selective endobronchial intubation, or with a jet ventilator.

Once the area of injury is identified, the proximal and distal airway is dissected free enough so that a repair can be performed using well-vascularized tissues without tension. Care should be taken not to dissect anymore than is necessary, especially in the lateral peritracheal planes. This will avoid recurrent laryngeal nerve injuries and minimize devascularization of the trachea. Devitalized tissue should be debrided and the mucosa should be approximated, with 3-0 or 4-0 interrupted absorbable sutures. We rarely, if ever, find it advisable to encircle the cartilaginous rings above and below an area of injury. When large amounts of tissue require debridement, repair of the tracheobronchial tree can be facilitated by dissecting and mobilizing the hilum and incising the inferior pulmonary ligament. Methods to enhance mobilization of the trachea and bronchi, which are sometimes needed for the management of acute injuries, have been described in detail (see Chapter 34).

Following completion of a repair, a strip of pleura, an intercostal muscle pedicle, or an omental pedicle should be used to buttress the suture line. It is best to avoid using any periosteum from the ribs when mobilizing the intercostal muscle pedicle because this can recalcify and lead to stenosis of the airway. Interposing a strip of viable tissue between the trachea and esophagus is especially important when both structures are injured. As pointed out by Flynn and colleagues (1989), this will decrease the incidence of postoperative leak and of tracheoesophageal fistula formation. Injuries to the large airways distal to the lobar divisions are best treated by lobectomy because these injuries are rarely isolated. Typically, they are associated with major vascular injuries that can be controlled simultaneously with the pulmonary resection.

Most victims with major airway injuries die shortly following their accident due to asphyxia; however, overall morbidity and mortality for tracheobronchial trauma depends on the associated injuries. Of victims evaluated and treated, the best prognosis is associated with isolated airway injuries, injuries to the cervical trachea, and penetrating injuries. Long-term functional results following tracheobronchial repair are good.

PROCEDURES FOR THE MANAGEMENT OF THORACIC TRAUMA

The surgical techniques used are standard for thoracic surgery, and therefore the following comments are intended only to give our references and recommendations.

Tube Thoracostomy

For most cases, we recommend insertion at the fourth or fifth intercostal space — nipple line — between the anterior and midaxillary lines. In hemodynamically stable patients, a short subcutaneous tunnel is made before penetrating the pleural cavity; in the critically injured patients, however, no subcutaneous tract is formed, because this may delay insertion of the tube. In adult patients we recommend a No. 36 French tube. Insertion of chest tubes with a trocar should be avoided in trauma patients. If, according to immediate follow-up radiograph, evacuation of a hemothorax or pneumothorax is incomplete, remedial action appropriate for the underlying injury should be immediately pursued.

Thoracotomy

Resuscitative thoracotomy, in the emergency department — ED, is indicated in victims of penetrating thoracic injuries suffering recent cardiopulmonary arrest. The use of resuscitative ED thoracotomy in blunt trauma victims is arguable, because survival for blunt trauma victims suffering cardiac arrest is dismal, as emphasized by Bodai and associates (1983). Therefore, we rarely use ED thoracotomy in blunt trauma victims with cardiac arrest. Cardiac arrest resulting from penetrating trauma, especially stab wounds to the heart, is associated with significant survival, averaging approximately 30% in several series reviewed by Ivatury and Rohman (1987). An aggressive approach to the victim with penetrating thoracic trauma with cardiac arrest therefore is recommended.

Urgent thoracotomy is indicated in patients with large or persistent hemothorax, or with air leaks that preclude adequate ventilation. When an air leak is the major indication for urgent operation, and circumstances permit, preoperative bronchoscopy is done. Its role, however, remains to be determined.

Techniques of Pulmonary Resections

Standard lung resections, according to anatomic divisions, are infrequently required for the management of trauma. If they are needed, segmental resections should be used in preference to lobectomies, and pneumonectomies should be avoided whenever possible. Damaged pulmonary parenchyma has a remarkable ability to recover, and pleural surfaces with troublesome oozing of blood or air leaks may be effectively treated in some instances with use of the Argon beam coagulator or fibrin glue. We believe it is better to re-operate promptly, if necessary, than to sacrifice potentially functioning lung tissue.

Bronchoscopy

Both flexible and rigid instruments should be available. We use rigid bronchoscopy when massive bleeding is present in the airways or when needed to establish an airway. Large foreign bodies such as broken teeth, which have been aspirated and are obstructing a bronchus, are also best removed endoscopically with a rigid bronchoscope. For diagnostic exams or clearing secretions, we prefer to use flexible instruments.

Methods of Tracheobronchial Reconstruction

Tracheobronchial repair of major airways has been discussed previously. The technical principles that apply are as follows: 1) prompt repair of an acute injury is better than delayed repair; 2) debridement of nonviable tissues, and approximation of viable edges, without tension is needed; 3) tissue conservation is an important goal, even in young, healthy patients, 4) the use of fine absorbable suture materials is recommended; monofilament suture materials, with knots tied outside the airway lumen are acceptable alternatives.

COMPLICATIONS FOLLOWING THORACIC TRAUMA

Empyema

The incidence of empyema following thoracic trauma, is approximately 3% in the experience of Helling (1989) and LeRoux (1986) and their colleagues. This incidence can be minimized by using meticulous sterile techniques while inserting thoracostomy tubes and by ensuring good apposition of the pleural surfaces so that no space remains for the accumulation of fluid or blood. The risk of empyema increases with persistent bronchopleural fistula and with residual clotted hemothorax.

Empyema rarely manifests itself with overt septic shock. It mostly presents as an indolent infectious process. CT scans aid in defining the size and location of loculated collections (Fig. 64–6). A visceral pleural peel can be identified by the characteristic "split pleura sign" described by Hanna (1991) and Waite (1990) and their associates, which represents intravenous contrast enhancement of the parietal and visceral pleurae.

Thoracentesis with appropriate culture of the fluid obtained assists antibiotic selection, because it will often identify the offending organisms. The most common organisms are skin flora such as staphylococcus or streptococcus. Gram-negative enteric organisms should be suspected when the initial trauma involved combined thoracic and abdominal injuries. Although initial antibiotic coverage should be broad, it should be promptly focused based on the results of culture and sensitivity studies. This will avoid the development of resistant organisms or opportunistic fungal infections.

The treatment of empyema depends on the clinical stage of development. The initial phase is an exudative state that is often amenable to drainage with thora-

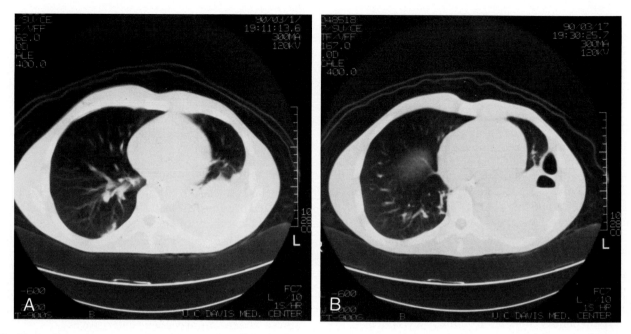

Fig. 64–6. Post-traumatic empyema. CT scans. *A*, Well-localized fluid collection, separated from adjacent pulmonary parenchyma and persistent despite chest tube placement. *B*, air-fluid level consistent with bronchopleural fistula and empyema.

costomy tube and intravenous antibiotic administration. During this time the pleural space has relatively few adhesions, and the likelihood that the collections are loculated is low. At this stage, video-assisted thoracotomy — VATS — can be very helpful in establishing adequate drainage of the infected pleural fluid. However, the diagnosis is more commonly established beyond the early exudative phase, in the fibrinopurulent phase. This transitional or fibrinopurulent phase is characterized by loculated collections of gelatinous material and the early development of a pleural peel. Subsequently, the chronic phase or organizing phase demonstrates the development of a thick, fibrotic pleural rind that entraps the lung. The latter stages typically require surgical intervention. Thoracotomy with decortication is associated with a lower morbidity and mortality than other treatment modalities, and early intervention is recommended by us as well as by Villalba (1979) and Smith (1991) and their colleagues, among others.

Alternative treatment modalities that have been proposed in the management of posttraumatic empyema but have not been well studied include the use of intracavitary fibrinolytic agents, which have been suggested by K.S. Lee (1991) and Moulton (1989) and their associates. We are skeptical that either fibrinolytic therapy or VATS will be anything more than valuable adjuncts to open drainage and decortication.

Clotted Hemothorax

Incompletely evacuated or clotted hemothorax following thoracic trauma is best prevented with early, effective tube thoracostomy drainage. Unfortunately, as

reported by Kish (1976) and Helling (1989) and their co-workers, incomplete drainage has been reported in approximately 15% of cases. Patients with significant volume loss that is due to residual hemothorax should undergo operative drainage. If performed within a week of the original trauma, VATS can be useful in avoiding rib-spreading thoracotomy in some cases. Effective and complete drainage greater than a week following the injury will almost certainly require a standard, open thoracotomy because of adhesions between the visceral and parietal pleurae and a tenacious inflammatory peel that envelops the lung.

Bronchopleural Fistula

Persistent air leak is an unusual complication following thoracic trauma. When a persistent bronchopleural fistula is present, injury to the proximal airways should be suspected and surgically repaired if present. Rarely, a thoracostomy tube may be lodged within the pulmonary parenchyma. If this is suspected, the tube should be immediately replaced, after allowing the lung to collapse temporarily to facilitate placement of the new tube into the pleural space.

Bronchopleural fistulas also occur in the intensive care unit as a result of the barotrauma of mechanical ventilation. In such cases treatment should be limited to draining any pneumothorax present — most of which are loculated — and to supporting the patient's ventilatory status. Most of these air leaks will improve as the patient's pulmonary compliance improves. Care should be taken in placing thoracostomy tubes in such patients because numerous adhesions are usually present in the thoracic cavity and the lung can be quite firm and vulnerable to injury because of the inflammatory process. Patients with stiff lungs and large air leaks may require intubation of each lung with dual ventilators to optimize their pulmonary status. This permits improved ventilation of the lungs by compensating for the large air leak. In spite of this theoretical advantage, in our experience, these patients have a poor prognosis, which is due to the severity of their underlying ARDS.

Treatment of a persistent bronchopleural air leak, other than from a major airway injury, rarely requires operative intervention. Occasionally, we discharge patients with chronic bronchopleural fistulas from the hospital with chest tubes and Heimlich valves. Usually, the air leaks stop by the time of the patient's first return visit. Rarely, the thoracostomy tube is placed to open drainage, and it is then advanced along its fibrous tract slowly over days until it is out. Even more rarely, if the bronchopleural fistula persists in spite of the aforementioned treatment to a pulmonary resection or an Eloesser flap may be required.

Bronchial Stenosis

Partial bronchial tears may often go undiagnosed at first presentation if the index of suspicion is not high. In such cases the partial tear will permit ventilation and re-expansion of the lung following the acute injury; however, as the bronchus heals, a stricture may form, leading to distal collapse of the lung (Fig. 64–7). If the distal lung is not infected, the atelectatic lung may not give rise to any symptoms and will remain undiagnosed until a subsequent chest radiograph is obtained. Distal infection will present with findings consistent with a pneumonia or pulmonary abscess. Bronchoscopy is diagnostic and should be performed whenever there is evidence of lobar collapse in the post-traumatic patient. Computed tomographic scanning of the chest may be helpful in determining whether there is distal infection.

The decision to repair the bronchus or to resect the involved lung should be based on whether distal infection is present. It is clear that an atelectatic lung can be aerated even after long periods of time with excellent functional results (Fig. 64–7), as one of us (J.R.B., 1958) and Eastridge (1970) and associates have reported. This requires resection of the bronchial stenosis with primary repair using fine absorbable sutures in an interrupted fashion, as previously described. A suppurative infection of the distal lung, however, precludes repair because of the acute morbidity associated with advanced infection. This infection will often spill over into the normal lung following repair of the stenosis. In addition the infected lung, distal to the stenosis is usually severe damage, as manifested by bronchiectasis. This poses a risk for chronic recurrent infections in the affected lung segment. Grossly infected lung distal to a bronchial stricture therefore should be resected, with bronchial repair being reserved for patients with atelectatic lung.

Chylothorax

The accumulation of chyle in the thorax, following injury to the thoracic duct, is a rare complication that

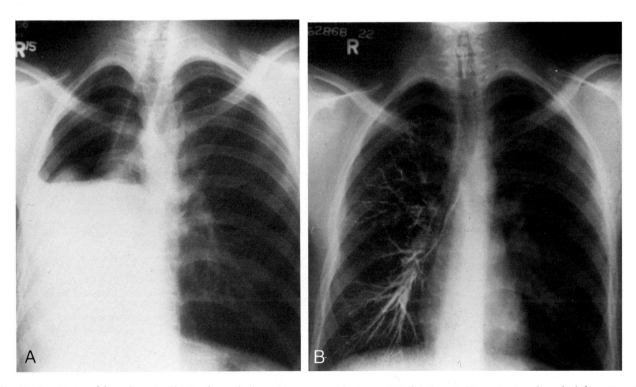

Fig. 64–7. Ruptured bronchus. *A*, Chest radiograph shows hemopneumothorax associated with complete main stem bronchial disruption. *B*, Bronchogram following repair of a transected bronchus reveals excellent longterm results.

can occur following blunt trauma, as recorded by Dulchavsky and colleagues (1988), and more commonly following penetrating injury. Findings on presentation include large and persistent chest tube drainage — 500 to 2000 ml/day — that is milky in character when the patient is taking an oral diet. These findings may not be present early in the posttraumatic period, which is due to the reduced lymph flow and the clear appearance of the chyle in the fasting state. Analysis of the fluid will reveal a high triglyceride level and will stain positive with the fat stain Sudan III. Infection is rare because of the bacteriostatic nature of chyle.

Once the diagnosis is established, initial treatment should consist of adequate drainage of the chest, bowel rest, and total parenteral nutrition for nutritional support. If significant drainage persists beyond 2 weeks of observation, then operative management should be pursued. Milson and associates (1985) have reviewed the current surgical management in the patients who have failed nonoperative management; insertion of a pleuroperitoneal shunt or transthoracic ligation of the thoracic duct at the diaphragmatic hiatus will, as a rule, successfully treat this difficult clinical problem. As a result of the infrequent occurrence of this problem, the ideal treatment is not well established (see Chapter 59).

REFERENCES

Ammons MA, Moore EE, Rosen P: Role of the observation unit in the management of thoracic trauma. J Emerg Med 4:279, 1986.

Anel D: L'Art de Succet les Plaies. Amsterdam: Francois Ander Plaats. 1707, p 13.

Armstrong CP, Van der Spuy J: The fractured scapula: importance and management based on a series of 62 patients. Injury 15:324, 1983.

Avery EE, Mörch ET, Benson DW: Critically crushed chests. J Thorac Surg 32:291, 1956.

Benfield JR, et al: The reversibility of chronic atelectasis. Surg Forum 8:473, 1958.

Besson A, Saegesser F: Color Atlas of Chest Trauma and Associated Injuries. Vol 1. Oradell, NJ: Medical Economics Company, 1983, p 9.

Bodai BI, et al: Emergency thoracotomy in the management of trauma: a review. JAMA 249:1891, 1983.

Bowling R, et al: Emergency pneumonectomy for penetrating and blunt trauma. Am Surg 51:136, 1985.

Buckman R, et al: The significance of stable patients with sternal fractures. Surg Gyn Obstet 164:261, 1987.

Burford TH, Burbank B: Traumatic wet lung. J Thorac Surg 14:415, 1945.

Campbell DB: Trauma to the chest wall, lung, and major airways. Semin Thorac Cardiovasc Surg 4:234, 1992.

Clark GC, Schecter WP, Trunkey DD: Variables affecting outcome in blunt chest trauma: flail chest vs. pulmonary contusion. J Trauma 28:298, 1988.

Conn JH, et al: Thoracic trauma: analysis of 1022 cases. J Trauma 3:22, 1963.

Dulchavsky SA, Ledgerwood AM, Lucas CE: Management of chylothorax after blunt chest trauma. J Trauma 28:1400, 1988.

Eastridge CE, et al: Tracheobronchial injury caused by blunt trauma. Ann Rev Respir Dis 101:230, 1970.

Fischer RP, Geiger JP, Guernsey, JM: Pulmonary resections for severe pulmonary contusions secondary to high-velocity missile wounds. J Trauma 14:293, 1974.

Flynn AE, Thomas AN, Schecter WP: Acute tracheobronchial injury. J Trauma 29:1326, 1989.

Freedland M, et al: The management of flail chest injury: factors affecting outcome. J Trauma 30:1460, 1990.

Galan G, et al: Blunt chest injuries in 1696 patients. Eur J Cardiothorac Surg 6:284, 1992.

Garcia VF, et al: Rib fractures in children: a marker of severe trauma. J Trauma 30:695, 1990.

Glinz W: Symposium paper: priorities in diagnosis and treatment of blunt chest injuries. Injury 17:318, 1986.

Glinz W: Causes of early death in thoracic trauma. In Webb WR, Besson A (eds): Thoracic Surgery: Surgical Management of Chest Injuries. Vol. 7. St Louis: Mosby Year Book, 1991.

Guttentag IJ, Rechtine GR: Fractures of the scapula: a review of the literature. Orthop Rev 17:147, 1988.

Haasler GB: Open fixation of flail chest after blunt trauma. Ann Thorac Surg 49:993, 1990.

Hanna JW, Reed JC, Choplin RH: Pleural infections: a clinical-radiologic review. J Thorac Imaging 6:68, 1991.

Hara KS, Prakash UBS: Fiberoptic bronchoscopy in the evaluation of acute chest and upper airway trauma. Chest 96:627, 1989.

Helling TS, et al: Complications following blunt and penetrating injuries in 216 victims of chest trauma requiring tube thoracostomy. J Trauma 29:1367, 1989.

Henley MB, et al: External fixation of the sternum for thoracic trauma. J Orthop Trauma 5:493, 1991.

Ivatury RR, Rohman M: Emergency department thoracotomy for trauma: a collective review. Resuscitation 15:23, 1987.

Karanfilian R, Machiedo GW, Bolanowski PJ: Management of non-penetrating stab and gunshot wounds of the chest. Surg Gynecol Obstet 153:395, 1981.

Kemmerer WT, et al: Patterns of thoracic injuries in fatal traffic accidents. J Trauma 1:595, 1961.

Kish G, et al: Indications for early thoracotomy in the management of chest trauma. Ann Thorac Surg 22:23, 1976.

Kulshrestha P, et al: Chest injuries: a clinical and autopsy profile. J Trauma 28:844, 1988.

Landercasper J, Cogbill TH, Lindesmith LA: Long-term disability after flail chest injury. J Trauma 24:410, 1984.

Landreneau RJ, Hinson JM, Hazelrigg SR: Strut fixation of an extensive flail chest. Ann Thorac Surg 51:473, 1991.

Lee KS, et al: Treatment of thoracic multiloculated empyemas with intracavitary urokinase: a prospective study. Radiology 179:771, 1991.

Lee MC, et al: Traumatic asphyxia. Ann Thorac Surg 51:86, 1991.

LeRoux BT, et al: Suppurative diseases of the lung and pleural space. Part I: Empyema thoracis and lung abscess. Curr Probl Surg 23:1, 1986.

LoCicero J, Mattox KL: Epidemiology of chest trauma. Surg Clin North Am 69:15, 1989.

Mackersie RC, et al: Continuous epidural fentanyl analgesia: ventilatory function improvement with routine use in treatment of blunt chest injury. J Trauma 27:1207, 1987.

MaGahan JP, Rab GT, Dublin A: Fractures of the scapula. J Trauma 20:880, 1980.

Milson JW, et al: Chylothorax: an assessment of current surgical management. J Thorac Cardiovasc Surg 89:221, 1985.

Moulton JS, Moore PT, Mencini RA: Treatment of loculated pleural effusions with transcatheter intracavitary urokinase. Am J Roentgenol 153:941, 1989.

Nakayama DK, Ramenofsky ML, Rowe MI: Chest injuries in childhood. Ann Surg 210:770, 1989.

Ordog GJ, Balasubramanium S, Wasserberger J: Outpatient management of 3757 gunshot wounds to the chest. J Trauma 23:832, 1983.

Otremski I, et al: Fracture of the sternum in motor vehicle accidents and its association with mediastinal injury. Injury 21:81, 1990.

Paris F, Tarrazona V, Garcia-Zarza A: Controversial aspects of surgical fixation for traumatic flail chest. In Webb WR, Besson A (eds): Thoracic Surgery: Surgical Management of Chest Injuries. Vol 7. St Louis: Mosby Year Book, 1991.

Playfair: Case of empyema treated by repeated aspiration and subsequently by drainage: recovery. Br Med J 1:45, 1875.

Poole GV: Fracture of the upper ribs and injury to the great vessels. Surg Gynecol Obstet 169:275, 1989.

Richardson JD, McElvein RB, Trinkle JK: First rib fracture: a hallmark of severe trauma. Ann Surg 181:251, 1975.

Scultetus J: The Surgeon's Storehouse. London: Starkey, 1674 p 159.

Shackford SR: Blunt chest trauma: the intensivists's perspective. J Int Care Med 1:125, 1986.

Shackford SR, et al: The management of flail chest: a comparison of ventilatory and nonventilatory treatment. Am J Surg 132:759, 1976.

Shorr RM, et al: Blunt thoracic trauma: analysis of 515 patients. Ann Surg 206:200, 1987.

Shorr RM, et al: Blunt chest trauma in elderly. J Trauma 29:234, 1989.

Smith JA, et al: Empyema thoracis: 14-years experience in a teaching center. Ann Thoracic Surg 51:39, 1991.

Stellin G: Survival in trauma victims with pulmonary contusion. Am Surg 57:780, 1991.

Swanson J, Trunkey DD: Trauma to the chest wall, pleura and thoracic viscera. In Shields TW (ed): General Thoracic Surgery. 3rd Ed. Philadelphia: Lea & Febiger, 1989.

Thomas AH, Roe BB: Air embolism following penetrating lung injuries. J Thorac Cardiovasc Surg 66:533, 1973.

Thomas AN, Blaisdell FW, Lewis FR Jr, Schlobohm RM: Operative stabilization for flail chest after blunt trauma. J Thorac Cardiovasc Surg 75:793, 1978.

Thompson DA, et al: Urgent thoracotomy for pulmonary or tracheobronchial injury. J Trauma 28:276, 1988.

Thompson DA, Flynn TC, Miller PW: The significance of scapular fractures. J Trauma 25:974, 1985.

Toombs BD, Sandler CM, Lester RG: Computed tomography of chest trauma. Radiology 140:733, 1981.

Trinkle JK, et al: Management of flail chest without mechanical ventilation. J Thoracic Surg 19:355, 1975.

Unger JM, Schuchmann GG, Grossman JE: Tears of the trachea and main bronchi caused by blunt trauma: radiologic findings. AJR Am J Roentgenol 153:1175, 1989.

Villalba M, et al: The etiology of post-traumatic empyema and the role of decortication. J Trauma 19:414, 1979.

Velly JF, et al: Post traumatic tracheobronchial lesions: a follow-up study of 47 cases. Eur J Cardiothorac Surg 5:352, 1991.

Wagner RB, Crawford WO, Schimpf PP: Classification of parenchymal injuries of the lung. Radiology 167:77, 1988.

Wagner RB, Jamieson PM: Pulmonary contusion: evaluation and classification by computed tomography. Surg Clin North Am 69:31, 1989.

Waite, RJ, et al: Parietal pleural changes in empyema: appearances at CT. Radiology 175:145, 1990.

Weigelt JA, et al: Management of asymptomatic patients following stab wounds to the chest. J Trauma 22:291, 1982.

Williams JS, Minken SL, Adams JT: Traumatic asphyxia — reappraised. Ann Surg 167:384, 1968.

Wilson RF, Murray C, Antonenko DR: Nonpenetrating thoracic injuries. Surg Clin North Am 57:17, 1977.

Winslow WH: Rupture of bronchus from wild duck. Philadelphia Med Times p 22, April 15, 1874.

Wisner DH: A stepwise logistic regression analysis of factors affecting morbidity and mortality after thoracic trauma: effect of epidural analgesia. J Trauma 30:799, 1990.

Wisner DH, Reed WH, Riddick RS: Suspected myocardial contusion. Ann Surg 212:82, 1990.

Worthley LIG: Thoracic epidural in the management of chest trauma: a study of 161 cases. Int Care Med 11:312, 1985.

Yee FS, Thomas AN, Wilson R: Management of air embolism in blunt and penetrating thoracic trauma. J Thorac Cardiovasc Surg 85:661, 1983.

READING REFERENCES

Beaumont W: Experiments and Observations on the Gastric Juice and the Physiology of Digestion. New York: Dover, 1959. (Original work published 1825).

Breadsted JH: The Edwin Smith Surgical Papyrus. Vol 1. Chicago: University of Chicago Press, 1930, p 391.

Johnston JR, McCaughey W: Epidural morphine: a method of management of multiple fractured ribs. Anaesthesia 35:155, 1980.

Meade RH: A History of Thoracic Surgery. Springfield, IL: Bannerston House, 1961, p 3.

Rovenstine EA, Byrd ML: The use of nerve block during treatment for fractured ribs. Am J Surg 46:303, 1939.

Theodoric: Surgery (AD 1267). Vol 1. Campbell E, Colton J (trans.). Norwalk, CT: Appleton-Century-Crofts, 1955.

CHAPTER 65

BAROTRAUMA AND INHALATION INJURIES

Joseph LoCicero, III

Occasionally, the thoracic surgeon is called on to assist in the management of patients with complex pulmonary problems in the intensive care unit — ICU. Two of the more common are barotrauma and inhalation injuries. To adequately manage these conditions, it is important to understand the underlying mechanisms of injury. Support and specific therapies then can be administered properly.

BAROTRAUMA

Cullen and Caldera (1979) noted the incidence of pneumothorax in ventilated ICU patients to range between 0.5 and 15%. Macklin and Macklin (1944) described the most common mechanism of injury. A small airway or alveolus ruptures and the air dissects through the bronchovascular connective tissue proximally into the mediastinum, ultimately rupturing into the pleural space.

Etiology

Although it is obvious that an air sack must rupture to produce a pneumothorax, the mechanism of that rupture is a subject of debate (Table 65–1). Most theories are based on overdistension or pressurization of the alveolus. Peevy and associates (1990) studied isolated perfused rabbit lungs, examining various methods of ventilation. They ventilated four sets of lungs with either a low or high gas flow rate while holding the peak inspiratory pressure either low — 27 cm H_2O — or high — 50 cm H_2O. They found that the high peak inspiratory pressure group produced significant microvascular injuries. Injury occurred in the higher flow rate

Table 65–1. Potential Causes of Barotrauma

High peak airway pressures
High mean airway pressures
Alveolar overdistension — increased volume
Positive end expiratory pressure — PEEP

and low-pressure group but not to the same extent as the high-pressure low flow rate group. They concluded that the peak airway pressure was the most important mechanism of injury.

Conversely, Marini and Ravenscraft (1992) used geometric and mathematic modeling to evaluate mean airway pressure. They found that under conditions of passive inflation, mean arterial pressure correlated with arterial oxygenation, hemodynamic performance, and barotrauma.

Two groups recently evaluated alveolar distensibility — a measure of alveolar energetics — as a precursor to barotrauma. Adkins and colleagues (1991) varied peak inspiratory pressure while ventilating young and old rabbits. They found that the young rabbits were more susceptible to pneumothorax and concluded that for the same inspiratory pressure, higher volumes would be presented in the young lungs and that overdistention was the etiologic factor. In an intriguing report, Colebatch and Ng (1991) studied 14 men who developed pneumothoraces during shallow water diving and compared their pulmonary mechanics to 34 healthy nonsmokers and 10 age-matched healthy male divers. They found that those who had developed pneumothoraces had stiffer airways and smaller air spaces. They concluded that such a situation would magnify the elastic stresses in the peribronchial alveolar tissue, which would increase the likelihood of interstitial gas dissection. It is known that patients with adult respiratory distress syndrome have markedly decreased compliance associated with smaller thickened alveoli, and this clinical situation might be analogous to the observed findings in the divers who developed pneumothoraces.

In another human study, Ranieri and associates (1991) looked at the effects of positive end-expiratory pressure — PEEP — on alveolar recruitment in patients with respiratory distress syndrome. Observing the pressure-volume loops on zero end-expiratory pressure — ZEEP — and PEEP, they found two populations of patients. Some patients showed evidence of alveolar recruitment as evidenced by an upward concavity of the pressure-volume curve during ZEEP ventilation, which increased with PEEP. Other patients demonstrated an upward convexity, noting volume displacement without alveolar recruitment. This was aggravated with PEEP. They believed that this sub-population of patients would be susceptible to baro-trauma.

Presentation

One of the earliest radiographic signs of barotrauma is mediastinal air. Although this finding is often a precursor of pneumothorax, not all patients with pneu-momediastinum develop a pneumothorax. In addition, pneumomediastinum usually does not give a clue as to the side of origin. Once pneumomediastinum develops, vigilance is important to discover early signs of pneu-mothorax.

Often, the first sign of barotrauma is not seen on routine chest radiographs but presents as an acute change in hemodynamics or oxygenation. Any patient with poor compliance on positive pressure ventilation and PEEP becomes acutely hypotensive or hypoxemic and may have a pneumothorax. In patients who have severe respiratory distress syndrome, the pneumothorax may not be large. The loss of even a small amount of lung volume may be sufficient to alter the steady state. Auscultation of the chest in pneumothorax may dem-onstrate disparate breath sounds, which may be con-firmed by the chest radiographs.

Management

In a patient who has acutely developed barotrauma and is hemodynamically unstable, a needle catheter thoracostomy may be diagnostic as well as life saving. A sterile needle placed through the second or third intercostal space lateral to the midclavicular lung will allow the air to escape and should stabilize the patient until a more definitive catheter or tube can be placed. A large tube — preferably a No. 28 or 32 French — should be placed in the fifth or sixth intercostal space at the anterior axillary line. The large tube is used to sufficiently remove any high-volume leak produced. Because many of these severely ill patients also have associated effusions, the tube should be directed pos-teriorly.

Sometimes the surgeon is notified of a critically ill ventilated patient when they develop a pneumomedi-astinum. Because the side of origin cannot be deter-mined in such a case, the choice is observation or bilateral tube thoracostomy. My preference is to as-semble in the room the equipment necessary for both a needle and a tube thoracostomy but to await the development of a pneumothorax and treat only that side.

Because of the underlying disease, the lungs are stiff and may not completely re-expand. However, positive pressure ventilation is being used on these patients. Because of these two facts, negative suction on the drainage system is unnecessary. Air from the air leak will escape through the water seal. Tubes should be left in place until the compliance significantly im-proves and the PEEP levels are consistently below 10 cm H_2O.

Prevention

Adjustment of ventilation to prevent barotrauma is as varied as the theories concerning its etiology. Because the major pulmonary mechanical changes in respiratory distress syndrome are decreased compliance and defect in diffusion, ventilation must be adjusted to optimize these values. Both pressure and volume determine alveolar distention and compliance. Theories show that peak airway pressure and PEEP are the major con-tributors to barotrauma. Optimal management is ac-complished by delivering the tidal volume — 10 to 15 ml/kg — at a rate sufficient to maintain a normal PCO_2 at the lowest flow rates possible. This will decrease the peak airway pressure and mean airway pressures yet deliver relatively normal lung volumes, thus optimizing compliance. The slower breath delivered by lower flow rates may also allow accommodation of the alveolar wall, thus decreasing local wall tension. As suggested by Shapiro and colleagues (1984) PEEP should be adjusted to the least levels necessary as measured by the best improvement in shunt fraction and oxygen delivery with the lowest dead space ventilation and inspired oxygen concentration.

INHALATION INJURIES

Two major types of pulmonary injuries occur in victims: inhalation injury at the time of acute trauma and pulmonary injury secondary to the management of cutaneous burns. The latter includes a wide variety of injuries from pulmonary edema secondary to massive crystalloid fluid resuscitation to acute lung injury and respiratory distress from sepsis and multiple organ failure. These are no different from any other critically ill patient. Management of these conditions are covered elsewhere and will not be discussed here.

Etiology of Inhalation Injury

The term "pulmonary burn" is a misnomer. The lungs are rarely burned secondary to inhalation injury. The oropharynx, nasopharynx, and upper airway sufficiently cool the gases that are inhaled so that thermal injury is minimal in the lungs. When a burn does occur, it is almost always fatal. Two circumstances in which this occurs are steam injuries in a closed space and over-heated gases in ventilated patients. I have personally managed a patient who received superheated — 45°C — ventilator gases for 8 hours from a faulty heating unit. This patient exhibited severe bronchorrhea and acute lung injury resistant to ventilator therapy and suc-cumbed within 48 hours. The heating elements have no alarms and must be checked on a regular basis by nursing and respiratory staff to prevent this unfortunate complication.

The most common pulmonary injury associated with burns is smoke inhalation. This is a serious problem and according to Demling (1989) accounts for at least 50% of the burn deaths at the accident scene. Death occurs by lethal chemical inhalation. Davies (1986) identified more than 50 chemicals in the blood of inhalation victims who died at the scene of fires.

The magnitude of the inhalation problem is illustrated by the studies of the deadly fire that occurred in the Stardust Nightclub in Dublin in 1981. Woolley (1984) reported on a re-enactment. A portion of the nightclub was re-created and monitored during a controlled fire. Within minutes of starting the fire, smoke production exceeded 1000 m^3/min and visibility dropped to less than 1 m. Near the fire, the oxygen concentration was only 2% with a 3% carbon monoxide level. Other toxic chemicals in lethal concentrations were hydrogen-cyanide and hydrogen-chloride. Near the exit, the oxygen concentration averaged 13%, while other toxic chemicals remained in lethal concentrations.

Pathophysiology

Common household items produce a variety of toxic chemicals (Table 65–2). Carbon monoxide, a colorless gas, binds avidly to hemoglobin with over 200 times the affinity of oxygen. It causes severe tissue hypoxia. Hydrogen cyanide is a product of incomplete combustion of plastics and blocks oxidative metabolism. Its effects are not seen for up to 40 minutes after exposure and are dose dependent. Ammonia combines with water on contact with mucosa to form ammonium hydroxide, a very strong alkali that produces liquefaction necrosis. Aldehydes, produced by combustion of wood, initiate severe pulmonary edema. Exposure to greater than 30 parts per million can produce death in 10 minutes. Hydrogen chloride released in combustion of plastics produces glottic and pulmonary edema. Nitrogen dioxide produced from combustion of cellulose usually causes no immediate problems. However, within a few hours, it can cause severe respiratory epithelial damage and pulmonary edema. It can also react with the blood to produce methemoglobin. Carbonyl-chloride — Phosgene — produced in the combustion of polyvinyl chloride, causes necrosis of epithelium and pulmonary edema. Because of its low concentration in fires, it usually produces only chest tightness and mucosal irritation.

Diagnosis

Many times, patients present with carbonaceous material around the nose and mouth or inside the oropharynx, making the diagnosis of smoke inhalation easy. Other times manifestations may be subtle, and only a high index of suspicion and laboratory testing lead to the diagnosis.

Clark and Nieman (1988) describe a variety of situations. The severe cases will cause death at the scene. Some patients may respond initially to resuscitation, only to die of severe hypoxia. Less severe cases may enter the hospital in respiratory distress that is due to airway edema and bronchorrhea. These patients may have stridor, wheezing, and decreased breath sounds. The mildest group may appear relatively comfortable but deteriorate within the first 24 hours, developing severe respiratory compromise.

To confirm injury, particularly in the mild cases, one must rely on laboratory evaluation. Arterial blood gases are usually diagnostic. Although the Po_2 — may be normal, carboxyhemoglobin and cyanmethemoglobin levels will be elevated. Mildly elevated carboxyhemoglobin may be not diagnostic, because it may be elevated in smokers. Elevated cyanmethemoglobin levels, however, are quite diagnostic.

Treatment

In management of inhalation injury, one must constantly reassess the patency of the airway and the adequacy of ventilation. Even at the scene of the accident, intubation may be required. Haponik and Summer (1987b) noted that as many as 50% of surviving inhalation victims may require intubation. Bronchoscopy is rarely required to make a diagnosis of inhalation injury or determine the need for intubation.

Oxygen is an important component of early therapy. Because of the mucosal edema that is present high, inspired concentrations may help to improve arterial oxygenation. Because carbon monoxide has such a great affinity for hemoglobin, a high Po_2 is required to displace it.

Florid respiratory failure is present in some victims. Patients with marginal oxygenation who fail to improve rapidly are treated vigorously because alveolar volume loss and total atelectasis is such a prominent feature in this illness. It is easier to prevent collapse than it is to restore alveolar volume. Clark (1992) recommends that these individuals be given intermittent mandatory positive pressure ventilation with PEEP. This may be the best way to maintain the necessary alveolar distention.

As resuscitation of a large cutaneous burn progresses, pulmonary edema worsens. This may be quite significant in patients with associated inhalation injury, even when the cutaneous burns are small. Aggressive ventilatory support is necessary through this transient period.

Table 65–2. Toxic Elements in Common Fire Smoke

Source	Toxin	Effect
Any organic matter	Carbon monoxide	Tissue hypoxia
	Carbon dioxide	Narcosis
Wood, wallpaper	Nitrogen dioxide	Bronchial irritation
		Pulmonary edema
	Aldehydes	Mucosal damage
Nylon	Ammonia	Mucosal irritation
Petroleum plastics	Benzene	Mucosal irritation
Polyvinyl chloride	Hydrogen chloride	Mucosal irritation
	Carbonyl chloride	Mucosal irritation

Corticosteroids have not been shown to improve survival.

According to Clark (1992), patients surviving the acute accident scene with isolated smoke inhalation injury usually experience illness for only several days and then begin to improve, allowing cautious withdrawal of support. Long-term sequelae directly from smoke inhalation are uncommon.

REFERENCES

Adkins WK et al: Age affects susceptibility to pulmonary barotrauma in rabbits. Crit Care Med 19:390, 1991.

Clark WR: Smoke inhalation: diagnosis and treatment. World J Surg 16:24, 1992.

Clark WR, Nieman GF: Smoke inhalation. Burn 14:473, 1988.

Colebatch HJ, Ng CK: Decreased pulmonary distensibility and pulmonary barotrauma in divers. Resp Phys 96:293, 1991.

Cullen DJ, Caldera DL: The incidence of ventilation-induced pulmonary barotrauma in critically ill patients. Anaesthesia 50:185, 1979.

Davies JWL: Toxic chemicals versus lung tissue — an aspect of inhalation injury revisited. J Burn Care Rehab 7:213, 1986.

Demling RH: Management of the burn patient. In Schumaker et al. (eds): Textbook of Critical Care. 2nd Ed. Philadelphia: WB Saunders, 1989.

Haponik ER, Summer WR: Respiratory complications in burn patients: diagnosis and management of inhalation injury. J Crit Care 2:121, 1987a.

Haponik ER, Summer WR: Respiratory complications in burn patients: pathogenesis and spectrum of inhalation injuries. J Crit Care 2:49, 1987b.

Macklin MT, Macklin CC: Malignant interstitial emphysema of the lungs and mediastinum. Medicine 23:281, 1944.

Marini JJ, Ravenscraft SA. Mean airway pressure: physiologic determinants and clinical importance. Part 2, clinical implications. Crit Care Med 20:1604, 1992.

Peevy KG, et al: Barotrauma and microvascular injury in lungs of non-adult rabbits: effect of ventilation pattern. Crit Care Med 18:634, 1990.

Ranieri VM, et al: The effects of positive inexpiratory pressure on alveolar recruitment and gas exchange in patients with adult respiratory distress syndrome. Am Rev Respir Dis 144:544, 1991.

Shapiro BA, Kane RD, Harrison RA: Positive end expiratory therapy in adults with special reference to acute lung injury: review of the literature and suggested clinical correlation. Crit Care Med 12:127, 1984.

Woolley WB: The Stardust Disco fire: Dublin 1981: studies of combustion products during simulation experiments. Fire Safe J 7:267, 1984.

CHAPTER 66

ADULT RESPIRATORY DISTRESS SYNDROME

R. Bernard Rochon, Charles L. Rice, and C. James Carrico

Adult respiratory distress syndrome — ARDS — is a relatively common presentation of acute respiratory failure. Although its exact *cause* is unknown, the conditions with which it is associated are now widely appreciated. Most involve forms of direct or indirect injury to the lung that results in diffuse injury to the alveolar capillary endothelium, pulmonary interstitium, and alveolar epithelium. The injury is characterized by increased capillary permeability and nonhydrostatic pulmonary edema, hypoxemia resistant to supplemental oxygen, decreased pulmonary compliance, and diffuse pulmonary infiltrates.

At a consensus conference sponsored by the National Heart, Lung, and Blood Institute — NHLBI, it was estimated that the incidence of ARDS in the United States was about 150,000 cases per year (1979). That incidence appears to have remained constant over the ensuing two decades.

Despite advances in critical care, the mortality rate of patients who develop ARDS remains greater than 50% in most studies, such as those of the NHLBI (1979), Divertie (1982), and Fowler and associates (1983). Fein (1983) and Montgomery (1985) and their colleagues noted that when ARDS is accompanied by other organ system failures or sepsis, mortality rates increase dramatically. In the NHLBI multicenter study (1979), the mortality rate increased from 45% with ARDS alone to 56%, 72%, 84%, and 100%, respectively, with the failure of one, two, three, or four other systems in addition to ARDS. Kaplan and co-workers (1979) reported that in patients with sepsis and ARDS, the mortality rate reached 90%. A similar mortality rate has been reported in patients with ARDS and renal failure.

ANATOMY

In normal lung tissue, the alveolar surface is lined by type I and type II pneumocytes, supported by a basement membrane. Type I pneumocytes are highly differentiated and cannot replicate. These are flattened squamous epithelial cells, and according to Bachofen and Weibel (1982), they cover approximately 95% of the alveolar surface (Fig. 66–1).

Type II pneumocytes are cuboidal and have microvilli on the alveolar surface (Fig. 66–2). Surfactant, a lipoprotein responsible for lowering surface tension and, hence, impending alveolar collapse, is produced by type II pneumocytes. These cells are more resistant to injury than are type I cells, and they can replicate as well as differentiate to form type I pneumocytes. Both types of cells are joined by tight junctions that are normally impermeable to water.

Alveolar capillaries lie in alveolar walls between adjacent alveoli and are lined by endothelial cells attached to a basement membrane by fibronectin (Fig. 66–3). In some areas, the capillary and epithelial basement membranes fuse to form a thin membrane that facilitates gas exchange. In other areas, the membranes are separated by the interstitial space. This space contains connective tissue elements — notably, elastin — as well as fibroblasts and fluid. Capillary endothelial cells are joined by loose junctions that allow small amounts of fluid and nutrients into the interstitium. Excess interstitial fluid is drained by the pulmonary lymphatics.

PATHOPHYSIOLOGY

The most widely held view of the pathophysiology of ARDS is based on the concept of capillary endothelial injury. This injury may result from the direct action of an agent in the plasma, or from the interaction of cellular elements of the blood with the endothelium. One candidate for such a role is the neutrophil — polymorphonuclear leukocyte, or PMN. The PMN contains within it proteases such as cathepsin G — whose substrate is fibronectin; elastase — substrate, elastin; and collagenase. It also contains granules capable of generating toxic oxygen metabolites, such as superoxide radical, hydrogen peroxide, and hypochlorous acid. Both of these categories of agents are normally employed by the PMN to destroy bacteria but may, under certain

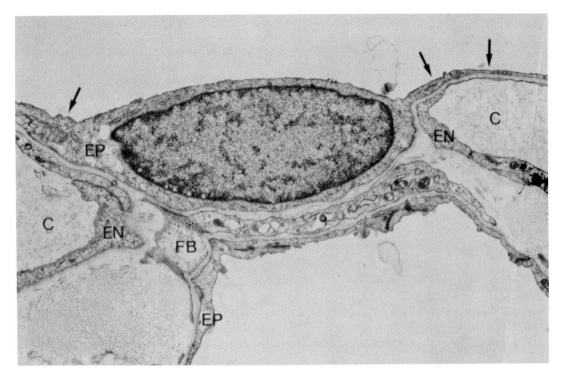

Fig. 66–1. Type I alveolar cell with thin cytoplasmic extensions (arrows). C = alveolar capillary; EP = Type I pneumocyte; EN = endothelial cell lining of capillary; FB = fibroblast process with an intracytoplasmic bundle of contractile filaments (*). ×8600.

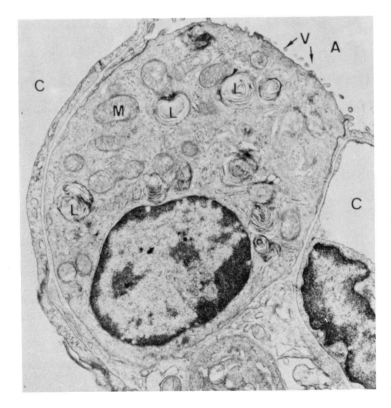

Fig. 66–2. Type II alveolar cell with osmiophilic lamellated bodies (L) and mitochrondria (M) in cytoplasm, and short microvilli (V) at surface toward alveolus (A). Note type I cell in vicinity. ×8600.

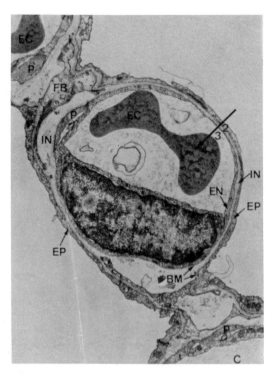

Fig. 66–3. Electron micrograph of alveolar capillary (C) from monkey lung with erythrocyte (EC). Note endothelial cell lining of capillary (EN), processes of pericytes (P) and the thin extensions of squamous alveolar epithelial cells (EP) covering the alveolar surface. The interstitial space (IN) is bounded by two basement membranes (BM) and contains some fibroblast processes (FB) as well as a few connective tissue fibrils. This lung was fixed by instillation of fixative into airways, which resulted in a loss of the surface lining layer; hence only parts 2 (tissue barrier), 3 (blood plasma), and 4 (erythrocyte) of the gas exchange pathway are preserved. ×8600. *From* Weibel ER: Morphometric estimation of pulmonary diffusion capacity. I. Model and method. Respir Physiol *11*:54, 1970/71.

circumstances, use them to attack the host. If the PMN is bound to the endothelial cells, natural defense mechanisms contained in the plasma may not be present in sufficient concentrations to protect the endothelial cell and its basement membrane from injury. This process is discussed in more detail subsequently in this chapter.

By whatever mechanism it occurs, this injury to the endothelium results in increased gap formation between the cells, leading to the leakage of fluid, protein, and cells into the interstitium. If the capacity of the lymphatics is exceeded, fluid begins to accumulate, collecting first around the bronchi and large pulmonary vessels, and resulting in the characteristic radiographic appearance of interstitial pulmonary edema. Edema then spreads to involve the areas around the alveolar capillaries.

When the capacity of the interstitial space is exceeded, alveolar flooding occurs. Type I cells are damaged and sloughed, leaving behind a denuded basement membrane. The alveoli are filled with protein-rich fluid containing erythrocytes, leukocytes, debris from type I cells, and fibrin strands. This material may

form sheets that adhere to the denuded basement membrane, forming hyaline membranes. The protein-rich fluid inactivates surfactant, leaving the alveolus vulnerable to flooding and collapse, and producing the radiographic pattern of diffuse alveolar infiltrate.

Before alveolar flooding occurs, the gas-exchange surfaces remain intact. Iliff and associates (1972) reported that with the increase in interstitial fluid, however, pulmonary compliance is reduced and work of breathing increased, leading to tachypnea. Ralph and colleagues (1985) documented that when alveoli are flooded air spaces are lost and areas of low ventilation-perfusion ratio — V/Q — are increased.

The net effect of these events is a decrease in — FRC, decreased static and dynamic pulmonary compliance, an increase in low V/Q alveoli, and an increase in shunting — Qs/Qt. These changes result in hypoxemia resistant to increases in inspired oxygen concentration. The excretion of carbon dioxide, a highly diffusible gas, however, is not usually impaired.

These events represent the early, or exudative, phase of ARDS. Within a few days of the initial injury, this exudative phase is followed by a proliferative phase. Type II pneumocytes proliferate to replace the lost type I cells. Because these type II cells are approximately 10 times the thickness of the type I cells they replace, diffusion distance is increased, as Bachofen and Wiebel (1977) pointed out. Fibroblasts in the interstitium show cytologic features consistent with an activated state. Such breaks in the alveolar basement membrane, as suggested by Zapol and associates (1983), may allow these activated fibroblasts into the alveolus. The polymorphonuclear leukocytes in the interstitium also begin to destroy elastin, thus markedly increasing the work necessary to expand the lung.

Pulmonary vascular resistance is also markedly increased at this phase. Several explanations for this increase have been advanced. Zapol and associates (1977) showed that the alveolar capillaries filled with microemboli and thrombi. Jones and colleagues (1985) suggested that these capillaries may also have been completely destroyed. Circulating thromboxane, elaborated by hepatic macrophages, is also a potent vasoconstrictor, as pointed out by Harlan and co-workers (1983). Last, recent studies by Rossaint and colleagues (1993) have shown that endothelial relaxation depends critically on nitric oxide and that nitric oxide synthetase is decreased during many of the conditions associated with ARDS. As pulmonary fibrosis and vascular constriction advance, pulmonary architecture becomes severely deranged. Separation between air spaces and vasculature develops, resulting in increased dead space and shunting. Fibrosis also greatly decreases pulmonary compliance, necessitating mechanical ventilation with high airway pressures. Lamy and colleagues (1976) reported that high airway pressures may cause over-distention of the terminal airways, leading to the formation of cavities, or pneumatoceles. Also contributing to this process is ischemia, necrosis, and autolysis. Such areas may contribute to increased dead space —

Vd/Vt. These cavities may also rupture from high ventilatory pressure — barotrauma, leading to pneumothorax; tension pneumothorax; or the formation of a bronchopleural fistula (see Chapter 65).

Not all patients with ARDS pass through this sequence of progressive destruction of the pulmonary system. Even with significant pulmonary fibrosis, recovery can occur. In patients who do recover, type II pneumocytes differentiate into type I pneumocytes to regenerate the alveolar epithelium. Much of the interstitial fibrosis resolves over time, and several studies have shown remarkable recovery of pulmonary function. According to the study of Elliott and associates (1981), lung mechanics and volumes usually recover or are only mildly reduced within 6 to 12 months after the acute phase. Patients who did not have pre-existing lung disease returned to normal physical activity, although most have persistently reduced exercise tolerance.

MECHANISMS OF PULMONARY ENDOTHELIAL INJURY

As previously noted, the final common pathway to ARDS includes the development of increased alveolar capillary permeability. Therefore, a great deal of effort has been devoted to defining the mechanisms of endothelial injury and the mediators involved in the injury process. Because of the diversity of the conditions that are associated with the development of ARDS (Table 66–1), Maunder (1986) and Winn (1987) and their colleagues suggested that there are multiple mechanisms of injury.

Growing evidence suggests that one mechanism involves the activation of PMNs, which aggregate and adhere to the capillary endothelium. Pathologic examinations of lungs from patients with early ARDS have demonstrated large numbers of neutrophils sequestered in the pulmonary vasculature and interstitium. Bronchoalveolar lavage in early ARDS generally demonstrates a substantial increase in the number of PMNs in the lavage fluid.

A variety of events may cause increased neutrophil adhesiveness and activation. Endotoxemia, trauma, burns, immune complexes, pancreatitis, and sepsis all lead to activation of complement, and complement is a potent activator of PMNs. Prostaglandins, leukotrienes, and lymphokines also cause neutrophil migration. Neutrophils can release proteases, reactive oxygen metabolites, arachidonic acid metabolites, platelet-activating factor, and other agents that are potentially injurious to the host. A number of investigators, including Sacks (1978), Weiss (1981), and Martin (1981) and their associates, have shown that superoxide, peroxide, and other reactive oxygen metabolite species released by activated neutrophils can damage endothelial cells, parenchymal cells, membranes, and enzymes. Others, such as Bruce and associates (1981) as well as Carp and Janoff (1980), have observed that these species inactivate alpha-proteinase inhibitor, a globulin normally present in plasma that protects the lung and

Table 66–1. Some Conditions Associated with Adult Respiratory Distress Syndrome

Conditions Associated with Direct Lung Injury
Pneumonia
  Viral
  Bacterial
  Myocoplasma
  Fungal
  Legionnaire's
Aspiration
  Gastric contents
  Near-drowning with water aspiration
Toxic Inhalation
  Smoke
  Chemical fumes
  Oxygen toxicity
Pulmonary contusion
Radiation Pneumonitis

Conditions Associated with Indirect Lung Injury
Shock
  Septic
  Anaphylactic
  Cardiogenic*
  Hemorrhagic†
Embolism
  Fat
  Air
  Amniotic fluid
Disseminated Intravascular Coagulation
Trauma
  Extrathoracic
  Head
  Burns
Metabolic
  Diabetic ketoacidosis
  Uremia
Pancreatitis
Post Cardiopulmonary Bypass
  Drugs
    Narcotics — heroin, methadone, darvon, codeine
    Barbiturates
    Salicylates
    Ethchlorvynol
    Thiazides
    Propoxyphene
    Colchicine
    Paraquat

*See Edelman NH, et al: Experimental cardiogenic shock: pulmonary performance after acute myocardial infarction. Am J Physiol 219:1723, 1970.

†See Buckberg GD, et al: Pulmonary changes following hemorrhagic shock and resuscitation in baboons. J Thorac Cardiovasc Surg 59:450, 1970.

other tissues from damage by proteolytic enzymes, particularly elastase.

Polymorphonuclear leukocyte-derived elastase is one of several proteases that have been found by Janoff and colleagues (1979), among others, to digest structural proteins, including collagen, elastin, and fibronectin. These proteases also activate complement, cleave fibrinogen and Hageman factor, and thereby lead to a multifaceted amplification of inflammation and lung injury.

As described previously, there is destruction of the capillary architecture in ARDS. Platelet-activating factor, as noted by Hechtman and co-workers (1984), is synthesized and released by activated PMNs, leading to platelet aggregation and thrombosis. Disseminated intravascular coagulopathy has been reported by Bone and associates (1976) in nearly one fourth of patients with ARDS, and the fibrin-degradation products thus released, according to Manwaring and colleagues (1978), may alter microvascular permeability. Although Greene and associates (1981) presented angiographic evidence of clot formation in the pulmonary microvasculature, Binder and colleagues (1980) showed that anticoagulants are not effective in reversing this process.

Polymorphonuclear leukocytes also increase the production of arachidonic acid metabolites, including prostaglandins and leukotrienes. The prostaglandins, especially thromboxane, are potent pulmonary vasoconstrictors, as noted by Harlan (1983) and Winn (1983) and their associates, and may cause both pulmonary hypertension and an increase in lymphatic flow. Thromboxane A_2 may cause not only platelet aggregation but bronchoconstriction as well.

Leukotrienes cause bronchoconstriction and increased pulmonary endothelial permeability, as well as being potent chemotactic agents attracting still more PMNs.

These data strongly implicate the PMN as at least one important agent in the pathogenesis of ARDS, but other studies strongly argue that they are not solely responsible. In both clinical studies, such as that of Ognibene and colleagues (1986), and laboratory experiments such as that conducted by Winn and co-workers (1987), ARDS occurs in the presence of severe neutropenia. Even the complete inhibition of PMN-endothelial cell binding by a monoclonal antibody to one of the leukocyte adhesion molecules, as demonstrated by Vedder and associates (1988), fails to prevent lung injury.

Direct damage to the alveolar capillary interface occurs with acid aspiration, with the inhalation of toxic substances — particularly hydrocarbons, and with fat embolization. Almost certainly, other mechanisms of injury are still to be elucidated, and these may include other cellular or chemical mediators.

CLINICAL CHARACTERISTICS

The development of ARDS is initiated with a predisposing injury or illness. The first clinical findings are only those associated with that process. Petty and Ashbaugh (1971) reported that the signs of progressive respiratory failure generally begin within 12 to 24 hours, although it is not uncommon for the presentation to occur at 4 to 5 days. Tachypnea and tachycardia, as noted by Pepe and colleagues (1983), progress to dyspnea and hypoxemia as interstitial edema and alveolar flooding, respectively, develop. The edema may result in severe hypoxemia, decreased static and dynamic compliance, diffuse bilateral infiltrates, pulmonary hypertension, and

a decrease in functional residual capacity (Fig. 66–4). However, it is essential to realize, as emphasized by Gattinoni and associates (1988), that these processes are not uniformly distributed through the lung. This fact has profound implications for clinical management.

In the initial phase, dead space is only moderately increased. As the process progresses to severe pulmonary fibrosis with widespread destruction of normal pulmonary architecture, dead space is markedly elevated and compliance is markedly reduced. In this phase, unlike the early phase, oxygenation is less of a problem, while CO_2 elimination becomes more difficult.

TREATMENT

Although ARDS was first described as a distinct clinical entity in 1967 by Ashbaugh and colleagues (1967) and has been the subject of considerable basic and clinical investigation during the intervening years, definitive treatment remains elusive, and therapeutic efforts are still largely supportive. Agents that may interrupt some of the pathologic processes are being developed and tested. In addition to the provision of supportive care, identification and treatment of the underlying disease process is essential. In general, unless this is accomplished, continuing assault on the lung with progression of respiratory and other organ system failure is likely. Vigilance in preventing and treating infections and other organ system dysfunction that frequently occurs in patients with ARDS is crucial, because concurrent sepsis or the failure of additional organs markedly increases mortality.

The goals of supportive care for patients with ARDS are to ensure adequate tissue oxygen delivery; support adequate nutrition for wound repair and anabolism; provide adequate patient comfort; and minimize the risk of further damage to the lung or to other organ systems.

Support of Gas Exchange

Patients with severe respiratory failure require some form of support of gas exchange to ensure adequate ventilation and oxygenation. Patients with ARDS will have increased work of breathing as a result of decreased compliance. Patients unable to support this additional work themselves will become hypercarbic and, thus, will require mechanical ventilatory assistance for adequate oxygenation and ventilation.

The hypoxemia of ARDS is generally not responsive to supplemental oxygenation alone. When adequate oxygenation — $Po_2 > 60$ — cannot be maintained with a — presumably — nontoxic concentration of inspired oxygen — $Fio_2 < 0.5$ — measures to increase FRC are required. Available techniques include continuous positive airway pressure — CPAP and PEEP, either alone or combined with mechanical ventilatory support.

As described previously, early ARDS is characterized by alveolar flooding, airway closure, and a decrease in compliance and in FRC. The decrease in FRC results in an increase in intrapulmonary shunt and, hence,

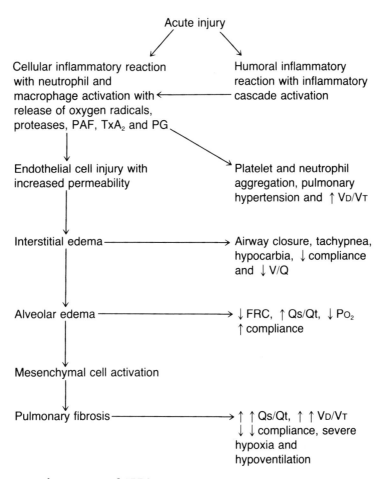

Fig. 66–4. Clinical characteristics and progression of ARDS.

hypoxemia. Because a substantial fraction of pulmonary artery blood flow is routed through areas of the lung that are not ventilated, supplemental oxygen alone is unlikely to produce a meaningful increase in systemic arterial oxygenation. Positive end-expiratory pressure and CPAP, however, increase FRC by shifting tidal ventilation to above the critical closing pressure, resulting in an opening of previously closed or partially closed airway units. According to Suter (1985), this opening may also improve compliance.

Positive end-expiratory pressure increases intrathoracic trauma and may cause barotrauma or impede cardiac filling, or both, causing a decrease in cardiac output. The hemodynamic effect can usually be offset by fluid administration but must be done with a flow-directed, thermistor-tipped pulmonary artery catheter in place to permit objective measurement of cardiac output. Therefore, PEEP must be carefully titrated to allow adequate arterial oxygenation — $Pa_{O_2} > 60$, $F_{I_{O_2}} < 0.5$, while still allowing adequate cardiac output. It is essential that the clinician understand that PEEP and CPAP are *supportive* measures only. Seen in this light, it will be clear that there is no benefit to be achieved — but considerable risk incurred — by pushing PEEP to levels beyond the minimum necessary for adequate oxygenation at safe inspired oxygen con-

centrations. Similarly, there is no prophylactic benefit from PEEP. Pepe and colleagues (1984) advised that its use in patients at risk to develop ARDS is not beneficial and carries a risk of morbidity.

As parenchymal consolidation, fibrosis, and severe derangements of the pulmonary architecture occur in the later stages of ARDS, PEEP may be less effective and may not alter the severely decreased static and dynamic compliance. The hemodynamic effect of PEEP may be lessened, because pressure is transmitted less well through stiffened lungs. This is, however, unpredictable, as noted by Marini (1990), because ARDS is a very heterogeneous process and affects the lung in a patchy pattern.

Other modes of ventilatory support have also been studied. High-frequency ventilation is a technique that limits inflation pressure and tidal volume and, by extrapolation, hyperinflation of the lung. Although it has been shown to be safe by the work of Carlon and associates (1983), it seems to offer no benefit over conventional, volume-cycled ventilation. In fact, according to Enderson and Rice (1987), it may well be less effective in sustaining oxygenation.

Pressure-controlled inverse ratio ventilation — PcIRV — is another approach. It is also pressure-cycled and reverses the inspiratory-to-expiratory ratio, producing a much longer inspiratory phase, which presumably permits a greater length of time for gas mixing in distal lung units, as well as keeping the lung inflated for a much longer fraction of the respiratory cycle. Lain and co-workers (1989) have noted that it appears to result in improved oxygenation and lower peak airway pressures but may markedly affect cardiac output by decreasing venous return. Its role in the management of patients with severe ARDS awaits clarification by a prospective clinical trial.

Nonspecific Support

Fluid replacement therapy in ARDS has been controversial. Some advocate the use of colloids, arguing that plasma oncotic pressure is thus increased, minimizing fluid movement across the capillary membrane. This line of argument, however, ignores the fact that in ARDS, the capillary membrane becomes more or less freely permeable, and that oncotic pressure cannot, therefore, be sustained. Protein moves across the capillary and into the interstitium. Any increase in oncotic pressure is, thus, as noted by Sibbald (1983) and Metildi (1984) and their associates, very transitory. To date, there has been no study to demonstrate that either colloids or crystalloids are superior to the other. Because the cost of colloids is quite great in comparison to crystalloids, routine use of colloids would appear to be unjustified.

The goal of fluid therapy in ARDS is to ensure adequate cardiac output and tissue perfusion while keeping cardiac filling pressures as low as possible to minimize any hydrostatic component of pulmonary edema. The pulmonary artery catheter may provide useful guidance by permitting the measurement of cardiac output and filling pressure, and by allowing measurement of mixed venous oxygenation. A further refinement of the pulmonary artery catheter is the incorporation of a rapid-response thermistor that, combined with an electrode to detect the cardiac cycle, permits the measurement of right ventricular end-systolic and end-diastolic volumes. In some settings, where high airway pressures may make the interpretation of pulmonary artery occlusion pressure difficult, Eddy and colleagues (1993) suggest that using end-diastolic volume of the right ventricle as a guide to fluid therapy may be extremely helpful.

Although there has been enthusiasm for the use of diuretics, based on their utility in cardiogenic pulmonary edema, most observers have not found them to be helpful. In fact, diuretics are most likely to result in the depletion of intravascular blood volume, leaving extravascular lung water unaffected.

In patients with severe hypoxemia, minimizing oxygen consumption may become necessary. Fever should be treated, because it increases metabolism and oxygen consumption. Both sedation and the careful use of neuromuscular paralysis may also assist in minimizing oxygen consumption.

General Support

As previously discussed, concurrent infection or multiorgan system failure greatly increases the morbidity and mortality associated with ARDS. The clinician must, therefore, be vigilant in efforts to protect other organ systems and prevent infection. For example, prophylaxis against stress-related gastric bleeding by the use of antacids, H_2 blocking agents, or — of preference — sucralfate, is strongly indicated. Strict adherence to sterile technique — especially meticulous handwashing — and careful surveillance for possible sites of infection is crucial. Infections that are identified should be promptly treated: with surgical drainage where indicated and with appropriate antimicrobial therapy.

Several studies, such as those of Stontenbeck (1984) and Ledingham (1988) and their associates, have suggested that selective decontamination of the gastrointestinal tract may diminish the likelihood of secondary bacterial pneumonia. Other studies, including that of Cerra and colleagues (1992), however, have been unable to confirm these results, and a large multicenter trial is underway to clarify the issue.

Nutritional support is essential, because starvation impairs wound healing and respiratory function. Nutrition may be administered either parenterally or, whenever possible, enterally. The latter route is preferred because of cost and because it appears, as noted by Border and co-workers (1987), to decrease both gastrointestinal hemorrhage and septic complications.

New Directions

Extracorporeal Membrane Oxygenation

The provision of adequate arterial oxygenation in the face of severe lung injury can become virtually impossible by conventional means. Extrapolating from its use in cardiac surgery, extracorporeal membrane oxygenation — ECMO — has been seen as a potentially useful approach for nearly 20 years. The NHLBI (1979) study conducted in the 1970s, however, although demonstrating improvement in hypoxemia and hypercarbia, failed to demonstrate any improvement in patient survival. Techniques have been improved subsequently, and there is renewed enthusiasm for its use. In children, particularly neonates and infants, Bartlett and associates (1986) reported that its use seems to definitely result in improved survival. Whether this finding will hold true in adults awaits further study, although initial results are discouraging.

A related technique is that of using low-frequency ventilation coupled with extracorporeal removal of CO_2. Although some workers including Gattinoni and colleagues (1980, 1986), have shown promising results, the technique has not been widely adopted.

Steroids

Although steroids have been widely used in treating ARDS, their efficacy has not been established. There is considerable theoretical support for their use: stabilization of lysosomal membranes, decreased neutrophil chemotaxis, decreased complement activation, decreased availability of arachidonic acid, preservation of endothelial integrity, and scavenging of reactive oxygen metabolites. Several trials reported by Weigelt (1985) and Luce (1988) and their associates, however, have failed to show any beneficial effect of steroids in interrupting the progression of the acute phase of ARDS. It is possible, however, as noted by Ashbaugh and Maier (1985), that steroids may be useful in the later stage of ARDS in those patients with progressive pulmonary fibrosis. Because of the substantial risks associated with steroid therapy, however, its proponents emphasize the importance of obtaining an open lung biopsy to exclude secondary infection and confirm the suspected histologic process before proceeding.

Eicosanoids

Nunn (1987) has pointed out that nonsteroidal anti-inflammatory agents inhibit cyclo-oxygenase, interfering with the synthesis of thromboxane A_2 and thromboxane, and as reported by Bernard and Brigham (1986), modulate PMN activation and margination. Price (1986) and Winn (1983) and their colleagues noted that they also block the development of pulmonary hypertension. In addition, Demling and LaLonde (1990) have shown that lipid peroxidation caused by reactive oxygen metabolites can be prevented by pretreatment with ibuprofen. Although these effects are of potential benefit in ARDS, to date, no clinical study has demonstrated their utility in the clinical setting.

Prostaglandin E_1

As described previously, ARDS produces intense pulmonary arteriolar vasoconstriction and accompanying pulmonary hypertension. Prostaglandin E_1 — PGE_1, another product of arachidonic acid metabolism, has certain actions that might be of benefit to the patient with ARDS. Prostaglandin E_1 has been shown by Craddock (1978) to cause pulmonary vasodilation; by Riukin and coworkers (1975), to cause suppression of neutrophil prophylaxis; by Zurier and associates (1974), to cause blockage of lysosomal enzyme release; and by Lehmeyer and Johnston (1978), to cause suppression of superoxide production. For these reasons, a study of its use in patients with ARDS reported by Holcroft and associates (1989) suggested that mortality might be improved. A subsequent study by Bone and colleagues (1989), however, failed to confirm these results.

Nitric Oxide

One of the major disadvantages of any vasodilation strategy delivered intravenously is that it will affect both those capillaries that are adjacent to ventilated alveoli — which should be beneficial to oxygenation — *and* those that are adjacent to nonventilated alveoli — which will worsen arterial oxygenation. A new approach has been recently described and may address this problem.

Nitric oxide is a potent gaseous vasodilator synthesized from L-arginine. It is produced in vivo by the vascular endothelium and is the principal endothelial-derived relaxing factor. It is rapidly metabolized.

In a study by Rossaint and associates (1993) of 10 patients with severe ARDS, nitric oxide was delivered by inhalation. Pulmonary artery pressure and pulmonary vascular resistance were markedly reduced, while systemic pressures and resistance were unaffected. Arterial oxygenation improved, and seven patients who received long-term treatment survived. Although this is a very early observation and awaits confirmation by larger, prospective, controlled trial, the rationale for the use of nitric oxide by this route is sound, and the likelihood of side effects is low.

PREVENTION

Many clinical, physiologic, and laboratory parameters have been surveyed in attempts to identify those patients likely to develop ARDS. To date, identification by predisposing clinical events has been the most useful. High-risk events include sepsis syndrome, aspiration of gastric contents, multiple blood transfusions, multiple fractures, and shock. Multiple risk events increase the chances of developing ARDS. Wherever possible, it is important to prevent or minimize the likelihood of development of sepsis, avoid airway contamination, and minimize blood transfusion. Early fixation of fractures in trauma victims is clearly beneficial.

The single most useful laboratory study in the identification of patients at risk for ARDS is sequential arterial blood gas analysis. Weigelt and colleagues (1981) pointed out that decreasing arterial oxygen tension necessitating increases in inspired oxygen concentration may indicate pulmonary deterioration. Several substances have been proposed as markers or mediators of lung injury, but the measurement of these substances has proven to be neither sensitive nor specific.

CONCLUSION

The high mortality rate associated with ARDS has changed little since 1967, when ARDS was first described. Current therapy remains primarily supportive, although as our understanding of the cellular and biochemical events that characterize this syndrome become increasingly well understood, definitive therapy to abort or prevent its development is more and more likely.

REFERENCES

Andreadis N, Petty TL: Adult respiratory distress syndrome: problems and progress. Am Rev Respir Dis 132:1344, 1985.
Appel PJ, Shoemaker WC: Hemodynamic and oxygen transport effects

of prostaglandin E_1 in patients with adult respiratory distress syndrome. Crit Care Med 12:528, 1984.

Ashbaugh DG, et al: Acute respiratory distress in adults. Lancet 2:319, 1967.

Ashbaugh DG, Maier RV: Idiopathic pulmonary fibrosis in adult respiratory distress syndrome: diagnosis and treatment. Arch Surg 120:350, 1985.

Bachofen M, Weibel ER: Alterations of the gas exchange apparatus in adult respiratory insufficiency associated with septicemia. Am Rev Respir Dis 116:589, 1977.

Bachofen M, Weibel ER: Structural alterations of lung parenchyma in the adult respiratory distress syndrome. Am J Surg 144:124, 1982.

Bartlett RH, et al: Extracorporeal membrane oxygenation (ECMO) in neonatal respiratory failure. Ann Surg 204:236, 1986.

Becker EL, Ward PA: Chemotaxis. In Parker CW (ed): Clinical Immunology. Philadelphia: WB Saunders, 1980, p 272.

Bernard GR, Brigham KL: Pulmonary edema: pathophysiologic mechanisms and new approaches to therapy. Chest 89:594, 1986.

Binder AS, et al: Effect of heparin on fibrinogen depletion on lung fluid balance in sheep after emboli. J Appl Physiol 48:414, 1980.

Bone RC, Francis PB, Pierce AK: Intravascular coagulation associated with the adult respiratory distress syndrome. Am J Med 61:585, 1976.

Bone RC, Maunder R, Hyers TM, Urspring JJ: Randomized double-blind, multicenter study of prostaglandin E_1 in patients with the adult respiratory distress syndrome. Chest 96:114, 1989.

Border JR, et al: The gut-origin septic states in blunt multiple trauma (ISS-40) in the ICU. Ann Surg 206:427, 1987.

Bruce MC, et al: Inactivation of alpha$_1$-proteinase inhibitor in infants exposed to high concentrations of oxygen (abstract). Am Rev Respir Dis 123(Suppl):166, 1981.

Carlon GC, et al: High frequency jet ventilation: a prospective randomized evaluation. Chest 84:551, 1983.

Carp H, Janoff A: Potential mediator of inflammation: phagocyte-derived oxidants suppress the elastase-inhibitory capacity of alpha$_1$-proteinase inhibitor in vitro. J Clin Invest 66:987, 1980.

Cerra FB, et al: Selective gut decontamination reduces nosocomial infections and length of stay but not mortality or organ failure in surgical intensive care patients. Arch Surg 127:163, 1992.

Clermont HG, Williams JS, Adams JT: Steroid effect on the release of the lysosomal enzyme acid phosphatase in shock. Ann Surg 179:917, 1974.

Craddock PR: Corticosteroid-induced lymphopenia, immuno-suppression, and body defense. Ann Intern Med 88:564, 1978.

Demling RH, LaLonde C: Early postburn lipid peroxidation: Effect of ibuprofen and allopurinol. Surgery 107:85, 1990.

Divertie MB: The adult respiratory distress syndrome. Mayo Clin Proc 57:371, 1982.

Douglas ME, Downs JB: Pulmonary function following severe acute respiratory failure and high levels of positive end-expiratory pressure. Chest 71:18, 1977.

Eddy CA, Rice CL, Amardi DM: Right ventricular dysfunction in multiple trauma victims. Am J Surg (in press) 1993.

Elliott CG, Morris AH, Cengiz M: Pulmonary function and exercise gas exchange in survivors of adult respiratory distress syndrome. Am Rev Respir Dis 123:492, 1981.

Enderson BL, Rice CL: High frequency ventilation. World J Surg 11:167, 1987.

Fein AM, et al: The risk factors, incidence, and prognosis of the adult respiratory distress syndrome following septicemia. Chest 83:40, 1983.

Fowler AA, et al: Adult respiratory distress syndrome: risk with common predispositions. Ann Intern Med 98:593, 1983.

Gattinoni L, et al: Treatment of acute respiratory failure, with low-frequency positive-pressure ventilation and extracorporeal removal of CO_2. Lancet 2:292, 1980.

Gattinoni L, et al: Low-frequency positive pressure ventilation with extracorporeal CO_2 removal in severe acute respiratory failure. JAMA 256:881, 1986.

Gattinoni L, et al: Relationships between lung computed tomographic density, gas exchange, and PEEP in acute respiratory failure. Anesthesiology 69:824, 1988.

Glauser FL, Millen JE, Falls R: Effects of acid aspiration on pulmonary alveolar epithelial membrane permeability. Chest 76:201, 1979.

Greene R, et al: Early bedside detection of pulmonary vascular occlusion during acute respiratory failure. Am Rev Respir Dis 124:593, 1981.

Hammerschmidt DE, et al: Corticosteroids inhibit complement-induced granulocyte aggregation: a possible mechanism for their efficacy in shock states. J Clin Invest 63:798, 1979.

Hammerschmidt EE, et al: Association of complement activation and elevated plasma C_5 with adult respiratory distress syndrome. Lancet 1:947, 1980.

Harlan J, et al: Selective inhibition of thromboxane synthesis during experimental endotoxemia in the goat: effects on pulmonary hemodynamics and lung lymph flow. Br J Clin Pharmacol 1:1235, 1983.

Hasleton PS: Adult respiratory distress syndrome — a review. Histopathology 7:307, 1983.

Hechtman HB, Valeri CR, Shepro D: Role of hormonal mediators in adult respiratory distress syndrome. Chest 86:623, 1984.

Holcroft JW, et al: Increased survival of patients with acute respiratory failure (ARDS) resulting from shock, trauma, or sepsis treated with prostin VR sterile solution (PGE 1; Alprostadil). Unpublished manuscript. Investigation data. University of California and The Upjohn Company, 1989.

Iliff LD, Greene RE, Hughes IMB: Effects of interstitial edema on distribution of ventilation and perfusion in isolated lung. J Appl Physiol 33:462, 1972.

Janoff A, et al: Lung injury induced by leukocytic proteases. Am J Pathol 97:111, 1979.

Janoff A: Proteases and lung injury, state of the art mini-review. Chest 83:548, 1983.

Jones R, et al: Pulmonary vascular pathology. In Zapol WM, Falke KJ (eds): Acute Respiratory Failure. New York: Marcel Dekker, 1985, p 23.

Kaplan RL, Sahn SA, Petty TL: Incidence and outcome of the respiratory distress syndrome in gram-negative sepsis. Arch Intern Med 139:867, 1979.

Klein JJ, et al: Pulmonary function after recovery from adult respiratory distress syndrome. Chest 69:350, 1976.

Lain DC, DiBenedetto R, Nguyen AV, Causey D: Pressure control inverse ratio ventilation as a method to reduce peak inspiratory pressure and provide adequate ventilation and oxygenation. Chest 95:1081, 1989.

Lakshminarayan S, Stanford RL, Petty TL: Prognosis after recovery from adult respiratory distress syndrome. Am Rev Respir Dis 113:7, 1976.

Lamy M, et al: Pathologic features and mechanisms of hypoxemia in adult respiratory distress syndrome. Am Rev Respir Dis 114:267, 1976.

Ledingham IM, et al: Triple regimen of selective decontamination of the digestive tract, systemic cefotaxime, and microbiological surveillance for prevention of acquired infection in intensive care. Lancet 1:785, 1988.

Lehmeyer JE, Johnston RB Jr: Effect of anti-inflammatory drugs and agents that elevate intracellular ABP on the release of toxic oxygen metabolites by phagocytes: studies in a model of tissue-bound I$_a$G. Clin Immunol Immunopathol 9:482, 1978.

Lowe RJ, et al: Crystalloid vs. colloid in the etiology of pulmonary failure after trauma: a randomized trial in man. Surgery 81:676, 1977.

Luce JM, et al: Ineffectiveness of high-dose methylprednisolone in preventing parenchymal lung injury and improving mortality in patients with septic shock. Am Rev Respir Dis 138:62, 1988.

Lung Program, National Heart and Lung Institute: Respiratory Diseases: Task Force on Problems. Research Approaches, Needs. Bethesda, MD: National Institutes of Health, 1972.

MacDonnell KF, Fahey PJ, Segal MS (eds): Respiratory Intensive Care. Boston: Little, Brown, 1987, p 423.

Malo J, et al: How does PEEP reduce Qs/Qt in pulmonary edema? Fed Proc 39:280, 1980.

Manwaring D, Thorning D, Curreri PW: Mechanisms of acute pulmonary dysfunction induced by fibrinogen degradation product C. Surgery 84:45, 1978.

Marini JJ: Lung mechanics in the adult respiratory distress syndrome: recent conceptual advances and implications for management. Clin Chest Med. *11*:673, 1990.

Martin WJ, et al: Oxidant injury of lung parenchymal cells. J Clin Invest *68*:1277, 1981.

Maunder RJ: Clinical prediction of the adult respiratory distress syndrome. Clin Chest Med 6:413, 1985.

Maunder RJ, et al: Occurrence of the adult respiratory distress syndrome in neutropenic patients. Am Rev Respir Dis *133*:3113, 1986.

Metildi LA, et al: Crystalloid versus colloid in fluid resuscitation of patients with severe pulmonary insufficiency. Surg Gynecol Obstet *158*:207, 1984.

Meyrick BO: Pathology of pulmonary edema. Semin Respir Med *4*:267, 1983.

Montgomery AB, et al: Causes of mortality in patients with the adult respiratory distress syndrome. Am Rev Respir Dis *132*:485, 1985.

National Heart, Lung, and Blood Institute, Division of Lung Diseases: Extracorporeal Support for Respiratory Insufficiency. Bethesda, MD: National Institutes of Health, 1979, p 243.

Nunn JF: Applied Respiratory Physiology. Boston, Butterworths, 1987, p 290.

Ognibene FP, et al: Adult respiratory distress syndrome in patients with severe neutropenia. N Engl J Med *315*:548, 1986.

Pepe PE, et al: Clinical predictors of the adult respiratory distress syndrome. Am J Surg *144*:124, 1982.

Pepe PE, et al: Early prediction of the adult respiratory distress syndrome by a simple scoring method. Ann Emerg Med *12*:749, 1983.

Pepe PE, Hudson LD, Carrico CJ: Early application of positive end-expiratory pressure in patients at risk for the adult respiratory distress syndrome. N Engl J Med *311*:281, 1984.

Petty TL, Ashbaugh DG: The adult respiratory distress syndrome. Chest *60*:233, 1971.

Price S, et al: Indomethacin, dazoxiben and extravascular lung water after E. coli infusion. J Surg Res *41*:189, 1986.

Ralph DD, et al: Distribution of ventilation and perfusion during positive end-expiratory pressure in the adult respiratory distress syndrome. Am Rev Respir Dis *131*:54, 1985.

Rossaint R, et al: Inhaled nitric oxide for the adult respiratory distress syndrome. N Engl J Med *328*:399, 1993.

Riukin I, Rosenblatt J, Becker E: The role of cyclic ABP in the chemotactic responsiveness and spontaneous mobility of rabbit neutrophil. J Immunol *115*:1126, 1975.

Sacks T, et al: Oxygen radicals mediate endothelial cell damage by complement-stimulated granulocytes: an in vitro model of immune vascular damage. J Clin Invest *61*:1161, 1978.

Said S, et al: Pulmonary surface activity in induced pulmonary edema. J Clin Invest *44*:458, 1965.

Sibbald WJ, et al: The short-term effects of increasing plasma colloid osmotic pressure in patients with noncardiac pulmonary edema. Surgery *93*:620, 1983.

Stontenbeck CP, et al: The prevention of superinfection in multiple trauma patients. J Antimicrob Chemother *14*(Suppl B):B203, 1984.

Suter PM: Assessment of respiratory mechanics in ARDS. *In* Zapol WM, Falke KJ (eds): Acute Respiratory Failure. New York: Marcel Dekker, 1985, p 507.

Sibbald WJ, et al: The short-term effects of increasing plasma colloid osmotic pressure in patients with noncardiac pulmonary edema. Surgery *93*:620, 1983.

Vedder NB, et al: A monoclonal antibody to the adherence-promoting leukocyte glycoprotein, CD18, reduces organ injury and improves survival from hemorrhagic shock and resuscitation in rabbits. J Clin Invest *81*:939, 1988.

Weigelt JA, Snyder WH III, Mitchell RA: Early identification of patients prone to develop adult respiratory distress syndrome. Am J Surg *142*:687, 1981.

Weigelt JA, et al: Early steroid therapy for respiratory failure. Arch Surg *120*:536, 1985.

Weiland JE, et al: Lung neutrophils in the adult respiratory distress syndrome: clinical and pathophysiologic significance. Am Rev Respir Dis *133*:218, 1986.

Weiss SJ, et al: Role of hydrogen peroxide in neutrophil-mediated destruction of cultured endothelial cells. J Clin Invest *68*:714, 1981.

Winn R, et al: Thromboxane A_2 mediates lung vasoconstriction but not permeability after endotoxin. J Clin Invest *72*:911, 1983.

Winn R, et al: Neutrophil depletion does not prevent lung edema after endotoxin infusion in goats. J Appl Physiol *62*:116, 1987.

Yahav J, Liberman P, Molho M: Pulmonary function following the adult respiratory distress syndrome. Chest *74*:457, 1978.

Zapol WM, et al: Vascular obstruction causes pulmonary hypertension in severe acute respiratory failure. Chest *71*:307, 1977.

Zapol WM, et al: Pulmonary fibrosis in severe acute respiratory failure. Am Rev Respir Dis *119*:547, 1979.

Zapol WM, et al: Pathophysiologic pathways of the adult respiratory distress syndrome. *In* Tinker J, Rapin M (eds): Care of the Critically Ill Patient. New York: Springer-Verlag, 1983, p 341.

Zapol WM, Falke KJ (eds): Acute Respiratory Failure. Vol 24. New York: Marcel Dekker, 1985, p 423.

Zurier RB, et al: Mechanisms of lysosomal enzyme release from human leukocytes. J Clin Invest *53*:297, 1974.

READING REFERENCES

Buckberg GD, et al: Pulmonary changes following hemorrhagic shock and resuscitation in baboons. J Thorac Cardiovasc Surg *59*:450, 1970.

Edelman NH, et al: Experimental cardiogenic shock: pulmonary performance after acute myocardial infarction. Am J Physiol *219*:1723, 1970.

Pleet AB: "Shock lung" syndrome following diabetic ketoacidosis; treatment with heparin. Chest *63*:434, 1973.

CHAPTER 67

MANAGEMENT OF FOREIGN BODIES OF THE TRACHEOBRONCHIAL TREE

Lauren D. Holinger

Techniques of endoscopic manipulation and extraction of foreign objects and preoccupation with technical expertise have often overshadowed the broader clinical aspects of foreign body management. The collection of recovered foreign bodies at the Children's Memorial Hospital in Chicago, accumulated over 5000 objects. This is indeed impressive but is perhaps placed in a more realistic perspective if one realizes that this collection was amassed over a period of more than 35 years. The National Safety Council tells us that each year in the United States there are approximately 1000 deaths from ingestion of foreign bodies. The discrepancy, of course, lies in the fact that those foreign bodies that cause death usually do so quickly. Often such patients are examined by no physician other than the coroner or medical examiner.

ETIOLOGY

The propensity of small children to put whatever comes into their grasp into their mouths is well-known. To this may be added their tendency to imitate adults. The parent who holds pins, screws, or nails in his mouth should not be surprised when an infant puts such an object in his own mouth at the first opportunity.

Foreign body ingestion may be encouraged by failure of the patient's protective mechanisms in several ways. Most common of these is probably the loss of tactile sense in the hard palate when the patient wears a full upper denture. Diminution of perception and reflex action when the person is in a state of alcoholic intoxication, epileptic seizure, deep sleep, or unconsciousness is also a contributing cause.

Carelessness may contribute to foreign body ingestion in many ways: improper preparation of food, hasty eating and drinking, permitting children to play while eating, talking with food in the mouth, giving food such as peanuts to children who do not have the molar teeth to chew them, and improper supervision of small children playing near infants. Small children have been seen to deliberately feed an object they knew to be dangerous — such as a safety pin — to an infant sibling. Such primitive solutions to the problem of sibling rivalry can be eliminated only by careful supervision.

Some foreign bodies are made to resemble objects that would normally be put in or near the mouth and are physically easy to ingest, such as light, slippery, plastic imitation lipsticks and doll bottle caps. The plastic tip from a Bic pen can be aspirated by older children and even by adults.

Marketing trends also affect the type of foreign body ingested. Rarely today does one see safety pins as foreign bodies because of the popularity of disposable diapers. Disc battery ingestion has been reported since the mid-1970s because of the increased use of calculators, cameras, watches, and hearing aids. This is one of the few true foreign body emergencies, because, as Maves and associates (1984) noted, esophageal perforation can occur within 4 hours of the ingestion. Jacks have been replaced by attractively colored Lite Brite pegs and other nonradiopaque plastic toys that now challenge the endoscopist.

RADIOGRAPHIC AIDS

Radiographic studies provide valuable assistance to the endoscopist, not only in documenting presence of a foreign body but also as an aid in extraction. Incomplete studies may lead to errors in diagnosis. An ingested object may lodge anywhere from the base of the skull to the floor of the perineum. Although many foreign bodies are radiolucent, special techniques such as inspiration-expiration films and fluoroscopy — with or without contrast material — may help to establish the diagnosis.

Appropriate study and proper technique are needed to accurately locate the foreign body. The relationship of the foreign object to surrounding structures must be understood and visualized to properly plan the endoscopic procedure.

The lateral soft tissue film of the neck is one of the most useful single studies available to the endoscopist. Even without supplementary contrast material, the caliber of the airway is often readily appreciated. Holinger (1962) suggested an "endoscopic" lateral film, in which the arms and shoulders are held backward and downward. A profile of the air column in the larynx and trachea is thus visible in a single film (Fig. 67–1).

In addition to the anteroposterior and lateral films of the chest normally taken during inhalation (Fig. 67–2A), similar films taken at the end of exhalation are helpful (Fig. 67–2B). Such studies are especially useful in delineating obstructive emphysema because the trapping of air behind the foreign object — and the failure of the trapped air to empty on exhalation — is most apparent on this film. Some radiologists prefer lateral decubitus films. A dynamic demonstration of this phenomenon can be obtained by fluoroscopy, during which the motion of the chest throughout the entire respiratory cycle can be continuously observed.

Contrast material such as barium is used with great caution and only after plain films have been inadequate to delineate the specific problem. An object such as a chicken or pork bone may be apparent in the lateral soft tissue film of the neck. Administration of contrast material in such a situation necessitates delay of the endoscopic procedure until the material has passed beyond the stomach. Contrast material retained above an obstructive foreign body not only complicates the removal of the foreign object but also might be aspirated into the respiratory tract.

Bronchography has occasionally been useful to demonstrate the relationship of a foreign object to the bronchial tree or to localize a radiolucent plastic foreign object. If contrast material must be used, Lipiodol is preferable because it is translucent and less likely to obscure the object during endoscopy.

LARYNGEAL FOREIGN BODY

Laryngeal foreign bodies that cause complete obstruction result in sudden death unless removed immediately at the scene of the incident. Objects that are only partially obstructive may cause hoarseness, aphonia, croupy cough, odynophagia, hemoptysis, wheezing, and varying degrees of dyspnea. These symptoms may be caused by the foreign body itself or by a residual laryngeal reaction from a foreign body that has migrated to the trachea. Such symptoms can also be caused by attempts at removal. If the foreign body is in fact lodged in the esophagus, there may still be sufficient periesophageal reaction and obstruction to cause secretions to overflow into the larynx and cause the laryngeal symptoms as secondary manifestations of the presence of a foreign body.

TRACHEAL FOREIGN BODY

Signs of tracheal foreign bodies include: stridor, audible slap, palpatory thud, and asthmatoid wheeze. The diagnosis is made by radiographic studies, auscultation, palpation, and bronchoscopy.

Esclamado and Richardson (1987) have reported that soft tissue neck films are the most helpful radiographic studies.

BRONCHIAL FOREIGN BODY

The most common symptoms of bronchial foreign bodies are coughing and wheezing. There may be a history of aspiration or of tooth extraction. Obstructive

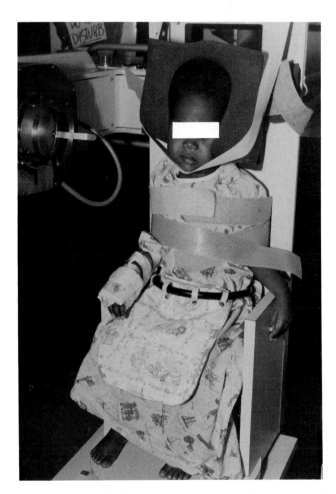

Fig. 67–1. Specially built chair used at the Children's Memorial Hospital in Chicago for soft tissue lateral radiographs of the neck and airway. The chin is held up, and the shoulders are down for consistently high-quality studies.

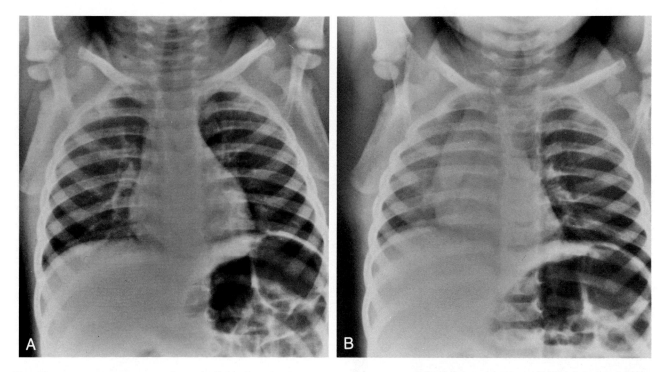

Fig. 67–2. *A,* Anteroposterior radiograph of the chest during inspiration. *B,* Anteroposterior radiograph of the chest during expiration. Note the trapping of air in the left lung field caused by a peanut in the left main stem bronchus.

foreign bodies cause emphysema, atelectasis, pulmonary edema, and eventually, pulmonary abscess. Organic materials are more apt to cause a relatively violent reaction, with the symptoms of laryngotracheal bronchitis, cough, and irregular fever. Any of these late manifestations may be obscured by prior treatment with antibiotics or steroids.

The physical signs of bronchial foreign bodies vary. Co-existing pathology, tracheobronchial anatomy, and type and location of the foreign body vary from one patient to another. Secretions, whether normal or pathological, may shift from one location to another. The foreign body itself may shift position and cause, from time to time, a variation in the aeration distal to the foreign object. Foreign bodies in the lower trachea may give rise to a variety of signs and symptoms localized in either or both lungs as the foreign body shifts its position in the region of the tracheal carina.

Radiographic examination should be made in conjunction with a careful physical examination. Obstructive emphysema, which may be apparent only on a good expiratory radiograph, sometimes can be discerned more readily by watching the patient's chest rise and fall with respiration and noting the lag in emptying on the obstructed side. Localization of the site of lodgement on the chest film depends on an accurate knowledge of the segments of the lung and the orifices of the segmental bronchi. The current medical practice of treating "asthmatic" or croupy children with antibiotics and steroids can obscure signs and symptoms that would normally be expected with a retained foreign object.

Clearing of symptoms with these agents cannot always be assumed to be diagnostic of a specific disease process. The fact that a wheeze disappears or that a pneumonic process clears may merely mean that a patient's reaction to the presence of the foreign object has been temporarily controlled. The recurrence of "asthma" after the withdrawal of therapy should heighten the physician's suspicion of a foreign object as the possible underlying cause of distress.

TREATMENT

In general, the treatment of choice for foreign bodies of the airway is reasonably prompt endoscopic removal under conditions of maximum safety and minimum trauma. Too often, foreign body aspirations are considered emergencies, leading to hasty, inadequate study, and poorly prepared, improper attempts at removal. The majority of patients with foreign bodies have already passed the acute phase. When there is no urgent danger to the patient's life, the problem can be approached with a complete and thoughtful consideration of the physiologic and mechanical factors involved. Endoscopic removal can be scheduled when trained personnel are available, instruments have been checked, and techniques have been tested.

The presence of a sharp or pointed foreign object, threateningly dramatized on a radiograph and compounded by parents' and referring physician's anxiety, must not be permitted to exert pressure on the endoscopist to act precipitously before necessary preparations have been made. However, untoward delay in removing the foreign body can also be harmful. Endoscopy, therefore, is deferred only until preparative studies have been performed and the patient has been prepared optimally for the operation by adequate hydration, emptying of the stomach, and so forth.

The three situations that are considered urgent are as follows: 1) Actual or potential airway obstruction. Foreign bodies in the larynx or tracheobronchial tree are removed the same day the diagnosis is made. 2) Aspiration of dried beans or peas into the airway. A major bronchus may be obstructed for a day until absorbed moisture finally bursts the capsule, and the child asphyxiates as the bean rapidly swells to occlude the trachea. 3) Disc battery ingestion with esophageal lodgement. Within 4 hours of ingestion, leakage of caustic battery contents may lead to erosion through the esophageal wall, as noted by Maves and colleagues (1984).

Heimlich Maneuver

Complete airway obstruction by a foreign body can be recognized in the conscious victim when a person who has been eating or has had a foreign body in his mouth is suddenly unable to speak or cough, even when asked, "can you speak?" Reflexively, or as a result of training, the victim may use the "distress signal of choking," which is the gesture of clutching the neck between the thumb and open palm. The Heimlich maneuver is indicated.

Finger Probing

Foreign objects that do not immediately cause complete obstruction but present with gagging, coughing, sputtering, wheezing, and so forth, place the physician in a position in which he may inadvertently make the patient worse. In such situations, probing the hypopharynx with the finger may impact a foreign body that is loose in the hypopharynx tightly into the larynx, thus transforming partial obstruction into complete obstruction; force the foreign body into the esophagus, where it may compress the trachea against the upper sternum, causing an obstruction that cannot be relieved even by tracheotomy; or — as the physician originally intended — remove the foreign body through the mouth or allow it to be carried harmlessly through the alimentary tract (Fig. 67–3).

Inhalation-Postural Drainage Technique

Burrington and Cotton (1972) introduced a controversial alternative to bronchoscopic extraction, consisting of inhalation of bronchodilator followed by postural drainage and percussion. This technique was continued up to 4 days before resorting to bronchoscopy.

Law and Kosloske (1976), however, found this technique had only a 25% success rate, compared to an 89%

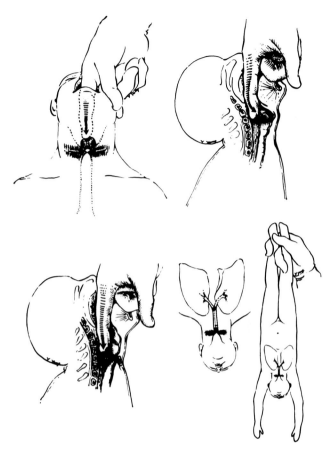

Fig. 67–3. Possible methods of impaction of a foreign body by ill-advised first aid. *From* Tucker GF Jr: Laryngeal and tracheobronchial foreign bodies. Trans Am Bronchoesoph Assoc 49:181, 1969.

success rate with bronchoscopy. They reported an episode of cardiopulmonary arrest secondary to migration of the foreign body from the bronchus to the trachea. This technique has been abandoned because of the greater risk of complication.

Flexible Bronchoscopy

Open-tube — rigid — bronchoscopy is the method of choice for removal of most foreign bodies from the tracheobronchial tree. Flexible fiber-optic bronchoscopy has no application in infants because there is no channel for ventilation, suction, or instrumentation. Thorburn and colleagues (1986) recommend flexible fiber-optic bronchoscopy in certain circumstances, including head and neck injury, patients with tracheotomy, and cases of peripheral foreign bodies.

Open-Tube — Rigid — Endoscopy

The open-tube bronchoscope is the instrument of choice for foreign body extractions. All other techniques should be discouraged unless the circumstances leave the physician no other choice.

The suspicion of the presence of a "foreign body" carries with it the unreasoning connotation that haste is always necessary. Deliberate speed is, of course, desirable in emergent situations. A properly trained endoscopic team with a full selection of instruments to meet the mechanical problems is of inestimable value in rising to the challenge presented by the true acute emergency. The experienced endoscopist also appreciates the value of careful preparation of himself, the patient, the instruments and the team before starting the procedure, because minimal morbidity and mortality depend on adequate preparation. If 2 hours are spent in such preparation, the safe endoscopic removal of the foreign body may take only 2 minutes. But if only 2 minutes are taken for preparation, the endoscopist may find himself attempting ineffective, makeshift procedures for the next frustrating 2 hours, as Holinger (1962) pointed out.

Following an unsuccessful attempt, for whatever reason, repeated instrumentation is not to be undertaken for several days, especially because the trauma of a second procedure might cause more edema, necessitating postoperative intubation. Such an interval might be used for steroid and antibiotic coverage to lessen laryngeal and bronchial reaction. Steroids should be withheld if there seems to be danger of esophageal perforation.

Time is also required to permit the stomach to empty of residual barium or food. Ideally, endoscopic procedures should be undertaken in the morning, when the team is at its best and a full range of ancillary services — anesthesia and radiology — is available. Children, especially, should be treated early in the day so that any untoward laryngeal reaction can be diagnosed and treated quickly.

Hospitals large enough to generate sufficient endoscopic treatment experience should concentrate this experience in the hands of those who are to handle foreign body problems. To request a doctor to remove foreign bodies but deny him the full range of endoscopic practice is a disservice to the patient. Even in the most specialized clinics, ingested foreign bodies constitute less than 5% of the overall endoscopic experience. Those hospitals that presume to offer this service to the patient must have available not only an experienced endoscopist but also a full team of nurse assistants, anesthesiologists, and radiologists, fully equipped to meet not only the apparent problems but also the unplanned complications.

Preliminary Study

The first step in the solution of the mechanical problem presented by the presence of any foreign body is the study of radiographs made in at least three planes: anteroposterior, lateral, and that corresponding to the greatest plane of the foreign body. The next step is to put a duplicate of the foreign body into a lung model and simulate the position shown by the radiographs to get an idea of the probable presentation. Because shifting may change the presentation, the duplicate foreign body is turned into as many different positions as possible to educate the eye in comprehending the possible presentations that may be encountered at bronchoscopy. For each presentation, a method of disimpaction, disengagement, disentanglement, or version and seizure should be worked out, as Jackson and Jackson (1936, 1959) emphasized.

Selection and Use of Forceps

Preliminary selection and test of forceps with a duplicate of the foreign body should be made in every case. It is sad to see a child arrive very ill or moribund from prolonged efforts elsewhere to remove a foreign body with forceps, the utter uselessness of which could have been determined in a moment by testing on a duplicate. In some cases, different forceps must be ready for different presentations. Forceps jaws must expand sufficiently to encompass the foreign body, if not in every diameter, at least in the diameter of the selected presentation.

Prepared by this practice and the radiographs, the endoscopist introduces the bronchoscope. The location of the foreign body is approached slowly and carefully to avoid overriding or displacement. A study of the presentation is as necessary for the bronchoscopist as for the obstetrician. The bronchoscopist should try to determine: the relation of the presenting part to the surrounding tissues and the probable position of the unseen portion, as determined by the appearance of the presenting part combined with the knowledge obtained by the radiographic studies.

The standard forward-grasping forceps has a powerful grip and is used on dense foreign bodies that require a very firm grip to prevent the forceps from slipping off. For more delicate manipulation, and particularly for friable foreign bodies, a lighter forceps, such as a fenestrated peanut forceps, is best. Forceps should be held in the right hand, the thumb in one ring and the third finger in the other ring. These fingers are used to open and close the forceps; all traction and pulsion is achieved by the right index finger, which is positioned on the forceps handle near the stylet (Fig. 67–4).

The bronchoscopist must resist the impulse to seize the foreign body as soon as he discovers it and must carefully study its size, shape, position, and relation to surrounding structures before making any attempt at extraction. When the most favorable point and position for grasping have been ascertained, the closed forceps is inserted through the bronchoscope. The forceps is advanced until it lightly touches the foreign body, then is allowed to expand. It is advanced far enough to grasp the object. If there are no sharp points on the foreign body, it is held, and the tube mouth is advanced against it. If it is too large to come out through the tube, it is held against the tube mouth,

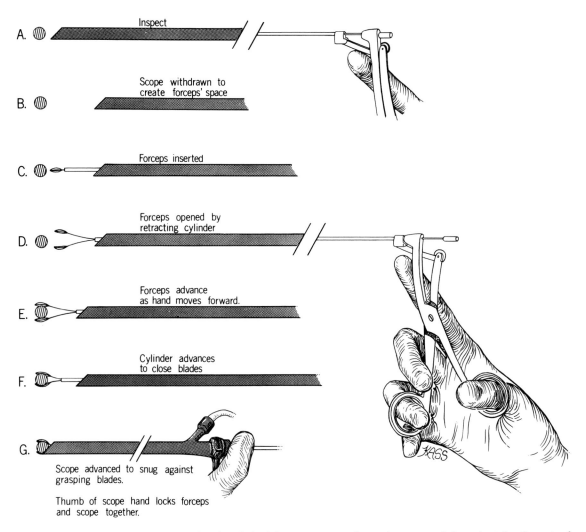

A. Inspect

B. Scope withdrawn to create forceps' space

C. Forceps inserted

D. Forceps opened by retracting cylinder

E. Forceps advance as hand moves forward.

F. Cylinder advances to close blades

G. Scope advanced to snug against grasping blades.

Thumb of scope hand locks forceps and scope together.

Fig. 67–4. Proper grasp of forceps. The right thumb and third finger are inserted into the rings and the right index finger is placed high on the handle. All traction is made with the index finger, the ring finger being used only to open and close the forceps. If any pushing is deemed safe, it may be done by placing the index finger behind the thumbnut on the eyelet. *From* Jackson C, Jackson CL: Diseases of the Air and Food Passages of Foreign Body Origin. Philadelphia: WB Saunders, 1936.

the grasp of the forceps being firmly maintained by the fingers on the right hand while all traction for withdrawal is made by the left hand, which firmly clamps forceps and bronchoscope as one piece. Thus, the three units are brought out as one, the endoscope keeping the vocal cords apart until the foreign body has entered the glottis.

Pins, needles, and similar pointed objects fall into two groups: 1) bendable pins and 2) breakable pins and needles. It is often desirable to bend a pin but less desirable to break it. When searching for pointed or sharp objects, special care must be taken not to override them. Pins are almost always found point upward.

Jackson's dictum states: "look not for the foreign body; look for the point." If the point is free, it should be worked into the lumen of the bronchoscope by manipulation with forceps and the lip of the tube. It then may be seized with the forceps and withdrawn. Should

the pin be grasped by the shaft, it is almost certain to turn across the tube mouth, where one pull may cause perforation, enormously increasing the difficulties of removal and perhaps resulting in serious trauma (Fig. 67–5).

Extraction of pointed, radiopaque foreign bodies in the lung periphery is attempted only under simultaneous biplane fluoroscopic guidance.

The sheathing and protective methods for the removal of pins apply also to the removal of tacks and other double-pointed objects. Tacks and staples are best managed with a special staple bronchoscope and forceps.

Hollow metallic objects are best held with one of the forceps jaws inside and one outside, or removed with hollow object — internal expansion — forceps. Hard, smooth, globular objects such as ball-bearings are best held with the ball-bearing forceps.

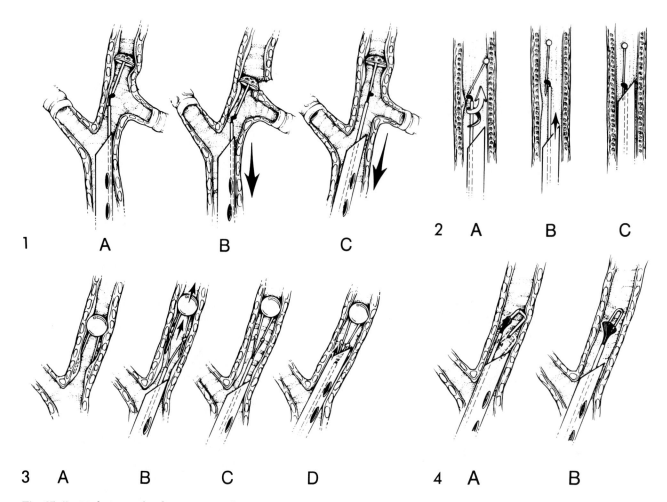

Fig. 67–5. Techniques of endoscopic removal. *1,* Long axis traction is particularly important for pointed objects with large heads. Point may be easily located *(A),* but greater hazard lies in risk of tearing bronchial wall with head of tack *(B).* Positioning patient's head toward opposite side straightens axis of airway, permitting relatively safe, slow, steady withdrawal of object *(C). 2,* Inward rotation method is used for pins or needles with imbedded point. Side-grasping forceps captures pin near point *(A).* Corkscrew motion is used to push pin distally while rotating it clockwise, freeing point and aligning shaft with long axis of forceps *(B).* Scope is advanced over point to sheathe *(C)* for extraction. *3,* Technique of managing bendable double-pointed objects. Points buried in mucosal wall *(A)* are released by moving them distally *(B).* Points are approximated *(C)* then sheathed for extraction by advancing rigid scope *(D). 4,* Tucker staple forceps *(A)* is angled to permit sheathing of both points within beveled tip of bronchoscope. Jackson broad-staple forceps *(B)* grasps and protects both points during advancement of bronchoscope to sheathe them. *From* Holinger LD: Management of sharp and penetrating foreign bodies of the upper aerodigestive tract. Ann Otol Rhinol Laryngol 99:684, 1990.

REFERENCES

Bendig DW: Removal of blunt esophageal foreign bodies by flexible endoscopy without general anesthesia. Am J Dis Child *140*:789, 1986.

Bigler FC: The use of a Foley catheter for removal of blunt foreign bodies from the esophagus. J Thorac Cardiovasc Surg *51*:759, 1966.

Burrington JD, Cotton EK: Removal of foreign bodies from the tracheobronchial tree. J Pediatr Surg 7:119, 1972.

Esclamado RN, Richardson MA: Laryngotracheal foreign bodies in children. Am J Dis Child *141*:259, 1987.

Hamman L: Spontaneous interstitial emphysema of the lungs. Trans Assoc Am Physicians 52:311, 1937.

Holinger LD: Management of sharp and penetrating foreign bodies of the upper aerodigestive tract. Ann Otol Rhinol Laryngol 99:684, 1990.

Holinger PH: Foreign bodies in the air and food passages. Trans Am Acad Ophthalmol Otolaryngol 66:193, 1962.

Jackson C, Jackson CL: Diseases of the air and food passages of foreign body origin. Philadelphia: WB Saunders, 1936.

Jackson C, Jackson CL: Diseases of the nose, throat, and ear. 2nd Ed. Philadelphia: WB Saunders, 1959.

Law DK, Kosloske AM: Management of tracheobronchial foreign bodies in children: a re-evaluation of postural drainage and bronchoscopy. Pediatrics 58:362, 1976.

Maves MD, Carithers JS, Birck HG: Esophageal burns secondary to disc battery ingestion. Ann Otol Rhinol Laryngol 93:364, 1984.

Thorburn JR, et al: A technique for foreign body removal from the airway. Endoscopy 18:71, 1986.

Tucker GF Jr: Laryngeal and tracheobronchial foreign bodies. Trans Pa Acad Ophthalmol Otolaryngol *19*(1):12, 1966.

CHAPTER 68

DIAPHRAGMATIC INJURIES

Panagiotis N. Symbas

Diaphragmatic lacerations may result from penetrating or blunt trauma to this musculotendinous structure that separates the thoracic and abdominal cavities. If the laceration is unrecognized and not promptly repaired, one or more of the abdominal viscera will herniate into the thoracic cavity, with resulting early or late compromise of ventilatory or gastrointestinal function. Immediate herniation is most often associated with a large tear in one of the diaphragmatic leaves, but the symptoms of the herniation usually are obscured by the symptoms of other associated injured organs or structures. Small rents such as those caused by stab wounds rarely are symptomatic early, but if they are unrepaired, progressive abdominal visceral herniation occurs because of the pressure gradient between the thoracic and peritoneal cavities. As the herniation of abdominal viscera progresses, the likelihood of ventilatory compromise or of mechanical obstruction, with or without strangulation, of a portion of the contained gastrointestinal tract increases.

Diaphragmatic injuries can be separated into two categories: those that are recognized at the time of initial hospitalization for the evaluation of an episode of trauma and those that are missed initially and recognized at some time remote from the first hospitalization.

RECOGNITION DURING INITIAL HOSPITALIZATION

The mechanism, symptoms, and other features of blunt and penetrating injuries are dissimilar. Therefore, the initial recognition and the management of these two types of injury are best discussed separately.

Blunt Diaphragmatic Trauma

Rupture of a portion of the diaphragm usually results from decelerating injuries suffered in motor vehicle accidents or from falls from great heights. Other crushing injuries to the lower chest or upper abdomen may also result in laceration of the diaphragm. Beal and McKennan (1988) reported an incidence of a ruptured

diaphragm of 3% in those patients suffering severe blunt trauma who survived long enough to be admitted to the hospital.

The rupture most commonly occurs in the left leaf. Contrary to common belief, the right hemidiaphragm is not immune from injury. The ratio of rupture of the left versus the right hemidiaphragm in my experience (1986) was 5:1, and Estrera and colleagues (1985) reported a 34% incidence of right-sided rupture. Brown and Richardson (1985) and Beal and McKennan (1988) also noted a similar incidence, as well as the occasional occurrence of bilateral rupture. Injuries on the right side are usually posterolateral to the central tendon. The pericardial or central portion of the diaphragm also may be ruptured, and avulsion of the diaphragm from the rib cage infrequently occurs.

Pathology

On the left side, the organs most commonly herniated into the chest are the stomach, spleen, large bowel, liver, small intestine, and omentum. On the right, when herniation occurs the liver is always present and the colon is occasionally herniated, as Brown and Richardson (1985) reported. Vascular injuries — tears of the juxtahepatic vena cava and hepatic vein injuries — as well as lacerations of the liver are frequently associated with rupture of the right hemidiaphragm.

Symptomatology

Symptoms and signs of diaphragmatic rupture — respiratory distress, cardiac disturbances, deviated trachea, and bowel sounds in the chest — are present in the minority of patients initially seen after the blunt injury; most symptoms present are related to other organ system injuries or to the presence of hypovolemic shock.

Radiographic Examinations

The routine radiograph of the chest is the most efficient study when the patient is stable enough to have

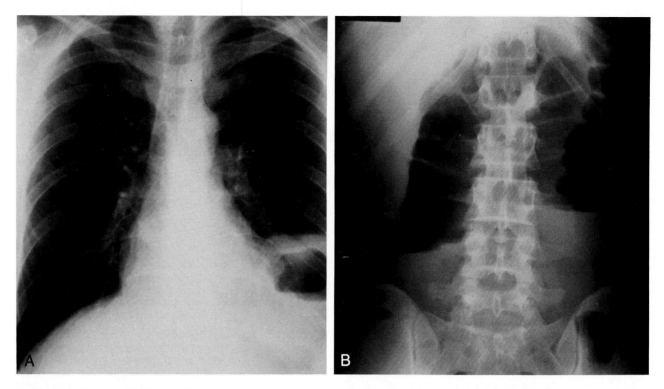

Fig. 68–1. Radiographs of a 30-year-old man following a vehicular accident. *A,* Frontal view of the chest shows abnormal diaphragmatic silhouette. *B,* Plain radiograph of the abdomen reveals upward displacement of the transverse colon. *From* Symbas PN, Vlasis SE, Hatcher C, Jr: Blunt and penetrating diaphragmatic injuries with or without herniation of organs into the chest. Ann Thorac Surg *42*:158, 1986.

the procedure done. It is abnormal in almost all and is diagnostic of rupture in over half of the patients. The abnormal radiograph of the chest shows an elevated, obscured, or irregular diaphragmatic dome on the side of the visceral herniation. The costophrenic angle is almost always blunted because of contained fluid. With lacerations on the left, one or more air-fluid levels and

radioluceny in the lower lung field, with or without shifting of the mediastinum away from the side of the hernia, appear (Fig. 68–1). Occasionally, the nasogastric tube can be seen to turn upward into the chest (Fig. 68–2). With right-sided injuries, the right leaf is markedly elevated with or without an associated fluid collection; air-fluid levels are less frequently observed.

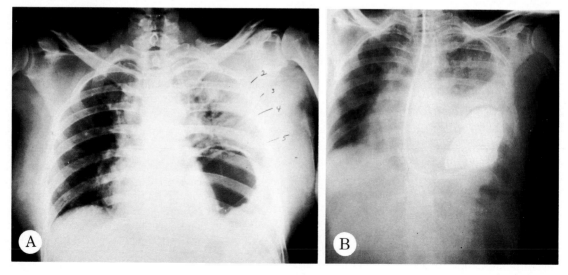

Fig. 68–2. *A,* Radiograph of chest made 12 hours after severe trauma, showing multiple rib fractures and a large gas bubble in the lower portion of the left side of the chest. *B,* Barium study revealed the large gas shadow to be the stomach, which had herniated through the ruptured diaphragm.

Occasionally, a rounded shadow protruding above the leaf appears on the lateral film; this is highly diagnostic for right-sided rupture (Fig. 68–3). Nondiagnostic findings of a pneumothorax or hydrothorax — hemothorax — or both, are also frequently present.

Diagnosis

The radiograph of the chest may be diagnostic, as noted. In those patients too ill to be moved, Ammann and colleagues (1983) suggested using bedside real-time sonographic examination. In patients not requiring emergency operation, the diagnosis may be confirmed with barium contrast studies of either the upper or lower gastrointestinal tract. Computed tomography — CT — as Heiberg (1980) and Toombs (1981) and their associates reported, can likewise be used to demonstrate the herniation. When right-sided injury is suspected and conditions permit, fluoroscopic examination and radionuclide liver scan, as well as ultrasonography and computed tomography, can be done to delineate the herniated portion of the liver. The use of diagnostic pneumoperitoneum is rarely indicated. In patients requiring emergency operation for control of bleeding or correction of other life-threatening injuries, the diagnosis must be made at operation. Both leaves of the diaphragm must, therefore, be adequately inspected in all patients with severe blunt chest and upper abdominal injuries who are operated on.

Treatment

Because of the danger of development of respiratory and even circulatory embarrassment or visceral obstruction, with incarceration or strangulation of the involved portion of the gastrointestinal tract, diaphragmatic injury should be repaired surgically as soon as possible after the diagnosis is established and when the patient's clinical condition permits. Although a diaphragmatic leaf may be best exposed through the chest, the approach chosen should be based on the clinical findings in each patient. Because the major source of massive bleeding is usually a lacerated abdominal viscus, Beal and McKennan (1988) prefer the abdominal approach. During the acute postinjury period, the diaphragmatic injury should be repaired through the incision required for the emergency repair of other organ injuries. In all the patients who were operated on by me and my associates (1986) shortly after the injury, laparotomy was the incision used.

Tears of the left hemidiaphragm are most often repaired through the abdomen because of frequently

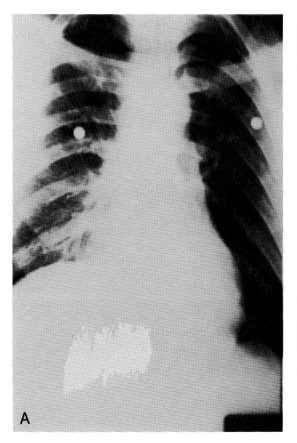
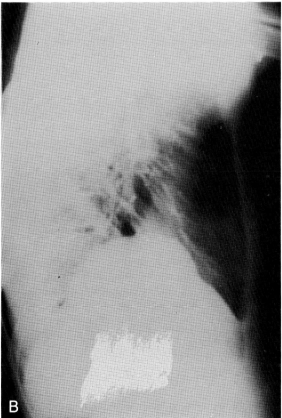

Fig. 68–3. Chest radiographs of a patient with ruptured right hemidiaphragm and partial herniation of the liver. *A,* Posteroanterior view suggested only minimal elevation of the right hemidiaphragm. *B,* Lateral view was fairly impressive. *From* Estrera A, et al: Blunt traumatic rupture of the right hemidiaphragm: experience in 12 patients. Ann Thorac Surg 39:525, 1985.

associated injuries to intra-abdominal organs, although in the absence of any symptoms suggesting such injury, a left thoracotomy is adequate. Tears of the right hemidiaphragm, when recognized preoperatively, are best repaired through a right thoracotomy, as Estrera and associates described in 1979. In 1985, however, these authors recommended that the approach be individualized, depending primarily on which cavity — thorax or abdomen — shows continued evidence of bleeding. When injury to the retrohepatic vena cava or hepatic veins is encountered during an abdominal approach, Estrera and associates (1985) extend the incision by a median sternotomy to place a temporary vena cava shunt to control the bleeding.

After control and repair of other associated visceral injuries, the diaphragmatic tear is closed with interrupted figure-of-eight No. 0 nonabsorbable sutures. Prosthetic material is rarely needed in acute blunt trauma injuries. Disruption of the repaired diaphragmatic leaf is rare.

Mortality

The mortality rates may be high in these patients, not as the result of the diaphragmatic injury per se but as the consequence of other severe visceral trauma. The author and associates (1986) reported a 22% mortality rate in this group of patients. Brooks (1978) and Brown and Richardson (1985) reported rates of 14% and 17%, respectively. Beal and McKennan (1988) reported a mortality rate of 40.5%. Ninety-seven percent of their patients had associated injuries, and 87% of those who died were in severe hypovolemic shock when admitted to the hospital.

Penetrating Diaphragmatic Injuries

These injuries usually result from stab wounds or gunshot wounds of the lower chest — below the nipples; the upper abdomen — epigastrium; the flanks; or the back; half of the patients treated by me and my associates (1986) had a wound of the chest below the nipples, but injuries of all other sites of the trunk were associated with a diaphragmatic wound. Injury to either diaphragmatic leaf occurs with almost equal frequency.

Pathology

The diaphragmatic injury is generally small, and herniation of the abdominal viscera into the chest is usually absent early. Only if the injury is missed does late herniation occur because of the different pressures in the two cavities.

Symptomatology

The history and physical exam per se do not indicate diaphragmatic injury. The presence of abdominal complaints or findings in a patient who has sustained a chest wound, however, is strongly suggestive of diaphragmatic injury, as is the presence of chest findings in one in whom the site of entrance of the wound is in the abdomen or flank. Many patients, however, have only findings associated with the cavity of entrance, and the diaphragmatic injury remains unsuspected until the time of exploration or, unfortunately, is occasionally missed entirely when exploration of either the chest or abdomen was thought not indicated. This latter event most often occurs with stab wounds, because patients with gunshot wounds of the trunk usually undergo either emergency abdominal or thoracic exploration.

Radiographic Findings

In 93 instances of penetrating injuries of the diaphragm, Miller and associates (1984) reported the radiograph of the chest to have been normal in 43% and abnormal in 57%. The abnormalities were a hemothorax or a pneumothorax, or both, in 96% and herniated abdominal contents or pneumoperitoneum in 2% each. The author and associates (1986) found the radiograph to be normal in one third of 185 patients with this type of injury.

Diagnosis

A high index of suspicion of the presence of a diaphragmatic injury must be present in all penetrating injuries of the trunk and particularly in those with wounds from the nipple line to the umbilicus. Miller and associates (1984), among others, have suggested that all such penetrating injuries, symptomatic or not, should be explored and complete inspection of both leaves of the diaphragm be carried out. In their series, 13% of the patients had no associated injuries. The author concurs with this policy for any gunshot wound, but at times a more conservative approach can be used in the management of stab wounds; most of which will, of course, be explored because of associated symptomatology. In the absence of any findings or suggestion of injury to the diaphragm or any visceral injury, however, exploration may not be mandatory. A few stab-wound injuries to the diaphragm will undoubtedly be missed with this approach, possibly as high as 13%, according to Miller and associates' (1984) report. Pneumoperitoneum and abdominal paracentesis, generally are of no aid in identifying these missed injuries early. Ultrasonography, CT examination, and barium studies, however, may lead to the discovery of some of these missed injuries. These tests should be performed when the chest radiographs show any, otherwise unexplained, persistent abnormality of the diaphragm or the lower lung field, or both.

Although peritoneoscopy or thoracoscopy have not been used for the diagnosis of diaphragmatic injury, they should be considered before the patient is discharged. Also, elective barium studies should be recommended in a 4- to 6-week period after the patient's discharge when routine exploration or thoracoscopy has not been done.

Treatment

In the absence of intrathoracic organ injury or major intrapleural bleeding, the abdominal approach is always preferred because it permits detection and treatment of nonevident intra-abdominal injury and enables the surgeon to examine both diaphragmatic leaflets, which is not possible through a transthoracic approach. Any injury to the diaphragm can be repaired readily with No. 0 nonabsorbable interrupted sutures.

Mortality

Diaphragmatic injury should not cause death. Associated organ injury, however, results in a variable number of deaths. In my series of 185 penetrating injuries, there were four deaths, a mortality rate of 2.2%.

LATE RECOGNITION

The initial injury to the diaphragm, from either blunt or penetrating trauma, may be undetected during the patient's first hospitalization and may only become manifest because of symptoms or signs related to a hernia of one or more abdominal viscera into the chest. Although no large body of data is available, it is most likely that more late diaphragmatic hernias result from missed stab wound injuries than from blunt trauma. In a small series reported by Hegarty and colleagues (1978), 22 of 25 late hernias were from previous stab wounds. Nonetheless, many examples of herniation caused by blunt injuries have been observed (Figs. 68–4, and 68–5).

These hernias may be recognized any time from a few weeks to over three or four decades after the original injury. The hernias resulting from blunt trauma tend to be larger, especially those involving the left hemidiaphragm, and to contain multiple abdominal viscera. In order of frequency, as the author and associates (1986) have noted, the stomach, colon, small bowel, omentum, and spleen herniate through a left diaphragmatic traumatic defect, whereas the colon and liver are the most commonly herniating organs through a right defect. Those from penetrating trauma tend to contain only colon or a portion of the stomach, or both.

Symptomatology

The larger hernias are more likely to produce ventilatory signs and symptoms caused by the reduction of the lung volume on the side of the hernia. Gastrointestinal problems caused by interference of the normal functioning of the contained viscera may also occur. The smaller hernias that contain only a loop of large bowel or stomach become symptomatic because of partial, and at times of complete, obstruction of the contained segment. When complete obstruction occurs, strangulation of the herniated visceral segment may develop and is an ominous complication.

Diagnosis

The diagnosis of traumatic diaphragmatic hernia should be suspected in any patient who sustained blunt or penetrating trauma of the trunk, particularly of the chest or epigastrium, and in whom the chest radiograph shows an abnormal diaphragmatic silhouette or lower lung field. The abnormality may include only an obscured or abnormal diaphragmatic shadow, a radiodensity, radiolucency, or one or more air-fluid levels in the lung fields with or without mediastinal shift. The radiographic examination of the chest, however, does not differentiate diaphragmatic hernia from various other conditions that cause these abnormalities, unless a nasogastric tube has been inserted and is seen in the chest cavity, which indicates the stomach is herniated in the thorax.

The most important studies for the diagnosis are either barium by mouth or a barium enema, as Felson (1973) pointed out. He noted that whichever of the organs is herniated — stomach or colon — the point of entry and exit through the torn diaphragmatic leaf is most often through a small single defect. Moreover, the edges of the defect are closely applied to the herniated viscus. Thus, the points of entry and exit are closely applied and constricted. This results in a side-by-side, beak-like narrowing of the barium column (Figs. 68–6 and 68–7). Carter and associates (1951) recorded that if the herniated bowel becomes obstructed, the number of beaks will be reduced to one; and dilatation proximal to the site of constriction will be observed (Fig. 68–8). The obstruction within the hernia is often of the closed-loop type, so distention of the loop within the hernia may be great. These authors also noted that the combination of a high left hemidiaphragm and the presence of splenic flexure obstruction is almost diagnostic of a traumatic diaphragmatic hernia.

Other diagnostic studies such as pneumoperitoneum, pneumothorax, and angiography are less rewarding than the barium studies. Ultrasonography and CT studies may be helpful at times but probably less so than they potentially are in the evaluation of patients thought to have acute injury of the diaphragm.

Treatment

Once the hernia is recognized, reduction of the hernia and repair of the diaphragmatic defect through the transthoracic route is indicated. The frequent presence of marked adhesions between the herniated viscus and thoracic contents necessitate this route. In the presence of obstruction, with or without strangulation of the contained viscus, the incarcerated diaphragmatic hernia must be approached by the transthoracic route. After mobilization of the obstructed or strangulated viscus, the abdomen may need to be entered through an abdominal incision to complete the necessary operative repair or resection and diversion of the involved viscus. Repair of the diaphragmatic

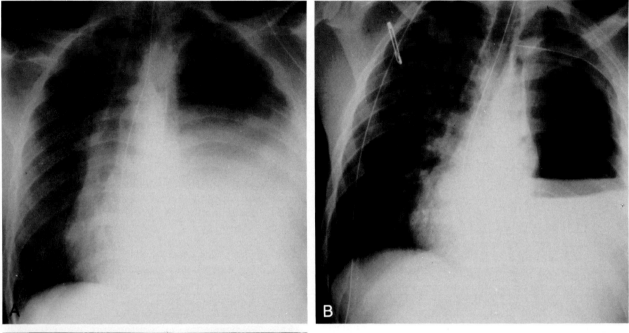

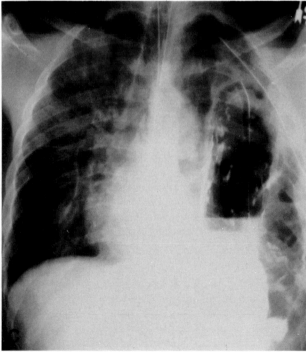

Fig. 68–4. Chest radiographs of a 46-year-old man who was involved in a car accident 6 years earlier. *A*, Supine chest radiograph shows radiodensity of the lower left lung field and radiolucency of the upper left field with displacement of the mediastinum. *B*, Erect frontal view shows two air-fluid levels. *C*, Upper gastrointestinal series and barium enema demonstrate both the stomach and large bowels in the left chest. *From* Symbas PN, Vlasis SE, Hatcher C Jr: Blunt and penetrating diaphragmatic injuries with or without herniation of organs into the chest. Ann Thorac Surg *42*:158, 1986.

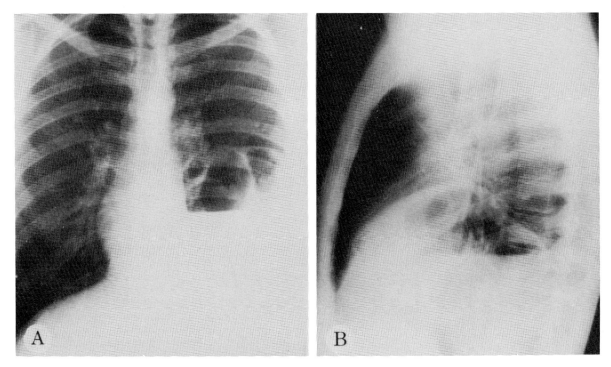

Fig. 68–5. Traumatic diaphragmatic hernia through the left paracardiac portion of the left hemidiaphragm discovered 15 years after the initial injury. *A,* PA radiograph of chest showing multiple air-fluid spaces in the lower half of the left chest. *B,* Lateral radiograph made with the patient in the upright position.

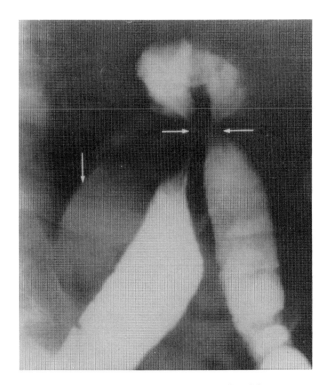

Fig. 68–6. Counter-incision breakdown after hiatal hernia repair. Nonobstructive hernia. The medial portion of the diaphragm is visible (vertical arrow). The lovebird sign is well shown. *From* Felson B: Chest Roentgenology. Philadelphia: WB Saunders, 1973, p 421.

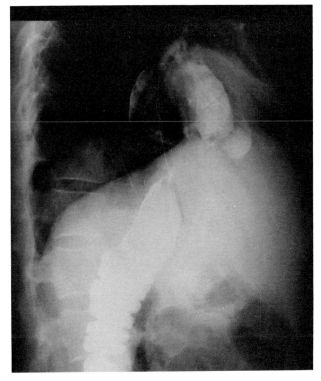

Fig. 68–7. Barium enema showing apposition of loops of large bowel herniating into the thorax through a previous stab wound of the diaphragm. *From* Symbas PN, Vlasis SE, Hatcher C Jr: Blunt and penetrating diaphragmatic injuries with or without herniation of organs into the chest. Ann Thorac Surg *42:*158, 1986.

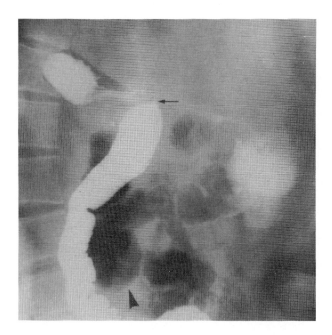

Fig. 68-8. Obstruction of the distal segment, lateral view. Note the single beak (arrow). The stomach, outlined with barium, is not herniated. The proximal colon shows moderate gaseous distention (arrowhead). *From* Felson B: Chest Roentgenology. Philadelphia: WB Saunders, 1973, p 421.

defect is accomplished by direct suture repair in almost all instances. Only rarely in the presence of large tears from original blunt trauma is a prosthetic graft necessary.

Morbidity and Mortality

The morbidity following repair of a diaphragmatic hernia that was recognized late is that seen after any major thoracotomy. The mortality, however, may vary greatly, depending on the status of the hernia at the time of its repair. When the procedure is done electively, the mortality rate should approach zero. In marked contrast, however, is the excessive mortality rate experienced in those patients who present with a strangulated, gangrenous viscus in the hernia. In such instances, the mortality may be as high as 80%, as Hegarty and associates (1978) reported. These missed hernias must therefore be recognized and repaired

before obstruction and gangrene of the contained visceral segment occur.

REFERENCES

Ammann AM, et al.: Traumatic rupture of the diaphragm: real time sonographic diagnosis. AJR *140*:915, 1983.

Beal SL, McKennan M: Blunt diaphragm rupture: a morbid injury. Arch Surg *123*:828, 1988.

Brooks JW: Blunt traumatic rupture of the diaphragm. Ann Thorac Surg *26*:199, 1978.

Brown GL, Richardson JD: Traumatic diaphragmatic hernia: a continuing challenge. Ann Thorac Surg *39*:170, 1985.

Carter BN, Giuseffi J, Felson B: Traumatic diaphragmatic hernia. AJR *65*:56, 1951.

Estrera AS, Platt MR, Mills LJ: Traumatic injuries of the diaphragm. Chest *75*:306, 1979.

Estrera AS, Landay MJ, McClelland RN: Blunt traumatic rupture of the right hemidiaphragm: experience in 12 patients. Ann Thorac Surg *39*:525, 1985.

Felson B: Chest Roentgenology. Philadelphia: WB Saunders, 1973, p 437.

Hegarty MM, et al.: Delayed presentation of traumatic diaphragmatic hernia. Ann Surg *188*:229, 1978.

Heiberg E, et al.: CT recognition of traumatic rupture of the diaphragm. AJR *135*:369, 1980.

Miller LW, et al.: Management of penetrating and blunt diaphragmatic injury. J Trauma *24*:403, 1984.

Symbas PN, Vlasis SE, Hatcher CR, Jr.: Blunt and penetrating diaphragmatic injuries with or without herniation of organs into the chest. Ann Thorac Surg *42*:158, 1986.

Toombs BD, Sandler CM, Lester RG: Computed tomography of chest trauma. Radiology *140*:733, 1981.

READING REFERENCES

Clay RC, Hanlon CR: Pneumoperitoneum in the differential diagnosis of diaphragmatic hernia. J Thorac Cardiovasc Surg *21*:57, 1951.

Ebert PA, Gaertner RA, Zuidema GD: Traumatic diaphragmatic hernia. Surg Gynecol Obstet *125*:59, 1967.

Fagan CJ, et al.: Traumatic diaphragmatic hernia into the pericardium: verification of diagnosis by computed tomography. J Comp Asst Tomogr *3*:405, 1979.

Hood RM: Traumatic diaphragmatic hernia (collective review). Ann Thorac Surg *12*:311, 1971.

Lucido JL, Wall CA: Rupture of the diaphragm due to blunt trauma. Arch Surg *86*:989, 1963.

Mansour KA, et al.: Diaphragmatic hernia caused by trauma: experience with 35 cases. Am Surg *41*:97, 1975.

Nelson JB, Jr et al.: Diaphragmatic injuries and posttraumatic hernia. J Trauma *2*:36, 1960.

Sutton JP, Carlisle RB, Stephenson SE, Jr.: Traumatic diaphragmatic hernia: a review of 25 cases. Ann Thorac Surg *3*:136, 1967.

Symbas PN: Blunt traumatic rupture of the diaphragm. Ann Thorac Surg *26*:193, 1978.

SECTION XIII
The Trachea

CHAPTER 69

MANAGEMENT OF NON-NEOPLASTIC DISEASES OF THE TRACHEA

Hermes C. Grillo

A wide spectrum of benign conditions that affect the trachea are described under the general headings of 1) lesions that are due to infection; 2) posttraumatic lesions, including iatrogenic injuries; 3) extrinsic lesions compressing the trachea; and 4) miscellaneous, including a variety of lesions largely of unknown origin. Additional topics that are dealt with in other chapters are congenital lesions of the trachea (Chapter 118) and acute traumatic injury (Chapter 64).

INFECTION

Tuberculosis

Tuberculosis of the upper airway appears principally to involve the lower trachea and/or the main bronchi. Acute ulcerative tuberculous tracheitis is treated medically. As the acute process heals, stenosis may evolve. Typically, the stenosis shows a pattern of submucosal fibrosis laid down in circumferential manner with marked narrowing or occlusion of the airway. The tracheal cartilages appear to be grossly intact, although there is peribronchial or peritracheal fibrosis. The lesions may be quite lengthy and thus present a marked or insuperable surgical challenge. Active tuberculosis should be arrested and controlled before surgical resection and reconstruction is performed. In one patient in whom surgery was forced because of acute disease obstructing both the distal trachea and the carina, healing was unsatisfactory, and fatal disruption occurred. In three patients who required carinal resection and reconstruction for excision of mature stenoses, two involved excision of the right upper lobe as well with reimplantation of the bronchus intermedius. Complete stenosis of the left main bronchus has been managed by total excision of that bronchus and advancement and reimplantation of the bifurcation of the left upper and lower lobes to the carina, as described by Newton and associates (1991).

Histoplasmosis

Histoplasmosis may affect the airways in several ways. It may produce massive mediastinal fibrosis with involvement of distal trachea, carina, and main bronchi, or it may involve principally the right bronchial tree in relation to the masses of lymph nodes in the right para- and pretracheal area and in the middle lobe sump. The fibrosing process may extend centrally to involve the right pulmonary artery up to its point of origin even within the pericardium. The lesions may be a composite of airway compression plus intrinsic fibrotic involvement. Massive histoplasmoma at the carina may compress the airway. In such lesions there may be central caseation with a fibrotic capsule that actually involves one or both main bronchial walls intimately. Another presentation is with densely fibrotic and calcified sub- and precarinal lymph nodes, which may invade and erode through the wall of the trachea, the carina, or the bronchi. Broncholiths also occur peripherally in the lobar bronchi. Secondary infection and hemorrhage may follow. In recent years, broncholithiasis has in general been associated with histoplasmosis rather than with tuberculosis, as it was in an earlier era. These clinical manifestations have been described by Mathisen and myself (1992). The organism *Histoplasma capsulatum* is more often identified by special stains in pathologic material removed at surgery rather than on cultures. Organisms have been identified in fewer than 50% of patients who are presumed to have disease originating from this source. It has been theorized that the continuing fibrotic process is a reaction to products of the infection rather than to viable organisms. Thus, diagnosis is often presumptive, based on pathologic and radiologic findings as well as on history of exposure and clinical evolution of the disease.

Other Inflammatory Disease Processes

A small number of patients has been seen who have suffered from diphtheria in childhood and presented many years later with tracheal stenosis or laryngotracheal stenosis. Because most of these patients had tracheostomies in infancy or early childhood for treatment of the acute disease, it is difficult to differentiate whether the late stenoses were due to the disease or to the treatment. Reconstruction may be possible.

Scleroma is a rare disease that may involve the airways as well as the nasopharynx. It is found in Mexico and Central America. A rare case of necrosing mucormycosis involving the trachea or carina as well as the lungs may be seen in diabetic patients or in people who are immunosuppressed or undergoing chemotherapy, particularly for lymphomas. Prompt and radical surgical excision with the protection of vigorous and prolonged treatment with amphotericin may save some of these patients, as noted by Tedder and associates (1993).

POSTTRAUMATIC LESIONS

Blunt Trauma

Ruptures of the trachea, carina, or main bronchi that are due to blunt trauma may go unrecognized. Such patients almost always have a history of pneumothorax treated by tube drainage, often bilateral in the case of tracheal rupture. They present with shortness of breath or wheezing. The trachea or bronchus may be reduced to only a tiny opening when the diagnosis is at last made. Treatment consists of prompt excision of stenosis and surgical repair. When the bronchus is injured, every effort is made to salvage the distal lung. This is usually possible unless severe infection has ensued. Deslauriers and associates (1982) have demonstrated adequate function of reimplanted lungs. Functional return appears to be roughly inversely proportional to the length of time that the lung was defunctioned.

In patients who have suffered tracheal separation that is due to blunt injury in the neck and who have been treated by tracheostomy only, total stenosis of the area of separation follows. Both recurrent laryngeal nerves are usually at least temporarily paralyzed and often permanently. Such patients must be carefully evaluated some months following their injury when the local inflammation has subsided. Laryngeal reconstruction where necessary, with stabilization of the glottic aperture, is generally accomplished first. The larynx is then reconnected to the trachea, as described by Mathisen and myself (1987). An effective although unmodulated voice is obtained. Pharyngoesophageal separation that was not repaired initially is reconstructed at the same time.

Inhalation Burns

Inhalation burns of the larynx, trachea, and bronchi are particularly difficult injuries to manage. The agent may have been chemical, thermal, or a combination of both. These patients often show little damage to the pharynx or supraglottic larynx once the immediate injury has subsided. Persistent damage often commences in the subglottis just below the vocal cords and extends down the airway in a gradually diminishing intensity of injury. The depth of injury as well as the length of airway injured probably relate to the dose received as well as to the actual injury potential of the agent. Gaissert and I and our colleagues (1993) found that in 18 patients treated for tracheal stenosis that was due to inhalation injury, 14 had subglottic strictures as well and two had main bronchial stenosis. Although it is sometimes difficult to differentiate later injuries from the intubation with which the patients were treated acutely, 3 of our patients had laryngotracheal strictures without any history of intubation.

In most cases, the tracheal rings were not destroyed and the injuries were confined to various depths of mucosal and submucosal damage. Attempts at resection of injuries, especially in the early phase, should not be made. First, involvement often commences immediately below the cords and involves the entire subglottic larynx, making repair almost impossible. Second, the burned airway responds poorly to early surgery, even where the lesion appears to be limited, much in the way that burned skin elsewhere in the body does — by the reformation of massive scarring. With appropriately placed splinting, silicone T-tubes, and a great deal of patience, a stable and open airway may usually be obtained in most of these patients in time.

Postoperative Stenosis

Stenosis of the trachea following tracheal reconstruction is due in most cases to excessive tension on the anastomosis, and this is related to overzealous resection of too great a length of trachea. Dangerous tensions in tracheal resection may be reached at about the 50% level of length of resection in the adult and at the 30 to 40% level in the child. Carinal resections are particularly at risk because of their complex nature. Patients chronically on high doses of prednisone are especially at risk if extensive tracheal resection is performed. Unnecessary disturbance of the blood supply to the trachea by extensive circumferential dissection will also lead to stenosis or separation. Profuse, hypertrophic granulations at the anastomosis, which were seen when nonabsorbable sutures were used for tracheal repair, have vanished since the introduction of Vicryl sutures.

Stenoses may also result from *radiation therapy* and *laser injury*. Brachytherapy has also contributed a number of main bronchial stenoses. The contribution of lasering to tracheal damage is more difficult to assess because the lasering is often applied for attempted treatment of pre-existing lesions and in conjunction with a tracheostomy performed to "safeguard" the airway. Whereas laser injury may often be dealt with by subsequent resectional surgery, irradiation injuries may either be surgically incorrectable when first seen or correctable only with considerable risk.

Postintubation Damage

Intubation either with oral or nasal endotracheal tubes or with tracheostomy tubes is most commonly used to deliver mechanical ventilatory support in respiratory failure. Assistance supplied through cuffed tubes has thus far proved to be the only practicable method of management for adults with poor pulmonary or chest wall compliance. High-flow respirators with uncuffed tubes, electrophrenic respirators, and negative pressure tank respirators have not been satisfactory for managing these severe problems. High-frequency ventilation for long-term use remains developmental. A whole spectrum of tracheal lesions resulting from such treatment was discerned by Andrews and Pearson (1971) and by me (1969, 1970) (Fig. 69–1). The most common lesions, and those most amenable to definitive treatment, are those responsible for airway obstruction. Because a single patient may have more than one lesion and because the treatment of these lesions differs, precise definition of the pathologic state is essential in planning treatment. Lindholm (1970) showed that endotracheal tubes may cause obstruction at the laryngeal level even after only 48 hours of intubation: glottic edema, vocal cord granulomas, erosions particularly over the arytenoids, formation of granulation tissue, polypoid obstructions, and actual stenosis, particularly at the subglottic intralaryngeal level. Subglottic injury is also produced by cricothyroidotomy and by cricoid erosion caused by high tracheostomy in the presence of kyphosis. Montgomery (1968) noted that subglottic stenosis may be difficult to correct. Sometimes it is impossible.

At the tracheostomy site, granulomas that can obstruct the airway may form during healing. If the tracheostomy stoma has been made too large by turning a large flap or excising a large window in the initial tracheostomy, or if erosion is caused by sepsis and heavy prying equipment, cicatricial healing may produce an anterior A-shaped stenosis that can severely compromise the airway. The posterior wall of the trachea may be relatively intact in these patients. At the level of the inflatable cuff, whether placed on a tracheostomy tube or an endotracheal tube, circumferential erosion of the tracheal wall may occur. If this erosion is deep enough, all the anatomic layers of the trachea may be destroyed, so that cicatricial repair results in a tight circumferential stenosis (Fig. 69–2). Malacia may also result. Below this level at the point where the tip of the tube may pry against the tracheal wall, additional erosion may occur with formation of granuloma, especially in children, for whom uncuffed tubes are used. In the segment between the stomal and cuff level, varying degrees of chondromalacia with resulting tracheomalacia may occur. Here, the cartilages are not totally destroyed but only thinned. Bacterial infection in this segment of the trachea during the period of ventilatory support probably contributes to this process.

The etiologic basis of the cuff stenosis has been variously attributed to pressure necrosis by the cuff, irritative quality of materials in rubber and plastic cuffs and tubes, irritant materials produced by gas sterilization, hypotension, and bacterial infection. Studies by Cooper and me (1969a), as well as by Florange and colleagues (1965), of autopsy specimens of patients who had been on ventilators with inflated cuffs (Fig. 69–3), prospective studies of similar patients by Andrews and Pearson (1971), and analysis of surgically removed lesions caused by cuffs and experimental reproduction of these lesions under controlled conditions by Cooper and me (1969a, 1969b) point to pressure necrosis as the principal etiologic agent. As my associates and I (1971) showed, if standard Rusch cuffs are inflated to just provide a seal at ventilatory pressures of about 25 cm H_2O, intracuff pressures rise to 180 to 250 mmHg. Carroll and associates (1969) noted that, although these pressures are not exactly those exerted on the tracheal mucous membrane, high pressures are indeed exerted. The trachea has an elliptic form, so it becomes deformed at the point where a seal is obtained. If perfusion pressures in the patient are lower than normal, necrosis

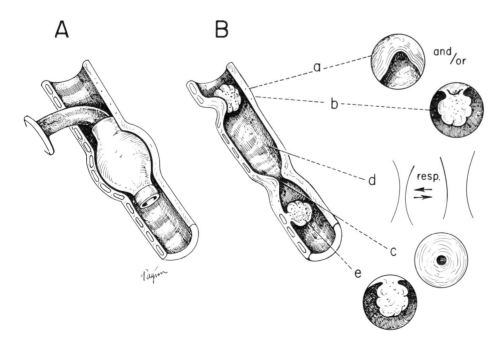

Fig. 69–1. Diagram of inflammatory lesions related to cuffed tracheostomy tubes. A, Location of the stoma and the distorting effect of a conventional cuff. B, Lesions developing at corresponding sites of injury. At the stoma, an anterior stricture (a) or a granuloma (b), or a combination may occur. At the cuff site (c), circumferential stricture occurs. Between the stoma and such a stricture, varying degrees of tracheal malacia may result, with functional occlusion (d). At the site of erosion by the tip of the tube (e), a granuloma may occur. Innominate erosion and a tracheoesophageal fistula are seen at both cuff level and tip level.

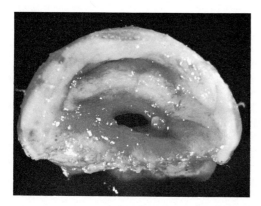

Fig. 69–2. Circumferential stenosis at cuff level. This surgical specimen shows the narrow size to which the lumen may be reduced before recognition of symptoms.

can occur even more easily. The mucosa overlying the cartilage is initially destroyed. The bared cartilages become necrotic and ultimately slough. Attempts at repair following full-thickness damage to the tracheal wall lead only to scar formation. Because the erosion is circumferential, the resultant strictures are also. Even further erosive damage can lead to tracheoesophageal fistula posteriorly or to perforation of the innominate artery anteriorly.

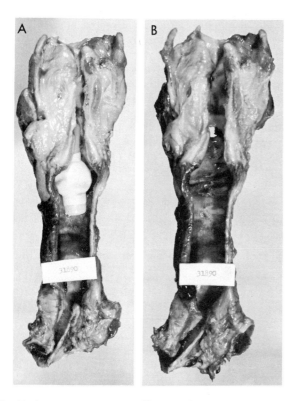

Fig. 69–3. Autopsy specimen of larynx and trachea reveals tracheal injury caused by cuffed tracheostomy tube. *A*, Portex tracheostomy tube had been in place for 19 days. Note the dilatation of the trachea where the cuff had been inflated. *B*, Inflammatory erosive changes have bared multiple cartilages. Note also a distal erosion caused by the tip of the tube. Similar injuries occur with metal or rubber tubes. *From* Grillo HC: Surgery of the trachea. Curr Probl Surg *July*:3, 1970.

Patients with stenosis and malacia develop symptoms and signs of airway obstruction consisting of dyspnea on exertion, stridor, cough, and obstructive episodes. Hemoptysis does not occur. In a few patients, pneumonia, sometimes bilateral, has been noted. On occasion, a patient while still intubated begins to develop obstruction from formation of granulations around the tip of the tube. In most instances, the obstruction appears only after extubation, because the tube splints a cuff stenosis or potential stomal stenosis as long as it remains in place. *Any patient who develops symptoms of airway obstruction who has been intubated for over 24 hours or more within the previous 2 years must be considered to have organic obstruction until proved otherwise.* Many such patients have been treated for varying lengths of time with the incorrect diagnosis of asthma. Such errors resulted from lack of awareness of these lesions and the fact that in most patients routine radiographs of the chest show normal lung fields.

Symptoms occurred in a few patients within 2 days of extubation; most demonstrated symptoms between 10 and 42 days after extubation, and few at greater intervals, usually within a few months. If a patient remains sedentary while recovering from his original disease, the airway may shrink to a critical diameter of 4 to 5 mm before symptoms become obvious. At this aperture, fatal obstruction may occur at any time.

Although general improvement has occurred with design of large-volume cuffs, most of these cuffs can still produce tracheal injury if slightly overinflated beyond their resting maximal volume, because of their relatively inextensible materials. Stomal injuries continue to occur for the reasons described. Cricothyroidotomy may lead to severe or irreparable subglottic injury.

Three additional and particularly severe injuries to the airway may occur from intubation. These are 1) tracheoesophageal fistula, 2) tracheoinnominate artery fistula, and 3) subglottic laryngeal or laryngotracheal stenosis. Tracheoesophageal fistula occurs most commonly in patients who have a ventilating cuff in the trachea for a long period of time along with a feeding tube in the esophagus. The two foreign bodies pincer the "party wall" between trachea and esophagus, leading first to inflammation, which seals one against the other, and then perforation, which may enlarge to include the entire membranous wall of the trachea. Concomitant circumferential injury to the trachea is usually present as well because this is basically a cuff lesion.

Anterior erosion of the trachea may lead to a fistula into the innominate artery. A small number of anterior erosions was seen in the past, which was due to angulation of a tube tip or a high-pressure cuff itself directly eroding through into the artery. More common, although fortunately still rare, are erosions of the artery, which occur at the inferior margin of a low-placed tracheostomy stoma, which is in immediate contiguity with the artery. The inner curve of the tube erodes its way through the arterial wall. It is seen most often in children and young adults in whom tracheostomy is placed too low, because on hyperextension more than half the trachea rises up into the neck. If the stoma is placed with respect to the sternal notch rather than to the cricoid cartilage, the tracheostomy will then reside just above the elevated innominate artery. Deslauriers and colleagues (1975) called attention to this complication.

Stenosis of the upper trachea may be associated with a severe subglottic stenosis as well. Stenosis of the subglottic larynx arises from three causes. The principal one is from erosion, which is due to an endotracheal tube that has been left in place for some time. The principal factor at fault may be use of a tube that has a bore too large for the patient. One of the narrowest parts of the upper airway is at the level of the cricoid cartilage. The second most common cause is erosion by a tracheostomy tube upward through the cricoid cartilage to affect the lower anterior larynx. This occurs most commonly in older patients who are kyphotic and in whom the cricoid cartilage is close to the sternal notch. A third cause of subglottic stenosis is the deliberate use of cricothyroidostomy for ventilation. If damage occurs at the stomal level, it is by surgical selection within the larynx. Lesions that involve the subglottic larynx as well as the upper trachea are much more difficult to repair surgically, although single-staged techniques have been devised by myself (1982) and by Pearson (1975) and by Couraud (1979) and their associates.

Tracheoesophageal fistula becomes manifest by sudden increase in tracheal secretions and the appearance of any ingested material in the trachea. If the patient is on a respirator, gastric distention may appear. Tracheoinnominate arterial fistulas are rare but may be announced by premonitory hemorrhage or by massive initial hemorrhage. In treating bleeding from a tracheostomy, it is important to differentiate between erosion of tracheal granulations or mucosa and arterial fistula. Sometimes an angiogram will demonstrate a false aneurysm that will soon bleed massively.

EXTRINSIC LESIONS

Goiter

Large goiters, either cervical or mediastinal, may gradually compress the airway sufficiently to cause symptoms. The slow growth of the goiter may deform cartilaginous rings without destroying them. When the goiter is removed, the trachea may remain distorted in shape and narrowed, but clinically significant airway obstruction is rarely present. Quite frequently, removal of the goiter leads to immediate improvement in respiratory symptoms. If, however, sufficient softening of the cartilages has occurred that is due to the prolonged compression, removing the supporting mass of thyroid tissue actually allows the trachea to collapse with respiratory effort. This is determined by intraoperative bronchoscopy, local examination and palpation in the operative field, and finally, by observation of the patient in the operating room following extubation.

Several methods of managing this problem have evolved, including intubation with an uncuffed tube followed by tracheostomy, preferably with insertion of a silicone T-tube several days later when the wound is sealed, immediate buttressing of the trachea with specially made polypropylene plastic rings, or in Europe, by using traction sutures from the tracheal wall tied over either internal or external buttons.

An anterior substernal goiter usually does not exert pressure on the trachea because of its position in front of the great vessels. Katlic and colleagues (1985) reported that the trachea was more likely to be compressed by posterior descending goiters that enter the thoracic strait lateral to the esophagus and trachea.

Vascular Compression

Symptoms of tracheal compression may be produced by congenital vascular rings or by aneurysms of the innominate artery or of an anomalous subclavian artery that passes behind the trachea and esophagus. In children, compression may be produced by the innominate artery itself (see Chapter 71).

Mediastinal Masses

Most mediastinal masses that compress the trachea are malignant neoplasms. On rare occasions, however, my colleagues and I have seen a large bronchogenic cyst located at the carina actually compress the airway and also have seen an infant trachea compressed by a large thymic cyst.

Postpneumonectomy Syndrome

Following right pneumonectomy, the mediastinum may move completely over to the right axilla and posteriorly, and in so doing, the aortic arch becomes rotated horizontally. This may lead to angulation and compression of the remaining tracheobronchial tree with obstruction either at the carina or in the proximal left main bronchus. The bronchus is actually compressed between the pulmonary artery, which is stretched in front of it, and either the aorta or the vertebral bodies posteriorly. It is unpredictable which patient will suffer this distortion following pneumonectomy. It was formerly thought that this was principally a syndrome seen in children, but my colleagues and I (1992) recently described a number of patients in whom the problem appeared following pneumonectomy in adulthood. The reverse situation may be seen after left pneumonectomy in the presence of a right aortic arch. The patient's symptoms may be rapidly progressive and lead to total disability (see Chapter 28).

MISCELLANEOUS LESIONS

Relapsing Polychondritis

This is a disease of unknown origin and uncertain course. Cartilaginous structures in the body may be affected, most prominently the nasal and ear cartilages and those of the tracheobronchial tree. The airway changes may precede the more diagnostic changes in the nose and ears, sometimes by years. When the lower trachea and bronchi are affected first, the disease manifests itself by progressive airway obstruction with difficulty in clearing secretions and ultimately pulmonary infections. The disease may extend into the segmental bronchi. Relapsing polychondritis may also affect the larynx and uppermost trachea. Here, the cartilages become inflamed and thickened, and there is constrictive narrowing of the subglottic and subcricoid airways. The disease may then progress distally, but without predictability. Surgical therapy is usually not applicable. Sometimes it is necessary to provide an airway with a tracheostomy tube, and at times stenting with a silicone T-tube or T-Y tube may provide palliation for a time. The disease is unrelenting.

Wegener's Granulomatosis

Wegener's granulomatosis may affect the larynx and trachea with inflammatory lesions that lead to airway obstruction. The rate and extent of involvement are highly unpredictable. With response to medical treatment, an apparently stable stenosis may result.

Sarcoidosis

Sarcoidosis may produce airway obstruction through the mechanism of massive enlargement of mediastinal lymph nodes compressing the airway and distorting it and, also, by intrinsic fibrotic changes in the wall of the trachea and bronchi. A circumferential stenosis results that usually involves a long segment of trachea and main bronchi. Indeed, it may involve bronchi more distally also. These lesions are not amenable to surgical treatment because of diffuseness and extent, but periodic dilatation will tide the patient over for some time.

Amyloid

Amyloid disease on rare occasions involves the trachea and main bronchi in a very extensive process leading to narrowing throughout the tracheobronchial tree. The lesion is too extensive to permit surgical resection and reconstruction.

Tracheopathia Osteoplastica

Tracheopathia osteoplastica manifests itself pathologically by the formation of calcified nodules beneath the mucosa, adjacent to but not actually originating from the cartilages, as described by Young and associates (1980). The involvement may commence in the subglottic larynx and extend throughout the trachea and more distally into the bronchial tree. It appears in adults, progressing insidiously. Patients have difficulty in raising their tenacious secretions as the disease progresses. Ultimately, severe obstructive symptoms may ensue. In some patients, however, the disease remains a curiosity and does not seriously impair them. Some reported cases have been discovered incidentally on autopsy. I have seen two patients who have required surgical relief.

Tracheobronchiomegaly

Tracheobronchiomegaly — Mounier-Kuhn syndrome — is probably of congenital origin, although it usually becomes clinically manifest in adulthood. The symptoms are progressive dyspnea on exertion and difficulty in raising secretions. The trachea may be hugely widened on radiographic examination with both unusually elongated cartilages, which are markedly deformed, and a redundant membranous wall. The cartilages tend gradually to assume a reverse curve, which brings the redundant membranous wall up against the cartilages, causing obstruction. The main bronchi are also involved.

Saber-Sheath Trachea

This is a deformity that is seen usually as an incidental finding in patients with varying degrees of chronic obstructive pulmonary disease later in their life — fifties and sixties. The radiologic presentation was detailed by Greene and Lechner (1975). The lower two thirds of the trachea — the intrathoracic trachea — gradually assumes a configuration in which the side-to-side diameter diminishes progressively and the anteroposterior diameter increases. The cartilages are not malacic. The configuration of the airway changes. In early stages it causes no difficulty, but as it become more and more marked, the posterior part of the cartilages approximate with attempts to cough and breathe deeply, and the patient finds that he cannot clear his secretions. The proximal cervical portion of the trachea usually appears quite normal.

Idiopathic Tracheal Stenosis

Idiopathic stenosis presents over a wide spectrum of age, almost exclusively in women, with progressive dyspnea on exertion and wheezing. These patients are usually found to have a short stenosis — about 2 to 3 cm — involving the uppermost trachea, and in many cases, the subglottic larynx as well. Distally, the trachea appears quite normal. The patients have no history of trauma, infection, inhalation injury, intubation for ventilation, or any other tracheal or airway disease. In a series of 49 patients that my colleagues and I described (1993), only three had any systemic symptoms. Two had mild arthralgias, and one had poorly defined arteritis. Many who had been followed for as long as 15 years had never developed any other systemic symptoms. The stricture itself is roughly circumferential and pathologically shows only chronic inflammation with marked submucosal fibrosis. The cartilages are uninvolved. The pathology is distinct from polychondritis, Wegener's granulomatosis, or any of the aforementioned conditions. The patients do not have mediastinal fibrosis or pathologic processes involving mediastinal lymph nodes. Of the patients in whom ANCA test was done, only the patient with polyarteritis had a positive antinuclear cytoplasmic antibody — ANCA. Interestingly, only one patient showed progression of stenosis following surgical resection.

In addition to this quite well-defined lesion, I have seen a small number of patients with stenosis involving a large part of the trachea and others where the carina or main bronchi, or both, were involved in an undefined inflammatory fibrotic process. In this small group of patients also there were no other incriminating signs, symptoms, or laboratory findings to implicate any known disease or syndrome.

Tracheal Malacia

Tracheal and tracheobronchial malacia remains poorly defined for the most part. A segmental area of malacia may result from postintubation injury either at the level of a cuff lesion or in the segment between the stoma and the cuff lesion. With chronic obstructive pulmonary disease, including emphysema and chronic bronchitis, malacia may develop in the lower trachea, main bronchi, and sometimes the more distal bronchi. In this situation the tracheal rings take on the shape of an archer's bow with elongation of the membranous wall. When the patient attempts to expire forcefully or to cough, the membranous wall approximates to the anterior softened and flattened cartilage, causing nearly total obstruction. Herzog and associates (1987) have carefully defined this entity. This is entirely different from the characteristics of sabre-sheath trachea. A smaller number of patients have been seen who have malacia involving a large portion or even the entire trachea wherein the rings are thinned to a point where they no longer support the airway. The airway takes on almost the appearance of the esophagus. In these patients, the malacia is total in contrast with the picture just described of antero-posterior collapse. The limited malacia that may result from compression by a goiter or thyroid adenoma has been previously mentioned.

DIAGNOSTIC STUDIES

Tracheal lesions often are recognized late despite a prolonged period of symptoms. As physicians become aware of the possibility of tracheal lesions, they are increasingly suspicious of a diagnosis of adult-onset asthma. Appropriate radiographic examinations are used to rule out the possibility of a tracheal lesion in any patient who has obstructive airway symptoms with radiographic demonstration of normal lung fields. Rarely, even specialized techniques fail to reveal an unusual lesion, and bronchoscopic examination is required.

Radiographic Examination of the Trachea

Radiographic studies of the trachea are used not only to rule in or out the presence of a tracheal lesion but also to define the location, extent, and sometimes the character of the lesion (Fig. 69-4). Further, these studies demonstrate the involvement of paratracheal structures by neoplastic lesions. I (1970) have found the following radiographs to be helpful.

Lateral films of the neck with the chin raised demonstrate most lesions of the upper half of the trachea.

Careful technique shows the cartilaginous structures of the larynx as well as the trachea and the relationship of the trachea to the vertebral column posteriorly. If the patient has an existing tracheostomy stoma or has a tracheostomy scar, a radiopaque marker placed on the skin at this level helps to identify its relationship to inflammatory posttracheostomy lesions.

Anteroposterior views of the airway from larynx to carina, using a copper filter, provide useful overall assessment.

Oblique views throw the tracheal air column into relief.

Fluoroscopy will demonstrate malacia and clarify vocal cord function.

Tracheal laminograms help give precise measurement of the extent of lesions and their relative distances from landmarks such as the vocal cords and the carina. A magnifying effect occurs in the radiographs, but at the same time the trachea is somewhat foreshortened because of its oblique passage through the chest. When viewing all radiographs, as well as during bronchoscopy, it should be noted that the level of the vocal cords is not that of the lowermost portion of the larynx. There are approximately 1.5 to 2 cm of larynx between the vocal cords and the inferior border of the cricoid cartilage. Planning for operative procedures must take this into account.

Contrast studies of the trachea add little information except with tracheoesophageal fistula, and this is better shown by barium esophagogram.

Computed tomography — CT — is valuable only in showing the mediastinal extent of a tumor. It is of little use in assessing benign stenosis except in special cases such as goiter, vascular lesions, or histoplasmosis. Inspiratory and expiratory CT scans help to clarify dynamic states such as tracheobronchomalacia and postpneumonectomy syndrome.

If a patient with tracheal stenosis still has a tracheostomy tube in place, it must be removed during radiographic examination to obtain useful information. Even if a tube has been in place for many months, it should be removed cautiously, with provision made for immediate reinsertion. Emergency equipment including suctioning devices and a range of replacement tubes should be available. The physician must be competent to perform such intubation under slight difficulty. The airway often becomes nearly totally obstructed within 20 to 40 minutes following removal of such a tube. Occasionally, considerable force is required for reinsertion of an airway. Weber and I (1978) described the radiographic findings in tracheal tumors and stenosis.

Bronchoscopy

Bronchoscopic examination is required, sooner or later, in all of these patients. When a lesion is known to be present, whether it is neoplastic or inflammatory, and when all else points to its surgical correctability, bronchoscopy is best deferred until preparations have been made for definitive treatment of the lesion. The trauma of bronchoscopy in a patient who is subtotally

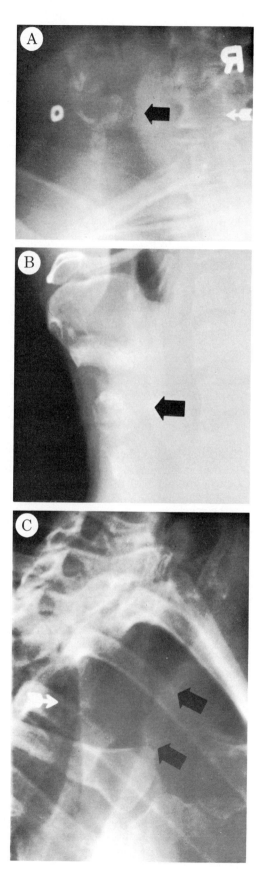

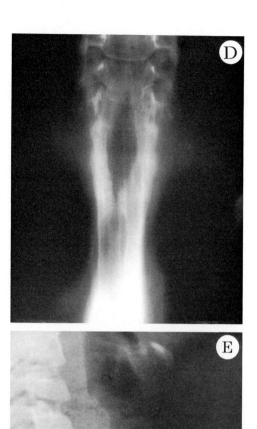

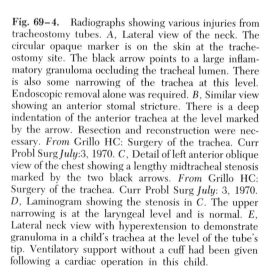

Fig. 69–4. Radiographs showing various injuries from tracheostomy tubes. *A*, Lateral view of the neck. The circular opaque marker is on the skin at the tracheostomy site. The black arrow points to a large inflammatory granuloma occluding the tracheal lumen. There is also some narrowing of the trachea at this level. Endoscopic removal alone was required. *B*, Similar view showing an anterior stomal stricture. There is a deep indentation of the anterior trachea at the level marked by the arrow. Resection and reconstruction were necessary. *From* Grillo HC: Surgery of the trachea. Curr Probl Surg *July*:3, 1970. *C*, Detail of left anterior oblique view of the chest showing a lengthy midtracheal stenosis marked by the two black arrows. *From* Grillo HC: Surgery of the trachea. Curr Probl Surg *July*: 3, 1970. *D*, Laminogram showing the stenosis in *C*. The upper narrowing is at the laryngeal level and is normal. *E*, Lateral neck view with hyperextension to demonstrate granuloma in a child's trachea at the level of the tube's tip. Ventilatory support without a cuff had been given following a cardiac operation in this child.

obstructed may precipitate complete obstruction. Little is lost by delaying the bronchoscopy until the time of definitive operation. Frozen sections may be obtained for histologic diagnosis. In the presence of most obstructive lesions, the requirements for resection are clear at the outset. The bronchoscopy is done with the patient under general anesthesia, permitting unhurried, atraumatic examination and manipulation. Bronchoscopic examination and removal are all that is required in patients with polypoid granulomas at the stomal site or at the site of the tube tip. Esophagoscopy is also performed when neoplasms are examined. Rigid bronchoscopy, under general inhalation anesthesia, using pediatric bronchoscopes serially, is used to dilate severe stenosis for emergency relief. Urgent operation is almost never required. Obstructing tumors may similarly be relieved in an emergency situation or if time is needed to assess a patient, by "coring out" tumor tissue with the tip of the bronchoscope assisted with biopsy forceps. In 30 years, I have never encountered dangerous bleeding or obstruction. The use of laser has been unnecessary for either benign or malignant lesions.

Other Diagnostic Studies

Pulmonary function studies in patients with obstructing lesions of the trachea confirm a high degree of airway obstruction. Measurements are sometimes useful in clarifying the presence of parenchymal disease and may alter the extent of the operative approach. Obstructing lesions generally require surgical relief. Function studies provide a useful basis for measurement of results, especially FEV_1, peak expiratory flow rate — PEFR, and flow-volume loops.

Bacteriologic cultures are made of tracheal secretions and of tracheostomy wounds. Antibiotic sensitivities guide the prophylactic program for perioperative protection.

OPERATIVE VERSUS NONOPERATIVE TREATMENT

The preferred treatment of benign obstruction of the trachea is resection and reconstruction when the patient can tolerate it. With careful evaluation, planning, and execution, most patients with lesions such as postintubation tracheal stenosis can be successfully treated operatively when they have recovered from the primary disease that led to the stenosis. A properly conducted anesthesia and operative repair from the anterior approach do not have a great physiologic impact on the patient. Nonoperative methods of temporizing are, however, available. When the disease is not malignant, undue risks must not be taken. Rarely, the medical condition may not permit even the relatively benign procedure required. If the patient has serious neurologic or psychiatric deficits that will prevent cooperation in the postoperative phase, reconstruction is best deferred. The patient and anesthesia must be selected to avoid the need for ventilatory support postoperatively. If

ventilatory support is needed postoperatively in a shortened trachea, the cuff may rest against the anastomosis and may lead to dehiscence.

The temporizing methods available are repetitive bronchoscopic dilatation of a stenosis or reinstitution of a tracheostomy, dilatation of the stricture, and passage of a tracheostomy tube or a silicone T-tube through the lesion to splint the airway. Lesions in the immediate supracarinal position are not easily managed in this way. A tube long enough to remain seated often causes episodes of obstruction when it is near the carina, and a T-Y tube may lead to bronchial granulations. Generally, however, it is wiser to use a T-tube for permanent airway than to undertake a hazardous reconstruction which has a high risk for failure. Gaissert and I (1993) and Cooper (1989) and colleagues have detailed the uses and results of T-tube management of complex airway problems.

Repeated dilatation and splinting have been proposed as definitive methods for treating tracheal stenosis. In most severe lesions in which the whole thickness of the tracheal wall has been converted to scar tissue, even prolonged stenting for many years will not lead to permanent recovery. Numerous patients have been treated this way. Despite repeated trials, it has been impossible, with only rare exceptions, to remove the splinting tube. When lesser degrees of damage have occurred, either in the completeness of a stricture of the circumference of the trachea or in the depth of the tracheal wall, a period of prolonged splinting, on occasion, may result in an adequate airway after removal of the splint. Such a result has been reported in children. Toty (1987) pointed out that laser treatment can lead to cure only in granuloma — also easily removed by bronchoscopy — and thin, weblike stenosis. Such stenoses are very rare. In the usual postintubation stenosis, definitive opening by laser lead to tracheal perforation. The principal effect of the laser in these lesions has been to delay definitive treatment and, sometimes, to worsen the lesion. Particularly to be deplored is re-establishment of tracheostomy to permit laser treatment, which is usually ineffective.

Few, if any, patients with postintubation tracheal stenosis cannot be repaired successfully when first identified. It is only successive failed or inappropriate therapies that make such patients nonreconstructible.

Prevention of Postintubation Tracheal Stenosis

The incidence of stenosis at the stomal level can be reduced by careful placement of the stoma, avoidance of large apertures, elimination of heavy and prying ventilatory connecting equipment, and meticulous care of the tracheostomy.

Many proposals have been made to reduce the formerly inevitable occurrence of some stenoses at the cuff level. These methods included use of double-cuff tubes, changes in materials and sterilization techniques, attempts to avoid cuffs altogether, use of disk and sponge seals instead of cuffs, use of spacers to relocate the cuff

A

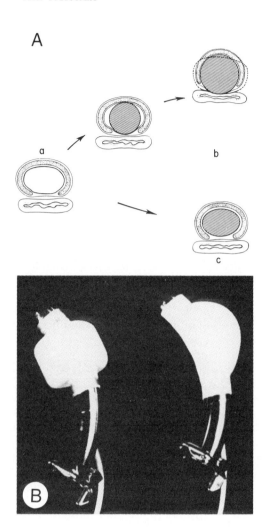

Fig. 69–5. *A*, Diagram of the mechanism of pressure necrosis by a tracheostomy cuff and its avoidance. *a-* Normal elliptic shape of the trachea. When a conventional cuff is inflated, it may expand in circular fashion in its widest diameter but at this point fails to occlude the basically irregularly elliptic shape of the trachea. *b-* Further distention has been required to effect a seal. At this point the trachea is deformed by the cuff, and much of the considerable intracuff tension is transmitted to the tracheal wall. *c-*A large-volume low-pressure cuff has been inflated with a minimal amount of air. The cuff conforms to the irregular shape of the lumen and provides a seal at low intracuff pressures. Correspondingly low pressures are transmitted to the tracheal wall. *B*, Comparison of a standard cuff and a large-volume low-pressure cuff. On the left, the large-volume cuff is shown spontaneously filled with air. No stretch has been placed on the rubber of the cuff wall at this point. The volume is sufficient to occlude most adult tracheas. On the right, a Rusch cuff has been distended with 8 ml of air. It is tense and eccentric. The stretching of the rubber has created a hard structure that exerts considerable pressure on the trachea, which it must deform to provide a seal. *From* Grillo HC, et al: A low pressure cuff for tracheostomy tubes to minimize tracheal injury: a comparative clinical trial. J Thorac Cardiovasc Surg 62:898, 1971.

level periodically, and prestretching of plastic cuffs. The only promising methods, accepting the present need for cuffs in management of adult patients in severe respiratory failure, have been intermittent inflation of cuffs cycled to the respirator, described by Arens and colleagues (1969), and more simply, the development of

large-volume, low-pressure cuffs that conform to the shape of the trachea rather than deforming it, described by Cooper and me (1969b) and by me and my co-workers (1971) (Fig. 69–5). Such a cuff provided a seal at intracuff pressures of 33 mmHg compared with 270 mmHg in a comparative Rusch standard cuff. Thus, in a series of 45 patients in whom such a cuff was compared, on a randomized basis, with standard cuffs, 25 patients with the soft cuff showed half as much damage — scaled on the basis of endoscopic observations at the time of deflation of the cuff — as 20 patients with standard cuffs. All severe damage was in the standard group. Incidence of cuff stenosis has dropped markedly as equipment has improved but low-pressure cuffs must be inflated carefully to avoid converting them to high-pressure cuffs. Failure to do so has continued to produce a steady flow of stenoses requiring reconstruction.

Cricothyroidostomy should be avoided. Although laryngeal injury is rare, it may not be correctible when it occurs. Tracheal injuries — also rare — are reparable when they first occur. Inappropriate treatment has served to make some incorrectible.

This section on operative versus nonoperative treatment and on prevention of lesions has been confined to the most frequent lesion — postintubation stenosis. Space does not permit consideration of each of the other varied benign lesions described earlier.

RESULTS OF TREATMENT

I reported (1979) 208 patients who underwent reconstruction for *postintubation tracheal injury* between 1965 and early 1979. In seven patients, a cuffed tube was inserted to prevent aspiration, and respirators were not used. Thirty-three of the referred patients had undergone prior reconstructive attempts or other major tracheal procedures. One hundred thirteen had postintubation stenoses at the site of an inflatable cuff — 23 of whom had only an endotracheal tube without subsequent tracheostomy. There were 78 stomal stenoses and 13 stomal and cuff stenoses, and in 4 the origin was uncertain. Nine patients with tracheoesophageal fistula were corrected by the technique I reported with my colleagues (1976). One presented with tracheoinnominate arterial cuff fistula. Corrective reconstructive surgery was effected through the cervical route alone in 126 of these patients, with the addition of an upper sternotomy in 83, through the transthoracic route in 6, and a skin tube replacement was constructed in one patient — a total of 216 operations in 208 patients (see Chapter 34).

In 168 of 203 patients followed, the results were good or excellent. An "excellent" result denotes an anatomically and functionally normal airway. The patient suffers no limitation whatsoever because of his airway, and on either radiographic or bronchoscopic examination, or both, essentially no narrowing is demonstrated at the anastomotic site. Patients classified as "good" have no functional difficulty whatsoever but may have a minimal anatomic narrowing that is definable on either radiographic study or bronchoscopic examination.

The results in 21 patients were classified as "satisfactory." These patients are able to carry out all of their normal daily activities but do have enough narrowing of their airway to limit major physical effort.

Nine patients were listed as failures. Causes of failure included inadequate appreciation of existing neurologic dysphagia, cardiac decompensation requiring postoperative ventilation, unappreciated severe laryngeal dysfunction, and restenosis. Five deaths occurred. In 4 of the patients who died, the patients were sent to us on respirators and hence reconstruction was contraindicated but undertaken because no therapeutic alternative existed. The other developed bilateral pneumonia and could not be weaned from postoperative need for respiratory support. My colleagues and I (1986) described the complications of tracheal surgery for both benign stenosis and neoplasms in detail. Over 600 patients have now undergone surgical repair of postintubation stenosis; these results are being analyzed.

Pearson and Andrews (1971) reported 60 patients with tracheal stenosis. In 34 the stenosis was at the stomal and in 26 at the cuff level. Thirty-seven segmental resections were performed. In 33 of the patients, the results were good, in 1 fair. There was 1 failure and 2 operative deaths. Six of the patients developed significant restenosis, and re-resection was performed with good results in all but 1 of the group. Laryngeal release was used as an adjunctive procedure in 5 of these patients.

The management of *acquired benign tracheoesophageal fistula* depends on whether the adjacent segment of trachea is circumferentially damaged — as it almost always is in postintubation lesions — or whether the posterior wall fistula is the sole tracheal pathology, as it usually is in fistulas that are due to foreign bodies. In the first case, concomitant tracheal resection is done with lateral excision of the fistula in the esophageal wall. In the latter, tracheal resection is unnecessary, and both membranous tracheal wall and esophageal wall are precisely repaired after division of the fistulae. Healthy tissue, such as strap muscles from the anterior approach or intercostal transthoracically, is always interposed between the two suture lines to prevent recurrence. Mathisen and associates (1991) noted excellent results following repair of 27 postintubation fistulas, with 1 death following anastomotic separation consequent to a very extensive tracheal resection. Three deaths also occurred after transthoracic repair of very distal posttraumatic fistulas in the presence of established mediastinal sepsis. All three required postoperative ventilation. Prompt recognition and repair following the initial injury would likely have been successful.

I reported the results, with my colleagues (1992), of single-stage laryngotracheal resection and repair of *postintubation subglottic stenosis* involving larynx and upper trachea in 50 patients. An additional 30 patients had stenoses in the same location from other causes: trauma, 7; idiopathic, 19; miscellaneous, 4. Long-term results were excellent in 18 patients, good in 51, satisfactory in 8, failed in 2. One died of acute myocardial infarction. Maddaus (1992) and Couraud (1979) and their colleagues have produced similar encouraging results.

Mathisen and I (1987) found that 16 of 17 patients treated for *laryngotracheal stenosis resulting from trauma* attained good airways and voices, despite the initial presence of vocal cord paralysis in 14. Four also had esophageal injury requiring repair. Eight needed intralaryngeal procedures before laryngotracheal repair.

Gaissert and co-workers (1993) found that complex *laryngotracheal strictures due to burns* responded well in many cases to prolonged stenting — mean 28 months — with recovery of a functional airway and voice in most patients. In a few resection of subglottic stenosis was necessary. Early tracheal resection was best avoided. Of 16 patients treated, 9 require no airway support, 4 have permanent tracheal tubes, 2 died — 1 from respiratory failure and 1 from unrelated cause, and 1 was lost to follow-up.

Following a failed attempt at tracheal reconstruction, with *postoperative stenosis*, it is best to wait for a prolonged period of time to permit resolution of the scar and inflammation in the operative field. A minimum of 4 months and preferably 6 months should be allowed. In the meanwhile it may be necessary to insert a tracheal T-tube or tracheostomy tube to maintain the airway. Reoperation is often extremely difficult. It is surprising, however, to find in some situations where there appeared to be tension at the original anastomosis, re-resection of a limited stricture may be done with the finding that there is no apparent tension at the time of the second repair. This, however, is not universally true. The greatest enemy of secondary resection is the possibility of anastomotic tension, which may have led to the first failure. Much therefore depends on the individual history of the patient.

Histoplasmosis can present nearly insuperable problems in airway management. In the description of the manifestations of mediastinal fibrosis and histoplasmosis, Mathisen and I (1992) listed nine patients who had undergone tracheobronchoplastic procedures: right carinal pneumonectomy four, carinal reconstruction one, sleeve lobectomy three, main bronchial sleeve resection one. Three died postoperatively, one from anastomotic separation after extended resection, and two from postpneumonectomy ARDS.

With my colleagues, I (1992) presented the results of surgical attempts to treat severe *postpneumonectomy syndrome* in 11 adults. Ten underwent mediastinal repositioning. Five who had not also developed tracheobronchomalacia did well. Another died from presumed pulmonary embolism. Four suffered malacic obstruction unrelieved by repositioning. Aortic division with bypass to relieve compression and resection of malacic airway in these desperately ill patients produced only one success. Clearly, correction must be done early, before malacia develops.

Extrinsic compression that is due to *substernal or intrathoracic goiter* is generally relieved, without need for tracheal procedures, by thyroidectomy, as shown by Katlic and colleagues (1985) in a series of 80 patients. Dyspnea was present preoperatively in 28% and stridor in 16%; 79% had tracheal deviation. Flow-volume loops showed tracheal obstruction. There were no deaths. The procedure is well tolerated even by frail and aged patients: Only a few required tracheal splinting. There is no effective medical treatment.

I and my associates (1993) defined the clinical and pathologic characteristics of *idiopathic laryngotracheal stenosis* and reported results of surgical treatment in 35 patients. Twenty-nine underwent single-stage laryngotracheal resection and reconstruction, and 6 underwent cricotracheal segmental resection and reconstruction. Thirty-two achieved good or excellent results in voice and airway, 2 needed annual dilatations, and 1 has a permanent tracheostomy.

In two patients who have presented with severely obstructive *tracheopathia osteoplastica*, I performed a tracheal fissure from the cricoid to the carina and inserted a T-Y tube for splinting. Once the trachea has been divided anteriorly, because the membranous wall is not involved by the disease process, it is possible to hinge the two anterolateral walls on either side outward so that a wide lumen is created by the T-Y tube. The tracheal wall can then be sutured together again. The T-Y tube is allowed to remain in place for 4 to 6 months to allow firm healing of the trachea in a now open position. The tube is removed, having established an adequate airway. Prior attempts have been made to use the laser but failed. I presented the first patient in 1992.

An attempt at splinting and shortening the posterior membranous wall combined with an attempt to reshape the reverse curve of the cartilages failed in one patient with *Mounier-Kuhn disease* in whom it was attempted. It was necessary to insert an in-lying permanent tracheal T-tube. Two other patients have been treated in similar fashion since that time, and all have achieved satisfactory palliative results.

In two patients with such extreme *sabre-sheath trachea* that they were unable to clear secretions, the trachea was splinted with external special polypropylene ring splints. The tracheal wall was sutured to the splints, pulling it outward. The sternohyoid muscles were turned down to embed the rings against the tracheal wall to maintain correction after nonabsorbable sutures ultimately pull through. The procedure permitted the patients to clear secretions, which they had not been able to do before.

In patients with *tracheobronchial malacia* affecting the lower two thirds of the trachea and main bronchi, who have softened, splayed out cartilages in an archer's bow configuration and, also, redundant membranous tracheal wall, reshaping the trachea was proposed and described by Herzog and colleagues (1987). A strip of splinting material is placed along the membranous wall of the trachea in a width corresponding to estimated normal. The corners of the cartilages on either side are sutured to the splint, and the membranous wall is quilted to the splint as well. Pulling the two ends of the cartilages together posteriorly causes the cartilages to arch forward, re-creating a more nearly normal cross-sectional configuration. The redundant membranous wall is fixed to the splint posteriorly so that it cannot pout forward to obstruct the lumen. Herzog originally used fascia lata and eventually moved to use of Gore-Tex. Other materials that have been used include lyophilized bone and perforated plastic splints.

Gore-Tex, in my experience, gave an initially excellent result. In one patient, however, after some months, fluid accumulated between the Gore-Tex and the membranous wall where sutures had pulled through, because Gore-Tex does not become enmeshed in scar tissue. Since then I have used strips of pericardium harvested within the operative field and have found this to be quite satisfactory. A synthetic material with pores large enough to permit ingrowth of connective tissue to fuse it to the membranous wall should work equally well. Although this procedure does not correct the underlying obstructive pulmonary disease from which most of these patients suffer, it does improve the delivery of gases through the major airways and provide more effective cough. It is possible from the right thoracotomy approach to splint not only the lower two thirds of the trachea but also the right main bronchus and bronchus intermedius and the left main bronchus to its bifurcation.

REFERENCES

Andrews MJ, Pearson FG: The incidence and pathogenesis of tracheal injury following cuffed tube tracheostomy with assisted ventilation: an analysis of a two year prospective study. Ann Surg 173:249, 1971.

Arens JF, Oschner JL, Gee C: Volume-limited intermittent cuff inflation for long-term respiratory assistance. J Thorac Cardiovasc Surg 58:837, 1969.

Carroll R, Hedden M, Safar P: Intratracheal cuffs: performance characteristics. Anesthesia 31:275, 1969.

Cooper JD, Grillo HC: The evolution of tracheal injury due to ventilatory assistance through cuffed tubes: a pathologic study. Ann Surg 169:334, 1969a.

Cooper JD, Grillo HC: Experimental production and prevention of injury due to cuffed tracheal tubes. Surg Gynecol Obstet 129:1235, 1969b.

Cooper JD, et al.: Use of silicone stents in the management of airway problems. Ann Thorac Surg 47:371, 1989.

Couraud L, et al.: Intérêt de la résection cricoïdienne dans le traitement des sténoses cricotrachéales après intubation. Ann Chir Thorac Cardiovasc 33:242, 1979.

Couraud L, Velly JF, Martigne C, N'Diaye M: Posttraumatic disruption of the laryngo-tracheal junction. Eur J Cardio Thorac Surg 3:441, 1989.

Deslauriers J, et al.: Innominate artery rupture: a major complication of tracheal surgery. Ann Thorac Surg 20:671, 1975.

Deslauriers J, et al.: Diagnosis and long-term follow-up of major bronchial disruptions due to nonpenetrating trauma. Ann Thorac Surg 33:32, 1982.

Florange W, Muller J, Forster E: Morphologie de la nécrose trachéale après trachéotomie et l'utilisation d'une prosthèse respiratoire. Anesth Analg 22:693, 1965.

Gaissert HA, Grillo HC, Mathisen DJ, Wain JC: Temporary and permanent restoration of airway patency with the tracheal T-tube. J Thorac Cardiovasc Surg (in press), 1993.

Gaissert HA, Lofgren RH, Grillo HC: Upper airway compromise after inhalation injury: complex strictures of larynx and trachea and their management. Ann Surg (in press), 1993.

Greene RE, Lechner GL: "Saber-sheath" trachea: a clinical and functional study of marked coronal narrowing of the intrathoracic trachea. Radiology 115:265, 1975.

Grillo HC: The management of tracheal stenosis following assisted respiration. J Thorac Cardiovasc Surg 57:52, 1969.

Grillo HC: Surgery of the trachea. Curr Probl Surg July:3, 1970.

Grillo HC: Surgical treatment of post-intubation tracheal injuries. J Thorac Cardiovasc Surg 78:860, 1979.

Grillo HC: Primary reconstruction of airway after resection of subglottic laryngeal and upper tracheal stenosis. Ann Thorac Surg 33:3, 1982.

Grillo HC, et al.: A low pressure cuff for tracheostomy tubes to minimize tracheal injury: a comparative clinical trial. J Thorac Cardiovasc Surg 62:898, 1971.

Grillo HC, Mark EJ, Mathisen DJ, Wain JC: Idiopathic laryngotracheal stenosis: the entity and its management. Ann Thorac Surg (in press), 1993.

Grillo HC, Mathisen DJ, Wain JC: Laryngotracheal resection and reconstruction for subglottic stenosis. Ann Thorac Surg 53:54, 1992.

Grillo HC, Moncure AC, McEnany MT: Repair of inflammatory tracheoesophageal fistula. Ann Thorac Surg 22:112, 1976.

Grillo HC, Shepard JO, Mathisen DJ, Kanarek DJ: Postpneumonectomy syndrome: diagnosis, management and results. Ann Thorac Surg 54:638, 1992.

Grillo HC, Zannini P, Michelassi F: Complications of tracheal reconstruction. J Thorac Cardiovasc Surg 91:322, 1986.

Herzog H, Heitz M, Keller R, Graedel E: Surgical therapy for expiratory collapse of the trachea and large bronchi. In Grillo HC, Eschapasse (eds): International Trends in General Thoracic Surgery: Major Challenges. Philadelphia: WB Saunders, 1987, p 74.

Katlic MR, Grillo HC, Wang CA: Substernal goiter: analysis of 80 Massachusetts General Hospital cases. Am J Surg 149:283, 1985.

Lindholm CE: Prolonged endotracheal intubation. Acta Anaesth Scand 33(Suppl):1, 1970.

Maddaus MA, Toth JLR, Gullane PJ, Pearson FG: Subglottic tracheal resection and synchronous laryngeal reconstruction. J Thorac Cardiovasc Surg 104:1443, 1992.

Mark EJ, Patterson GA, Grillo HC: Case records of the Massachusetts General Hospital. N Engl J Med 327:1512, 1992.

Mathisen DJ, Grillo HC: Laryngotracheal trauma. Ann Thorac Surg 43:254, 1987.

Mathisen DJ, Grillo HC: Clinical manifestations of mediastinal fibrosis and histoplasmosis. Ann Thorac Surg 54:1053, 1992.

Mathisen DJ, Grillo HC, Wain JC, Hilgenberg AD: Management of acquired nonmalignant tracheoesophageal fistula. Ann Thorac Surg 52:759, 1991.

Montgomery WW: The surgical management of supraglottic and subglottic stenosis. Ann Otol 77:534, 1968.

Newton JR, Grillo HC, Mathisen DJ: Main bronchial sleeve resection with pulmonary conservation. Ann Thorac Surg 52:1272, 1991.

Pearson FG, Andrews MJ: Detection and management of tracheal stenosis following cuffed tube tracheostomy. Ann Thorac Surg 12:359, 1971.

Pearson FG, Cooper JD, Nelems JM, Van Nostrand AWP: Primary tracheal anastomosis after resection of the cricoid cartilage with preservation of recurrent laryngeal nerves. J Thorac Cardiovasc Surg 70:806, 1975.

Tedder M, et al: Pulmonary mucormycosis: results of medical and surgical therapy. J Thorac Cardiovasc Surg (in press), 1993.

Toty L, et al.: Laser treatment of postintubation lesions. In Grillo HC, Eschapasse H (eds): International Trends in General Thoracic Surgery. Vol. 2. Philadelphia: WB Saunders, 1987, p 31.

Weber AL, Grillo HC: Tracheal stenosis: an analysis of 151 cases. Radiol Clin North Am 16:291, 1978.

Young RH, Sandstrom RE, Mark EJ: Tracheopathia osteoplastica: clinical, radiologic, pathologic and histogenetic features. J Thorac Cardiovasc Surg 79:537, 1980.

CHAPTER 70

BENIGN AND MALIGNANT TUMORS OF THE TRACHEA

L. Penfield Faber, James R. Hemp, and William H. Warren

Tumors of the trachea are rare despite their histologic similarity to tumors of the main stem bronchus and lung. They are approximately 100 times less common than bronchial tumors and constitute only 2% of all upper respiratory tract tumors, as reported by Perelman and Koroleva (1987). Malignant tumors of the trachea are more common than those that are benign. Houston and associates (1969) reviewed 30 years of experience at the Mayo Clinic, and 53 of 90 tracheal tumors were malignant. Hajdu and colleagues (1970) reported a series of 41 primary malignancies of the trachea that were treated over a period of 33 years at a major cancer hospital. This number represents slightly more than one malignant tracheal tumor per year seen at a major referral center, which emphasizes the relative rarity of these tumors. The most common malignant tumors are squamous cell carcinoma and adenoid cystic carcinoma. In a review of 43 tracheal tumors occurring in infants and children, Gilbert and associates (1953) noted that 93% were benign. The predominant benign tumors in children are papillomas, fibromas, and hemangiomas.

Secondary tumors also involve the trachea. Direct extension into the trachea occurs from cancers of the thyroid, larynx, lung, and esophagus. Mediastinal tumors may directly invade the trachea and the most common is lymphoma. Metastasis to the trachea is uncommon, but breast cancer, melanoma, and sarcomas have all been found in the trachea.

SYMPTOMS AND FINDINGS

Cough is a common symptom associated with tracheal neoplasms, but no particular salient features are associated with the cough to indicate that it is caused by a tracheal tumor. As the airway becomes narrowed, the classic symptom of wheezing becomes apparent. Stridor is a more prominent form of wheezing and indicates significant compromise of the airway. Often a patient with a tracheal tumor is treated for asthma for a prolonged period. Dyspnea and shortness of breath on exertion are common presenting symptoms and, according to Perelman and Koroleva (1987), occur when the tracheal lumen has been reduced to one third of its normal cross-sectional area. It is important to note that the dyspnea associated with a tracheal tumor is usually inspiratory, unlike that of bronchial asthma or emphysema.

Hemoptysis occurs in approximately 25% of patients with tracheal neoplasms and is most commonly seen in patients with squamous cell carcinoma. Persons with benign tumors, rarely, if ever, present with hemoptysis. A change in voice quality can be related to paralysis of the vocal cord resulting from invasion of the recurrent laryngeal nerve or by direct extension of an upper tracheal tumor into the larynx. Recurrent pneumonitis, either unilateral or bilateral, can occur from obstruction of a main bronchus. Perelman and Koroleva (1987) reported that the interval between the onset of early symptoms and diagnosis was approximately 25 months for benign tumors and 8 months for malignant tumors. Dysphagia is an uncommon symptom that indicates esophageal compression by a large bulky neoplasm. Auscultation of the chest reveals a coarse wheeze that is enhanced by rapid and deep inspiration. The wheeze is more prominent on inspiration than on expiration and is different than the wheezing commonly associated with bronchial asthma. The obstruction from a tracheal tumor can also be heard if the examiner places an ear close to the patient's open mouth during deep and forceful breathing. This is a simple but major finding associated with laryngeal or tracheal obstruction. The neck should be examined carefully for evidence of enlarged lymph nodes that may indicate spread of a malignant tumor.

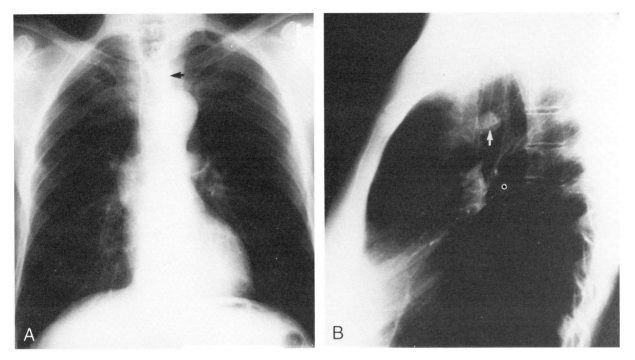

Fig. 70–1. *A*, A chondroma can be seen on this frontal chest radiograph (arrow). *B*, Tracheal hamartoma is clearly identified on this lateral chest radiograph (arrow).

DIAGNOSIS

Radiographic Features

Careful inspection of the tracheal air column on posteroanterior and lateral chest radiographs sometimes reveals the presence of a tracheal tumor (Fig. 70–1). Frequently, a tracheal tumor has been identified during a diagnostic bronchoscopy and more pertinent radiologic evaluation must then be obtained. Oblique views of the trachea and lateral neck radiographs in hyperextension reveal the presence of the tumor, but do not provide specific information necessary for a planned resection and reconstruction. Linear tomography, as described by Weber and Grillo (1992), provides excellent visualization of the extent of the tumor (Fig. 70–2). Tracheal tomograms, however, are not effective for determining extralumenal extension of the tumor or lymph node invasion.

Computed tomography — CT — is replacing linear tomography as the primary method of radiologic evaluation of a tracheal tumor. Mediastinal extension, esophageal compression, and tracheal lumen size are all seen clearly on the CT scan (Fig. 70–3). Using thin-cut CT sections and knowing the distance between the cuts can permit a moderately accurate measurement of the length of trachea that is involved by the tumor. Gross pathologic characteristics of the tumor are also identified on the CT scan. Benign lesions usually are round and smooth and approximately 2 cm in diameter. The tumor is generally inside the lumen of the trachea and the

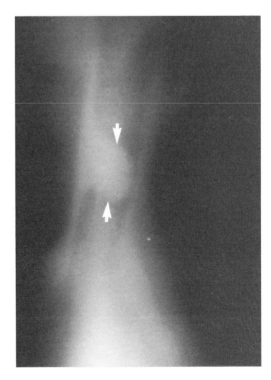

Fig. 70–2. Linear tomogram clearly depicts the length of involvement of a carcinoid tumor of the trachea (arrows).

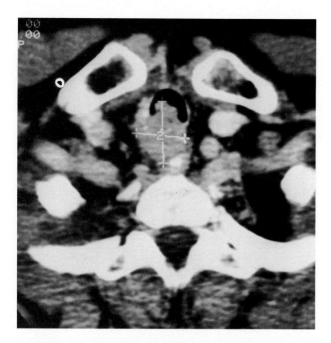

Fig. 70–3. Computed tomogram identifies posterior mediastinal extension of an adenoid cystic carcinoma.

ulcerated. The trachea wall is obviously invaded by the tumor at its base and extralumenal growth may be present. Enlarged lymph nodes usually indicate metastatic spread. The CT scan should always be done with infusion to delineate clearly the relationship of the tumor to the superior vena cava and other vascular structures in the mediastinum.

Magnetic resonance — MR — imaging does not offer significant advantages over CT. Its only advantage is that coronal, oblique, and sagittal views can be obtained that assist in better defining the length of tracheal involvement by the tumor.

If the patient complains of dysphagia, a barium examination of the esophagus will demonstrate compression or possibly invasion.

Pulmonary function studies reveal airway obstruction characterized by a reduced volume of air expired in 1 second, a significantly decreased peak flow rate, and a flattened expiratory flow volume loop. Maximum voluntary ventilation will be diminished. Pulmonary functions may also delineate the presence or absence of parenchymal lung disease.

Bronchoscopy

Bronchoscopy is a necessary step in the diagnosis and clinical evaluation of a patient with a tracheal tumor. Biopsy and manipulation of a tracheal tumor is potentially hazardous, however, as bleeding can cause complete tracheal obstruction. A sedated or anesthetized patient may be unable to maintain adequate ventilation and the passage of an endotracheal tube may not be possible because of the obstructing tumor. The bronchoscopic examination should be carried out by an

well-circumscribed nature of the tumor is clearly evident. Calcification is also a characteristic of benign lesions and is seen in tumors such as chondromas and hamartomas (Fig. 70–4). Calcification is also present, however, in a chondrosarcoma. Malignant tumors extend up and down the trachea for several centimeters and the surface of the tumor is irregular and possibly

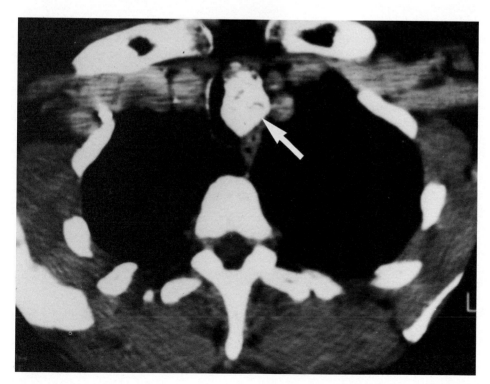

Fig. 70–4. The computed tomogram demonstrates almost total calcification of a tracheal chondroma (arrow).

experienced endoscopist who has the ability to insert an open tube bronchoscope through the tumor to establish an airway and manage any complications of hemorrhage.

A bronchoscopic examination is always conducted in the operating room where ventilating bronchoscopes and biopsy forceps are available and a trained anesthesiologist is close at hand. Grillo (1989) believes that when the indications for primary tracheal resection are clear cut, bronchoscopy can be deferred until the time of the operative procedure and frozen sections are used to determine histology. With the flexible fiberoptic bronchoscope, however, a careful examination and biopsy can be accomplished in the awake patient. A preresection bronchoscopy offers several advantages: 1) vocal cord function is evaluated and the entire larynx and cricoid cartilage are seen clearly; this visualization is particularly important for upper tracheal lesions in which a partial resection of the cricoid or laryngectomy may be required; 2) the gross characteristics of the tumor are noted and an impression can be gained whether the tumor is benign or malignant; 3) the size of the tracheal lumen is clearly noted, and this assessment is extremely helpful in planning anesthetic management of the airway during the initial phase of tracheal resection; 4) a biopsy sample can be obtained with the small biopsy forceps through the flexible instrument, and knowing the histology is of benefit in planning the treatment program; 5) frequently, the small, flexible fiberoptic bronchoscope can be inserted past the neoplasm and the distal airway can be carefully examined. The length of the tumor can be carefully measured and correlated with the radiologic measurements. These findings are all extremely helpful in planning the surgical approach and resection.

The bronchoscopy is performed with the flexible fiberscope passed through a topically anesthetized nasopharynx to a position above the larynx. Supplemental oxygen is provided through the mouth. Several aliquots of 4% lidocaine — Xylocaine — are instilled on and through the vocal cords until satisfactory topical anesthesia is achieved. The vocal cords and larynx are examined carefully and the bronchoscope is then passed into the trachea to visualize the tumor. Decision for biopsy depends on the vascularity of the tumor and the size of the tracheal lumen. The decision for biopsy requires careful judgment and the biopsy should not be done if there is any possibility of airway compromise (Fig. 70–5). Houston and colleagues (1969) reported that of 53 primary cancers of the trachea, the diagnosis was established by bronchoscopic biopsy without complication in 47 patients.

Lifethreatening airway obstruction by a tracheal tumor can be relieved by the coring out of a tumor with the use of the rigid bronchoscope and biopsy forceps, as described by Mathisen and Grillo, (1989). The maintenance of adequate oxygenation by the use of the technique of jet ventilation may be beneficial in this situation, as noted in Chapter 22. The YAG laser can

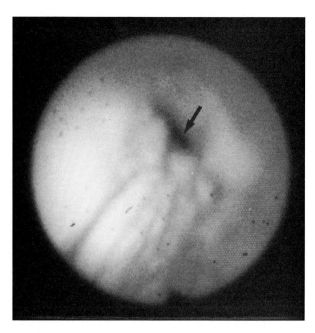

Fig. 70–5. A trachea almost totally occluded by adenoid cystic carcinoma (arrow). Bleeding from biopsy or manipulation could be life-threatening.

also be of significant benefit in the removal of an obstructing tumor.

BENIGN TUMORS

Gilbert and associates (1953) reported that the common benign tumors of the trachea are chondroma, papilloma, fibroma, and hemangioma (Table 70–1).

Table 70–1. Benign Tracheal Tumors*

Tumor Type	Perelman and Korolewa (1987)	Grillo and Mathisen (1990)
Squamous papillomata	9	5
Multiple	—	(4)
Solitary	—	(1)
Pleomorphic adenoma	4	2
Granular cell tumor	—	2
Fibrous histiocytoma	—	1
Leiomyoma	1	2
Chondroma	—	2
Chondroblastoma	—	1
Nerve sheath tumor	6	2
Paraganglioma	—	2
Vascular tumor	4	1
Vascular malformation	—	2
Myoblastoma	1	—
Lipoma	1	—
Xanthoma	1	—
Pseudosarcoma	—	1
Total	27	23

*Some of the tumors listed have been reclassified from the original source (Editor).

Benign tumors most often occur in the upper one third of the trachea in children and are more common in the lower one third in adults, frequently arising from the membranous portion of the trachea.

Chondroma

The most common benign mesenchymal tumor of the trachea, as noted by Mark (1983), is a chondroma (Fig. 70–6). These tumors histologically duplicate normal cartilage and can exhibit vascular invasion. Endoscopically, a chondroma appears as a firm, white nodule projecting into the lumen of the trachea. There is a preponderance of four to one in men, and the tumor is more common in adults than in children. No definite etiology for this lesion has been described. A chondroma occurs more frequently in the larynx than in the trachea. Biopsy of the lesion can be difficult because of its firm consistency, and this characteristic can indicate the diagnosis. Vascularity is minimal and the lesion can be removed easily through the bronchoscope. Recurrence after endoscopic removal has been observed, however, and malignant transformation to chondrosarcoma has also been reported by Salminen and colleagues (1990). Recommended treatment is segmental tracheal resection.

Papilloma

A solitary papilloma of the trachea is rare, but this lesion does occur in adults. A solitary benign papilloma is easily removed through the bronchoscope and the base of the tumor can be ablated with the YAG laser. Periodic endoscopic surveillance is indicated and recurrence can again be treated with laser ablation.

Juvenile laryngotracheal papillomatosis is common in children and is seen more frequently when compared to the incidence of solitary papilloma of the trachea. It accounts for 60% of benign tracheal tumors in children, according to Beattie and associates (1992). It has been linked with the human papilloma virus of types 6 and 11. Papillomatosis more commonly involves the larynx, but it is found in the tracheobronchial tree in 20% of patients. It follows a relatively benign course, requiring repeated endoscopic removal with recurrence rates as high as 90%. Complications include chronic cavitary respiratory papillomatosis resulting from proliferation of the virus in the distal bronchial tree, as noted by Karley and colleagues (1989). Malignant transformation of papillomatosis has been reported in patients with a history of radiation therapy or smoking, but it may also occur in nonsmokers, as noted by Guillou and associates (1991). The types of therapy for the more invasive form of the disease include photodynamic therapy with sensitization of papilloma cells using hematoporphyrin diacetate, as described by Kavuru (1990) and Basheda (1991) and their colleagues. Leventhal and associates (1991) reported successful treatment with the use of lymphoblastoid interferon α-N1.

Fibroma

A fibroma accounts for approximately 20% of all benign tumors in adults, according to Beattie and colleagues (1992). Mark (1983) reported that a fibroma is more common than fibrous sarcoma and can be difficult to distinguish from a fibrous histiocytoma. A benign fibroma is easily removed through the bronchoscope, followed by careful laser ablation of the base of the tumor. Local recurrence would be unusual, but if it does occur, segmental tracheal resection would then be indicated.

Hemangioma

Mark (1983) noted that the tracheal lesion is similar to the hemangioma of the skin in infants, with an increase in size at 1 month of age followed by a spontaneous decrease in size at 1 year. It may arise in the trachea or extend into the tracheal lumen from a hemangioma located in the mediastinum. Treatment may require tracheostomy to provide an adequate airway followed by repeated small doses of radiation to shrink the tumor. Steroids have been used by Weber and co-workers (1990) to cause regression. Many lesions require no treatment and natural regression frequently occurs. Larger hemangiomas of the lower trachea may require direct surgical intervention. In this instance, a careful plan must be developed for airway control during excision of the tumor. Franks and Rothera (1990) used cardiopulmonary bypass to resect a low-lying tracheal hemangioma.

Other Benign Tumors

The granular cell tumor occurs less frequently in the trachea than it does in the tongue, neck, or larynx. Burton and associates (1992) summarized the reported experience with this tumor in the trachea and identified 24 cases. The tumor is thought to be of neurogenic origin and is derived from Schwann cells. Malignant transformation of the granular cell tumor does occur in other sites, but it has never been reported in the trachea. Both endoscopic and partial tracheal resection have been successful as a form of treatment of this lesion. Burton and associates (1992), however, described a case of local recurrence following endoscopic resection that then required partial tracheal resection. Daniel and colleagues (1980) recommended that tumors larger than 1 cm should be removed by a segmental tracheal resection because of the increased risk for full-thickness wall involvement with tumors of this size. Smaller lesions — less than 1 cm — are easily ablated by endoscopic YAG laser therapy. Cunningham and co-workers (1989) recommend the use of bipolar cautery. Endoscopic therapy would certainly be applicable to larger tumors, as well, with resection reserved for local recurrence, because malignant transformation of this tumor in the trachea has yet to be reported.

The fibrous histiocytoma is a histologically benign tumor of the trachea, but it can be locally infiltrative (Fig. 70–7). An associated prominent inflammatory component can cause the tumor to be termed an inflammatory pseudotumor. The behavior of this tumor in the trachea appears to be benign, but because of its local infiltration, segmental resection is the treatment

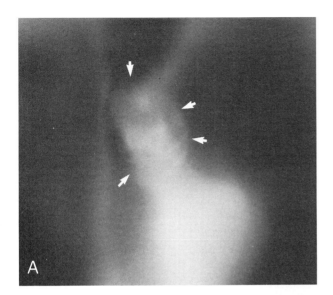

Fig. 70-6. *A*, Linear tomogram depicts a calcified chondroma (arrows). *B*, The benign chondroma is removed by segmental tracheal resection. *C*, Microscopic examination reveals areas of ossification in a largely cartilaginous tumor.

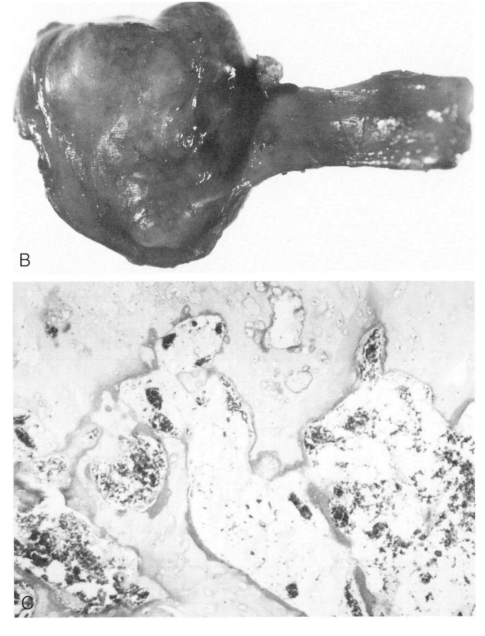

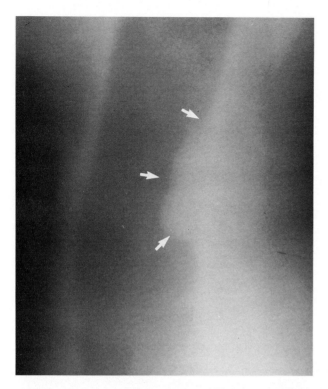

Fig. 70–7. A broad-based fibrous histiocytoma (arrows) removed by segmental tracheal resection.

of choice. Resection of a malignant fibrous histiocytoma of the trachea was reported by Randleman and associates (1990) with identification of one other case in the literature.

The glomus tumor is a benign neoplasm arising from specialized cells surrounding arterial venous anastomoses. Garcia-Prats and colleagues (1991) reviewed the literature and found six cases of tracheal origin. All of the tumors were treated by segmental tracheal resection.

Tracheal lipoma is a rare lesion, with five cases reported previously (Fig. 70–8). Chen (1990) described a patient with a tracheal lipoma requiring major tracheal resection for complete removal. Other authors describe endoscopic removal. It is only logical to approach this tumor with endoscopic removal as it is a completely benign tumor and any local recurrence can be treated successfully with laser therapy.

A leiomyoma may occur as a primary tracheal tumor and, according to Mark (1983), it usually occurs in the distal one third of the trachea. Both tracheal resection and endoscopic removal have been described in rare case reports.

The neurofibroma can occur in the trachea as a primary tumor, but it is not associated with generalized neurofibromatosis. This tumor can invade the wall of the trachea and segmental resection would be the treatment of choice.

Pang (1989) presented two cases of primary neurilemmoma — Schwannoma — of the trachea. His review identified 14 other reported cases. These tumors are derived from the Schwann cell and are typically slow growing. The tumor usually has a broad base and complete removal by bronchoscopy would be difficult. These tumors can recur with malignant potential, and segmental tracheal resection is the treatment of choice.

A hamartoma is a benign tumor composed of tissues normally found in that organ or structure, but the normal appearing tissues are not in their normal histologic pattern. Most hamartomas are found in the pulmonary parenchyma, but 10% are located in the main bronchus or trachea. They are polypoid in appearance and can cause symptoms of respiratory obstruction. The CT scan can be diagnostic in detecting fat and calcification in a smooth and rounded lesion. They do not become malignant and endoscopic resection is the treatment of choice (Fig. 70–9).

MALIGNANT PRIMARY TRACHEAL TUMORS

The most frequent malignant primary tracheal tumors in the adult are squamous cell carcinoma and adenoid cystic carcinoma. Manninen and associates (1991) reported a national registry study from Finland of tracheal carcinoma that demonstrated the overall rarity of this malignancy. They noted that primary carcinoma of the trachea accounted for 0.03% of all detected malignancies registered in Finland between the years 1967 and 1985. Tracheal malignancy accounted for less than 0.2% of all malignancies of the respiratory tract over the same period, and squamous cell carcinoma was the most common tumor. In a review of 198 patients with tracheal tumors, Grillo and Mathisen (1990) reported 80 patients with adenoid cystic carcinoma and 70 with squamous cell carcinoma. In a series of 90 patients, Perelman and Koroleva (1987) recorded 56 adenoid cystic carcinomas and 20 squamous cell carcinomas (Table 70–2).

Squamous Cell Carcinoma

Squamous cell carcinoma of the trachea occurs most commonly in the distal one third of the trachea and originates frequently along the posterior wall (Fig. 70–10). It affects men approximately four times more frequently than women, spreads to regional lymph nodes, and invades adjacent mediastinal structures. It accounts for approximately 50% of all primary tracheal malignancies and most patients are heavy smokers. It is not unusual for these patients to develop or have had a second primary cancer of the larynx or lung. At the time of diagnosis, Mark (1983) states that invasion into the tracheal wall has occurred in 50% of patients, extension into the mediastinum in 33%, and metastasis to cervical lymph nodes in 33%. Grillo and Mathisen (1992) noted that in approximately two thirds of patients with squamous cell carcinoma, the lesion is resectable at the time of presentation. Limitations to resectability include an excessive linear extent of the tumor leaving insufficient trachea for reconstruction, invasion of critical mediastinal structures, and distant metastasis. In patients with squamous cell carcinoma, the status of lymph nodes in the mediastinum at the time of resection and

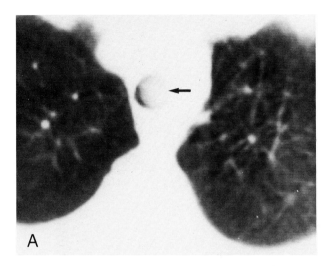
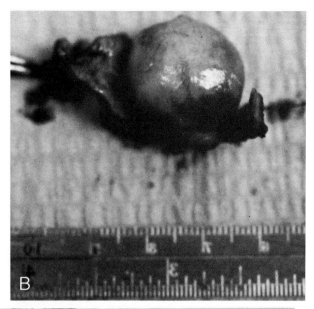
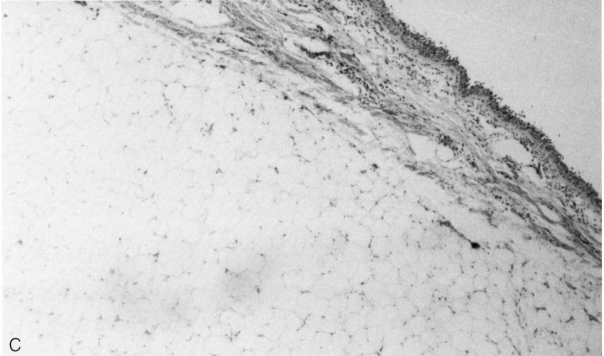

Fig. 70–8. *A,* Computed tomogram shows almost total tracheal obstruction by a lipoma (arrow). *B,* Tracheal resection was required for the removal of the broad-based lesion. *C,* On microscopic examination, the fatty tumor is seen in the submucosa of the trachea.

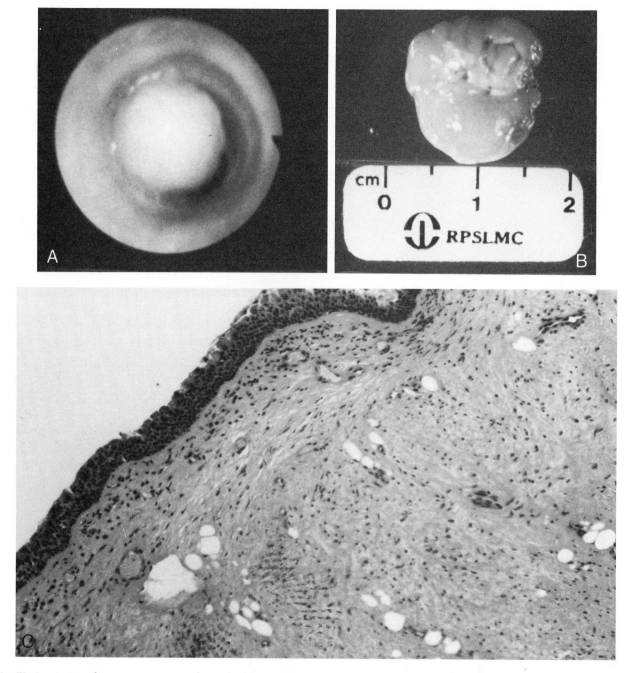

Fig. 70–9. A, Bronchoscopic appearance of a tracheal hamartoma. B, Resection was accomplished through a rigid, open bronchoscope. C, Fibrous hamartoma. Microscopic examination reveals dense connective tissue, fat, and smooth muscle in tracheal submucosa.

Table 70–2. Malignant Tumors of the Trachea*

Tumor Type	Perelman and Koroleva (1987)	Grillo and Mathisen (1990)	Eschapasse (1983)
Adenoid cystic carcinoma	56	80	4
Squamous cell carcinoma	20	70	16
Carcinoid tumors	21	11	—
Typical	(15)	(10)	—
Atypical	(6)	(1)	—
Mucoidepidermoid tumor	3	4	—
Hemangiopericytoma	2	—	—
Adenocarcinoma	2	1	2
Small cell carcinoma	1	1	—
Fibrosarcoma	1	—	—
Melanoma	—	1	—
Chondrosarcoma	—	1	—
Spindle cell sarcoma	—	2	—
Rhabdomyosarcoma	—	1	—
Adenosquamous cell	—	1	—
Others	—	—	5
Total	106	173	27

*Some of the tumors have been reclassified from the original source (Editor).

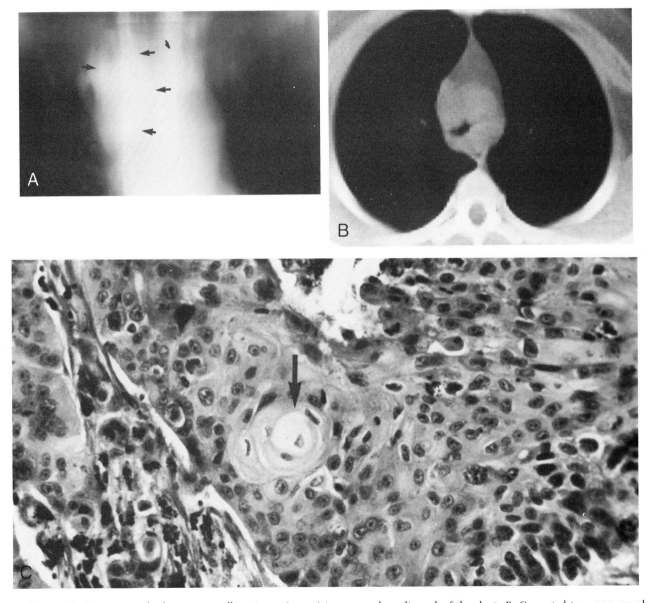

Fig. 70–10. *A*, Extensive tracheal squamous cell carcinoma (arrows) is seen on the radiograph of the chest. *B*, Computed tomogram reveals significant involvement of the tracheal lumen. *C*, Biopsy revealed a squamous carcinoma. A keratin pearl is seen (arrow) in the center of the microscopic section.

the presence of tumor at the margin of surgical resection serve as major determinants of prognosis.

Adenoid Cystic Carcinoma

Adenoid cystic carcinoma more commonly arises in the upper one third of the trachea in contrast to squamous cell carcinoma (Fig. 70–11). In many series, it is the most common tracheal malignancy and, according to Mark (1983), it is proportionately more prevalent in the trachea than in a main stem bronchus. This tumor is frequently referred to as a cylindroma, but this terminology should be abandoned, as it implies

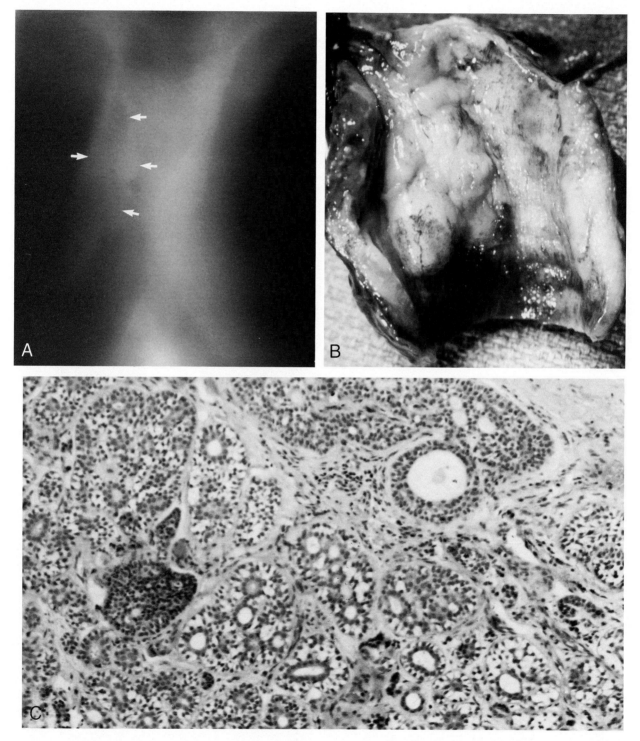

Fig. 70–11. *A,* Adenoid cystic carcinoma is seen on a linear tomogram (arrows). *B,* Six centimeters of trachea were resected for the adenoid cystic carcinoma seen in *A. C,* Adenoid cystic carcinoma. Microscopic examination reveals a cribiform pattern within nests of tumor cells separated by a hyalinized stroma.

that the tumor is benign. The adenoid cystic carcinoma is a slow-growing neoplasm and patients frequently have experienced symptoms for longer than 1 year before diagnosis is made. This tumor arises from bronchial glands and is histologically identical to those that arise in the salivary glands. Tobacco exposure is not a risk factor. It classically infiltrates the submucosa of the trachea for a distance greater than is grossly apparent. This pathologic feature accounts for an increased likelihood of a positive microscopic surgical margin at the time of tracheal resection (Fig. 70–12). The tumor grows through the tracheal cartilaginous rings and also infiltrates the sheath of nerves adjacent to the trachea. It frequently pushes adjacent mediasti-

nal structures aside, rather than directly invading them. The adenoid cystic carcinoma less commonly spreads to regional lymph nodes but does metastasize to the lung or other distant organs. Local recurrence after resectional therapy can occur many years later and these patients should be followed for the rest of their life. Because of the relatively slow growth of these tumors, significant palliation can be achieved by resections that are associated with a positive margin. Postoperative radiation is a determinant in achieving long-term control. Grillo and Mathisen (1990) reported that prognosis did not appear to depend on a positive resection margin or the presence of positive lymph nodes.

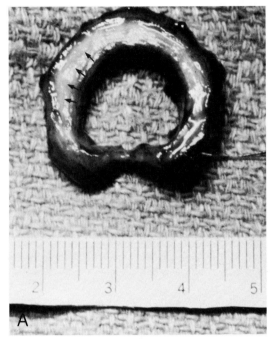

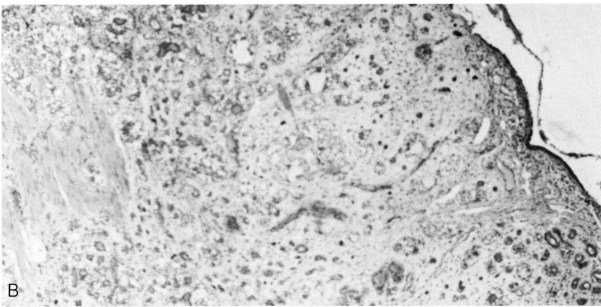

Fig. 70–12. *A*, Gross examination reveals submucosal extension of adenoid cystic carcinoma at the distal margin of resection. *B*, Microscopic examination reveals submucosal infiltration of the tumor at the margin of resection.

Carcinoid Tumors

Carcinoid tumors are the third most common malignant tumors of the trachea. Briselli and colleagues (1978) published a review of the occurrence of this tumor in the trachea. Tracheal carcinoids may be of the typical or atypical histologic types. The former is the more common and behaves in a "benign" fashion; only minimal margins beyond the tumor are required at the time of resection. The atypical carcinoids are of greater malignant potential and may invade tissues beyond the trachea. Lymph node metastases may be present. In such cases, more aggressive resection is required.

Other Primary Malignant Tumors

Tracheal adenocarcinoma accounts for approximately 10% of all primary tracheal malignancies, as reported by Mark (1983) (Fig. 70–13); this does not include adenocarcinomas arising from a main stem bronchus that extend to the lower trachea or carina. Adenocarcinoma carries a poor long-term prognosis because of its propensity to spread directly into the mediastinum and to metastasize to the regional lymph nodes. Therapy is primary resection, if technically feasible.

Small cell carcinoma of the trachea is rare when compared to its more common bronchial presentation. Prognosis is extremely poor and its natural history parallels that of small cell carcinoma of the lung. Primary treatment is chemotherapy and local radiation therapy.

Other malignant tumors include mucoepidermoid tumor, which was reported by Heitmiller and associates (1989), mixed tumor, and various mesenchymal tumors, including chondrosarcoma and fibrosarcoma. Thedinger and co-workers (1991) reported a patient with a tracheal leiomyosarcoma. Primary lymphoma of the trachea was described by Kaplan and associates (1992). Treatment of lymphoma depends on stage of the disease, as well as histologic subtype. A localized lymphoma responds to primary radiation therapy. Plasma cell tumor of the trachea has been reported, and when the diagnosis is established, therapy is initial endoscopic removal and subsequent radiation therapy. The patient should be monitored closely for the late development of multiple myeloma.

SECONDARY MALIGNANT TRACHEAL TUMORS

The trachea is subject to invasion by adjacent malignancies, including laryngeal, thyroid, lung, and esophageal cancer. Metastasis from distant primary tumors is also possible, including melanoma as well as tumors of the breast, kidney, and stomach.

Extension of laryngeal carcinoma into the upper portion of the trachea is a common phenomenon and is treated by surgical excision during the course of laryngectomy with end tracheostomy formation. Recurrence of the cancer at the stoma is rarely resectable for cure and is best treated with palliative radiation therapy, chemotherapy, or both. Sisson (1975) and Krespi (1985) and their colleagues used an aggressive surgical approach in the treatment of tracheal stomal recurrences. The morbidity and mortality rates, however, are high. Ujiki and associates (1987) recorded the major and, unfortunately, frequent problems attendant with the associated reconstruction of gastrointestinal continuity with transposition of the stomach and a pharyngogastric anastomosis in a previously irradiated field.

Invasion into the wall of the trachea is estimated to occur in 12% of patients afflicted with thyroid cancer (Fig. 70–14). In a review by Grillo and associates (1992), the most common presentation was that of a patient with previous thyroid resection in whom the cancerous gland had to be "shaved" off the underlying trachea. This group of patients was often treated with radioactive iodine or external radiation therapy postoperatively, seldom with success. Recurrence in this area is particularly troublesome with recurrent airway bleeding and eventual suffocation from tumor progression. Therefore, as emphasized by Grillo and associates (1992), palliation and in some instances, cure, can be achieved by segmental tracheal resection at the site of recurrence.

Carcinoma of the lung involves the trachea and tracheal carina by either proximal extension from tumors arising from a main stem bronchus or extrinsic compression and invasion from disease in the paratracheal or subcarinal lymph nodes. Most if not all patients with local invasion from metastatic disease in mediastinal lymph nodes are not candidates for resection. Electrocautery or laser ablation and brachytherapy, however, may be palliative in the management of intraluminal obstructive growth. The role of neoadjuvant

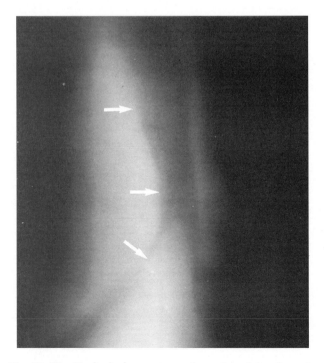

Fig. 70–13. Tracheal adenocarcinoma (arrows) involving the main stem bronchus and carina.

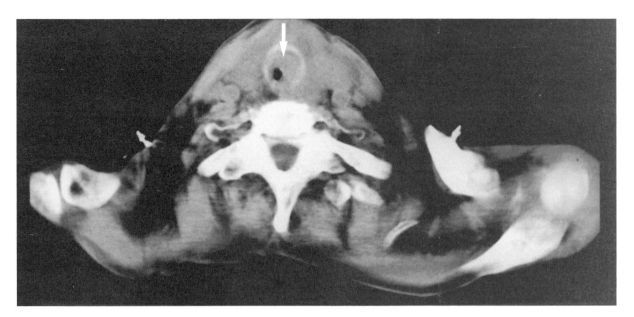

Fig. 70–14. Recurrent thyroid carcinoma (arrow) invading the trachea. Clinical signs were hemoptysis and severe stridor.

multimodality therapy followed by excision needs to be evaluated. Direct involvement of the tracheal carina by proximal extension of a main stem bronchial tumor without mediastinal lymph node involvement may be considered for possible resection — tracheal sleeve pneumonectomy — especially if the postoperative mortality can be kept in the range of 10% (see Chapter 35).

Invasion of esophageal malignancy into the trachea often results in esophagorespiratory fistula. Burt and co-workers (1991) reviewed the extensive experience with this problem at the Memorial Hospital in New York. The approach to this problem has varied with many people advocating esophageal stents or gastrostomy for feeding purposes. Esophageal exclusion with gastric or colon bypass is a major operative procedure that is associated with a high operative mortality and most often only brief postoperative survival.

Metastasis to the trachea from distant sites is usually treated with endoscopic resection and YAG laser ablation to debulk the lesion. Systemic chemotherapy or radiation therapy is used as indicated.

PRINCIPLES AND RESULTS OF SURGICAL TREATMENT

History

Belsey (1950) reported experience with tracheal resection and listed 2 cm as the maximal length of trachea that could be circumferentially resected. Resection of part of the tracheal wall with reconstruction by autologous or synthetic material was reported by Rob and Bateman (1949). These procedures frequently were complicated by fistula, mediastinal infection, and stenosis. In subsequent years, some authors described successful resection of longer lengths of trachea. The

door was opened to extended and aggressive tracheal surgery by Grillo and associates (1964) when they thoroughly and systematically described the amount of trachea that could be removed from thoracic and cervical mediastinal approaches. The landmark conclusion was that approximately one half of the trachea could be removed and reapproximated. The many reports by Grillo and colleagues (1964, 1983, 1989, 1990, 1992) on techniques and results of resection of tracheal tumors and stenosis paved the way for modern techniques of tracheal resection. Pearson and associates (1975) were among the first to describe resection techniques for high tracheal lesions that involved the cricoid.

Prosthetic Replacement of the Trachea

A significant number of animal experiments have been carried out in an attempt to develop a prosthesis that could replace a long segment of the trachea. Tube grafts of stainless steel, plastic, and glass have all met with failure. This failure is related to granulation tissue that obstructs or results in strictures at the anastomosis and to migration of the prosthesis leading to erosion of mediastinal vessels. Neville and associates (1990) reported 19 years of experience with the use of a silicone tube to re-establish airway continuity in cases of malignant and benign tracheal obstruction. In some patients, the silicone tube was used as a stent and in others, resection of the trachea with primary anastomosis of the tube to the proximal and distal trachea was accomplished. Successful use of such prosthesis has not been duplicated in other centers and its use is not recommended.

Selection of Surgical Procedure

Tracheal resection and end-to-end anastomosis using various release techniques to minimize tension is the primary form of therapy for tracheal neoplasms. The standard techniques are discussed in Chapter 34.

Benign tumors must be approached with a full knowledge of the pathology of the tumor to be treated. Benign tumors that are broad based and have a likelihood of local recurrence are best managed by tracheal resection. These tumors usually involve the trachea for a distance of 1 or 2 cm and the resection and anastomosis is accomplished without difficulty. Benign tumors, such as lipoma, solitary papilloma, and hamartoma can be removed through the rigid bronchoscope. The YAG laser has facilitated the total ablation of these tumors, and after endoscopic removal, the base of the tumor is ablated with the laser. Endoscopic surveillance is indicated to be certain that local recurrence does not occur.

Malignant primary tumors of the trachea should be treated by primary resection when the clinical findings indicate that the tumor most likely can be removed and tracheal reconstruction can be accomplished safely. Grillo and Mathisen (1990) reported 147 resections in 198 tracheal tumors seen from 1962 to 1989. These resections included laryngotracheal resection, staged reconstruction, as well as carinal resection. There were 82 "pure" tracheal resections and of these, 32 were for squamous carcinoma and 22 for adenoid cystic carcinoma. The operative mortality in the tracheal reconstructions was 1% — 1 in 82.

Squamous Cell Carcinoma

Grillo and associates (1992) reported that in approximately two thirds of patients with squamous cell carcinoma, the lesion is resectable on presentation. Because resection margins are frequently limited and wide en-bloc dissection is not possible, however, Grillo and Mathisen (1990) recommend postoperative radiation for all patients undergoing tracheal resection for squamous cell carcinoma.

Adenoid Cystic Carcinoma

Prognosis is not dependent on a positive resection margin or the finding of positive lymph nodes. This factor is important to keep in mind at the time of the surgical resection, as patients who have grossly negative resection margins, but a positive frozen section margin, do not require more aggressive resection with the attendant higher risk of anastomotic separation. Grillo and Mathisen (1990) also recommend postoperative radiation of approximately 5000 cGy for all patients with adenoid cystic carcinoma.

Other Malignant Tumors

All other types of primary tracheal malignant tumors should be resected, if it is technically feasible. The majority of these patients should have postoperative radiation. An exception to this therapeutic program would be the patient with a carcinoid tumor with negative margins at resection.

Prognosis

Grillo and Mathisen (1990) reported that 49% — 20 of 41 — of patients with squamous cell cancer are alive without evidence of tumor following resection. These results included those patients who also had a carinal resection. Negative factors that affected long-term survival in patients with squamous cell carcinoma were positive nodes and microscopic tumor at the resection margin. Grillo (1990) states that, "resection combined with irradiation provides a tripled survival time for squamous cell carcinoma," when compared to radiation alone. Median survival of resected squamous cell carcinoma with postoperative radiation was 34 months. Perelman and Koroleva (1987) reported a survival for resected tracheal squamous cell carcinoma of 27% at 3 years and 13% at 5 and 10 years. Pearson and co-workers (1984) identified four of six patients with tracheal squamous cell carcinoma who were alive at 6 months following resection.

Adenoid cystic carcinoma is a malignant tumor of the trachea that can recur many years following a resection. Therefore, reporting the true results is somewhat difficult given the possibility of local recurrence at 10 or 15 years postoperatively. Despite an increased incidence of tumor at the resection margin, however, Grillo and colleagues (1990) reported 75% — 39 of 52 — of patients were alive and disease-free. Median survival was 118 months. Perelman and Koroleva (1987) reported an overall survival for resected adenoid cystic carcinoma of the trachea of 71% at 3 years, 66% at 5 years, and 56% at 10 and 15 years. Pearson and associates (1984) reported resection in 14 patients with adenoid cystic carcinoma; 9 were free of disease, 3 were dead of disease, and 2 were alive with disease. Long-term prognosis for patients with adenoid cystic carcinoma is obviously better than that for those with squamous cell carcinoma.

RADIATION THERAPY

In patients with a primary malignant tumor of the trachea that does not meet the criteria for resection, radiation therapy can be an alternative form of therapy, although it does not appear to be as effective as primary resection for providing long-term control. Rostom and Morgan (1978) reported radiation therapy for 39 patients with primary malignant tumors of the trachea of which 28 were squamous cell carcinomas and 3 were adenoid cystic carcinomas. Of these 31 patients, five were reported to be free of disease at 4 to 11 years after treatment, six died of nonrelated causes, and the remainder expired from local recurrence or metastatic cancer. Radiation dose varied from 5000 to 7000 cGy. Patients with disease limited to the trachea had a better prognosis and 58% — 11 of 19 — with tumors confined to the trachea were controlled locally at the time of death or at the last followup evaluation — 3 to 16 years. Fields and colleagues (1989) reported on 24 patients with primary malignant tumors of the trachea who received radiation therapy as all or part of their treatment. This group included 13 with squamous cell carcinomas and 4 with adenoid cystic carcinomas. The median actuarial survival was 10 months with 5-year and 10-year survival of 25 and 13%, respectively. For patients treated with radiation therapy alone, response was related to dose, and a dose of over 6000 cGy was statistically significant in achieving a complete response. Five patients developed serious complications, however, including innominate artery rupture, tracheoesophageal fistula, and esophageal stricture. In this series, it appeared that no survival advantage of radiation therapy over surgery was achieved for localized lesions and primary tumor control was infrequent with the more advanced lesions. Survival was significantly better for patients with adenoid cystic carcinoma than for those with squamous carcinoma. Median survivals were 126 months and 6.5 months, respectively. Grillo and Mathisen (1990) compared their patients who underwent resection and postoperative radiation therapy with those that underwent irradiation alone. Significantly better results were achieved with resection and postoperative irradiation. Computed tomographic treatment planning and neutron therapy with modern techniques of deliverance may enhance the radiation treatment of primary tracheal malignancies. At present, however, radiation is to be considered only as a primary form of therapy when the tumor cannot be technically resected or the patient is medically unfit for surgery.

ENDOSCOPIC MANAGEMENT

Palliation of obstructing or bleeding tracheal malignancies can be achieved with current endoscopic procedures. Modern intravenous anesthetic techniques permit spontaneous ventilation during open tube bronchoscopy, which provides safety for the compromised airway. Dumon and colleagues (1982) described the use of a specially designed bronchoscope through which the YAG laser fiber is passed, along with debridement forceps. YAG laser resection is particularly valuable in establishing an open airway in a patient with an obstructing tracheal neoplasm. The laser controls hemorrhage following tumor debridement with biopsy forceps or the end of the open tube bronchoscope (Fig. 70–15). Gelb and colleagues (1988) described 13 patients who underwent palliative YAG laser treatment for relief of malignant tracheal obstruction. Tracheal diameter was significantly increased after single or multiple laser treatments with improvement of inspiratory flow rates. Symptomatic relief occurred for 4 to 48 months.

Cryotherapy and photodynamic therapy with hematoporphyrin derivative offers no benefit over YAG laser ablation of the tumor.

Brachytherapy is effective in providing high dose radiation in a localized radiation field. The high activity isotope iridium-192 is placed into a catheter that is

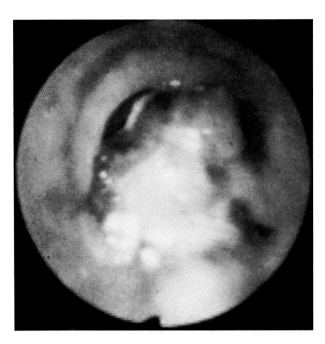

Fig. 70–15. Large upper tracheal adenoid cystic carcinoma causing severe airway compromise. An adequate airway was established with YAG laser ablation of the tumor.

appropriately positioned in the lumen of the tumor. Specific afterloading radiation machines are also available for this type of therapy. Hetzel and Smith (1991) reported that brachytherapy is complementary to laser resection and effective palliation of the airway can be achieved. Fritz and associates (1991) described a new applicator to position the afterloading catheter centrally to minimize irregular dose distribution.

Following endoscopic ablation of an intraluminal tumor and radiation therapy either by external beam or brachytherapy, an endobronchial stent can be used to maintain an adequate airway, as suggested by Cooper and co-workers (1989). Tracheal stents made of Silastic are commercially available. Using various endoscopic techniques, they are positioned properly with the aid of the open rigid-tube bronchoscope. Stents have afforded significant airway palliation for both intrinsic and extrinsic neoplasms. Stainless steel stents have been used for maintenance of a major airway, but placement and repositioning are particularly difficult and the tumor can also grow through the interstices of the stent. The stainless steel stent cannot be removed once it has been expanded into position.

MANAGEMENT OF SECONDARY TUMORS INVOLVING THE TRACHEA

Thyroid cancer can invade the trachea, and Grillo and associates (1992) described 34 patients who underwent some form of tracheal resection for thyroid carcinoma. The majority of the tumors were papillary carcinoma. Ten tracheal sleeve resections and ten complex laryngeal and tracheal procedures were performed. Fourteen patients were alive up to 4 years postoperatively. Ishihara and colleagues (1991) described 60 patients with advanced thyroid cancer in whom the tumor was resected along with a portion of the trachea. A complete resection was achieved in 34 patients and 5-year actuarial survival in this group was 78%. In the patients undergoing incomplete resection, the 5-year actuarial survival was 44%. Resection of a portion of the trachea or larynx, or both, in patients with invading thyroid carcinoma can offer significant palliation from bleeding and obstruction and, possibly, cure.

In a rare instance, tracheal involvement is the only extramural spread of the esophageal malignancy, and partial tracheal resection with musculocutaneous flap reconstruction of the trachea has been accomplished. This operation is often in association with total laryngoesophagectomy, in which the reconstruction is part of a cervical or mediastinal tracheostomy construction, as reported by Sodeyama and co-workers (1990).

REFERENCES

Basheda SG, et al: Endobronchial and parenchymal juvenile laryngotracheobronchial papillomatosis. Effect of photodynamic therapy. Chest 100:5, 1458, 1991.

Beattie EJ, Bloom ND, Harvey JC: Trachea. In Beattie EJ, Bloom ND, Harvey JC (eds): Thoracic Surgical Oncology. New York: Churchill Livingstone, 1992, pp. 273–281.

Belsey R: Resection and reconstruction of the intrathoracic trachea. Br J Surg 38:200, 1950.

Briselli M, Mark GJ, Grillo HC: Tracheal carcinoids. Cancer 42:2870, 1978.

Burt M, et al: Malignant esophagorespiratory fistula: Management options and survival. Ann Thorac Surg 52:1222, 1991.

Burton DM, Heffner DK, Paptow CA: Granular cell tumors of the trachea. Laryngoscope 102:807, 1992.

Chen TF, et al: Obstructing tracheal lipoma: Management of a rare tumor. Ann Thorac Surg 49:137, 1990.

Cooper JD, et al: Use of silicone stents in the management of airway problems. Ann Thorac Surg 47:371, 1989.

Cunningham L, et al: Treatment of tracheobronchial granular cell myoblastomas with endoscopic bipolar cautery. Chest 96:427, 1989.

Daniel TM, et al: Transbronchoscopic versus surgical resection of tracheobronchial granular cell myoblastomas. J Thorac Cardiovasc Surg 80:598, 1980.

Dumon JF, et al: Treatment of tracheo-bronchial lesions by laser photoresection. Chest 81:278:284, 1982.

Eschapasse H: Primary tumors of the trachea. In Grillo HC, Eschapasse H (eds): International Trends in General Thoracic Surgery. Vol. 2. Philadelphia: WB Saunders, 1987, p. 107.

Fields JN, Rigaud G, Emami BN: Primary tumors of the trachea. Results of radiation therapy. Cancer 63:2429, 1989.

Franks R, Rothera M: Cardiopulmonary bypass for resection of low tracheal hemangioma. Arch Dis Child 65:630, 1990.

Fritz P, et al: A new applicator, positionable to the center of tracheobronchial lumen for HDR-1R-192-afterloading of tracheobronchial tumors. Int J Radiat Oncol Biol Phys 20:1061, 1991.

Garcia-Prats MD, et al: Glomus tumour of the trachea; report of a case with microscopic, ultrastructural and immunohistochemical examination and review of the literature. Histopathology 19:459, 1991.

Gelb AF, et al: Diagnosis and Nd-YAG laser treatment of unsuspected malignant tracheal obstruction. Chest 94:767, 1988.

Gilbert JG, Mazzarella LA, Geit LJ: Primary tracheal tumors in the infant and adult. Arch Otolaryngol Head Neck Surg 58:1, 1953.

Grillo HC: Tracheal tumors: Diagnosis and management. In Choi NC, Grillo HC (eds): Thoracic Oncology. New York: Raven Press, 1983, pp. 271–278.

Grillo HC: Benign and malignant disease of the trachea. In Shields TW (ed): General Thoracic Surgery. 3rd Ed. Philadelphia: Lea & Febiger, 1989.

Grillo HC: Tracheal replacement. Ann Thorac Surg 49:864, 1990.

Grillo HC, Mathisen DJ: Primary tracheal tumors: Treatment and results. Ann Thorac Surg 49:69, 1990.

Grillo HC, Dignan EF, Mirua T: Extensive resection and reconstruction of mediastinal trachea without prosthesis or graft: An anatomical study in man. J Thorac Cardiovasc Surg 48:471, 1964.

Grillo HC, Mathisen DJ, Wain JC: Management of tumors of the trachea. Oncology 6:3:61, 1992.

Grillo HC, et al: Resectional management of thyroid carcinoma invading the airway. Ann Thorac Surg 54:3, 1992.

Guillou L, et al: Squamous cell carcinoma of the lung in a nonsmoking, nonirradiated patient with juvenile laryngotracheal papillomatosis. Am J Surg Pathol 15:891, 1991.

Hajdu SI, et al: Carcinoma of the trachea. Clinicopathologic study of 41 cases. Cancer 25:1448, 1970.

Heitmiller RF, et al: Mucoepidermoid lung tumors. Ann Thorac Surg 47:394, 1989.

Hetzel MR, Smith SGT: Endoscopic palliation of tracheobronchial malignancies. Thorax 46:325, 1991.

Houston HE, et al: Primary cancers of the trachea. Arch Surg 99:132, 1969.

Ishihara T, et al: Surgical treatment of advanced thyroid carcinoma invading the trachea. J Thorac Cardiovasc Surg 102:717, 1991.

Kaplan MA, et al: Primary lymphoma of the trachea with morphologic and immunophenotypic characteristics of low-grade B-cell lymphoma of mucosa-associated lymphoid tissue. Am J Surg Pathol 16:71, 1992.

Karley SW, et al: Chronic cavitary respiratory papillomatosis. Arch Pathol Lab Med 113:1166, 1989.

Kavuru MS, Mehta AC, Eliachar I: Effect of photodynamic therapy and external beam radiation therapy on juvenile laryngotracheobronchial papillomatosis. Am Rev Respir Dis 141:509, 1990.

Krespi YP, Wurster CF, Sisson GA: Immediate reconstruction after total laryngopharyngoesophagectomy and mediastinal dissection. Laryngoscope 95:156, 1985.

Leventhal BG, et al: Long-term response of recurrent respiratory papillomatosis to treatment with lymphoblastoid interferon Alfa-NI. N Engl J Med 325:613, 1991.

Manninen MO, et al: Occurrence of tracheal carcinoma in Finland. Acta Otolaryngeal (Stockh) 111:1162, 1991.

Mark E: Pathology of tracheal neoplasms. In Choi NC, Grillo HC (eds): Thoracic Oncology. New York: Raven Press, 1983, pp. 256–269.

Mathisen DJ, Grillo HC: Endoscopic relief of malignant airway obstruction. Ann Thorac Surg 48:469, 1989.

Neville WE, Bolanowski PJ, Kotia GG: Clinical experience with the silicone tracheal prosthesis. J Thorac Cardiovasc Surg 99:604, 1990.

Pang LC: Primary neurilemmoma of the trachea. South Med J 82:785, 1989.

Pearson FG, Todd TRJ, Cooper JD: Experience with primary neoplasms of the trachea and carina. J Thorac Cardiovasc Surg 88:511, 1984.

Pearson FG, et al: Primary tracheal anastomosis after resection of the cricoid cartilage with preservation of recurrent laryngeal nerves. J Thorac Cardiovasc Surg 70:806, 1975.

Perelman MI, Koroleva NS: Primary tumors of the trachea. In Grillo HC, Eschapasse H (eds): International Trends in General Thoracic Surgery. Philadelphia: WB Saunders, 1987, pp. 91–110.

Randleman CD, Unger ER, Mansour KA: Malignant fibrous histiocytoma of the trachea. Ann Thorac Surg 50:458, 1990.

Rob CG, Bateman GH: Reconstruction of the trachea and cervical esophagus. Br J Surg 36:202, 1949.

Rostom AY, Morgan RL: Results of treating primary tumors of the trachea by irradiation. Thorax *33*:387, 1978.

Salminen U, et al: Recurrence and malignant transformation of endotracheal chondroma. Ann Thorac Surg *49*:830, 1990.

Sisson GA, Bytelle E, Edison BD: Transternal radical neck dissection for control of stomal recurrence — end results. Laryngoscope *85*:1504, 1975.

Sodeyama H, et al: Platysma musculocutaneous flap for reconstruction of trachea in esophageal cancer. Ann Thorac Surg *50*:485, 1990.

Thedinger BA, et al: Leiomyosarcoma of the trachea. Ann Otol Rhinol Laryngol *100*:337, 1991.

Ujiki GT, et al: Mortality and morbidity of gastric pull-up for replacement of the pharyngoesophagus. Arch Surg *122*:644, 1987.

Weber AL, Grillo HC: Tracheal lesions — assessment by conventional films, computed tomography and magnetic resonance imaging. Israel J Med Sci *28*:233, 1992.

Weber TR, et al: Complex hemangiomas of infants and children. Arch Surg *125*:1017, 1990.

CHAPTER 71

COMPRESSION OF THE TRACHEA
BY VASCULAR RINGS

Carl L. Backer

The phrase "vascular ring" refers to a group of developmental malformations of the aortic arch complex that form an anatomic "ring" that constricts and compresses the trachea, or esophagus, or both. Hommel, cited by Turner (1962) described the first vascular ring — a double aortic arch in 1737. Gross (1945) reported the first successful operation for a vascular ring when he divided a double aortic arch causing tracheal obstruction in a 1-year-old infant. Almost all clinically significant vascular rings become symptomatic in infants or young children and present with airway obstruction from tracheal compression. Esophageal compression and obstruction usually becomes apparent later when solid foods are started. The classification of vascular rings that is used at Children's Memorial Hospital in Chicago is based on anatomic and clinical features, particularly the location of the aortic arch (Table 71–1). As indicated, some of these anomalies are anatomically complete rings, or true vascular rings; others are anatomically incomplete, or partial vascular rings, but present with similar symptoms because of the tracheoesophageal compression.

Table 71–1. Classification of Vascular Rings

Complete Vascular Rings
  Double aortic arch
    Right arch dominant
    Left arch dominant
    Balanced arches
  Right aortic arch with left ligamentum arteriosum
    Retroesophageal left subclavian artery
    Mirror-image branching

Partial Vascular Rings
  Innominate artery compression syndrome
  Pulmonary artery sling
  Left aortic arch
    Aberrant right subclavian artery
    Right ligamentum arteriosum, right descending aorta

EMBRYOLOGY

Congdon (1922) reported an extensive experience with the embryonic development of the human aortic arch system, showing that six pairs of aortic arches connect the two primitive ventral and dorsal aortae (Fig. 71–1). Most portions of the first, second, and fifth arches

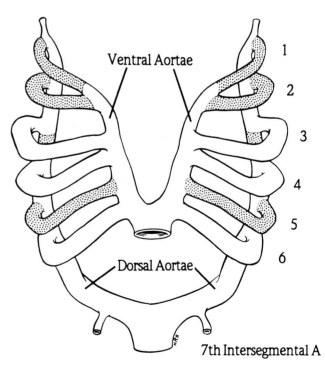

Fig. 71–1. The embryonic aortic arches. Six pairs of aortic arches develop between the dorsal and ventral aortae. Areas that are shaded regress. The seventh intersegmental arteries migrate cephalad to form the subclavian arteries. *From* Lowe GM, Donaldson JS, Backer CL: Vascular rings: 10-year review of imaging. RadioGraphics *11*:637, 1991.

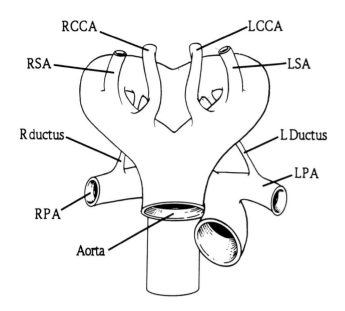

Fig. 71–2. Edwards' double aortic arch system. A double aortic arch is formed when both the right and left fourth arches persist. RPA = right pulmonary artery; RSA = right subclavian artery; RCCA = right common carotid artery; LCCA = left common carotid artery; LSA = left subclavian artery; LPA = left pulmonary artery. *From* Lowe GM, Donaldson JS, Backer CL: Vascular rings: 10-year review of imaging. RadioGraphics *11*:637, 1991.

regress. The third arches become the carotid arteries. A branch from the ventral bud of the sixth arch meets the lung bud to form the pulmonary artery. On the right side, the dorsal contribution to the sixth arch disappears, on the left it persists as the ductus arteriosus. The formation of a vascular ring depends on preservation or deletion of specific segments of the embryonic aortic arch complex. To help visualize this, Edwards (1948) proposed a schematic model with a double aortic arch system and bilateral ductus arteriosus (Fig. 71–2). By definition, the location of the arch is determined by its relationship to the trachea. In the normal arch formation, the right fourth arch regresses, leaving a left aortic arch system — apex of aortic arch to left of trachea. If both fourth arches persist, a double aortic arch is formed. If the left fourth arch regresses, a right aortic arch system is created — apex of aortic arch to right of trachea.

CLINICAL FEATURES, DIAGNOSES, AND SURGICAL TREATMENT

Double Aortic Arch

This is the most common complete vascular ring that causes tracheoesophageal compression. Potts and associates (1948) noted that patients typically present in the first months of life with symptoms of stridor, respiratory distress, and a cough that sounds like a seal's bark. A simple "cold" may precipitate severe respiratory difficulty. The ascending aorta divides into two arches that pass around the trachea and esophagus and join

posteriorly to form the descending aorta (see Fig 71–2). I and my associates (1989) showed that in two thirds of these infants, the right-sided — posterior — arch is dominant, and in one third, the left-sided — anterior — arch is dominant. Rarely, the arches are of equal size — balanced arches. The carotid and subclavian arteries originate symmetrically and separately from each arch. The tight, constricting ring thus formed compresses the trachea and esophagus.

The diagnosis can be suspected on examination of the chest radiograph because the location of the aortic arch in relation to the trachea is indeterminate. Ideally, the next study is a barium esophagogram, which Arciniegas (1979) has shown to be the most reliable study for diagnosis of vascular rings. The double aortic arch on an anteroposterior esophagogram appears as bilateral indentations of unequal size that persist in location (Fig. 71–3). At the Children's Memorial Hospital of Chicago, it is believed that this provides sufficient information to plan for surgical intervention; however, many clinicians will also obtain a computed tomogram — CT — or magnetic resonance — MR — imaging be-

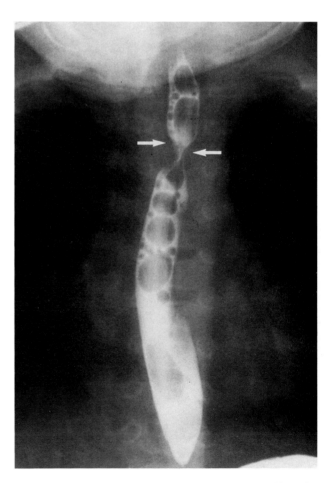

Fig. 71–3. Anteroposterior esophagogram of a 4-month-old boy who presented with stridor and was found to have a double aortic arch. *From* Backer CL, Ilbawi MN, Idriss FS, DeLeon SY: Vascular anomalies causing tracheoesophageal compression. Review of experience in children. J Thorac Cardiovasc Surg 97:725, 1989.

fore surgical referral. McLoughlin and co-workers (1981) have shown that CT scanning is very accurate in the identification of vascular anomalies of the aortic arch and great vessels. A double aortic arch is diagnosed with certainty when both limbs are patent and enhanced with the administration of contrast material (Fig. 71–4). As described by Lowe and associates (1991), one clue to an arch anomaly — specifically a double aortic arch or a right aortic arch with retroesophageal subclavian artery and a ligamentum arteriosum — is the "four artery sign." This is seen on sections cephalad to the aortic arch and consists of two dorsal subclavian arteries and two ventral carotid arteries spaced evenly around the trachea. The sign is present when the two dorsal subclavian arteries arise directly from the aorta and not from a brachiocephalic artery (Fig. 71–5). Cardiac catheterization is recommended now only for infants with associated congenital cardiac anomalies. Bronchoscopy is obtained sometimes as the initial study because of the severe stridor and shows external compression of the trachea.

All infants with double aortic arch should be operated on; a narrowed trachea, when further compromised by mucosal edema from even a mild upper respiratory infection, can cause sudden respiratory arrest. Surgical approach is through a left thoracotomy, except in cases of associated intracardiac lesions, in which simultaneous repair can be effected through a median sternotomy. The left thoracotomy can be performed with a muscle-sparing technique, elevating the serratus anterior and the latissimus dorsi and entering the thorax through the fourth intercostal space. The vascular ring caused by the double aortic arch is released by dividing the lesser of the two arches, usually where it inserts into the descending aorta (Fig. 71–6). In 30 to 40% of the

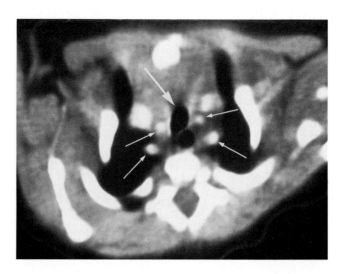

Fig. 71–5. Same infant as in Figure 71–4. The small arrows point to the four brachiocephalic vessels; large arrow points to trachea.

patients, this portion of the arch will be atretic. After applying the vascular clamps, the anesthesiologist carefully checks the carotid and radial pulses on both sides, to ensure blood flow is not interrupted. The arch is then divided between the vascular clamps, and the stumps are oversewn with prolene sutures; simple ligation should not be done. The ligamentum arteriosum is also divided. Careful dissection is then performed around the trachea and esophagus to lyse any residual adhesive bands. The recurrent laryngeal and phrenic nerves are identified and protected throughout the procedure.

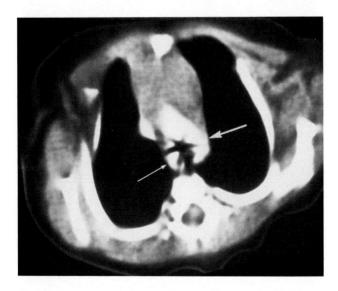

Fig. 71–4. Contrast-enhanced CT scan of a 3-week-old girl presenting with severe stridor shows a double aortic arch, left arch dominant. The right arch was successfully divided through a left thoracotomy. The large arrow points to the dominant left (anterior) arch. The small arrow points to the smaller right (posterior) arch.

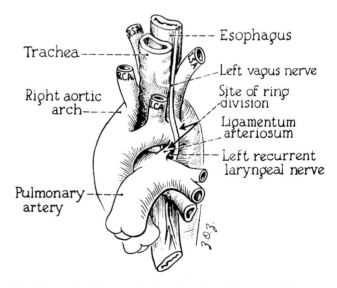

Fig. 71–6. Double aortic arch with right arch dominant. The vascular ring is divided at the sites shown by the arrows. LCA = left carotid artery; RCA = right carotid artery. *From* Backer CL, Idriss FS: Tracheoesophageal compressive syndromes of vascular origin: rings and slings. *In* Baue AE, et al (eds): Glenn's Thoracic and Cardiovascular Surgery. 5th Ed. Norwalk, CT: Appleton-Century-Crofts, 1991.

The postoperative care includes high humidity to loosen secretions, oxygen therapy when needed as monitored by pulse oximetry, vigorous chest physiotherapy, and nasopharyngeal suctioning. Results of surgical intervention are excellent and no surgical mortality has resulted at Children's Memorial Hospital from a double aortic arch procedure since 1952. As Nikaidoh and associates (1972) reported, many children have residual noisy breathing for 6 months to 2 years, but this gradually resolves.

Right Aortic Arch

Right aortic arch with a left ligamentum arteriosum completing the vascular ring is almost as common as a double aortic arch. The ring, however, is usually not as tight, and children typically present somewhat later in life — 6 to 12 months of age. Symptoms are similar to those in infants with double aortic arch, with stridor

and respiratory distress. In older children, dysphagia may be present. Some of these children eat very slowly and tend to be the last child to leave the table because they have to carefully chew their food as a learned procedure to prevent choking. Embryologically, depending on the exact site or sites of interruption of the left fourth arch and the branching pattern to the left subclavian artery, left carotid artery, and ductus arteriosus, different configurations of right aortic arch are possible. Felson and Palayew (1963) showed that the two common variations are retroesophageal left subclavian artery — 65% — and mirror-image branching — 35% (Fig. 71–7A and B). In either case it is the left ligamentum arteriosum between the descending aorta and the left pulmonary artery that completes the ring. Although D'Cruz and associates (1966) have reported that one third of patients with tetralogy of Fallot and truncus arteriosus

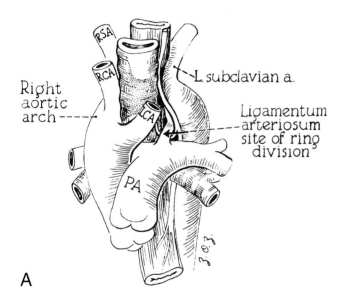

Fig. 71–7. *A*, With a right aortic arch and retroesophageal left subclavian artery, the ring is divided by dividing the ligamentum arteriosum, which extends from the aorta opposite the origin of the left subclavian artery to the left pulmonary artery (PA). *B*, With a right aortic arch and mirror-image branching of the great vessels, it is the ligamentum between the descending aorta and pulmonary artery, which is divided to release the ring. *C*, With a right aortic arch and mirror-image branching, if the ligamentum connects the innominate artery to the pulmonary artery, a vascular ring is not formed, and the child would have no symptoms.

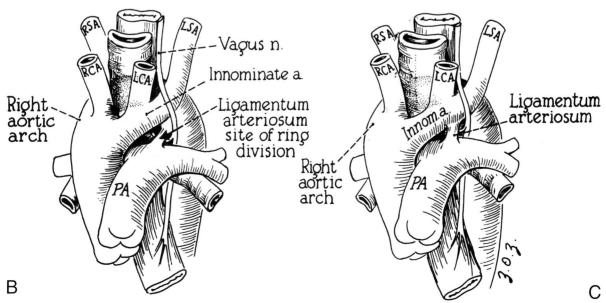

have a right aortic arch, our group did not find a reverse association with a specific cardiac defect when a vascular ring is formed by a right arch. In most infants with a cardiac defect and a right aortic arch, there is mirror-image branching with the ligamentum from the innominate artery to the pulmonary artery, so a vascular ring is not formed (Fig. 71–7C).

The diagnosis is suggested by the chest radiograph, which shows an aortic arch to the right of the tracheal air column. The single most effective diagnostic examination is the barium esophagogram (Fig. 71–8). Again, the referring clinician will often obtain a CT or MR imaging before referring the patient for surgery. Bisset and associates (1987) have shown that MR imaging, like CT, is useful for identification of vascular rings. Axial images provide the same information as CT without ionizing radiation or the need for intravenously administered contrast material. In addition, coronal and sagittal sections or images can be helpful in confusing cases. A disadvantage to MR imaging is the length of time required for the study and thus necessitating sedation. An example of an MR image in

a patient with a right aortic arch, left ligamentum, and retroesophageal left subclavian artery is shown in Figure 71–9.

The surgical approach is through a left thoracotomy, reserving median sternotomy for those patients with associated intracardiac lesions. After careful dissection and identification of the configuration of the aortic arch, the ligamentum arteriosum is identified as compressing the esophagus. The ring is released by dividing the ligamentum between vascular clamps and oversewing the stumps. Any adhesive bands are lysed. Chun and associates (1992) have emphasized the importance of an associated Kommerell's (1936) diverticulum. This diverticulum is embryologically a remnant of the left fourth aortic arch that did not undergo complete involution. The diverticulum may independently compress the esophagus or trachea even with the ring divided. This aneurysmal dilatation should either be resected or pexed to the thoracic wall or spinal column to prevent this complication. The results of surgical intervention for this anomaly are very good. At Children's Memorial Hospital there has been no mortality

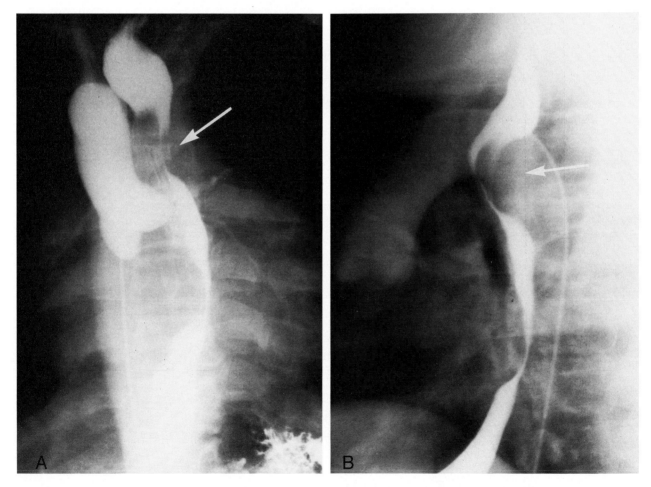

Fig. 71–8. Anteroposterior (A) and lateral (B) views of simultaneous esophagogram and aortogram in a patient with a right aortic arch and left ligamentum. The origin of the left subclavian artery is aneurysmal, forming a Kommerell's diverticulum. The combination of the tight ligamentum and the diverticulum (arrow) severely compresses the esophagus. In particular, the lateral film shows a classic deep posterior indentation from the large right arch.

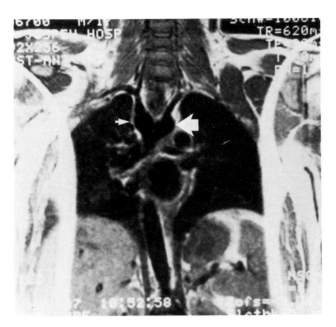

Fig. 71–9. A 17-year-old patient with dysphagia. Magnetic resonance imaging shows a right aortic arch (small arrow) and a Kommerell diverticulum (large arrow) at the origin of the left subclavian artery. *From* Backer CL, Ilbawi MN, Idriss FS, DeLeon SY: Vascular anomalies causing tracheoesophageal compression. Review of experience in children. J Thorac Cardiovasc Surg 97:725, 1989.

following surgery for an isolated right aortic arch since 1959.

Innominate Artery Compression Syndrome

This syndrome results from anterior compression of the trachea by the innominate artery. There is usually a "normal" left aortic arch. The innominate artery appears to originate somewhat more posteriorly and leftward on the aortic arch than usual. Ardito and associates (1980) have described how, as the artery then courses to the right, upward, and posterior to reach the thoracic outlet, it compresses the trachea anteriorly. These infants present with stridor, respiratory distress, cyanosis, and apnea with feeding. The infant may hold the head hyperextended to splint the trachea and improve breathing. Apnea or cyanosis may be precipitated by swallowing a bolus of food that presses on the soft posterior trachea with the innominate artery compressing the anterior trachea.

Enthusiasm for this diagnosis increased in the late 1970s when bronchoesophagologists switched from local to general anesthesia for bronchoscopy. As experience with these patients was gained, the selection criteria for surgery became more stringent. The diagnosis is made with rigid bronchoscopy, and this should demonstrate a pulsatile anterior compression of the trachea extending from left to right, with at least a 70% obstruction of the tracheal lumen. Anterior compression of the tracheal wall by the bronchoscope may compress the innominate artery and temporarily obliterate the right radial pulse. The diagnosis can be confirmed by CT scan, which will demonstrate flattening and obliteration of the tracheal

lumen by the contrast-filled innominate artery (Fig. 71–10). Radionuclide studies for gastroesophageal reflux, sleep studies, and neurologic evaluation — including CT of the brain and electroencephalograms — should all be performed to rule out other causes of apnea. Barium esophagogram is normal in these infants.

When indicated, the management of compression of the trachea by the innominate artery classically has been with suspension of the innominate artery to the posterior aspect of the sternum, as originally described by Gross and Neuhauser (1948). At Children's Memorial Hospital we have preferred a small right submammary thoracotomy. The right lobe of the thymus is excised, taking care not to injure the right phrenic nerve. The innominate artery is secured with pledget-supported sutures to the posterior periosteum of the sternum to lift the innominate artery away from the trachea, simultaneously pulling the anterior tracheal wall open. Hawkins and colleagues (1992) have described using a median sternotomy with division of the innominate artery and reimplantation into the ascending aorta at a site more to the right and anterior to the original site. This technique seems to sacrifice the active suspending mechanism on the tracheal wall provided by the classic technique and to have some risk of cerebrovascular accident.

At the Children's Memorial Hospital, the author and colleagues (1992) reported suspension for 76 children with 2 — 3% — undergoing reoperation, 71 — 93% — relieved of symptoms, and no deaths related to the actual procedure. Innominate artery compression of the

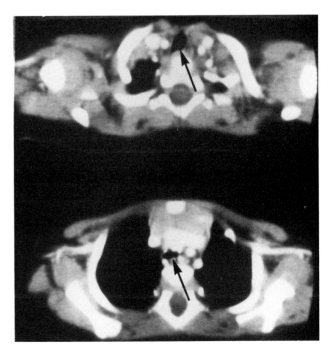

Fig. 71–10. CT scan with contrast of an infant with innominate artery compression syndrome. The superior cut shows a normal-size trachea (arrow). The inferior cut shows the trachea (arrow) compressed by the innominate artery.

trachea historically has been well managed by innominate artery suspension through a right anterolateral thoracotomy, and I continue to recommend this approach.

Pulmonary Artery Sling

A pulmonary artery sling is a rare vascular anomaly in which the left pulmonary artery originates from the right pulmonary artery and encircles the right main stem bronchus and distal trachea before coursing anterior to the esophagus and descending aorta to enter the hilum of the left lung. This anomaly was first reported by Glaevecke and Doehle (1897) as a postmortem finding in a 7-month-old infant with severe respiratory distress. Sade (1975) reported that embryologically a pulmonary artery sling occurs when the developing left lung captures its arterial supply from derivatives of the *right* sixth aortic arch through capillaries *caudad* rather than cephalad to the developing tracheobronchial tree. The "sling" compresses and compromises the distal trachea and right main stem bronchus. In addition, Cosentino and associates (1991) have shown that 30 to 40% of these infants also will have complete tracheal rings, which Berdon and colleagues (1984) have appropriately referred to as the "ring-sling" complex. The membranous portion of the trachea is absent and the cartilages are circumferential.

Nearly all infants with this diagnosis present within the first months of life with respiratory distress, particularly if there are associated complete tracheal rings. A chest radiograph may show unilateral hyperaeration of the right lung field. A barium esophagogram shows anterior compression of the esophagus on the lateral views (Fig. 71–11). Diagnosis requires either CT or MR imaging; angiography is no longer recommended, unless an associated congenital cardiac anomaly is suspected. Both CT and MR imaging will show clearly the left pulmonary artery originating from the right pulmonary artery, encircling the trachea, and coursing to the hilum of the left lung (Fig. 71–12). Bronchoscopy should be performed in all these infants to check for associated complete tracheal rings. Tracheograms are indicated only in select cases and must be done with extreme caution to avoid further ventilatory compromise.

Surgical intervention should be undertaken as soon as the diagnosis is made because of the usual tenuous respiratory status. The first successful operation for pulmonary artery sling was performed by Potts and co-workers (1954) at Children's Memorial Hospital, through a right thoracotomy. Chronologically, the next several patients operated on at Children's Memorial Hospital were reported by Koopot and associates (1975), with the approach through a left thoracotomy. The pericardium is opened and the left pulmonary artery is clamped and divided at its origin from the right pulmonary artery. It is then transposed anterior to the trachea and anastomosed to the main pulmonary artery (Fig. 71–13). This procedure recently was reported by Pawade and associates (1992) to have good results, except in infants with associated tracheal stenosis.

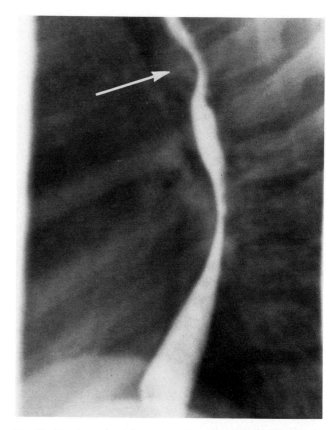

Fig. 71–11. Lateral esophagogram of an 18-month-old with chronic upper respiratory tract infections. Arrow points to the anomalous left pulmonary artery compressing the esophagus anteriorly.

Because between 30 and 40% of patients with pulmonary artery sling will have associated complete tracheal rings, the "ring-sling" complex, my associates and I (1992) now advocate an approach with median sternotomy and the

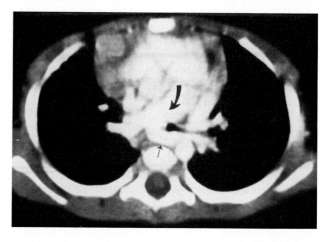

Fig. 71–12. CT scan with contrast material from a 14-month-old girl with pulmonary artery sling and complete tracheal rings from the fourth tracheal ring to the carina. Curved arrow points to main pulmonary artery. Small arrow points to left pulmonary artery, which is wrapping around the trachea from right to left. Note that the tracheal lumen is small from complete tracheal rings.

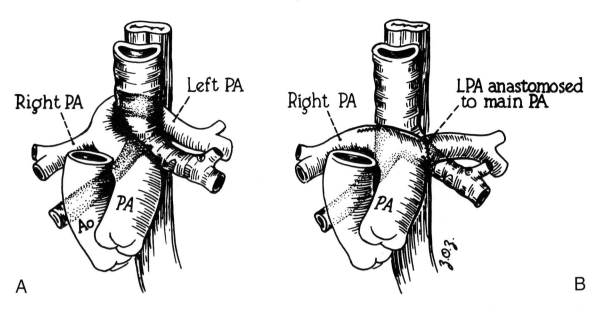

Fig. 71–13. Operative technique. *A*, Left pulmonary artery encircles and compresses distal area of trachea and right main stem bronchus. *B*, Repair is by transecting left pulmonary artery at its origin from right pulmonary artery and anastomosing left pulmonary artery to main pulmonary artery at a site that approximates the usual anatomic configuration. *From* Backer CL, Idriss FS: Tracheoesophageal compressive syndromes of vascular origin: rings and slings. *In* Baue A.E. et al (eds): Glenn's Thoracic and Cardiovascular Surgery. 5th Ed. Norwalk, CT: Appleton-Century-Crofts, 1991, p 963.

use of extracorporeal circulation. This allows accurate ligation and division of the left pulmonary artery with implantation into the main pulmonary artery anterior to the trachea. The operation can be performed without respiratory compromise, and enough time and care can be taken to ensure patency of the left pulmonary artery. If there are associated complete tracheal rings, then simultaneous pericardial patch tracheoplasty, as originally described by Idriss (1984), can be performed. Our group has operated on 10 infants with isolated pulmonary artery sling, and 5 infants with pulmonary artery sling and complete tracheal rings. There have been no early deaths, but two late deaths have resulted from airway complications. The patency rate of the left pulmonary artery using the technique of median sternotomy and extracorporeal circulation approaches 100%.

The technique of tracheoplasty uses a median sternotomy with extracorporeal circulation (Fig. 71–14). If a pulmonary artery sling is present, this is repaired first. The innominate artery and vein, and the trachea, are dissected free. A pericardial patch is harvested. After initiation of cardiopulmonary bypass with an aortic and single atrial venous cannula, under bronchoscopic guidance, an anterior incision is made in the trachea through the complete tracheal rings (Fig. 71–15). Bronchoscopy is used to identify the extent of the complete tracheal rings. The pericardial patch is then inserted using interrupted absorbable suture (Fig. 71–16). The patient then undergoes bronchoscopy to aspirate secretions and to ensure that the stenosis has been relieved. The patch is stented with an endotracheal tube for 1 week, during which time the child is placed under respiratory paralysis and is oxygenated by mechanical ventilation. Follow-up bronchoscopy is performed to remove gran-

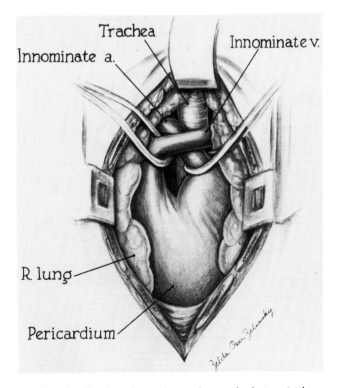

Fig. 71–14. For the infant with complete tracheal rings (with or without pulmonary artery sling), median sternotomy is performed, and the innominate artery, innominate vein, and trachea are dissected free. *From* Idriss FS, et al: Tracheoplasty with pericardial patch for extensive tracheal stenosis in infants and children. J Thorac Cardiovasc Surg 88:527, 1984.

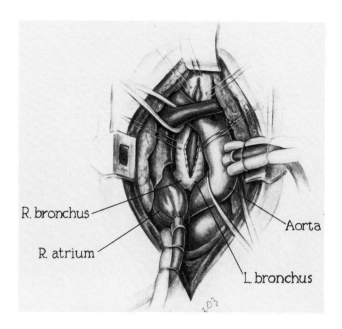

Fig. 71–15. The infant is placed on cardiopulmonary bypass to provide respiratory support while an anterior incision is made in the trachea through the complete rings, under bronchoscopic guidance. *From* Idriss FS, et al: Tracheoplasty with pericardial patch for extensive tracheal stenosis in infants and children. J Thorac Cardiovasc Surg 88:527, 1984.

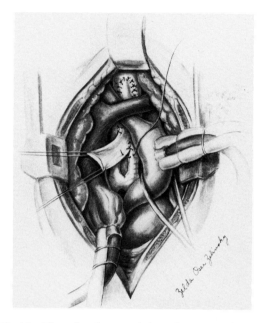

Fig. 71–16. The tailored pericardial patch is inserted with interrupted absorbable suture, completing the repair. *From* Idriss FS, et al: Tracheoplasty with pericardial patch for extensive tracheal stenosis in infants and children. J Thorac Cardiovasc Surg 88:527, 1984.

ulation tissue, clear secretions, and identify any residual stenosis. The child is then weaned from the ventilator and extubated. In the Children's Memorial Hospital series of 20 patients undergoing pericardial patch tracheoplasty — including 5 with simultaneous pulmonary artery sling repair, there have been 4 deaths. The other infants are essentially asymptomatic, except for 2, who still require tracheostomies.

Aberrant Right Subclavian Artery

A left aortic arch with aberrant right subclavian artery arising from the descending aorta may cause posterior indentation of the esophagus (Fig. 71–17). Gross (1946) described this as the cause of dysphagia lusoria. Abbott (1936) reported that this is the most common vascular anomaly of the aortic arch system — 0.5% of humans. As Beabout and associates (1964) showed, however, it is usually not a source of symptoms severe enough to cause surgical intervention, unless there is aneurysmal dilatation of the subclavian origin. We have not operated on a child with this diagnosis since 1973.

In adults, however, the base of the aberrant right subclavian artery may become dilated and aneurysmal, compressing the esophagus and causing symptoms of dysphagia. In that case the right subclavian artery should be divided, the aneurysm resected, and the right subclavian artery implanted into the aorta or right common carotid artery. Pifarre and associates (1971) described this as a one-stage procedure with a left thoracotomy approach. More recently, van Son and associates (1990) have recommended a surgical approach

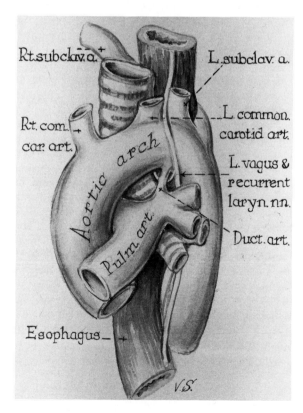

Fig. 71–17. Aberrant right subclavian artery originating as the last branch from the aortic arch. The artery courses posterior to the esophagus up to the right arm. *From* Idriss FS, et al: Surgery for vascular anomalies causing obstruction of the trachea and esophagus. *In* Tucker BL, Lindesmith GG (eds): Congenital Heart Disease. New York: Grune & Stratton, 1979, 125.

through a *right* thoracotomy. Esposito and associates (1988) found only 26 cases of aneurysm of an aberrant subclavian artery in the world literature, and only 16 patients had been operated on. They recommended an initial approach through a right cervical incision to divide the right subclavian distal to the aneurysmal dilatation and anastomosis of the distal end to the right carotid artery to preserve blood flow to the distal distribution of the artery. The patient is then placed in a right lateral decubitus position, and the aneurysm is excised through a left thoracotomy approach. These authors believe this approach obviates the possible complications of upper limb ischemia, cerebral embolization, and intraoperative hemorrhage.

Miscellaneous Vascular Compression

A cervical aortic arch may ascend into the neck and compress the trachea and esophagus. An anomalous left carotid artery may compress the trachea as it courses from right to left across the trachea. Whitman and associates (1982) reported that a left aortic arch with right-sided ligamentum and right-sided descending aorta is another unusual cause of tracheoesophageal compression. This is one of the very rare vascular rings that, as McFaul and associates (1981) reported, may necessitate a right thoracotomy for successful correction. These infants often have associated cardiac anomalies, and the diagnosis is made by cardiac catheterization. The esophagogram also has a very distinctive appearance with extrinsic indentation in the upper left posterior aspect of the esophagus at the level of the second thoracic vertebra. Binet and colleagues (1978) described a single case report of a ductus arteriosus traversing from the right pulmonary artery to the descending aorta between the trachea and esophagus with an aberrant right subclavian artery. The ductus was compressing the trachea and right bronchus in a manner analogous to pulmonary artery sling.

RESULTS AND CONCLUSIONS

Since 1947 a total of 251 patients have undergone surgery for relief of tracheoesophageal compression from vascular rings or associated tracheoesophageal compression syndromes at Children's Memorial Hospital in Chicago. The results are shown in Table 71–2. Seventeen patients have expired of complications following operation for an overall mortality rate of 7%. Since 1967 there have been no deaths from an isolated vascular ring. Nine of the 17 deaths occurred in infants with major associated cardiac or respiratory anomaly.

The diagnosis of vascular ring should be suspected in any infant or child who presents with symptoms of respiratory distress. The diagnosis is best established by esophagogram for double aortic arch or right aortic arch with left ligamentum. CT scanning and MR imaging are used for diagnosis of pulmonary artery slings or in unusual cases. Bronchoscopy is required for the diag-

Table 71–2. Vascular Rings/Slings/Tracheal Rings: Results from Children's Memorial Hospital, October 1947 to December 1992

	Patients	Death	%
Double aortic arch	76	6	8
Right aortic arch/left ligamentum	66	5	8
Innominate compression	79	3	4
Tracheal rings/tracheoplasty	15	3	20
Pulmonary artery sling	10	1	10
Simultaneous pulmonary artery sling repair and tracheoplasty	5	1	20
Total	251	19	7.6

nosis of innominate artery compression, which can be confirmed by CT. The surgical technique employed is a left thoracotomy with a muscle-sparing approach for both double aortic arch and right aortic arch with left ligamentum. A right thoracotomy is best for innominate artery suspension. A median sternotomy and the use of extracorporeal circulation is recommended for the repair of pulmonary artery sling and patients who have associated complete tracheal rings. Surgical intervention successfully provides relief of tracheoesophageal compression from vascular structures in over 95% of infants and children.

REFERENCES

Abbott ME: Atlas of Congenital Cardiac Disease. New York: The American Heart Association, 1936, p 16.

Arciniegas E, et al.: Surgical management of congenital vascular rings. J Thorac Cardiovasc Surg 77:721, 1979.

Ardito JM, et al.: Innominate artery compression of the trachea in infants with reflex apnea. Ann Otol 89:401, 1980.

Backer CL, et al.: Vascular anomalies causing tracheoesophageal compression. J Thorac Cardiovasc Surg 97:725, 1989.

Backer CL, et al.: Pulmonary artery sling. J Thorac Cardiovasc Surg 103:683, 1992.

Backer CL, Holinger LD, Mavroudis C: Invited letter concerning: innominate artery compression — division and reimplantation versus suspension. J Thorac Cardiovasc Surg 103:817, 1992.

Beabout JW, Stewart JR, Kincaid OW: Aberrant right subclavian artery, dispute of commonly accepted concepts. AJR Am J Roentgenol 92:855, 1964.

Berdon WE, et al.: Complete cartilage-ring tracheal stenosis associated with anomalous left pulmonary artery: the ring-sling complex. Radiology 152:57, 1984.

Binet JP, et al.: Ductus arteriosus sling: Report of a newly recognized anomaly and its surgical correction. Thorax 33:72, 1978.

Bisset GS, et al.: Vascular rings: MR imaging. AJR Am J Roentgenol 149:251, 1987.

Chun KF, et al.: Diagnosis and management of congenital vascular rings: a 22-year experience. Ann Thorac Surg 53:597, 1992.

Congdon ED: Transformation of the aortic arch system during the development of the human embryo. Contrib Embryol 14:47, 1922.

Cosentino CM, et al.: Pericardial patch tracheoplasty for severe tracheal stenosis in children: intermediate results. J Pediatr Surg 26:879, 1991.

D'Cruz IA, et al.: Right-sided aorta. Br Heart J 28:722, 1966.

Edwards JE: Anomalies of derivatives of aortic arch system. Med Clin North Am 32:925, 1948.

Esposito RA, et al.: Surgical treatment for aneurysm of aberrant subclavian artery based on a case report and review of the literature. J Thorac Cardiovasc Surg 95:888, 1988.

Felson B, Palayew MJ: The two types of right aortic arch. Radiology 81:745, 1963.

Glaevecke, Doehle: Ueber eine seltene angeborene Anomalie der Pulmonalarterie. Munch Med Wochenschr 44:950, 1897.

Gross RE: Surgical relief for tracheal obstruction from a vascular ring. N Engl J Med 233:586, 1945.

Gross RE: Surgical treatment for dysphagia lusoria. Ann Surg 124:532, 1946.

Gross RE, Neuhauser EBD: Compression of the trachea by an anomalous innominate artery: an operation for its relief. Am J Dis Child 75:570, 1948.

Hawkins JA, Bailey WW, Clark SM: Innominate artery compression of the trachea: treatment by reimplantation of the innominate artery. J Thorac Cardiovasc Surg 103:678, 1992.

Idriss FS, et al.: Tracheoplasty with pericardial patch for extensive tracheal stenosis in infants and children. J Thorac Cardiovasc Surg 88:527, 1984.

Kommerell B: Verlagerung des Osophagus durch eine abnorm verlaufende Arteria Subclavia Dextra (Arteria Lusoria). Fortsch Geb Rontgenstr 54:590, 1936.

Koopot R, Nikaidoh H, Idriss FS: Surgical management of anomalous left pulmonary artery causing tracheobronchial obstruction: pulmonary artery sling. J Thorac Cardiovasc Surg 69:239, 1975.

Lowe GM, Donaldson JS, Backer CL: Vascular rings: 10-year review of imaging. RadioGraphics 11:637, 1991.

McFaul R, Millard P, Nowicki E: Vascular rings necessitating right thoracotomy. J Thorac Cardiovasc Surg 82:306, 1981.

McLoughlin MJ, Weisbrod G, Wise DJ, Young HPH: Computed tomography in congenital anomalies of the aortic arch and great vessels. Radiology 138:399, 1981.

Nikaidoh H, Riker WL, Idriss FS: Surgical management of "vascular rings." Arch Surg 105:327, 1972.

Pawade A, et al.: Pulmonary artery sling. Ann Thorac Surg 54:967, 1992.

Pifarre R, Niedballa RG, Dieter RA Jr: Definitive surgical treatment of the aberrant retroesophageal right subclavian artery in the adult. J Thorac Cardiovasc Surg 61:154, 1971.

Potts WJ, Gibson S, Rothwell R: Double aortic arch: report of two cases. Arch Surg 57:227, 1948.

Potts WJ, Holinger PH, Rosenblum AH: Anomalous left pulmonary artery causing obstruction to right main bronchus: report of a case. JAMA 155:1409, 1954.

Sade RM, et al.: Pulmonary artery sling. J Thorac Cardiovasc Surg 69:333, 1975.

Turner W: On irregularities of the pulmonary artery, arch of the aorta and the primary branches of the arch with an attempt to illustrate their mode of origin by a reference to development. Br Foreign Med Chir Rev 30:173, 1962.

van Son JAM, et al.: Anatomic support of surgical approach of anomalous right subclavian artery through a right thoracotomy. J Thorac Cardiovasc Surg 99:1115, 1990.

Whitman G, Stephenson LW, Weinberg P: Vascular ring: left cervical aortic arch, right descending aorta, and right ligamentum arteriosum. J Thorac Cardiovasc Surg 83:311, 1982.

Index

rib fractures in, 771
thoracic trauma in, 767
thymic rebound after malignancy treatment in, 1736
tuberculosis in, 968, 971
surgery in, 982-983, *982*
ventilatory changes after pneumonectomy in, 398
Chlorambucil (Leukeran), 1223t
2-Chlorodeoxyadenosine (2-CDA), 1224t, 1225
Chloroquine, for amebiasis, 1019, 1020t
Chlorpromazine, interactions of, during anesthesia, 302t
Chlorthiazide, interactions of, during anesthesia, 301t
Choking, "distress signal of," 801
Cholecystitis, acalculous candidal, 1005
Cholecystokinin, lower esophageal sphincter function and, 1550
Cholesterol, pleural fluid, in pleural effusion diagnosis, 678
Cholesterol pleural effusion(s), chylothorax vs., 717
Cholesterol pneumonitis, 952, *953*
Cholinergic crisis, 1777
Chondrogladiolar deformity, 540, *540*, 540t
Chondroma, of rib, 581-582
pulmonary, 1314. See also Hamartoma(s), pulmonary
tracheal, *829, 830*, 832, *833*
Chondromanubrial deformity, 540-541, 540t, *541, 542*
surgical repair of, 542, *544*
Chondromyxoid hamartoma. See Hamartoma(s), pulmonary
Chondrosarcoma, of esophagus, 1689
of lung, 1322
of rib, 583-585, *583-585, 587*
Chordoma(s), of spine, 1728
Choriocarcinoma, 1740
esophageal adenocarcinoma and, 1683
pulmonary metastases from, 1343
treatment of, 1806
Choristoma, tracheobronchial, 1689
Chromogranin, in differential diagnosis of thymoma, 1786
Chromoscopy, with esophagoscopy, 1424
Chromosome(s), abnormalities of, in lung cancer, 1101, 1242
radiation damage to, 1198-1199
Chronic granulomatous disease of childhood, pulmonary infections in, 953
Chronic obstructive pulmonary disease (COPD), diaphragm pacing in, 614, 626
lung cancer with, radiation therapy and, 1213
lung transplantation for, 1066
postoperative management after, 1076
results of, *1086*, 1087, *1087, 1088*
rise in cigarette consumption and, 280, *281*
spontaneous pneumothorax in, 663
thoracotomy effect in, 281
tracheobronchial malacia in, 821
treatment of, 826
Churg-Strauss syndrome, 1054
Chyle, 714-715, 714t
Chylothorax, 714-721
after pulmonary resection, 410-411
after transhiatal esophagectomy, 1465
causes of, 715-716, 715t
congenital, 715-716
management of, 719
conservative therapy for, 718, 719-720
diagnosis of, 717
management of, 717-720, 717t, *718-720*
neoplastic, 716
nontraumatic, management of, 719
pathophysiology of, 716-717

pseudochylothorax vs., 678, 717
traumatic, 716, 781-782
due to operative injury, 716
management of, 719
Chylous fistula, operative therapy of, 718-719, *718, 719*
Cicatricial bronchial stenosis, after sleeve resection, 458
Cicatrization atelectasis, 145
CIE (countercurrent immunoelectrophoresis), in pleural effusion diagnosis, 678
Cigarette(s). See Smoking
Cilastatin, imipenem with, for cystic fibrosis, 881
Cilia, development of, 46
in airway epithelium, 58-60, *59, 60*
in respiratory bronchioles, 61
Cimetidine, drug interactions with, 301t
Cine-esophagography, 1404
limitations of, 1413
for reflux diagnosis, 1415
Ciprofloxacin, for cystic fibrosis, 881
Cirrhosis, pleural effusion due to, 680
Cisplatin, 1222, 1223t
for esophageal adenocarcinoma, surgery with, 1668
for esophageal carcinoma, radiation therapy with, 1697, 1698, 1698t
squamous cell, 1651
for lung cancer, α-interferon with, 1267-1268
non–small cell, 1235, 1235t
small cell, 1247t
for malignant thymoma, 1807
for mesothelioma, 745
for nonseminomatous malignant germ cell tumor, 1805-1806, 1806t
for seminoma, 1804, *1804*
peripheral neuropathy due to, 1270
radiation synergism with, 1210, *1210*
radiation therapy with, for esophageal carcinoma, 1697, 1698, 1698t
for non–small cell lung cancer, 1235, 1235t
side effects of, 1227
Cisterna chyli, 105, 106
Clagett procedure, modified, for postpneumonectomy empyema, 696
Clagett window, for empyema after lung transplantation, 1081, *1081*
"Clam shell" incision, 388
Clara cell(s), in airway epithelium, 49, 58, *60*, 61
Clara cell adenoma, 1312-1313
Clavicle(s), 15, *16*
fracture of, 772-773
tumors of, 586
Clear cell carcinoma, of lung, 1108
Clear cell tumor, of lung, 1315
"Clearance," for surgery, 304-305
Cleft sternum, 546-548, *549*, 549t
Clindamycin, for anaerobic parapneumonic empyema, 688
for aspiration lung abscess, 942
Clinical trials of chemotherapy, design of, 1220
Clofazimine, for atypical mycobacterial infection in AIDS, 978
Clonidine, interactions of, during anesthesia, 301t
management of surgical patient on, 290
Closing volume, 117, *117*
Clubbing, 724-725
in lung cancer, 1126
with neurogenic tumors of diaphragm, 652
CMV infection. See Cytomegalovirus (CMV) infection
Coagulopathy, postoperative hemorrhage due to, 402
Coal worker's pneumoconiosis, 1051
Cobalt, diffuse lung disease due to, 1051
⁶⁰Cobalt teletherapy unit, 1197
Cocaine, diffuse lung disease due to, 1055

Coccidioidomycosis, 992-995, *992-994*
diagnosis of, 242, 995
in immunocompromised host, 1059
pleural, 708
treatment of, 987t, *994*, 995
Coil embolization, selective, of pulmonary arteriovenous fistulas, 901, *901*, 902
Coin lesion. See Pulmonary nodule(s)
Colitis, peptic, after esophageal reconstruction using colon, 1491
Collagen vascular disease (CVD). See also specific disorders
esophageal stricture in, 1598-1599, *1599*
pulmonary involvement in, 1047-1048
Collis gastroplasty, for Barrett's ulcer, 1618
for esophageal stricture, peptic, 1605-1607, *1606, 1607*
with Barrett's esophagus, 1617
Colloid solution(s), for fluid replacement during thoracic surgery, 318
Colocolic anastomosis, in esophageal reconstruction using colon, 1486-1487
Coloesophageal anastomosis. See Esophagocolic anastomosis
Cologastric anastomosis, in esophageal reconstruction using colon, 1487
Colon, arterial supply of, *1485*
esophageal bypass using, for palliation in esophageal cancer, 1672, *1674*
esophageal reconstruction using. See under Esophageal reconstruction
sluggish, esophageal reconstruction using, 1491
Colony-stimulating factor(s). See Hematopoietic growth factor(s)
Colorectal carcinoma, pulmonary metastases from, 1341-1342, *1341*, 1348t
Columnar epithelium, in esophagus. See also Barrett's esophagus
potential difference measurements for detection of, 1398
sources of, 1682, *1682*, 1683
Complement deficiency(ies), bronchiectasis in, 931t
Complement fixation test, for paragonimiasis, 1035
Compliance, in mechanically ventilated patient, 128
of chest wall, 122
of lung, 120-121, *121*
Complication(s), defined, 279
postoperative, 279t
predicting occurence of, 303-304, 304t. See also Operative risk
pulmonary, physical therapy for prevention of, 371-378
Compression atelectasis, 145
Compression index, in bullous emphysema assessment, 918, *919, 920*
Computed tomography (CT), 137, *138*
high-resolution (HRCT), 159
in asymptomatic solitary pulmonary nodule assessment, 1148-1149
in diffuse lung disease diagnosis, 1044-1045
in bullous emphysema assessment, 917-918, *917*
in diffuse lung disease diagnosis, 1044-1045
in esophageal cancer diagnosis, 1640-1642, *1641*
in lung cancer, for detection of distant metastases, 1143-1144
for diagnosis, 1136-1138, *1136, 1137*
for staging, 265, 1244
in pulmonary metastasis diagnosis, 1335-1336
in pulmonary nodule assessment, 151, 1148-1149
phantom study for, 166, *168*
in superior vena cava syndrome assessment, 1718
in tracheal tumor diagnosis, 829-830, *830*
of esophagus, 1407, *1408, 1409*

radiolabeled, imaging using, 223-224, 1140, 1282
sputum cytology using, in lung cancer screening, 1157, 1242
to small cell cancer antigens, 1268
Mononucleosis, infectious, 246
Monosporosis. *See* Pseudallescheriasis
Montgomery salivary tube, for esophageal intubation, 1674, *1676*
Moon sign. *See* Crescent sign
Morphine, for postoperative pain, continuous intravenous infusion of, 342
epidural administration of, 343
Mounier-Kuhn syndrome, 820
treatment of, 826
MRI. *See* Magnetic resonance imaging
Mucinous cystadenoma(s), of lung, 1312
Mucocele, with bronchial atresia, 860
Mucociliary clearance, postoperative, 347
Mucociliary escalator, 58-60
Mucoepidermoid carcinoma, of esophagus, 1682-1683
prognosis in, 1684
of lung, 1303-1305, *1303-1305*
Mucoepidermoid tumor, of trachea, 840
Mucormycosis, 1005-1006, *1006*
airway involvement in, 816
in immunocompromised host, 1059
medical treatment of, 987t
Mucous gland adenoma, 1311-1312, *1312, 1313*
Multi-drug resistance, 1220
Multiple inert gas technique, 114
Multiple myeloma, pulmonary involvement in, 1330
Multiple sclerosis, esophageal dysfunction in, 1552
Mural fibrosing alveolitis, 1041-1042, 1042t, *1043*
Muscle relaxant(s), drug interactions with, 301t, 302t
in neonatal anesthesia, 331
Muscle transposition, for chest wall reconstruction, 591-594, *592-595*
for postpneumonectomy empyema space closure, 697-698, *697-699*
with surgery for tuberculosis, 983
Muscle-sparing thoracotomy, 383-384, *385-386*
Muscular dystrophy, oropharyngeal dysphagia due to, 1543
Mushroom worker's lung, 1050
Mutamycin. *See* Mitomycin C
MVV. *See* Maximum voluntary ventilation
Myasthenia. *See also* Myasthenia gravis
ocular, 1777
transient neonatal, 1775
Myasthenia gravis (MG), 1774-1781
clinical aspects of, 1774-1775
clinical classification of, 1774t
congenital, 1775
defined, 1774
diagnosis of, 1775, *1776,* 1776t
immunobiologic classification of, 1776t
juvenile, 1775
results of treatment in, 1781
oropharyngeal dysphagia due to, 1543, *1544*
pathology of, 1776
pathophysiology of, 1775-1776, *1775*
prognosis in, 1777
treatment of, 1776-1781
medical, 1776-1777
surgical, 1777-1781, *1778-1780,* 1781t
video-assisted thoracic surgery for thymectomy in, 522n, 1812, *1813*
with thymoma, 1776, 1776t, 1786-1787
prognosis in, 1781
Myasthenic crisis, 1777
Myasthenic syndrome. *See* Lambert-Eaton syndrome

myc gene(s), 1099-1100, 1101
in small cell lung cancer, 1242
Mycetoma. *See* Fungus ball
Mycobacteria. *See also* Tuberculosis; *specific species*
atypical, 969
classification of, 237, 239t
identification of, 239-240
Mycobacterial infection(s), 237-240, 239t, *240,* 968-985. *See also* Tuberculosis; *specific species*
atypical, in cystic fibrosis, 881
in immunocompromised host, 1058-1059
medical therapy for, 978
clinical manifestations of, 972-973
in immunocompromised host, 1058-1059
pathology of, 971
radiographic features of, 975
Mycobacterium avium complex (MAC), 969
identification of, 240
infection with, gallium imaging of chest in, 220, *220*
in AIDS, 240, 978, 1058-1059
in immunocompromised host, 1058-1059
mediastinal, 1706, *1708*
medical therapy for, 978, 979
morbidity and mortality after surgical treatment of, 983
pathology of, 971
Mycobacterium chelonei infection, medical therapy for, 978
failure of, 979
Mycobacterium fortuitum, 969
medical therapy for infection with, 978
Mycobacterium gordonae, 969
identification of, 240
Mycobacterium intracellulare. See Mycobacterium avium complex
Mycobacterium kansasii, 969
infection with, clinical manifestations of, 973
medical therapy for, 978, 979
Mycobacterium scrofulaceum, 969
Mycobacterium tuberculosis, 968. *See also* Tuberculosis
drug resistance in, 239, *240*
identification of, 239-240
Mycobacterium xenopi, 969
infection with, failure of medical therapy for, 979
morbidity and mortality after surgical treatment of, 983
Mycosis. *See* Fungal infection(s); *specific diseases*
Mycostatin (nystatin), for candidal esophagitis, 1555
Myeloma. *See* Plasmacytoma
Myelopathy, radiation, 1202-1203, 1214, 1264
Myelosuppression, due to chemotherapy, 1227
management of, 1227, 1251-1252, 1267, 1269
Myenteric plexus, esophageal motility disorders due to metastatic carcinomatous involvement of, 1552
in Chagas' disease, 1559
Myleran. *See* Busulfan
Myoblastoma(s). *See* Granular cell tumor(s)
Myocardial dysfunction, primary, perioperative low cardiac output syndrome due to, 294
Myocardial infarction, after pulmonary resection, 406
operative risk and, 288-289, 303, 345
perioperative, 345
Myocardial ischemia, after pulmonary resection, 406
Myoclonus, in lung cancer, 1125, 1126t
Myocutaneous flap, for chest wall reconstruction, after osteoradionecrosis, 562, *562*
after trauma, 773, *774*
Myoid cell(s), of thymus, 1773

Myopathy, carcinomatous, 1125
Myxosarcoma, pulmonary, 1322t

Nadolol, interactions of, during anesthesia, 301t
Naked heart, 550-552, *550, 551,* 551t, 552t
Narcotic(s). *See also* Opioid(s)
for premedication, 307
Nasal polyposis, in cystic fibrosis, 876
Nasogastric intubation, esophageal stricture due to, 1597
Nasotracheal intubation. *See also* Endotracheal intubation
postoperative, method for, 354
Nausea, due to chemotherapy, 1227
management of, 1268
NCAM (neural cell adhesion molecule), monoclonal antibodies reacting with, 1120
Nd:YAG laser. *See* Neodymium:YAG (Nd:YAG) laser
Nebulization, sputum induction using, 231, 233
therapy with, for cystic fibrosis, 880
Neck, cancer of, pulmonary metastases from, 1345
cross section of, *1704*
infection in, extension of, to mediastinum, 1703-1705, *1704, 1705*
structures and fascial planes of, esophagus' relationship to, 1361-1362, *1363*
Necrotizing sarcoid granulomatosis (NSG), 1049
Needle aspiration, 233
for hydatid cyst, 1029-1030
for pneumothorax, 666
percutaneous transthoracic, 269-272, *270, 271*
in asymptomatic solitary pulmonary nodule assessment, 1149-1150
in lung cancer diagnosis, 1141
tumor cell implantation after, 1150
transbronchial (TBNA), in carcinoid tumor diagnosis, 1290
in lung cancer diagnosis, 1140-1141
indications for, 254
technique for, 257, *257-259*
Needle biopsy, of pleura, 273
in lung cancer diagnosis, 1141
in malignant pleural effusion, 760
in pleural effusion diagnosis, 679
in pleural tuberculosis diagnosis, 702
Negative inspiratory force (NIF), measurement of, prior to weaning from ventilator, 362
Negative pi-meson(s), 1195
Negative predictive index, 265n
Nematode(s), intestinal, 242-243
Neodymium:YAG (Nd:YAG) laser. *See also* YAG (yttrium aluminum garnet) laser
endoscopic therapy with, for adenoid cystic carcinoma of lung, 1302
for carcinoid tumor, 1294, *1295*
for malignant esophageal obstruction, 1425, 1678, 1679t
for pulmonary metastasectomy, 1338
pulmonary resection using, 467-468, *467*
thoracoscopic pleurodesis using, for apical blebs, 925
video-assisted thoracoscopic surgery using, 510-512, *512*
for pulmonary nodule resection, 522, *522*
Neomycin, for postpneumonectomy empyema, 696
Neon, 114
Neonate(s), anesthesia in, 328-334
drugs for, 331-332
monitoring in, 332-333
cardiovascular adaptation in, 328-329, *328-330,* 330t
lungs of, 45, *46, 47*
metabolic adaptation in, 331, 331t
pharmacologic considerations in, 331-332